"At last! An authoritative reference on the ma
How to separate the good from the bad and the
work that will become the stand

Vincent T. DeVita
The Amy and Joseph Perella P
Yale Cancer Center, Yale Sc
Former Director, National

"Natural Standard *provides exceptionally high-quality, authoritative, rigorous scientific reviews on complementary and alternative medicine treatments. The resource is invaluable for healthcare providers and consumers alike. The sections on precautions/contraindications and interactions offer useful, easy-to-use information that will help to guide the safe use of herbal products and supplements."*

Lorenzo Cohen, PhD
Director, Integrative Medicine Program
The University of Texas M.D. Anderson Cancer Center

"Natural Standard *is simply the best resource for high-quality, up-to-date, evidence-based information. I continue to be impressed with the comprehensive job they've done in this challenging, rapidly evolving field. I can say from personal experience that their evidence-based expert opinion and many layered review are invaluable and not available anywhere else. NS is way ahead of the pack."*

Ellen Hughes, MD
Clinical Professor of Medicine
Director of Education, Osher Center for Integrative Medicine
University of California, San Francisco

"Natural Standard *provides a critical and transparent review of the evidence regarding herbs and supplements. As such, it is an extremely valuable resource for both clinicians and investigators."*

David Eisenberg, MD
Director, Osher Institute
Division for Research and Education in Complementary and Integrative Medical Therapies
Harvard Medical School

"A fabulous resource for clinicians who wish to practice in an informed and responsible manner when working with patients who use herbs and supplements. By expertly evaluating traditional uses in the light of up-to-date scientific evidence, both clinicians and their patients will benefit immensely from this guide."

Karl Berger, ABT, LMT
President, Integrative Medicine Alliance
Shiatsu Therapist

"Natural Standard *has provided just what the doctor ordered—an evidence-based review to tell us what is known and what is not. Given the clear imperative to talk with our patients about CAM, here's the evidence summary you need."*

Harley Goldberg, DO
Medical Director, Complementary and Alternative Medicine
Kaiser Permanente

"Natural Standard *is a very useful resource for any healthcare practitioner who is looking for evidence-based medical perspective on herbs, dietary supplements, and other complementary therapies. I incorporate the* Natural Standard's *results into my routine drug information searches at our center and also make sure that our students are familiar with this resource."*

Lana Dvorkin, PharmD
Acting Director, Center for Complementary and Alternative Pharmacotherapy
Associate Professor of Pharmacy Practice
Massachusetts College of Pharmacy and Health Sciences

"The authors have conducted a systematic and careful review of the scientific literature, providing clear summaries of what is known about the risks and benefits of herbs and supplements."

Anthony L. Komaroff, MD
Professor of Medicine, Harvard Medical School
Editor-in-Chief, Harvard Health Publications

"Natural Standard's *guides could not come at a better time. Systematic reviews of this kind remain essential to resolution of the U.S. healthcare crisis, even as gaps in the national health information infrastructure begin to be addressed. These reviews support interim comparisons of the economic, health, health-related quality of life, and patient satisfaction outcomes of conventional, complementary, and alternative care to advance the nation's best practices. Expect to see these guides applied to a broad variety of health policy challenges, ranging from eliminating disparities in ethnic and minority health to supporting consumer choice and consumer-driven health plans."*

Synthia Laura Molina, BS, MBA
Chief Executive Officer
Alternative Link

"Natural Standard's *evidence-based review articles are a must for all physicians, nurses, and pharmacists who need an unbiased review of nutritional supplements. The reviews are comprehensive, up-to-date, and easy to maneuver for the information you need."*

Joseph Pepping, PharmD
Assistant Director, Integrative Medicine Service
Kaiser Permanente
Alternative Medicine Contributing Editor, *American Journal of Health-System Pharmacy*

"Natural Standard *is unsurpassed as a source of high-quality, unbiased information about complementary and alternative therapies. They have built a sound reputation for thorough, up-to-date research. This book will be a welcome adjunct to the Natural Standard website as a trustworthy source of information."*

Miriam S. Wetzel, PhD
Medical Content Analyst, InteliHealth
Assistant Professor of Medicine (Ret.)
Harvard Medical School

"The reviews published by Natural Standard *are the most reliable source of up-to-date, balanced information on herbs and supplements I have found. Knowing that the information is based on a comprehensive review of the scientific evidence, considers the historic/folkloric perspective, is developed by experts in the field, and peer-reviewed makes* Natural Standard *my top choice for information on herbs and supplements. When* The Rx Consultant *develops an issue on herbs or supplements,* Natural Standard *is a key resource."*

Terry M. Baker, PharmD
Editor, The Rx Consultant

"Natural Standard *has created an important evidence-based database to objectively evaluate a number of complementary therapies. This is incredibly important, given their widespread use in our society. This field is rapidly changing, so it is the first place I look to for obtaining unbiased, current, and accurate information for cancer patients and their families to help them make informed decisions."*

Deborah K. Mayer, RN, MSN, AOCN, FAAN
Program Manager
Institute for Clinical Research and Health Policy Studies
Tufts–New England Medical Center

"There is a critical need among healthcare providers for an evidence-based, continuously updated, and practical database on complementary and alternative medicine (CAM). With a large percentage of the U.S. population employing CAM therapies, healthcare providers in this country must be able to quickly grasp the clinical significance of these therapies with regard to the overall management of patients' health. Natural Standard *provides a credible, rigorously researched, unbiased source of information on an ever-expanding number of complementary and alternative therapies. Boston University School of Medicine Continuing Medical Education has partnered with* Natural Standard *to sponsor many of the NS modules for AMA PRA Category 1 credit for physicians."*

Julie L. White, MS
Administrative Director
Continuing Medical Education
Boston University School of Medicine

"This resource has my highest recommendation."

Jane D. Saxton
Director of Library Services
Bastyr University

"National Standard *provides a critical resource for clinicians and researchers, as well as patients and the general public. Using standardized, rigorous research methodology, this multidisciplinary collaboration of experts has set a new standard, literally, for the field. All clinicians and CAM researchers should have access to these evidence-based monographs on complementary and alternative medicine."*

Mary Ann Richardson, DrPH
Vice President, Research and Development
National Foundation for Alternative Medicine

"There is a growing popularity for an "evidence-based" approach to CAM. Unfortunately, not everyone takes the time to critically appraise what is out there. As a consequence, some "tomes" regarding natural health product information are surprisingly thick, given the scarcity of good quality information. Natural Standard's *success is due to adopting a rigorous approach to the systematic review of evidence regarding natural health products and its careful selection of leaders in the field to review/edit/collaborate so that well-conducted reviews are paired with clinical experts in the field to assess clinical relevance."*

Dr. Sunita Vohra
Director of The Complementary and Alternative
Research and Evaluation (CARE) Program
Stollery Children's Hospital
University of Alberta, Canada

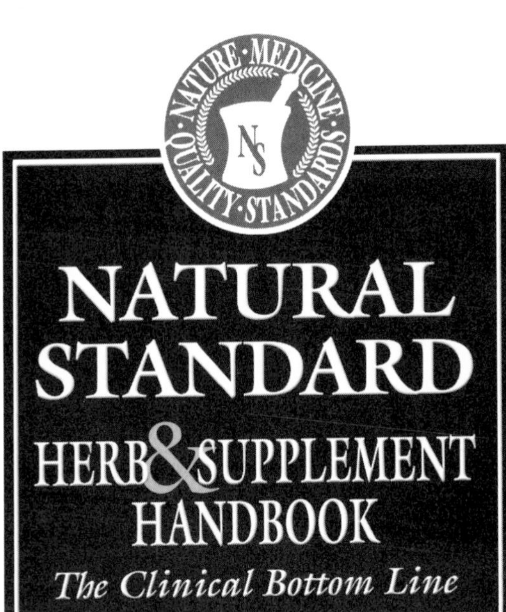
NATURE·MEDICINE·QUALITY·STANDARDS
NS
NATURAL STANDARD
HERB & SUPPLEMENT HANDBOOK
The Clinical Bottom Line

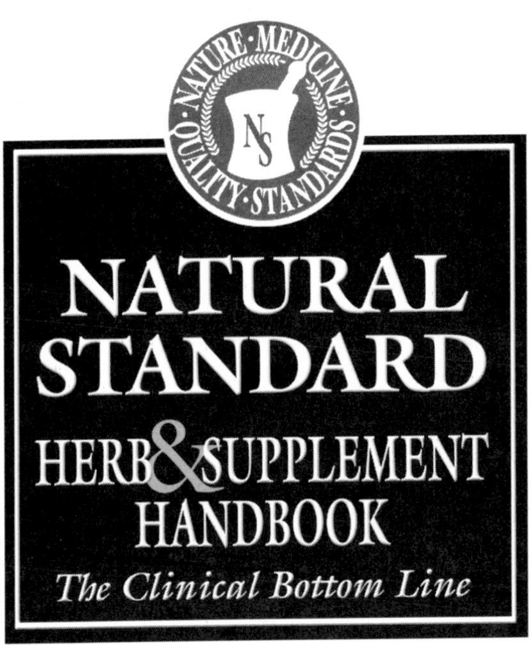

Ethan M. Basch, MD, MPhil
Chief Editor

Natural Standard Research Collaboration
Cambridge, Massachusetts
www.naturalstandard.com
Department of Medicine
Memorial Sloan-Kettering Cancer Center
New York, New York

Catherine E. Ulbricht, PharmD
Chief Editor

Natural Standard Research Collaboration
Cambridge, Massachusetts
www.naturalstandard.com
Department of Pharmacy
Massachusetts General Hospital
Boston, Massachusetts

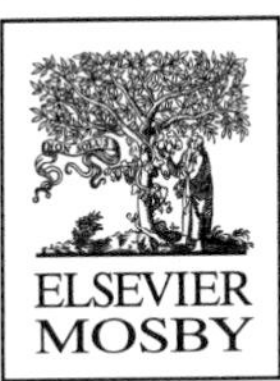

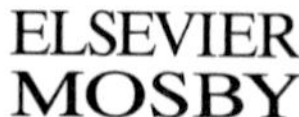

11830 Westline Industrial Drive
St. Louis, Missouri 63146

NATURAL STANDARD HERB & SUPPLEMENT HANDBOOK: THE CLINICAL BOTTOM LINE

ISBN 0-323-02993-0

NOTICE

Pharmacology is an ever-changing field. Standard safety precautions must be followed, but as new research and clinical experience broaden our knowledge, changes in treatment and drug therapy may become necessary or appropriate. Readers are advised to check the most current product information provided by the manufacturer of each drug to be administered to verify the recommended dose, the method and duration of administration, and contraindications. It is the responsibility of the licensed prescriber, relying on experience and knowledge of the patient, to determine dosages and the best treatment for each individual patient. Neither the publisher nor the author assumes any liability for any injury and/or damage to persons or property arising from this publication.

The Publisher

International Standard Book Number 0-323-02993-0

Acquisitions Editor: Kellie White
Senior Developmental Editor: Kim Fons
Publishing Services Manager: Patricia Tannian
Project Manager: John Casey
Book Design Manager: William Drone

Printed in United States of America

Last digit is the print number: 9 8 7 6 5 4 3 2 1

Disclaimer

The content in this book is for general informational purposes only and is not intended as a substitute for medical advice, treatment, or diagnosis. You should consult a physician or other competent medical provider for specific advice applicable to you. If you think you are ill or in need of medical attention, you should seek immediate medical care. Any use of this book or reliance on its content or information is solely at your own risk.

Although some complementary and alternative techniques have been studied scientifically, high-quality data regarding safety, effectiveness, dosage, and mechanism of action are limited or controversial for most therapies. Whenever possible, a practitioner of complementary and alternative techniques should be licensed by a recognized professional organization that adheres to clearly published and generally accepted standards. Before starting any new technique or engaging such a practitioner, an individual should consult with his or her own primary healthcare provider(s). Among other factors, you and your healthcare provider should evaluate the potential risks, benefits, costs, scientific and evidence-based support, and alternatives for the proposed complementary and alternative technique.

As of the date of this publication, the U.S. Food and Drug Administration does not strictly regulate herbs and supplements. There is no guarantee of strength, purity, or safety of unregulated products, and the effects of any such products may vary. Always read product labels fully. If you have a medical condition or are taking a prescription drug or other drugs, herbs, or supplements, you should speak with a qualified healthcare provider about contraindications, interactions, side-effects, and other adverse reactions before starting any new therapy. Immediately consult with a healthcare provider if you experience any unintended side effects or adverse reactions. In reading and using this book, you agree that the book and its content are provided "as is, where is" and with all faults and that Natural Standard, its shareholders, officers, directors, staff, editors, authors, contributors, and consultants (the "affiliated parties") make no representations or warranties of any kind with respect to the book and its content, including without limitation, as to matters of safety, effectiveness, accuracy, reliability, completeness, timeliness, or results. To the fullest extent allowed by law, Natural Standard and the affiliated parties hereby expressly disclaim any and all representations, guarantees, conditions, and warranties of any and every kind, express or implied or statutory, including without limitation, warranties of title or infringement, and implied warranties of merchantability or fitness for a particular purpose. Readers and users of this book assume full responsibility for the appropriate use of the information it contains and agree to hold Natural Standard and the affiliated parties harmless from and against any and all liabilities, claims, and actions arising from the reader's or user's use of the work or its content. Some jurisdictions do not allow exclusions or limitations of implied warranties, so certain of the above exclusions might not apply.

Natural Standard Editorial Board and Contributors

Because so many individuals contribute to the formation of each Natural Standard monograph, it is not practical to list all who have written, edited, or reviewed each document individually. In many cases, individuals listed below have participated in the writing or editing of the full systematic reviews on which the "Bottom Line" pieces in this book are based. Therefore a list is provided below of the Natural Standard Editors, who are all considered as co-editors of this book.

CHIEF EDITORS

Ethan Basch, MD, MPhil

Dr. Basch received his medical degree from Harvard Medical School, internal medicine training at Massachusetts General Hospital, and graduate degree in literature from Oxford University. He has held faculty appointments at Harvard Medical School, Northeastern University, University of Rhode Island, University of Missouri, and Massachusetts General Hospital. His background in healthcare decision-support, informatics, and policy includes the design of clinical effectiveness programs and decision-support utilities for multiple healthcare systems. He serves on the editorial board of Harvard Health Publications, the publishing arm of Harvard Medical School, as well as editorial boards of multiple CAM peer-reviewed journals including the *Journal of Herbal Pharmacotherapy*, *Journal of Cancer Integrative Medicine*, *Alternative Medicine Research Report*, and *Journal of the American Nutraceutical Association*. He is chief editor of the *Massachusetts General Hospital Primer of Outpatient Medicine* (Lippincott, Williams & Wilkins) and serves as an advisor to the Integrative Medicine Alliance and Cancer Source.

Catherine Ulbricht, PharmD

Dr. Ulbricht serves as senior attending pharmacist, Massachusetts General Hospital and assistant clinical professor at eight universities. She serves on the editorial board of Harvard Health Publications, *Journal of the American Nutraceutical Association, Journal of Integrative Cancer Medicine,* and *Pharmacy Practice News* and is the editor-in-chief of the *Journal of Herbal Pharmacotherapy.* Her background includes experience in the areas of quality improvement, healthcare informatics, and drug therapy decision-support. Dr. Ulbricht has also been trained in physical therapy and chiropractic care.

SENIOR EDITORIAL BOARD (ALPHABETICAL ORDER)

Ernie-Paul Barrette, MD, FACP

Dr. Barrette received his medical degree from Harvard Medical School, his MA from Harvard University in Organic Chemistry, and conducted his internal medicine training at Massachusetts General Hospital. He has served as an attending physician and assistant professor at the University of Washington School of Medicine and at Massachusetts General Hospital and is currently on faculty at MetroHealth Medical Center (Ohio) and Case Western Reserve University School of Medicine. He is an expert in complementary and alternative therapies, has contributed to multiple textbooks, and serves as an author and editorial advisor for the newsletter *Alternative Medicine Alert.*

Samuel Basch, MD

Dr. Samuel Basch is an associate clinical professor of psychiatry at Mount Sinai Medical School (NY) and a psychoanalyst. He received his training at Mount Sinai Hospital, where he served as chief resident and at Columbia University Psychoanalytic Clinic. His subspecialties include psychopharmacology and the psychiatric treatment of people with medical illness; he has served as consultant to the cancer unit, the hemodialysis unit, and the organ transplantation unit. His subspecialties also include transcultural psychiatry, and he has worked and taught in Nigeria, Kenya, and Iran, where he studied indigenous treatments and healthcare traditions. Dr. Basch serves on the admissions committee and the board of directors of the Association of Attending Staff at Mount Sinai Hospital and on the Medical Committee of the Riverdale Mental Health Association. He serves on multiple other committees and has published on a wide variety of subjects, including cross-cultural psychiatry, the psychiatric aspects of hemodialysis, and organ transplantation.

William Benda, MD, FACEP, FAAEM

Dr. Benda received his professional training at Duke University, University of Miami School of Medicine, Harbor-UCLA Medical Center, and the Program in Integrative Medicine at the University of Arizona under Dr. Andrew Weil. He has served as director of emergency medical services and assistant clinical professor of medicine at UCLA, as the sole physician in Eastern Rwanda during the 1994 genocide and subsequent cholera epidemic, and as medical director of the Big Sur Health Center. His research and clinical work has focused on patients with breast cancer, animal-assisted therapy, and physician health and well-being. Dr. Benda is a co-founder of the National Integrative Medicine Council, a nonprofit organization for which he has served as Director of Medical and Public Affairs. He is an editor, contributor, and medical advisory board member for several conventional and alternative medicine journals, and he lectures extensively on a variety of topics in the integrative arena.

Stephen Bent, MD

Graduate of Duke University and Vanderbilt University School of Medicine, residency in internal medicine, and fellowship in general internal medicine/clinical epidemiology at the University of California, San Francisco (UCSF), Dr. Bent is an assistant professor of medicine and attending physician at UCSF, where he conducts research evaluating the safety and effectiveness of alternative therapies. He is the project director of an NIH-funded, randomized controlled trial of the herb saw palmetto and the principal investigator of a study evaluating a commonly used Chinese herbal remedy. Dr. Bent is a co-author of textbooks in evidence-based medicine and internal medicine, and he is an expert in the systematic evaluation of alternative therapies.

Heather Boon, BSc Phm, PhD

As an author and researcher, Dr. Boon has gained an international reputation, evidenced by her membership on the prestigious international editorial board of the British journal, *Focus on Alternative and Complementary Therapies* (FACT). She founded and chairs the Toronto CAM Research Network and is an advisor to multiple government and private organizations. In addition, she chaired the Canadian Society for Hospital Pharmacists (CSHP) Task Force to Develop Guidelines for Handling Alternative Medication/Therapy. Dr. Boon has been the principal investigator for myriad large studies focusing on CAM therapies used to treat cancer and on emerging CAM practice patterns. She is widely published as the author of primary research and reviews and maintains a faculty position at the University of Toronto.

Stefan Bughi, MD

Dr. Bughi is president of the Southern California Society of Clinical Hypnosis and a fellow of the American Institute of Stress. He is board certified in internal medicine and endocrinology and serves as assistant professor of clinical medicine at the Keck School of Medicine, University of Southern California in Los Angeles. Presently he works as a physician specialist in the endocrine/diabetes service at Rancho Los Amigos National Rehabilitation Center and at the University of Southern California. Dr. Bughi received his medical degree from the University of Bucharest School of Medicine, Romania, internal medicine training at NE Pennsylvania Affiliated Programs, and endocrinology fellowship at the University of Southern California. His research interests include stress and psychosomatic disorders. He has organized and presented seminars on stress to health professionals and at national and international scientific meetings.

Richard Philip Cohan, DDS, MS, MBA

After Dr. Cohan received an AB in bacteriology from University of California, Berkeley, he engaged in molecular genetic research at Stanford Medical School and Syntex Laboratories. Subsequently, he completed a master's degree in (oral) biology at Southern Methodist University and a DDS at Case Western Reserve University. He joined the faculty of the University of the Pacific (UOP) School of Dentistry in San Francisco in 1972 and became section head of oral diagnosis and treatment planning in 1984. Dr. Cohan has attained both a master's degree in educational psychology and an MBA from UOP during his tenure there. Since 1989, his research, new course development, publishing, editing, and consulting activities have focused primarily on integrative medicine in dentistry. Most recently, he co-authored and submitted for publication a chapter on complementary and alternative medicine for the leading dental pharmacology textbook. He maintains a private dental practice at the California Pacific Medical Center in San Francisco.

William Collinge, MPH, PhD

Dr. Collinge received his MPH and PhD from the University of California, Berkeley, and clinical training at Harvard's Mind/Body Medical Institute. He has served as a peer-review panelist at the National Institutes of Health, National Center for Complementary and Alternative Medicine (NCCAM) and has taught at the UC Berkeley School of Public Health and several other universities. He has conducted research in integrative programs for cancer, HIV, and chronic fatigue syndrome and has extensive clinical background in behavioral, mind/body, and energy medicine. He consults in patient-centered approaches to program development in integrative medicine. He is on the editorial boards of *Subtle Energies & Energy Medicine* and *The International Journal of Healing and Caring*. His books include *Subtle Energy* and *The American Holistic Health Association Complete Guide to Alternative Medicine*.

Cathi Dennehy, PharmD

Dr. Dennehy is an assistant clinical professor in the department of clinical pharmacy in the School of Pharmacy at the University of California, San Francisco (UCSF). Her areas of specialty are herbal medicine and anticoagulation. Dr. Dennehy co-coordinates an evidence-based course in herbal remedies and dietary supplements at UCSF. She has co-authored book chapters on herbs and dietary supplements in various medical and pharmacy textbooks. Dr. Dennehy serves as a consultant to various organizations and journal publications in the area of herbal medicine. In addition, she has coordinated various continuing education programs for state and national pharmacy societies on herbs and dietary supplements and speaks statewide and nationally on this subject.

J. Donald Dishman, DC, MSc

Dr. Dishman is an associate professor in the departments of anatomy and research at the New York Chiropractic College (NYCC) in Seneca Falls, NY. He serves as director of the chiropractic clinic of Monroe Community Hospital in Rochester, NY. In addition to his DC, he was awarded a master of science degree in neurophysiology from the Institute for Sensory Research at Syracuse University. His research has focused on the neurophysiology of spinal manipulative therapy. He maintains a full-time research laboratory at NYCC in which neurophysiological techniques (e.g., H-reflexes, transcranial magnetic stimulation, electromyography) are employed in the investigation of the effects of spinal manipulation on the nervous system. Dr. Dishman also maintains an appointment as adjunct associate professor of bioengineering and neuroscience at the Institute for Sensory Research of Syracuse University. He has published numerous manuscripts in the field of neurophysiology of spinal manipulation, including in the international journal, *Spine*. He also serves as a reviewer for the *Journal of Manipulative and Physiological Therapeutics* and the *Journal of the Neuromusculoskeletal System*.

Joan Engebretson, DrPH, RN

Dr. Engebretson is an associate professor at the University of Texas Health Science Center at Houston, School of Nursing and the School of Public Health. Her background is in maternal child health and community health. She has taught in maternal/child health, women's health, and community health. She is co-editor of the *Maternal, Neonatal and Women's Health Nursing* textbook. Dr. Engebretson has conducted and supervised ethnographic studies examining cultural issues and approaches to healing, as well as clinical research with traditional healers and recipients of touch therapies. She has published numerous articles and book chapters on complementary and alternative therapies, serves on several advisory boards, and consults with many organizations regarding the use of complementary therapies. She teaches a course on culture and complementary therapies at the University of Texas.

Edzard Ernst, MD, PhD, FRCP

Dr. Ernst is one of the best-known worldwide figures in complementary and alternative medicine research, and he has published over 500 major articles and books in this area. His work has focused on the systematic production of rigorous and trustworthy information. He is currently director of the department of complementary medicine at Exeter University, England, which is a premier global center for scientific research in this field.

Mitchell A. Fleisher, MD, DHt, FAAFP, DcABCT

Dr. Fleisher is a board-certified family physician specializing in classical homeopathy, nutritional and botanical medicine, and chelation therapy with over 20 years of clinical experience in integrative medicine. He serves as an active member of the clinical faculty of the National Center for Homeopathy and is clinical instructor for the University of Virginia Health Sciences Center and at the Medical College of Virginia, where he teaches homeopathy in the complementary medicine program. He has lectured throughout the United States and internationally on classical homeopathy and nutritional therapy and regularly contributes as an author and editor to medical journals and popular magazines. Dr. Fleisher attended Stanford University School of Medicine. He has served on the faculty of the New England School of Homeopathy, is currently a clinical preceptor at the Hahnemann College of Homeopathy, and is a graduate of both of these institutions. He is a former assistant clinical professor of family medicine at the Medical College of Virginia and former associate medical director of the MCV/Blackstone Family Practice Residency Training Program, of which he is a graduate. Dr. Fleisher is a fellow of the American Academy of Family Physicians, a diplomate of the American Board of Family Practice and American Board of Homeotherapeutics, and a diplomate candidate of the American Board of Chelation Therapy.

Harley Goldberg, DO

Dr. Goldberg is the director of complementary and alternative medicine for Kaiser Permanente Northern California Medical Care Program and the chief of complementary medicine at Santa Teresa Medical Center in San Jose, California. A graduate of the University of Osteopathic Medicine and Health Sciences, he completed a family medicine residency at Oregon Health Sciences University, Portland, Oregon. He is board certified in family medicine, a fellow of the American Academy of Family Practice, and board certified in neuromusculoskeletal and osteopathic manipulative medicine. Dr. Goldberg has written or edited over 20 systematic reviews of CAM modalities, which are widely used in the Kaiser Permanente system, and he serves on the editorial board of *FACT: Focus on Alternative and Complementary Therapies,* and *Alternative Therapies in Health and Medicine.*

Joerg Gruenwald, PhD

Dr. Gruenwald is primary author of the *PDR for Herbal Medicines* and is a leading European expert in the field of botanicals/phytomedicines. He is the president of Phytopharm Consulting, a unit of analyze & realize ag, Berlin, Germany, a specialized consulting company for natural medicine and dietary supplements. His activities range from market analysis, product development, to R&D, licensing, and medical writing. His main focus is the international exchange of information with an emphasis on Europe and the United States, based on his long experience as medical director of Lichtwer Pharma and on several years as president of Phytopharm Consulting. Dr. Gruenwald has published over 180 scientific articles, five books, and the CD-ROM "Herbal Remedies." He is a regular chairman of international conferences.

Paul Hammerness, MD

Dr. Hammerness is a graduate of Dartmouth Medical School, with postgraduate training in psychiatry and child and adolescent psychiatry at Massachusetts General Hospital and McLean Hospital. He has clinical, administrative, and editorial experience within numerous evidence-based research groups. Dr. Hammerness is committed to continuous quality improvement, particularly when applied to the evaluation of CAM and psychiatric therapies. He is the author of multiple CAM review articles and serves on the editorial board for Harvard Health Publications, the publishing arm of Harvard Medical School.

Charles Holmes, MD, MPH

Dr. Holmes trained in internal medicine at Massachusetts General Hospital and is presently a fellow in infectious disease at Massachusetts General Hospital/Brigham and Women's Hospital and a clinical fellow at Harvard Medical School. Following a graduate degree in epidemiology and international health from the University of Michigan, Dr. Holmes practiced infectious disease epidemiology at the World Health Organization in Geneva, Switzerland. He is currently engaged in HIV research in Boston and sub-Saharan Africa.

Courtney Jarvis, PharmD

Dr. Jarvis serves as an assistant professor in the department of pharmacy practice, Massachusetts College of Pharmacy and Health Sciences (MCPHS), where she teaches graduate level courses involving traditional and complementary medicine. In particular, Dr. Jarvis co-coordinates the therapeutics sequence and an evidence-based course in women's health, which incorporates herbs and dietary supplements into the curriculum. Dr. Jarvis practices clinical pharmacy at UMASS/Memorial Health Care Medical Center with the family medicine residency program.

Karta Purkh Singh Khalsa, CDN, RH (AHG)

KP Khalsa teaches Ayurvedic and botanical medicine in the naturopathic doctoral program and the herbal sciences bachelor's program at Bastyr University, the foremost naturopathic medicine educational institution in the United States. He is a leading member of The American Herbalists Guild, having served two terms on the board of directors. He continues to act as a national association officer. He is a certified dietitian-nutritionist and one of the first registered herbalists in the United States. Author or editor of over a dozen books, he recently co-authored *Herbal Defense* (Warner Books). He is a frequent contributor to mainstream and professional publications in the natural healing field. KP Khalsa is on the faculty of several professional training programs and is the founder of The Professional Herbalist Certificate Course, a 2-year postsecondary curriculum that trains professional herbalists, now being offered at several colleges in Washington and New Mexico. He is a frequent lecturer and presenter to professional healthcare organizations throughout the United States.

Catherine DeFranco Kirkwood, MPH, CCCJS-MAC

Catherine Kirkwood serves as program education coordinator for the Complementary/Integrative Medicine Education Resources (CIMER) Program of the Office of Educational Programs at MD Anderson Cancer Center. She previously served as the director of clinical education and training for the AIDS Education and Training Center for Texas and Oklahoma, a program of the University of Texas School of Public Health. Ms. Kirkwood received her master's degree in public health from the University of Texas. She has more than 20 years of experience in education of healthcare professionals at the Texas Medical Center. She is an appointed member of the Ryan White Planning Council and serves as a senior member of the Advances in Medications and Treatment subcommittee.

David J. Kroll, PhD

Former research director of the Duke University Center for Integrative Medicine, Dr. Kroll is nationally recognized for his work in alternative medicine education and research. He recently joined the Natural Products Program of Research Triangle Institute where the anticancer drug Taxol was first isolated. He was recently named a president's teaching scholar of the University of Colorado. He has co-authored reference books for clinical and lay audiences on evidence-based evaluation of phytomedicinals and has served as series co-editor for 16 consumer books on alternative medicine. He is a graduate of the Philadelphia College of Pharmacy and Science and of the University of Florida College of Medicine, department of pharmacology and therapeutics, with a postdoctoral fellowship in molecular oncology at the University of Colorado School of Medicine, divisions of endocrinology and medical oncology. Dr. Kroll has spent most of his academic career as an associate professor of pharmacology and toxicology at the University of Colorado School of Pharmacy, where he has conducted NIH-funded research on the molecular pharmacology of natural product drugs that target DNA topoisomerases, herbal remedies that interact with these antitumor drugs, and the molecular mechanisms of cytochrome P-450 induction by botanicals.

Richard Liebowitz, MD

Dr. Liebowitz is the director of clinical services for the Duke University Center for Integrative Medicine. Before his current position, he served as director of education for Dr. Andrew Weil's program in integrative medicine, as well as general medicine section chief at the University of Arizona. He has received multiple honors and awards for excellence in teaching at these institutions. Dr. Liebowitz is a graduate of Robert Wood Johnson (Rutgers) Medical School and of the internal medicine residency program at the University of Massachusetts. In addition to his other responsibilities, he currently directs a community-based program in Durham, NC, to improve health in an underserved population. He serves on the editorial board of *Archives of Internal Medicine*.

Ann M. Lynch, RPh, AE-C

Ann Lynch serves as a clinical instructor in the department of pharmacy practice, Massachusetts College of Pharmacy and Health Sciences (MCPHS). She received her BS in pharmacy from Northeastern University and graduate level training at MCPHS. Her professional focus is in the area of herbal medicine and interactions, as well as in community practice with specialty interests in asthma, diabetes, and women's health. Ms. Lynch coordinates on-site screenings and community educational clinics regarding conventional and complementary medicine practices at Fallon Clinic Pharmacies and co-coordinates courses in drug interactions and pharmaceutical care at MCPHS.

Ed Mills DPH, MSc (Oxon)

Dr. Mills is director of research at the Canadian College of Naturopathic Medicine. He is the author of numerous publications, reviews, and original research related to evidence-based complementary and alternative medicine. He has also authored original research articles on issues surrounding risk and risk perception in complementary and alternative medicine. His academic interests and clinical trial work focus on improving the methodology of herb-drug interaction studies. He is the chair of the Evidence-Based Complementary and Alternative Medicine (EBCAM) Working Group.

Shri Kant Mishra, ABMS (BHU), MD, MS, FAAN, FIAA

Dr. Mishra is professor of neurology and coordinator of the integrative medicine program at the Keck School of Medicine, University of Southern California, and staff neurologist at the VA Greater Los Angeles Healthcare System and Olive View UCLA Medical Center. He graduated Ayurveda Charya, bachelor of medicine and surgery (ABMS) from Banaras Hindu University in Varanasi, India, and received his master's of science (anatomy) from Queens University, Kingston, Ontario, Canada, his medical degree from the University of Toronto, and his master's degree in administrative medicine from the University of Wisconsin. He is a member of numerous neuroscience and integrative medicine societies and editorial boards and is president of the American Academy of Ayurvedic Medicine (AAAM). He has been chair of an NCCAM (NIH) study section. He is a practicing neurologist, Ayurvedist, and yoga teacher. He has served as president and chair of the Indian Medical Association of Southern California, FIA of Southern California, and as regional director of AAPI.

Howard Moffet, MS, MPH

Howard Moffet serves as a research program manager at the Kaiser Permanente (KP) Division of Research in Oakland, California, and is a member of the KP Complementary and Alternative Medicine Research Group. He currently teaches in the Department of Health Education, Institute for Holistic Healing Studies, San Francisco State University, and was appointed by former governor Gray Davis to the California Acupuncture Board. He received his graduate degrees from the Harvard School of Public Health and the American College of Traditional Chinese Medicine. He is a licensed acupuncturist, and his research interest is in the physiological mechanisms of acupuncture.

Adrianne Rogers, MD

Dr. Rogers received her medical degree from Harvard Medical School and pathology training at the Mallory Institute of Pathology (Boston City Hospital) and the Peter Bent Brigham Hospital. She is professor and associate chair of pathology and laboratory medicine and director of the Office of Medical Education at Boston University School of Medicine and is on the pathology staff at Boston Medical Center. She is the author of numerous articles on experimental studies of dietary and nutritional effects on chemical carcinogenesis, is a diplomate and member of the American Board of Toxicology, on which she just completed a term as chair of the examination committee, and is a member of the editorial boards of the *Journal of Nutritional Biochemistry, Toxicology,* and *Nutrition and Cancer.* She is a member of the expert panel of the Research Institute for Fragrance Materials (RIFM), which reviews publications and data related to safety of materials used in fragrances, and of the Beryllium Industries Scientific Advisory Committee (BISAC), which reviews basic science and clinical studies of beryllium toxicity. For many years she served on and chaired the grants review panel for the American Institute for Cancer Research (AICR), which supports research in diet and cancer.

Aviva Romm, BSc, RH (AHG), CPM

Aviva Romm has been in clinical practice as an herbalist and midwife since 1986. She is currently president of the American Herbalists Guild (AHG). The author of six books on botanical medicine, Aviva is also the executive editor of the peer-reviewed *Journal of the American Herbalists Guild.* She serves as primary editor for the *Textbook of Botanical Medicine for Women,* to be published by Churchill/Elsevier in 2004. Her policy work has focused on developing national standards for botanical medicine education and practice in the United States. She regularly writes for national health magazines and peer-reviewed publications, is on the advisory board for Bastyr University's bachelor of science program in botanical medicine, and regularly presents at national conferences.

Michael Rotblatt, MD, PharmD

Dr. Rotblatt began his career as a pharmacist, receiving his PharmD from UC San Francisco, and worked as a drug information and clinical pharmacist at Stanford University Hospital. He received his medical degree from UC Irvine and completed internal medicine residency training at a UCLA program. He is currently an associate professor of medicine at UCLA and an attending physician at the Sepulveda VA Ambulatory Care Center and the Olive View–UCLA Medical Center. His area of interest is evaluating herbal medicines and other dietary supplements and educating health care professionals in this field. He is co-author of the book, *Evidence-Based Herbal Medicine*, has lectured nationally to health professional groups, and serves on the editorial board for *Focus on Alternative and Complementary Therapies* (FACT).

Andrew L. Rubman, ND

Dr. Rubman received his naturopathic medical degree from National College of Naturopathic Medicine in Portland, Oregon. A founder and lifetime member of the American Association of Naturopathic Physicians, he has been active in national media and organizations advocating the evolution of a responsible medical continuum among all licensed physicians. He has served as an advisor and lecturer for the White House Commission for Complementary and Alternative Medical Policy and medical schools across the United States. An adjunct associate professor of clinical medicine at the College of Naturopathic Medicine, University of Bridgeport, and an adjunct professor of medicine at the Florida College of Integrative Medicine, he is widely published. Dr. Rubman serves as the content provider in naturopathic medicine for the North American Menopause Society and is an editorial advisor to numerous publications.

Kenneth Sancier, PhD

Dr. Sancier is the founder and chairman of the board of directors of the Qigong Institute. He is a professor at the American College of Traditional Medicine, San Francisco. He received a doctorate from Johns Hopkins University, and his research has focused on basic and applied chemistry. Dr. Sancier developed the computerized Qigong Research Database, has written multiple reviews of qigong scientific investigations, and has published numerous qigong clinical studies. He has participated in international qigong conferences in China, Japan, Canada, and the United States. He is an editor of the *Journal of the International Society of Life Information Science* (JISLIS), director of the California Information Center of ISLIS, on the advisory board of the *Journal Of Alternative Therapies*, and is on the Council of the World Academic Society of Medical Qigong.

Elad Schiff, MD

Dr. Schiff received his internal medicine training at B'nai Zion Medical Center in Israel. He has served as chairman of the Committee for Regulation of Complementary Medicine Studies, Ministries of Education and Health, Israel. He has published multiple articles in the areas of acupuncture and pain medicine and is currently a residential fellow at the Program in Integrative Medicine at the University of Arizona under Dr. Andrew Weil. In addition to practicing internal medicine, he teaches in leading schools of complementary medicine in Israel and is involved with a complementary medicine clinic that provides reflexology, shiatsu, and acupuncture services.

Robb Scholten, MSLIS

Robb Scholten serves as the information officer at the Division for Research and Education on Complementary and Integrative Medical Therapies, Harvard Medical School. Before that he worked as an academic representative at PaperChase, a pioneer organization in consumer-accessible database interfaces. He conducted his graduate work in information science at the University of Tennessee, where he helped design one of the first web-controlled online remote access database services in the state. Robb is also the secretary for the division's three major continuing education courses, which focus on integrative medical therapies.

Michael Smith, MRPharmS, ND

Dr. Smith serves as associate dean for research at the Canadian College of Naturopathic Medicine. He is the author of numerous review articles and texts on the safety and uses of natural products, including *Herbs to Homeopathy*, published by Prentice Hall Canada in 2002. He has served as principal investigator for multiple studies, including a prospective controlled study of echinacea published in the *Archives of Internal Medicine* (2000), studies of alternative therapies in cancer, and studies of alternative therapies in pregnancy. As a recognized authority in Canada, he serves on multiple national and international panels, including the National Advisory Group on Complementary and Alternative Medicine and HIV/AIDS, and the International Editorial Board for Focus on Alternative and Complementary Therapies (FACT).

David Sollars, MAc, HMC

David Sollars holds a master's degree in oriental medicine from the New England School of Acupuncture (NESA). He is currently an adjunct professor of biology at Merrimack College, where he lectures on integrated approaches to sports medicine. He is a diplomat of the National Commission for the Certification of Acupuncturists, NESA's Chinese Herbal Medical Program, the North American Homeopathic Master's Clinician Course, and the International Federation of Homeopathy. He is certified in Japanese Shiatsu, Sotai, and Chinese Tui-Na massage. He has been practicing in the Boston area for over 16 years, has authored books on acupuncture, fitness, and homeopathy, and is a frequent lecturer and consultant for colleges, hospitals, insurance companies, and patient support groups.

Philippe Szapary, MD

Dr. Szapary is a graduate of Brown University and the University of Chicago Pritzker School of Medicine. He conducted his internship and residency in primary care internal medicine at the University of California, San Francisco. Dr. Szapary is an assistant professor of medicine in the division of general internal medicine at the University of Pennsylvania, where he conducts clinical trials in complementary and alternative therapies in cardiovascular disease. He is the principal investigator of a randomized clinical trial of gugulipid in hypercholesterolemia and has participated in several industry-sponsored trials of plant stanol esters in hyperlipidemia. Dr. Szapary has also recently been awarded a career development award from the NIH to study the effects of Ayurvedic botanicals in atherosclerosis. He has authored several chapters in ambulatory medicine, evidence-based medicine, and CAM therapies in cardiovascular disease. Dr. Szapary is also a regular contributor to the publication *Alternative Medicine Alert.*

Candy Tsourounis, PharmD

Dr. Tsourounis is the acting director of the Drug Information Analysis Service at the University of California, San Francisco (UCSF). She also serves as an assistant clinical professor in the department of clinical pharmacy at UCSF. Dr. Tsourounis co-coordinates an evidence-based course in herbal remedies and dietary supplements, sponsored by the Osher Center for Integrative Medicine. She has co-authored multiple book chapters on herbs and dietary supplements in medical and pharmacy textbooks. Dr. Tsourounis serves as a clinical consultant and editor for several drug information publications and computer software programs, particularly in the areas of herbal remedies and dietary supplements. She has coordinated continuing education programs for national pharmacy societies on herbs and dietary supplements and lectures nationally.

Andrew Weil, MD

Andrew Weil is an internationally recognized expert on medicinal plants, alternative medicine, and the reform of medical education. Dr. Weil received his undergraduate degree in biology (botany) from Harvard University, medical degree from Harvard Medical School, and completed a medical internship at Mt. Zion Hospital in San Francisco. In the 1970s, as a fellow of the Institute of Current World Affairs, Dr. Weil traveled widely in North and South America and Africa collecting information on drug use in other cultures, medicinal plants, and alternative methods of treating disease. He subsequently conducted research on medicinal and psychoactive plants at the Harvard Botanical Museum. Dr. Weil currently serves as director of the Program in Integrative Medicine of the College of Medicine, University of Arizona, where he holds appointments as clinical professor of medicine and clinical assistant professor of family and community medicine. The Program in Integrative Medicine aims to change U.S. medical education by including information on alternative therapies, mind-body interactions, healing, and other subjects not currently emphasized in the training of physicians. Dr. Weil is the author of numerous scientific and popular articles, as well as seven books, including the international best sellers *Spontaneous Healing* and *Eight Weeks to Optimum Health.* His most recent books include *Eating Well for Optimum Health: The Essential Guide to Food, Diet, and Nutrition* and *The Healthy Kitchen: Recipes for a Better Body, Life, and Spirit* (with Rosie Daley).

Roger Wood, LMT, Dipl. ABT (NCCAOM)

Roger Wood is a shiatsu practitioner. He received his training at the Boston Shiatsu School and 2 years of advanced training in North Yorkshire, England. He is the founder and president of the American Organization for Bodywork Therapies of Asia (MA), a professional organization for shiatsu and other Asian bodywork therapists. He is a diplomate of the National Certification Commission for Acupuncture and Oriental Medicine. In addition to his clinical practice, he supervises students at the Boston Shiatsu School Student Clinic and participates in NIH-sponsored research on low back pain at the Beth Israel Deaconess Medical Center, Harvard Medical School.

Robert Zori, MD

Dr. Zori is an associate professor, chief of the division of genetics, and director of cytogenetics in the department of pediatrics at the University of Florida. He is a graduate of Odense University Medical School in Denmark and the Baystate Medical Center Residency Program in Massachusetts. He has practiced medicine in both Denmark and the United States.

AUTHORS/CONTRIBUTORS

Clement Abedamowo, MD: Harvard School of Public Health
Winnie Abrahamson, ND: Private practice
Tracee Abrams, PharmD: University of Rhode Island
Imtiaz Ahmad, MD: Harvard School of Public Health
Jennifer Armstrong, PharmD: University of Rhode Island
Rawan Barakat, PharmD: Massachusetts College of Pharmacy
James P. Barassi, DC, DACBSP: Harvard Medical School
Steve Bediakoh, PharmD: Northeastern University
Karl Berger, ABT, LMT: Harvard Vanguard Alternative Paths to Health
Anja Bevens, PharmD: Northeastern University
Michael Bodock, RPh: Massachusetts General Hospital
Jay Bradner, MD: Brigham & Women's Hospital
Larry Callanan, MD: Beth Israel Deaconess Healthcare
Carolyn Carley, PharmD: Northeastern University
John Clark, PharmD: Massachusetts General Hospital
Colleen Collins, PharmD: Massachusetts General Hospital
Jeffrey Collins, MD, PhD: Brigham and Women's Hospital
Michelle Corrado, PharmD: Harvard Vanguard Medical Association
Mary Couillard, PhD, RN, FNP: North County Children's Clinic
Renn Crichlow, MD: Harvard Medical School
Cynthia Dacey, PharmD: Natural Standard Research
Alicia Dalton, PhD: Harvard University
Sean Dalton, MD, MPH, PhD: University of Cambridge (UK)
Theresa Davies-Heerema, PhD: Boston School of Medicine
Kamal Dhanota, PharmD: Northeastern University
Diana Do, MD: Johns Hopkins University Medical School
Mary Dulay, PharmD: Northeastern University
Samantha Duong, PharmD: Massachusetts General Hospital
Benjamin Ebert MD, PhD: Harvard Medical School
Sarah Elshama, PharmD: Massachusetts College of Pharmacy

Carla Falkson, MD: University of Alabama
Ivo Foppa, MD, PhD: University of South Carolina
Steve Gabardi, PharmD: Brigham and Women's Hospital
Levi Garraway, MD, PhD: Harvard Medical School
Anait Gasparyan, PharmD: Northeastern University
Cristina Gavriel, PharmD: Massachusetts College of Pharmacy
Gerald Gianutsos, PhD, JD: University of Connecticut
Peter Glickman, MD: Harvard Medical School
Penelope Greene, PhD: Harvard School of Public Health
Jaspal Gujral, MBBS: Medical College of Georgia
Rita Guldbrandsen, PharmD: Northeastern University
Adarsh Gupta, RPh: Children's Hospital
Shlomit Halachmi, MD: Harvard Vanguard
Michelle Harrison, PharmD: University of Rhode Island
Sadaf Hashmi, MD, MPh: Harvard School of Public Health
Jo Hermanns, PhD: Naresuan University: Thailand
Charissa Hodgeboom, PhD, Lac: Private practice
Taras Hollyer, ND: Canadian College of Natural Medicine
Kathy Iglesias, PharmD: Northeastern University
Jason Jang, Bs.C., DC: Palmer Chiropractic West
Sun Kang, PharmD: Northeastern University
Kelly Karpa, BSPharm, PhD: Penn State University College of Medicine
Beth Kerbel PharmD: New England Medical Center
Helena Kim: PharmD: Northeastern University
Eileen Kingsbury, PharmD: University of Rhode Island
Mitchell Knutson, MPH: Harvard School of Public Health
Paul Kraus, PharmD: Northeastern University
Brad Kuo, MD: Massachusetts General Hospital
Grace Kuo, PharmD: Baylor College of Medicine
James Lake, MD: Pacific Grove
Rebecca Lawrence, ND: Lawrence Natural Medicine
Anh Le, PhD: Emory University
Melissa Leck, PharmD: Massachusetts College of Pharmacy
Erik Letko, MD: Massachusetts Eye and Ear Infirmary
Nikos Linardakis, MD: Private practice
Anita Lipke, PharmD: Natural Standard Research
Anthony Lisi, DC: Palmer College of Chiropractic West
Nicole Maisch, PharmD: St. John's University
Timothy McCall, MD: Author, *Examining Your Doctor*
Michelle Mele, PharmD: Northeastern University
Victor Mendoza, MD: Washington University Medical Center
Arielle Mizrahi-Arnaud, MD: Children's Hospital Boston
Jamie Nelsen, PharmD: University of Rhode Island
Ly Nguyen, PharmD: Northeastern University
David Olson, MD: Boston Medical Center
Carolyn Williams Orlando, MA: Private practice
Kimberly Pacitto, PharmD: Massachusetts College of Pharmacy
Regina Pacor, ND, MW: Private practice
George Papaliodis, MD: Massachusetts Eye and Ear Infirmary

Jeff Peppercorn, MD: Harvard Medical School
An T Pham, PharmD: Northeastern University
Cam Pham, PharmD: Massachusetts College of Pharmacy
Karen Powell, PharmD: Private practice
Venessa Price, PharmD: Harvard Vanguard Medical Associates
Carol Rainville, ND: Private practice
Victoria Rand, MD: University of California San Francisco
Swathi Reddy, PharmD: Massachusetts College of Pharmacy
J. Daniel Robinson, PharmD: University of Florida
Andrew Ross, MD: Harvard Medical School
Haleh Sadig, PharmD: Massachusetts College of Pharmacy
Anabela Santos, PharmD: Northeastern University
Lisa Scully, PharmD: Massachusetts College of Pharmacy
Huaihai Shan, Qigong Master, MD: Shanghai University, China
Natalia Shcherbak, PhD: St. Petersburg State Medical University
Elizabeth Sheehan, PharmD: Northeastern University
Scott Shurmur, MD: Nebraska Medical Center
Charlene So, PharmD: University of Michigan
Carolyn Soo, PharmD: Northeastern University
Anne Spencer, PharmD, BCPS: Medical University of South Carolina
Nancy Tannous, PharmD: Northeastern University
Kellie Taylor, PharmD: Northeastern University
Vera Terry, PhD, LLB: Children's Hospital, Westmead, Australia
Huy N. Tran, PharmD: Northeastern University
My Le Truong, PharmD: Northeastern University
Verda Tunaligil, MD, MPh: Harvard School of Public Health
Dietrich von Stechow, MD: Harvard Medical School
Mamta Vora, PharmD: Natural Standard Research
Kirstin Wadewitz, PharmD: Massachusetts General Hospital
Deborah Wexler, MD: Harvard Medical School
Peter Wolsko, MD: Harvard Medical School
Jerod Work, PharmD, MBA: University of Minnesota
Jack Wylie, MD: Harvard Medical School
Monica Zangwill, MD, MPH: Beth Israel Deaconess Medical Center
Meng Yeng, PharmD: ACS-Consultec, Inc.

TRANSLATORS

Alata Brys (Polish)
Baochong Chang, MD, PhD (Chinese)
Elif Cindik, MD, MPH (German)
Raquel Domínguez, MD (Spanish, German)
Amaia Egues, PharmD (Spanish)
Ivo Foppa, MD, PhD (German, French, Italian)
Irina Gladkikh, RN, JD (French, Russian)
Silvia Goldstein (Spanish)
Regina Gorenshteyn (Russian)
Francesco Graziano, MD (Italian)
Jens Hasskarl, MD (German)
Shahidul Islam, MD, PhD (Swedish)

Acknowledgments

Many individuals have contributed significantly to the content and effort underlying this book and the Natural Standard Research Collaboration in general.

We are grateful to John Martinson, without whose support this project would not have been possible. Our close colleague and friend Paul Hammerness has shouldered significant editorial responsibility, as has Charles Holmes, a fellow co-founder of Natural Standard. Early contributors to Natural Standard provided the solid methodological and editorial foundation that has distinguished the organization, in particular, Michael Smith, Heather Boon, David Sollars, Philippe Szapary, E-P Barrette, and Steve Bent. We would also like to thank several individuals—Adrianne Rogers, Candy Tsourounis, and Cathi Dennehy—who have continued to contribute significantly to the collaboration, including materials in this book.

Invaluable has been the contribution of Chris Wisdo, whose technical aptitude has facilitated the functionality of Natural Standard. Members of the Research Team over the past years have fostered a productive and collegial work environment, and we are particularly grateful for the commitment of Regina Gorenshteyn and Michelle Nhuch.

There are several trailblazers in the field of evidence-based/academic CAM who have defined an environment in which the work of Natural Standard is valued. We are thankful to David Eisenberg, who has continued to provide us with valuable guidance and enthusiasm, as has his Information Officer, our friend Robb Scholten. Edzard Ernst has given insights as an editor for Natural Standard and continues to push this field ahead through publishing. Ellen Hughes has persistently provided guidance and support. Harley Goldberg remains a champion of this field, as well as a friend.

We would especially like to thank Kellie White, Kim Fons, Inta Ozols, and Linda Duncan at Elsevier, who have shared our enthusiasm for Natural Standard print projects and have been a pleasure as colleagues. All of the editors and authors of Natural Standard have helped forge this unique multidisciplinary collaboration, yielding a unique consensus and center in an otherwise fractured field. We look forward to our continued work together. Finally, we would like to thank our families and friends, who have supported us through this and other arduous projects.

Kate and Ethan

Contents

Introduction

Since its establishment in 1999, the Natural Standard Research Collaboration has become one of the world's premier sources of scientifically based information on complementary and alternative medicine (CAM). This international collaborative effort has involved more than 300 contributors from multiple healthcare disciplines across numerous countries. Editors and reviewers range from the most well-known researchers and clinicians in this field to private practitioners.

Natural Standard maintains an online database of evidence-based CAM reviews, including coverage of herbs, supplements, modalities (such as chiropractic or massage), daily news briefings, continuing education, and conditions-based cross-referencing. Subscriptions to this database are available for individuals or institutions at www.naturalstandard.com. In addition, Natural Standard provides CAM information for hospitals, healthcare institutions, HMOs, research organizations, manufacturers, journals, magazines, and textbooks worldwide. Millions of clinicians and patients have relied on Natural Standard content.

This book includes comprehensive systematic reviews of selected herbs and supplements, designed for use by clinicians and researchers. The topics covered in this first volume have been selected based on utilization data, sales trends, frequency of information requests by institutional/ individual users of Natural Standard, and safety concerns. Tremendous time, labor, and cost are involved with the creation of each piece, involving numerous individuals via an extensive methodology (described below). We are constantly adding new topics and expanding this database.

These pieces demonstrate the growing body of literature regarding the efficacy and safety of CAM therapies, although research for many of these therapies is still in its early phases. It is our hope that this information will serve as a helpful guide to these selected agents.

NATURAL STANDARD BACKGROUND

Natural Standard aims to provide high-quality, reliable information about CAM therapies to clinicians, patients, and healthcare institutions. Through systematic aggregation and analysis of scientific data (see below), incorporation of historic and folkloric perspectives, consultation with multidisciplinary editorial experts, use of validated grading scales (see Table 1), and blinded peer-review processes, Natural Standard builds evidence-based and consensus-based content. This content is designed to support safer and more informed therapeutic decisions.

As the volume of CAM safety concerns and scientific research increases, clinicians and patients are faced with progressively complex therapeutic decisions. These issues, coupled with a growing consciousness among practitioners that many patients use CAM therapies, has created a need for high-quality information services and decision support utilities.

However, rigorous, peer-reviewed, evidence-based resources in this area are scarce. Sources of CAM information are often not updated with appropriate frequency, rely on anecdotal evidence rather than an evidence-based approach, are not rooted in academic health centers, are not scientifically rigorous, and do not encompass a multidisciplinary approach.

In response to this need, the Natural Standard Research Collaboration was formed as a multidisciplinary, multi-institution initiative in 1999. Natural Standard content and rigorous methodology are designed to address issues of safety and efficacy that directly pertain to the questions raised by clinicians, patients, and healthcare institutions.

CAM is one part of a larger healthcare context that is becoming progressively integrated. Natural Standard aspires to raise the standards for CAM information, toward improving the quality of healthcare delivery overall.

MONOGRAPH METHODOLOGY: SYSTEMATIC AGGREGATION, ANALYSIS, AND REVIEW OF THE LITERATURE

Search Strategy

To prepare each Natural Standard monograph, electronic searches are conducted in 10 databases, including AMED, CANCERLIT, CINAHL, CISCOM, the Cochrane Library, EMBASE, HerbMed, International Pharmaceutical Abstracts, Medline, and NAPRALERT. Search terms include the common name(s), scientific name(s), and all listed synonyms for each topic. Hand searches are conducted of 20 additional journals (not indexed in common databases) and of bibliographies from 50 selected secondary references. No restrictions are placed on language or quality of publications. Researchers in the CAM field are consulted for access to additional references or ongoing research.

Selection Criteria

All literature is collected pertaining to efficacy in humans (regardless of study design, quality, or language), dosing, precautions, adverse effects, use in pregnancy/lactation, interactions, alteration of laboratory assays, and mechanism of action (*in vitro,* animal research, human data). Standardized inclusion/exclusion criteria are used in the selection.

Data Analysis

Data extraction and analysis are performed by healthcare professionals conducting clinical work and research at academic centers, using standardized instruments that pertain to each monograph section (defining inclusion and exclusion criteria and analytic techniques, including validated measures of study quality). Data are verified by a second reviewer.

Review Process

Blinded review of monographs is conducted by multidisciplinary research-clinical faculty at major academic centers with expertise in epidemiology and biostatistics, pharmacology, toxicology, CAM research, and clinical practice. In cases of editorial disagreement, a three-member panel of the editorial board addresses conflicts and consults experts when applicable. Authors of studies are contacted when clarification is required.

Update Process

Natural Standard regularly monitors scientific literature and industry warnings. When clinically relevant new data emerge, best efforts are made to update content immediately. In addition, regular updates with renewed searches occur every 3 to 18 months, varying by topic.

NATURAL STANDARD EVIDENCE-BASED VALIDATED GRADING RATIONALE

Multiple grading scales have been developed over the past decade to evaluate the level of available scientific evidence supporting the efficacy of medical interventions. Based on existing grading scales, as well as the unique challenges involved in the evaluation of CAM therapies, the Natural Standard grading scale was developed through a multidisciplinary consensus group, widely reviewed, then piloted and validated. This scale has been found to have a high level of inter-rater reliability, has been used in numerous publications, and has been presented for discussion at the Agency for Healthcare Research and Quality (AHRQ).

These grades are used in all Natural Standard reviews (monographs). Specific grades reflect the level of available scientific evidence in support of the efficacy of a given therapy for a specific indication. Expert opinion and folkloric precedent are not included in this assessment and are reflected in a separate section of each monograph. Evidence of harm is considered separately, and the grades apply only to evidence of benefit (Table 1).

Table 1
Natural Standard Evidence-Based Validated Grading Rationale

Level of Evidence Grade	Criteria
A (Strong scientific evidence)	Statistically significant evidence of benefit from more than two properly randomized, controlled trials (RCTs), *or* evidence from one properly conducted RCT *and* one properly conducted meta-analysis, or evidence from multiple RCTs with a clear majority of the properly conducted trials showing statistically significant evidence of benefit *and* with supporting evidence in basic science, animal studies, or theory.
B (Good scientific evidence)	Statistically significant evidence of benefit from one or two properly RCTs, *or* evidence of benefit from one or more properly conducted meta-analysis *or* evidence of benefit from more than one cohort/case-control/non-randomized trials *and* with supporting evidence in basic science, animal studies, or theory.

Continued

Natural Standard Evidence-Based Validated Grading Rationale—*cont'd*

C (Unclear or conflicting scientific evidence)	Evidence of benefit from one or more small RCT(s) without adequate size, power, statistical significance, or quality of design by objective criteria,* *or* conflicting evidence from multiple RCTs without a clear majority of the properly conducted trials showing evidence of benefit or ineffectiveness, *or* evidence of benefit from more than one cohort/case-control/non-randomized trials *and* without supporting evidence in basic science, animal studies, or theory, *or* evidence of efficacy only from basic science, animal studies, or theory.
D (Fair negative scientific evidence)	Statistically significant negative evidence (i.e., lack of evidence of benefit) from cohort/case-control/non-randomized trials, *and* evidence in basic science, animal studies, or theory suggesting a lack of benefit.
F (Strong negative scientific evidence)	Statistically significant negative evidence (i.e. lack of evidence of benefit) from one or more properly randomized adequately powered trial(s) of high-quality design by objective criteria.*
Lack of evidence[†]	Unable to evaluate efficacy due to lack of adequate or available human data.

*Objective criteria are derived from validated instruments for evaluating study quality, including the 5-point scale developed by Jadad et al., in which a score below 4 is considered to indicate lesser quality methodologically (Jadad AR, Moore RA, Carroll D, et al. Assessing the quality of reports of randomized clinical trials: is blinding necessary? *Controlled Clinical Trials* 1996; 17[1]:1–12).
[†]Listed separately in monographs in the section, "Historical or Theoretical Uses That Lack Sufficient Evidence."

CAM IN THE UNITED STATES: A BRIEF BACKGROUND

Various definitions have been assigned to the term "complementary and alternative medicine (CAM)," but it is generally regarded as encompassing a broad group of healing philosophies, diagnostic approaches, and therapeutic interventions that do not belong to the politically dominant (conventional) health system of a particular society.[1,2] Some authors separately define *alternative* therapies as those used in place of conventional practices, whereas *complementary* or *integrative* medicine can be combined with mainstream approaches.[2,3] Other terms used to refer to CAM include folkloric, holistic, irregular, non-conventional, non-Western, traditional, unconventional, unorthodox, and unproven medicine.

In the United States and other Western countries, CAM therapies are often defined functionally as interventions neither taught in medical schools nor available in hospital-based practices.[4] Examples include dietary supplements (amino acids, herbal products/botanicals, minerals, vitamins, and substances that increase total dietary intake),[5] modalities (manipulative therapies, mind-body medicine, and energy/bioelectromagnetic-based approaches), spiritual healing, and nutritional/dietary alteration. Boundaries between CAM and conventional therapies are not always clear and often change over time. Scientific evidence has led to broader mainstream acceptance of some CAM therapies and rejection of others.

CAM Research

The safety and efficacy of many CAM approaches are not well studied, although the body of research is growing. In 1992, the U.S. Congress established the Office of Alternative Medicine (OAM) within the National Institutes of Health (NIH), with a budget of $2 million to "investigate and evaluate promising unconventional medical practices." In 1998, Congress elevated the status of the OAM to a NIH Center, becoming the National Center for Complementary and Alternative Medicine (NCCAM).

The budget of NCCAM has progressively increased, from $50 million in fiscal year 1999 to $114 million in 2003, toward its mission to "support rigorous research on CAM, to train researchers in CAM, and to disseminate information to the public and professionals on which CAM modalities work, which do not, and why."

Prevalence

In the United States, an estimated 44% of the population used at least one CAM therapy in 1997.[4,6-8] Utilization in specific chronic diseases appears to be even higher. For example, surveys published since 1999 suggest that between 25% to 83% of U.S. cancer patients have used CAM therapies at some point after diagnosis, with variations in use rates depending on geographic area and type of cancer.[9-24] These reports suggest use of high-dose vitamins among cancer patients to be 21% to 81%, herbs and supplements 9% to 60%, combination herbal teas (such as Essiac) 7% to 25%, and lifestyle diets (such as vegan or macrobiotic) 9% to 24%.

Earlier studies generally report lower overall prevalence of CAM use (9% to 54%), possibly due to increasing rates of utilization or to broadening of the definition of CAM in survey questionnaires and in the views of respondents.[25,26]

CAM use appears to be more common among those with higher educational level, higher income, female sex, younger age, use of chemotherapy or surgery, or history of CAM use before diagnosis.[12,15,18] Overall, surveys vary in terms of definitions of CAM and of specific types of therapy included in questionnaires, complicating assessment of overall prevalence.

Safety Concerns

Significant potential morbidity and cost have been indirectly associated with herb/supplement-drug interactions, including increased emergency room visits, outpatient clinic visits, and perioperative complications.[27-29] However, the true direct and indirect costs, morbidity, and mortality associated with CAM-related interactions or adverse effects are not known or well studied.

Systematic study or published data regarding potential interactions between specific herbs and vitamins and prescription drugs is limited.[30-38] (See Appendix A for a list of agents with potentially concerning properties, such as bleeding risk, sedation, hepatotoxicity, estrogenic effects, P450 inhibition or induction, or hypoglycemic effects.)

Standardization

Preparation of herbs and supplements may vary from manufacturer to manufacturer and from batch to batch within one manufacturer. Because it is often not clear what are the active components of a product, standardization may not be possible, and the clinical effects of different brands may not be comparable.

Patient-Clinician Communication

Some research reports that neither adult[23] nor pediatric[39] patients receive sufficient information or discuss CAM therapies with a physician, pharmacist, nurse, or CAM practitioner, whereas other studies find more than 60% of patients discuss CAM with their physician.[20] These discrepancies likely reflect an overall heterogeneity in clinicians' styles of managing patients who use CAM.

Most physicians do not receive formal training regarding the safety and effectiveness of CAM and have limited knowledge in this area.[40] There appears to be significant concern among practitioners about potential safety risks and patient out-of-pocket expenses associated with CAM use.[41,42] Surveys suggest a desire by clinicians for access to quality CAM information, both to improve quality of care and to enhance communication with patients.[43,44] Due to potential adverse effects and interactions associated with CAM use, clinicians are often encouraged to ask patients about CAM use, although it is not known if beneficial outcomes result from this practice. Recommended approaches for clinicians to patients who use CAM have been published[45,46] and generally include suggestions to encourage patients to discuss their reasons for seeking CAM, to provide patients with evidence-based information about specific CAM therapies (or explain when available evidence is insufficient), to explain known safety concerns and note that "natural" does not always equate with safety, to support patients emotionally and psychologically even if they choose a CAM therapy with which the clinician does not agree, and to provide close clinical follow-up of patients using CAM therapies. Several evidence-based CAM informational resources are available online for clinicians and patients and can be used as a starting point for discussions in this area (Table 2).

Table 2
Evidence-Based Online CAM Resources (For Clinicians and Patients)

Resource	Description
Natural Standard Collaboration (www.naturalstandard.com)	The online counterpart to this book, containing hundreds of reviews of herbs, supplements, modalities (chiropractic, massage, etc), patient information, and monthly news briefs.
M. D. Anderson CIMER (www.mdanderson.org/departments/CIMER)	An informational site maintained by M. D. Anderson Cancer Center with information on CAM therapies relevant to cancer patients and access to other resources.
National Center for Complementary and Alternative Medicine (NCCAM) (http://nccam.nih.gov)	A site maintained by NCCAM, the NIH Center dedicated to primary CAM research.
Office of Dietary Supplements (http://ods.od.nih.gov/index.aspx)	A federal agency that supports research and disseminates research results in the area of dietary supplements.
Cochrane Collaboration (www.cochrane.org)	An international collaboration that prepares systematic reviews of numerous medical therapies, including many CAM approaches.
ConsumerLab (www.consumerlab.com)	An organization that evaluates commercially available products for constituents and adulterants, and publishes online lists of these test results.

References

1. Panel on Definition and Description, Office of Alternative Medicine, National Institutes of Health, CAM Research Methodology Conference, Bethesda, MD, April 1995.
2. Zollman C, Vickers A. ABC of complementary medicine: What is complementary medicine? Br Med J 1999;319:693-696.
3. Cassileth BR. "Complementary" or "alternative"? It makes a difference in cancer care. Complement Ther Med 1999;44:22.
4. Eisenberg DM, Davis, RB, Ettner SL, et al. Trends in alternative medicine use in the United States, 1990-1997. Results of a follow-up national survey. JAMA 1998;280(18): 1569-1575.
5. Dietary Supplement Health and Education Act of 1994 (DSHEA), Public Law 103-417, October 25, 1994 (103rd Congress).

6. Wolsko PM, Eisenberg DM, Davis RB, et al. Insurance coverage, medical conditions, and visits to alternative medicine providers. Results of a national survey. Arch Intern Med 2002;162:281-287.
7. Astin JA. Why patients use alternative medicine: results of a national survey. JAMA 1998;279:1548-1553.
8. Druss B. Association between use of unconventional therapies and conventional medical services. JAMA 1999;282:651-656.
9. White JD. The National Cancer Institute's perspective and agenda for promoting awareness and research on alternative therapies for cancer (keynote address). J Altern Complement Med 2002;8(5):545-550.
10. Adler SR, Fosket JR. Disclosing complementary and alternative medicine use in the medical encounter: A qualitative study in women with breast cancer. J Fam Pract 1999;48:453-458.
11. Bernstein BJ, Grasso T. Prevalence of complementary and alternative medicine use in cancer patients. Oncology (Huntington) 2001;15(10):1267-1272.
12. Burstein HJ, Gelber S, Guadagnoli E, at al. Use of alternative medicine by women with early-stage breast cancer. N Engl J Med 1999;340(22):1733-1739.
13. Gotay CC, Hara W, Issel BF, et al. Use of complementary and alternative medicine in Hawaii cancer patients. Hawaii Med J 1999;58(4):94-98.
14. Kao GD, Devine P. Use of complementary health practices by prostate carcinoma patients undergoing radiation therapy. Cancer 2000;88(3):615-619.
15. Lee MM, Chang JS, Jacobs B, et al. Complementary and alternative medicine use among men with prostate cancer in four ethnic populations. Am J Public Health 2002;92(10): 1606-1609.
16. Lippert MC, McClain R, Boyd JC, et al. Alternative medicine use in patients with localized prostate carcinoma treated with curative intent. Cancer 1999;86(12):2642-2648.
17. Maskarinec G, Shumay DM, Kakai H, et al. Ethnic differences in complementary and alternative medicine use among cancer patients. J Altern Complement Med 2000;6(6): 531-538.
18. Morris KT, Johnson N, Homer L, et al. A comparison of complementary therapy use between breast cancer patients and patients with other primary tumor sites (abstract). Am J Surg 2000;179:407-411.
19. Patterson RE, Neuhouser ML, Hedderson MM, et al. Types of alternative medicine used by patients with breast, colon, or prostate cancer: predictors, motives, and costs. J Altern Complement Med 2002;8(4):477-485.
20. Richardson MA, Sanders T, Palmer JL, et al. Complementary/alternative medicine use in a comprehensive cancer center and the implications for oncology. J Clin Oncol 2000; 18(13):2505-2514.
21. Shumay DM, Maskarinec G, Gotay CC, et al. Determinants of the degree of complementary and alternative medicine use among patients with cancer. J Altern Complement Med 2002;8(5):661-671.
22. Sparber A, Bauer L, Curt G, et al. Use of complementary medicine by adult patients participating in cancer clinical trials. Oncol Nurs Forum 2000;27(4):623-630.
23. Swisher EM, Cohn DE, Goff BA, et al. Use of complementary and alternative medicine among women with gynecologic cancers. Gynecol Oncol 2002;84:363-367.
24. VandeCreek L, Rogers E, Lester J. Use of alternative therapies among breast cancer outpatients compared with the general population. Altern Ther Health Med 1999;5(1): 71-76.
25. Ernst E, Cassileth BR. The prevalence of complementary/alternative medicine in cancer. A systematic review. Cancer 1998;83(4):777-782.
26. Sparber A, Wooten JC. Surveys of complementary and alternative medicine. II. Use of alternative and complementary cancer therapies. J Altern Complement Med 2001; 7(3):281-287.
27. Rogers EA, Gough JE, Brewer KL. Are emergency department patients at risk for herb-drug interactions? Acad Emerg Med 2001;8(9):932-934.
28. Farah MH, Edwards R, Lindquist M, et al. International monitoring of adverse health effects associated with herbal medicines. Pharmacoepidemiol Drug Safety 2000;9:105-112.

29. Ang-Lee MK, Moss J, Yuan CS. Herbal medicines and perioperative care. JAMA 2001; 286:208-216.
30. Palmer ME, Haller C, McKinney PE, et al. Adverse events associated with dietary supplements: an observational study. Lancet 2003;361(9352):101-106.
31. Fugh-Berman A. Herb-drug interactions. Lancet 2000;355(9198):134-138.
32. Abebe W. Herbal medication: potential for adverse interactions with analgesic drugs. J Clin Pharm Ther 2002;27(6):391-401.
33. Ernst E. Possible interactions between synthetic and herbal medicinal products. 1. A systematic review of the indirect evidence. Perfusion 2000;13:4-15.
34. Ernst E. Interactions between synthetic and herbal medicinal products. 2. A systematic review of the direct evidence. Perfusion 2000;13:60-70.
35. Piscitelli SC, Burstein AH. Herb-drug interactions and confounding in clinical trials. J Herbal Pharmacother 2002;2(1):23-26.
36. Izzo AA, Ernst E. Interactions between herbal medicines and prescribed drugs: a systematic review. Drugs 2001;61(15):2163-2175.
37. Hardy ML. Herb-drug interactions: An evidence-based table. Alternative Medicine Alert 2000;June:64-69.
38. Lambrecht J, Hamilton W, Rabinovich A. A review of herb-drug interactions: documented and theoretical. U S Pharmacist 2000;25(8):1-12.
39. Friedman T, Slayton WB, Allen LS, et al. Use of alternative therapies for children with cancer. Pediatrics 1997;100(6):E1(2-6).
40. Jonas WB. Alternative medicine—learning from the past, examining the present, advancing to the future. JAMA 1998;280:1616-1618.
41. Angell M. Alternative medicine—the risks of untested and unregulated remedies. N Engl J Med 1998;339(123):839-841.
42. Studdert DM. Medical malpractice implications of alternative medicine. JAMA 1998;280(18):1610-1615.
43. Winslow LC, Shapiro H. Physicians want education about complementary and alternative medicine to enhance communication with their patients. Arch Intern Med 2002;162(10): 1176-1181.
44. Kroll DJ. Concerns and needs for research in herbal supplement pharmacotherapy and safety. J Herbal Pharmacother 2001;1(2):3-23.
45. Weiger WA, Smith M, Boon H, et al. Advising patients who seek complementary and alternative medical therapies for cancer. Ann Intern Med 2002;137(11):889-903.
46. Eisenberg DM. Advising patients who seek alternative medical therapies. Ann Intern Med 1997;127:61.

Acidophilus (Lactobacillus)

(*Lactobacillus acidophilus*)

RELATED TERMS

- Acidophilus, Acidophilus Extra Strength, acidophilus milk, Actimel, Bacid, DDS-Acidophilus, Enpac, Fermalac, Florajen, Gynoflor, Kala, Kyo-Dophilus, *L. acidophilus* milk, *L. acidophilus* yogurt, Lacteol Fort, Lactinex, Lactobacillaceae, lactobacillus (lactobacilli), Lacto Bacillus, MoreDophilus, Narine, Probiata, Pro-Bionate, probiotic, Superdophilus, yogurt.

BACKGROUND

- Lactobacilli are bacteria that normally live in the human small intestine and vagina. *Lactobacillus acidophilus* is considered to be beneficial because it produces vitamin K, lactase, and antimicrobial substances such as acidolin, acidolphilin, lactocidin, and bacteriocin. Multiple trials in humans report the benefits of acidophilus for bacterial vaginosis. Other medicinal uses of acidophilus have not been sufficiently studied to form clear conclusions.
- The term *probiotic* is used to describe organisms that are used medicinally, including bacteria such as *L. acidophilus* and yeast such as *Saccharomyces boulardii.*
- Although it is generally believed to be safe with few side effects, oral *L. acidophilus* should be avoided in people with intestinal damage, a weakened immune system, or overgrowth of intestinal bacteria.

USES BASED ON SCIENTIFIC EVIDENCE	Grade*
Bacterial vaginosis Multiple studies in humans report that *L. acidophilus* vaginal suppositories are effective in the treatment of bacterial vaginosis. A small number of studies suggest that eating yogurt enriched with *Lactobacillus acidophilus* may be similarly beneficial. Additional research is necessary before a firm conclusion can be reached. Persons with persistent vaginal discomfort are advised to seek medical attention.	B
Asthma There is limited research in this area, with unclear results.	C
Diarrhea prevention Limited research studies in humans suggest that *L. acidophilus* may not be effective when used to prevent diarrhea in travelers or in people taking antibiotics. Several studies reported that the related species *Lactobacillus GG* was helpful in the prevention of diarrhea in children and travelers. Additional study is needed in these areas before a firm conclusion can be drawn.	C

Continued

Diarrhea treatment (in children) A small amount of studies in children, using different forms of acidophilus, report no improvement in diarrhea. Future studies should use a viable *L. acidophilus* culture to assess its effects. Multiple studies in humans using *Lactobacillus GG*, a different species, suggest that this species may be a safe and effective treatment for diarrhea in otherwise healthy infants and children. *L. acidophilus* may be helpful in the management of chronic or persistent diarrhea and bacterial-overgrowth related diarrhea. Further research is needed to determine potential safe and effective dosing.	C
Hepatic encephalopathy There have been limited studies of *L. acidophilus* as therapy for hepatic encephalopathy, a liver disorder with symptoms including confused thinking. Results were inconclusive.	C
High cholesterol There is conflicting information from several studies in humans regarding the effect of *L. acidophilus*–enriched dairy products on decreasing blood levels of total cholesterol or low-density lipoprotein ("bad cholesterol").	C
Irritable bowel syndrome Studies in humans report mixed results in the improvement of bowel symptoms in patients taking *L. acidophilus* by mouth.	C
Lactose intolerance Several studies in humans examined whether *L. acidophilus* given by mouth improves digestion of lactose. Results were inconclusive, and more research is needed in this area.	C
Necrotizing enterocolitis prevention One study using *L. acidophilus* in combination with another bacterium (*Bifidobacterium infantis*) in infants reported fewer cases of necrotizing enterocolitis (severe inflammation of the gut), and no complications related to treatment. Additional research is necessary in this area before conclusions can be drawn.	C
Vaginal candidiasis (yeast infection) In some studies, *L. acidophilus* has been taken by mouth or as a vaginal suppository for the prevention or treatment of vaginal yeast infections. The results have not been adequately assessed, and more research is needed in this area before a conclusion can be drawn.	C

*Key to grades: *A:* Strong scientific evidence for this use; *B:* Good scientific evidence for this use; *C:* Unclear scientific evidence for this use; *D:* Fair scientific evidence against this use (it may not work); *F:* Strong scientific evidence against this use (it likely does not work). For a more detailed explanation of efficacy criteria, see "Natural Standard Evidence-Based Validated Grading Rationale" in the Introduction.

Uses Based on Tradition, Theory, or Limited Scientific Evidence

Acne, AIDS, allergies, cancer, canker sores, colitis, colon cancer prevention, constipation, diaper rash, Crohn's disease, diverticulitis, *Escherichia coli* infection in cancer patients, fever blisters, heart disease, heartburn, hives, immune enhancer, indigestion, infection, overgrowth of bacteria in the small bowel, preoperative prevention of infections or gut bacteria loss, stomach ulcer, thrush, ulcerative colitis, urinary tract infection.

DOSING

The following doses are based on scientific research, publications, traditional use, or expert opinion. Many herbs and supplements have not been thoroughly tested, and their safety and effectiveness may not be proven. Brands may be made differently, with variable ingredients even within the same brand. The doses shown may not apply to all products. It is important to always read product labels and discuss doses with a qualified healthcare provider before therapy is started.

Standardization

- Standardization involves measuring the amount of certain chemicals in products to try to make different preparations similar to each other. It is not always known if the chemicals being measured are the "active" ingredients. *L. acidophilus* is commercially prepared as a concentrate, in a freeze-dried form, or as viable cultures. For all formulations, the dose is based on the number of living organisms. Standardization of *L. acidophilus* has been a challenge because it is difficult to assess which products contain live bacteria and are free from contaminants. Significant variations in effectiveness and shelf life have been observed. Storage conditions and the length of time that the product is stored can alter the effectiveness, and refrigeration is recommended for *L. acidophilus* products. Pasteurization kills *L. acidophilus.*

Adults (18 Years and Older)

- **Tablets/capsules/liquid/yogurt:** A dose between 1 billion and 10 billion viable (live) *L. acidophilus* bacteria taken daily in divided doses is considered sufficient for most people. Higher doses may cause mild abdominal discomfort, and smaller doses may not establish a stable population in the gut. For vaginal bacterial infections, a dose that has been used is 8 ounces of yogurt containing *L. acidophilus* in a concentration of 100 million colony-forming units (10^8 CFU) in each milliliter. In one study, capsules containing 1.5 g of *L. acidophilus* were used.
- **Vaginal suppository:** Doses used for vaginal infections include 1 to 2 tablets (containing 10 million to 1 billion CFU in each tablet), inserted into the vagina once or twice daily.

Children (Younger Than 18 Years)

- **Tablets/capsules/liquid:** Some natural medicine textbooks and experts suggest that one-quarter teaspoon or one-quarter capsule of commercially available *L. acidophilus* may be safe for use in children for the replacement of gut bacteria destroyed by antibiotics. Up to 12 billion lyophilized heat-killed *L. acidophilus* has been given every 12 hours for up to 5 days. It is often recommended that

L. acidophilus supplements be taken at least 2 hours after antibiotic doses, because antibiotics may kill *L. acidophilus* if they are taken at the same time. A qualified healthcare practitioner should be consulted before *L. acidophilus* is given to children. Special caution should be used in children younger than 3 years of age.

- **Topical (applied to the skin):** Acidophilus liquid preparations have been used on the diaper area to treat yeast infections; however, safety and effectiveness have not been well studied. A qualified healthcare practitioner should be consulted before using *L. acidophilus* in children. Special caution should be used in children younger than three years of age.

SAFETY

The U.S. Food and Drug Administration does not strictly regulate herbs and supplements. There is no guarantee of the strength, purity, or safety of products, and effects may vary. It is important to always read product labels. People who have a medical condition, or are taking other drugs, herbs, or supplements, should consult a qualified healthcare provider before starting a new therapy. A healthcare provider should be contacted immediately about any side effects.

Allergies

- Lactose-sensitive people may experience abdominal discomfort from dairy products containing *L. acidophilus.*

Side Effects and Warnings

- Studies report few side effects from *L. acidophilus* when it is used at recommended doses. The most common complaint is abdominal discomfort (gas), which usually resolves with continued use. To reduce the risk of abdominal discomfort, some experts recommend limiting the daily dose to fewer than 10 billion live *L. acidophilus* organisms. Some women have reported a burning sensation in the vagina after using *L. acidophilus* vaginal tablets.
- There have been rare reports of *L. acidophilus* infection of heart valves, and the risk may be greater in people with artificial heart valves. People with severely weakened immune systems (due to disease, cancer chemotherapy drugs, or organ transplant immunosuppressants) may develop serious infections or bacteremia (bacteria in the blood) after taking *L. acidophilus.* Therefore, *L. acidophilus* should be avoided in such individuals. People with intestinal damage or recent bowel surgery also should avoid taking lactobacilli.

Pregnancy and Breastfeeding

- There are not enough scientific studies available to establish safety during pregnancy. Pregnant women should use *L. acidophilus* cautiously and under medical supervision, if at all. A small number of pregnant women have taken part in studies investigating the use of *L. acidophilus* vaginal tablets and a culture of *L. acidophilus*; no negative effects were reported, but further research is needed in this area.

INTERACTIONS

Most herbs and supplements have not been thoroughly tested for interactions with other herbs, supplements, drugs, or foods. The interactions listed here are based on reports in scientific publications, laboratory experiments, or traditional use. It is important to always read product labels. People who have a medical condition, or are taking other drugs, herbs, or supplements, should consult a qualified healthcare provider before starting a new therapy.

Interactions with Drugs

- Some experts believe that *L. acidophilus* taken by mouth should be used 2 to 3 hours after antibiotic doses to prevent killing the acidophilus organisms. It has also been suggested that lactobacilli are damaged by alcohol, and therefore alcohol should be avoided when taking acidophilus products. Scientific research is limited in these areas.
- In theory, *L. acidophilus* taken by mouth may not survive the acidic environment of the stomach. Some experts suggest that antacids should be taken 30 to 60 minutes before taking lactobacilli. However, this has not been well studied in humans.
- In theory, *L. acidophilus* may prolong the effects of some drugs, including birth control pills and benzodiazepines such as diazepam (Valium). Based on laboratory experiments, *L. acidophilus* may reduce the effectiveness of sulfasalazine (Azulfidine), a drug used for inflammatory bowel disease.

Interactions with Herbs and Dietary Supplements

- Fructo-oligosaccharides (FOS, also called *probiotics*) are non-digestible sugar chains that are nutrients for lactobacilli. FOS, taken by mouth at a dose of 2000 to 3000 mg, may stimulate the growth of lactobacilli. Natural food sources of FOS include bananas, Jerusalem artichokes, onions, asparagus, and garlic.
- *Lactobacillus casei*, *Saccharomyces boulardii*, and other probiotics may add to the effects of *L. acidophilus.*

Selected References

Natural Standard developed the preceding evidence-based information based on a systematic review of more than 200 scientific articles. For comprehensive information about alternative and complementary therapies on the professional level, go to www.naturalstandard.com. Selected references are listed here.

Agerholm-Larsen L, Raben A, Haulrik N, et al. Effect of 8 week intake of probiotic milk products on risk factors for cardiovascular diseases. Eur J Clin Nutr 2000;54(4):288-297.

Alm L. [Acidophilus milk for therapy in gastrointestinal disorders.] Nahrung 1984; 28(6-7):683-684.

Anderson JW, Gilliland SE. Effect of fermented milk (yogurt) containing *Lactobacillus acidophilus* L1 on serum cholesterol in hypercholesterolemic humans. J Am Coll Nutr 1999;18(1):43-50.

Arvola T, Laiho K, Torkkeli S, et al. Prophylactic *Lactobacillus GG* reduces antibiotic-associated diarrhea in children with respiratory infections: a randomized study. Pediatrics 1999; 104(5):e64

Bayer AS, Chow AW, Betts D, et al. Lactobacillemia—report of nine cases. Important clinical and therapeutic considerations. Am J Med 1978;64(5):808-813.

Berman S, Spicer D. Safety and reliability of lactobacillus dietary supplements in Seattle, Washington. American Public Health Association 130th Annual Meeting, November 9-13 2002;A37244.

Boulloche J, Mouterde O, Mallet E. Management of acute diarrhea in infants and young children: controlled study of the antidiarrheal efficacy of killed *L. acidophilus* (LB strain) versus a placebo and a reference drug (loperamide). Ann Pediatr 1994;41(7):457-463.

Chomarat M, Espinouse D. *Lactobacillus rhamnosus* septicemia in patients with prolonged aplasia receiving ceftazidime-vancomycin. Eur J Clin Microbiol Infect Dis 1991;10(1):44.

Clements ML, Levine MM, Ristaino PA, et al. Exogenous lactobacilli fed to man—their fate and ability to prevent diarrheal disease. Prog Food Nutr Sci 1983;7(3-4):29-37.

D'Souza AL, Rajkumar C, Cooke J, et al. Probiotics in prevention of antibiotic associated diarrhoea: meta-analysis. BMJ 2002;324(7350):1361.

Davies AJ, James PA, Hawkey PM. Lactobacillus endocarditis. J Infect 1986;12(2):169-174.

de Roos NM, Schouten G, Katan MB. Yoghurt enriched with *Lactobacillus acidophilus* does not lower blood lipids in healthy men and women with normal to borderline high serum cholesterol levels. Eur J Clin Nutr 1999;53(4):277-280.

Dehkordi N, Rao DR, Warren AP, et al. Lactose malabsorption as influenced by chocolate milk, skim milk, sucrose, whole milk, and lactic cultures. J Am Diet Assoc 1995;95(4):484-486.

dios Pozo-Olano J, Warram JH Jr, Gomez RG, et al. Effect of a lactobacilli preparation on traveler's diarrhea. A randomized, double blind clinical trial. Gastroenterology 1978; 74(5 Pt 1):829-830.

Friedlander A, Druker MM, Schachter A. *Lactobacillus acidophilus* and vitamin B complex in the treatment of vaginal infection. Panminerva Med 1986;28(1):51-53.

Gaon D, Garcia H, Winter L, et al. Effect of *Lactobacillus* strains and *Saccharomyces boulardii* on persistent diarrhea in children. Medicina (B Aires) 2003;63(4):293-298.

Gaon D, Garmendia C, Murrielo NO, et al. Effect of *Lactobacillus* strains (*L. casei* and *L. Acidophillus* strains cerela) on bacterial overgrowth–related chronic diarrhea. Medicina (B Aires) 2002;62(2):159-163.

Gotz V, Romankiewicz JA, Moss J, et al. Prophylaxis against ampicillin-associated diarrhea with a lactobacillus preparation. Am J Hosp Pharm 1979;36(6):754-757.

Griffiths JK, Daly JS, Dodge RA. Two cases of endocarditis due to *Lactobacillu*s species: antimicrobial susceptibility, review, and discussion of therapy. Clin Infect Dis 1992;15(2): 250-255.

Hallen A, Jarstrand C, Pahlson C. Treatment of bacterial vaginosis with lactobacilli. Sex Transm Dis 1992;19(3):146-148.

Halpern GM, Prindiville T, Blankenburg M, et al. Treatment of irritable bowel syndrome with Lacteol Fort: a randomized, double-blind, cross-over trial. Am J Gastroenterol 1996;91(8): 1579-1585.

Hilton E, Isenberg HD, Alperstein P, et al. Ingestion of yogurt containing *Lactobacillus acidophilus* as prophylaxis for candidal vaginitis. Ann Intern Med 1992;116(5):353-357.

Hoyos AB. Reduced incidence of necrotizing enterocolitis associated with enteral administration of *Lactobacillus acidophilus* and *Bifidobacterium infantis* to neonates in an intensive care unit. Int J Infect Dis 1999;3(4):197-202.

Kim HS, Gilliland SE. *Lactobacillus acidophilus* as a dietary adjunct for milk to aid lactose digestion in humans. J Dairy Sci 1983;66(5):959-966.

Kostiuk OP, Chernyshova LI, Slukvin II. [Protective effect of *Lactobacillus acidophilus* on development of infection, caused by *Klebsiella pneumoniae*.] Fiziol Zh 1993;39(4):62-68.

Larvol L, Monier A, Besnier P, et al. [Liver abscess caused by *Lactobacillus acidophilus*.] Gastroenterol Clin Biol 1996;20(2):193-195.

Lidbeck A, Nord CE, Gustafsson JA, et al. Lactobacilli, anticarcinogenic activities and human intestinal microflora. Eur J Cancer Prev 1992;1(5):341-353.

Lin SY, Ayres JW, Winkler W Jr, et al. Lactobacillus effects on cholesterol: in vitro and in vivo results. J Dairy Sci 1989;72(11):2885-2899.

Macbeth WA, Kass EH, McDermott WV. Treatment of hepatic encephalopathy by alteration of intestinal flora with lactobacillus acidophilus. Lancet 1965;191:399-403.

Michielutti F, Bertini M, Presciuttini B, et al. [Clinical assessment of a new oral bacterial treatment for children with acute diarrhea.] Minerva Med 1996;87(11):545-550.

Neri A, Sabah G, Samra Z. Bacterial vaginosis in pregnancy treated with yoghurt. Acta Obstet Gynecol Scand 1993;72(1):17-19.

Newcomer AD, Park HS, O'Brien PC, et al. Response of patients with irritable bowel syndrome and lactase deficiency using unfermented acidophilus milk. Am J Clin Nutr 1983;38(2): 257-263.

Ozmen S, Turhan NO, Seckin NC. *Gardnerella*-associated vaginitis: comparison of three treatment modalities. Turkish J Med Sci 1998;28(2):171-173.

Parent D, Bossens M, Bayot D, et al. Therapy of bacterial vaginosis using exogenously-applied Lactobacilli acidophili and a low dose of estriol: a placebo-controlled multicentric clinical trial. Arzneimittelforschung 1996;46(1):68-73.

Patel R, Cockerill FR, Porayko MK, et al. Lactobacillemia in liver transplant patients. Clin Infect Dis 1994;18(2):207-212.

Read AE, McCarthy CF, Heaton KW, et al. *Lactobacillus acidophilus* (enpac) in treatment of hepatic encephalopathy. BMJ 1966;5498:1267-1269.

Reuman PD, Duckworth DH, Smith KL, et al. Lack of effect of *Lactobacillus* on gastrointestinal bacterial colonization in premature infants. Pediatr Infect Dis 1986;5(6):663-668.

Saltzman JR, Russell RM, Golner B, et al. A randomized trial of *Lactobacillus acidophilus* BG2FO4 to treat lactose intolerance. Am J Clin Nutr 1999;69(1):140-146.

Satta A, Delplano A, Cossu P, et al. [Treatment of enterocolitis and other intestinal disorders with a *Bifidobacterium bifidum* and *Lactobacillus acidophilus* combination.] Clin Ter 1980; 94(2):173-184.

Schaafsma G, Meuling WJ, van Dokkum W, et al. Effects of a milk product, fermented by *Lactobacillus acidophilus* and with fructo-oligosaccharides added, on blood lipids in male volunteers. Eur J Clin Nutr 1998;52(6):436-440.

Shalev E, Battino S, Weiner E, et al. Ingestion of yogurt containing *Lactobacillus acidophilus* compared with pasteurized yogurt as prophylaxis for recurrent candidal vaginitis and bacterial vaginosis. Arch Fam Med 1996;5(10):593-596.

Siboulet A. [Vaccination against nonspecific bacterial vaginosis. Double-blind study of Gynatren.] Gynakol Rundsch 1991;31(3):153-160.

Simakachorn N, Pichaipat V, Rithipornpaisarn P, et al. Clinical evaluation of the addition of lyophilized, heat-killed *Lactobacillus acidophilus* LB to oral rehydration therapy in the treatment of acute diarrhea in children. J Pediatr Gastroenterol Nutr 2000;30(1):68-72.

Sussman JI, Baron EJ, Goldberg SM, et al. Clinical manifestations and therapy of *Lactobacillus* endocarditis: report of a case and review of the literature. Rev Infect Dis 1986;8(5):771-776.

Tankanow RM, Ross MB, Ertel IJ, et al. A double-blind, placebo-controlled study of the efficacy of Lactinex in the prophylaxis of amoxicillin-induced diarrhea. DICP 1990;24(4): 382-384.

Unoki T, Nakamura I, Fujisawa T, et al. [Infective endocarditis due to *Lactobacillus acidophilus* group. Report of a case and review of the literature.] Kansenshogaku Zasshi 1988;62(9): 835-840.

Van Niel CW, Feudtner C, Garrison MM, et al. Lactobacillus therapy for acute infectious diarrhea in children: a meta-analysis. Pediatrics 2002;109(4):678-684.

Wheeler JG, Shema SJ, Bogle ML, et al. Immune and clinical impact of *Lactobacillus acidophilus* on asthma. Ann Allergy Asthma Immunol 1997;79(3):229-233.

Witsell DL, Garrett CG, Yarbrough WG, et al. Effect of *Lactobacillus acidophilus* on antibiotic-associated gastrointestinal morbidity: a prospective randomized trial. J Otolaryngol 1995; 24(4):230-233.

Alfalfa

(*Medicago sativa* L.)

RELATED TERMS

- Al-fac-facah, arc, buffalo herb, California clover, Chilean clover, Fabaceae, feuille de luzerne, isoflavone, jatt, kaba yonca, Leguminosae, lucerne, medicago, mielga, mu su, phytoestrogen, purple medic (purple medick, purple medicle), sai pi li ka, saranac, Spanish clover, team, weevelchek, yonja.

BACKGROUND

- Alfalfa has a long history of dietary and medicinal use. A small number of animal and preliminary human studies report that alfalfa supplements may lower blood levels of cholesterol and glucose. However, most research studies have not been well designed, and thus there is not enough reliable evidence to form clear conclusions in these areas.
- Alfalfa supplements taken by mouth appear to be generally well tolerated. However, ingestion of alfalfa tablets has been associated with reports of a lupus-like syndrome or lupus flares. These reactions may be due to the amino acid L-canavanine, which appears to be present in alfalfa seeds and sprouts but not in the leaves. There are also reports of rare cases of pancytopenia (low blood cell count), dermatitis (skin inflammation), and gastrointestinal upset.

USES BASED ON SCIENTIFIC EVIDENCE	Grade*
Atherosclerosis (cholesterol plaques in arteries) Several studies in animals report reductions in cholesterol plaques of the arteries after use of alfalfa. Well-designed research studies in humans are necessary before a conclusion can be drawn.	C
Diabetes A small number of studies in rats report reductions in blood sugar levels following ingestion of alfalfa. Human data are limited, and it remains unclear if alfalfa can aid in the control of sugar levels in patients with diabetes or hyperglycemia.	C
High cholesterol Reductions in blood levels of total cholesterol and low-density lipoprotein ("bad cholesterol") have been reported in animal studies and in a small number of human cases. High-density lipoprotein ("good cholesterol") has not been altered in these cases. Although this evidence is promising, better research is needed before a firm conclusion can be reached.	C

*Key to grades: *A:* Strong scientific evidence for this use; *B:* Good scientific evidence for this use; *C:* Unclear scientific evidence for this use; *D:* Fair scientific evidence against this use (it may not work); *F:* Strong scientific evidence against this use (it likely does not work). For a more detailed explanation of efficacy criteria, see "Natural Standard Evidence-Based Validated Grading Rationale" in the Introduction.

Uses Based on Tradition, Theory, or Limited Scientific Evidence

Allergies, appetite stimulant, asthma, bladder disorders, blood clotting disorders, boils, cough, convalescence, diuresis (increasing urination), estrogen replacement, gastrointestinal tract disorders, gum healing after dental procedures, hay fever, increasing breast milk, indigestion, inflammation, insect bites, jaundice, kidney disorders, menopausal symptoms, nutritional support, prostate disorders, rheumatoid arthritis, scurvy, skin damage from radiation, stomach ulcers, thrombocytopenic purpura, uterine stimulant, vitamin supplementation (vitamins A, C, E, and K).

DOSING

The listed doses are based on scientific research, publications, traditional use, or expert opinion. Many herbs and supplements have not been thoroughly tested, and their safety and effectiveness may not have been proven. Brands may be made differently, with variable ingredients even within the same brand. The doses shown may not apply to all products. It is important to always read product labels and discuss doses with a qualified healthcare provider before therapy is started.

Standardization

- There are no standard or well-studied doses of alfalfa, and many different doses are used traditionally. Safety of use beyond 8 weeks has not been proven in studies.

Adults (18 Years and Older)

- **Dried herb:** 5 to 10 g of dried herb taken by mouth three times daily has been used.
- **Tablets:** A regimen of two 1-g tablets of Cholestaid (esterin-processed alfalfa) taken by mouth three times daily for up to 2 months, and then one tablet three times daily, has been recommended by the manufacturer.
- **Liquid extract:** 5 to 10 ml (1 to 2 teaspoonfuls) of a 1:1 solution in 25% alcohol taken by mouth three times daily has been used.
- **Seeds:** For lowering high cholesterol, 40 g of heated seeds prepared three times daily and taken by mouth with food has been used.

Children (Younger Than 18 Years)

- Scientific data are too limited to recommend alfalfa supplements for use in children, and such preparations are not recommended because of potential side effects.

SAFETY

The U.S. Food and Drug Administration does not strictly regulate herbs and supplements. There is no guarantee of the strength, purity, or safety of products, and effects may vary. It is important to always read product labels. People who have a medical condition, or are taking other drugs, herbs, or supplements, should consult a qualified healthcare provider before starting a new therapy. A healthcare provider should be contacted immediately about any side effects.

Allergies

- Alfalfa should be avoided by people with allergies to members of the Fabaceae or Leguminosae plant family. It remains unclear whether alfalfa cross-reacts with grass, and caution is warranted in persons with grass allergies.

Side Effects and Warnings

- Alfalfa appears to be well tolerated by most people, although rarely, serious adverse effects have been reported.
- Mild gastrointestinal symptoms may occur, such as stomach discomfort, diarrhea, gas, or larger/more frequent stools. Dermatitis (skin inflammation/redness) has been reported and may be due to alfalfa allergy.
- Blood sugar levels may be reduced, according to animal studies and a human case report. Caution is advised in persons with diabetes or hypoglycemia, and in those taking drugs, herbs, or supplements that affect blood sugar levels. Serum glucose levels may need to be monitored by a healthcare provider, and medication adjustments may be necessary.
- Lupus-like effects have been associated with alfalfa use, including antinuclear antibodies in the blood, muscle pains, fatigue, abnormal immune system function, and kidney abnormalities. Therefore, people with a history of lupus (systemic lupus erythematosus) or with a family history of lupus should avoid alfalfa supplements.
- Other reported rare adverse effects include abnormal blood cell counts (pancytopenia) and decreased potassium levels (hypokalemia). In theory, thyroid hormone levels may be increased, gout flares may be stimulated, and estrogen-like effects may occur.
- Contamination of alfalfa products with potentially dangerous bacteria (including *Escherichia coli* O157:H7, *Salmonella,* and *Listeria monocytogenes*) has been reported.
- Tinctures/liquid extracts may contain high levels of alcohol and should be avoided in people who will be driving or operating heavy machinery.

Pregnancy and Breastfeeding

- Alfalfa supplements are not recommended during pregnancy and breastfeeding because of insufficient evidence and a theoretical risk of birth defects or spontaneous abortion. Amounts found in food generally are believed to be safe. Traditionally, alfalfa is believed to stimulate breast milk production, although this effect has not been well studied.
- Tinctures/liquid extracts may contain high levels of alcohol and should be avoided during pregnancy.

INTERACTIONS

Most herbs and supplements have not been thoroughly tested for interactions with other herbs, supplements, drugs, and foods. The interactions listed here are based on reports in scientific publications, laboratory experiments, or traditional use. It is important to always read product labels. People who have a medical condition, or are taking other drugs, herbs, or supplements, should speak with a qualified healthcare provider before starting a new therapy.

Interactions with Drugs

- Blood sugar levels may be reduced, according to animal studies and a human case report. Caution is advised with use of medications that also may lower blood sugar. Persons who are taking drugs for diabetes by mouth or insulin should be monitored closely by a qualified healthcare provider. Medication adjustments may be necessary.
- Alfalfa contains vitamin K and therefore may reduce the "blood-thinning" effect of the drug warfarin (Coumadin). Alfalfa may add to the effects of cholesterol-lowering medications such as atorvastatin (Lipitor) and simvastatin (Zocor).

- Alfalfa may increase the risk of severe sunburn when used with drugs that increase sun sensitivity, such as chlorpromazine (Thorazine). Because of estrogen-like chemicals in alfalfa, the side effects of drugs that contain estrogens (such as birth control pills and hormone replacement therapy) may be increased. In theory, alfalfa may increase thyroid hormone levels and may alter the effects of thyroid drugs such as thyroxine (Synthroid, Levoxyl).
- Many tinctures/liquid extracts contain high levels of alcohol and may cause nausea or vomiting when taken with metronidazole (Flagyl) or disulfiram (Antabuse).

Interactions with Herbs and Dietary Supplements

- Blood sugar levels may be reduced, according to animal studies and a human case report. Caution is advised with use of herbs or supplements that also may lower blood sugar. Possible examples are *Aloe vera*, American ginseng, bilberry, bitter melon, burdock, fenugreek, fish oil, gymnema, horse chestnut seed extract (HCSE), maitake mushroom, marshmallow, milk thistle, *Panax ginseng*, rosemary, shark cartilage, Siberian ginseng, stinging nettle, and white horehound. Blood glucose levels may require monitoring, and doses may need adjustment.
- Alfalfa may add to the effects of cholesterol-lowering agents such as fish oil, garlic, guggul, red yeast, and niacin.
- Because alfalfa contains estrogen-like chemicals, the effects of other agents believed to have estrogen-like properties may be altered. Possible examples are black cohosh, bloodroot, burdock, hops, kudzu, licorice, pomegranate, red clover, soy, thyme, white horehound, and yucca.

Selected References

Natural Standard developed the preceding evidence-based information based on a systematic review of more than 150 articles. For comprehensive information about alternative and complementary therapies on the professional level, go to www.naturalstandard.com. Selected references are listed here.

Alcocer-Varela J, Iglesias A, Llorente L, et al. Effects of L-canavanine on T cells may explain the induction of systemic lupus erythematosus by alfalfa. Arthritis Rheum 1985;28(1):52-57.

Anon. From the Centers for Disease Control and Prevention. Outbreaks of *Escherichia coli* O157:H7 infection associated with eating alfalfa sprouts—Michigan and Virginia, June-July 1997. JAMA 1997;278(10):809-810.

Backer HD, Mohle-Boetani JC, Werner SB, et al. High incidence of extra-intestinal infections in a *Salmonella* Havana outbreak associated with alfalfa sprouts. Public Health Rep 2000; 115(4):339-345.

Bengtsson AA, Rylander L, Hagmar L, et al. Risk factors for developing systemic lupus erythematosus: a case-control study in southern Sweden. Rheumatology (Oxford) 2002 May; 41(5):563-571.

Boue SM, Wiese TE, Nehls S, et al. Evaluation of the estrogenic effects of legume extracts containing phytoestrogens. J Agric Food Chem 2003 Apr 9;51(8):2193-2199.

Dong Y, Iniguez AL, Ahmer BM, Triplett EW. Kinetics and strain specificity of rhizosphere and endophytic colonization by enteric bacteria on seedlings of *Medicago sativa* and *Medicago truncatula*. Appl Environ Microbiol 2003 Mar;69(3):1783-1790.

Elakovich SD, Hampton JM. Analysis of coumestrol, a phytoestrogen, in alfalfa tablets sold for human consumption. J Agric Food Chem 1984;32(1):173-175.

Farber JM, Carter AO, Varughese PV, et al. Listeriosis traced to the consumption of alfalfa tablets and soft cheese. N Engl J Med 1990;322(5):338.

Farnsworth NR. Alfalfa pills and autoimmune diseases. Am J Clin Nutr 1995;62(5): 1026-1028.

Gill CJ, Keene WE, Mohle-Boetani JC, et al. Alfalfa seed decontamination in a *Salmonella* outbreak. Emerg Infect Dis 2003 Apr;9(4):474-479.

Howard MB, Hutcheson SW. Growth dynamics of *Salmonella enterica* strains on alfalfa sprouts and in waste seed irrigation water. Appl Environ Microbiol 2003 Jan;69(1):548-553.

Hwang J, Hodis HN, Sevanian A. Soy and alfalfa phytoestrogen extracts become potent low-density lipoprotein antioxidants in the presence of acerola cherry extract. J Agric Food Chem 2001;49(1):308-314.

Jackson IM. Abundance of immunoreactive thyrotropin-releasing hormone–like material in the alfalfa plant. Endocrinology 1981;108(1):344-346.

Kaufman W. Alfalfa seed dermatitis. JAMA 1954;155(12):1058-1059.

Liao CH, Fett WF. Isolation of *Salmonella* from alfalfa seed and demonstration of impaired growth of heat-injured cells in seed homogenates. Int J Food Microbiol 2003 May 15;82(3): 245-253.

Mahon BE, Ponka A, Hall WN, et al. An international outbreak of *Salmonella* infections caused by alfalfa sprouts grown from contaminated seeds. J Infect Dis 1997;175(4):876-882.

Malinow MR, Bardana EJ Jr, Goodnight SH Jr. Pancytopenia during ingestion of alfalfa seeds. Lancet 1981;1(8220 Pt 1):615.

Malinow MR, Bardana EJ Jr, Pirofsky B, et al. Systemic lupus erythematosus–like syndrome in monkeys fed alfalfa sprouts: role of a nonprotein amino acid. Science 1982;216(4544): 415-417.

Malinow MR, McLaughlin P, Naito HK, et al. Effect of alfalfa meal on shrinkage (regression) of atherosclerotic plaques during cholesterol feeding in monkeys. Atherosclerosis 1978a; 30(1):27-43.

Malinow MR, McLaughlin P, Naito HK, et al. Regression of atherosclerosis during cholesterol feeding in *Macaca fascicularis*. Am J Cardiol 1978b;41:396.

Malinow MR, McLaughlin P, Stafford C. Alfalfa seeds: effects on cholesterol metabolism. Experientia 1980;36(5):562-564.

Mohle-Boetani J, Werner B, Polumbo M, et al. From the Centers for Disease Control and Prevention. Alfalfa sprouts—Arizona, California, Colorado, and New Mexico, February-April, 2001. JAMA 2002;287(5):581-582.

Molgaard J, von Schenck H, Olsson AG. Alfalfa seeds lower low density lipoprotein cholesterol and apolipoprotein B concentrations in patients with type II hyperlipoproteinemia. Atherosclerosis 1987;65(1-2):173-179.

Morimoto I, Shiozawa S, Tanaka Y, et al. L-canavanine acts on suppressor-inducer T cells to regulate antibody synthesis: lymphocytes of systemic lupus erythematosus patients are specifically unresponsive to L-canavanine. Clin Immunol Immunopathol 1990;55(1):97-108.

Ponka A, Andersson Y, Siitonen A, et al. *Salmonella* in alfalfa sprouts. Lancet 1995; 345:462-463.

Prete PE. The mechanism of action of L-canavanine in inducing autoimmune phenomena. Arthritis Rheum 1985;28(10):1198-1200.

Roberts JL, Hayashi JA. Exacerbation of SLE associated with alfalfa ingestion. N Engl J Med 1983;308(22):1361.

Srinivasan SR, Patton D, Radhakrishnamurthy B, et al. Lipid changes in atherosclerotic aortas of *Macaca fascicularis* after various regression regimens. Atherosclerosis 1980;37(4): 591-601.

Story JA, LePage SL, Petro MS, et al. Interactions of alfalfa plant and sprout saponins with cholesterol in vitro and in cholesterol-fed rats. Am J Clin Nutr 1984;39(6):917-929.

Swanston-Flatt SK, Day C, Bailey CJ, et al. Traditional plant treatments for diabetes. Studies in normal and streptozotocin diabetic mice. Diabetologia 1990;33(8):462-464.

Taormina PJ, Beuchat LR, Slutsker L. Infections associated with eating seed sprouts: an international concern. Emerg Infect Dis 1999;5(5):626-634.

Van Beneden CA, Keene WE, Strang RA, et al. Multinational outbreak of *Salmonella enterica* serotype Newport infections due to contaminated alfalfa sprouts. JAMA 1999;281(2): 158-162.

Winthrop KL, Palumbo MS, Farrar JA, et al. Alfalfa sprouts and *Salmonella* Kottbus infection: a multistate outbreak following inadequate seed disinfection with heat and chlorine. J Food Prot 2003 Jan;66(1):13-17.

Aloe
(*Aloe vera*)

RELATED TERMS

- Acemannan, *Aloe africana*, *Aloe arborescens* Miller, *Aloe barbadensis*, *Aloe capensis*, *Aloe ferox*, aloe latex, aloe mucilage, *Aloe perfoliata*, *Aloe perryi* Baker, *Aloe spicata*, *Aloe vulgari*, Barbados aloe, bitter aloe, burn plant, Cape aloe, Carrisyn, hirukattali, Curaçao aloe, elephant's gall, first-aid plant, Ghai kunwar, Ghikumar, hsiang-dan, jelly leek, kumari, lahoi, laloi, lily of the desert, lu-hui, medicine plant, Mediterranean aloe, miracle plant, Mocha aloes, musabbar, natal aloes, nohwa, plant of immortality, plant of life, rokai, sabilla, Savila, Socotrine aloe, subr, true aloe, Venezuela aloe, Za'bila, Zanzibar aloe.

BACKGROUND

- Transparent gel from the pulp of the meaty leaves of *Aloe vera* has been used topically for thousands of years to treat wounds, skin infections, burns, and numerous other dermatologic conditions. Dried latex from the inner lining of the leaf has traditionally been used as an oral laxative.
- There is strong scientific evidence in support of the laxative properties of aloe latex, based on the well-established cathartic properties of anthraquinone glycosides (found in aloe latex). However, aloe's therapeutic value compared with other approaches to constipation remains unclear.
- Preliminary *in vitro*, animal, and human studies suggest that topical aloe gel has immunomodulatory properties that may improve wound healing and skin inflammation.

USES BASED ON SCIENTIFIC EVIDENCE	Grade*
Constipation (laxative) Dried latex from the inner lining of aloe leaves has been used traditionally as an oral laxative. Although few studies have been conducted to assess this effect in humans, the laxative properties of aloe components such as aloin are well supported by scientific evidence. A combination herbal remedy containing aloe was found to be an effective laxative, although it is not clear if this effect was caused by aloe or by other ingredients in the product. Further studies are needed to establish dosages and to compare the effectiveness and safety of aloe with commonly used laxatives.	A
Genital herpes Limited evidence from studies in humans suggests that a 0.5% extract from *Aloe vera* in a hydrophilic cream may be an effective treatment of genital herpes in men (better than aloe gel or placebo). Although seemingly well designed, there may have been problems with the way in	B

Continued

which these studies were conducted. Additional research is needed before a strong recommendation can be made.	
Psoriasis vulgaris Evidence from one trial in humans suggests that a 0.5% extract from *aloe vera* in a hydrophilic cream is an effective treatment for psoriasis vulgaris. However, there may have been problems with the way in which this study was conducted. Additional research is needed before a strong recommendation can be made.	**B**
Seborrheic dermatitis (seborrhea, dandruff) One study using a 30% aloe lotion suggests effectiveness for treating seborrheic dermatitis when applied to the skin twice daily for 4 to 6 weeks. Further study is needed in this area before a strong recommendation can be made.	**B**
Cancer prevention Preliminary evidence from a small case-control study suggests that oral aloe may reduce the risk of developing lung cancer. Further study is needed to clarify whether aloe itself or other factors are responsible for this benefit.	**C**
Canker sores (aphthous stomatitis) Weak evidence from two studies suggests that treatment of recurrent aphthous ulcers of the mouth with aloe gel reduces pain and increases the amount of time between the appearance of new ulcers. Further study is needed before a recommendation can be made.	**C**
Diabetes (type 2—adult onset) Laboratory studies show that aloe can stimulate insulin release from the pancreas and lower blood glucose levels in mice. Results from two poorly conducted human trials in humans suggest that oral aloe gel may be effective in lowering blood glucose levels, although a third, smaller study found no effect. More research is needed to explore the effectiveness and safety of aloe in persons with diabetes.	**C**
HIV infection Acemannan, a component of aloe gel, has been shown in laboratory tests to have immune-stimulating and antiviral activities. Results from early studies in humans are mixed, and because of flaws in the way these studies were designed, firm conclusions are not possible. Further trials are needed before the evidence can be considered convincing either in favor or against this use of aloe.	**C**
Radiation dermatitis Reports in the 1930s of topical aloe's beneficial effects on skin after radiation exposure led to the widespread use of aloe in skin products. Currently, aloe gel is sometimes recommended for radiation-induced dermatitis, although results from two studies in humans are inconclusive.	**C**

Continued

Skin burns Preliminary evidence suggests that aloe may be effective in promoting healing of mild to moderate skin burns. However, the existing studies are small and poor in quality, and therefore no clear conclusion can be drawn. Further study is needed in this area.	C
Infected surgical wounds In one study, application of aloe gel to surgical wounds after abdominal surgery was found to prolong wound-healing time. Further study is needed, because wound healing is a popular use of topical aloe. Aloe cannot be recommended for application to surgical wounds at this time.	D
Pressure ulcers A well-designed human trial found no benefit of topical acemannan hydrogel (a component of aloe gel) in the treatment of pressure ulcers.	D

*Key to grades: *A:* Strong scientific evidence for this use; *B:* Good scientific evidence for this use; *C:* Unclear scientific evidence for this use; *D:* Fair scientific evidence against this use (it may not work); *F:* Strong scientific evidence against this use (it likely does not work). For a more detailed explanation of efficacy criteria, see "Natural Standard Evidence-Based Validated Grading Rationale" in the Introduction.

Uses Based on Tradition, Theory, or Limited Scientific Evidence

Alopecia (hair loss), antimicrobial, arthritis, asthma, bacterial skin infections, bowel disorders, chemoprotectant, chronic fatigue syndrome, chronic leg wounds, congestive heart failure, damaged blood vessels, elevated cholesterol or other lipids, frostbite, heart disease prevention, hepatitis, kidney and bladder stones, leukemia, lichen planus, stomach ulcers, parasitic worm infections, scratches or superficial wounds of the eye, skin protection during radiation therapy, sunburn, systemic lupus erythematosus, tic douloureux, untreatable tumors, vaginal contraceptive, wound healing after cosmetic dermabrasion, yeast infections of the skin.

DOSING

The following doses are based on scientific research, publications, traditional use, and expert opinion. Many herbs and supplements have not been thoroughly tested, and safety and effectiveness may not be proven. Brands may be made differently, with variable ingredients even within the same brand. The doses shown may not apply to all products. It is important to read product labels and discuss doses with a qualified healthcare provider before therapy is started.

Standardization

- Standardization involves measuring the amount of certain chemicals in products when attempting to make different preparations similar to each other. It is not always known if the chemicals being measured are the "active" ingredients.
- Standardized aloe products are not widely available. Although this is likely not a concern in the use of aloe gel on the skin, it may pose dangers with aloe taken

orally (because of the potential lowering of blood sugar levels). Oral aloe preparations often contain 10 to 30 mg of hydroxyanthracene derivatives per daily dose, calculated as anhydrous aloin.

Adults (18 Years and Older)

Topical (on the Skin)

- **General use:** Pure *Aloe vera* gel is often used liberally on the skin. There are no reports that using aloe on the skin causes absorption of chemicals into the body that might cause significant side effects. Skin products are available that contain aloe alone or aloe combined with other active ingredients.
- **Psoriasis vulgaris:** Hydrophilic cream of 0.5% (by weight) of a 50% ethanol extract of aloe, combined with mineral and castor oils, three times daily for 5 consecutive days per week for up to 4 weeks, has been studied.
- **Genital herpes:** Hydrophilic cream of 0.5% (by weight) of a 50% ethanol extract, combined with liquid paraffin and castor oil, three times daily on lesions for five consecutive days per week for up to 2 weeks, has been studied.

Oral (by Mouth)

- **Constipation:** The dose often recommended is the minimum amount to maintain a soft stool, typically 0.04 to 0.17 g of dried juice (corresponding to 10 to 30 mg of hydroxyanthraquinones). As an alternative, in combination with celandine (300 mg) and psyllium (50 mg), 150 mg of the dried juice of aloe taken daily has been effective as a laxative in research studies.
- **Diabetes (type 2—adult onset):** 5 to 15 ml of aloe juice twice daily has been used; however, the safety and efficacy of this regimen have not been proven.
- **HIV infection:** 1000 to 1600 mg of acemannan taken orally in four equal doses has been used as therapy for HIV infection; however, the safety and efficacy of this regimen have not been proven.
- **Intravenous (IV)/intramuscular (IM) therapy:** Four deaths have been associated with *Aloe vera* injections under unclear circumstances. Therefore, IV and IM administration of aloe compounds is not recommended.

Children (Younger Than 18 Years)

- Topical use of aloe gel in children is common and appears to be well tolerated.

SAFETY

The U.S. Food and Drug Administration does not strictly regulate herbs and supplements. There is no guarantee of strength, purity or safety of products, and effects may vary. It is important to always read product labels. People who have a medical condition, or are taking other drugs, herbs, or supplements, should consult a qualified healthcare provider before starting a new therapy. A healthcare provider should be contacted immediately about any side effects.

Allergies

- People with known allergy to garlic, onions, tulips, or other plants of the *Liliaceae* family may have allergic reactions to aloe. Individuals using aloe gel for prolonged times have developed allergic reactions, including hives and an eczema-like rash.

Side Effects and Warnings

- The use of aloe on surgical wounds has been reported to slow healing and, in one case, to cause redness and burning after aloe juice was applied to the face after a skin-peeling procedure (dermabrasion). Application of aloe prior to sun exposure may lead to rash in sun-exposed areas.

- The use of aloe or aloe latex by mouth as a laxative may cause cramping or diarrhea. Use for more than 7 days may cause dependency or worsening of constipation after treatment is stopped. Ingestion of aloe for longer than 1 year has been reported to increase the risk of colorectal cancer. Persons experiencing severe abdominal pain, appendicitis, ileus (temporary paralysis of the bowel), or a prolonged period without bowel movements should not take aloe.
- Electrolyte imbalances in the blood, including low potassium levels, may be caused by the laxative effect of aloe. This effect may be greater in people with diabetes or kidney disease. Low potassium levels can lead to abnormal heart rhythms or muscle weakness. People with heart disease, kidney disease, or electrolyte abnormalities should not take aloe by mouth. Healthcare providers should monitor for changes in potassium and other electrolytes in persons who take aloe by mouth for more than a few days.
- Based on a small number of studies in humans, aloe taken by mouth may lower blood sugar levels. Caution is advised in people with diabetes or hypoglycemia, and in those taking drugs, other herbs, or supplements that affect blood sugar. Serum glucose levels may need to be monitored by a healthcare provider, and dosing adjustments may be necessary.
- Intravenous (IV) and intramuscular (IM) injections of aloe have been associated with cases of death under unclear circumstances. Therefore IV and IM administration of aloe compounds is not recommended.

Pregnancy and Breastfeeding

- Although topical use of aloe is unlikely to be harmful during pregnancy or breastfeeding, oral use is not recommended because of the theoretical stimulation of uterine contractions. It is not known whether active ingredients of aloe may be present in breast milk. The dried juice of aloe leaves should not be consumed by breastfeeding mothers.

INTERACTIONS

Most herbs and supplements have not been thoroughly tested for interactions with other herbs, supplements, drugs, and foods. The interactions listed here are based on reports in scientific publications, laboratory experiments, and traditional use. It is important to always read product labels. People who have a medical condition, or are taking other drugs, herbs, or supplements, should consult a qualified healthcare provider before starting a new therapy.

Interactions with Drugs

- Based on a small number of studies in humans, aloe taken by mouth may lower blood sugar levels. Persons taking medications that also lower blood sugar levels, such as drugs for diabetes by mouth or insulin, should be monitored closely by a qualified healthcare provider. Medication adjustments may be necessary. In addition, insulin may add to the decrease in blood potassium levels that can occur with aloe.
- Because of lowering of potassium levels that may occur when aloe is taken by mouth, the effectiveness of heart medications such as digoxin and digitoxin, and of other medications used for heart rhythm disturbances, may be reduced. The risk of adverse effects may be increased with these medications because of low potassium levels.

- Caution should be used by persons taking loop diuretics, such as furosemide (Lasix), which increase the elimination of both fluid and potassium in the urine. Use of aloe combined with such agents may increase the risk of potassium depletion and dehydration.
- Use of aloe with laxative drugs may increase the risk of dehydration, potassium depletion, electrolyte imbalance, and changes in blood pH.
- Application of aloe to the skin may increase the absorption of steroid creams such as hydrocortisone. In addition, oral use of aloe and steroids such as prednisone may increase the risk of potassium depletion.
- Preliminary reports suggest that levels of AZT, a drug prescribed for HIV infection, may be increased by intake of aloe.

Interactions with Herbs and Dietary Supplements

- Based on the laxative properties of oral aloe, prolonged use may result in potassium depletion. This may be worsened by the use of licorice root.
- Theoretically, use of oral aloe and other laxative herbs may increase the risk of dehydration, potassium depletion, electrolyte imbalance, and changes in blood pH. Other herbs with potential laxative qualities are alder buckthorn, black root, blue flag rhizome, butternut bark, dong quai, European buckthorn, eyebright, cascara bark, castor oil, chasteberry, colocynth fruit pulp, dandelion, gamboges bark, horsetail, jalap root, manna bark, plantain leaf, podophyllum root, psyllium, rhubarb, senna, wild cucumber fruit, and yellow dock root.
- Based on preliminary data from studies in humans, oral aloe can reduce blood sugar levels. Caution is advised when using aloe with other herbs or supplements that may also lower blood sugar. Blood glucose levels may require monitoring, and doses may need adjustment. Possible examples include American ginseng, bilberry, bitter melon, burdock, fenugreek, fish oil, gymnema, horse chestnut seed extract, marshmallow, milk thistle, *Panax ginseng*, rosemary, Siberian ginseng, stinging nettle, and white horehound.

Interactions with Foods

- Aloe taken by mouth may interfere with absorption of foods and orally administered drugs.
- Prolonged oral use of aloe may lead to poor absorption of nutrients in the intestine.

Selected References

Natural Standard developed the preceding evidence-based information based on a systematic review of more than 250 scientific articles. For comprehensive information about alternative and complementary therapies on the professional level, go to www.naturalstandard.com. Selected references are listed here.

Bosley C, Smith J, Baratti P, et al. A phase III trial comparing an anionic phospholipid-based (APP) cream and aloe vera-based gel in the prevention and treatment of radiation dermatitis. Int J Radiat Oncol Biol Phys 2003;57(Suppl 2):S438.

Choi S, Kim KW, Choi JS, et al. Angiogenic activity of beta-sitosterol in the ischaemia/reperfusion-damaged brain of Mongolian gerbil. Planta Med 2002;68(4):330-335.

Chung JG, Li YC, Lee YM, et al. Aloe-emodin inhibited *N*-acetylation and DNA adduct of 2-aminofluorene and arylamine *N*-acetyltransferase gene expression in mouse leukemia L1210 cells. Leuk Res 2003;27(9):831-840.

Ernst E, Pittler MH, Stevinson C. Complementary/alternative medicine in dermatology: evidence-assessed efficacy of two diseases and two treatments. Am J Clin Dermatol 2002; 3(5):341-348.

Ferro VA, Bradbury F, Cameron P, et al. In vitro susceptibilities of Shigella flexneri and *Streptococcus pyogenes* to inner gel of *Aloe barbadensis* Miller. Antimicrob Agents Chemother 2003;47(3):1137-1139.

Furukawa F, Nishikawa A, Chihara T, et al. Chemopreventive effects of *Aloe arborescens* on *N*-nitrosobis(2-oxopropyl)amine–induced pancreatic carcinogenesis in hamsters. Cancer Lett 2002;178(2):117-122.

Grover JK, Yadav S, Vats V. Medicinal plants of India with anti-diabetic potential. J Ethnopharmacol 2002;81(1):81-100.

Heggie S, Bryant GP, Tripcony L, et al. A Phase III study on the efficacy of topical aloe vera gel on irradiated breast tissue. Cancer Nurs 2002;25(6):442-451.

Kaufman T, Kalderon N, Ullmann Y, et al. Aloe vera gel hindered wound healing of experimental second-degree burns: a quantitative controlled study. J Burn Care Rehabil 1988;9(2): 156-159.

Montaner JS, Gill J, Singer J, et al. Double-blind placebo-controlled pilot trial of acemannan in advanced human immunodeficiency virus disease. J Acquir Immune Defic Syn Hum Retrovirol 1996;12:153-157.

Olsen DL, Raub W Jr., Bradley C, et al. The effect of aloe vera gel/mild soap versus mild soap alone in preventing skin reactions in patients undergoing radiation therapy. Oncol Nurs Forum 2001;28(3):543-547.

Schmidt JM, Greenspoon JS. Aloe vera dermal wound gel is associated with a delay in wound healing. Obstet Gynecol 1991;78(1):115-117.

Syed TA, Afzal M, Ashfaq AS. Management of genital herpes in men with 0.5% *Aloe vera* extract in a hydrophilic cream: a placebo-controlled double-blind study. J Derm Treatment 1997;8(2):99-102.

Syed TA, Ahmad SA, Holt AH, et al. Management of psoriasis with *Aloe vera* extract in a hydrophilic cream: a placebo-controlled, double-blind study. Trop Med Int Health 1996;-1(4):505-509.

Syed TA, Cheema KM, Ahmad SA, et al. Aloe vera extract 0.5% in hydrophilic cream versus aloe vera gel for the measurement of genital herpes in males: a placebo-controlled, double-blind, comparative study. J Eur Acad Derm Veneriol 1996;7(3):294-295.

Thomas DR, Goode PS, LaMaster K, et al. Acemannan hydrogel dressing versus saline dressing for pressure ulcers: a randomized, controlled trial. Adv Wound Care 1998;11(6):273-276.

Vardy AD, Cohen AD, Tchetov T. A double-blind, placebo-controlled trial of *Aloe vera* (*A. barbadensis*) emulsion in the treatment of seborrheic dermatitis. J Derm Treatment 1999; 10(1):7-11.

Vogler BK, Ernst E. Aloe vera: a systematic review of its clinical effectiveness. Br J Gen Pract 1999;49(447):823-828.

Williams MS, Burk M, Loprinzi CL, et al. Phase III double-blind evaluation of an *Aloe vera* gel as a prophylactic agent for radiation-induced skin toxicity. Int J Radiation Oncol Biol Phys 1996;36(2):345-349.

Antineoplastons
(Phenylacetate)

RELATED TERMS

- A1, A2, A3, A4, A5, A10, A10-1, AS2-1, AS2-5, AS5, antineoplaston A, antineoplaston H, antineoplaston L, antineoplaston O, antineoplaston F, antineoplaston Ch, antineoplaston K, 3-*N*-phenylacetylaminopiperidine-2,6 dione, phenylacetylglutamine (PAG), phenylacetylisoglutamine (PAIG), phenylacetic acid (PAA), 3-phenylacetylamino-2,6-piperidinedione, sodium phenylacetate.

BACKGROUND

- Antineoplastons are a group of naturally occurring peptide fractions that were observed by Stanislaw Burzynski in the late 1970s to be absent in the urine of cancer patients. It was hypothesized that these substances might have anti-tumor properties. In the 1980s, Burzynski identified chemical structures for several of these antineoplastons and developed a process to prepare them synthetically. Antineoplaston A10, identified as 3-phenylacetylamino-2,6-piperidinedione may have similar benefits and was the first to be synthesized.
- The use of antineoplastons for the treatment of various types of cancer has been studied in the laboratory, in animals, and in limited preliminary human research. In 1991, the Cancer Therapy Evaluation Program of the National Cancer Institute (NCI) examined records of seven patients with brain tumors treated at the Burzynski Clinic in Texas. Based on their findings, the NCI sponsored a brain tumor clinical trial. However, because of difficulty recruiting patients and disagreement over study design, this research was canceled. The results in nine patients who were included prior to cancellation were reported but were not conclusive. In 1997, Dr. Burzynski encountered legal problems because of permitting antineoplastons to be shipped out of Texas.
- Evidence from randomized, controlled trials is lacking in support of antineoplastons as a cancer treatment, and antineoplaston therapy is not approved by the U.S. Food and Drug Administration. Antineoplastons are not widely available in the United States, and their safety and efficacy has not been proven, although multiple studies of antineoplastons in treatment for various cancers have been sponsored by the Burzynski Research Institute. In recent years, antineoplastons have been suggested as therapy for other conditions such as Parkinson's disease, sickle cell anemia, and thalassemia.

USES BASED ON SCIENTIFIC EVIDENCE	Grade*
Cancer Scientific evidence regarding the effectiveness of antineoplastons in cancer therapy is inconclusive. Several preliminary studies in humans (case series, phase I/II trials) have examined antineoplaston types A2, A5, A10, AS2-1, and AS2-5 as treatment for a variety of cancer types. It remains unclear whether antineoplastons are effective, or what doses may be safe. Until better research is available, no clear conclusion can be drawn.	C

Continued

HIV infection A small preliminary study published by Burzynski and colleagues in 1992 reported increased energy and weight in patients with HIV infection, a decreased number of opportunistic infections, and increased CD4+ counts overall. These patients were treated with antineoplaston AS2-1. However, this evidence cannot be considered conclusive. Currently, drug therapy regimens are available for HIV infections with clearly demonstrated effects (HAART, or highly active anti-retroviral therapy), and patients with HIV infection should consult a physician about treatment options.	C
Sickle cell anemia/thalassemia A small preliminary study of the use of antineoplastons as therapy for sickle cell anemia/thalassemia reported positive findings, but there is currently insufficient evidence to make a clear recommendation in this area.	C

*Key to grades: *A:* Strong scientific evidence for this use; *B:* Good scientific evidence for this use; *C:* Unclear scientific evidence for this use; *D:* Fair scientific evidence against this use (it may not work); *F:* Strong scientific evidence against this use (it likely does not work). For a more detailed explanation of efficacy criteria, see "Natural Standard Evidence-Based Validated Grading Rationale" in the Introduction.

Uses Based on Tradition, Theory, or Limited Scientific Evidence

Acute lymphocytic leukemia, adenocarcinoma, aging, astrocytoma, basal cell epithelioma, bladder cancer, brain/central nervous system tumors, cholesterol/triglyceride abnormalities, chronic lymphocytic leukemia, colon cancer, encephalitis, glioblastoma, hepatocellular carcinoma, leukocytosis, malignant melanoma, medulloblastoma, metastatic synovial sarcoma, Parkinson's disease, promyelocytic leukemia, prostate cancer, rectal cancer, skin cancer, thrombocytosis.

DOSING

The following doses are based on scientific research, publications, traditional use, and expert opinion. Many herbs and supplements have not been thoroughly tested, and safety and effectiveness may not be proven. Brands may be made differently, with variable ingredients even within the same brand. The doses shown may not apply to all products. It is important to always read product labels and discuss doses with a qualified healthcare provider before therapy is started.

Adults (18 Years and Older)

- Various doses of antineoplastons have been used in preliminary studies. Safety and effectiveness have not been established for any specific dose or use. In studies, oral doses of antineoplaston A10 in studies range from 10 to 40 g, or 100 to 288 mg per kg of body weight, daily. Duration of use has varied. Antineoplaston AS2-1 has been studied at doses of 12 to 30 g, or 97 to 130 mg per kg of body weight, daily. Antineoplastons also have been studied applied to the skin and administered by intravenous (IV) or intramuscular (IM) routes.

Children (Younger Than 18 Years)

- There are insufficient data available to recommend the use of antineoplastons in children.

SAFETY

The U.S. Food and Drug Administration does not strictly regulate herbs and supplements. There is no guarantee of strength, purity, or safety of products, and effects may vary. It is important to always read product labels. People who have a medical condition, or are taking other drugs, herbs, or supplements, should consult a qualified healthcare provider before starting a new therapy. A healthcare provider should be contacted immediately about any side effects.

Allergies

- Allergic skin rash has been reported after injection of antineoplaston AS2-1. Persons who have reacted to antineoplastons in the past should avoid this therapy.

Side Effects and Warnings

- Adverse effects have been reported in several preliminary studies. It is not clear how common these reactions are, or if they occur more frequently than with placebo. Because many patients taking antineoplastons have been diagnosed with serious illnesses such as advanced cancer, it is not clear whether these effects may be caused by the illnesses themselves or by the antineoplastons.
- Antineoplaston therapy has been associated with drowsiness, headache, fatigue, mild dizziness/vertigo, and confusion. Antineoplaston A10 is retained in the brain tissue of animals; the importance of this in humans is not known. Weakness, nausea, vomiting, upset stomach, abdominal pain, and increased flatulence (gas) have been reported.
- Various types of antineoplastons administered for a period of weeks to years have been associated with sore throat, fever, chills, reduced blood albumin levels, liver function test abnormalities, low blood sugar levels (hypoglycemia), low potassium levels, and a strong body odor similar to that of urine.
- Palpitations, high blood pressure (hypertension), and mild peripheral edema (water retention) have been noted. Chest pressure and irregular or fast heart beat have also been observed. Joint swelling, muscle/joint pain, muscle contractions in the throat, weakness, and finger rigidity have been reported in clinical trials.
- Decreases in blood platelets, red blood cells, and white blood cells have been observed. Other serious reported effects include slow or abnormal breathing, metabolic/electrolyte abnormalities, cerebral edema (brain swelling), dangerously low blood pressure (hypotension), and death.

Pregnancy and Breastfeeding

- The safety of antineoplastons during pregnancy or breastfeeding is not known, and therefore antineoplastons are not recommended.

INTERACTIONS

Most herbs and supplements have not been thoroughly tested for interactions with other herbs, supplements, drugs, and foods. The interactions listed here are based on reports in scientific publications, laboratory experiments, and traditional use. It is important to always read product labels. People who have a medical condition, or are taking other drugs, herbs, or supplements, should consult a qualified healthcare provider before starting a new therapy.

Interactions with Drugs, Herbs, and Dietary Supplements

- Limited information is available about interactions with antineoplastons. Agents with adverse effects similar to antineoplastons may have additive effects, such as lowering blood potassium and glucose levels and causing liver abnormalities. It is not known whether antineoplastons add to the effects of chemotherapeutic drugs.

Selected References

Natural Standard developed the preceding evidence-based information based on a systematic review of more than 100 scientific articles. For comprehensive information about alternative and complementary therapies on the professional level, go to www.naturalstandard.com. Selected references are listed here.

Badria F, Mabed M, El Awadi M, et al. Immune modulatory potentials of antineoplaston A-10 in breast cancer patients. Cancer Lett 2000;157(1):57-63.

Badria F, Mabed M, Khafagy W, et al. Potential utility of antineoplaston A-10 levels in breast cancer. Cancer Lett 2000;157(1):67-70.

Buckner JC, Malkin MG, Reed E, et al. Phase II study of antineoplastons A10 (NSC 648539) and AS2-1 (NSC 620261) in patients with recurrent glioma. Mayo Clin Proc 1999;74(2): 137-145.

Burzynski R. Treatment of bladder cancer with antineoplaston formulations. Adv Exp Clin Chemother 1988;2:37-46.

Burzynski SR, Conde AB, Peters A, et al. Retrospective study of antineoplastons A10 and AS2-1 in primary brain tumors. Clin Drug Invest 1999;18:1-10.

Burzynski SR, Kubove E, Burzynski B. Phase I clinical studies of antineoplaston A5 injections. Drugs Exp Clin Res 1987;13 Suppl 1:37-43.

Burzynski SR, Kubove E, Burzynski B. Phase II clinical trials of antineoplaston A10 and AS2-1 infusion in astrocytoma. In: Adam D, Buchner T, Rubinstein E, editors. Recent Advances in Chemotherapy. Munich, Futuramed Publishers, 1991:2506-2507.

Burzynski SR, Kubove E, Burzynski B. Treatment of hormonally refractory cancer of the prostate with antineoplaston AS2-1. Drugs Exp Clin Res 1990;16(7):361-369.

Burzynski SR, Kubove E, Szymkowski B, et al. Phase II clinical trials of novel differentiation inducer—antineoplaston AS2-1 in AIDS and asymptomatic HIV infection [abstract]. Int Conf AIDS 1992;8(3):61 (abstract no. Pub 7074).

Burzynski SR, Kubove E. Initial clinical study with antineoplaston A2 injections in cancer patients with five years' follow-up. Drugs Exp Clin Res 1987;13(Suppl 1):1-11.

Burzynski SR, Kubove E. Phase I clinical studies of antineoplaston A3 injections. Drugs Exp Clin Res 1987;13(Suppl 1):17-29.

Burzynski SR, Kubove E. Toxicology studies on antineoplaston A10 injections in cancer patients. Drugs Exp Clin Res 1986;12(Suppl 10):47-55.

Burzynski SR. Potential of antineoplastons in diseases of old age. Drugs Aging 1995;7(3): 157-167.

Burzynski SR. Toxicology studies on antineoplaston AS2-5 injections in cancer patients. Drugs Exp Clin Res 1986;12(Suppl 1):17-24.

Burzynski R. Isolation, purification, and synthesis of antineoplastons. Int J Exper Clin Chemother 1989;2:63-69.

Choi BG. Synthesis of antineoplaston A10 as potential antitumor agents. Arch Pharm Res 1998; 21(2):157-163.

Green S. "Antineoplastons." An unproved cancer therapy. JAMA 1992;267(21):2924-2928.

Juszkiewicz M, Chodkowska A, Burzynski SR, et al. The influence of antineoplaston A5 on particular subtypes of central dopaminergic receptors. Drugs Exp Clin Res 1995;21(4): 153-156.

Kumabe T. Antineoplaston treatment for advanced hepatocellular carcinoma. Oncology Rep 1998;5(6):1363-1367.

Liau MC, Szopa M, Burzynski B, et al. Quantitative assay of plasma and urinary peptides as an aid for the evaluation of cancer patients undergoing antineoplaston therapy. Drugs Exp Clin Res 1987;13(Suppl 1):61-70.

Soltysiak-Pawluczuk D, Burzynski SR. Cellular accumulation of antineoplaston AS21 in human hepatoma cells. Cancer Lett 1995;88(1):107-112.

Sugita Y, Tsuda H, Maruiwa H, et al. The effect of Antineoplaston, a new antitumor agent on malignant brain tumors. Kurume Med J 1995;42(3):133-140.

Tsuda H, Hara H, Eriguchi N, et al. Toxicological study on antineoplastons A-10 and AS2-1 in cancer patients. Kurume Med J 1995;42(4):241-249.

Tsuda H, Iemura A, Sata M, et al. Inhibitory effect of antineoplaston A10 and AS2-1 on human hepatocellular carcinoma. Kurume Med J 1996;43(2):137-147.

Tsuda H, Sata M, Kumabe T, et al. Quick response of advanced cancer to chemoradiation therapy with antineoplastons. Oncol Rep 1998;5(3):597-600.

Tsuda H, Sata M, Saitsu H, et al. Antineoplaston AS2-1 for maintenance therapy in liver cancer. Oncol Rep 1997;4:1213-1216.

Tweddle S, James N. Lessons from antineoplaston. Lancet 1997;349(9054):741.

Arginine

(L-Arginine)

RELATED TERMS

- Arg, arginine, arginine hydrochloride (intravenous formulation), ibuprofen-arginate (Spedifen), 2-amino-5-guanidinopentanoic acid.
- *Note:* Arginine vasopressin has an entirely different mechanism than arginine/L-arginine. NG-monomethyl-L-arginine also is different from arginine/L-arginine and functions as an inhibitor of nitric oxide synthesis.
- **Dietary sources of arginine:** Almonds, barley, Brazil nuts, brown rice, buckwheat, cashews, cereals, chicken, chocolate, coconut, corn, dairy products, filberts, gelatin, meats, oats, peanuts, pecans, raisins, sesame and sunflower seeds, walnuts.

BACKGROUND

- L-Arginine was first isolated in 1886. In 1932, L-arginine was found to be required for the generation of urea, which is necessary for the removal of toxic ammonia from the body. In 1939, L-arginine was also shown to be required for the synthesis of creatine. Creatine degrades to creatinine at a constant rate and is cleared from the body by the kidney.
- Arginine is considered a semi-essential amino acid, because although it is normally synthesized in sufficient amounts by the body, supplementation is sometimes required (for example, because of inborn errors of urea synthesis, protein malnutrition, excess ammonia production, excessive lysine intake, burns, infection, peritoneal dialysis, rapid growth, and sepsis). Symptoms of arginine deficiency include poor wound healing, hair loss, skin rash, constipation, and fatty liver.
- Arginine is a precursor of nitric oxide, which causes blood vessel relaxation (vasodilation). Preliminary evidence suggests that arginine may be useful in the treatment of medical conditions that are improved by vasodilation, such as angina, atherosclerosis, coronary artery disease, erectile dysfunction, heart failure, intermittent claudication/peripheral vascular disease, and vascular headache. Arginine also stimulates protein synthesis and has been studied for its role in wound healing, bodybuilding, enhancement of sperm production (spermatogenesis), and prevention of wasting in people with critical illness.
- Arginine hydrochloride has a high chloride content and has been used for the treatment of metabolic alkalosis. This use should be under the supervision of a qualified healthcare professional.
- Most people likely do not need to take arginine supplements because the body usually makes sufficient amounts.

USES BASED ON SCIENTIFIC EVIDENCE	Grade*
Growth hormone reserve test/pituitary disorder diagnosis Intravenously administered arginine can be used to evaluate growth hormone reserve in individuals with suspected growth hormone deficiency (for example, in patients with suspected panhypopituitarism, growth/stature abnormalities, gigantism/acromegaly, or pituitary adenoma). This is a U.S. Food and Drug Administration (FDA)–labeled indication for arginine.	A
Inborn errors of urea synthesis In patients with inborn errors of urea synthesis, high blood ammonia levels and metabolic alkalosis may occur, particularly in patients with ornithine carbamoyl transferase (OCT) deficiency or carbamoyl phosphate synthetase (CPS) deficiency. Arginine can be helpful by shifting the way that the body processes nitrogen but should be avoided in patients with hyperargininemia (high arginine blood levels). Other drugs, such as citrulline, sodium benzoate, and sodium phenylbutyrate, may have similar benefits, although dialysis may be necessary initially. This use of arginine should be supervised by a qualified healthcare professional.	A
Adrenoleukodystrophy Adrenoleukodystrophy (ALD) is a rare inherited metabolic disorder characterized by the loss of fatty coverings (myelin sheaths) on nerve fibers in the brain, and progressive destruction of the adrenal glands. ALD is inherited as an X-linked genetic trait that results in dementia and adrenal failure. Injections of arginine have been proposed to help manage this disorder, although most study results are inconclusive. Further research is needed to evaluate the use of arginine in ALD.	C
Burns A randomized, controlled clinical trial designed to evaluate immune function of patients given 15 mg of arginine orally suggests that arginine may aid in the recovery of immune function and protein function in partial-thickness burn patients. Further research is necessary to confirm these findings.	C
Coronary artery disease/angina Initial evidence from several studies suggests that arginine administered orally or by injection improves exercise tolerance and blood flow in arteries of the heart. Benefits have been shown in some patients with coronary artery disease and angina. A small, randomized, controlled clinical trial studied the effects of a nutritional bar enriched with L-arginine and a combination of other nutrients in the management of chronic stable angina. The authors found that this arginine-rich medical food, when used with traditional therapy, improved vascular function, exercise capacity, and other aspects of quality of life in these patients. However, further research is needed to confirm these findings and to establish safe and effective doses.	C

Continued

Critical illness C

Some studies suggest that arginine may provide benefits when added to nutritional supplements during critical illnesses (for example, in patients being treated in intensive care units [ICUs]). However, the specific role of arginine in improving recovery is unclear. A randomized, controlled clinical trial was designed to study the effects of a high-protein formula enriched with arginine, fiber, and antioxidants in early nutrition therapy of critically ill patients. The study measured infections in the ICU, length of hospital stay, and death rates. Patients fed the high-protein formula–enriched diet developed fewer hospital infections than patients fed a standard high-protein diet. There was no difference in length of ICU hospital stay or death rate.

Dental pain (ibuprofen arginate) C

A well-designed multicenter, randomized controlled clinical trial found that ibuprofen arginate (Spedifen) reduced pain faster after dental surgery compared with conventional ibuprofen alone. The study included 498 patients who were given ibuprofen arginate, ibuprofen, or placebo after dental surgery. The degree of the relief of pain, onset of action, and tolerability of both ibuprofen arginate and ibuprofen were compared. It was found that ibuprofen arginate relieved pain faster, and adverse events with ibuprofen arginate were similar to those seen with ibuprofen alone. Another, similar trial concluded that patients treated with ibuprofen arginate rated its overall effectiveness higher than those treated with ibuprofen alone. Adverse event profiles were similar across all treatment groups. Further research is merited in this area.

Erectile dysfunction C

Early studies suggested that arginine supplements are useful for managing erectile dysfunction (ED) in men with low levels of nitrates in blood or urine. A randomized, controlled clinical trial reported improvements in patients with mild-to-moderate ED following use of a combination of L-arginine, glutamate, and yohimbine hydrochloride. Notably, yohimbine hydrochloride is an FDA-approved therapy for this condition, and the effects caused by arginine alone in this combination therapy are difficult to determine. It is not clear what doses of arginine may be safe or effective in treating this condition, and comparisons have not been made with other agents used for ED.

Gastrointestinal cancer surgery C

Supplementation with an oral combination of arginine and omega-3 fatty acids may reduce length of hospital stay and infections after surgery in gastrointestinal cancer patients. There is conflicting evidence about whether to give the combination before or after surgery. Both strategies have been reported as superior to conventional treatment (no artificial nutrition) in reducing infections after surgery and of hospital stay.

In a large, randomized, controlled clinical trial, malnourished cancer patients were given oral enteral nutrition supplemented by arginine,

Continued

omega-3 fatty acids, and RNA before surgery. It was found that supplementation with the combination given before surgery reduced complications after surgery and hospital stay. Another randomized, controlled clinical trial in patients with gastrointestinal cancer studied the effects of an enteral diet supplemented with arginine, omega-3 fatty acids, and glutamine (administered after surgery) on immune function and inflammatory response. This study reported the supplement to be well tolerated with positive effects on immune and inflammatory response. Further research is needed to determine the effects of arginine alone.	
Congestive heart failure (CHF) Studies of arginine in patients with CHF have shown mixed results. Some studies reported improved exercise tolerance. Additional studies are needed to confirm these findings.	C
Heart protection during coronary artery bypass grafting (CABG) Arginine-supplemented "blood cardioplegic solution" is proposed to have protective properties. A randomized, controlled clinical trial using this solution in patients undergoing heart surgery (CABG) reported improved heart protection. Further research is needed before a firm conclusion can be drawn.	C
High blood pressure A small study suggested that arginine taken by mouth may help to dilate the arteries and temporarily reduce blood pressure in hypertensive patients with type 2 diabetes. Larger, high-quality studies are needed before a recommendation can be made.	C
Migraine headache Preliminary studies suggest that adding arginine to ibuprofen therapy may decrease migraine headache pain.	C
Peripheral vascular disease/claudication Intermittent claudication is a condition characterized by leg pain and fatigue due to buildup of cholesterol plaques or clots in leg arteries. A small number of studies reported that arginine therapy may improve walking distance in patients with claudication. Further research is needed before a firm conclusion can be drawn.	C
Recovery after surgery One study suggests that arginine provides benefits when used as a supplement after surgery. It is not clear what the specific role of arginine may be in improving immune function, and safe and effective doses have not been determined.	C
Wound healing Arginine has been suggested to improve the rate of wound healing in elderly individuals. A randomized, controlled clinical trial reported improved wound healing after surgery in patients with head and neck	C

Continued

cancer, following the use of an enteral diet supplemented with arginine and fiber. Arginine has also been used topically (on the skin) to improve wound healing. Further research is necessary in this area before a firm conclusion can be drawn.

Cyclosporine toxicity — D

Studies in animals showed that arginine blocked the toxic effects of cyclosporine, a drug used to prevent organ transplant rejection. However, results from studies in humans did not show that arginine offered any protection from cyclosporine-induced toxicity.

Infertility — D

Although there have been several studies in this area, it is not clear what effects arginine has on improving the likelihood of getting pregnant. Early evidence does not support the finding that arginine has any benefits in women who are undergoing in vitro fertilization or in men with abnormal sperm.

Interstitial cystitis — D

Arginine has been proposed as a treatment for interstitial cystitis (inflammation of the bladder). However, most well-designed studies in humans have not found that arginine offers any benefit in treating symptoms such as urinary frequency or urgency.

Kidney disease — D

It has been suggested that arginine may be a useful supplement in people diagnosed with kidney failure. However, results from available studies do not support this claim. A small, randomized, controlled clinical trial studied the ability of L-arginine to improve dilation of blood vessels in children with chronic renal failure. Results showed that blood vessel dilation (endothelial function) was not improved with oral L-arginine, suggesting that dietary supplementation is not a beneficial or useful clinical approach in children with chronic renal failure.

Kidney protection during angiography — D

The contrast media or dye used during angiography to map a patient's arteries (or during some CT scans) can be toxic to the kidneys, especially in people with pre-existing kidney disease. A randomized, parallel, double-blind clinical trial studied the use of L-arginine to protect kidneys in patients with chronic renal failure undergoing angiography. The authors found no evidence that injections of L-arginine protect the kidney from damage due to contrast media.
Other therapies, such as *N*-acetylcysteine (NAC), have been found beneficial in protecting the kidneys from contrast-induced damage, particularly in patients at high risk, such as those with diabetes.

Asthma — F

Although arginine has been suggested as a treatment for asthma, studies in humans have found that arginine actually *worsens* inflammation in the

Continued

lungs and *contributes* to asthma symptoms. Therefore, taking arginine by mouth or by inhalation is not recommended for people with asthma.

*Key to grades: *A:* Strong scientific evidence for this use; *B:* Good scientific evidence for this use; *C:* Unclear scientific evidence for this use; *D:* Fair scientific evidence against this use (it may not work); *F:* Strong scientific evidence against this use (it likely does not work). For a more detailed explanation of efficacy criteria, see "Natural Standard Evidence-Based Validated Grading Rationale" in the Introduction.

Uses Based on Tradition, Theory, or Limited Scientific Evidence

AIDS/HIV, ammonia toxicity, anti-aging, beta-hemoglobinopathies, cancer, cardiac syndrome X, cold prevention, cystic fibrosis, dementia, diabetes, enhanced athletic performance, enhanced immune function, glaucoma, growth hormone stimulation, heart attack, hemolytic uremic syndrome (HUS), hepatic encephalopathy, immunomodulation, infection, pulmonary hypertension (high blood pressure in the lungs), high cholesterol, increased muscle mass, infantile necrotizing enterocolitis, inflammatory bowel disease, ischemic stroke, liver disease, lower esophageal sphincter relaxation, low sperm count, metabolic acidosis, obesity, osteoporosis, pain, peritonitis, preeclampsia, pre-term labor contractions, Raynaud's phenomenon, sepsis, sickle cell anemia, stomach motility disorders, stomach ulcer, stroke, supplementation to a low protein diet, thrombotic thrombocytopenic purpura (TTP).

DOSING

The following doses are based on scientific research, publications, traditional use, and expert opinion. Many herbs and supplements have not been thoroughly tested, and safety and effectiveness may not be proven. Brands may be made differently, with variable ingredients even within the same brand. The doses shown may not apply to all products. It is important to always read product labels and discuss doses with a qualified healthcare provider before therapy is started.

Standardization

- Intravenous arginine hydrochloride is available as a 10% solution (950 mOsm/L), with 47.5 mEq chloride ion per 100 ml. There is no established standardization for oral arginine products.
- *Note:* Most people likely do not need to take arginine supplements because the body usually makes sufficient amounts.

Adults (18 Years and Older)

- **Tablets/capsules:** There are no standard or well-established doses for arginine, and many different doses have been used and studied. A dose studied for treating coronary artery disease is 2 to 3 g taken by mouth three times daily for 3 to 6 months. A dose studied for treatment of heart failure is 5.6 to 12.6 g, divided into two or three equal doses, taken by mouth daily for 6 weeks. For erectile dysfunction, 1.6 g taken by mouth three times daily for 6 weeks has been studied. For low sperm count, 4 g daily taken by mouth for 3 months has been used. For women undergoing *in*

vitro (test tube) fertilization, an oral dose of 16 g per day has been used; however, this therapy should be discussed with the healthcare provider coordinating the in vitro program. For interstitial cystitis, 500 mg taken by mouth three times daily for six weeks has been used. For the long-term management of inborn disorders of the urea cycle, oral doses of 0.5 to 2 g daily have been used.
- **Intravenous:** Intravenous administration of arginine depends on specific institutional dosing guidelines and should be given under the supervision of a qualified healthcare provider.

Children (Younger Than 18 Years)

- Arginine supplements are not recommended for children because scientific information is lacking about this therapy in children and because of potential side effects.

SAFETY

The U.S. Food and Drug Administration does not strictly regulate herbs and supplements. There is no guarantee of strength, purity, or safety of products, and effects may vary. It is important to always read product labels. People who have a medical condition, or are taking other drugs, herbs, or supplements, should consult a qualified healthcare provider before starting a new therapy. A healthcare provider should be contacted immediately about any side effects.

Allergies

- Anaphylaxis (severe allergic reaction) has occurred after arginine injections. People with a known allergy should avoid arginine. Signs of allergy include rash, itching, and shortness of breath.

Side Effects and Warnings

- Arginine has been well tolerated by most people in studies lasting up to 6 months; however, there is the possibility of serious adverse effects in some individuals.
- Stomach discomfort, including nausea, stomach cramps, and an increased number of stools, may occur. People with asthma may experience a worsening of symptoms if arginine is inhaled, which may be related to allergy.
- Other potential side effects include low blood pressure and changes in numerous chemicals and electrolytes in the blood. Examples are high potassium, high chloride, low sodium, low phosphate, high blood urea nitrogen, and high creatinine levels. People with liver or kidney disease may be especially susceptible to these complications and should avoid using arginine except under medical supervision. After injections of arginine, low back pain, flushing, headache, numbness, restless legs, venous irritation, and death of surrounding tissues have been reported.
- In theory, arginine may increase the risk of bleeding. Persons using anticoagulants (blood thinners) or antiplatelet drugs, and those with underlying bleeding disorders, should consult a qualified healthcare provider before using arginine and should be monitored.
- Arginine may increase blood sugar levels. Caution is advised in patients taking prescription drugs to control sugar levels.

Pregnancy and Breastfeeding

- Arginine cannot be recommended as a supplement during pregnancy and breastfeeding because insufficient scientific information is available.

INTERACTIONS

Most herbs and supplements have not been thoroughly tested for interactions with other herbs, supplements, drugs, and foods. The interactions listed here are based on reports in scientific publications, laboratory experiments, and traditional use. It is important to always read product labels. People who have a medical condition, or are taking other drugs, herbs, or supplements, should consult a qualified healthcare provider before starting a new therapy.

Interactions with Drugs

- Because arginine increases the activity of some hormones in the body, many possible drug interactions may occur. The prescription drug aminophylline and the sweetening agent xylitol can decrease the effects of arginine on glucagon.
- Estrogens (found in birth control pills and hormone replacement therapies) may increase the effects of arginine on growth hormone, glucagon and insulin. In contrast, progestins (also found in birth control pills and some hormone replacement therapies) may decrease the responsiveness of growth hormone to arginine.
- When used with arginine, some diuretics such as spironolactone (Aldactone) and ACE-inhibitor blood pressure drugs such as enalapril (Vasotec) may cause elevated potassium levels in the blood. Monitoring of blood potassium levels may be required.
- Arginine should be used carefully with drugs such as nitroglycerin and sildenafil (Viagra) because blood pressure may fall too low. Other adverse effects such as headache and flushing may occur when arginine is used with these drugs.
- Because arginine can cause the stomach to make more acid, it may reduce the effectiveness of drugs that block stomach acid, such as ranitidine (Zantac) and esomeprazole (Nexium).
- In theory, arginine may increase the risk of bleeding when used with anticoagulants (blood thinners) or antiplatelet drugs. Examples are warfarin (Coumadin), heparin, and clopidogrel (Plavix). Some pain relievers may also increase the risk of bleeding if used with arginine. Examples include aspirin, ibuprofen (Motrin, Advil) and naproxen (Naprosyn, Aleve, Anaprox).
- Arginine may raise blood sugar levels. People using arginine and also taking oral drugs for diabetes or using insulin should be monitored closely by a qualified health care provider. Dosing adjustments may be necessary.
- Studies suggest that a combination of ibuprofen and arginine (ibuprofen-arginate [Spedifen]) has a faster onset of pain relief than ibuprofen alone. Use of other ibuprofen-based pain relievers such as Motrin or Advil with ibuprofen-arginate may increase the risk of toxic effects. People should consult their healthcare provider before combining these medications.

Interactions with Herbs and Dietary Supplements

- Arginine may block the benefits of lysine in treating cold sores.
- Arginine may increase the activity of growth hormone if used with ornithine.
- In theory, arginine may further increase the risk of bleeding when taken with herbs and supplements that are believed to increase the risk of bleeding. Multiple cases of bleeding have been reported with the use of *Ginkgo biloba*, and fewer cases have been reported with the use of garlic and saw palmetto. Numerous other agents may theoretically increase the risk of bleeding, although this has not been proven in most cases. Examples are alfalfa, American ginseng, angelica, anise, *Arnica montana*, asafetida, aspen bark, bilberry, birch, black cohosh, bladderwrack, bogbean,

boldo, borage seed oil, bromelain, capsicum, cat's claw, celery, chamomile, chaparral, clove, coleus, cordyceps, danshen, devil's claw, dong quai, EPA (eicosapentaenoic acid, found in fish oils), evening primrose oil, fenugreek, feverfew, fish oil, flaxseed/flax powder (not a concern with flaxseed oil), ginger, grapefruit juice, grapeseed, green tea, guggul, gymnestra, horse chestnut, horseradish, licorice root, lovage root, male fern, meadowsweet, nordihydroguaiaretic acid (NDGA), omega-3 fatty acids, onion, papain, *Panax ginseng*, parsley, passion flower, poplar, prickly ash, propolis, quassia, red clover, reishi, Siberian ginseng, sweet clover, rue, sweet birch, sweet clover, turmeric, vitamin E, white willow, wild carrot, wild lettuce, willow, wintergreen, and yucca.

- Because arginine may raise blood sugar level, people taking arginine and also using other herbs or supplements that may raise blood sugar levels (for example, cocoa, dehydroepiandrosterone [DHEA], ephedra [when combined with caffeine], and melatonin) should be monitored closely by their healthcare provider. Dosing adjustments may be necessary.

Selected References

Natural Standard developed the above evidence-based information based on a systematic review of more than 550 articles. For comprehensive information about alternative and complementary therapies on the professional level, go to www.naturalstandard.com. Selected references are listed below.

Bath PM, Willmot M Leonardi-Bee J, et al. Nitric oxide donors (nitrates), L-arginine, or nitric oxide synthase inhibitors for acute stroke. Cochrane Database Syst Rev 2002;(4): CD000398.

Beale RJ, Bryg DJ, Bihari DJ. Immunonutrition in the critically ill: a systematic review of clinical outcome. Crit Care Med 1999;27(12):2799-2805.

Bennett-Richards KJ, Kattenhorn M, Donald AE, et al. Oral L-arginine does not improve endothelial dysfunction in children with chronic renal failure. Kidney Int 2002;62(4):1372-1378.

Black P, Max MB' Desjardins P, Norwood T, et al. A randomized, double-blind, placebo-controlled comparison of the analgesic efficacy, onset of action, and tolerability of ibuprofen arginate and ibuprofen in postoperative dental pain. Clin Ther 2002;24(7):1072-1089.

Boger RH, Bode-Boger SM, Thiele W, et al. Restoring vascular nitric oxide formation by L-arginine improves the symptoms of intermittent claudication in patients with peripheral arterial occlusive disease. J Am Coll Cardiol 1998;32(5):1336-1344.

Braga M, Gianotti L, Nespoli L, Radaelli G, et al. Nutritional approach in malnourished surgical patients: a prospective randomized study. Arch Surg 2002;137(2):174-180.

Caparros T, Lopez J, Grau T. Early enteral nutrition in critically ill patients with a high-protein diet enriched with arginine, fiber, and antioxidants compared with a standard high-protein diet. The effect on nosocomial infections and outcome. JPEN J Parenter Enteral Nutr 2001;25(6):299-308; discussion 308-309.

Carrier M, Pellerin M, Perrault LP, et al. Cardioplegic arrest with L-arginine improves myocardial protection: results of a prospective randomized clinical trial. Ann Thorac Surg 2002; 73(3):837-841; discussion 842.

Cartledge JJ, Davies AM, Eardley I. A randomized double-blind placebo-controlled crossover trial of the efficacy of L-arginine in the treatment of interstitial cystitis. BJU Int 2000;85(4): 421-426.

Cen Y, Luo XS, Liu XX. Effect of L-arginine supplementation on partial-thickness burned patients. Zhongguo Xiu Fu Chong Jian Wai Ke Za Zhi 1999;13(4):227-231.

Chen J, Wollman Y, Chernichovsky T, et al. Effect of oral administration of high-dose nitric oxide donor L-arginine in men with organic erectile dysfunction: results of a double- blind, randomized, placebo-controlled study. BJU Int 1999;83(3):269-273.

Chuntrasakul C, Siltharm S, Sarasombath S, et al. Metabolic and immune effects of dietary arginine, glutamine and omega-3 fatty acids supplementation in immunocompromised patients. J Med Assoc Thai 1998;81(5):334-343.

de Luis DA, Aller R, Izaola O, et al. Postsurgery enteral nutrition in head and neck cancer patients. Eur J Clin Nutr 2002;56(11):1126-1129.
de Luis DA, Izaola O, Cuellar L, et al. Effects of c-reactive protein and interleukin blood levels in postsurgery arginine-enhanced enteral nutrition in head and neck cancer patients. Eur J Clin Nutr 2003;57(1):96-99.
Desjardins P, Black P, Papageorge M, et al. Ibuprofen arginate provides effective relief from postoperative dental pain with a more rapid onset of action than ibuprofen. Eur J Clin Pharmacol 2002;58(6):387-394.
Gianotti L, Braga M, Nespoli L, et al. A randomized controlled trial of preoperative oral supplementation with a specialized diet in patients with gastrointestinal cancer. Evid Based Nurs 2003;6(2):47.
Huynh NT, Tayek JA. Oral arginine reduces systemic blood pressure in type 2 diabetes: its potential role in nitric oxide generation. J Am Coll Nutr 2002;21(5):422-427.
Klotz T, Mathers MJ, Braun M, et al. Effectiveness of oral L-arginine in first-line treatment of erectile dysfunction in a controlled crossover study. Urol Int 1999;63(4):220-223.
Korting G, Smith S, Wheeler M, et al. A randomized double-blind trial of oral L-arginine for treatment of interstitial cystitis. J Urol 1999;161(2):558-565.
Lebret T, Herve JM, Gorny P, et al. Efficacy and safety of a novel combination of L-arginine, glutamate, and yohimbine hydrochloride: a new oral therapy for erectile dysfunction. Eur Urol 2002;41(6):608-613.
Lekakis JP, Papathanassiou S, Papioannou TG, et al. Oral L-arginine improves endothelial dysfunction in patients with essential hypertension. Int J Cardiol 2002;86(2-3):317-323.
Maxwell AJ, Zapien MP, Pearce GL, et al. Randomized trial of a medical food for the dietary management of chronic, stable angina. J Am Coll Cardiol 2002;39(1):37-45.
McGovern MM, Wasserstein MP, Aron A, et al. Biochemical effect of intravenous arginine butyrate in X-linked adrenoleukodystrophy. J Pediatr. 2003;142(6):709-713.
Mehlisch DR, Ardia A, Pallotta T. A controlled comparative study of ibuprofen arginate versus conventional ibuprofen in the treatment of postoperative dental pain. J Clin Pharmacol 2002;42(8):904-911.
Miller HI, Dascalu A, Rassin TA, et al. Effects of an acute dose of L-arginine during coronary angiography in patients with chronic renal failure: a randomized, parallel, double-blind clinical trial. Am J Nephrol 2003;23(2):91-95.
Sandrini G, Franchini S, Lanfranchi S, et al. Effectiveness of ibuprofen-arginine in the treatment of acute migraine attacks. Int J Clin Pharmacol Res 1998;18(3):145-150.
Wu GH, Zhang YW, Wu ZH. Modulation of postoperative immune and inflammatory response by immune-enhancing enteral diet in gastrointestinal cancer patients. World J Gastroenterol 2001;7(3): 357-362.

Astragalus

(*Astragalus membranaceus*)

RELATED TERMS

- *Astragalus trigonus, Astragalus gummifera, Astragalus mollissimus, Astragalus lentiginosus,* astragel, baak kei (beg kei, bei qi, buck qi), Fabaceae, goat's horn (goat's thorn), green dragon, gum dragon, gum tragacanthae (gummi tragacanthae), hoang ky, hog gum, huang-chi (huang qi, huangoi, huangqi, hwanggi), ji cao, Leguminosae, locoweed, membranous milk vetch, milk vetch, mongolian milk, mongolian milk vetch, neimeng huangqi, ogi (ougi), radix astragali, spino santo, Syrian tragacanth, tai shen, tragacanth, wong kei, yellow vetch, zhongfeng-naomitong.
- **Selected combination products that include this herb:** Astragalus-Power, Baoyuan Dahuang, Biomune OSF Plus, Bu Zhong Yi Qi Tang, CH-100, Chi Power, Chinese Thermo-Chi, Deep Defense, Energy Boost Tincture, Equi-lizer Fast Start, Excel Energy, Fast Start, Fit America Natural Weight Control Aid, Formula One, Formula 3, Formula 3 Cell Activator, Fu-Zheng, Han-Dan-Gan-Le, Herbal Balance, Intra, Jian Yan Ling (JYL), Jiangtangjia, Magic Herb Diet Plus Formula + Chromium Picolinate, Man-Shen-Ling (MSL), Master Herb with Chromium Picolinate, Megawatt, Nature's Nutrition Formula One, Nature's Power Trim Super Fat Burner, New Image, New Image Plus, Sanhuang, Shengxue Mixture (SXM), Shen-Qi, Shi-quan-da-bu-tang (SQT), Thermojetics Beige, Tri-Chromaleane, Ultra Energy Now, Vita Chromaleane, Yi-qi Huo-xue Injection (YHI), Yogi Herbal Tea.

BACKGROUND

- Astragalus products are derived from the roots of *Astragalus membranaceus* or related species, which are native to China. In traditional Chinese medicine, astragalus is commonly found in mixtures with other herbs and is used in the treatment of numerous ailments, including heart, liver, and kidney diseases, as well as cancer, viral infections, and immune system disorders. Western herbalists began using astragalus in the 1800s as an ingredient in various tonics. The use of astragalus became popular in the 1980s based on theories about anti-cancer properties, although these proposed effects have not been clearly demonstrated in studies in humans.
- Some medicinal uses of astragalus are based on its proposed immunostimulatory properties, reported in preliminary laboratory and animal experiments, but not conclusively demonstrated in humans. Most astragalus research has been conducted in China and has not been well designed or reported.
- The gummy sap (tragacanth) from astragalus is used as a thickener (ice cream), emulsifier, denture adhesive, and anti-diarrheal agent.

USES BASED ON SCIENTIFIC EVIDENCE	Grade*
Antiviral activity Antiviral activity has been reported with the use of astragalus in laboratory and animal studies. Limited human research has examined the use of astragalus for viral infections in the lung, heart (pericarditis), liver (hepatitis B and C), cervix (papillomavirus), and for HIV infection. Studies have included combinations of astragalus with the drug interferon and astragalus as a component of herbal mixtures. However, most studies have been small and poorly designed. Because of a lack of well-designed research studies, no firm conclusions can be drawn.	C
Cancer Although early laboratory and animal studies reported increased immune cell function and reduced cancer cell growth associated with the use of astragalus, there is no reliable human evidence in these areas. Because of a lack of well-designed research studies, a firm conclusion cannot be drawn.	C
Chemotherapy side effects In Chinese medicine, astragalus-containing herbal mixtures are sometimes used to reduce the side effects of cancer treatments. Because of the lack of well-designed research studies, a firm conclusion cannot be drawn.	C
Coronary artery disease In Chinese medicine, herbal mixtures containing astragalus have been used to treat coronary artery disease. Several studies in humans report reduced symptoms and improved heart function, although these are not well described. High-quality research studies in humans are necessary before a conclusion can be drawn.	C
Heart failure In Chinese medicine, herbal mixtures containing astragalus have been used to treat various heart diseases. There are several human case reports of reduced symptoms, improved heart function, and diuretic ("water pill") effects, although these are not well described. High-quality research studies in humans are necessary before conclusions can be drawn.	C
Immunostimulation Astragalus has been suggested as an immunostimulant in preliminary laboratory and animal research, and in traditional accounts. Published studies from China report increases in white blood cell counts with the use of astragalus preparations, but details are limited. High-quality research studies in humans are necessary before a firm conclusion can be drawn.	C

Continued

Liver protection Several animal and human studies report that astragalus may protect the liver from damage related to toxins or hepatitis B and C. Overall, this research has been poorly designed and reported. Astragalus alone has not been well evaluated. Better-quality research studies are necessary before a conclusion can be drawn.	**C**
Myocarditis/endocarditis (heart infections) Antiviral activity has been reported in laboratory studies and animal models of myocarditis/endocarditis. Research studies in humans are limited in this area, and further research is necessary before a conclusion can be drawn.	**C**
Renal failure Several animal and human studies report that kidney damage from toxins and kidney failure may be improved with the use of astragalus-containing herbal mixtures. Overall, this research has been poorly designed and reported. Astragalus alone has not been well evaluated. Better quality research is necessary before a conclusion can be drawn.	**C**
Upper respiratory tract infection Astragalus is often used in Chinese medicine as a part of herbal mixtures to prevent or treat upper respiratory tract infections. Antiviral activity has been reported in laboratory and animal studies and in limited reports of studies in humans. However, most studies have been small and poorly designed. Because of a lack of well-designed research studies, no firm conclusions can be drawn.	**C**

*Key to grades: *A:* Strong scientific evidence for this use; *B:* Good scientific evidence for this use; *C:* Unclear scientific evidence for this use; *D:* Fair scientific evidence against this use (it may not work); *F:* Strong scientific evidence against this use (it likely does not work). For a more detailed explanation of efficacy criteria, see "Natural Standard Evidence-Based Validated Grading Rationale" in the Introduction.

Uses Based on Tradition, Theory, or Limited Scientific Evidence

Adrenal insufficiency (Addison's disease), aging, AIDS/HIV, allergies, Alzheimer's disease, anemia, angina, ankylosing spondylitis, anorexia, antifungal, antimicrobial, antioxidant, asthma, blood thinner, bone-marrow suppression from cancer or HIV, bronchitis, cervicitis, "chi deficiency" (fatigue, weakness, loss of appetite), chronic fatigue syndrome, chronic hepatitis, cleanser, cyclosporine-induced immunosuppression, dementia, demulcent, denture adhesive (astragalus sap), diabetes, diabetic foot ulcers, diabetic neuropathy, diarrhea, digestion enhancement, diuretic (urination stimulant), edema, fatigue, fever, gangrene, gastrointestinal disorders, genital herpes, graft-versus-host disease, hearing damage from toxins/gentamicin, heart attack, hemorrhage (bleeding), hemorrhoids, high cholesterol, high blood pressure, hyperthyroidism, insomnia, joint pain, laxative, leprosy,

Continued

Uses Based on Tradition, Theory, or Limited Scientific Evidence ***(cont'd)***

leukemia, liver disease, low blood-platelet levels, lung cancer, memory, menstrual disorders, metabolic disorders, minimal brain dysfunction, myalgia (muscle pain), myasthenia gravis, nephritis, night sweats, palpitations, pelvic congestion syndrome, postpartum fever, postpartum urinary retention, prostatitis, rectal prolapse, rotavirus enterocolitis (in infants), shortness of breath, sperm motility, stamina/endurance enhancement, stomach ulcer, stroke, sweating (excessive), systemic lupus erythematosus (SLE), tissue oxygenation, uterine prolapse, uterine bleeding, weight loss, wound healing.

DOSING

The listed doses are based on scientific research, publications, traditional use, and expert opinion. Many herbs and supplements have not been thoroughly tested, and safety and effectiveness may not be proven. Brands may be made differently, with variable ingredients even within the same brand. The doses shown may not apply to all products. It is important to always read product labels, and discuss doses with a qualified healthcare provider before therapy is started.

Standardization

- Standardization involves measuring the amount of certain chemicals in products when attempting to make different preparations similar to each other. It is not always known if the chemicals being measured are the "active" ingredients.
- Anecdotal reports have recommended the standardization of astragalus to a minimum of 0.4% 4-hydroxy-3-methoxy-isoflavone-7-glycoside per dose. However, because astragalus is often added to herbal mixtures with unclear amounts of astragalus used, standardization is not always possible.

Adults (18 Years and Older)

- **General use by mouth:** In Chinese medicine, astragalus is used in soups, teas, extracts, and pill form. In practice and in most scientific studies, astragalus is one component of multi-herb mixtures. Therefore, precise dosing of astragalus alone is unclear. Safety and effectiveness are not clearly established for any particular dose. Various doses of astragalus that have been used or studied include 250 to 500 mg of extract taken four times daily, 1 to 30 g of dried root taken daily (doses as high as 60 g have been reported), and 500 to 1000 mg of root capsules taken 3 times daily. Dosing of tinctures and fluid extracts depends on the strength of preparations.
- *Note:* In theory, tragacanth (the gummy sap derived from astragalus) may reduce absorption of drugs taken by mouth and thus should not be taken at the same time.

Children (Younger Than 18 Years)

- There is insufficient scientific data to recommend astragalus for use in children.

SAFETY

The U.S. Food and Drug Administration does not strictly regulate herbs and supplements. There is no guarantee of strength, purity, or safety of products, and effects may vary. It is important to always read product labels. People who have a medical condition, or are taking other drugs, herbs, or supplements, should consult a qualified healthcare provider before starting a new therapy. A healthcare provider should be contacted immediately about any side effects.

Allergies

- In theory, patients with allergies to members of the Leguminosae family may react to astragalus. Cross-reactivity with Quillaja bark (soap bark) has been reported for astragalus gum tragacanth.

Side Effects and Warnings

- Some species of astragalus cause poisoning in livestock, although these species are not usually present in human preparations (which primarily include *Astragalus membranaceus*). Livestock toxicity, referred to as "locoweed" poisoning, has occurred with species that contain swainsonine (*Astragalus lentiginosus, Astragalus mollissimus, Astragalus nothrosys, Astragalus pubentissimus, Astragalus thuseri, Astragalus wootoni*) and in species that accumulate selenium (*Astragalus bisulcatus, Astragalus flavus, Astragalus praelongus, Astragalus saurinus, Astragalus tenellus*).
- Overall, it is difficult to determine the side effects or toxicity of astragalus, because it is most commonly used in combination with other herbs. There are numerous reports of side effects, ranging from mild to deadly, in the U.S. Food and Drug Administration computer database, although most of these occur with multi-ingredient products and cannot be attributed to astragalus specifically. Astragalus used alone and in recommended doses is traditionally considered to be safe, although this herb's safety has not been well studied. The most common side effects appear to be mild stomach upset and allergic reactions. In the United States, tragacanth (astragalus gummy sap) has been classified as GRAS (generally recognized as safe) for food use, but astragalus itself does not have GRAS status.
- Based on preliminary animal studies and limited human research, astragalus may decrease blood sugar levels. Caution is advised in patients with diabetes or hypoglycemia and in those taking drugs, herbs, or supplements that affect blood sugar levels. Serum glucose levels may need to be monitored by a healthcare professional, and dosing adjustments may be necessary.
- Based on anecdotal reports and preliminary laboratory research, astragalus may increase the risk of bleeding. Caution is advised in patients with bleeding disorders and in people taking drugs that may increase the risk of bleeding. Dosing adjustments may be necessary.
- Preliminary reports of use in China have noted decreased blood pressure at doses of less than 15 g and increased blood pressure at doses above 30 g. Animal research suggests possible blood pressure–lowering effects. Because of a lack of well-designed studies, no firm conclusions can be drawn. Nonetheless, people with abnormal blood pressure or taking blood pressure medications should use caution when taking astragalus and should be monitored by a qualified healthcare professional. Palpitations have been noted in human reports in China.
- Based on studies of animals, astragalus may act as a diuretic and increase urination. In theory, this may lead to dehydration or metabolic abnormalities. There is one report of pneumonia in an infant who had "breathed in" (inhaled) a combination herbal medicine powder that included *Astragalus sarcocolla*.
- Astragalus may increase growth hormone levels.

Pregnancy and Breastfeeding

- There is insufficient scientific evidence to recommend the use of *Astragalus membranaceus* during pregnancy or breastfeeding. Studies of toxic astragalus species, such as *Astragalus lentiginosus* and *Astragalus mollissimus* (locoweed) have reported harmful effects in pregnant animals, leading to abortions or abnormal heart development.

INTERACTIONS

Most herbs and supplements have not been thoroughly tested for interactions with other herbs, supplements, drugs, and foods. The interactions listed here are based on reports in scientific publications, laboratory experiments, and traditional use. It is important to always read product labels. People who have a medical condition, or are taking other drugs, herbs, or supplements, should consult a qualified healthcare provider before starting a new therapy.

Interactions with Drugs

- Based on preliminary animal studies and limited human research, astragalus may decrease blood sugar levels. Caution is advised in patients with diabetes or hypoglycemia and in people taking drugs that affect blood sugar levels. Serum glucose levels may need to be monitored by a healthcare provider, and dosing adjustments may be necessary.
- Preliminary reports of use in China have noted decreased blood pressure at doses of less than 15 g and increased blood pressure at doses above 30 g. Research in animals suggests possible blood pressure–lowering effects. Although well-designed studies are not available, people taking drugs that affect blood pressure should use caution when taking astragalus and should be monitored by a qualified healthcare professional. It has been suggested that beta-blocker drugs such as propranolol (Inderal) and atenolol (Tenormin) may reduce the effects of astragalus on the heart, although this has not been well studied.
- Based on anecdotal reports, astragalus may further increase the risk of bleeding when taken with drugs that increase the risk of bleeding. Examples are aspirin, anticoagulants ("blood thinners") such as warfarin (Coumadin) and heparin, antiplatelet drugs such as clopidogrel (Plavix), and non-steroidal anti-inflammatory drugs such as ibuprofen (Motrin, Advil) and naproxen (Naprosyn, Aleve).
- Based on animal research and traditional use, astragalus may act as a diuretic and increase urination. In theory, this may lead to dehydration or metabolic abnormalities (low blood levels of sodium or potassium), particularly when used in combination with diuretic drugs such as furosemide (Lasix), chlorothiazide (Diuril), and spironolactone (Aldactone).
- Based on laboratory and animal studies, astragalus may possess immunostimulating properties, although research in humans is not conclusive. Some research suggests that astragalus may interfere with the effects of drugs that suppress the immune system, such as steroids and agents used in organ transplants. Better research is necessary before a firm conclusion can be reached.
- Although there is no reliable scientific evidence in this area, some sources suggest other potential drug interactions. These include reduced effects of astragalus when used with sedative drugs (e.g., phenobarbital) and hypnotic agents (e.g., chloral hydrate), increased effects of astragalus when taken with colchicine, increased effects of paralytics such as pancuronium or succinylcholine when used with astragalus, increased effects of stimulants such as ephedrine or epinephrine, increased side effects of dopamine antagonists such as haloperidol (Haldol), and increased side effects of the cancer drug procarbazine.
- In theory, tragacanth (the gummy sap derived from astragalus) may reduce absorption of drugs taken by mouth and thus should be taken at a different time.

Interactions with Herbs and Dietary Supplements

- Based on preliminary animal studies and limited human research, astragalus may decrease blood sugar levels. Caution is advised in patients with diabetes or hypoglycemia and in people taking herbs or supplements that affect blood sugar levels. Examples are *Aloe vera*, American ginseng, bilberry, bitter melon, burdock, fenugreek, fish oil, gymnema, horse chestnut seed extract (HCSE), marshmallow, milk thistle, *Panax ginseng*, rosemary, Siberian ginseng, stinging nettle and white horehound. Serum glucose levels may need to be monitored by a healthcare provider, and dosing adjustments may be necessary.
- Preliminary reports of human use in China have noted decreased blood pressure at doses of less than 15 g and increased blood pressure at doses above 30 g. Animal research suggests possible blood pressure–lowering effects. Although well-designed studies are not available, people taking herbs or supplements that affect blood pressure should use caution when taking astragalus and should be monitored by a qualified healthcare professional. Herbs that may lower blood pressure include aconite/monkshood, arnica, baneberry, betel nut, bilberry, black cohosh, bryony, calendula, California poppy, coleus, curcumin, eucalyptol, eucalyptus oil, ginger, goldenseal, green hellebore, hawthorn, Indian tobacco, jaborandi, mistletoe, night blooming cereus, oleander, pasque flower, periwinkle, pleurisy root, shepherd's purse, Texas milkweed, turmeric, and wild cherry.
- Based on anecdotal reports, astragalus may further increase the risk of bleeding when taken with herbs or supplements that increase the risk of bleeding. Multiple cases of bleeding have been reported with the use of *Ginkgo biloba*, and fewer cases have been reported with the use of garlic and saw palmetto. Theoretically, numerous other agents may increase the risk of bleeding, although this has not been proven in most cases. Examples are alfalfa, American ginseng, angelica, anise, *Arnica montana*, asafetida, aspen bark, bilberry, birch, black cohosh, bladderwrack, bogbean, boldo, borage seed oil, bromelain, capsicum, cat's claw, celery, chamomile, chaparral, clove, coleus, cordyceps, danshen, devil's claw, dong quai, evening primrose, fenugreek, feverfew, flaxseed/flax powder (not a concern with flaxseed oil), ginger, grapefruit juice, grapeseed, green tea, guggul, gymnestra, horse chestnut, horseradish, licorice root, lovage root, male fern, meadowsweet, nordihydroguaiaretic acid (NDGA), onion, papain, *Panax ginseng*, parsley, passion flower, poplar, prickly ash, propolis, quassia, red clover, reishi, rue, Siberian ginseng, sweet birch, sweet clover, turmeric, vitamin E, white willow, wild carrot, wild lettuce, willow, wintergreen, and yucca.
- Based on animal research and traditional use, astragalus may act as a diuretic and increase urination. In theory, this may lead to dehydration or metabolic abnormalities (low blood levels of sodium or potassium), particularly when used in combination with other herbs or supplements that may possess diuretic properties. Examples are artichoke, celery, corn silk, couch grass, dandelion, elder flower, horsetail, juniper berry, kava, shepherd's purse, uva ursi, and yarrow.
- Based on laboratory and animal studies, astragalus may possess immunostimulating properties, although research in humans is not conclusive. It is not known if astragalus interacts with other agents proposed to affect the immune system. Examples are bromelain, calendula, coenzyme Q10, echinacea, ginger, ginseng, goldenseal, gotu kola, lycopene, maitake mushroom, marshmallow, polypodium, propolis, and tea tree oil.

- In theory, tragacanth (the gummy sap derived from astragalus) may reduce absorption of other herbs or supplements taken by mouth and thus should be taken at a different time.

Selected References

Natural Standard developed the preceding evidence-based information based on a systematic review of more than 200 publications. For comprehensive information about alternative and complementary therapies on the professional level, go to www.naturalstandard.com. Selected references are listed here.

Al-Fakhri SA. Herbal medicine: possible cause of aspiration pneumonia: a case report. Saudi Pharm J 1998;6(1):88-91.

Batey RG, Bensoussan A, Fan YY, et al. Preliminary report of a randomized, double-blind placebo-controlled trial of a Chinese herbal medicine preparation CH-100 in the treatment of chronic hepatitis C. J Gastroenterol Hepatol 1998;13(3):244-247.

Bedir E, Pugh N, Calis I, et al. Immunostimulatory effects of cycloartane-type triterpene glycosides from astragalus species. Biol Pharm Bull 2000;23(7):834-837.

Bisignano G, Iauk L, Kirjavainen S, et al. Anti-inflammatory, analgesic, antipyretic and antibacterial activity of Astragalus siculus biv. Int J Pharm 1994;32(4):400-405.

Burack JH, Cohen MR, Hahn JA, et al. Pilot randomized controlled trial of Chinese herbal treatment for HIV-associated symptoms. J Acquir Immune Defic Syndr Hum Retrovirol 1996;12(4):386-393.

Chen KT, Su CH, Hsin LH, et al. Reducing fatigue of athletes following oral administration of huangqi jianzhong tang. Acta Pharmacol Sin 2002 Aug;23(8):757-761.

Chen LX, Liao JZ, Guo WQ. [Effects of Astragalus membranaceus on left ventricular function and oxygen free radical in acute myocardial infarction patients and mechanism of its cardiotonic action.] Zhonghuo Zhong Xi Yi Jie He Za Zhi 1995;15(3):141-143.

Chu DT, Lepe-Zuniga J, Wong WL, et al. Fractionated extract of *Astragalus membranaceus*, a Chinese medicinal herb, potentiates LAK cell cytotoxicity generated by a low dose of recombinant interleukin-2. J Clin Lab Immunol 1988;26(4):183-187.

Chu DT, Lin JR, Wong W. [The in vitro potentiation of LAK cell cytotoxicity in cancer and AIDS patients induced by F3—a fractionated extract of *Astragalus membranaceus*.] Zhonghua Zhong Liu Za Zhi 1994;16(3):167-171.

Chu DT, Sun Y, Lin JR. [Immune restoration of local xenogeneic graft-versus-host reaction in cancer patients in vitro and reversal of cyclophosphamide-induced immune suppression in the rat in vivo by fractionated *Astragalus membranaceus*.] Zhong Xi Yi Jie He Za Zhi 1989; 9(6):351-354, 326.

Chu DT, Wong WL, Mavligit GM. Immunotherapy with Chinese medicinal herbs. II. Reversal of cyclophosphamide-induced immune suppression by administration of fractionated *Astragalus membranaceus* in vivo. J Clin Lab Immunol 1988;25(3):125-129.

Coppes MJ, Anderson RA, Egeler RM, et al. Alternative therapies for the treatment of childhood cancer. N Engl J Med 1998;339(12):846-847.

Cuellar M, Giner RM, Recio MC, et al. Screening of antiinflammatory medicinal plants used in traditional medicine against skin diseases. Phytother Res 1998;12:18-23.

Cui R, He J, Wang B, Zhang F, et al. Suppressive effect of *Astragalus membranaceus* Bunge on chemical hepatocarcinogenesis in rats. Cancer Chemother Pharmacol. 2003;51(1):75-80. Epub 2002 Nov 26.

Dai CF, Zhang ZZ, Qi XL, et al. [Clinical and experimental study of treatment of nanmiqing capsule for chronic prostatitis.] Zhonghua Nan Ke Xue 2002;8(5):379-382.

Duan P, Wang ZM. [Clinical study on effect of *Astragalus* in efficacy enhancing and toxicity reducing of chemotherapy in patients of malignant tumor.] Zhongguo Zhong Xi Yi Jie He Za Zhi 2002;22(7):515-517.

el Sebakhy NA, Asaad AM, Abdallah RM, et al. Antimicrobial isoflavans from *Astragalus* species. Phytochemistry 1994;36(6):1387-1389.

Fu QL. [Experimental study on Yiqi-huoxue therapy of liver fibrosis.] Zhongguo Zhong Xi Yi Jie He Za Zhi 1992;12(4):228-229, 198.

Gariboldi P, Pelizzoni F, Tato M, et al. Cycloartane triterpene glycosides from *Astragalus trigonus*. Phytochem 1995;40(6):1755-1760.

Gu W, Yang YZ, He MX. [A study on combination therapy of Western and traditional Chinese medicine of acute viral myocarditis.] Zhongguo Zhong Xi Yi Jie He Za Zhi 1996;16(12): 713-716.

Guo SK, Chen KJ, Yu FR, et al. Treatment of acute myocardial infarction with AMI-mixture combined with Western medicine. Planta Med 1983;48(1):63-64.

He Z, Findlay JA. Constituents of *Astragalus membranaceus*. J Natural Prod 1991;54(3): 810-815.

Hikino H, Funayama S, Endo K. Hypotensive principle of Astragalus and Hedysarum roots. Planta Med 1976;30:297-302.

Hirotani M, Zhou Y, Rui H, et al. Cycloartane triterpene glycosides from the hairy root cultures of Astragalus membranaceus. Phytochem 1994;37(5):1403-1407.

Hong CY, Lo YC, Tan FC, et al. *Astragalus membranaceus* and *Polygonum multiflorum* protect rat heart mitochondria against lipid peroxidation. Am J Chinese Med 1994;22(1):63-70.

Hong GX, Qin WC, Huang LS. [Memory-improving effect of aqueous extract of Astragalus membranaceus (Fisch.) Bge.] Zhongguo Zhong Yao Za Zhi 1994;19(11):687-688, 704.

Hou YD, Ma GL, Wu SH, et al. Effect of Radix Astragali seu Hedysari on the interferon system. Chin Med J (Engl) 1981;94(1):35-40.

Huang WM, Yan J, Xu J. [Clinical and experimental study on inhibitory effect of Sanhuang mixture on platelet aggregation.] Zhongguo Zhong Xi Yi Jie He Za Zhi 1995;15(8):465-467.

Huang ZQ, Qin NP, Ye W. [Effects of *Astragalus membranaceus* on T-lymphocyte subsets in patients with viral myocarditis.] Zhongguo Zhong Xi Yi Jie He Za Zhi 1995;15(6): 328-330.

Jin R, Wan LL, Mitsuishi T, et al. [Immunomodulative effects of Chinese herbs in mice treated with anti-tumor agent cyclophosphamide.] Yakugaku Zasshi 1994;114(7):533-538.

Kajimura K, Takagi Y, Ueba N, et al. Protective effect of astragali radix by oral administration against Japanese encephalitis virus infection in mice. Biol Pharm Bull 1996;19(9): 1166-1169.

Khoo KS, Ang PT. Extract of *Astragalus membranaceus* and *Ligustrum lucidum* does not prevent cyclophosphamide-induced myelosuppression. Singapore Med J 1995;36(4):387-390.

Kim C, Ha H, Kim JS, Kim YT, et al. Induction of growth hormone by the roots of *Astragalus membranaceus* in pituitary cell culture. Arch Pharm Res 2003;26(1):34-39.

Lau BH, Ruckle HC, Botolazzo T, et al. Chinese medicinal herbs inhibit growth of murine renal cell carcinoma. Cancer Biother 1994;9(2):153-161.

Lei ZY, Qin H, Liao JZ. [Action of *Astragalus membranaceus* on left ventricular function of angina pectoris.] Zhongguo Zhong Xi Yi Jie He Za Zhi 1994;14(4):199-202.

Li C, Luo J, Li L, et al. The collagenolytic effects of the traditional Chinese medicine preparation, Han-Dan-Gan-Le, contribute to reversal of chemical-induced liver fibrosis in rats. Life Sci 2003;72(14):1563-1571.

Li CX, Li L, Lou J, et al. The protective effects of traditional Chinese medicine prescription, Han-dan-gan-le, on CCl4-induced liver fibrosis in rats. Am J Chin Med 1998;26(3-4): 325-332.

Li L, Wang H, Zhu S. [Hepatic albumin's mRNA in nephrotic syndrome rats treated with Chinese herbs.] Zhonghua Yi Xue Za Zhi 1995;75(5):276-279.

Li NQ. [Clinical and experimental study on shen-qo injection with chemotherapy in the treatment of malignant tumor of digestive tract.] Zhongguo Zhong Xi Yi Jie He Za Zhi 1992;12(10):579, 588-592.

Li X, et al. Pharmacological study of APS-G: Part 1—effect on reaction to stress. Zhong Cheng Yao 1989;11(3):27-29.

Li X, et al. Pharmacological study of APS-G: Part 3—effect on blood glucose and glycogen content in liver. Zhong Cheng Yao 1989;11(9):32-33.

Liu ZG, Xiong ZM, Yu XY. [Effect of astragalus injection on immune function in patients with congestive heart failure.] Zhongguo Zhong Xi Yi Jie He Za Zhi 2003;23(5):351-353.

Luo HM, Dai RH, Li Y. [Nuclear cardiology study on effective ingredients of *Astragalus membranaceus* in treating heart failure.] Zhongguo Zhong Xi Yi Jie He Za Zhi 1995; 15(12):707-709.

Ma J, Peng A, Lin S. Mechanisms of the therapeutic effect of *Astragalus membranaceus* on sodium and water retention in experimental heart failure. Chin Med J 1998;111(1):17-23.

Ma Y, Tian Z, Kuang H, et al. Studies of the constituents of *Astragalus membranaceus* Bunge. III. Structures of triterpenoidal glycosides, huangqiyenins A and B, from the leaves. Chem Pharm Bull 1997;45(2):359-361.

Ning L, Chen CX, Jin RM, et al. [Effect of components of dang-gui-bu-xue decoction on hematopenia.] Zhongguo Zhong Yao Za Zhi. 2002 Jan;27(1):50-53.

Pan SY. [Pharmacological action of *Astragalus membranaceus* on the central nervous system in mice.] Zhong Yao Tong Bao 1986;11(9):47-49.

Qian ZW, Li YY. [Synergism of *Astragalus membranaceus* with interferon in the treatment of cervical erosion and their antiviral activities.] Zhong Xi Yi Jie He Za Zhi 1987;7(5):268-269, 287, 259.

Raghuprasad PK, Brooks SM, Litwin A, et al. Quillaja bark (soap bark)–induced asthma. J Allergy Clin Immunol 1980;65(4):285-287.

Rios JL, Waterman PG. A review of the pharmacology and toxicology of astragalus. Phytother Res 1997;11:411-418.

Rittenhouse JR, Lui PD, Lau BH. Chinese medicinal herbs reverse macrophage suppression induced by urological tumors. J Urol 1991;146(2):486-490.

Sheng ZL, Li NY, Ge XP. [Clinical study of baoyuan dahuang decoction in the treatment of chronic renal failure.] Zhongguo Zhong Xi Yi Jie He Za Zhi 1994;14(5):268-270, 259.

Shirataki Y, Takao M, Yoshida S, et al. Antioxidative components isolated from the roots of *Astragalus membranaceus* Bunge (Astragali Radix). Phytother Res 1997;11:603-605.

Su ZZ, He YY, Chen G. [Clinical and experimental study on effects of Man-shen-ling oral liquid in the treatment of 100 cases of chronic nephritis.] Zhongguo Zhong Xi Yi Jie He Za Zhi 1993;13(5):269-260.

Sun Y, Hersh EM, Lee S, et al. Preliminary observations on the effects of the Chinese medicinal herbs *Astragalus membranaceus* and *Ligustrum lucidum* on lymphocyte blastogenic responses. J Biol Response Mod 1983;2(3):227-237.

Sun Y, Hersh EM, Talpax M, et al. Immune restoration and/or augmentation of local graft versus host reaction by traditional Chinese medicinal herbs. Cancer 1983;52(1):70-73.

Sun Y. The role of traditional Chinese medicine in supportive care of cancer patients. Recent Results Cancer Res 1988;108:327-334.

Tianqing P, Yingzhen Y, Riesemann H, et al. The inhibitory effect of *Astragalus membranaceus* on Coxsackie B-3 virus RNA replication. Chin Med Sci J 1995;10(3):146-150.

Wang D, Shen W, Tian Y, et al. [Protective effect of total flavonoids of radix Astragali on mammalian cell damage caused by hydroxyl radical.] Zhongguo Zhong Yao Za Zhi 1995; 20(4):240-242.

Wang F. Twenty-eight cases of diabetic foot ulcer and gangrene treated with the Chinese herbal medicine combined with injection of ahylsantinfarctase. J Tradit Chin Med 2002;22(1):3-4.

Wang Q. [Inotropic action of *Astragalus membranaceus* Bge. saponins and its possible mechanism.] Zhongguo Zhong Yao Za Zhi 1992;17(9):557-559.

Wei H, Sun R, Xiao W, et al. Traditional Chinese medicine Astragalu*s* reverses predominance of Th2 cytokines and their up-stream transcript factors in lung cancer patients. Oncol Rep 2003;10(5):1507-1512.

Weng XS. [Treatment of leucopenia with pure Astragalus preparation—an analysis of 115 leucopenic cases.] Zhongguo Zhong Xi Yi Jie He Za Zhi 1995;15(8):462-464.

Wu XS, Chen HY, Li M. [Clinical observation on effect of combined use of Astragalus and compound salviae injection in treating acute cerebral infarction.] Zhongguo Zhong Xi Yi Jie He Za Zhi. 2003;23(5):380-381.

Xiangzhe J. A clinical investigation on 30 cases of senile benign renal arteriosclerosis treated by Huang qi gu jing yin. J Tradit Chin Med 2001;21(3):177-180.

Xu XY, Li LH, Wu LS, Zhao CL, Lin HY. [Adjustment effect of Dadix Astragalus and Dadix Angelicae sinensis on TNF-alpha and bFGF on renal injury induced by ischemia reperfusion in rabbit.] Zhongguo Zhong Yao Za Zhi. 2002;27(10):771-773.

Xuan W, Dong M, Dong M. Effects of compound injection of *Pyrola rotundifolia* L. and *Astragalus membranaceus* Bge on experimental guinea pigs' gentamicin ototoxicity. Ann Otol Rhinol Laryngol 1995;104(5):374-380.

Yan HJ. [Clinical and experimental study of the effect of kang er xin-I on viral myocarditis.] Zhong Xi Yi Jie He Za Zhi 1991;11(8):468-470, 452.

Yang Y, Jin P, Guo Q, et al. Effect of *Astragalus membranaceus* on natural killer cell activity and induction of alpha- and gamma-interferon in patients with Coxsackie B viral myocarditis. Chin Med J 1990;103(4):304-307.

Yang Y, Jin P, Guo Q, et al. Treatment of experimental Coxsackie B-3 viral myocarditis with *Astragalus membranaceus* in mice. Chin Med J 1990;103(1):14-18.

Yin X, Zhang S, Kong Y, et al. Observation on efficiency of Jiangtang capsule in treating diabetes mellitus type 2 with hyperlipidemia. Chin J Integ Tradit West Med 2001; 7(3): 214-216.

Yu L, Lu Y, Li J, Wang H. Identification of a gene associated with astragalus and angelica's renal protective effects by silver staining mRNA differential display. Chin Med J (Engl) 2002 Jun; 115(6):923-927.

Yuan WL, Chen HZ, Yang YZ, et al. Effect of *Astragalus membranaceus* on electric activities of cultured rat beating heart cells infected with Coxsackie B-2 virus. Chin Med J 1990;103(3): 177-182.

Zee-Cheng RK. Shi-quan-da-bu-tang (ten significant tonic decoction), SQT. A potent Chinese biological response modifier in cancer immunotherapy, potentiation and detoxification of anticancer drugs. Methods Find Exp Clin Pharmacol 1992;14(9):725-736.

Zhang BZ, Ding F, Tan LW. [Clinical and experimental study on Yi-gan-ning granule in treating chronic hepatitis B.] Zhongguo Zhong Xi Yi Jie He Za Zhi 1993;13(10):597-599, 580.

Zhang H, Huang J. [Preliminary study of traditional Chinese medicine treatment of minimal brain dysfunction: analysis of 100 cases.] Zhong Xi Yi Jie He Za Zhi 1990;10(5):278-279, 260.

Zhang HE, et al. Treatment of adult diabetes with Jiangtangjia tablet. J Tradit Chin Med 1986;27(4):37-39.

Zhang JG, Gao DS, Wei GH. [Clinical study on effect of Astragalus injection on left ventricular remodeling and left ventricular function in patients with acute myocardial infarction.] Zhongguo Zhong Xi Yi Jie He Za Zhi. 2002;22(5):346-348.

Zhang WJ, Wojta J, Binder BR. Regulation of the fibrinolytic potential of cultured human umbilical vein endothelial cells: Astragaloside IV downregulates plasminogen activator inhibitor-1 and upregulates tissue-type plasminogen activator expression. J Vasc Res 1997; 34:273-280.

Zhang YD, Shen JP, Zhu SH, et al. [Effects of astragalus (ASI, SK) on experimental liver injury.] Yao Xue Xue Bao 1992;27(6):401-406.

Zhang ZL, Wen QZ, Liu CX. Hepatoprotective effects of astragalus root. J Ethnopharmacol 1990;30(2):145-149.

Zhao KS, Mancini C, Doria G. Enhancement of the immune response in mice by *Astragalus membranaceus* extracts. Immunopharmacol 1990;20(3):225-233.

Zhao KW, Kong HY. [Effect of Astragalan on secretion of tumor necrosis factors in human peripheral blood mononuclear cells.] Zhongguo Zhong Xi Yi Jie He Za Zhi 1993;13(5): 263-265, 259.

Zhao XZ. [Effects of *Astragalus membranaceus* and *Tripterygium hypoglancum* on natural killer cell activity of peripheral blood mononuclear in systemic lupus erythematosus.] Zhongguo Zhong Xi Yi Jie He Za Zhi 1992;12(11):669-671, 645.

Zhou Y, Hirotani M, Rui H, et al. Two triglycosidic triterpene astragalosides from hairy root cultures of *Astragalus membranaceus.* Phytochemistry 1995;38(6):1407-1410.

Zhou Y, Huang Z, Huang T, et al. Clinical study of Shengxue Mixture in treating aplastic anemia. Chin J Integ Trad West 2001;7(3):186-189.

Zong PP, Yan TY, Gong MM. [Clinical and experimental studies of effects of Huayu decoction on scavenging free radicals.] Zhongguo Zhong Xi Yi Jie He Za Zhi 1993;13(10):591-593, 579.

Zuo L, Guo H. [Quantitative study on synergistic effect of radix astragali A6 and acyclovir against herpes simplex virus type I by polymerase chain reaction.] Zhongguo Zhong Xi Yi Jie He Za Zhi 1998;18(4):233-235.

Barley

(*Hordeum vulgare* L., Germinated Barley Foodstuff [GBF])

RELATED TERMS

- Barley malt, barley oil, brewers spent grain, dietary fiber, germinated barley, high-protein barley flour (HPBF), Gramineae, high-fiber barley, hordeum, *Hordeum distychum*, *Hordeum dislichon*, *Hordeum murinum*, mai ya, pearl barley, Poaceae, pot barley, scotch barley, wild barley grass.
- *Note:* Most scientific studies have been of foods containing barley rather then barley supplements.

BACKGROUND

- Barley is a cereal used as a staple food in many countries. It is commonly used as an ingredient in baked products and soup in Europe and the United States. Barley malt is used to make beer and as a natural sweetener called malt sugar or barley jelly sugar.
- Recent data suggest that barley may reduce total cholesterol and low-density lipoprotein (LDL) in mildly hyperlipidemic patients. Barley has a high fiber content; in a recent large prospective cohort study, a modest inverse association was observed between dietary fiber intake and cardiovascular disease, although results were not statistically significant.
- Germinated barley foodstuff (GBF) is derived from the aleurone and scutellum fractions of germinated barley. GBF may play a role in the management of ulcerative colitis, although further controlled studies are warranted. GBF has also been suggested as a treatment for mild constipation.
- Barley bran flour accelerates gastrointestinal transit and increases fecal weight. High-fiber barley may be useful in the diets of patients with diabetes, because of its low glycemic index and ability to reduce glucose levels after eating.

USES BASED ON SCIENTIFIC EVIDENCE	Grade*
High cholesterol Several small studies suggest that high-fiber barley, barley bran flour, and barley oil may reduce cholesterol by increasing the elimination of cholesterol from the body. Scientific research supports the use of barley in a cholesterol-lowering diet in mild cases of high cholesterol. Larger and longer studies are needed to determine the safety and effectiveness of doses.	B
Constipation Barley has been used traditionally as a treatment for constipation because of its high fiber content. However, there is limited scientific evidence in this area. Further research is necessary in order to establish safety and dosing recommendations.	C

Continued

High blood sugar/glucose intolerance Preliminary evidence suggests that barley meal may improve glucose tolerance. Better research is necessary before a firm conclusion can be drawn.	C
Ulcerative colitis GBF, which is derived from maturing barley, has been suggested as potentially helpful in patients with ulcerative colitis. Scientific evidence in this area is preliminary, and further research is needed before GBF can be recommended for ulcerative colitis.	C

*Key to grades: *A:* Strong scientific evidence for this use; *B:* Good scientific evidence for this use; *C:* Unclear scientific evidence for this use; *D:* Fair scientific evidence against this use (it may not work); *F:* Strong scientific evidence against this use (it likely does not work). For a more detailed explanation of efficacy criteria, see "Natural Standard Evidence-Based Validated Grading Rationale" in the Introduction.

Uses Based on Tradition, Theory, or Limited Scientific Evidence

Antimicrobial, appetite suppressant, asthma, boils, bowel/intestinal disorders, bronchitis, celiac disease, colon cancer, diabetes, diarrhea, improved blood circulation, kidney disease, nutritional supplement, stamina/strength enhancer, sweetener, weight loss.

DOSING

The doses listed are based on scientific research, publications, traditional use, or expert opinion. Many herbs and supplements have not been thoroughly tested, and their safety and effectiveness may not be proven. Brands may be made differently, with variable ingredients, even within the same brand. The doses shown may not apply to all products. It is important to always read product labels and discuss doses with a qualified healthcare provider before therapy is started.

Adults (18 Years and Older)

- **High cholesterol:** 1.5 ml of barley oil twice daily or 30 g of barley bran flour daily by mouth has been used in studies.
- **Ulcerative colitis (mild to moderate):** 10 g of GBF taken three times daily has been studied and reported as well tolerated.
- **Constipation:** In limited research studies, 9 g of GBF daily for up to 20 days has been used.

Children (Younger Than 18 Years)

- There is insufficient scientific information to recommend barley for use in children.

SAFETY

The U.S. Food and Drug Administration does not strictly regulate herbs and supplements. There is no guarantee of the strength, purity, or safety of products, and effects may vary. It is important to always read product labels. People who have a medical condition, or are taking other drugs, herbs, or supplements, should consult a qualified healthcare provider before starting a new therapy. A healthcare provider should be contacted immediately about any side effects.

Allergies

- People with known allergy or hypersensitivity to barley flour or beer should avoid barley products. Severe allergic reactions (anaphylaxis) and skin rashes have been reported in persons who drank beer made with malted barley. People with allergy/hypersensitivity to grass pollens or wheat allergy may also react to barley.
- "Bakers' asthma" is an allergic response caused by breathing in cereal flours that occurs in workers in the baking and milling industries and can result from barley flour exposure. If a person is allergic to one cereal (like barley), it is possible that other cereals may cause similar symptoms.

Side Effects and Warnings

- Barley appears to be well tolerated in non-allergic, healthy adults in recommended doses for short periods of time, as a cereal or in the form of beer. Individuals with celiac disease (wheat allergy) may have an increased risk of developing gastrointestinal (stomach) upset with barley products. Barley may cause a feeling of "fullness." Five infants fed with a formula containing barley water, whole milk, and corn syrup developed malnutrition and anemia, possibly due to vitamin deficiencies.
- Theoretically, eating large amounts of barley may lower blood sugar levels. Caution is advised in patients with diabetes or hypoglycemia, and in those taking drugs, herbs, or supplements that affect blood sugar levels. Serum glucose levels may need to be monitored by a healthcare provider, and dosing adjustments may be necessary.
- Hordenine, a chemical in the root of developing barley, may stimulate the sympathetic nervous system. The effects of hordenine in humans are not clear, although theoretically, increased heart rate and wakefulness can occur.
- Eye, nasal, and sinus irritation or asthmatic reactions can occur from exposure to barley dust. Some persons may experience inflammation or irritation of the skin, eyelids, arms, or legs. Contact with the malt in beer may cause skin rash. Evening "feverish episodes" have been reported in dockworkers and silo operators who have handled barley products or dust.
- Contamination of barley with fungus has been associated with Kashin-Beck disease (KBD), a bone disorder estimated to affect 1 to 3 million people in rural China and Tibet. Another contaminant that has been found in barley is ochratoxin A.

Pregnancy and Breastfeeding

- Traditionally, women have been advised against eating large amounts of barley sprouts during pregnancy. Infants fed with a formula containing barley water, whole milk, and corn syrup developed malnutrition and anemia, possibly as a result of vitamin deficiencies.

INTERACTIONS

Most herbs and supplements have not been thoroughly tested for interactions with other herbs, supplements, drugs, or foods. The interactions listed here are based on reports in scientific publications, laboratory experiments, and traditional use. It is important to always read product labels. People who have a medical condition, or are taking other drugs, herbs, or supplements, should consult a qualified healthcare provider before starting a new therapy.

Interactions with Drugs

- Fiber in barley may decrease the absorption of medications taken by mouth and prevent full beneficial effects. Eating barley in large quantities may lower blood sugar levels. Caution is advised when using medications that may also lower blood sugar levels. Persons taking drugs for diabetes by mouth or insulin should be monitored closely by a qualified healthcare provider. Medication adjustments may be necessary.
- Barley has been associated with decreased total cholesterol and LDL concentrations, and it may act additively with other cholesterol-lowering agents such as lovastatin (Mevacor) and atorvastatin (Lipitor). Hordenine, a chemical in the root of the developing barley, stimulates the sympathetic nervous system. In theory, taking hordenine with stimulant drugs may result in additive effects such as increased heart rate and wakefulness.

Interactions with Herbs and Dietary Supplements

- Fiber in barley may reduce the absorption of some herbs and supplements that are taken by mouth. In theory, barley may lower blood sugar levels. Caution is advised when using herbs or supplements that may also lower blood sugar levels. Blood glucose levels may require monitoring, and doses may need adjustment. Examples are *Aloe vera*, American ginseng, bilberry, bitter melon, burdock, fenugreek, fish oil, gymnema, horse chestnut seed extract (HCSE), marshmallow, milk thistle, *Panax ginseng*, rosemary, Siberian ginseng, stinging nettle, and white horehound.
- Barley has been associated with decreased total cholesterol and LDL concentrations, and it may add to the effects of cholesterol-lowering agents such as fish oil, garlic, guggul, and niacin. Hordenine, a chemical in the root of the developing barley, stimulates the sympathetic nervous system. In theory, taking hordenine with stimulant agents such as ephedra or caffeine may result in additive effects such as increased heart rate and wakefulness.

Selected References

Natural Standard developed the preceding evidence-based information based on a systematic review of more than 160 scientific articles. For comprehensive information about alternative and complementary therapies on the professional level, go to www.naturalstandard.com. Selected references are listed here.

Armentia A, Rodriguez R, Callejo A, et al. Allergy after ingestion or inhalation of cereals involves similar allergens in different ages. Clin Exp Allergy 2002;32(8):1216-1222.

Bamba T, Kanauchi O, Andoh A, et al. A new prebiotic from germinated barley for nutraceutical treatment of ulcerative colitis [review]. J Gastroenterol Hepatol 2002;17(8):818-824.

Bonadonna P, Crivellaro M, Dama A, et al. Beer-induced anaphylaxis due to barley sensitization: two case reports. J Investig Allergol Clin Immunol 1999;9(4):268-270.

Callaway TR, Elder RO, Keen JE, et al. Forage feeding to reduce preharvest *Escherichia coli* populations in cattle, a review. J Dairy Sci 2003;86(3):852-860.

Czerwiecki L, Czajkowska D, Witkowska-Gwiazdowska A. On ochratoxin A and fungal flora in Polish cereals from conventional and ecological farms—Part 1: occurrence of ochratoxin A and fungi in cereals in 1997. Food Addit Contam 2002;19(5):470-477.

Gabrovska D, Fiedlerova V, Holasova M, et al. The nutritional evaluation of underutilized cereals and buckwheat. Food Nutr Bull 2002;23(Suppl 3):246-249.

Ivarsson A, Hernell O, Stenlund H, et al. Breast-feeding protects against celiac disease. Am J Clin Nutr 2002;75(5):914-921.

Jenkins DJ, Kendall CW, Marchie A, et al. Type 2 diabetes and the vegetarian diet [Review]. Am J Clin Nutr 2003;78(Suppl 3):610S-616S.
Kanauchi O, Mitsuyama K, Saiki T, et al. Germinated barley foodstuff increases fecal volume and butyrate production in humans. Int J Mol Med 1998a;1(6):937-941.
Kanauchi O, Mitsuyama K, Saiki T, et al. Germinated barley foodstuff increases fecal volume and butyrate production at relatively low doses and relieves constipation in humans. Int J Mol Med 1998b;2(4):445-450.
Lupton JR, Robinson MC, Morin JL. Cholesterol-lowering effect of barley bran flour and oil. J Am Diet Assoc 1994;94(1):65-70.
McIntosh GH, Whyte J, McArthur R, et al. Barley and wheat foods: influence on plasma cholesterol concentrations in hypercholesterolemic men. Am J Clin Nutr 1991;53(5):1205-1209.
Mitsuyama K, Saiki T, Kanauchi O, et al. Treatment of ulcerative colitis with germinated barley foodstuff feeding: a pilot study. Aliment Pharmacol Ther 1998;12(12):1225-1230.

Belladonna

(*Atropa belladonna* L. or its variety *Atropa acuminata* Royle ex Lindley)

RELATED TERMS

- Beladona, belladone, belladonnae herbae pulvis standardisatus, belladonna herbum, belladonna leaf, belladonna pulvis normatus, belladonnae folium, belladonna radix, belladonne, deadly nightshade, deadly nightshade leaf, devil's cherries, devil's herb, die Belladonna, die Tollkirsche, divale, dwale, dwayberry, galnebaer, great morel, herba belladonna, hoja de belladonna, naughty man's cherries, poison black cherries, powdered belladonna, Solanaceae, *solanum mortale, solanum somniferum,* strygium, stryshon, tollekirsche, tollkirschenblatter.
- **Selected Combination Products:** Bellergal, Bellergal to S, Bellergil, Bel to Phen to Ergot S, B&O Supprettes, Cafergot to PB, Distovagal, Phenerbel to S, PMS to Opium & Beladonna.

BACKGROUND

- Belladonna is an herb that has been used for centuries for a variety of indications, including headache, menstrual symptoms, peptic ulcer disease, inflammation, and motion sickness. Belladonna is known to contain active agents with anticholinergic properties, such as the tropane alkaloids atropine, hyoscine (scopolamine) and hyoscyamine.
- There are few available studies of belladonna monotherapy for any indication. Most research studies have evaluated belladonna in combination with other agents such as ergot alkaloids or barbiturates, or in homeopathic (diluted) preparations. Preliminary evidence suggests possible efficacy in combination with barbiturates for the management of symptoms associated with irritable bowel syndrome. However, there is currently insufficient scientific evidence regarding the use of belladonna for this or any other indication.
- There is extensive literature on the adverse effects and toxicity of belladonna, related principally to its known anticholinergic actions. Common adverse effects include dry mouth, urinary retention, flushing, papillary dilation, constipation, confusion, and delirium. Many of these effects may occur at therapeutic doses.

USES BASED ON SCIENTIFIC EVIDENCE	Grade*
Airway obstruction Belladonna can cause relaxation of the airways and reduce the amount of mucus produced. A study in infants demonstrated possible beneficial effects of belladonna on airway obstruction during sleep. However, because of lack of high-quality research studies in humans in this area, there is not enough evidence to form a clear conclusion.	**C**

Continued

Ear infections Little reliable research is available on the use of belladonna for ear infections. Other therapies have been shown to be effective and are recommended for this condition.	C
Headache The available studies of belladonna in the treatment of headache are not well designed and do not show a clear benefit. More, better-designed studies are needed to test the ability of belladonna alone (not in multi-ingredient products) to treat or prevent headache.	C
Irritable bowel syndrome Belladonna has been used historically for the treatment of irritable bowel, and in theory its mechanism of action should be effective for some of the symptoms. However, of the few studies that are available, none clearly shows that belladonna alone (not as part of a mixed product) provides this effect.	C
Nervous system disorders The autonomic nervous system, which helps control basic body functions like sweating and blood flow, is affected in several disorders. To date, studies in humans have shown no benefit from belladonna in treating these disorders.	C
Premenstrual syndrome (PMS) Bellergal (a combination of phenobarbital, ergot, and belladonna) has been used historically to treat PMS symptoms. Limited studies have reported improvement in symptoms. More studies are needed before a strong recommendation can be made.	C
Radiation therapy rash (radiation burn) There is little reliable scientific evidence available for the effectiveness of belladonna for rash after radiation therapy. Further study is needed before a recommendation can be made.	C

*Key to grades: *A:* Strong scientific evidence for this use; *B:* Good scientific evidence for this use; *C:* Unclear scientific evidence for this use; *D:* Fair scientific evidence against this use (it may not work); *F:* Strong scientific evidence against this use (it likely does not work). For a more detailed explanation of efficacy criteria, see "Natural Standard Evidence-Based Validated Grading Rationale" in the Introduction.

Uses Based on Tradition, Theory, or Limited Scientific Evidence

Abnormal menstrual periods, anesthetic, anxiety, arthritis, asthma, bedwetting, chickenpox, colds, colitis, conjunctivitis (inflamed eyes), difficulty passing urine, diverticulitis, diuretic (use as a "water pill"), earache, encephalitis (inflammation of the brain), excessive sweating, excessive unintentional muscle movements, fever, flu, glaucoma, gout, hay fever, hemorrhoids, inflammation, kidney stones,

Continued

Uses Based on Tradition, Theory, or Limited Scientific Evidence *(cont'd)*

measles, motion sickness, mumps, muscle and joint pain, pupil dilation, nausea and vomiting during pregnancy, pain from nerve disorders, Parkinson's disease, pancreatitis, poisoning (especially by insecticides), rash, scarlet fever, sciatica (back and leg pain), sedative, sore throat, stomach ulcers, teething, toothache, ulcerative colitis, warts, whooping cough.

DOSING

The following doses are based on scientific research, publications, traditional use, or expert opinion. Many herbs and supplements have not been thoroughly tested, and their safety and effectiveness may not be proven. Brands may be made differently, with variable ingredients even within the same brand. The doses shown may not apply to all products. It is important to always read product labels and discuss doses with a qualified healthcare provider before therapy is started.

Standardization

- Standardization involves measuring the amount of certain chemicals in products when attempting to make different preparations similar to each other. It is not always known if the chemicals being measured are the "active" ingredients. There is currently no widely used standardization for the preparation of belladonna. Doses of belladonna are often calculated in mg of total alkaloids. *Atropa belladonna* contains up to 20 different tropane alkaloid compounds. The leaves and roots contain different amounts of the individual tropane alkaloids. Non-homeopathic dilutions of belladonna should be clearly labeled with the amount of the ingredient group "tropane alkaloid."

Adults (18 Years and Older)

Oral (by Mouth)

- **Traditional dosing:** A traditional dose of belladonna leaf powder is 50 to 100 mg, with a maximum single dose of 200 mg (0.6 mg of total alkaloids, calculated as the ingredient hyoscyamine) and a maximum daily dose of 600 mg. A traditional dose of belladonna root is 50 mg, with a maximum single dose of 100 mg (0.5 mg of total alkaloids, calculated as hyoscyamine) and a maximum daily dose of 300 mg. A traditional dose of belladonna extract is 10 mg, with a maximum single dose of 100 mg (0.5 mg of total alkaloids, calculated as hyoscyamine) and a maximum daily dose of 150 mg. The expert German panel, the Commission E, suggests these doses mainly for the treatment of "gastrointestinal spasm." For tincture of belladonna (composed of 27 to 33 mg of belladonna leaf alkaloids in 100 ml of alcohol), informal reports suggest either a total dose of 1.5 mg daily (divided into 3 doses daily, with a double dose at bedtime) or a dose of 0.6 to 1 ml (0.18 to 0.3 mg of belladonna leaf alkaloids) taken 3 or 4 times daily.
- **Irritable bowel syndrome:** Studies report several doses and preparations of belladonna for irritable bowel syndrome, including Hyoscine butylbromide (10 mg by mouth, taken four times daily), a combination preparation containing 0.25 mg levorotatory alkaloids of belladonna and 50 mg of phenobarbital, and Donnatal tablets (0.1037 mg of hyoscyamine sulfate, 0.0194 mg of atropine sulfate, 0.0065 mg of hyoscine hydrobromide, and 16.2 mg of phenobarbital). One study used a higher

dose (8 mg of belladonna and 30 mg of phenobarbital), but because belladonna is potentially dangerous in high doses, this dose is not recommended.

- **Nervous system disorders:** One study in humans used a dose of a combination formula (15 mg of belladonna, 60 mg of ergot alkaloids, 15 mg of propranolol, and 25 mg of amobarbital), taken three times daily for 2 weeks.
- **Headache:** Studies have been carried out using the combination product Bellergal (40 mg of phenobarbital, 0.6 mg of ergotamine tartrate, and 0.2 mg of levorotatory alkaloids of belladonna), taken by mouth twice daily.
- **Menopausal symptoms:** A study using Bellergal Retard (total daily dose: 80 mg of phenobarbital, 1.2 mg of ergotamine tartrate, and 0.4 mg levorotatory alkaloids of belladonna) for 4 weeks reported no benefit.
- **Premenstrual syndrome:** One study used Bellergal (40 mg of phenobarbital, 0.6 mg of ergotamine tartrate, and 0.2 mg of levorotatory alkaloids of belladonna), taken by mouth twice daily for 10 days before the menstrual period was expected.
- **Homeopathic dosing:** Homeopathic doses often depend on the symptom being treated and the style of the prescribing provider. Dosing practices may therefore vary widely. Usually, a homeopathic product is diluted several times. For example, belladonna may be diluted by 100 (one teaspoon belladonna added to 99 teaspoons water) in the first round, and this new, dilute mixture may be diluted 30-fold (1 teaspoon of the dilute mixture added to 29 teaspoons water). The naming of these dilutions follows a complicated set of definitions. For example, when a supplement is diluted by 10 and this mix is then diluted by 30, it has a strength of *30X*, or *30D*. When a supplement is first diluted by 100 and then diluted again by 30, it is referred to as *30C*. "Proving studies" have been conducted to observe the effects of homeopathic belladonna in healthy volunteers. These studies have used preparations of Belladonna 30CH (Deutsche Homöopathie Union, Karlsruhe, Germany) and Belladonna C30 (Ainsworth's Homeopathic Pharmacy, London, England), given as 1 tablet by mouth twice daily.
- **Radiation burns:** A study of patients treated with radiation for cancer reported that a dose of Belladonna 7CH (Laboratoires Boiron, Sainte-Fey-Les-Lyon, France), taken as 3 granules under the tongue twice daily, failed to reduce rash severity.

Topical (Applied to the Skin)

- **Muscle and bone aches:** A belladonna plaster produced by Cuxson Gerrard (Oldsbury West Midlands, England) containing 0.25% belladonna alkaloids (hyoscine 2% and atropine 1%) was described in a case report. Long-term use may cause a rash at the site of the plaster.

Children (Younger Than 18 Years)

Oral (by Mouth)

- **Traditional dosing:** Informal reports described a typical dose of 0.03 ml for each kilogram of body weight, taken by mouth three times daily. Another dose used 0.8 ml for each square meter of body surface area, taken by mouth three times daily (27 to 33 mg of belladonna leaf alkaloids in 100 ml). The maximum dose is reported as 3.5 ml daily. Safety and effectiveness have not been proven.
- **Airway obstruction:** A study in infants used a tincture of belladonna, in a dose equal to 0.01 mg of atropine for each kg of body weight, at bedtime.
- *Note:* Death in children may occur as the result of a dose of 0.2 mg of atropine for each kg 92.2 lb) of body weight. Because 2 mg of atropine are often found in a fruit berry, just two fruits may be deadly for a small child.

- **Homeopathic dosing:** Homeopathic doses often depend on the symptom being treated and the style of the prescribing provider. Dosing practices may therefore vary widely. Usually, a homeopathic product is diluted several times. For example, belladonna may be diluted by 100 (one teaspoon of belladonna added to 99 teaspoons water) in the first round; this new, dilute mixture may then be diluted 30-fold (1 teaspoon of the dilute mixture added to 29 teaspoons water). The naming of these dilutions follows a complicated set of definitions. For example, when a supplement is diluted by 10 and this mix is then diluted by 30, it has a strength of *30X*, or *30D*. When a supplement is first diluted by 100 and then diluted again by 30, it is referred to as *30C*.
- **Ear infections:** A study in children compared homeopathic prescription medications using belladonna 30X globules (brand and dose were not specified).

SAFETY

The U.S. Food and Drug Administration does not strictly regulate herbs and supplements. There is no guarantee of the strength, purity, or safety of products, and effects may vary. It is important to always read product labels. People who have a medical condition, or are taking other drugs, herbs, or supplements, should consult a qualified healthcare provider before starting a new therapy. A healthcare provider should be contacted immediately about any side effects.

Allergies

Use of belladonna should be avoided in people who have had significant reactions to belladonna or anticholinergic drugs, or who are allergic to belladonna or other members of the *Solanaceae* (nightshade) family, such as bell peppers, potatoes, and eggplants. Long-term use of *belladonna* on the skin can lead to allergic rashes.

Side Effects and Warnings

- At a dose of up to 1.5 mg daily, belladonna is traditionally thought to be safe, but it may cause frequent side effects such as dilated pupils, blushing of the skin, dry mouth, rapid heartbeat, confusion, nervousness, and hallucinations. High doses can cause death.
- In children, death can be caused by as little as 0.2 mg of atropine (one of the active ingredients of belladonna) per kilogram (2.2 lb) of body weight. Because the fruit (berry) of the belladonna plant contains about 2 mg of atropine, ingestion of only two berries can be deadly for a small child. Several reports of accidental belladonna overdose and death have been reported. In one case, the poisoning was caused by eating a rabbit that had been feeding on belladonna plant. Adults and children have died or been seriously ill after eating the berries of deadly nightshade (*Atropa belladonna*) or woody nightshade (*Solanum dulcamara*), a relative of belladonna. In one report, eating tomatoes grown from a plant grafted to Jimson weed (*Datura stramonium*) led to death.
- Belladonna overdose can occur when it is applied to the skin. Belladonna overdose is highly dangerous and should be treated by qualified medical professionals. Because belladonna can slow the movement of food and drugs through the stomach and gut, side effects can occur long after the belladonna has been swallowed.
- Belladonna may cause redness of the skin, flushing, dry skin, sun sensitivity, hives and allergic rashes, even at dilute concentrations, and a serious, potentially life-threatening rash called Stevens-Johnson syndrome. This syndrome is characterized by red, at times blistered or painful spots on the skin. The mouth, eyes, and genitals

may be affected. Severe cases may require hospitalization. Other side effects are headache, hyperactivity, nervousness, dizziness, lightheadedness, drowsiness or sedation, unsteady walking, confusion, hallucinations, slurred speech, exaggerated reflexes, convulsions, and coma. The eyes may be dilated or sensitive to light, and vision may be blurred. If parts of a belladonna plant are put into the eyes, the pupils may be dilated permanently.

- There have been case reports of hyperventilation, coma with loss of breathing, rapid or abnormal heart rate, and abnormally high blood pressure. Other reports include dry mouth, abdominal fullness, difficult urination, decreased perspiration, slow release of breast milk while nursing, muscle cramps or spasms, and tremors. People who have difficulty passing urine, enlarged prostate, kidney stones, dry mouth, Sjögren syndrome, dry eyes, or glaucoma should avoid using belladonna. Caution should be used if a person has a fever. People with myasthenia gravis (a disorder of nerves and muscles) or Down syndrome may be especially sensitive to belladonna.
- Older adults and children should avoid using belladonna, because there are many reports of serious side effects in these age groups. Belladonna products should not be combined with prescribed anticholinergic agents. It is important to check with the healthcare provider who is prescribing medications to see whether any of the medications are anticholinergic. People who have had a heart attack and those with heart disease, fluid in the lungs, high blood pressure, or abnormal heart rhythms should avoid the use of belladonna. Because belladonna can affect the activity of the stomach and intestines, people with ulcers, reflux, hiatal hernia, obstruction of the bowel, poor movement of the intestines, constipation, colitis, or an ileostomy or colostomy also should avoid the use of belladonna after surgery.

Pregnancy and Breastfeeding

- Belladonna is not recommended for women who are pregnant or who are breast-feeding because of the risks of side effects and poisoning. Belladonna is listed under category C by the U.S. Food and Drug Administration (FDA category C includes drugs for which no thorough studies have been published). In nursing women who use belladonna, belladonna ingredients are found in breast milk, possibly endangering infants.

INTERACTIONS

Most herbs and supplements have not been thoroughly tested for interactions with other herbs, supplements, drugs, or foods. The interactions listed below are based on reports in scientific publications, laboratory experiments, or traditional use. It is important to always read product labels. People who have a medical condition, or are taking other drugs, herbs, or supplements, should consult a qualified healthcare provider before starting a new therapy.

Interactions with Drugs

- Belladonna may slow the movement of food and medication through the gut, and therefore may retard the absorption of other medications. Many prescribed medications can interact with anticholinergic drugs that have similar effects to those of belladonna. Examples are acetophenazine, amantadine, amitriptyline, atropine, benztropine, bethanechol, biperiden, brompheniramine, carbinoxamine, chlorpromazine, clemastine, clozapine, cyclopentolate, cyproheptadine, dicyclomine, diphenhydramine, dixyrazine, ethopropazine, fenotherol, fluphenazine, haloperidol, homatropine, hyoscyamine, ipratropium, loxapine, mesoridazine, methdilazine, methotrimeprazine, olanzapine, oxybutynin, perazine, periciazine, perphenazine, pimozide, pipotiazine, prochlorperazine, procyclidine, promazine, promethazine, propiomazine, quinidine, scopolamine, thiethylperazine, thioridazine, thiothixene, trifluoperazine, triflupromazine, trihexyphenidyl, trimeprazine, and triprolidine.

- Atropine is an ingredient in belladonna, and theoretically, drugs that interact with atropine may also interact with belladonna. Examples are ambenonium, arbutamine, cisapride, cromolyn, halothane, methacholine, and procainamide. Some antidepressant medications (tricyclic drugs) can interact with belladonna. The effects of the drug cisapride, used to increase the movement of food through the stomach, may be blocked. Medications that can increase heart rate, especially procainamide, can cause an exaggerated increase in heart rate if given with belladonna. The use of alcohol with belladonna can cause extreme slowing of brain function. Some of the effects that belladonna has on the brain may be treatable with the prescription drug tacrine (Cognex).

Interactions with Herbs and Dietary Supplements

- Belladonna may slow the movement of food and medication through the gut, and therefore some supplements may be absorbed more slowly. The use of belladonna with supplements that have anticholinergic activity may increase its desired effects and worsen its side effects. Examples of anticholinergic herbs are bittersweet (*Solanum dulcamara*), henbane (*Hyoscyamus niger*), and Jimson weed (*Datura stramonium*).

Selected References

Natural Standard developed the preceding evidence-based information based on a systematic review of more than 150 scientific articles. For comprehensive information about alternative and complementary therapies on the professional level, go to www.naturalstandard.com. Selected references are listed below.

Balzarini A, Felisi E, Martini A, et al. Efficacy of homeopathic treatment of skin reactions during radiotherapy for breast cancer: a randomised, double-blind clinical trial. Br Homeopath J 2000;89(1):8-12.

Bergmans M, Merkus J, Corbey R, et al. Effect of Bellergal Retard on climacteric complaints: a double-blind, placebo-controlled study. Maturitas 1987;9:227-234.

Bettermann H, Cysarz D, Portsteffen A, et al. Bimodal dose-dependent effect on autonomic, cardiac control after oral administration of *Atropa belladonna*. Auton Neurosci 2001; 90(1-2):132-137.

Ceha LJ, Presperin C, Young E, et al. Anticholinergic toxicity from nightshade berry poisoning responsive to physostigmine. J Emerg Med 1997;15(1):65-69.

Duncan G, Collison DJ. Role of the non-neuronal cholinergic system in the eye: a review. Life Sci 2003;72(18-19):2013-2019.

Friese KH, Kruse S, Ludtke R, et al. The homeopathic treatment of otitis media in children: comparisons with conventional therapy. Int J Clin Pharm Ther 1997;35(7):296-301.

Jellema K, Groeneveld GJ, van Gijn J. [Fever, large eyes and confusion; the anticholinergic syndrome.] Ned Tijdschr Geneeskd 2002:146(46):2173-2176.

Kahn A., Rebuffat E, Sottiaux M, et al. Prevention of airway obstructions during sleep in infants with breath-holding spells by means of oral belladonna: a prospective double-blind crossover evaluation. Sleep 1991;14(5):432-438.

King JC. Anisotropine methylbromide for relief of gastrointestinal spasm: double-blind crossover comparison study with belladonna alkaloids and phenobarbital. Curr Ther Res Clin Exp 1966;8(11):535-541.

Lichstein J, Mayer JD. Drug therapy in the unstable bowel (irritable colon). A 15-month double-blind clinical study in 75 cases of response to a prolonged-acting belladonna alkaloid-phenobarbital mixture or placebo. J Chron Dis 1959;9(4):394-404.

Rhodes JB, Abrams JH, Manning RT. Controlled clinical trial of sedative-anticholinergic drugs in patients with the irritable bowel syndrome. J Clin Pharmacol 1978;18(7):340-345.

Ritchie JA, Truelove SC. Treatment of irritable bowel syndrome with lorazepam, hyoscine butylbromide, and ispaghula husk. Br Med J 1979;1(6160):376-378.

Robinson K, Huntington KM, Wallace MG. Treatment of the premenstrual syndrome. Br J Obstet Gynaecol 1977;84(10):784-788.

Shanafelt TD, Barton DL, Adjei AA, et al. Pathophysiology and treatment of hot flashes. Mayo Clin Proc 2002;77(11):1207-1218.

Stieg RL. Double-blind study of belladonna-ergotamine-phenobarbital for interval treatment of recurrent throbbing headache. Headache 1977;17(3):120-124.

Walach H, Koster H, Hennig T, et al. The effects of homeopathic belladonna 30CH in healthy volunteers: a randomized, double-blind experiment. J Psychosom Res 2001;50(3):155-160.

Whitmarsh TE, Coleston-Shields DM, Steiner TJ. Double-blind randomized placebo-controlled study of homeopathic prophylaxis of migraine. Cephalalgia 1997;17(5):600-604.

Betel Nut

(*Areca catechu* L.)

B

RELATED TERMS

- Amaska, areca nut, arecoline, arequier, betal, betelnusspalme, betel quid, chavica etal, gutkha, hmarg, maag, marg, mava, mawa, pan, paan, Palmaceae, pan masala, pan parag, pinang, pinlang, *Piper betel* Linn. (leaf of vine used to wrap betel nuts), L. pugua, quid, Sting (Tantric Corporation), supai, ugam.

BACKGROUND

- Betel nut use refers to a combination of three ingredients: the nut of the betel palm (*Areca catechu*), part of the *Piper betel* vine (the leaf of which is used to wrap betel nuts), and lime. Anecdotal reports have indicated that small doses generally lead to euphoria and increased flow of energy, whereas large doses often result in sedation. Although all three ingredients may contribute to these effects, most experts attribute the psychoactive effects to the alkaloids found in betel nuts.
- Betel nut is reportedly used by a substantial portion of the world's population as a recreational drug because of its central nervous system stimulant activity. Found originally in tropical southern Asia, betel nut has been introduced to the communities of east Africa, Madagascar, and the West Indies. There is little evidence from adequately controlled studies to support clinical use of betel, but its constituents have demonstrated pharmacologic actions. The main active component, the alkaloid arecoline, has potent cholinergic activity.
- Constituents of *Areca* are potentially carcinogenic. Long-term use has been associated with oral submucous fibrosis (OSF), pre-cancerous oral lesions, and squamous cell carcinoma. Acute effects of betel chewing include asthma exacerbation, hypotension, and tachycardia.

USES BASED ON SCIENTIFIC EVIDENCE	Grade*
Anemia Preliminary poor-quality research studies report that betel nut chewing may lessen anemia in pregnant women. The reasons for this finding are not clear, and betel nut use may be unsafe during pregnancy.	C
Dental cavities In the past, toothpaste that contained betel nut was believed to offer protection against tooth decay and strengthen gums. Poor-quality research studies have reported fewer cavities in betel nut chewers, and laboratory studies have shown action of betel nut against some bacteria. However, betel nut chewing may actually have a harmful effect on the gums. Because of the known toxicities of betel nut and the availability of other safe and effective products for dental hygiene, the use of betel nut is not recommended.	C

Continued

Saliva stimulant Betel nut chewing may increase salivation. However, it is not clear whether this is helpful for any specific health condition. Based on the known toxicities of betel nut, the risks may outweigh any potential benefits.	C
Schizophrenia Preliminary poor-quality studies in humans suggest improvements in symptoms of schizophrenia with betel nut chewing. Effects may be due to arecoline, a chemical in betel nut that acts on the brain as a neuro-transmitter. However, side effects such as tremors and stiffness have been reported. More research is necessary before a firm conclusion can be made.	C
Stimulant Betel nut use refers to a combination of three ingredients: the nut of the betel palm (*Areca catechu*), part of the *Piper betel* vine, and lime. It is believed that small doses can lead to stimulant and euphoric effects, and betel nut chewing is popular because of these effects. Although all three ingredients may contribute to betel's stimulant properties, most experts believe that alkaloids in the betel nuts are responsible. Other substances that may be combined with betel nut chewing, such as tobacco, may also contribute to its effects. Chronic use of betel nuts may increase the risk of some cancers, and immediate effects may include asthma exacerbation, high or low blood pressure, and abnormal heart rate. Based on the known toxicities of betel nut, the risks may outweigh any potential benefits.	C
Stroke recovery Several poor-quality studies report the use of betel nut taken by mouth in patients recovering from stroke. In light of the potential toxicities of betel nut, additional evidence is needed in this area before a recommendation can be made.	C
Ulcerative colitis Currently, there is a lack of satisfactory evidence to recommend the use of betel nut for ulcerative colitis. Based on the known toxicities of betel nut, the risks may outweigh any potential benefits.	C

*Key to grades: *A:* Strong scientific evidence for this use; *B:* Good scientific evidence for this use; *C:* Unclear scientific evidence for this use; *D:* Fair scientific evidence against this use (it may not work); *F:* Strong scientific evidence against this use (it likely does not work). For a more detailed explanation of efficacy criteria, see "Natural Standard Evidence-Based Validated Grading Rationale" in the Introduction.

Uses Based on Tradition, Theory, or Limited Scientific Evidence

Alcoholism, aphrodisiac, appetite stimulant, asthma, blindness from methanol poisoning, cough, dermatitis (used on the skin), intestinal worms, digestive aid, diphtheria, diuretic, ear infection, excessive thirst, excessive menstrual flow, fainting, flatulence (gas), glaucoma, impotence, joint pain and swelling, leprosy, respiratory stimulant, toothache, veterinary use (intestinal worms).

DOSING

The following doses are based on scientific research, publications, traditional use, or expert opinion. Many herbs and supplements have not been thoroughly tested, and their safety and effectiveness may not be proven. Brands may be made differently, with variable ingredients even within the same brand. The doses shown may not apply to all products. It is important to always read product labels and discuss doses with a qualified healthcare provider before therapy is started.

Adults (18 Years and Older)

- **Oral (by mouth):** Betel nut can be chewed alone but is often chewed in combination with other ingredients (called a "quid") such as calcium hydroxide, water, catechu gum, cardamom, cloves, anise seeds, cinnamon, tobacco, nutmeg, and gold or silver metal. The combined ingredients may be wrapped in a betel leaf, which is then placed in the side of the mouth. It has been reported that ingestion of 8 to 30 g of *Areca* (betel nut) may be deadly.

Children (Younger Than 18 Years)

- Betel nut is not recommended in children because of the risks associated with its use, including worsening symptoms of asthma, adverse effects on the heart, and cancer.

SAFETY

The U.S. Food and Drug Administration does not strictly regulate herbs and supplements. There is no guarantee of the strength, purity or safety of products, and effects may vary. It is important to always read product labels. People who have a medical condition, or are taking other drugs, herbs, or supplements, should consult a qualified healthcare provider before starting a new therapy. A healthcare provider should be contacted immediately about any side effects.

Allergies

- Breathing problems with betel nut use have been reported, although no allergic reactions are noted in the available scientific literature. Caution is warranted in people with allergies to other members of the Palmaceae family.

Side Effects and Warnings

- Betel nut cannot be considered safe for human use by mouth because of the toxic effects associated with short- and long-term chewing or eating of betel nut.
- Chemicals in betel nut and betel leaves may cause skin color changes, dilated pupils, blurred vision, wheezing and difficulty breathing, and increased breathing rate. Tremors, slow movements, and stiffness have been reported in people also taking

anti-psychotic medications. Worsening of spasmodic movements has occurred in patients with Huntington's disease. Seizure has been reported with high doses.

- "Cholinergic" toxicity symptoms of betel use include salivation, increased tearing, lack of urinary control (incontinence), sweating, diarrhea, and fever. Other potential problems are confusion, eye movement disorders, psychosis, amnesia, stimulant effects, and a feeling of euphoria. Long-term users may form a dependence on betel, and discontinuing use may be accompanied by signs of withdrawal such as anxiety and memory lapse.
- Chewing betel nuts can cause nausea, vomiting, diarrhea, stomach cramps, chest pain, irregular heart beats, and abnormally high or low blood pressure. A heart attack occurred in a man immediately after chewing betel nut. It is not clear whether betel was the cause.
- Betel nut chewing has been shown to have a harmful effect on the gums. The nut may cause the teeth, mouth, lips, and stool to become red-stained. Burning and dryness of the mouth may occur.
- Studies of Asian populations have linked pre-cancerous conditions of the mouth and esophagus to betel use (oral submucous fibrosis). There is an increased risk of cancers of the liver, mouth, stomach, prostate, cervix, and lung with regular betel use.
- A chemical in betel nut lowers blood sugar levels in animals. Although studies in humans are lacking in this area, caution is advised in people with diabetes or glucose intolerance, and in those taking drugs, herbs, or supplements that affect blood sugar levels. Serum glucose levels should be monitored by a healthcare provider, and dosing adjustments may be necessary. Studies in animals reported mixed effects on thyroid function, as well as increased skin temperature. Other problems may include increased blood calcium levels and kidney disease (milk alkali syndrome), possibly caused by the calcium carbonate paste sometimes used for preparing betel nuts for chewing.
- Some betel nuts may be contaminated with harmful substances, including aflatoxin and lead.

Pregnancy and Breastfeeding

- Betel nut is not recommended during pregnancy and breastfeeding because of the risk of birth defects and spontaneous abortion.

INTERACTIONS

Most herbs and supplements have not been thoroughly tested for interactions with other herbs, supplements, drugs, or foods. The interactions listed here are based on reports in scientific publications, laboratory experiments, or traditional use. It is important to always read product labels. People who have a medical condition, or are taking other drugs, herbs, or supplements, should consult a qualified healthcare provider before starting a new therapy.

Interactions with Drugs

- The effects of anticholinergic drugs may be decreased when they are used in combination with betel nut or its constituent arecoline. Use with cholinergic drugs may cause toxicity (salivation, increased tearing, incontinence, sweating, diarrhea, vomiting, and fever). Betel nut may slow or raise the heart rate, and may alter the effects of drugs that slow the heart, such as beta-blockers, calcium channel blockers, and digoxin.

- Based on studies in animals, betel nut may lower blood sugar levels. Caution is advised when using medications that may also lower blood sugar. People who are taking drugs for diabetes by mouth or insulin should be monitored closely by a qualified healthcare provider. Dosing adjustments may be necessary.
- Based on laboratory and animal research studies, betel nut may increase the effects of monoamine oxidase inhibitors (MAOIs), angiotensin-converting enzyme (ACE) inhibitors, phenothiazines, cholesterol-lowering drugs, and stimulant drugs. Betel may increase or decrease the effects of anti-glaucoma eye drops. Reliable studies in humans are needed in these areas.

Interactions with Herbs and Dietary Supplements

- Taking betel with other cholinergic herbs may cause toxicity (salivation, tearing, urinary incontinence, sweating, diarrhea, vomiting, facial flushing. and fever) due to the chemical arecoline. Examples are American hellebore, jaborandi, lobelia, pulsatilla, and snakeroot. Betel may reduce the effects of herbs with possible anticholinergic properties, such as belladonna, henbane, hyoscyamine, and *Swertia japonica* Makino.
- Based on research studies in animals, betel may lower blood sugar levels. Caution is advised when using herbs or supplements that may also lower blood sugar. Blood glucose levels may require monitoring, and doses may need adjustment. Examples are *Aloe vera*, American ginseng, bilberry, bitter melon, burdock, fenugreek, fish oil, gymnema, horse chestnut seed extract (HCSE), maitake mushroom, marshmallow, milk thistle, *Panax ginseng*, rosemary, shark cartilage, Siberian ginseng, stinging nettle, and white horehound.
- Based on studies in animals, betel may inhibit the action of monoamine oxidase and therefore may increase the effects of herbs and supplements that have similar effects on monoamine oxidase, such as 5-hydroxytryptophan (5-HTP), California poppy, chromium, dehydroepiandrosterone (DHEA), DL phenylalanine (DLPA), ephedra, evening primrose oil, fenugreek, *Ginkgo biloba*, hops, mace, St. John's wort, *S*-adenosylmethionine (SAMe), sepia, tyrosine, valerian, vitamin B_6, and yohimbe bark extract.
- Betel nut extracts may lower blood cholesterol levels in studies of animals, and they may increase the effects of agents that lower cholesterol levels, such as fish oil, garlic, guggul, and niacin.
- The stimulant and euphoric effects of betel may add to the effects of stimulants such as caffeine, guarana, and ephedra (ma huang).
- Betel has been reported to deplete the essential vitamin thiamine. Theoretically, betel may cause neurologic disorders including Wernicke-Korsakoff syndrome (confusion, poor muscle coordination, eye movement problems, and amnesia). Simultaneous long-term use of betel and alcohol may lead to an increased risk of oral cancer.

Selected References

Natural Standard developed the preceding evidence-based information based on a systematic review of more than 200 scientific articles. For comprehensive information about alternative and complementary therapies on the professional level, go to www.naturalstandard.com. Selected references are listed here.

Deng JF, Ger J, Tsai WJ, et al. Acute toxicities of betel nut: rare but probably overlooked events. J Toxicol Clin Toxicol 2001;39(4):355-360.

Huang Z, Xiao B, Wang X, et al. Betel nut indulgence as a cause of epilepsy. Seizure. 2003;12(6):406-408.

Jeng JH, Chang MC, Hahn LJ. Role of areca nut in betel quid-associated chemical carcinogenesis: current awareness and future perspectives. Oral Oncol 2001;37(6):477-492.

Kuruppuarachchi KA, Williams SS. Betel use and schizophrenia. Br J Psychiatry 2003;182:455.

Lee CN, Jayanthi V, McDonald B, et al. Betel nut and smoking. Are they both protective in ulcerative colitis? A pilot study. Arq Gastroenterol 1996;33(1):3-5.

Mannan N, Boucher BJ, Evans SJ. Increased waist size and weight in relation to consumption of *Areca catechu* (betel-nut); a risk factor for increased glycaemia in Asians in east London. Br J Nutr 2000;83(3):267-273.

Phukan RK, Ali MS, Chetia CK, et al. Betel nut and tobacco chewing; potential risk factors of cancer of oesophagus in Assam, India. Br J Cancer 2001;85(5):661-667.

Shiu MN, Chen TH, Chang SH, et al. Risk factors for leukoplakia and malignant transformation to oral carcinoma: a leukoplakia cohort in Taiwan. Br J Cancer 2000;82(11):1871-1874.

Stoopler ET, Parisi E, Sollecito TP. Betel quid-induced oral lichen planus: a case report. Cutis 2003;71(4):307-311.

Sullivan RJ, Allen JS, Otto C, et al. Effects of chewing betel nut (Areca catechu) on the symptoms of people with schizophrenia in Palau, Micronesia. Br J Psychiatry 2000;177:174-178.

Tsai JF, Chuang LY, Jeng JE, et al. Betel quid chewing as a risk factor for hepatocellular carcinoma: a case-control study. Br J Cancer 2001;84(5):709-713.

Bilberry
(*Vaccinium myrtillus*)

RELATED TERMS

- Airelle, black whortle, bleaberry, blueberry, burren myrtle, dwarf bilberry, dyeberry, *Ericaceae,* European blueberry, heidelberry, huckleberry, hurtleberry, Myrtilli fructus, trackleberry, *Vaccinium myrtillus* anthocyanoside (VMA) extract, VME, whortleberry, wineberry.

BACKGROUND

- Bilberry, a close relative of blueberry, has a long history of medicinal use. The dried fruit has been popular for the symptomatic treatment of diarrhea, topical relief of minor mucous membrane inflammation, and various eye disorders, including poor night vision, eyestrain, and myopia.
- Bilberry fruit and its extracts contain a number of biologically active components, including a class of compounds called anthocyanosides. These have been the focus of recent research in Europe.
- Bilberry extract has been evaluated for efficacy as an antioxidant, mucostimulant, hypoglycemic, anti-inflammatory, vasoprotectant, and lipid-lowering agent. Although pre-clinical studies have been promising, human data are limited and largely of poor quality. At this time, there is insufficient evidence in support of (or against) the use of bilberry for most indications. Notably, the evidence suggests a lack of benefit of bilberry for the improvement of night vision.
- Bilberries are commonly used to make jams, pies, cobblers, syrups, and alcoholic and non-alcoholic beverages. Fruit extracts are used as a coloring agent in wines.

USES BASED ON SCIENTIFIC EVIDENCE	Grade*
Atherosclerosis, peripheral vascular disease Bilberry has sometimes been used traditionally to treat heart disease and atherosclerosis ("hardening of the arteries"). There has been some laboratory research in this area, but there is no clear information about the use of bilberry for this purpose in humans.	C
Cataracts Bilberry extract has been used for a number of eye problems, including the prevention of cataract worsening. At this time, there is limited scientific information in this area.	C
Chronic venous insufficiency Chronic venous insufficiency, a condition more commonly diagnosed in Europe than in the United States, may include leg swelling, varicose	C

Continued

veins, leg pain, itching, and skin ulcers. A standardized extract of bilberry called *Vaccinium myrtillus* anthocyanoside (VMA) is popular in Europe for the treatment of chronic venous insufficiency. However, there is only preliminary research in this area, and more studies are needed before a recommendation can be made.	
Diabetes mellitus Bilberry has been used traditionally in the treatment of diabetes, and animal research suggests that bilberry leaf extract can lower blood sugar levels. Studies in humans are needed in this area before a recommendation can be made.	**C**
Diarrhea Bilberry is used traditionally to treat diarrhea, but there are no reliable research data in this area.	**C**
Fibrocystic breast disease Limited research studies suggest a possible benefit of bilberry in the treatment of fibrocystic breast disease. More research is needed before a recommendation can be made.	**C**
Painful menstruation (dysmenorrhea) Preliminary evidence suggests that bilberry may be helpful for relief of menstrual pain, although more research is necessary before a firm conclusion can be drawn.	**C**
Retinopathy Based on animal research and several small studies in humans, bilberry may be useful in the treatment of retinopathy in patients with diabetes or high blood pressure. However, this research is limited, and it is still unclear whether bilberry is beneficial for this condition.	**C**
Stomach ulcers (peptic ulcer disease) Bilberry extract has been suggested as a treatment for stomach ulcers. There is some support for this use from studies in animals, but there is no reliable human evidence from research in humans.	**C**
Night vision Traditional use and several unclear studies from the 1960s and 1970s suggest beneficial effects of bilberry on night vision. However, more recent, better-designed studies reported no benefits. Based on this evidence, it does not appear that bilberry is helpful for improving night vision.	**D**

*Key to grades: *A:* Strong scientific evidence for this use; *B:* Good scientific evidence for this use; *C:* Unclear scientific evidence for this use; *D:* Fair scientific evidence against this use (it may not work); *F:* Strong scientific evidence against this use (it likely does not work). For a more detailed explanation of efficacy criteria, see "Natural Standard Evidence-Based Validated Grading Rationale" in the Introduction.

Uses Based on Tradition, Theory, or Limited Scientific Evidence

Angina, angiogenesis, antioxidant, arthritis, bleeding gums, cancer, cardiovascular disease, chemoprotectant, common cold, cough, dermatitis, dysentery, eye disorders, fevers, glaucoma, gout, heart disease, hemorrhoids, high blood pressure, high cholesterol, kidney disease, leukemia, liver disease, oral ulcers, pharyngitis, poor circulation, prevention/stopping of lactation (breast milk flow), retinitis pigmentosa, scurvy, skin infections, stomach upset, urine blood, urinary tract infection, vision improvement.

DOSING

The following doses are based on scientific research, publications, traditional use, or expert opinion. Many herbs and supplements have not been thoroughly tested, and their safety and effectiveness may not be proven. Brands may be made differently, with variable ingredients even within the same brand. The doses shown may not apply to all products. It is important to always read product labels and discuss doses with a qualified healthcare provider before therapy is started.

Standardization

- Standardization involves measuring the amounts of certain chemicals in products to try to make different preparations similar to each other. It is not always known if the chemicals being measured are the "active" ingredients. A component from bilberry extract called VMA (*Vaccinium myrtillus* anthocyanoside) is standardized to contain 25% anthocyanidin and has been used in many European studies. However, the strength and dosing of preparations available in the United States may differ from those used in European studies.

Adults (18 Years and Older)

- **General use:** Oral doses recommended by some experts based on traditional use include 55 to 115 g of fresh berries three times daily, or 80 to 160 mg of aqueous extract three times daily (standardized to 25% anthocyanosides).
- **Circulatory and eye use:** Oral doses of VMA extract ranging from 80 to 480 mg daily in 2 to 3 divided doses by mouth have been used in studies. A common dose is 80 mg of extract twice daily (standardized to contain 25% anthocyanidin).
- **Diarrhea:** Dried fruit, 4 to 8 g, taken with water two times per day has been used traditionally or a decoction of dried fruit (made by boiling 5 to 10 g of crushed dried fruit in 150 ml of water for 10 minutes and straining while hot), taken by mouth three times per day, or a cold macerate of dried fruit (made by soaking dried crushed fruit in 150 ml of water for several hours), taken by mouth three times per day. Experts advise people to use dried bilberry preparations, because the fresh fruit may actually worsen diarrhea.
- **Painful menstruation (dysmenorrhea):** There is limited research using 160 mg of bilberry VMA extract taken by mouth twice daily for 8 days, beginning 3 days before the start of the menstrual period.
- **Peptic ulcer disease:** Half a cup of fresh bilberries or 20 to 40 mg of standardized anthocyanidin extract three times per day by mouth has been used.
- **Mucous membrane swelling:** Some experts recommend using a mouthwash gargle of 10% dried fruit decoction as needed.

Children (Younger Than 18 Years)

- There is not enough scientific evidence to recommend the use of bilberry in children.

SAFETY

The U.S. Food and Drug Administration does not strictly regulate herbs and supplements. There is no guarantee of the strength, purity, or safety of products, and effects may vary. It is important to always read product labels. People who have a medical condition, or are taking other drugs, herbs, or supplements, should consult a qualified healthcare provider before starting a new therapy. A healthcare provider should be contacted immediately about any side effects.

Allergies

- People with allergies to plants of the *Ericaceae* family or to anthocyanosides may have reactions to bilberry. However, there are no available reliable published cases of serious allergic reactions to bilberry.

Side Effects and Warnings

- Bilberry is generally believed to be safe in recommended doses for short periods of time, based on its history as a foodstuff. There are no known reports of serious toxicity or side effects, although if bilberry is taken in large doses, there is an increased risk of bleeding, upset stomach, and hydroquinone poisoning.
- Based on human use, fresh bilberry fruit may cause diarrhea or have a laxative effect. Based on animal studies bilberry may lower blood sugar levels. Caution is therefore advised in people with diabetes or hypoglycemia, and in those taking drugs, herbs, or supplements that affect blood sugar levels. Serum glucose levels may need to be monitored by a healthcare provider, and medication adjustments may be necessary. In theory, bilberry may decrease blood pressure. In theory, there is an increased risk of bleeding with the use of bilberry leaf extract, although there are no reliable published human reports of bleeding available. Caution is advised in people who have bleeding disorders or are taking drugs that may increase the risk of bleeding before some surgeries and dental procedures.

Pregnancy and Breastfeeding

- There is not enough scientific evidence to recommend the use of bilberry during pregnancy or when breastfeeding, although eating bilberry fruit is believed to be safe based on its history of use as a foodstuff. One study used bilberry extract to treat pregnancy-induced leg swelling (edema), and no adverse effects were reported.

INTERACTIONS

Most herbs and supplements have not been thoroughly tested for interactions with other herbs, supplements, drugs, or foods. The interactions listed here are based on reports in scientific publications, laboratory experiments, or traditional use. It is important to always read product labels. People who have a medical condition, or are taking other drugs, herbs, or supplements, should consult a qualified healthcare provider before starting a new therapy.

Interactions with Drugs

- Based on animal research, bilberry may lower blood sugar levels. There are no reliable human studies in this area. Caution is advised when using medications that may also lower blood sugar. People taking drugs for diabetes by mouth or insulin should be monitored closely by a qualified healthcare provider. Medication adjustments may be necessary.

- Based on human use, bilberry may increase diarrhea when taken with drugs that cause or worsen diarrhea, such as laxatives and some antibiotics. Bilberry theoretically may increase the risk of bleeding when taken with drugs that also increase the risk of bleeding. Examples are aspirin, anticoagulants ("blood thinners") such as warfarin (Coumadin) and heparin, anti-platelet drugs such as clopidogrel (Plavix), and nonsteroidal anti-inflammatory drugs such as ibuprofen (Motrin, Advil) and naproxen (Naprosyn, Aleve). There are no reliable published human reports of bleeding with the use of bilberry. Theoretically, bilberry may further lower blood pressure when taken with drugs that decrease blood pressure.

Interactions with Herbs and Dietary Supplements

- Based on animal research, bilberry may lower blood sugar levels. Although there are no reliable studies of humans available in this area, caution is advised when using herbs or supplements that may also lower blood sugar. Examples are *Aloe vera*, American ginseng, bitter melon, burdock, fenugreek, fish oil, gymnema, horse chestnut seed extract (HCSE), marshmallow, milk thistle, *Panax ginseng*, rosemary, Siberian ginseng, stinging nettle, and white horehound. Blood glucose levels may require monitoring, and doses may need adjustment.
- In theory, bilberry may further lower blood pressure when taken with herbs or supplements that decrease blood pressure. Herbs that may have this effect include aconite/monkshood, arnica, baneberry, betel nut, black cohosh, bryony, calendula, California poppy, coleus, curcumin, eucalyptol, eucalyptus oil, ginger, goldenseal, green hellebore, hawthorn, Indian tobacco, jaborandi, mistletoe, night-blooming cereus, oleander, pasque flower, periwinkle, pleurisy root, shepherd's purse, Texas milkweed, turmeric, and wild cherry.
- Bilberry theoretically may increase the risk of bleeding when taken with herbs and supplements that are believed to also increase the risk of bleeding. Multiple cases of bleeding have been reported with the use of *Ginkgo biloba*, fewer cases with garlic, and two cases with saw palmetto. Numerous other agents may increase the risk of bleeding, although this has not been proven in most cases. Examples are alfalfa, American ginseng, angelica, anise, *Arnica montana*, asafetida, aspen bark, birch, black cohosh, bladderwrack, bogbean, boldo, borage seed oil, bromelain, capsicum, cat's claw, celery, chamomile, chaparral, clove, coleus, cordyceps, danshen, devil's claw, dong quai, evening primrose, fenugreek, feverfew, flaxseed/flax powder (not a concern with flaxseed oil), ginger, grapefruit juice, grapeseed, green tea, guggul, gymnestra, horse chestnut, horseradish, licorice root, lovage root, male fern, meadowsweet, nordihydroguaiaretic acid (NDGA), onion, papain, *Panax ginseng*, parsley, passion flower, poplar, prickly ash, propolis, quassia, red clover, reishi, Siberian ginseng, sweet clover, rue, sweet birch, sweet clover, turmeric, vitamin E, white willow, wild carrot, wild lettuce, willow, wintergreen, and yucca.
- Based on traditional use, bilberry may increase diarrhea or laxative effects when taken with herbs and supplements that are believed to also have laxative effects. Examples are alder buckthorn, aloe dried leaf sap, black root, blue flag rhizome, butternut bark, dong quai, European buckthorn, eyebright, cascara bark, castor oil, chasteberry, colocynth fruit pulp, dandelion, gamboges bark, horsetail, jalap root, manna bark, plantain leaf, podophyllum root, psyllium, rhubarb, senna, wild cucumber fruit, and yellow dock root.

- Consuming bilberry with quercetin supplements may result in additive effects, based on one small study in which bilberry consumption resulted in higher serum concentrations of quercetin.

Selected References

Natural Standard developed the preceding evidence-based information based on a systematic review of more than 130 scientific articles. For comprehensive information about alternative and complementary therapies on the professional level, go to www.naturalstandard.com. Selected references are listed here.

Bomser J, Madhavi D, Singletary K, et al. In vitro anticancer activity of fruit extracts from *Vaccinium* species. Planta Med 1996;62(3):212-216.

Erlund I, Marniemi J, Hakala P, et al. Consumption of black currants, lingonberries and bilberries increases serum quercetin concentrations. Eur J Clin Nutr. 2003;57(1):37-42.

Hou DX. Potential mechanisms of cancer chemoprevention by anthocyanins. Curr Mol Med. 2003;3(2):149-159. Review.

Katsube N, Iwashita K, Tsushida T, et al. Induction of apoptosis in cancer cells by Bilberry (*Vaccinium myrtillus*) and the anthocyanins. J Agric Food Chem 2003;51(1):68-75.

Laplaud PM, Lelubre A, Chapman MJ. Antioxidant action of *Vaccinium myrtillus* extract on human low density lipoproteins in vitro: initial observations. Fundam Clin Pharmacol 1997;11(1):35-40.

Levy Y, Glovinsky Y. The effect of anthocyanosides on night vision. Eye 1998;12 Pt 6):967-969.

Muth ER, Laurent JM, Jasper P. The effect of bilberry nutritional supplementation on night visual acuity and contrast sensitivity. Altern Med Rev 2000;5(2):164-173.

Rasetti FRM, Caruso D, Galli G, et al. Extracts of *Ginkgo biloba* L. leaves and *Vaccinium myrtillus* L. fruits prevent photo induced oxidation of low density lipoprotein cholesterol. Phytomed 1997;3:335-338.

Roy S, Khanna S, Alessio HM, et al. Anti-angiogenic property of edible berries. Free Radic Res 2002;36(9):1023-1031.

Savickiene N, Dagilyte A, Lukosius A, Zitkevicius V. [Importance of biologically active components and plants in the prevention of complications of diabetes mellitus.] Medicina (Kaunas) 2002;38(10):970-975.

Viana M, Barbas C, Bonet B, et al. In vitro effects of a flavonoid-rich extract on LDL oxidation. Atherosclerosis 1996;123(1-2):83-91.

Zadok D, Levy Y, Glovinsky Y. The effect of anthocyanosides in a multiple oral dose on night vision. Eye 1999;13(Pt 6):734-736.

Bitter Almond

(*Prunus amygdalus* Batsch var. amara [DC.] Focke)

RELATED TERMS

- Aci badem, almendra amara, amande amere, amendoa amarga, *Amygdala amara*, *Amygdalis dulcis amara*, bitter almond oil, bittere amandel, bittermandel, gorkiy mindal, karvasmanteli, keseru mandula, ku wei bian tao, ku xing ren, lawz murr, mandorla amara, *Prunus communis amara*, *Prunus dulcis* (Mill.) D.A. Webb var. *amara* (DC.) H.E. Moore, *Prunus amygdalus amara*, Rosaceae, volatile almond oil.
- *Note:* Bitter almond should not be confused with "sweet almond." Sweet almond seeds do not contain amygdalin and are edible, whereas bitter almonds can be toxic.

BACKGROUND

- The almond is closely related to the peach, apricot, and cherry (all classified as drupes). In contrast to the others, however, the outer layer of the almond is not edible. The edible portion of the almond is the seed. A compound called amygdalin differentiates the bitter almond from the sweet almond. In the presence of water (hydrolysis), amygdalin yields glucose and the chemicals benzaldehyde and hydrocyanic acid (HCN). HCN, the salts of which are known as cyanide, is poisonous. In order for almond to be used in food or as a flavoring agent, the HCN must be removed from the bitter almond oil. Once the HCN is removed, the oil is called volatile almond oil and is considered to be almost pure benzaldehyde. Volatile almond oil also can be toxic in large amounts.
- *Laetrile*, an alternative cancer drug marketed in Mexico and other countries outside the United States, is derived from amygdalin, which is present in the pits of fruits and nuts such as the bitter almond. Multiple cases of cyanide poisoning, some resulting in death, have been associated with laetrile therapy.

USES BASED ON SCIENTIFIC EVIDENCE	Grade*
Cancer (Laetrile) Multiple animal studies in animals and preliminary studies in humans suggest that laetrile is not beneficial in the treatment of cancer. In 1982, the U.S. National Cancer Institute concluded that laetrile was not effective for cancer therapy. Nonetheless, people continue to travel to Mexico and other countries to be able to use this therapy. Many cases of cyanide poisoning, some resulting in death, have been associated with laetrile therapy.	**D**

*Key to grades: *A:* Strong scientific evidence for this use; *B:* Good scientific evidence for this use; *C:* Unclear scientific evidence for this use; *D:* Fair scientific evidence against this use (it may not work); *F:* Strong scientific evidence against this use (it likely does not work). For a more detailed explanation of efficacy criteria, see "Natural Standard Evidence-Based Validated Grading Rationale" in the Introduction.

Uses Based on Tradition, Theory, or Limited Scientific Evidence

Antibacterial, anti-inflammatory, anti-itch, cough suppressant, local anesthetic, muscle relaxant, pain suppressant, sedative.

DOSING

The following doses are based on scientific research, publications, traditional use, or expert opinion. Many herbs and supplements have not been thoroughly tested, and their safety and effectiveness may not be proven. Brands may be made differently, with variable ingredients even within the same brand. The doses shown may not apply to all products. It is important to always read product labels and discuss doses with a qualified healthcare provider before therapy is started.

Standardization

- Standardization involves measuring the amounts of certain chemicals to try to make different preparations similar to each other. It is not always known if the chemicals being measured are the "active" ingredients. Hydrocyanic acid (HCN), the salts of which are known as cyanide, is present in bitter almond and is poisonous. In order for bitter almond to be used in food or as a flavoring agent, HCN must be removed from bitter almond oil. Once it is removed, the oil is called volatile almond oil. Volatile almond oil can still be toxic in large amounts.
- Mexico supplies the majority of laetrile used by U.S. citizens, and standardization has been unreliable. Laetrile samples from Mexico have been tested for strength and contamination and were found to include lower concentrations of the compound than the labeled amount, and to be contaminated with other chemicals.

Adults (18 Years and Older)

- Because of its potential toxicity, no widely accepted standard dose has been established for bitter almond.

Children (Younger Than 18 Years)

- Because of its potential toxicity, bitter almond should be avoided in children.

SAFETY

The U.S. Food and Drug Administration does not strictly regulate herbs and supplements. There is no guarantee of the strength, purity, or safety of products, and effects may vary. It is important to always read product labels. People who have a medical condition, or are taking other drugs, herbs, or supplements, should consult a qualified healthcare provider before starting a new therapy. A healthcare provider should be contacted immediately about any side effects.

Allergies

- Allergies to almonds are common and have led to severe reactions, including throat swelling that interferes with breathing and painful swelling under the skin (angioedema). People who are allergic to other nuts should probably avoid almonds. In one case report, after 3 weeks of laetrile therapy, a patient developed redness of the skin with a spotted rash. Within 2 days after stopping laetrile and receiving treatment with cortisone, the rash subsided.

Side Effects and Warnings

- Laetrile is considered unsafe in any form because of its potential for causing cyanide toxicity. Reactions are more severe when laetrile is taken by mouth than when injected into a vein or muscle. Side effects include dilated pupils, dizziness, drooping eyelids, drowsiness, headache, increased breathing, muscle weakness, nausea, stomach pain, and vomiting. High doses of bitter almond or laetrile may lead to a slowing of brain functions or breathing. Several cases of cyanide poisoning (some fatal) have been reported.
- In one case, a woman who had been taking laetrile for 5 years developed a low white blood cell count; when she stopped taking laetrile, the condition disappeared. Another case involved a 22-year-old man who took 12 to 18 laetrile tablets at once in order to make up for missed doses, developed seizures, and was admitted to the hospital for cyanide poisoning. An "odor" that smelled like almonds was noted by the hospital staff. Life support measures and treatment for poisoning allowed the patient to fully recover. In another case, an 11-month-old girl swallowed one to five 500-mg laetrile tablets; after 30 minutes she was brought to the hospital in a coma with shock and irregular breathing. Four days later, the child died.
- Most cases of laetrile overdose have been treated with supportive care, lavage of the stomach, hydration, oxygen therapy (with respiratory assistance), and medications such as amyl nitrite, sodium nitrite, and sodium thiosulfate to decrease cyanide levels.
- Drowsiness or sedation may occur with bitter almond. Caution is advised in people who are driving or operating heavy machinery.

Pregnancy and Breastfeeding

- Bitter almond compounds are not recommended because of insufficient available data and the potential risk of birth defects. One study reported that laetrile given by mouth to pregnant hamsters caused abnormal skeleton formation in the offspring, although intravenous laetrile did not.

INTERACTIONS

Most herbs and supplements have not been thoroughly tested for interactions with other herbs, supplements, drugs, or foods. The interactions listed here are based on reports in scientific publications, laboratory experiments, or traditional use. It is important to always read product labels. People who have a medical condition, or are taking other drugs, herbs, or supplements, should consult a qualified healthcare provider before starting a new therapy.

Interactions with Drugs

- In theory, bitter almond may increase the amount of drowsiness caused by some drugs. Examples are benzodiazepines such as lorazepam (Ativan) and diazepam (Valium), barbiturates such as phenobarbital, narcotics such as codeine, some antidepressants, and alcohol. Caution is advised while driving or operating machinery. Avoid the use of alcohol, since almond oil was shown in mice to cause a toxic reaction (nausea, vomiting, increased breathing, sweating) when taken with alcohol.

Interactions with Herbs and Dietary Supplements

- In theory, bitter almond may increase the amount of drowsiness caused by some herbs or supplements. Examples are calamus, calendula, California poppy, capsicum, catnip, celery, couch grass, dogwood, elecampane, German chamomile, goldenseal, gotu kola, hops, kava (may help sleep without drowsiness), lavender aromatherapy, lemon balm, sage, sassafras, skullcap, shepherd's purse, Siberian ginseng, St. John's wort, stinging nettle, valerian, wild carrot, wild lettuce, withania root, and yerba mansa. Caution is advised in people who are driving or operating machinery.

Interactions with Foods

- There are no reliable published reports of interactions of bitter almond with food.

Selected References

Natural Standard developed the preceding evidence-based information based on a systematic review of more than 75 scientific articles. For comprehensive information about alternative and complementary therapies on the professional level, go to www.naturalstandard.com. Selected references are listed here.

Beamer WC, Shealy RM, Prough DS. Acute cyanide poisoning from laetrile ingestion. Ann Emerg Med 1983;12(7):449-451.

Liegner KB, Beck EM, Rosenberg A. Laetrile-induced agranulocytosis. JAMA 1981;246(24): 2841-2842.

Moertel CG, Fleming TR, Rubin J, et al. A clinical trial of amygdalin (Laetrile) in the treatment of human cancer. N Engl J Med 1982;306(4):201-206.

Shragg TA, Albertson TE, Fisher CJ Jr. Cyanide poisoning after bitter almond ingestion. West J Med 1982;136(1):65-69.

Willhite CC. Congenital malformations induced by laetrile. Science 1982;215(4539): 1513-1515.

Black Cohosh
(*Cimicifuga racemosa* [L.] Nutt.)

B

RELATED TERMS

- *Actaea macrotys, Actaea racemosa* L., actee a grappes, Amerikanisches Wanzenkraut, baneberry, black snakeroot, botrophis serpentaria, bugwort, cohosh bugbane, Cimicifuga, *Cimicifugae racemosae* rhizoma, cimicifugawurzelstock, herbe au punaise, macrotys, Macrotys actaeoides, Ranunculaceae, rattle root, rattle snakeroot, rattle top, rattle weed, richweed, schwarze schlangenwurzel, solvlys, squaw root, *Thalictrodes racemosa*, traubensilberkerze, wanzwenkraut.
- *Note:* Do not confuse black cohosh with blue cohosh (*Caulophyllum thalictroides*), which contains chemicals that may damage the heart and raise blood pressure. Do not confuse black cohosh (*Cimicifuga racemosa*) with *Cimicifuga foetida*, bugbane, fairy candles, or sheng ma; these are species from the same family (Ranunculaceae) with different effects.

BACKGROUND

- Black cohosh is popular as an alternative to hormonal therapy in the treatment of menopausal (climacteric) symptoms such as hot flashes, mood disturbances, diaphoresis, palpitations, and vaginal dryness. Several controlled trials and case series have reported that black cohosh improved menopausal symptoms for up to 6 months. Although these initial studies are suggestive, they have been few in number and have universally suffered from methodological weaknesses.
- The mechanism of action of black cohosh remains unclear, and the effects (if any) on estrogen receptors and hormonal levels have not been fully elucidated. Recent publications suggest that there may be no direct effects on estrogen receptors, although this is an area of active controversy. Safety and efficacy data beyond 6 months are not available, although recent reports suggest safety of short-term use, including in women experiencing menopausal symptoms for whom estrogen replacement therapy is contraindicated. Nonetheless, because of the lack of long-term follow-up, caution is advised until better-quality safety data are available. Use of black cohosh in high-risk populations (such as in women with a history of breast cancer) should be under the supervision of a licensed healthcare professional.

USES BASED ON SCIENTIFIC EVIDENCE	Grade*
Menopausal symptoms Black cohosh is a popular alternative to prescription hormonal therapy for treatment of menopausal symptoms such as hot flashes, mood problems, perspiration, heart palpitations, and vaginal dryness. Initial research in humans suggests that black cohosh may improve some of these symptoms for up to 6 months. However, most studies were not well designed and results were inconclusive. Most research has used	B

Continued

a specially designed questionnaire to measure menopausal symptoms that does not consider some of the important symptoms of menopause, such as vaginal dryness, but does measure other symptoms which are not commonly associated with menopause, such as tingling sensations and dizziness. Well-designed studies using black cohosh for longer than 6 months are needed.	
Joint pain There is not enough human research to make a clear recommendation about the use of black cohosh for painful joints in rheumatoid arthritis or osteoarthritis.	**C**

*Key to grades: *A:* Strong scientific evidence for this use; *B:* Good scientific evidence for this use; *C:* Unclear scientific evidence for this use; *D:* Fair scientific evidence against this use (it may not work); *F:* Strong scientific evidence against this use (it likely does not work). For a more detailed explanation of efficacy criteria, see "Natural Standard Evidence-Based Validated Grading Rationale" in the Introduction.

Uses Based on Tradition, Theory, or Limited Scientific Evidence

Anti-itch, anxiety, aphrodisiac, appetite stimulant, asthma, back pain, breast disease, breast pain/inflammation (mastitis), bone diseases, bronchitis, cervical dysplasia (abnormal pap smear), childbirth (labor induction), cough remedy, decreased blood platelets, depression, diarrhea, dizziness, edema, endometriosis, fever, gallbladder disorders, headache, heart disease/palpitations, high blood pressure, infertility, inflammation, insect repellent, kidney inflammation, liver disease, malaria, menstrual period problems, miscarriage, muscle pain, muscle spasms, ovarian cysts, pancreatitis, perspiration, pertussis (whooping cough), polycystic breast disease, polycystic ovarian syndrome, premenstrual syndrome (PMS), ringing in the ears, sleep disorders, snakebites, sore throat, tamoxifen-related hot flashes, uterine diseases and bleeding, vaginal discharge, yellow fever.

DOSING

The following doses are based on scientific research, publications, traditional use, or expert opinion. Many herbs and supplements have not been thoroughly tested, and their safety and effectiveness may not be proven. Brands may be made differently, with variable ingredients even within the same brand. The doses shown may not apply to all products. It is important to always read product labels and discuss doses with a qualified healthcare provider before therapy is started.

Standardization

- Standardization involves measuring the amounts of certain chemicals in products to try to make different preparations similar to each other. It is not always known if the chemicals being measured are the "active" ingredients. The dose of black cohosh is often based on the amount of the chemical 27-deoxyactein. The German product Remifemin, used in most studies in humans, contains an alcoholic extract of black cohosh standardized to contain 1 mg of 27-deoxyactein in each 20-mg tablet. The manufacturing process and dosing recommendations for Remifemin have changed over the past 20 years, and doses used in different studies are not always the same. A standardized liquid formulation of Remifemin has also been used in some studies.

Adults (18 Years and Older)

- **Tablets:** For menopausal symptoms, some studies have used 20 mg or 40 mg of Remifemin tablets (containing 1 or 2 mg of 27-deoxyactein) twice daily or 40 drops of a liquid extract. Other clinical studies have used 20 mg taken twice daily.
- **Dried rhizome (root):** The British Herbal Compendium recommends 40 to 200 mg of dried rhizome daily in divided doses, although traditional doses have been as high as 1 g taken three times daily.
- **Tincture/liquid:** The British Herbal Compendium recommends 0.4 to 2 ml of a (1:10) 60% ethanol tincture daily.

Children (Younger Than 18 Years)

- There is not enough scientific information to recommend black cohosh in children.

SAFETY

The U.S. Food and Drug Administration does not strictly regulate herbs and supplements. There is no guarantee of the strength, purity, or safety of products, and effects may vary. It is important to always read product labels. People who have a medical condition, or are taking other drugs, herbs, or supplements, should consult a qualified healthcare provider before starting a new therapy. A healthcare provider should be contacted immediately about any side effects.

Allergies

- People who are allergic to other members of the Ranunculaceae (buttercup or crowfoot) family should avoid black cohosh products. In nature, black cohosh contains small amounts of salicylic acid (which is found in aspirin), but it is not clear how much (if any) is present in commercially available products. Black cohosh should be used cautiously in people allergic to aspirin or other salicylates.

Side Effects and Warnings

- Black cohosh is generally well tolerated in recommended doses and has been studied in trials as long as 6 months. High doses of black cohosh may cause frontal headache, dizziness, perspiration, or visual disturbances. Several side effects have been noted in studies, including constipation, intestinal discomfort, loss of bone mass (leading to osteoporosis), irregular or slow heart beat, low blood pressure, and nausea and vomiting.
- It is not clear whether black cohosh is safe in persons with hormone-sensitive conditions such as breast cancer, uterine cancer, and endometriosis. There is controversy as to whether black cohosh is similar to estrogen in its mechanism, although recent studies suggest that this may not be true. The influence of black cohosh on anti-estrogen drugs (e.g., tamoxifen) and hormone replacement therapy is unclear. It is not known if black cohosh possesses the beneficial effects that estrogen is believed to have on bone mass, or the potential harmful effects, such as increased risk of stroke or hormone-sensitive cancers.
- Australian cases of hepatitis (liver damage) in persons who used combination herbal products containing black cohosh; liver transplantation for severe liver failure was

necessary in two of these patients. These case reports have been criticized as being inadequately substantiated. Nonetheless, persons with liver disease should consult a licensed healthcare professional before using black cohosh.

- Black cohosh should be used cautiously in persons with a history of blood clots or stroke, seizure disorder, high blood pressure requiring medication, known allergy to aspirin/salicylates, liver disease, or hormone-sensitive cancers.

Pregnancy and Breastfeeding

- Safety during pregnancy and breastfeeding has not been established. Black cohosh may relax the muscular wall of the uterus, and some nurse-midwives in the United States use black cohosh to stimulate labor. There has been one report of severe multi-organ damage in an infant delivered with the aid of both black cohosh and blue cohosh (*Caulophyllum thalictroides*), who was not breathing at the time of birth. The child survived but had permanent brain damage. Blue cohosh is known to have effects on the heart and blood vessels and may have been responsible for these effects.
- Tinctures are not recommended during pregnancy because of potentially high alcohol content.

INTERACTIONS

Most herbs and supplements have not been thoroughly tested for interactions with other herbs, supplements, drugs, or foods. The interactions listed here are based on reports in scientific publications, laboratory experiments, or traditional use. It is important to always read product labels. People who have a medical condition, or are taking other drugs, herbs, or supplements, should consult a qualified healthcare provider before starting a new therapy.

Interactions with Drugs

- The potential estrogen-like effects of black cohosh continue to be debated, and the active chemical contents of black cohosh have not been clearly identified. Although recent studies suggest no significant effects of black cohosh on estrogen receptors in the body, caution is warranted in people taking both black cohosh and estrogens. The influence of black cohosh in combination with tamoxifen is unclear, and it is not known if tamoxifen counteracts the effects of black cohosh. One trial suggests that black cohosh may not be useful in the short-term treatment of tamoxifen-related hot flashes, although further study is needed in this area.
- Black cohosh may lower blood pressure, and therefore should be used cautiously with other hypotensive agents, including beta-blockers such as metoprolol (Lopressor, Toprol) and propranolol (Inderal) and calcium-channel blockers such as diltiazem (Cardizem, Tiazac) and verapamil (Isoptin, Calan). Black cohosh may contain small amounts of salicylic acid, and may increase the anti-platelet effects of other agents such as aspirin.
- In theory, because of the possible alcohol content in some tinctures of black cohosh, combination with disulfiram (Antabuse) or metronidazole (Flagyl) may cause nausea and vomiting.

Interactions with Herbs and Dietary Supplements

- Black cohosh should be used cautiously in people taking herbs with possible estrogen-like effects, such as alfalfa, bloodroot, burdock, hops, kudzu, licorice, pomegranate, red clover, soy, thyme, white horehound, and yucca. Information in this area is limited. In nature, black cohosh contains small amounts of salicylic acid, and may increase the anti-platelet effects of agents such as aspen bark, birch, poplar, willow bark, and wintergreen. This is a theoretical concern, and it is not clear if the amounts of salicylates present in commercial or processed black cohosh products have significant effects in humans.

- In one study, seizures were reported in a woman taking a combination of black cohosh, chaste tree (berries and seeds), and evening primrose oil for 4 months, while also consuming alcohol. The cause of the seizures was unclear.
- Both black cohosh and blue cohosh (*Caulophyllum thalictroides*) are used by nurse-midwives in the United States to assist birth. There was one report of severe multi-organ damage in an infant delivered with the aid of both black cohosh and blue cohosh, who was not breathing at the time of birth. The child survived with permanent brain damage. Blue cohosh is known to have effects on the heart and blood vessels and may have been responsible for these effects. Pennyroyal and black cohosh should not be used together because of the possibility of increased toxicity and death.
- Black cohosh may lower blood pressure. Other herbs that may lower blood pressure include aconite/monkshood, arnica, baneberry, betel nut, bilberry, bryony, calendula, California poppy, coleus, curcumin, eucalyptol, eucalyptus oil, flax/flaxseed oil, garlic, ginger, ginkgo, goldenseal, green hellebore, hawthorn, Indian tobacco, jaborandi, mistletoe, night blooming cereus, oleander, pasque flower, periwinkle, pleurisy root, shepherd's purse, Texas milkweed, turmeric, and wild cherry.
- In theory, black cohosh may increase the risk of bleeding when taken with herbs and supplements that are believed to also increase the risk of bleeding. Multiple cases of bleeding have been reported with the use of *Ginkgo biloba*, fewer cases with garlic, and two cases with saw palmetto. Numerous other agents may theoretically increase the risk of bleeding, although this has not been proven in most cases. Examples are alfalfa, American ginseng, angelica, anise, *Arnica montana*, asafetida, aspen bark, bilberry, birch, bladderwrack, bogbean, boldo, borage seed oil, bromelain, capsicum, cat's claw, celery, chamomile, chaparral, clove, coleus, cordyceps, danshen, devil's claw, dong quai, evening primrose, fenugreek, feverfew, flaxseed/flax powder (not a concern with flaxseed oil), ginger, grapefruit juice, grapeseed, green tea, guggul, gymnestra, horse chestnut, horseradish, licorice root, lovage root, male fern, meadowsweet, nordihydroguaiaretic acid (NDGA), onion, papain, *Panax ginseng*, parsley, passion flower, poplar, prickly ash, propolis, quassia, red clover, reishi, rue, Siberian ginseng, rue, sweet birch, sweet clover, turmeric, vitamin E, white willow, wild carrot, wild lettuce, willow, wintergreen, and yucca.

Selected References

Natural Standard developed the preceding evidence-based information based on a systematic review of more than 100 scientific articles. For comprehensive information about alternative and complementary therapies on the professional level, go to www.naturalstandard.com. Selected references are listed here.

Anderson IB, Mullen WH, Meeker JE, et al. Pennyroyal toxicity: measurement of toxic metabolite levels in two cases and review of the literature. Ann Intern Med 1996;124(8): 726-734.

Anon. *Cimicifuga racemosa*—Monograph. Altern Med Rev 2003;8(2):186-189.

Baillie N, Rasmussen P. Black and blue cohosh in labour. N Z Med J 1997;110(1036):20-21.
Beuscher N, Reichert R. *Cimicifuga racemosa* L.—black cohosh. Zeit Phytother 1995;16: 301-310.
Boblitz N, Schrader E, Henneicke-von Zepelin HH, et al. Benefit of a fixed drug combination containing St. John's wort and black cohosh for climacteric patients—results of a randomised clinical trial (poster presentation from 6th Annual Symposium on Complementary Health Care, Exeter, England, December 2-4, 1999). Focus Alt Comp Ther (FACT) 2000;5(1): 85-86.
Bodinet C, Freudenstein J. Influence of *Cimicifuga racemosa* on the proliferation of estrogen receptor–positive human breast cancer cells. Breast Cancer Res Treat 2002;76(1):1-10.
Borrelli F, Ernst E. *Cimicifuga racemosa*: a systematic review of its clinical efficacy. Eur J Clin Pharmacol 2002;58(4):235-241.
Borrelli F, Izzo AA, Ernst E. Pharmacological effects of *Cimicifuga racemosa*. Life Sci 2003; 73(10):1215-1229.
Burdette JE, Liu J, Chen SN, et al. Black cohosh acts as a mixed competitive ligand and partial agonist of the serotonin receptor. J Agric Food Chem 2003;51(19):5661-5670.
Daiber W. Menopause symptoms: success without hormones. Arztl Praxis 1983;35:1946-1947.
Dixon-Shanies D, Shaikh N. Growth inhibition of human breast cancer cells by herbs and phytoestrogens. Oncol Rep 1999;6(6):1383-1387.
Dog TL, Powell KL, Weisman SM. Critical evaluation of the safety of *Cimicifuga racemosa* in menopause symptom relief. Menopause 2003;10(4):299-313.
Duker EM, Kopanski L, Jarry H, et al. Effects of extracts from *Cimicifuga racemosa* on gonadotropin release in menopausal women and ovariectomized rats. Planta Med 1991; 57(5):420-424.
Einer-Jensen N, Zhao J, Andersen KP, et al. *Cimicifuga* and Melbrosia lack oestrogenic effects in mice and rats. Maturitas 1996;25(2):149-153.
Freudenstein J, Bodinet C. Influence of an isopropanolic aqueous extract of *Cimicifugae racemosae* rhizoma on the proliferation of MCF-7 cells. 23rd International LOF-Symposium on Phytoestrogens, University of Ghent, Belgium (January 15, 1999).
Genazzani E, Sorrentino L. Vascular action of acteina: active constituent of *Actaea racemosa* L. Nature 1962;194(4828):544-545.
Gunn TR, Wright IM. The use of black and blue cohosh in labour. N Z Med J 1996; 109(1032):410-411.
Hailemeskel B, Lee HJ, Thomhe H. Incidence of potential herb-drug interactions among herbal users. ASHP Midyear Clinical Meeting 2000;35:p-267e.
Hemmi H, Kitame F, Ishida N, et al. Inhibition of thymidine transport into phytohemagglutinin-stimulated lymphocytes by triterpenoids from *Cimicifuga* species. J Pharm Dyn 1979;2: 339-349.
Hemmi H, Kusano G, Ishida N. Selective inhibition of nucleoside transport into mouse lymphoma L-5178Y cells by cimicfugoside. J Pharmacobiodyn 1980;3(12):636-642.
Hernandez MG, Pluchino S. *Cimicifuga racemosa* for the treatment of hot flushes in women surviving breast cancer. Maturitas 2003;44(Suppl 1):S59-S65.
Hunter A. *Cimicifuga racemosa*: pharmacology, clinical trials and clinical use. Eur J Herbal Med 1999;5(1):19-25.
Huntley A, Ernst E. A systematic review of the safety of black cohosh. Menopause 2003; 10(1):58-64.
Jacobson JS, Troxel AB, Evans J, et al. Randomized trial of black cohosh for the treatment of hot flashes among women with a history of breast cancer. J Clin Oncol 2001;19(10): 2739-2745.
Jarry H, Harnischfeger G. [Endocrine effects of constituents of *Cimicifuga racemosa*. 1. The effect on serum levels of pituitary hormones in ovariectomized rats.] Planta Med 1985;51(1):46-49.
Jarry H, Harnischfeger G, Duker E. [The endocrine effects of constituents of *Cimicifuga racemosa*. 2. In vitro binding of constituents to estrogen receptors.] Planta Med 1985; 51(4):316-319.
Jarry H, Metten M, Spengler B, et al. In vitro effects of the *Cimicifuga racemosa* extract BNO 1055. Maturitas 2003;44(Suppl 1):S31-S38.

Johnson BM, van Breemen RB. In vitro formation of quinoid metabolites of the dietary supplement *Cimicifuga racemosa* (black cohosh). Chem Res Toxicol 2003;16(7):838-846.

Kligler B. Black cohosh. Am Fam Physician 2003;68(1):114-116.

Koeda M, Aoki Y, Sakurai N, et al. Studies on the Chinese crude drug "shoma." IX. Three novel cyclolanostanol xylosides, cimicifugosides H-1, H-2 and H-5, from cimicifuga rhizome. Chem Pharm Bull (Tokyo) 1995;43(5):771-776.

Korn WD. Six month oral toxicity study with remifemin-granulate in rats followed by an 8-week recovery period. International Bioresearch, Hannover, Germany 1991;1.

Lehmann-Willenbrock E, Riedel HH. [Clinical and endocrinologic studies of the treatment of ovarian insufficiency manifestations following hysterectomy with intact adnexa.] Zentralbl Gynakol 1988;110(10):611-618.

Li W, Sun Y, Liang W, et al. Identification of caffeic acid derivatives in *Actea racemosa* (*Cimicifuga racemosa*, black cohosh) by liquid chromatography/tandem mass spectrometry. Rapid Commun Mass Spectrom 2003;17(9):978-982.

Lieberman S. A review of the effectiveness of *Cimicifuga racemosa* (black cohosh) for the symptoms of menopause. J Womens Health 1998;7(5):525-529.

Liske E. Therapeutic efficacy and safety of *Cimicifuga racemosa* for gynecologic disorders. Adv Ther 1998;15(1):45-53.

Liske E, Hanggi W, Henneicke-von Zepelin HH, et al. Physiological investigation of a unique extract of black cohosh (*Cimicifugae racemosae* rhizoma): a 6-month clinical study demonstrates no systemic estrogenic effect. J Womens Health Gend Based Med 2002;11(2):163-174.

Liske E, Wüstenberg P, Boblitz N. Human-pharmacological investigations during treatment of climacteric complaints with *Cimicifuga racemosa* (Remifemin): No estrogen-like effects. ESCOP 2001;1:1.

Liske E, Wüstenberg P. Efficacy and safety of phytomedicines with particular references to *Cimicifuga racemosa*. J Med Assoc Thai 1998;Jan:s108.

Liske E, Wüstenberg P. Therapy of climacteric complaints with Cimicifuga racemosa: herbal medicine with clinically proven evidence [poster presentation]. Menopause 1998; 5(4):250.

Liu J, Burdette JE, Xu H, et al. Evaluation of estrogenic activity of plant extracts for the potential treatment of menopausal symptoms. J Agric Food Chem 2001;49(5):2472-2479.

Liu Z, Yang Z, Zhu M, et al. [Estrogenicity of black cohosh (*Cimicifuga racemosa*) and its effect on estrogen receptor level in human breast cancer MCF-7 cells.] Wei Sheng Yan Jiu 2001; 30(2):77-80.

Lontos S, Jones RM, Angus PW, et al. Acute liver failure associated with the use of herbal preparations containing black cohosh. Med J Aust 2003;179(7):390-391.

Lupu R, Mehmi I, Atlas E, et al. Black cohosh, a menopausal remedy, does not have estrogenic activity and does not promote breast cancer cell growth. Int J Oncol 2003;23(5):1407-1412.

Mahady GB. Is black cohosh estrogenic? Nutr Rev 2003;61(5 Pt 1):183-186.

McFarlin BL, Gibson MH, O'Rear J, et al. A national survey of herbal preparation use by nurse-midwives for labor stimulation. Review of the literature and recommendations for practice. J Nurse Midwifery 1999;44(3):205-216.

McKenna DJ, Jones K, Humphrey S, et al. Black cohosh: efficacy, safety, and use in clinical and preclinical applications. Altern Ther Health Med 2001;7(3):93-100.

Mills SY, Jacoby RK, Chacksfield M, et al. Effect of a proprietary herbal medicine on the relief of chronic arthritic pain: a double-blind study. Br J Rheumatol 1996;35(9):874-878.

Nesselhut T, Schellhase C, Dietrich R, et al. [Investigations into the growth-inhibitive efficacy of phytopharmacopia with estrogen-like influences on mammary gland carcinoma cells] (translated from German). Arch Gynecol Obstet 1993;254:817-818.

Pepping J. Black cohosh: *Cimicifuga racemosa*. Am J Health Syst Pharm 1999;56(14): 1400-1402.

Popp M, Schenk R, Abel G. Cultivation of *Cimicifuga racemosa* (L.) nuttal and quality of CR extract BNO 1055. Maturitas 2003;44(Suppl 1):S1-S7.

Pritchard JB, French JE, Davis BJ, Haseman JK. The role of transgenic mouse models in carcinogen identification. Environ Health Perspect 2003;111(4):444-454

Seidlova-Wuttke D, Hesse O, Jarry H, et al. Evidence for selective estrogen receptor modulator activity in a black cohosh (*Cimicifuga racemosa*) extract: comparison with estradiol-17beta. Eur J Endocrinol 2003;149(4):351-362.

Seidlova-Wuttke D, Jarry H, Becker T, et al. Pharmacology of *Cimicifuga racemosa* extract BNO 1055 in rats: bone, fat and uterus. Maturitas 2003;44(Suppl 1):S39-S50.

Shuster J. Heparin and thrombocytopenia. Black Cohosh root? Chasteberry tree? Seizures! Hosp Pharm 1996;31:1553-1554.

Siess VM, Seybold G. [Studies on the effects of *Pulsatilla pratensis*, *Cimicifuga racemosa* and *Aristolochia clematitis* on the estrus in infantile and castrated white mice.] Arzneimittelforschung 1960;10:514-520.

Stoll W. Phytotherapeutikum beeinflusst atrophisches Vaginal epithel. Doppelblindversuch *Cimicifuga* vs. Oestrogenpraeparat [Phytopharmaceutical influences on atrophic vaginal epithelium. Double-blind study on *Cimicifuga* vs. an estrogen preparation]. Therapeutickon 1987;1:23-32.

Stolze H. [An alternative to treat menopausal complaints.] Gynecologie 1982;1:14-16.

Struck D, Tegtmeier M, Harnischfeger G. Flavones in extracts of *Cimicifuga racemosa*. Planta Med 1997;63:289-290.

Takahira M, Kusano A, Shibano M, et al. Antimalarial activity and nucleoside transport inhibitory activity of the triterpenic constituents of *Cimicifuga* spp. Biol Pharm Bull 1998;21(8):823-828.

Thomsen M, Schmidt M. Hepatotoxicity from *Cimicifuga racemosa*? Recent Australian case report not sufficiently substantiated. J Altern Complement Med 2003;9(3):337-340.

Vitetta L, Thomsen M, Sali A. Black cohosh and other herbal remedies associated with acute hepatitis. Med J Aust 2003;178(8):411-412.

Vorberg G. Treatment of menopause symptoms. ZFA (Stuttgart) 1984;60:626-629.

Warnecke G. Using phyto-treatment to influence menopause symptoms. Med Welt 1985; 36:871-874.

Whiting PW, Clouston A, Kerlin P. Black cohosh and other herbal remedies associated with acute hepatitis. Med J Aust 2002;177(8):440-443.

Zava DT, Dollbaum CM, Blen M. Estrogen and progestin bioactivity of foods, herbs, and spices. Proc Soc Exp Biol Med 1998;217(3):369-378.

Zierau O, Bodinet C, Kolba S, et al. Antiestrogenic activities of *Cimicifuga racemosa* extracts. J Steroid Biochem Mol Biol 2002;80(1):125-130.

Black Tea

(*Camellia sinensis*)

B

RELATED TERMS

- *Camellia assamica,* camellia tea, camellia, catechin, Chinese tea, tea for America, theifers, *Thea sinensis, Thea bohea, Thea viridis.*
- *Note:* Also see the chapter on green tea.

BACKGROUND

- Black tea is made from the dried leaves of *Camellia sinensis,* a perennial evergreen shrub. Black tea has a long history of use, dating back to China approximately 5000 years ago. Green tea, black tea, and oolong tea are all derived from the same plant.
- Black tea is a source of caffeine, a methylxanthine which stimulates the central nervous system, relaxes smooth muscle in the airways to the lungs (bronchioles), stimulates the heart, and acts on the kidney as a diuretic (increasing urine flow). One cup of tea contains approximately 50 mg of caffeine, depending on the strength and size of cup (compare with coffee, which contains 65 to 175 mg of caffeine per cup). Tea also contains polyphenols (catechins, anthocyanins, and phenolic acids), tannin, trace elements, and vitamins.
- The tea plant is native to Southeast Asia and can grow to a height of 40 feet but is usually maintained at a height of 2 to 3 feet by regular pruning. The first spring leaf buds, called the *first flush,* are considered the highest-quality leaves. When the first flush leaf bud is picked, another one grows, which is called the *second flush;* this sequence continues until an *autumn flush.* The older leaves picked farther down the stems are considered to be of poorer quality.
- Tea varieties reflect the growing region (e.g., Ceylon or Assam), the district (e.g., Darjeeling), the form (e.g., pekoe is cut, gunpowder is rolled), and the processing method (e.g., black, green, and oolong). India and Sri Lanka are the major producers of black tea.
- Historically, tea has been served as a part of various ceremonies, and people have used tea to stay alert during long meditations. A legend in India describes the story of Prince Siddhartha Gautama, the founder of Buddhism, who tore off his eyelids in frustration at his inability to stay awake during meditation while journeying through China. A tea plant is said to have sprouted from the spot where his eyelids fell, providing him with the ability to stay awake, meditate, and reach enlightenment.
- Turkish traders reportedly introduced tea to Western cultures in the 6th century. By the 18th century, tea was commonly consumed in England, where it became customary to drink tea at 5 o'clock in the afternoon.
- Black tea reached the Americas with the first European settlers in 1492. Black tea gained notoriety in the America in 1773 when American colonists, protesting unfair taxation, tossed a shipload of black tea overboard during what is now known as the *Boston Tea Party.*

USES BASED ON SCIENTIFIC EVIDENCE	Grade*
Asthma Research has shown that caffeine causes improvements in airflow to the lungs (bronchodilation). However, it is unclear whether caffeine or tea use has significant clinical benefits in people with asthma. Better research is needed in this area before a conclusion can be drawn.	C
Cancer prevention Several studies have explored a possible association between regular consumption of black tea and rates of cancer in populations. This research has yielded conflicting results, with some studies suggesting benefits, and others reporting no effects. Laboratory studies have shown that components of tea such as polyphenols have antioxidant properties and effects against tumors. However, effects in humans remain unclear, and these components may be more common in green tea than in black tea. Some laboratory research and studies in animals suggest that components of black tea may be carcinogenic, although effects in humans are unclear. Overall, the relationship of black tea consumption and cancer in humans remains undetermined.	C
Dental cavity prevention There are limited studies of black tea as a mouthwash for the prevention of dental cavities (caries). It is not clear if this is a beneficial therapy.	C
Heart attack prevention/cardiovascular risk There is conflicting evidence from a small number of studies examining the relationship of tea intake and the risk of heart attack Tea may reduce the risk of platelet aggregation or endothelial dysfunction and is proposed to be beneficial against blockage of arteries in the heart. The long-term effects of tea consumption on cardiovascular risk factors such as cholesterol levels, blood pressure, and atherosclerosis are unknown. One study reports that drinking black tea regularly does not alter plasma homocysteine concentrations.	C
Memory enhancement Several preliminary studies have examined the effects of caffeine, tea, or coffee use on short- and long-term memory. It remains unclear whether tea is beneficial for this use.	C
Mental performance/alertness Limited, poor-quality research studies have reported that the use of black tea may improve cognition and sense of alertness (black tea contains caffeine, which is a stimulant).	C
Methicillin-resistant *Staphylococcus aureus* (MRSA) infection In one small study, inhaled tea catechin was reported to be temporarily effective in the reduction of MRSA infection and shortening of hospital stay in elderly patients with MRSA-infected sputum. Additional research is needed to further explore these results.	C

Continued

B

Osteoporosis prevention	C
Preliminary research suggests that regular use of black tea may improve bone mineral density in older women. Better research is needed in this area before a conclusion can be drawn.	

*Key to grades: *A:* Strong scientific evidence for this use; *B:* Good scientific evidence for this use; *C:* Unclear scientific evidence for this use; *D:* Fair scientific evidence against this use (it may not work); *F:* Strong scientific evidence against this use (it likely does not work). For a more detailed explanation of efficacy criteria, see "Natural Standard Evidence-Based Validated Grading Rationale" in the Introduction.

Uses Based on Tradition, Theory, or Limited Scientific Evidence

Acute pharyngitis, antioxidant, anxiety, cancer multidrug resistance, circulatory/blood flow disorders, "cleansing" colorectal cancer, Crohn's disease, diabetes, diarrhea, diuretic (increasing urine flow), energy metabolism, gum disease, headache, hyperactivity (in children), immune enhancement/improving resistance to disease, influenza, joint pain, kidney stone prevention, melanoma, obesity, osteoarthritis, pain, prostate cancer, stomach disorders, toxin/alcohol elimination from the body, trigeminal neuralgia, vomiting, weight loss.

DOSING

The following doses are based on scientific research, publications, traditional use, or expert opinion. Many herbs and supplements have not been thoroughly tested, and their safety and effectiveness may not be proven. Brands may be made differently, with variable ingredients even within the same brand. The doses shown may not apply to all products. It is important to always read product labels and discuss doses with a qualified healthcare provider before therapy is started.

Adults (18 Years and Older)

- Black tea has not been proven as an effective therapy for any condition, and benefits of specific doses are not established. Studies of the use of tea for heart disease prevention evaluated 250 to 900 ml of tea consumed daily for up to 4 weeks. In research studies of the effect of tea on cognitive performance, an example dose is 400 ml of black tea taken three times daily. In studies of the effect of tea on dental cavity prevention, 20 ml of black tea gargled for 60 seconds daily has been used.
- One cup of tea contains approximately 50 mg of caffeine, depending on tea strength and cup size.

SAFETY

The U.S. Food and Drug Administration does not strictly regulate herbs and supplements. There is no guarantee of the strength, purity, or safety of products, and effects may vary. It is important to always read product labels. People who have a medical condition, or are taking other drugs, herbs, or supplements, should consult a qualified healthcare provider before starting a new therapy. A healthcare provider should be contacted immediately if there are any side effects.

Allergies

- People with known allergy/hypersensitivity to caffeine or tannin should avoid black tea. Skin rash and hives have been reported following caffeine ingestion.

Side Effects and Warnings

- Studies of the side effects of black tea specifically are limited. However, black tea contains caffeine, from which multiple reactions have been reported.
- Caffeine is a stimulant of the central nervous system and may cause insomnia in adults, children, and infants (including nursing infants of mothers who take caffeine). Caffeine acts on the kidneys as a diuretic (increasing urine flow and urine sodium/potassium levels and potentially decreasing blood sodium/potassium levels) and may worsen urge incontinence. Caffeine-containing beverages may increase the production of stomach acid, and may worsen ulcer symptoms. Tannin in tea can cause constipation. Caffeine in doses of 250 to 350 mg can increase heart rate and blood pressure, although people who consume caffeine regularly do not seem to experience these effects over the long term.
- An increase in blood sugar levels may occur after drinking black tea containing the equivalent of 200 mg of caffeine (4 to 5 cups, depending on tea strength and cup size). Caffeine-containing beverages such as black tea should be used cautiously in persons with diabetes. People with severe liver disease should use caffeine cautiously, as levels of caffeine in the blood may accumulate and be long-lasting. Skin rashes have been associated with caffeine ingestion. In laboratory research studies and studies in animals, caffeine has been found to affect blood clotting, but effects in humans are unknown.
- **Caffeine toxicity/high doses:** When 500 mg of caffeine are consumed (usually more than 8 to 10 cups per day, depending on tea strength and cup size), symptoms of anxiety, delirium, agitation, psychosis, and detrusor instability (unstable bladder) may occur. Conception may be delayed in women who consume large amounts of caffeine. Seizures, muscle spasms, life-threatening muscle breakdown (rhabdomyolysis), and life-threatening abnormal heart rhythms have been reported with caffeine overdose. Doses greater than 1000 mg may be fatal.
- **Caffeine withdrawal:** Chronic use can result in tolerance and psychological dependence. Abrupt discontinuation may result in withdrawal symptoms such as headache, irritation, nervousness, anxiety, tremors, and dizziness. In people with psychiatric disorders such as affective disorder and schizoaffective disorder, caffeine withdrawal may worsen symptoms or cause confusion, disorientation, excitement, restlessness, violent behavior, or mania.
- **Chronic effects:** Several population studies initially suggested a possible association between caffeine use and fibrocystic breast disease, but more recent research has not confirmed this connection. Limited research studies have reported a possible relationship between caffeine use and multiple sclerosis, although evidence is not definitive in this area. Studies in animals reported that tannin fractions from tea plants may increase the risk of cancer, although it is not clear that the tannin present in black tea has significant carcinogenic effects in humans.
- Drinking tannin-containing beverages such as tea may contribute to iron deficiency, and, in infants, tea has been associated with impaired iron metabolism and microcytic anemia.

Pregnancy and Breastfeeding

- Large amounts of black tea should be used cautiously in pregnant women, as caffeine crosses the placenta and has been associated with spontaneous abortion, intrauterine growth retardation, and low birth weight. Heavy caffeine intake (400 mg per day or greater) during pregnancy may increase the risk of later developing SIDS (sudden infant death syndrome). Very high doses of caffeine (greater than or equal to 1100 mg daily) have been associated with birth defects, including limb and palate malformations.
- Caffeine is readily transferred in breast milk. Caffeine ingestion by infants can lead to sleep disturbances/insomnia. Infants nursing from mothers consuming greater than 500 mg of caffeine daily have been reported to experience tremors and heart rhythm abnormalities. Components present in breast milk may reduce an infant's ability to metabolize caffeine, resulting in higher than expected blood levels. Tea consumption by mothers of breastfeeding infants has been associated with anemia, reductions in iron metabolism, and irritability in these infants.

INTERACTIONS

Most herbs and supplements have not been thoroughly tested for interactions with other herbs, supplements, drugs, or foods. The interactions listed here are based on reports in scientific publications, laboratory experiments, or traditional use. It is important to always read product labels. People who have a medical condition, or are taking other drugs, herbs, or supplements, should consult a qualified healthcare provider before starting a new therapy.

Interactions with Drugs

Studies of the interactions of black tea with drugs are limited. However, black tea is an important source of caffeine, from which multiple interactions have been documented.

- The combination of caffeine with ephedrine, an ephedra alkaloid, has been implicated in numerous severe and life-threatening cardiovascular events such as abnormally high blood pressure, stroke, and heart attack. This combination is commonly used in over-the-counter weight loss products and may also be associated with other adverse effects, including abnormal heart rhythms, insomnia, anxiety, headache, irritability, poor concentration, blurred vision, and dizziness. Stroke has been reported after the nasal ingestion of caffeine with amphetamine.
- Caffeine may add to the effects of other stimulants, including nicotine, beta-adrenergic agonists such as albuterol (Ventolin), and other methylxanthines such as theophylline. Caffeine can counteract drowsy effects and mental slowness caused by benzodiazepines such as lorazepam (Ativan) and diazepam (Valium). Phenylpropanolamine and caffeine should not be used together because of reports of numerous, potentially serious adverse effects; oral phenylpropanolamine formulations have been removed from the United States market because of reports of bleeding into the head.
- When taken with caffeine, a number of drugs may increase caffeine blood levels or the length of time that caffeine acts on the body. Examples are disulfiram (Antabuse), oral contraceptives, hormone replacement therapy, ciprofloxacin (Cipro), norfloxacin, fluvoxamine (Luvox), cimetidine (Tagamet), verapamil, and mexiletine. Caffeine levels may be lowered by taking dexamethasone (Decadron)

The metabolism of caffeine by the liver (cytochrome P-450 isoenzyme 1A2) may be affected by multiple drugs, although the effects in humans are not clear.

- Caffeine may lengthen the effects of carbamazepine (Tegretol) and increase the effects of clozapine (Clozaril) and dipyridamole (Persantine, Aggrenox). Caffeine may affect serum lithium levels, and abrupt discontinuation of caffeine use by regular caffeine users taking lithium may result in high levels of lithium or lithium toxicity. Levels of aspirin or phenobarbital may be lowered in the blood, although clinical effects in humans are not clear.
- Although caffeine by itself does not appear to have pain-relieving properties, it is used in combination with ergotamine tartrate in the treatment of migraine or cluster headaches (e.g., Cafergot). It has been shown to increase the headache-relieving effects of other pain relievers such as acetaminophen and aspirin (e.g., Excedrin). Caffeine may also increase the pain-relieving effects of codeine and ibuprofen (Advil, Motrin).
- As a diuretic, caffeine increases urine and sodium losses through the kidneys and may add to the effects of other diuretics such as furosemide (Lasix).

Interactions with Herbs and Dietary Supplements

- Studies of black tea interactions with herbs and supplements are limited. However, black tea is a source of caffeine, from which multiple interactions have been documented.
- Caffeine may add to the effects and side effects of other stimulants. The combination of caffeine with ephedrine, which is present in ephedra (ma huang), has been implicated in numerous severe or life-threatening cardiovascular events such as abnormally high blood pressure, stroke, and heart attack. This combination is commonly used in over-the-counter weight loss products, and may also be associated with other adverse effects, including abnormal heart rhythms, insomnia, anxiety, headache, irritability, poor concentration, blurred vision, and dizziness.
- Cola nut, guarana (*Paullina cupana*), and yerba mate (*Ilex paraguariensis*) are also sources of caffeine, and may add to the effects and side effects of caffeine in black tea. A combination product containing caffeine, yerba mate, and damania (*Turnera difussa*) has been reported to cause weight loss, slowing of gastrointestinal tract motility, and a feeling of stomach fullness.
- As a diuretic, caffeine increases urine and sodium losses through the kidneys, and may add to the effects of other diuretic agents such as artichoke, celery, corn silk, couchgrass, dandelion, elder flower, horsetail, juniper berry, kava, shepherd's purse, uva ursi, and yarrow.

Selected References

Natural Standard developed the preceding evidence-based information based on a systematic review of more than 575 articles. For comprehensive information about alternative and complementary therapies on the professional level, go to www.naturalstandard.com. Selected references are listed here.

Arab L, Il'yasova D. The epidemiology of tea consumption and colorectal cancer incidence. J Nutr 2003;133(10):3310S-3318S.

Arts IC, Hollman PC, Feskens EJ, et al. Catechin intake might explain the inverse relation between tea consumption and ischemic heart disease: the Zutphen Elderly Study. Am J Clin Nutr 2001;74(2):227-232.

Birkett NJ, Logan AG. Caffeine-containing beverages and the prevalence of hypertension. J Hypertens Suppl 1988;6(4):S620-S622.

Blot WJ, Chow WH, McLaughlin JK. Tea and cancer: a review of the epidemiological evidence. Eur J Cancer Prev 1996;5(6):425-438.

Blot WJ, McLaughlin JK, Chow WH. Cancer rates among drinkers of black tea. Crit Rev Food Sci Nutr 1997;37(8):739-760.

Brinckmann J, Sigwart H, van Houten Taylor L. Safety and efficacy of a traditional herbal medicine (Throat Coat) in symptomatic temporary relief of pain in patients with acute pharyngitis: a multicenter, prospective, randomized, double-blinded, placebo-controlled study. J Altern Complement Med 2003;9(2):285-298.

Brown CA, Bolton-Smith C, Woodward M, et al. Coffee and tea consumption and the prevalence of coronary heart disease in men and women: results from the Scottish Heart Health Study. J Epidemiol Community Health 1993;47(3):171-175.

Brown SL, Salive ME, Pahor M, et al. Occult caffeine as a source of sleep problems in an older population. J Am Geriatr Soc 1995;43(8):860-864.

Cerhan JR, Putnam SD, Bianchi GD, et al. Tea consumption and risk of cancer of the colon and rectum. Nutr Cancer 2001;41(1-2):33-40.

Chow WH, Blot WJ, McLaughlin JK. Tea drinking and cancer risk: epidemiologic evidence. Proc Soc Exp Biol Med 1999;220(4):197.

Chow WH, Swanson CA, Lissowska J, et al. Risk of stomach cancer in relation to consumption of cigarettes, alcohol, tea and coffee in Warsaw, Poland. Int J Cancer 1999;81(6):871-876.

Clausson B, Granath F, Ekbom A, et al. Effect of caffeine exposure during pregnancy on birth weight and gestational age. Am J Epidemiol 2002;155(5):429-436.

Cnattingius S, Signorello LB, Anneren G, et al. Caffeine intake and the risk of first-trimester spontaneous abortion. N Engl J Med 2000;343(25):1839-1845.

Davies MJ, Judd JT, Baer DJ, et al. Black tea consumption reduces total and LDL cholesterol in mildly hypercholesterolemic adults. J Nutr 2003;133(10):3298S-3302S.

Dlugosz L, Belanger K, Hellenbrand K, et al. Maternal caffeine consumption and spontaneous abortion: a prospective cohort study. Epidemiology 1996;7(3):250-255.

Dora I, Arab L, Martinchik A, et al. Black tea consumption and risk of rectal cancer in Moscow population. Ann Epidemiol 2003;13(6):405-411.

Duffy SJ, Keaney JF, Jr., Holbrook M, et al. Short- and long-term black tea consumption reverses endothelial dysfunction in patients with coronary artery disease. Circulation 2001; 104(2):151-156.

Esimone CO, Adikwu MU, Nwafor SV, et al. Potential use of tea extract as a complementary mouthwash: comparative evaluation of two commercial samples. J Altern Complement Med 2001;7(5):523-527.

Fernandes O, Sabharwal M, Smiley T, et al. Moderate to heavy caffeine consumption during pregnancy and relationship to spontaneous abortion and abnormal fetal growth: a meta-analysis. Reprod Toxicol 1998;12(4):435-444.

Ford RP, Schluter PJ, Mitchell EA, et al. Heavy caffeine intake in pregnancy and sudden infant death syndrome. New Zealand Cot Death Study Group. Arch Dis Child 1998;78(1):9-13.

Geleijnse JM, Launer LJ, Van der Kuip DA, et al. Inverse association of tea and flavonoid intakes with incident myocardial infarction: the Rotterdam Study. Am J Clin Nutr 2002;75(5): 880-886.

Goldbohm RA, Hertog MG, Brants HA, et al. Consumption of black tea and cancer risk: a prospective cohort study. J Natl Cancer Inst 1996;88(2):93-100.

Grosso LM, Rosenberg KD, Belanger K, et al. Maternal caffeine intake and intrauterine growth retardation. Epidemiology 2001;12(4):447-455.

Hadeed A, Siegel S. Newborn cardiac arrhythmias associated with maternal caffeine use during pregnancy. Clin Pediatr (Phila) 1993;32(1):45-47.

Hakim IA, Harris RB, Brown S, et al. Effect of increased tea consumption on oxidative DNA damage among smokers: a randomized controlled study. J Nutr 2003;133(10):3303S-3309S.

Hodgson JM, Burke V, Beilin LJ, et al. Can black tea influence plasma total homocysteine concentrations? Am J Clin Nutr 2003;77(4):907-911.

Hodgson JM, Devine A, Puddey IB, et al. Tea intake is inversely related to blood pressure in older women. J Nutr 2003;133(9):2883-2886.

Jatoi A, Ellison N, Burch PA, et al. A phase II trial of green tea in the treatment of patients with androgen independent metastatic prostate carcinoma. Cancer 2003;97(6):1442-1446.

Lambert JD, Yang CS. Mechanisms of cancer prevention by tea constituents. J Nutr 2003; 133(10):3262S-3267S.

Lambert JD, Yang CS. Cancer chemopreventive activity and bioavailability of tea and tea polyphenols. Mutat Res 2003;523-524:201-208.

Mameleers PA, Van Boxtel MP, Hogervorst E. Habitual caffeine consumption and its relation to memory, attention, planning capacity and psychomotor performance across multiple age groups. Hum Psychopharmacol 2000;15(8):573-581.

Mei Y, Wei D, Liu J. Reversal of cancer multidrug resistance by tea polyphenol in KB cells. J Chemother 2003;15(3):260-265.

Hegarty VM, May HM, Khaw KT. Tea drinking and bone mineral density in older women. Am J Clin Nutr 2000;71(4):1003-1007.

Heilbrun LK, Nomura A, Stemmermann GN. Black tea consumption and cancer risk: a prospective study. Br J Cancer 1986;54(4):677-683.

Hindmarch I, Quinlan PT, Moore KL, et al. The effects of black tea and other beverages on aspects of cognition and psychomotor performance. Psychopharmacology (Berl) 1998; 139(3):230-238.

Hodgson JM, Puddey IB, Burke V, et al. Effects on blood pressure of drinking green and black tea. J Hypertens 1999;17(4):457-463.

Infante-Rivard C, Fernandez A, Gauthier R, et al. Fetal loss associated with caffeine intake before and during pregnancy. JAMA 1993;270(24):2940-2943.

James JE. Chronic effects of habitual caffeine consumption on laboratory and ambulatory blood pressure levels. J Cardiovasc Risk 1994;1(2):159-164.

Kinlen LJ, McPherson K. Pancreas cancer and coffee and tea consumption: a case-control study. Br J Cancer 1984;49(1):93-96.

Kinlen LJ, Willows AN, Goldblatt P, et al. Tea consumption and cancer. Br J Cancer 1988; 58(3):397-401.

Klatsky AL, Armstrong MA, Friedman GD. Coffee, tea, and mortality. Ann Epidemiol 1993;3(4):375-381.

Kohlmeier L, Weterings KG, Steck S, et al. Tea and cancer prevention: an evaluation of the epidemiologic literature. Nutr Cancer 1997;27(1):1-13.

Lawson DH, Jick H, Rothman KJ. Coffee and tea consumption and breast disease. Surgery 1981;90(5):801-803.

Nakagawa K, Ninomiya M, Okubo T, et al. Tea catechin supplementation increases antioxidant capacity and prevents phospholipid hydroperoxidation in plasma of humans. J Agric Food Chem 1999;47(10):3967-3973.

Ohno Y, Wakai K, Genka K, et al. Tea consumption and lung cancer risk: a case-control study in Okinawa, Japan. Jpn J Cancer Res 1995;86(11):1027-1034.

Rechner AR, Wagner E, Van Buren L, et al. Black tea represents a major source of dietary phenolics among regular tea drinkers. Free Radic Res 2002;36(10):1127-1135.

Santos IS, Victora CG, Huttly S, et al. Caffeine intake and pregnancy outcomes: a meta-analytic review. Cad Saude Publica 1998;14(3):523-530.

Sesso HD, Gaziano JM, Buring JE, et al. Coffee and tea intake and the risk of myocardial infarction. Am J Epidemiol 1999;149(2):162-167.

Shirlow MJ, Mathers CD. A study of caffeine consumption and symptoms; indigestion, palpitations, tremor, headache and insomnia. Int J Epidemiol 1985;14(2):239-248.

Stavchansky S, Combs A, Sagraves R, et al. Pharmacokinetics of caffeine in breast milk and plasma after single oral administration of caffeine to lactating mothers. Biopharm Drug Dispos 1988;9(3):285-299.

Stoner GD, Mukhtar H. Polyphenols as cancer chemopreventive agents. J Cell Biochem Suppl 1995;22:169-180.

Wrenn KD, Oschner I. Rhabdomyolysis induced by a caffeine overdose. Ann Emerg Med 1989;18(1):94-97.

Yamada H, Ohashi K, Atsumi T, et al. Effects of tea catechin inhalation on methicillin-resistant *Staphylococcus aureus* in elderly patients in a hospital ward. Hosp Infect 2003;53(3):229-231.

Yang CS, Wang ZY. Tea and cancer. J Natl Cancer Inst 1993;85(13):1038-1049.

Bladderwrack/Seaweed/Kelp

(*Fucus vesiculosus*)

B

RELATED TERMS

- Black-tang, bladder, bladder fucus, blasen-tang, common seawrack, cut weed, Dyers fucus, Fucus, hai-ts'ao, kelp, kelpware, knotted wrack, Meereiche, popping wrack, *Quercus marina*, red fucus, rockrack, rockweed, schweintang, sea kelp, sea oak, seatang, seaware, seaweed, sea wrack, swine tang, tang, *Varech vesiculeux*, vraic, wrack.

BACKGROUND

- *Fucus vesiculosus* is a brown seaweed that grows on the northern coasts of the Atlantic and Pacific oceans, and the North and Baltic seas. Its name is sometimes used for *Ascophyllum nodosum*, which is another brown seaweed that grows alongside *Fucus vesiculosus*. These species are often included in kelp preparations along with other types of seaweed.

USES BASED ON SCIENTIFIC EVIDENCE	Grade*
Antibacterial/antifungal Laboratory study suggests antifungal and antibacterial activity of bladderwrack. However, there are no reliable human studies to support use as an antibacterial or antifungal agent.	C
Anticoagulant (blood-thinner) Laboratory study has found anticoagulant properties in fucans and fucoidans, which are components of brown algae such as bladderwrack. However, there have been no studies to support this use in humans.	C
Antioxidant Laboratory study suggests antioxidant activity in fucoidans, which are components in some brown algae. However, no studies support use as an antioxidant in humans.	C
Cancer In laboratory research studies and studies in animals, several brown algae, including bladderwrack (*Fucus vesiculosus*), appear to suppress the growth of various cancer cells. However, currently no reliable studies in humans support a recommendation for use in cancer.	C
Diabetes Based on animal research data, extracts of bladderwrack may lower blood sugar levels. However, reliable studies in humans are unavailable to support a recommendation for use in hyperglycemic conditions, such as diabetes.	C

Continued

Goiter (thyroid disease) Bladderwrack contains variable levels of iodine (up to 600 mg of iodine per gram of bladderwrack). Because of this, it has been used to treat thyroid disorders such as goiter. Although there are case reports of seaweed/kelp products causing hyperthyroidism, there have been no studies of dosing, safety, or efficacy, and there is no widely accepted standardization of iodine content for these products. Although the evidence does suggest thyroid activity, there is not enough research to support this use of bladderwrack.	C
Weight loss Bladderwrack and other seaweed products are often marketed for weight loss. Theoretically, thyroid stimulation by bladderwrack may increase metabolism and cause weight loss. However, the safety and effectiveness of these products have not been studied in humans.	C

*Key to grades: *A:* Strong scientific evidence for this use; *B:* Good scientific evidence for this use; *C:* Unclear scientific evidence for this use; *D:* Fair scientific evidence against this use (it may not work); *F:* Strong scientific evidence against this use (it likely does not work). For a more detailed explanation of efficacy criteria, see "Natural Standard Evidence-Based Validated Grading Rationale" in the Introduction.

Uses Based on Tradition, Theory, or Limited Scientific Evidence

Atherosclerosis, arthritis, benign prostatic hypertrophy, bladder inflammatory disease, eczema, edema, enlarged glands, fatigue, hair loss, heart disease, heartburn, high cholesterol, kidney disease, laxative, lymphadenoid goiter, malnutrition, menstruation irregularities, obesity, parasites, psoriasis, radiation protection, rheumatism, sore throat, stomach upset, stool softener, swollen or painful testes, ulcers, urinary tract tonic.

DOSING

The following doses are based on scientific research, publications, traditional use, or expert opinion. Many herbs and supplements have not been thoroughly tested, and their safety and effectiveness may not be proven. Brands may be made differently, with variable ingredients even within the same brand. The doses shown may not apply to all products. It is important to always read product labels and discuss doses with a qualified healthcare provider before therapy is started.

Standardization

- Standardization involves measuring the amounts of certain chemicals in products to try to make different preparations similar to each other. It is not always known if the chemicals being measured are the "active" ingredients. There is no known standardization for bladderwrack. Because of the potential contamination of bladderwrack with heavy metals, its consumption should always be considered potentially unsafe.

Adults (18 Years and Older)

- **General use (by mouth):** Soft capsules (alcohol extract) in doses of 200 to 600 mg daily have been used. Tablets have also been used, initially taken 3 times daily and gradually increased to 24 tablets per day. A dose of 16 g of bruised plant mixed with 1 pint of water has been used, administered in 2 fluid ounce doses 3 times per day, or as an alcoholic liquid extract in a dose of 4 to 8 ml before meals.
- **Patch:** Bladderwrack and seaweed patches are sold commercially as weight loss products, although there are no commonly accepted or tested doses.

Children (Younger Than 18 Years)

- There is not enough scientific evidence to recommend safe use of bladderwrack in children. Because of bladderwrack's iodine content and potential for contamination with heavy metals, it is not recommended for use in children.

SAFETY

The U.S. Food and Drug Administration does not strictly regulate herbs and supplements. There is no guarantee of the strength, purity, or safety of products, and effects may vary. It is important to always read product labels. People who have a medical condition, or are taking other drugs, herbs, or supplements, should consult a qualified healthcare provider before starting a new therapy. A healthcare provider should be contacted immediately about any side effects.

Allergies

- Allergy/hypersensitivity to *Fucus vesiculosus* or any of its components, as well as iodine sensitivity, may occur.

Side Effects and Warnings

- Most adverse effects appear to be related to high iodine content, heavy metal or other contamination of bladderwrack preparations, rather than to the seaweed itself. Because of the potential contamination of bladderwrack with heavy metals, its consumption should always been considered potentially unsafe.
- Based on the known effects of iodine toxicity, the high iodine content in bladderwrack may lead to abnormal thyroid conditions. There have been reports of increased thyroid activity (hyperthyroidism) and decreased thyroid activity (hypothyroidism) from ingestion of seaweed/kelp products. In theory, bladderwrack may increase or decrease blood thyroid hormone levels. In addition, acne-type skin lesions may occur, and severe acne exacerbations with the use of kelp have been reported. Iodine may cause a brassy taste, increased salivation, and stomach irritation.
- Reports of kidney and nerve toxicity, attributed to high levels of arsenic, have occurred in persons taking seaweed/kelp. In one case report, abnormal bleeding and reduced blood platelet count were attributed to contaminants in a kelp product.
- Bladderwrack contains many vitamins and minerals, and people taking bladderwrack products may have increased blood levels of calcium, magnesium, potassium, and sodium.
- Based on animal study, bladderwrack may lower blood sugar levels. Caution is advised in people with diabetes or hypoglycemia, and in those taking drugs, herbs, or supplements that affect blood sugar levels. Serum glucose levels may need to be monitored by a healthcare provider, and medication adjustments may be necessary.
- Based on laboratory study, bladderwrack may have blood-thinning (anticoagulant) properties. Abnormal bleeding, petechiae, and autoimmune thrombocytopenic

purpura with dyserythropoiesis have been reported. Caution is advised in people with bleeding disorders or taking drugs that may increase the risk of bleeding. Dosing adjustments may be necessary.

- Laxative properties have traditionally been attributed to chronic use of bladderwrack and other brown seaweeds and may be due to the component alginic acid, which is present in many laxative agents.

Pregnancy and Breastfeeding

- Bladderwrack is not recommended during pregnancy or lactation because of the lack of reliable scientific information and the presence of high levels of iodine and possible heavy metal contamination.

INTERACTIONS

Most herbs and supplements have not been thoroughly tested for interactions with other herbs, supplements, drugs, or foods. The interactions listed here are based on reports in scientific publications, laboratory experiments, or traditional use. It is important to always read product labels. People who have a medical condition, or are taking other drugs, herbs, or supplements, should consult a qualified healthcare provider before starting a new therapy.

Interactions with Drugs

- In theory, the high iodine content of bladderwrack may interfere with the function of drugs that act on the thyroid such as levothyroxine (Synthroid, Levoxyl). The use of bladderwrack or kelp with amiodarone or lithium may alter thyroid function because of the high iodine levels in all these agents.
- Based on animal study, extracts of bladderwrack may cause lowered blood sugar levels. Caution is advised when using medications that may also lower blood sugar levels. People who are taking drugs for diabetes by mouth or insulin should be monitored closely by a qualified healthcare provider. Medication adjustments may be necessary.
- Based on laboratory study, bladderwrack may have blood-thinning (anticoagulant) properties. Therefore, bladderwrack may increase the risk of bleeding when taken with drugs that increase the risk of bleeding. Examples are aspirin, anticoagulants (blood thinners) such as warfarin (Coumadin) and heparin, antiplatelet drugs such as clopidogrel (Plavix), and nonsteroidal anti-inflammatory drugs such as ibuprofen (Motrin, Advil) and naproxen (Naprosyn, Aleve).
- Laxative properties have traditionally been attributed to chronic use of bladderwrack and other brown seaweeds. This effect may be due to the component alginic acid, which is present in many laxative agents. Combination of bladderwrack products with laxatives may have an additive effect. Theoretically, because of its thyroid-stimulating properties, bladderwrack may have additive effects when taken with other thyroid stimulants.
- The presence of heavy metal contaminants in bladderwrack preparations, including arsenic, cadmium, chromium, and lead, may increase the risk of kidney toxicity if taken with drugs that may cause kidney damage.

Interactions with Herbs and Dietary Supplements

- Based on animal study, extracts of bladderwrack may lower blood sugar levels. Caution is advised when using herbs or supplements that may also lower blood sugar levels. Examples are *Aloe vera*, American ginseng, bilberry, bitter melon, burdock, fenugreek, fish oil, gymnema, horse chestnut seed extract (HCSE), marshmallow, milk thistle, *Panax ginseng*, rosemary, Siberian ginseng, stinging nettle, and white horehound. Blood glucose levels may require monitoring, and doses may need adjustment.

- In theory, the high iodine content of bladderwrack may interfere with the function of herbs or supplements that act on the thyroid.
- Based on laboratory study, bladderwrack may increase the risk of bleeding when it is taken with herbs and supplements that are believed to increase the risk of bleeding. Multiple cases of bleeding have been reported with the use of *Ginkgo biloba*, and fewer cases with garlic and saw palmetto. Numerous other agents may theoretically increase the risk of bleeding, although this has not been proven in most cases. Examples are alfalfa, American ginseng, angelica, anise, *Arnica montana*, asafetida, aspen bark, bilberry, birch, black cohosh, bogbean, boldo, borage seed oil, bromelain, capsicum, cat's claw, celery, chamomile, chaparral, clove, coleus, cordyceps, danshen, devil's claw, dong quai, evening primrose, fenugreek, feverfew, flaxseed/flax powder (not a concern with flaxseed oil), ginger, grapefruit juice, grapeseed, green tea, guggul, gymnestra, horse chestnut, horseradish, licorice root, lovage root, male fern, meadowsweet, nordihydroguaiaretic acid (NDGA), onion, papain, *Panax ginseng*, parsley, passion flower, poplar, prickly ash, propolis, quassia, red clover, reishi, rue, Siberian ginseng, sweet birch, sweet clover, turmeric, vitamin E, white willow, wild carrot, wild lettuce, willow, wintergreen, and yucca.
- Laxative properties have traditionally been attributed to chronic use of bladderwrack and other brown seaweeds, and this effect may be due to the component alginic acid, which is present in many laxative agents. Combination with laxatives or with other herbs that have laxative properties may have an additive effect. Examples of such herbs are alder buckthorn, aloe dried leaf sap, black root, blue flag rhizome, butternut bark, cascara bark, castor oil, chasteberry, colocynth fruit pulp, dandelion, dong quai, European buckthorn, eyebright, gamboges bark, horsetail, jalap root, manna bark, plantain leaf, podophyllum root, psyllium, rhubarb, senna, wild cucumber fruit, and yellow dock root.
- In theory, because of its thyroid-stimulating properties, bladderwrack may have additive effects if taken with herbs or supplements with stimulant-type activity, such as caffeine, guarana, and ephedra (ma huang). The presence of heavy metal contaminants in bladderwrack preparations, including arsenic, cadmium, chromium, and lead, may increase the risk of kidney toxicity if taken with herbs or supplements that can cause kidney damage.
- In theory, bladderwrack may decrease iron absorption, especially if ingested for a prolonged period of time. Bladderwrack preparations contain variable levels of calcium, magnesium, potassium, sodium, vitamins, and minerals and may therefore increase blood levels of these substances.

Selected References

Natural Standard developed the preceding evidence-based information based on a systematic review of more than 60 scientific articles. For comprehensive information about alternative and complementary therapies on the professional level, go to www.naturalstandard.com. Selected references are listed here.

Anonymous. Kelp diets can produce myxedema in iodide-sensitive individuals. JAMA 1975;233(1):9-10.

Colliec S, Fischer AM, Tapon-Bretaudiere J, et al. Anticoagulant properties of a fucoidan fraction. Thromb Res 1991;64(2):143-154.

Clark CD, Bassett B, Burge MR. Effects of kelp supplementation on thyroid function in euthyroid subjects. Endocr Pract 2003;9(5):363-369.

Conz PA, La Greca G, Benedetti P, et al. *Fucus vesiculosus*: a nephrotoxic alga? Nephrol Dial Transplant 1998;13(2):526-527.

Criado MT, Ferreiros CM. Selective interaction of a *Fucus vesiculosus* lectin-like mucopolysaccharide with several *Candida* species. Ann Microbiol (Paris) 1983;134A(2):149-154.

Criado MT, Ferreiros CM. Toxicity of an algal mucopolysaccharide for *Escherichia coli* and *Neisseria meningitidis* strains. Rev Esp Fisiol 1984;40(2):227-230.

Durig J, Bruhn T, Zurborn KH, et al. Anticoagulant fucoidan fractions from *Fucus vesiculosus* induce platelet activation in vitro. Thromb Res 1997;85(6):479-491.

Eliason BC. Transient hyperthyroidism in a patient taking dietary supplements containing kelp. J Am Board Fam Pract 1998;11(6):478-480.

Ellouali M, Boisson-Vidal C, Durand P, et al. Antitumor activity of low molecular weight fucans extracted from brown seaweed *Ascophyllum nodosum*. Anticancer Res 1993;13(6A): 2011-2020.

Grauffel V, Kloareg B, Mabeau S, et al. New natural polysaccharides with potent antithrombic activity: fucans from brown algae. Biomaterials 1989;10(6):363-368.

Harrell BL, Rudolph AH. Letter: Kelp diet: a cause of acneiform eruption. Arch Dermatol 1976;112(4):560.

Hartman AA. [Hyperthyroidism during administration of kelp tablets.] Ned Tijdschr Geneeskd 1990;134(28):1373.

Lamela M, Anca J, Villar R, et al. Hypoglycemic activity of several seaweed extracts. J Ethnopharmacol 1989;27(1-2):35-43.

Le Tutour B, Benslimane F, Gouleau MP, et al. Antioxidant and pro-oxidant activities of the brown algae, *Laminaria digitata*, *Himanthalia elongata*, *Fucus vesiculosus*, *Fucus serratus* and *Ascophyllum nodosum*. J Applied Phycology 1998;10(2):121-129.

Maruyama H, Nakajima J, Yamamoto I. A study on the anticoagulant and fibrinolytic activities of a crude fucoidan from the edible brown seaweed *Laminaria religiosa*, with special reference to its inhibitory effect on the growth of sarcoma-180 ascites cells subcutaneously implanted into mice. Kitasato Arch Exp Med 1987;60(3):105-121.

Norman JA, Pickford CJ, Sanders TW, et al. Human intake of arsenic and iodine from seaweed-based food supplements and health foods available in the UK. Food Addit Contam 1987; 5(1):103-109.

Pye KG, Kelsey SM, House IM, et al. Severe dyserythropoiesis and autoimmune thrombocytopenia associated with ingestion of kelp supplements. Lancet 1992;339(8808):1540.

Riou D, Colliec-Jouault S, Pinczon du Sel D, et al. Antitumor and antiproliferative effects of a fucan extracted from *Ascophyllum nodosum* against a non–small-cell bronchopulmonary carcinoma line. Anticancer Res 1996;16(3A):1213-1218.

Rocha A, Rache LS, Rhoden CR. [Natural products utilized as alternative treatment for obesity.] Revist Brasil Med 1994;51(10):1454, 1456, 1459-1460, 1464.

Shilo S, Hirsch HJ. Iodine-induced hyperthyroidism in a patient with a normal thyroid gland. Postgrad Med J 1986;62(729):661-662.

Springer GF, Wurzel HA, McNeal GM, et al. Isolation of anticoagulant fractions from crude fucoidin. Proc Soc Exp Biol Med 1957;94:404-409.

Soeda S, Sakaguchi S, Shimeno H, et al. Fibrinolytic and anticoagulant activities of highly sulfated fucoidan. Biochem Pharmacol 1992;43(8):1853-1858.

Walkiw O, Douglas DE. Health food supplements prepared from kelp—a source of elevated urinary arsenic. Clin Toxicol 1975;8(3):325-331.

Yamamoto I, Nagumo T, Fujihara M, et al. Antitumor effect of seaweeds. II. Fractionation and partial characterization of the polysaccharide with antitumor activity from *Sargassum fulvellum*. Jpn J Exp Med 1977;47(3):133-140.

Blessed Thistle

(*Cnicus benedictus* L.)

RELATED TERMS

- Bitter thistle, *Carbenia benedicta*, cardin, cardo santo, *Carduus benedictus*, chardon benit, *Cnici benedicti* Herba, cnicus, holy thistle, kardo-benedictenkraut, spotted thistle, St. Benedict thistle.
- *Note:* Blessed thistle should not be mistaken for milk thistle (*Silybum marianus*) or other members of the thistle family.

BACKGROUND

- Blessed thistle leaves, stems, and flowers have traditionally been used in "bitter tonic" drinks and in other preparations taken by mouth to enhance appetite and digestion. It may be a component of the unproven anti-cancer herbal remedy Essiac. Blessed thistle has been tested in laboratory studies for its properties against infections, cancer, and inflammation with promising results. However, no high-quality trials have shown benefits in humans.

USES BASED ON SCIENTIFIC EVIDENCE	Grade*
Bacterial infections Laboratory studies reported that blessed thistle (specifically, chemicals in blessed thistle such as cnicin and polyacetylene) had activity against several types of bacteria, including *Bacillus subtilis*, *Brucella* species, *Escherichia coli*, *Proteus* species, *Pseudomonas aeruginosa*, *Staphylococcus aureus*, and *Streptococcus*. However, other studies have found no effects against *Klebsiella*, *Pseudomonas*, *S. aureus*, *Salmonella typhi*, or yeast. There are no reliable studies in humans. Further evidence is necessary in this area before a firm conclusion can be drawn.	C
Indigestion and flatulence Blessed thistle is traditionally believed to stimulate stomach acid secretion and has been used in treatment for indigestion and flatulence (gas). However, there has been limited scientific study in this area. Additional research is needed before a firm conclusion can be reached.	C
Viral infections In laboratory studies, blessed thistle had no activity against herpesviruses, influenza viruses, or poliovirus. The effects of blessed thistle (or chemicals in blessed thistle called lignans) against HIV are unclear. There have been no reliable research studies in humans of blessed thistle as treatment for viral infections.	C

*Key to grades: *A:* Strong scientific evidence for this use; *B:* Good scientific evidence for this use; *C:* Unclear scientific evidence for this use; *D:* Fair scientific evidence against this use (it may not work); *F:* Strong scientific evidence against this use (it likely does not work). For a more detailed explanation of efficacy criteria, see "Natural Standard Evidence-Based Validated Grading Rationale" in the Introduction.

Uses Based on Tradition, Theory, or Limited Scientific Evidence

Abortifacient, anorexia, appetite stimulant, astringent, bleeding, blood purifier, boils, breast milk stimulant, bubonic plague, cervical dysplasia, choleretic (bile flow stimulant), colds, contraceptive, diaphoretic (sweat stimulant), diarrhea, digestion enhancement, diuretic (increasing urine flow), expectorant, fever reducer, gallbladder disease, inflammation, jaundice, liver disorders, malaria, memory improvement, menstrual disorders, menstrual flow stimulant, painful menstruation, rabies, salivation stimulant, skin ulcers, wound healing, yeast infections.

DOSING

The following doses are based on scientific research, publications, traditional use, or expert opinion. Many herbs and supplements have not been thoroughly tested, and their safety and effectiveness may not be proven. Brands may be made differently, with variable ingredients even within the same brand. The doses shown may not apply to all products. It is important to always read product labels and discuss doses with a qualified healthcare provider before therapy is started.

Standardization

- Standardization involves measuring the amounts of certain chemicals in products to try to make different preparations similar to each other. It is not always known if the chemicals being measured are the "active" ingredients. There is no widely accepted standardization for blessed thistle, although laboratory tests are available to determine the presence of the "bitter" constituent cnicin. Pharmacopeial-grade blessed thistle is often assigned a "bitterness value" greater than 800.
- Blessed thistle herbal preparations are often obtained from the leaves and flowers of the plant.

Adults (18 Years and Older)

- **Tea:** Traditional doses include 1.5 to 3.0 g of dried flowering tops steeped in 150 ml of boiling water taken three times daily, or 1 to 3 teaspoons of the dried herb steeped in one cup of boiling water for 5 to 15 minutes and taken three times daily (sometimes recommended to be taken 30 minutes before meals). The tea may be bitter in taste.
- **Tincture** (1.5 g of blessed thistle per liter): 7.5 to 10 ml by mouth taken three times daily has been used.
- **Liquid extract** (1 gram of blessed thistle per 1 ml of 25% alcohol): 1.5 to 3.0 ml by mouth taken three times daily has been used.

Children (Younger Than 18 Years)

- Blessed thistle is not recommended for use in children because of the lack of reliable safety data.

SAFETY

The U.S. Food and Drug Administration does not strictly regulate herbs and supplements. There is no guarantee of the strength, purity, or safety of products, and effects may vary. It is important to always read product labels. People who have a medical condition, or are taking other drugs, herbs, or supplements, should consult a qualified healthcare provider before starting a new therapy. A healthcare provider should be contacted immediately about any side effects.

Allergies

- Allergic reactions to blessed thistle (including contact dermatitis) may occur, as well as cross-reactivity with mugwort and echinacea. Cross-reactivity may also occur with bitter weed, blanket flower, chrysanthemum, coltsfoot, daisy, dandelion, dwarf sunflower, goldenrod, marigold, prairie sage, ragweed, and other plants in the Asteraceae/Compositae family.

Side Effects and Warnings

- Blessed thistle is generally considered to be safe when used by mouth in recommended doses for short periods of time, and there have been few reported side effects. Direct contact with blessed thistle can cause skin irritation (contact dermatitis) or irritation of the eyes.
- Anecdotally, blessed thistle taken in high doses (for example, greater than 5 g per cup of tea) may cause stomach irritation and vomiting. Blessed thistle is traditionally believed to increase stomach acid secretion, and its use may be inadvisable in persons with stomach ulcers, reflux disease (heartburn), hiatal hernia, or Barrett's esophagus.
- Blessed thistle contains approximately 8% tannins. Long-term ingestion of plants containing greater than 10% tannins may cause gastrointestinal upset, liver disease, kidney toxicity, or increased risk of developing esophageal or nasal cancer. The effects of blessed thistle tannins on humans are unknown.
- Laboratory studies suggest that blessed thistle may increase the risk of bleeding, although this has not been confirmed in humans. Caution is advised in people with bleeding disorders or those taking other agents that may increase the risk of bleeding. Dosing adjustments may be necessary.
- Many tinctures contain high levels of alcohol, and their use should be avoided by people who are driving or operating heavy machinery.

Pregnancy and Breastfeeding

- Blessed thistle has been used traditionally to stimulate menstruation and abortion, and therefore its use should be avoided during pregnancy. Although blessed thistle has been used historically to stimulate breast milk flow, it is not recommended during breastfeeding because of limited safety information. There are no reliable research data available in these areas.
- Many tinctures contain high levels of alcohol, and their use should be avoided during pregnancy.

INTERACTIONS

Most herbs and supplements have not been thoroughly tested for interactions with other herbs, supplements, drugs, or foods. The interactions listed here are based on reports in scientific publications, laboratory experiments, or traditional use. It is important to always read product labels. People who have a medical condition, or are taking other drugs, herbs, or supplements, should consult a qualified healthcare provider before starting a new therapy.

Interactions with Drugs

- Traditionally, blessed thistle is believed to stimulate stomach acid secretion, and may reduce the effectiveness of drugs such as cimetidine (Tagamet), famotidine (Pepcid), nizatidine (Axid), and ranitidine (Zantac).
- Based on laboratory studies, blessed thistle may increase the risk of bleeding when taken with drugs that also may increase the risk of bleeding (although effects in

humans are not known). Examples of such agents are anticoagulants (blood thinners) such as warfarin (Coumadin) and heparin, antiplatelet drugs such as clopidogrel (Plavix), aspirin, and nonsteroidal anti-inflammatory drugs (NSAIDs) such as ibuprofen (Motrin, Advil) and naproxen (Naprosyn, Aleve).
- Many tinctures contain high levels of alcohol, and may cause nausea or vomiting when taken with metronidazole (Flagyl) or disulfiram (Antabuse).

Interactions with Herbs and Dietary Supplements

- Based on laboratory studies, blessed thistle may increase the risk of bleeding when taken with herbs or supplements that may also increase the risk of bleeding (although effects in humans are not known). Multiple cases of bleeding have been reported with the use of *Ginkgo biloba*, and fewer cases with garlic and saw palmetto. Numerous other agents may theoretically increase the risk of bleeding, although this has not been proven in most cases. Examples are alfalfa, American ginseng, angelica, anise, *Arnica montana*, asafetida, aspen bark, bilberry, birch, black cohosh, bladderwrack, bogbean, boldo, borage seed oil, bromelain, capsicum, cat's claw, celery, chamomile, chaparral, clove, coleus, cordyceps, danshen, devil's claw, dong quai, eicosapentaenoic acid (EPA, found in deep-sea fish oils), evening primrose oil, fenugreek, feverfew, fish oil, flaxseed/flax powder (not a concern with flaxseed oil), ginger, grapefruit, grapeseed, green tea, guggul, gymnestra, horse chestnut, horseradish, licorice root, lovage root, male fern, meadowsweet, nordihydroguaiaretic acid (NDGA), onion, *Panax ginseng*, papain, parsley, passion flower, poplar, prickly ash, propolis, quassia, red clover, reishi, rue, Siberian ginseng, sweet birch, sweet clover, turmeric, vitamin E, white willow, wild carrot, wild lettuce, willow, wintergreen, and yucca.

Selected References

Natural Standard developed the preceding evidence-based information based on a systematic review of more than 50 scientific articles. For comprehensive information about alternative and complementary therapies on the professional level, go to www.naturalstandard.com. Selected references are listed below.

Cobb E. Antineoplastic agent from *Cnicus benedictus*. Patent Brit 1973;335:181.

Eich E, Pertz H, Kaloga M, et al. (-)-Arctigenin as a lead structure for inhibitors of human immunodeficiency virus type-1 integrase. J Med Chem 1996;39(1):86-95.

Kataria H. Phytochemical investigation of medicinal plant *Cnicus wallichii* and *Cnicus benedictus* L. Asian J Chem 1995;7:227-228.

May G, Willuhn G. [Antiviral effect of aqueous plant extracts in tissue culture.] Arzneimittelforschung 1978;28(1):1-7.

Novitch M, Schweiker R. Orally administered menstrual drug products for over-the-counter human use. Federal Register 1982;47:55076-55101.

Perez C, Anesini C. In vitro antibacterial activity of Argentine folk medicinal plants against *Salmonella typhi*. J Ethnopharmacol 1994;44(1):41-46.

Perez C, Anesini C. Inhibition of *Pseudomonas aeruginosa* by Argentinean medicinal plants. Fitoterapia 1994;65(2):169-172.

Recio M, Rios J, Villar A. Antimicrobial activity of selected plants employed in the Spanish Mediterranean area. Part II. Phytother Res 1989;3:77-80.

Ryu SY, Ahn JW, Kang YH, et al. Antiproliferative effect of arctigenin and arctiin. Arch Pharm Res 1995;18(6):462-463.

Schimmer O, Kruger A, Paulini H, et al. An evaluation of 55 commercial plant extracts in the Ames mutagenicity test. Pharmazie 1994;49(6):448-451.

Schneider G, Lachner I. [Analysis and action of cnicin.] Planta Med 1987;53(3):247-251.

Ubelen A, Berkan T. Triterpenic and steroidal compounds of *Cnicus benedictus*. Planta Med 1977;31:375-377.
Vanhaelen M, Vanhaelen-Fastre R. Lactonic lignans from *Cnicus benedictus*. Phytochemistry 1975;14:2709.
Vanhaelen-Fastre R, Vanhaelen M. [Antibiotic and cytotoxic activity of cnicin and of its hydrolysis products. Chemical structure—biological activity relationship (author's transl).] Planta Med 1976;29(2):179-189.
Vanhaelen-Fastre R. [Antibiotic and cytotoxic activity of cnicin isolated from *Cnicus benedictus* L.] J Pharm Belg 1972;27(6):683-688.
Vanhaelen-Fastre R. [Constitution and antibiotical properties of the essential oil of *Cnicus benedictus*.] Planta Med 1973;24(2):165-175.
Vanhaelen-Fastre R. [Polyacetylen compounds from *Cnicus benedictus*.] Planta Med 1974;25:47-59.
Yang L, Lin S, Yang T, et al. Synthesis of anti-HIV activity of dibenzylbutyrolactone lignans. Bioorg Med Chem Lett 1996;6(8):941-944.
Zeller W, de Gols M, Hausen BM. The sensitizing capacity of Compositae plants. VI. Guinea pig sensitization experiments with ornamental plants and weeds using different methods. Arch Dermatol Res 1985;277(1):28-35.

Boron

RELATED TERMS

- Atomic number 5, B, Borax, boric acid, boric anhydride, boron aspartate, boron citrate, boron glycinate, boron oxide, boron sesquioxide, Dobill's solution, magnesium perborate, sodium biborate, sodium borate, sodium metaborate, sodium perborate, sodium pyroborate, sodium tetraborate, Tincal.

BACKGROUND

- Boron is a trace element that is found throughout the global environment. It has been suggested for numerous medicinal purposes, but there is no strong evidence for any specific use. Preliminary studies suggest that boron may not be helpful in commonly used therapies such as enhancing bodybuilding, reducing menopausal symptoms, and treating psoriasis.

USES BASED ON SCIENTIFIC EVIDENCE	Grade*
Improving cognitive function Preliminary studies in humans reported that boron supplements enhanced performance on tasks testing eye-hand coordination, attention, perception, and short- and long-term memory. However, additional research is needed before a firm conclusion can be drawn.	C
Osteoarthritis Based on human population research, in a boron-rich environment, people appear to have fewer joint disorders. It has also been proposed that boron deficiency may contribute to the development of osteoarthritis. However, there is no clear human evidence that supplementation with boron is beneficial as prevention against or as a treatment for osteoarthritis.	C
Osteoporosis Research in animals and preliminary studies in humans report that boron plays a role in mineral metabolism, with effects on calcium, phosphorus, and vitamin D. However, research of bone mineral density in women taking boron supplements does not clearly demonstrate benefits in osteoporosis. Additional study is needed before a firm conclusion can be drawn.	C
Vaginitis Inorganic boron (boric acid, Borax) has been used as an antiseptic, based on its proposed antibacterial and antifungal properties. It has been proposed that boric acid may have effects against candidal and	C

Continued

noncandidal vulvovaginitis. A limited amount of poor-quality research reports that boric acid capsules used in the vagina may be effective for vaginitis. Further evidence is needed before a recommendation can be made.	
Bodybuilding aid (increasing testosterone levels) There is preliminary negative evidence for the use of boron for improving performance in bodybuilding by increasing testosterone. Although boron is suggested to raise testosterone levels, in early human research, total lean body mass has not been affected by boron supplementation in bodybuilders. Additional research is necessary before a firm conclusion can be drawn.	**D**
Menopausal symptoms It has been proposed that boron affects estrogen levels in postmenopausal women. However, preliminary studies have found no changes in menopausal symptoms.	**D**
Prevention of blood clotting (coagulation effects) It has been proposed that boron may affect the activity of certain blood clotting factors. A small (15 healthy men 45 to 65 years of age), randomized, placebo-controlled, double-blind, crossover study concluded that there is no evidence of boron lowering clotting factor VIIa, and therefore that boron did not alter the risk of bleeding. Notably, a manufacturer of boron funded this study. There is not enough evidence in this area to form a clear conclusion.	**D**
Psoriasis (boric acid ointment) Preliminary studies in humans of an ointment containing boric acid reported no significant benefits in psoriasis.	**D**

*Key to grades: *A:* Strong scientific evidence for this use; *B:* Good scientific evidence for this use; *C:* Unclear scientific evidence for this use; *D:* Fair scientific evidence against this use (it may not work); *F:* Strong scientific evidence against this use (it likely does not work). For a more detailed explanation of efficacy criteria, see "Natural Standard Evidence-Based Validated Grading Rationale" in the Introduction.

Uses Based on Tradition, Theory, or Limited Scientific Evidence

Antiseptic, breast cancer, boron deficiency, diaper rash (avoid because of case reports of death in infants who had absorbed boron through the skin or when taken by mouth), cancer, eye cleansing, high cholesterol, increasing lifespan, leukemia, rheumatoid arthritis, vitamin D deficiency, wound care.

DOSING

The following doses are based on scientific research, publications, traditional use, or expert opinion. Many herbs and supplements have not been thoroughly tested, and their safety and effectiveness may not be proven. Brands may be made differently, with variable ingredients even within the same brand. The doses shown may not apply to all products. It is important to always read product labels and discuss doses with a qualified healthcare provider before therapy is started.

Standardization

- Standardization involves measuring the amounts of certain chemicals in products to try to make different preparations similar to each other. It is not always known if the chemicals being measured are the "active" ingredients. Most of the nutritional boron products available commercially are either sodium Borax or a boron-chelated agent combined with aspartate, glycinate, or citrate.
- Boron (as boric acid or Borax) can be easily absorbed by mouth, through the skin, or by breathing.

Adults (18 Years and Older)

Oral (by mouth)

- **Dietary intake:** The average reported boron intake in the usual American diet is 1.17 mg daily for men and 0.96 mg daily for women; the intake for vegetarians ranges from 1.29 to 1.47 mg daily. Foods high in boron include beans, grapes, peaches, peanut butter, and wine.
- **Osteoarthritis:** 3 to 6 mg of elemental boron (as sodium tetraborate decahydrate) taken by mouth daily for up to 8 weeks has been used.
- **Osteoporosis prevention:** 3 mg of boron taken by mouth per day for persons on a diet low in boron (limited fruit and vegetables) has been studied.
- **Improvement of cognitive function:** 3 mg of elemental boron taken by mouth daily has been studied.
- **Menopausal symptoms:** 2.5 to 3 mg of elemental boron taken by mouth daily has been studied.

Topical

- **Psoriasis:** In some studies,1.5% boric acid and 3% zinc oxide was applied to the skin as needed.
- **Vaginitis:** Boric acid powder capsules administered vaginally daily have been studied. Their safety and effectiveness are not established.

Children (Younger Than 18 Years)

- There are insufficient scientific data to recommend the safe use of boron in children. There are case reports of death in infants following the use of boron (taken by mouth or placed on the skin).

SAFETY

The U.S. Food and Drug Administration does not strictly regulate herbs and supplements. There is no guarantee of the strength, purity, or safety of products, and effects may vary. It is important to always read product labels. People who have a medical condition, or are taking other drugs, herbs, or supplements, should consult a qualified healthcare provider before starting a new therapy. A healthcare provider should be contacted immediately about any side effects.

Allergies

- Boron should be avoided in patients who have a history of reactions to boron, boric acid, Borax, citrate, aspartate, or glycinate.

Side Effects and Warnings

- Boron is potentially toxic, although humans tend not to accumulate high levels of boron because of the ability to rapidly excrete it. In adults, it is believed that adverse reactions in doses of less than 10 mg of boron per day in adults are less likely to occur and there are few reports of toxicity. Higher doses may result in acute poisoning. There are case reports of death in infants who were exposed to boron by mouth or on the skin. Historically, a honey and Borax solution has been used to clean infant pacifiers, and topical boric acid powder was used to prevent diaper rash. These practices were associated with several infant deaths.
- Boron toxicity may cause skin rash, nausea, vomiting (color may be blue-green), diarrhea (color may be blue-green), abdominal pain, and headache. Low blood pressure and metabolic changes in the blood (acidosis) have been reported. Agitation and irritability, or the opposite reaction (weakness, lethargy, depression) may occur. Fever, hyperthermia, tremors, and seizure have been reported.
- In studies of animals, excess amounts of boron ingestion have been shown to cause testicular toxicity, decreased sperm motility, and reduced fertility. Hair loss has been reported with boron poisoning. Chronic boron exposure may cause dehydration, seizures, low red blood cell count, and kidney or liver damage.
- Boron has been proposed to increase blood levels of estrogen and testosterone; research study results have been mixed. Boron may be associated with reduced blood levels of calcitonin, insulin, or phosphorus and with increased levels of vitamin D_2, calcium, copper, magnesium, or thyroxine. Exposure to boric acid or boron oxide dust can cause eye irritation, dryness of the mouth and nose, sore throat, and productive cough.

Pregnancy and Breastfeeding

- There is insufficient scientific evidence to recommend the safe use of boron by pregnant and breastfeeding women.

INTERACTIONS

Most herbs and supplements have not been thoroughly tested for interactions with other herbs, supplements, drugs, or foods. The interactions listed here are based on reports in scientific publications, laboratory experiments, or traditional use. It is important to always read product labels. People who have a medical condition, or are taking other drugs, herbs, or supplements, should consult a qualified healthcare provider before starting a new therapy.

Interactions with Drugs

- Magnesium may interfere with the effects of boron in the body. Sources of magnesium include antacids containing magnesium oxide or magnesium sulfate (milk of magnesia, Maalox).
- In theory, the use of boron with estrogen-active drugs such as birth control pills or hormone replacement therapy may result in increased estrogen effects. The use of boron with testosterone-active drugs such as Testoderm may result in increased testosterone effects.

Interactions with Herbs and Dietary Supplements

- Boron supplementation may result in increased calcium levels in the blood and may add to the effects of calcium and vitamin D supplementation. In theory, the use of boron with estrogen-active herbs or supplements may result in increased estrogen effects. Possible examples: alfalfa, black cohosh, bloodroot, burdock, hops, kudzu, licorice, pomegranate, red clover, soy, thyme, white horehound, and yucca.

Selected References

Natural Standard developed the preceding evidence-based information based on a systematic review of more than 300 scientific articles. For comprehensive information about alternative and complementary therapies on the professional level, go to www.naturalstandard.com. Selected references are listed here.

Anonymous. Antineoplastic effect of new boron compounds against leukemic cell lines and cells from leukemic patients. J Exp Clin Cancer Res 2002;(3):351-356.

Biquet I, Collette J, Dauphin JF, et al. Prevention of postmenopausal bone loss by administration of boron. Osteoporos Int 1996;6(Suppl 1):249.

Devarian TA, Volpe SL. The physiological effects of dietary boron. Crit Rev Food Sci Nutr 2003;43(2):219-231.

Green NR, Ferrando AA. Plasma boron and the effects of boron supplementation in males. Environ Health Perspect 1994;102(Suppl 7):73-77.

Guaschino S, De Seta F, Sartore A, et al. Efficacy of maintenance therapy with topical boric acid in comparison with oral itraconazole in the treatment of recurrent vulvovaginal candidiasis. Am J Obstet Gynecol 2001;184(4):598-602.

Hunt CD, Herbel JL, Nielsen FH. Metabolic responses of postmenopausal women to supplemental dietary boron and aluminum during usual and low magnesium intake: boron, calcium, and magnesium absorption and retention and blood mineral concentrations. Am J Clin Nutr 1997;65(3):803-813.

Kumar SK, Hager E, Pettit C, et al. Design, synthesis, and evaluation of novel boronic-chalcone derivatives as antitumor agents. J Med Chem 2003;46(14):2813-2815.

Limaye S, Weightman W. Effect of an ointment containing boric acid, zinc oxide, starch and petrolatum on psoriasis. Australas J Dermatol 1997;38(4):185-186.

Naghii MR. The significance of dietary boron, with particular reference to athletes. Nutr Health 1999;13(1):31-37.

Nielsen FH, Penland JG. Boron supplementation of peri-menopausal women affects boron metabolism and indices associated with macromineral metabolism, hormonal status and immune function. J Trace Elem Exp Med 1999;12(3):251-261.

Nielsen FH, Hunt CD, Mullen LM, et al. Effect of dietary boron on mineral, estrogen, and testosterone metabolism in postmenopausal women. FASEB J 1987;1(5):394-397.

Nzietchueng RM, Dousset B, Franck P, et al. Mechanisms implicated in the effects of boron on wound healing J Trace Elem Med Biol 2002;16(4):239-244.

Penland JG. Dietary boron, brain function, and cognitive performance. Environ Health Perspect 1994;102(Suppl 7):65-72.

Roig-Navarro AF, Lopez FJ, Serrano R, et al. An assessment of heavy metals and boron contamination in workplace atmospheres from ceramic factories. Sci Total Environ 1997; 201(3):225-234.

Travers RL, Rennie GC, Newnham RE. Boron and arthritis: the results of a double-blind pilot study. J Nutrit Med 1990;1:127-132.

Usuda K, Kono K, Yoshida Y. Serum boron concentration from inhabitants of an urban area in Japan: reference value and interval for the health screening of boron exposure. Biol Trace Elem Res 1997;56(2):167-178.

Van Slyke KK, Michel VP, Rein MF. The boric acid powder treatment of vulvovaginal candidiasis. J Am Coll Health Assoc 1981;30(3):107-109.

Van Slyke KK, Michel VP, Rein MF. Treatment of vulvovaginal candidiasis with boric acid powder. Am J Obstet Gynecol 1981;141(2):145-148.

Volpe SL, Taper LJ, Meacham S. The relationship between boron and magnesium status and bone mineral density in the human: a review. Magnes Res 1993;6(3):291-296.

Wallace JM, Hannon-Fletcher MP, Robson PJ, et al. Boron supplementation and activated factor VII in healthy men. Eur J Clin Nutr 2002;56(11):1102-1107.

Bromelain

(*Ananas comosus*)

RELATED TERMS

- *Ananas sativus*, Ananase, bromelainum, Bromeliaceae bromelin, bromeline, pineapple extract, plant protease concentrate, Traumanase.

BACKGROUND

- Bromelain is a digestive enzyme that is extracted from the stem and fruit of the pineapple.

USES BASED ON SCIENTIFIC EVIDENCE	Grade*
Cancer Scientific evidence is insufficient to recommend for or against the use of bromelain in the treatment of cancer, whether it is used alone or in addition to other therapies.	C
Chronic obstructive pulmonary disease (COPD) There is not enough information to recommend for or against the use of bromelain in COPD.	C
Digestive enzyme/pancreatic insufficiency Bromelain is an enzyme with the ability to digest proteins. However, there have been few reliable research studies on whether bromelain is helpful as a digestive aid. Better-quality and more extensive studies are needed before a firm conclusion can be made.	C
Inflammation Several preliminary studies suggest that bromelain, when taken by mouth, can reduce inflammation or pain caused by inflammation. Better-quality studies are needed to confirm these results.	B
Nutrition supplementation Scientific evidence is insufficient to recommend for or against the use of bromelain as a nutritional supplement.	C
Rheumatoid arthritis (RA) There is not enough information to recommend for or against the use of bromelain in rheumatoid arthritis (RA). Notably, most studies and case reports in this area have been published by the same authors.	C

Continued

Sinusitis It has been proposed that bromelain may be a useful addition to other therapies used for sinusitis (such as antibiotics) because of its ability to reduce inflammation and swelling. Studies report mixed results, although overall bromelain appears to be beneficial for reducing swelling and improving breathing. Better-quality studies are needed before a strong recommendation can be made.	**B**
Steatorrhea (fatty stools due to poor digestion) There is not enough information to recommend for or against the use of bromelain in the treatment of steatorrhea.	**C**
Urinary tract infection (UTI) There is not enough information to recommend for or against the use of bromelain in urinary tract infections.	**C**

*Key to grades: *A:* Strong scientific evidence for this use; *B:* Good scientific evidence for this use; *C:* Unclear scientific evidence for this use; *D:* Fair scientific evidence against this use (it may not work); *F:* Strong scientific evidence against this use (it likely does not work). For a more detailed explanation of efficacy criteria, see "Natural Standard Evidence-Based Validated Grading Rationale" in the Introduction.

Uses Based on Tradition, Theory, or Limited Scientific Evidence

Acquired immunodeficiency syndrome (AIDS), allergic rhinitis (hay fever), amyloidosis, angina, antibiotic absorption problems in the gut, appetite suppressant, atherosclerosis ("hardening of the arteries"), autoimmune disorders, back pain, blood clot treatment, bronchitis, bruises, burn and wound care, bursitis, cancer prevention, carpal tunnel syndrome, cellulitis/skin infections, colitis, common cold, cough, diarrhea, epididymitis, episiotomy pain (after childbirth), food allergies, food lodged in the esophagus, frostbite, gout, heart disease, hemorrhoids, immune system regulation, indigestion, infections, injuries, joint disease, "leaky gut" syndrome, menstrual pain, pain (general), pancreatic problems with food digestion, Peyronie's disease (abnormal curvature, pain, and scar tissue in the penis), platelet inhibition (blood thinner), pneumonia, poor absorption of digested food, poor blood circulation in the legs, sciatica, scleroderma, shingles pain/postherpetic neuralgia, shortening of labor, smooth muscle relaxation, sports-related or other physical injuries, staphylococcal bacterial infections, stimulation of muscle contractions, stomach ulcer prevention, swelling after surgery or injury, tendonitis, thick mucus, thrombophlebitis, treatment of scar tissue, ulcerative colitis, upper respiratory tract infection, varicose veins, wound healing.

DOSING

The following doses are based on scientific research, publications, traditional use, or expert opinion. Many herbs and supplements have not been thoroughly tested, and their safety and effectiveness may not be proven. Brands may be made differently, with variable ingredients even within the same brand. The doses shown may not apply to all products. It is important to always read product labels and discuss doses with a qualified healthcare provider before therapy is started.

Standardization

- Standardization involves measuring the amounts of certain chemicals in products to try to make different preparations similar to each other. It is not always known if the chemicals being measured are the "active" ingredients. Bromelain may be standardized to milk clotting units (MCU), gelatin digesting units (GDU), FIP units, or Rorer units (RU) per gram. The MCU is officially recognized by the Food Chemistry Codex. Some experts recommend using bromelain standardized to contain at least 2000 MCU per gram, whereas other sources recommend a range of 1200 to 1800 MCU per gram.

Adults (18 Years and Older)

- **Oral (by mouth):** A variety of doses have been used and studied. Research studies in the 1960s and 1970s used 120 to 240 mg of bromelain concentrate tablets daily (Traumanase or Ananase; 2500 RU per mg) in three or four divided doses for up to 1 week to treat inflammation. The German expert panel (Commission E) has recommended 80 to 320 mg (200 to 800 FIP units) taken two to three times daily. Some authors recommend 500 to 1000 mg of bromelain to be taken three times daily, and many manufacturers sell products standardized to 2000 GDU in 500-mg tablets. The effects of bromelain may occur at lower doses, and treatment may be started at a low dose and increased as needed.
- **Topical (applied to the skin):** Cream containing 35% bromelain in an oil-containing base has been used to clean wounds.

Children (Younger Than 18 Years)

- Scientific research evidence is insufficient to recommend the safe use of bromelain in children.

SAFETY

The U.S. Food and Drug Administration does not strictly regulate herbs and supplements. There is no guarantee of the strength, purity, or safety of products, and effects may vary. It is important to always read product labels. People who have a medical condition, or are taking other drugs, herbs, or supplements, should consult a qualified healthcare provider before starting a new therapy. A healthcare provider should be contacted immediately about any side effects.

Allergies

- There have been multiple reports of allergic and asthmatic reactions to bromelain products, including throat swelling and difficulty breathing. Allergic reactions to bromelain may occur in people who are allergic to pineapples or other members of the Bromeliaceae family, and in those who are sensitive or allergic to birch pollen, carrot, celery, cypress pollen, fennel, grass pollen, honeybee venom, latex, papain, rye flour, or wheat flour.

Side Effects and Warnings

- Few serious side effects have been reported with the use of bromelain at daily doses up to 10 g for each kilogram (2.2 pounds) of body weight. The most common side effects reported are stomach upset and diarrhea. Other reactions include increased heart rate, nausea, vomiting, irritation of mucous membranes, and menstrual problems.

- In theory, bromelain may increase the risk of bleeding. Caution is advised in people who have bleeding disorders or are taking drugs that increase the risk of bleeding. Dosing adjustments may be necessary. Bromelain should be used with caution in people with stomach ulcers, active bleeding, or a history of bleeding, in those who are taking medications that thin the blood or who are going to have certain dental or surgical procedures.
- Higher doses of bromelain may increase the heart rate, and it should be used cautiously in people with heart disease. Some experts warn against bromelain use by people with liver or kidney disease, although there is limited scientific information in this area. Bromelain may cause abnormal uterine bleeding or heavy/prolonged menstruation.

Pregnancy and Breastfeeding

- Bromelain is not recommended during pregnancy or when a woman is breastfeeding because information about its safety is limited.

INTERACTIONS

Most herbs and supplements have not been thoroughly tested for interactions with other herbs, supplements, drugs, or foods. The interactions listed here are based on reports in scientific publications, laboratory experiments, or traditional use. It is important to always read product labels. People who have a medical condition, or are taking other drugs, herbs, or supplements, should consult a qualified healthcare provider before starting a new therapy.

Interactions with Drugs

- In theory, bromelain may increase the risk of bleeding when taken with drugs that increase the risk of bleeding. Examples are anticoagulants (blood thinners) such as warfarin (Coumadin) and heparin, antiplatelet drugs such as clopidogrel (Plavix), aspirin, and nonsteroidal anti-inflammatory drugs (NSAIDs) such as ibuprofen (Motrin, Advil) and naproxen (Naprosyn, Aleve). In addition, bromelain theoretically may add to the anti-inflammatory effects of NSAIDs.
- Studies in humans suggest that bromelain may increase the absorption of some antibiotics, notably amoxicillin and tetracycline, and increase levels of these drugs in the body. Bromelain may increase the actions of the chemotherapy (anti-cancer) drugs 5-fluorouracil and vincristine, although reliable scientific research in this area is lacking. In theory, the use of bromelain with blood pressure medications in the "ACE inhibitor" class, such as captopril (Capoten) and lisinopril (Zestril), may cause larger decreases in blood pressure than expected.
- Some experts suggest that bromelain may cause drowsiness or sedation and may increase the amount of drowsiness caused by some drugs. Examples are alcohol, some antidepressants, barbiturates such as phenobarbital, benzodiazepines such as lorazepam (Ativan) and diazepam (Valium), and narcotics such as codeine. Caution is advised in people who are driving or operating machinery.

Interactions with Herbs and Dietary Supplements

- In theory, bromelain may increase the risk of bleeding when taken with herbs and supplements that are believed to increase the risk of bleeding. Multiple cases of bleeding have been reported with the use of *Ginkgo biloba*, and fewer cases with garlic and with saw palmetto. Numerous other agents may theoretically increase the risk of bleeding, although this has not been proven in most cases. Examples

are alfalfa, American ginseng, angelica, anise, *Arnica montana*, asafetida, aspen bark, bilberry, birch, black cohosh, bladderwrack, bogbean, boldo, borage seed oil, capsicum, cat's claw, celery, chamomile, chaparral, clove, coleus, cordyceps, danshen, devil's claw, dong quai, eicosapentaenoic acid (EPA), evening primrose, fenugreek, feverfew, fish oil, flaxseed/flax powder (not a concern with flaxseed oil), ginger, grapefruit juice, grapeseed, green tea, guggul, gymnestra, horse chestnut, horseradish, licorice root, lovage root, male fern, meadowsweet, nordihydroguaiaretic acid (NDGA), onion, *Panax ginseng*, papain, parsley, passion flower, poplar, prickly ash, propolis, quassia, red clover, reishi, rue, Siberian ginseng, sweet birch, sweet clover, turmeric, vitamin E, white willow, wild carrot, wild lettuce, willow, wintergreen, and yucca.
- Based on preliminary studies in animals, bromelain and the enzyme trypsin may have stronger anti-inflammatory effects when combined. It has been suggested that zinc may block the effects of bromelain in the body, whereas magnesium may increase the effects, although scientific research in this area is lacking.

Interactions with Foods

- Some studies suggest that potato protein and soybeans may reduce the effects of bromelain in the body. Some experts recommend taking bromelain on an empty stomach.

Selected References

Natural Standard developed the preceding evidence-based information based on a systematic review of more than 250 scientific articles. For comprehensive information about alternative and complementary therapies on the professional level, go to www.naturalstandard.com. Selected references are listed here.

Balakrishnan V, Hareendran A, Nair CS. Double-blind cross-over trial of an enzyme preparation in pancreatic steatorrhoea. J Assoc Phys India 1981; 29(3):207-209.

Cirelli MG. Five years of clinical experience with bromelains in therapy of edema and inflammation in postoperative tissue reaction, skin infections and trauma. Clin Med 1967;74(6):55-59.

Cohen A, Goldman J. Bromelains therapy in rheumatoid arthritis. Penn Med J 1964;67:27-30.

Cowie DH, Fairweather DV, Newell DJ. A double-blind trial of bromelains as an adjunct to vaginal plastic repair operations. J Obstet Gynaecol Br Commonw 1970;77(4):365-368.

Gerard G. [Anticancer treatment and bromelains.] Agressologie 1972;13(4):261-274.

Glade MJ, Kendra D, Kaminski MV. Improvement in protein utilization in nursing-home patients on tube feeding supplemented with an enzyme product derived from *Aspergillus niger* and Bromelain. Nutrition 2001;17(4):348-350.

Gylling U, Rintala A, Taipale S, et al. The effect of a proteolytic enzyme combinate (bromelain) on the postoperative oedema by oral application. A clinical and experimental study. Acta Chir Scand 1966;131(3):193-196.

Hotz G, Frank T, Zoller J, et al. [Antiphlogistic effect of bromelaine following third molar removal.] Dtsch Zahnarztl Z 1989;44(11):830-832.

Howat RC, Lewis GD. The effect of bromelain therapy on episiotomy wounds—a double blind controlled clinical trial. J Obstet Gynaecol Br Commonw 1972;79(10):951-953.

Hunter RG, Henry GW, Civin WH. The action of papain and bromelain on the uterus. Part III. The physiologically incompetent internal cervical os. Am J Obst Gynec 1957;73(4):875-880.

Korlof B, Ponten B, Ugland O. Bromelain—a proteolytic enzyme. Scand J Plast Reconstr Surg 1969;3(1):27-29.

Kugener H, Bergmann D, Beck K. [Efficacy of bromelain in pancreatogenic digestive insufficiency.] Zeitschrift fur Gastroenterologie 1968;6:430-433.

Mader H. [Comparative studies on the effect of bromelin and oxyphenbutazone in episiotomy pains.] Schweiz Rundsch Med Prax 1973;62(35):1064-1068.

Masson M. [Bromelain in blunt injuries of the locomotor system. A study of observed applications in general practice.] Fortschr Med 1995;113(19):303-306.
Miller JM, Ginsberg M, McElfatrick GC, et al. The administration of bromelain orally in the treatment of inflammation and edema. Exper Med Surg 1964;22:293-299.
Mori S, Ojima Y, Hirose T, et al. The clinical effect of proteolytic enzyme containing bromelain and trypsin on urinary tract infection evaluated by double blind method. Acta Obstet Gynaecol Jpn 1972;19(3):147-153.
Morrison AW, Morrison MC. Bromelain—a clinical assessment in the post-operative treatment of arthrotomies of the knee and facial injuries. Brit J Clin Pract 1965;19(4):207-210.
Mudrak J, Bobak L, Sebova I. Adjuvant therapy with hydrolytic enzymes in recurrent laryngeal papillomatosis. Acta Otolaryngol Suppl 1997;527:128-130.
Ryan RE. A double-blind clinical evaluation of bromelains in the treatment of acute sinusitis. Headache 1967;7(1):13-17.
Seligman B. Bromelain: an anti-inflammatory agent. Angiology 1962;13:508-510.
Seligman B. Oral bromelains as adjuncts in the treatment of acute thrombophlebitis. Angiology 1969;20(1):22-26.
Seltzer AP. Adjunctive use of bromelains in sinusitis: a controlled study. Eye Ear Nose Throat Mon 1967;46(10):1281, 1284, 1286-1288.
Spaeth GL. The effect of bromelains on the inflammatory response caused by cataract extraction: a double-blind study. Eye Ear Nose Throat Mon 1968;47(12):634-639.
Stange R, Schneider R, Maurer R, et al. Proteolytic enzyme bromelaine enhances zytotoxicity in patients with breast cancer [abstract]. Nat Scien Conf Compl Altern Integ Med Res, Boston, April 12-14, 2002.
Tassman GC, Zafran JN, Zayon GM. A double-blind crossover study of a plant proteolytic enzyme in oral surgery. J Dent Med 1965;20(2):51-54.
Tassman GC, Zafran JN, Zayon GM. Evaluation of a plant proteolytic enzyme for the control of inflammation and pain. J Dental Med 1964;19(2):73-77.
Taub SJ. The use of bromelains in sinusitis: a double-blind clinical evaluation. Eye Ear Nose Throat Mon 1967;46(3):361.
Weiss S, Scherrer M. [Crossed double-blind trial of potassium iodide and bromelain (Traumanase) in chronic bronchitis.] Schweiz Rundsch Med Prax 1972;61(43):1331-1333.
Zatuchni GI, Colombi DJ. Bromelains therapy for the prevention of episiotomy pain. Obstet Gynecol 1967;29(2):275-278.

Burdock
(*Arctium lappa*)

RELATED TERMS

- Akujitsu, anthraxivore, arctii, *Arctium minus*, *Arctium tomentosa*, *Asteraceae (Compositae)*, bardana, Bardanae radix, bardane, bardane grande, beggar's buttons, burdock root, burr, burr seed, chin, clot-burr, Clotbur, cocklebur, cockle button, cuckold, daiki kishi, edible burdock, fox's clote, grass burdock, great bur, great burdock, gobo, grosse klette, happy major, hardock, hare burr, hurrburr, kletterwurzel, lampazo, lappola, love leaves, niu bang zi, oil of lappa, personata, philanthropium, thorny burr, turkey burrseed, wild gobo, woo-bang-ja.

BACKGROUND

- Burdock has historically been used to treat a wide variety of ailments, including arthritis, diabetes, and hair loss. It is a principal herbal ingredient in the popular cancer remedies Essiac (rhubarb, sorrel, and slippery elm) and Hoxsey formula (red clover, poke, prickly ash, bloodroot, and barberry).
- Burdock fruit has been reported to cause hypoglycemia in animals, and preliminary studies in humans have examined the efficacy of burdock root for diabetes. Studies in both animals and in the laboratory have explored the use of burdock for bacterial infections, cancer, HIV infection, and nephrolithiasis. Currently, scientific evidence is insufficient regarding the efficacy of burdock for any indication in humans.

USES BASED ON SCIENTIFIC EVIDENCE	Grade*
Diabetes Research in animals and initial studies in humans suggest that burdock root and fruit may decrease blood sugar levels. However, the studies in humans were not well designed, and further research is needed before a clear recommendation can be made.	**C**

*Key to grades: *A:* Strong scientific evidence for this use; *B:* Good scientific evidence for this use; *C:* Unclear scientific evidence for this use; *D:* Fair scientific evidence against this use (it may not work); *F:* Strong scientific evidence against this use (it likely does not work). For a more detailed explanation of efficacy criteria, see "Natural Standard Evidence-Based Validated Grading Rationale" in the Introduction.

Uses Based on Tradition, Theory, or Limited Scientific Evidence

Abscesses, acne, anorexia nervosa, aphrodisiac, arthritis, back pain, bacterial infections, bladder disorders, blood thinner, boils, burns, cancer, canker sores, common cold, cosmetic uses, dandruff, detoxification, diuretic (increasing urine flow), eczema, fever, fungal infections, gout, hair loss, headache, hemorrhoids,

Continued

Uses Based on Tradition, Theory, or Limited Scientific Evidence (*cont'd*)
hives, HIV infection, hormonal effects, ichthyosis (skin disorder), impotence, inflammation, kidney diseases, kidney stones, laxative, lice, liver disease, liver protection, measles, pneumonia, psoriasis, respiratory infections, rheumatoid arthritis, ringworm, sciatica, scurvy, seborrhea (overactivity of sebaceous skin glands), skin disorders, skin moisturizer, sores, sterility, syphilis, tonsillitis, ulcers, urinary tract infections, venereal diseases, warts, wound healing.

DOSING

The following doses are based on scientific research, publications, traditional use, or expert opinion. Many herbs and supplements have not been thoroughly tested, and their safety and effectiveness may not be proven. Brands may be made differently, with variable ingredients even within the same brand. The doses shown may not apply to all products. It is important to always read product labels and discuss doses with a qualified healthcare provider before therapy is started.

Standardization

- Standardization involves measuring the amounts of certain chemicals in products to try to make different preparations similar to each other. It is not always known if the chemicals being measured are the "active" ingredients. Currently, there is no widely accepted standardization for burdock products, and traditionally various preparations and doses have been used.

Adults (18 Years and Older)

- **Oral use (by mouth):** No specific dose of burdock has been proven effective or safe, although a wide range of doses and types of preparations have been used. As a dried root, the doses used include 2 to 6 g of pure dried root daily and 2 to 6 g of dried root in the form of a decoction three times daily. Burdock is available in 425- to 475-mg capsules. In a decoction (1:20), 500 ml daily has been used. In a tincture, 8 to 12 ml (1:5) three times daily, 2 to 8 ml (1:10 in 25% alcohol) three times daily, or one quarter to 1 teaspoon (1:10 in 45% alcohol) up to three times daily has been used. Burdock fluid extract (1:1 in 25% alcohol), has been used in doses of 2 to 8 ml three times daily. Burdock has also been used as a root tea, with 2 to 6 g of dried burdock root in 500 ml of water taken three times daily, or 1 cup 3 to 4 times daily, or 1 teaspoon of dried burdock root boiled in 3 cups of water for 30 minutes (up to 3 cups daily). Burdock has been used as a diuretic (to increase urine flow), with preparations made from powdered burdock seeds as a yellow product called oil of lappa.
- **Topical (on the skin):** Burdock has been used on the skin as a compress or plaster for eczema, psoriasis, baldness, and warts.

Children (Younger Than 18 Years)

- Scientific information is insufficient to recommend the use of burdock in children.

SAFETY

The U.S. Food and Drug Administration does not strictly regulate herbs and supplements. There is no guarantee of the strength, purity, or safety of products, and effects may vary. It is important

to always read product labels. People who have a medical condition, or are taking other drugs, herbs, or supplements, should consult a qualified healthcare provider before starting a new therapy. A healthcare provider should be contacted immediately about any side effects.

Allergies

- Allergic reactions to burdock may occur in people with allergies to members of the Asteraceae/Compositae family, including ragweed, chrysanthemums, marigolds, and daisies. Severe allergic reactions (anaphylaxis) have been associated with burdock use. Allergic skin reactions have been associated with the use of burdock plasters on the skin.

Side Effects and Warnings

- Based on traditional use, burdock is generally believed to be safe when taken by mouth in recommended doses for short periods of time. Handling the plant or using preparations on the skin (such as plasters) has occasionally been reported to cause allergic skin reactions. Diuretic effects (increasing urine flow) and estrogen-like effects have been reported with oral burdock use in people with HIV infection. Although reports of symptoms such as dry mouth and slow heart rate have been noted in persons taking burdock products, it is believed that contamination with belladonna may be responsible for these reactions. Contamination may occur during harvesting.
- In theory, tannins present in burdock may be toxic, although toxicity has not been reported in studies in animals. Tannins may cause stomach upset and in high concentrations may cause kidney or liver damage. Long-term use of tannins may increase the risk of head and neck cancers, although this has not been seen in humans. Based on research in animals and limited studies in humans, burdock may increase or reduce blood sugar levels. Caution is advised in people with diabetes or hypoglycemia, and in those taking drugs, other herbs, or supplements that affect blood sugar levels. Blood glucose levels may need monitoring by a qualified healthcare provider, and medication adjustments might be necessary. In theory, burdock may also cause electrolyte imbalances (for example, changes in potassium or sodium levels in the blood) due to diuretic effects (increasing urine flow).

Pregnancy and Breastfeeding

- Based on animal studies that showed that components of burdock caused uterus stimulation, burdock is sometimes recommended to be avoided during pregnancy. Because of limited scientific studies in this area, burdock cannot be considered safe for women during pregnancy or when breastfeeding.

INTERACTIONS

Most herbs and supplements have not been thoroughly tested for interactions with other herbs, supplements, drugs, or foods. The interactions listed here are based on reports in scientific publications, laboratory experiments, or traditional use. It is important to always read product labels. People who have a medical condition, or are taking other drugs, herbs, or supplements, should consult a qualified healthcare provider before starting a new therapy.

Interactions with Drugs

- Based on research in animals and limited studies in humans, burdock may decrease or raise blood sugar levels. Caution is advised in people who are using medications that may also affect blood sugar levels. Persons who are taking drugs for diabetes by mouth or insulin should be monitored closely by a qualified healthcare provider. Medication adjustments may be necessary. Burdock has been associated with diuretic effects (increasing urine flow) in one human report and in theory may cause excess fluid loss (dehydration) or electrolyte imbalances (for example, changes in potassium or sodium levels in the blood). These effects may be increased when burdock is taken at the same time as diuretic drugs such as chlorothiazide (Diuril), furosemide (Lasix), hydrochlorothiazide (HCTZ), or spironolactone (Aldactone). Based on limited human evidence that is not entirely clear, burdock may have estrogen-like properties and may act to increase the effects of estrogenic agents including hormone replacement therapies such as Premarin or birth control pills. Research in animals suggests that burdock may increase the risk of bleeding when taken with drugs that increase the risk of bleeding (although human research is lacking). Some examples include anticoagulants ("blood thinners") such as warfarin (Coumadin) and heparin, antiplatelet drugs such as clopidogrel (Plavix), aspirin, and nonsteroidal anti-inflammatory drugs such as ibuprofen (Motrin, Advil) and naproxen (Naprosyn, Aleve). Tinctures of burdock may contain high concentrations of alcohol (ethanol) and if these tinctures are used with disulfiram (Antabuse) or metronidazole (Flagyl), vomiting may result.

Interactions with Herbs and Dietary Supplements

- Research in animals and limited studies in humans suggest that burdock may decrease or raise blood sugar levels. Caution is advised in people who are using other herbs or supplements that can alter blood sugar levels. Blood glucose levels may require monitoring, and doses may need adjustment. Possible examples of herbs that may lower blood sugar are *Aloe vera*, American ginseng, bilberry, bitter melon, fenugreek, fish oil, gymnema, horse chestnut seed extract (HCSE), marshmallow, milk thistle, *Panax ginseng*, rosemary, Siberian ginseng, stinging nettle, and white horehound. Agents that may raise blood sugar levels include arginine, cocoa, and ephedra (when combined with caffeine).
- Burdock has been associated with diuretic effects (increasing urine flow) in one human report, and in theory may cause excess fluid loss (dehydration) or electrolyte imbalances (for example, changes in potassium or sodium levels in the blood) when used with other diuretic herbs or supplements such as artichoke, celery, corn silk, couchgrass, dandelion, elder flower, horsetail, juniper berry, kava, shepherd's purse, uva ursi, and yarrow. Because burdock may contain estrogen-like chemicals, the effects of other agents believed to have estrogen-like properties may be altered. Possible examples include alfalfa, black cohosh, bloodroot, hops, kudzu, licorice, pomegranate, red clover, soy, thyme, white horehound, and yucca. These possible interactions are based on initial, unclear evidence.
- Studies in animals suggest that burdock may increase the risk of bleeding when taken with other herbs and supplements that are believed to increase the risk of bleeding. Multiple cases of bleeding have been reported with the use of *Ginkgo biloba*, fewer cases with garlic, and two cases with saw palmetto. Numerous other agents may theoretically increase the risk of bleeding, although this has not been proven in most cases. Examples of such agents are alfalfa, American ginseng, angelica, anise, *Arnica montana*, asafetida, aspen bark, bilberry, birch, black cohosh, bladderwrack, bogbean, boldo, borage seed oil, bromelain, capsicum, cat's claw, celery, chamomile, chaparral, clove, coleus, cordyceps, danshen, devil's claw, dong

quai, evening primrose, fenugreek, feverfew, flaxseed/flax powder (not a concern with flaxseed oil), ginger, grapefruit juice, grapeseed, green tea, guggul, gymnestra, horse chestnut, horseradish, licorice root, lovage root, male fern, meadowsweet, nordihydroguaiaretic acid (NDGA), onion, *Panax ginseng*, papain, parsley, passion flower, poplar, prickly ash, propolis, quassia, red clover, reishi, rue, Siberian ginseng, sweet birch, sweet clover, turmeric, vitamin E, white willow, wild carrot, wild lettuce, willow, wintergreen, and yucca.

Selected References

Natural Standard developed the preceding evidence-based information based on a systematic review of more than 60 scientific articles. For comprehensive information about alternative and complementary therapies on the professional level, go to www.naturalstandard.com. Selected references are listed here.

Anonymous. In vitro screening of traditional medicines for anti-HIV activity: memorandum from a WHO meeting. Bull World Health Org 1989;67(6):613-618.

Flickinger EA, Hatch TF, Wofford RC, et al. In vitro fermentation properties of selected fructooligosaccharide-containing vegetables and in vivo colonic microbial populations are affected by the diets of healthy human infants. J Nutr 2002;132(8):2188-2194.

Grases F, Melero G, Costa-Bauza A, et al. Urolithiasis and phytotherapy. Int Urol Nephrol 1994;26(5):507-511.

Holetz FB, Pessini GL, Sanches NR, et al. Screening of some plants used in the Brazilian folk medicine for the treatment of infectious diseases. Mem Inst Oswaldo Cruz 2002;97(7): 1027-1031.

Iwakami S, Wu JB, Ebizuka Y, et al. Platelet activating factor (PAF) antagonists contained in medicinal plants: lignans and sesquiterpenes. Chem Pharm Bull (Tokyo) 1992;40(5): 1196-1198.

Lin CC, Lu JM, Yang JJ, et al. Anti-inflammatory and radical scavenge effects of *Arctium lappa*. Am J Chin Med 1996;24(2):127-137.

Lin SC, Chung TC, Lin CC, et al. Hepatoprotective effects of *Arctium lappa* on carbon tetrachloride- and acetaminophen-induced liver damage. Am J Chin Med 2000;28(2): 163-173.

Lin SC, Lin CH, Lin CC, et al. Hepatoprotective effects of *Arctium lappa* Linné on liver injuries induced by chronic ethanol consumption and potentiated by carbon tetrachloride. J Biomed Sci 2002;9(5):401-409.

Morita K, Kada T, Namiki M. A desmutagenic factor isolated from burdock (*Arctium lappa* Linné). Mutat Res 1984;129(1):25-31.

Os'kina OA, Pashinskii VG, Kanakina TA, et al. The mechanisms of the anti-ulcer action of plant drug agents [Article in Russian]. Eksp Klin Farmakol 1999;62(4):37-39.

Rodriguez P, Blanco J, Juste S, et al. Allergic contact dermatitis due to burdock (*Arctium lappa*). Contact Dermatitis 1995;33(2):134-135.

Sasaki Y, Kimura Y, Tsunoda T, et al. Anaphylaxis due to burdock. Int J Dermatol 2003; 42(6):472-473.

Swanston-Flatt SK, Day C, Flatt PR, et al. Glycaemic effects of traditional European plant treatments for diabetes. Studies in normal and streptozotocin diabetic mice. Diabetes Res 1989;10(2):69-73.

Xie LH, Ahn EM, Akao T, et al. Transformation of arctiin to estrogenic and antiestrogenic substances by human intestinal bacteria. Chem Pharm Bull (Tokyo) 2003;51(4):378-384.

Yang L, Lin S, Yang T, et al. Synthesis of anti-HIV activity of dibenzylbutyrolactone lignans. Bioorganic Medicinal Chem Lett 1996;6:941-944.

Yao XJ, Wainberg MA, Parniak MA. Mechanism of inhibition of HIV-1 infection in vitro by purified extract of *Prunella vulgaris*. Virology 1992;187(1):56-62.

Calendula

(*Calendula officinalis* L., Marigold)

RELATED TERMS

- Asteraceae, bride of the sun, bull thistle flower, butterwort, *Caltha officinalis*, *Calendula arvensis* L., calendulae flos, calendula flower, calendulae herba, calendula herb, claveton, Compositae, cowbloom, death-flower, drunkard gold, fior d'ogni, flaminquillo, fleurs de tous les mois, gauche-fer, gold bloom, goldblume, golden flower of Mary, goulans, gouls, holligold, holygold, husband's dial, kingscup, maravilla, marigold, marybud, marygold, mejorana, poet's marigold, pot marigold, publican and sinner, ringelblume, ruddles, Scotch marigold, shining herb, solsequia, souci, souci des champs, souci des jardins, summer's bride, sun's bride, water dragon, yolk of egg.
- *Note:* Calendula, or marigold, should not be confused with the common garden or French marigold (*Tagetes*), African marigold (*T. erecta*), or Inca marigold (*T. minuta*).

BACKGROUND

- Calendula, also known as marigold, traditionally has been widely used on the skin to treat minor wounds, skin infections, burns, bee stings, sunburn, warts, and cancer. Most scientific evidence regarding its effectiveness as a wound-healing agent is based on laboratory research and studies in the laboratory and in animals, but studies in humans are limited.

USES BASED ON SCIENTIFIC EVIDENCE	Grade*
Ear infections Calendula has been studied for reducing pain caused by ear infections. Some randomized controlled trials in humans suggest that calendula may possess mild anesthetic (pain-relieving) properties equal to those of similar non-herbal ear drop preparations. Further studies are needed before a recommendation can be made in this area.	C
Skin inflammation Limited animal research suggests that calendula extracts may reduce inflammation when applied to the skin. Studies in humans are lacking in this area.	C
Wound and burn healing Calendula is commonly used on the skin to treat minor wounds. A small number of studies in animals and poor-quality studies in humans reported that calendula reduced healing time and increased the strength	C

Continued

of healed areas. Reliable human research studies are necessary before a firm conclusion can be drawn.

*Key to grades: *A:* Strong scientific evidence for this use; *B:* Good scientific evidence for this use; *C:* Unclear scientific evidence for this use; *D:* Fair scientific evidence against this use (it may not work); *F:* Strong scientific evidence against this use (it likely does not work). For a more detailed explanation of efficacy criteria, see "Natural Standard Evidence-Based Validated Grading Rationale" in the Introduction.

Uses Based on Tradition, Theory, or Limited Scientific Evidence

Abscesses, acne, anemia, antioxidant, antiviral agent, anxiety, appetite stimulant, atherosclerosis (clogged arteries), athlete's foot, bacterial infections, benign prostatic hypertrophy, bladder irritation, "blood purifier," blood vessel clots, bowel irritation, bruises, cholera, circulation problems, conjunctivitis, constipation, cough, cramps, diaper rash, diuretic, dizziness, eczema, edema, eye inflammation, fatigue, fever, frostbite, fungal infections, gastrointestinal tract disorders, gingivitis, gout, headache, heart disease, hemorrhoids, HIV infections, HSV infections, immune system stimulant, indigestion, influenza, insomnia, jaundice, liver cancer, liver dysfunction, menstrual period abnormalities, metabolic disorders, mouth and throat infections, muscle wasting, nausea, nervous system disorders, nosebleed, pain, prostatitis, ringing in the ears, skin cancer, sore throat, spasms, spleen disorders, stomach ulcers, syphilis, toothache, tuberculosis, ulcerative colitis, urinary retention, uterus problems, varicose veins, warts, yeast infections.

DOSING

The following doses are based on scientific research, publications, traditional use, or expert opinion. Many herbs and supplements have not been thoroughly tested, and their safety and effectiveness may not be proven. Brands may be made differently, with variable ingredients even within the same brand. The doses shown may not apply to all products. It is important to always read product labels and discuss doses with a qualified healthcare provider before therapy is started.

Adults (18 Years and Older)

- **Ointment applied to the skin:** According to two European expert panels (the German Commission E and the European Scientific Cooperative on Phytotherapy [ESCOP]), a 2% to 5% ointment has been used. Preparations have been applied 3 to 4 times daily as needed.
- **Tincture/compress applied to the skin:** A 1:1 tincture in 40% alcohol or a 1:5 tincture in 90% alcohol, diluted at least 1:3 with freshly boiled water, has been applied to the skin as a compress 3 to 4 times daily.
- **Ear drops:** For ear infections, the combination herbal product Otikon Otic (which includes calendula) has been used in a dose of 5 drops placed in the affected ear 3 times daily.

Children (Younger Than 18 Years)

- Currently, scientific evidence is insufficient to recommend the use of calendula in children.

SAFETY

The U.S. Food and Drug Administration does not strictly regulate herbs and supplements. There is no guarantee of the strength, purity, or safety of products, and effects may vary. It is important to always read product labels. People who have a medical condition, or are taking other drugs, herbs, or supplements, should consult a qualified healthcare provider before starting a new therapy. A healthcare provider should be contacted immediately about any side effects.

Allergies

- People with allergies to plants in the Asteraceae/Compositae family such as ragweed, chrysanthemums, marigolds, and daisies are likely to have an allergic reaction to calendula. One case has been reported of a person who had a severe allergic reaction (anaphylactic shock) after gargling with a calendula preparation.

Side Effects and Warnings

- Aside from allergic reactions, few severe reactions are found in published reports. In one small study in animals, calendula was associated with a fatal decrease in blood glucose levels, accompanied by decreased serum lipids and protein. Skin and eye irritation have been reported.

Pregnancy and Breastfeeding

- It is not clear whether calendula is safe for use during pregnancy or breastfeeding. In studies in animals, calendula had effects on the uterus. Traditionally, calendula has been believed to have harmful effects on sperm and to cause abortions. It is not clear whether these effects occur with the use of calendula on the skin.

INTERACTIONS

Most herbs and supplements have not been thoroughly tested for interactions with other herbs, supplements, drugs, or foods. The interactions listed here are based on reports in scientific publications, laboratory experiments, or traditional use. It is important to always read product labels. People who have a medical condition, or are taking other drugs, herbs, or supplements, should consult a qualified healthcare provider before starting a new therapy.

Interactions with Drugs

- In early studies in animals, high doses of calendula were reported to cause drowsiness. It is not clear if use of calendula on the skin of humans has this effect. In theory, calendula used in combination with sedative drugs may cause increased drowsiness. Examples of such drugs are alcohol, some antidepressants, barbiturates such as phenobarbital, benzodiazepines such as lorazepam (Ativan) and diazepam (Valium), and narcotics such as codeine. Caution is advised in people who are driving or operating machinery.
- In early studies in animals, high doses of calendula preparations were reported to lower blood pressure. It is not clear if use of calendula on the skin of humans has this effect. In theory, calendula used in combination with drugs that lower blood pressure may lead to increased effects.

- Other possible interactions include increases in the activity of hypoglycemic (diabetic) medications, insulin, and agents that decrease lipids and triglycerides (cholesterol-lowering drugs).

Interactions with Herbs and Dietary Supplements

- In early studies in animals, high doses of calendula were reported to cause drowsiness. It is not clear if use of calendula on the skin of humans has this effect. In theory, calendula used in combination with herbs or supplements that have possible sedative effects may lead to increased drowsiness. Examples are calamus, California poppy, capsicum, catnip, celery, couch grass, dogwood, elecampane, German chamomile, goldenseal, gotu kola, hops, kava (may help sleep without drowsiness), lavender aromatherapy, lemon balm, sage, sassafras, shepherd's purse, Siberian ginseng, skullcap, St. John's wort, stinging nettle, valerian, wild carrot, wild lettuce, withania root, and yerba mansa. Caution is advised in people who are driving or operating machinery.
- In early studies in animals, high doses of calendula preparations were reported to lower blood pressure. It is not clear if use of calendula on the skin of humans has this effect. In theory, calendula used in combination with herbs that may lower blood pressure may lead to increased effects. Examples are aconite/monkshood, arnica, baneberry, betel nut, bilberry, black cohosh, bryony, California poppy, coleus, curcumin, eucalyptol, eucalyptus oil, ginger, goldenseal, green hellebore, hawthorn, Indian tobacco, jaborandi, mistletoe, night-blooming cereus, oleander, pasque flower, periwinkle, pleurisy root, shepherd's purse, Texas milkweed, turmeric, and wild cherry.
- Other possible interactions include increases in the activity of hypoglycemic (diabetic) medications, insulin, and agents that decrease lipids and triglycerides (cholesterol-lowering agents).
- Because the stem and leaves of calendula contain lutein and beta-carotene, interaction of calendula preparations is possible with other products that contain these ingredients.

Selected References

Natural Standard developed the preceding evidence-based information based on a systematic review of more than 200 scientific articles. For comprehensive information about alternative and complementary therapies on the professional level, go to www.naturalstandard.com. Selected references are listed here.

Anonymous. Final report on the safety assessment of *Calendula officinalis* extract and *Calendula officinalis*. Int J Toxicol 2001;20(Suppl 2):13-20.

Cordova CA, Siqueira IR, Netto CA, et al. Protective properties of butanolic extract of the *Calendula officinalis* L. (marigold) against lipid peroxidation of rat liver microsomes and action as free radical scavenger. Redox Rep 2002;7(2):95-102.

Della Loggia R, et al. Topical anti-inflammatory activity of *Calendula officinalis* extracts. Planta Med 1990;56:658.

Hamburger M, Adler S, Baumann D, et al. Preparative purification of the major anti-inflammatory triterpenoid esters from Marigold (*Calendula officinalis*). Fitoterapia 2003; 74(4):328-338.

Kartikeyan S, Chaturvedi RM, Narkar SV. Effect of calendula on trophic ulcers. Lepr Rev 1990;61(4):399.

Krazhan IA, Garazha NN. [Treatment of chronic catarrhal gingivitis with polysorb-immobilized calendula.] Stomatologiia (Mosk) 2001;80(5):11-13.

Lavagna SM, Secci D, Chimenti P, et al. Efficacy of *Hypericum* and *Calendula* oils in the epithelial reconstruction of surgical wounds in childbirth with caesarean section. Farmaco 2001;56(5-7):451-453.
Lievre M, et al. Controlled study of three ointments for the local management of 2nd and 3rd degree burns. Clinical Trials and Meta-analysis 1992;28:9-12.
Sarrell EM, Mandelberg A, Cohen HA. Efficacy of naturopathic extracts in the management of ear pain associated with acute otitis media. Arch Pediatr Adolesc Med 2001;155(7):796-799.

Chamomile

(*Matricaria recutita, Chamaemelum nobile*)

C

Related Terms

- *Anthemis arvensis*, *Anthemis cotula*, *Anthemis nobile*, *Anthemis nobilis*, Asteraceae/Compositae, baboonig, babuna, babunah camomile, babunj, bunga kamil, camamila, camomile, camomile sauvage, camomilla, camomille allemande, Campomilla, *Chamaemelum nobile* L., Chamomilla, chamomilla recutita, chamomillae ramane flos, chamomille commune, classic chamomile, common chamomile, double chamomile, echte kamille, English chamomile, feldkamille, fleur de camomile, fleurs de petite camomille, flores anthemidis, flos chamomillae, garden chamomile, German chamomile, grosse kamille, grote kamille, ground apple, Hungarian chamomile, kamille, kamillen, Kamillosan, kamitsure, kamiture, kleine, kleme kamille, lawn chamomile, low chamomile, manzanilla, manzanilla chiquita, manzanilla comun, manzanilla dulce, *Matricaria chamomilla*, *Matricaria recutita*, *Matricaria suaveolens*, matricariae flos, matricariae flowers, matricaire, may-then, nervine, pin heads, rauschert, romaine, romaine manzanilla, Roman chamomile, romische kamille, single chamomile, sweet chamomile, sweet false chamomile, sweet feverfew, true chamomile, whig-plant, wild chamomile.

Background

- Chamomile has been used medicinally for thousands of years and is widely used in Europe. It is a popular treatment for numerous ailments, including sleep disorders, anxiety, diaper rash, digestion/intestinal conditions, infantile colic, skin infections/inflammation (including eczema), teething pains, and wound healing. In the United States, chamomile is best known as an ingredient in herbal tea preparations proposed to have mild sedating effects.
- German chamomile (*Matricaria recutita*) and Roman chamomile (*Chamaemelum nobile*) are the two major types of chamomile used for health conditions. They are believed to have similar effects on the body, although German chamomile may be slightly stronger. Most research has focused on German chamomile, which is more commonly used everywhere except in England, where Roman chamomile is more common.
- Although chamomile is widely used, there is not enough reliable research in humans to support its use for any condition. Despite its reputation as a gentle medicinal plant, there have been many reports of allergic reactions (including life-threatening anaphylaxis) in people after eating or coming into contact with chamomile preparations.

USES BASED ON SCIENTIFIC EVIDENCE	Grade*
Common cold One study reported that inhaling steam with chamomile extract improved common cold symptoms. More extensive and better-quality research is needed before a recommendation can be made.	C

Continued

Diarrhea in children One study reported that chamomile with apple pectin may reduce the length of time that children experience diarrhea. However, neither the design nor the results were well reported, and it is unclear whether the benefits reported were owing to the effects of chamomile or of the apple pectin.	C
Gastrointestinal conditions Chamomile is used traditionally for numerous gastrointestinal conditions, including digestion disorders, "spasm" or colic, upset stomach, flatulence (gas), ulcers, and gastrointestinal irritation. However, there have been no reliable studies in humans in these areas. In large doses, chamomile may cause vomiting.	C
Hemorrhagic cystitis (bladder irritation with bleeding) One poor-quality study reported that the combination of chamomile baths, chamomile bladder washes, and antibiotics was superior to antibiotics alone as therapy for hemorrhagic cystitis. Additional research is necessary before a conclusion can be reached. Hemorrhagic cystitis is a potentially serious condition for which medical attention should be sought.	C
Hemorrhoids One poor-quality study reported that chamomile ointment may improve hemorrhoids. Better evidence is needed before a recommendation can be made.	C
Mucositis from cancer treatment (mouth ulcers/irritation) Poor-quality studies have used chamomile mouthwash for the prevention or treatment of mouth mucositis caused by radiation therapy or cancer chemotherapy. Results are conflicting, and it remains unclear whether chamomile is helpful in this situation.	C
Quality of life in cancer patients A small amount of research suggests that massage using chamomile essential oil may improve anxiety and quality of life in patients with cancer. However, this evidence is not of high quality, and it is unclear whether this approach is superior to massage alone without essential oils. Additional study is needed before a firm conclusion can be reached.	C
Skin conditions (eczema/radiation damage/wound healing) Laboratory research and studies in animals have reported that chamomile has anti-inflammatory properties. Studies in humans suggest that chamomile ointment may work as well as hydrocortisone cream for eczema and that it may improve wound healing, but that chamomile cream may not work as well as almond oil for treating skin damage after radiation therapy. Relief of inflammation and itching has been observed in clinical trials. These studies were not well designed or reported, and better-quality research is needed before a firm conclusion can be reached.	C

Continued

Sleep aid/sedation Traditionally, chamomile preparations such as tea and essential oil aromatherapy have been used for insomnia and sedation (calming effects). Small, poor-quality studies have reported mild hypnotic effects of chamomile aromatherapy and possible sedative properties of tea. However, there are no well-designed trials in humans in these areas. Better-quality research is needed before a recommendation can be made.	**C**
Vaginitis (inflammation of the vagina) Symptoms of vaginitis include itching, discharge, and pain with urination. A small study reported that chamomile douche improved symptoms of vaginitis with few side effects. Because vaginitis can be caused by infection (including sexually transmitted diseases), poor hygiene, or nutritional deficiencies, people with this condition should consult a qualified healthcare provider. More extensive and better-quality research studies are needed before a conclusion can be drawn regarding the role of chamomile in the management of vaginitis.	**C**
Postoperative sore throat/hoarseness due to intubation A trial in humans compared chamomile extract spray with normal saline spray (control), administered before placement of a breathing (endotracheal) tube, to determine effects on postoperative sore throat and hoarseness. Results did not show that chamomile prevented postoperative sore throat and hoarseness any more effectively than normal saline.	**D**

*Key to grades: *A:* Strong scientific evidence for this use; *B:* Good scientific evidence for this use; *C:* Unclear scientific evidence for this use; *D:* Fair scientific evidence against this use (it may not work); *F:* Strong scientific evidence against this use (it likely does not work). For a more detailed explanation of efficacy criteria, see "Natural Standard Evidence-Based Validated Grading Rationale" in the Introduction.

Uses Based on Tradition, Theory, or Limited Scientific Evidence

Abdominal bloating, abrasions, abscesses, acne, anorexia, antibacterial, antifungal, anti-inflammatory, antioxidant, anxiety, arthritis, back pain, bedsores, blocked tear ducts, burns, cancer, carpal tunnel syndrome, chickenpox, constipation, contact dermatitis, convulsions, delirium tremens (DTs), diaper rash, diaphoretic, diuretic, (increasing urine flow), dysmenorrhea, ear infections, eye infections, fever, fistula healing, flatulence (gas), frostbite, fungal infections, gingivitis, gum irritation, hay fever, heartburn, heat rash, hives, impetigo, infantile colic, insect bites, irritable bowel syndrome, liver disorders, malaria, mastitis (breast inflammation), menstrual disorders, morning sickness, motion sickness, neuralgia (nerve pain), nausea, parasites/worms, poison ivy, psoriasis, restlessness, sciatica, sea sickness, seizure disorder, sinusitis, skin infections, teething pain (mouth rinse), uterine disorders.

DOSING

The following doses are based on scientific research, publications, traditional use, or expert opinion. Many herbs and supplements have not been thoroughly tested, and their safety and effectiveness may not be proven. Brands may be made differently, with variable ingredients even within the same brand. The doses shown may not apply to all products. It is important to always read product labels and discuss doses with a qualified healthcare provider before therapy is started.

Standardization

- Standardization involves measuring the amounts of certain chemicals in products to try to make different preparations similar to each other. It is not always known if the chemicals being measured are the "active" ingredients.
- Most American chamomile products are not standardized to any particular constituent. Many German chamomile products, such as Kamillosan, which contains 20 mg chamomile essential oil per 100 g of cream, are standardized to a minimum value of chamazulene and alpha-bisobolol. Tablets and capsules of chamomile may be standardized to contain 1.2% apigenin and 0.5% essential oil per dose. Examples of standardized chamomile preparations are Nutritional Dynamics German Chamomile (400 mg of chamomile flower per capsule, standardized to 1.25% apigenin and 0.5% essential oil), Nature's Way German chamomile (125 mg of extract standardized to 1.25% apigenin, and 350 mg of chamomile flower per capsule).

Adults (18 Years and Older)

- **Tea/infusion:** Traditional doses include tea made from 150 ml of boiling water poured over 2 to 4 g of fresh flower heads and steeped for 10 minutes, taken by mouth three times daily. One to 4 cups of chamomile tea (made from tea bags) taken daily has also been used.
- **Liquid extract/tincture:** As a liquid extract (1:1 in 45% alcohol), 1 to 4 ml taken by mouth three times daily has been used. As a tincture (1:5 in alcohol), 15 ml taken three or four times daily has been used.
- **Capsules/tablets:** 400 to 1600 mg taken by mouth daily in divided doses has been used.
- **Skin use:** There are no standard doses for chamomile used on the skin. Some natural medicine publications have recommended paste, plaster, or ointment containing 3% to 10% chamomile flower heads.
- **Douche:** There is no standard or well-studied dose for chamomile used as a douche. Some natural medicine publications have recommended a preparation containing 3% to 10% chamomile.
- **Mouth-rinse/gargle:** 1% fluid extract or 5% tincture has been used.
- **Bath:** 5 g of chamomile or 0.8 g of alcoholic extract per liter of water has been used.

Children (Younger Than 18 Years)

- Reliable scientific data are insufficient to recommend the safe use of chamomile products in children. Some natural medicine publications recommend that the dose of chamomile tea for children should be half of the adult dose.

SAFETY

The U.S. Food and Drug Administration does not strictly regulate herbs and supplements. There is no guarantee of the strength, purity, or safety of products, and effects may vary. It is important

to always read product labels. People who have a medical condition, or are taking other drugs, herbs, or supplements, should consult a qualified healthcare provider before starting a new therapy. A healthcare provider should be contacted immediately about any side effects.

Allergies

- There have been multiple reports of serious allergic reactions (including anaphylaxis, throat swelling, and shortness of breath) to chamomile taken by mouth or used as an enema. Skin allergic reactions have been reported frequently, including dermatitis and eczema. Chamomile eyewash can cause allergic conjunctivitis (pink eye).
- People with allergies to other plants in the Asteraceae/Compositae family should avoid chamomile. Examples are aster, chrysanthemum, mugwort, ragweed, and ragwort. Cross-reactions may occur with birch pollen, celery, chrysanthemum, feverfew, and tansy. Individuals with allergies to these plants should avoid chamomile.

Side Effects and Warnings

- Impurities (adulterants) in chamomile products are common and may cause adverse effects.
- Chamomile in various forms may cause drowsiness or sedation. Caution should be used in people who are driving or operating heavy machinery. In large doses, chamomile can cause vomiting.
- Because of its coumarin content, chamomile may theoretically increase the risk of bleeding. Caution is advised in people who have bleeding disorders or are taking drugs that may increase the risk of bleeding. Dosing adjustments may be necessary.
- One poor-quality study reported slight increases in blood pressure from chamomile, but the evidence is insufficient to make a firm conclusion.

Pregnancy and Breastfeeding

- In theory, chamomile may act as a uterine stimulant or lead to abortion. Therefore, its use should be avoided during pregnancy. There are insufficient scientific data to recommend the safe use of chamomile by women who are breastfeeding.

INTERACTIONS

Most herbs and supplements have not been thoroughly tested for interactions with other herbs, supplements, drugs, or foods. The interactions listed here are based on reports in scientific publications, laboratory experiments, or traditional use. It is important to always read product labels. People who have a medical condition, or are taking other drugs, herbs, or supplements, should consult a qualified healthcare provider before starting a new therapy.

Interactions with Drugs

- Interactions of chamomile with drugs have not been well studied.
- Chamomile may increase the level of drowsiness caused by some drugs. Examples are alcohol, some antidepressants, barbiturates such as phenobarbital, benzodiazepines such as lorazepam (Ativan) and diazepam (Valium), and narcotics such as codeine. Caution is advised in people who are driving or operating machinery.
- In theory, chamomile may increase the risk of bleeding when used with anticoagulants or antiplatelet drugs. Examples are anticoagulants (blood thinners) such as warfarin (Coumadin) and heparin, antiplatelet drugs such as clopidogrel (Plavix), aspirin, and nonsteroidal anti-inflammatory drugs (NSAIDs) such as ibuprofen (Motrin, Advil) and naproxen (Naprosyn, Aleve).

- Limited laboratory research and studies in animals suggest that chamomile may interfere with how the body uses the liver's cytochrome P450 enzyme system to process components of some drugs. As a result, blood levels of these components may be elevated and may cause increased effects or potentially serious adverse reactions. People who are using any medications should always read the package insert and consult with their healthcare provider or pharmacist about possible interactions. This effect of chamomile has not been reliably tested in humans.
- *Note*: Many tinctures contain high levels of alcohol and may cause vomiting when taken with metronidazole (Flagyl) and disulfiram (Antabuse).

Interactions with Herbs and Dietary Supplements

- Chamomile may increase the level of drowsiness caused by some herbs or supplements. Examples are calamus, calendula, California poppy, capsicum, catnip, celery, couch grass, dogwood, elecampane, goldenseal, gotu kola, hops, kava (may help sleep without drowsiness), lavender aromatherapy, lemon balm, sage, sassafras, scullcap, shepherd's purse, Siberian ginseng, stinging nettle, St. John's wort, valerian, wild carrot, wild lettuce, withania root, and yerba mansa. Caution is advised in people who are driving or operating machinery.
- In theory, chamomile may increase the risk of bleeding when taken with other products that are believed to increase the risk of bleeding. Multiple cases of bleeding have been reported with the use of *Ginkgo biloba*, and fewer cases with garlic and saw palmetto. Numerous other agents may theoretically increase the risk of bleeding, although this has not been proven in most cases. Examples are alfalfa, American ginseng, angelica, anise, *Arnica montana*, asafetida, aspen bark, bilberry, birch, black cohosh, bladderwrack, bogbean, boldo, borage seed oil, bromelain, capsicum, cat's claw, celery, chaparral, clove, coleus, cordyceps, danshen, devil's claw, dong quai, evening primrose, fenugreek, feverfew, flaxseed/flax powder (not a concern with flaxseed oil), ginger, grapefruit juice, grape seed, green tea, guggul, gymnestra, horseradish, licorice root, lovage root, male fern, meadowsweet, nordihydroguaiaretic acid (NDGA), onion, *Panax ginseng*, papain, parsley, passion flower, poplar, prickly ash, propolis, quassia, red clover, reishi, rue, Siberian ginseng, sweet birch, sweet clover, turmeric, vitamin E, white willow, wild carrot, wild lettuce, willow, wintergreen, and yucca.
- Limited laboratory research and studies in animals suggest that chamomile may interfere with how the body uses the liver's cytochrome P450 enzyme system to processes components of other herbs and supplements. As a result, blood levels of these components may be elevated. Chamomile may alter the effects of other herbs on the cytochrome P450 system. Examples of such herbs are bloodroot, cat's claw, chaparral, chasteberry, damiana, *Echinacea angustifolia*, goldenseal, grapefruit juice, licorice, oregano, red clover, St. John's wort, wild cherry, and yucca. People who are using any medications should always read the package insert and consult their healthcare provider or pharmacist about possible interactions.

Selected References

Natural Standard developed the preceding evidence-based information based on a systematic review of more than 160 articles. For comprehensive information about alternative and complementary therapies on the professional level, go to www.naturalstandard.com. Selected references are listed here.

Aertgeerts P, Albring M, Klaschka F, et al. [Comparative testing of Kamillosan cream and steroidal (0.25% hydrocortisone, 0.75% fluocortin butyl ester) and non-steroidal (5% bufexamac) dermatologic agents in maintenance therapy of eczematous diseases.] Z Hautkr 1985;60(3):270-277.

Balslev T, Moller AB. [Burns in children caused by camomile tea.] Ugeskr Laeger 1990; 152(19):1384.

Benetti C, Manganelli F. [Clinical experiences in the pharmacological treatment of vaginitis with a camomile-extract vaginal douche.] Minerva Ginecol 1985;37(12):799-801.

Benner MH, Lee HJ. Anaphylactic reaction to chamomile tea. J Allergy Clin Immunol 1973; 52(5):307-308.

Carl W, Emrich LS. Management of oral mucositis during local radiation and systemic chemotherapy: a study of 98 patients. J Prosthet Dent 1991;66(3):361-369.

Casterline CL. Allergy to chamomile tea. JAMA 1980;244(4):330-331.

de la Motte S, Bose-O'Reilly S, Heinisch M, et al. [Double-blind comparison of an apple pectin-chamomile extract preparation with placebo in children with diarrhea.] Arzneimittelforschung 1997;47(11):1247-1249.

de la Torre MF, Sanchez Machin I, Garcia Robaina JC, et al. Clinical cross-reactivity between *Artemisia vulgaris* and *Matricaria chamomilla* (chamomile). J Investig Allergol Clin Immunol 2001;11(2):118-122.

Fidler P, Loprinzi CL, O'Fallon JR, et al. Prospective evaluation of a chamomile mouthwash for prevention of 5-FU-induced oral mucositis. Cancer 1996;77(3):522-525.

Foti C, Nettis E, Panebianco R, et al. Contact urticaria from *Matricaria chamomilla*. Contact Dermatitis 2000;42(6):360-361.

Giordano-Labadie F, Schwarze HP, Bazex J. Allergic contact dermatitis from camomile used in phytotherapy. Contact Dermatitis 2000;42(4):247.

Gowania HJ, Raulin C, Swoboda M. [Effect of chamomile on wound healing—a clinical double-blind study.] Z Hautkr 1987;62(17):1262, 1267-1271.

Gould L, Reddy CV, Gomprecht RF. Cardiac effects of chamomile tea. J Clin Pharmacol 1973;13(11):475-479.

Jensen-Jarolim E, Reider N, Fritsch R, et al. Fatal outcome of anaphylaxis to camomile-containing enema during labor: a case study. J Allergy Clin Immunol 1998;102(6 Pt 1): 1041-1042.

Kagawa D, Jokura H, Ochiai R, Tokimitsu I, Tsubone H. The sedative effects and mechanism of action of cedrol inhalation with behavioral pharmacological evaluation. Planta Med 2003;69(7):637-641.

Kyokong O, Charuluxananan S, Muangmingsuk V, et al. Efficacy of chamomile-extract spray for prevention of post-operative sore throat. J Med Assoc Thai 2002;85(Suppl 1): S180-S185.

Maiche A, Grohn P, Maki-Hokkonen H. Effect of chamomile cream and almond ointment on acute radiation skin reaction. Acta Oncol 1991;30:395-397.

Maiche A, Maki-Hokkonen H, Grohn P. [Comparative trial of chamomile cream in radiotherapy.] Suomen Laakarilehti 1991;46(24):2206-2208.

Maliakal PP, Wanwimolruk S. Effect of herbal teas on hepatic drug metabolizing enzymes in rats. J Pharm Pharmacol 2001;53(10):1323-1329.

McGeorge BC, Steele MC. Allergic contact dermatitis of the nipple from Roman chamomile ointment. Contact Dermatitis 1991;24(2):139-140.

Patzelt-Wenczler R, Ponce-Poschl E. Proof of efficacy of Kamillosan cream in atopic eczema. Eur J Med Res 2000;5:171-175.

Paulsen E. Contact sensitization from Compositae-containing herbal remedies and cosmetics. Contact Dermatitis 2002;47(4):189-198.

Pereira F, Santos R, Pereira A. Contact dermatitis from chamomile tea. Contact Dermatitis 1997;36(6):307.

Reider N, Sepp N, Fritsch P, et al. Anaphylaxis to camomile: clinical features and allergen cross-reactivity. Clin Exp Allergy 2000;30(10):1436-1443.

Rodriguez B, Rodriguez A, de Barrio M, et al. Asthma induced by canary food mix. Allergy Asthma Proc 2003;24(4):265-268.

Ross SM. An integrative approach to eczema (atopic dermatitis). Holist Nurs Pract 2003;17(1): 56-62.

Rycroft RJ. Recurrent facial dermatitis from chamomile tea. Contact Dermatitis. 2003; 48(4):229.

Saller R, Beschomer M, Hellenbrecht D, et al. Dose dependency of symptomatic relief of complaints by chamomile steam inhalation in patients with common cold. Eur J Pharmacol 1990;183:728-729.

Seidler-Lozykowska K. Determination of the ploidy level in chamomile (*Chamomilla recutita* [L.] Rausch.) strains rich in alpha-bisabolol. J Appl Genet 2003;44(2):151-155.

Smolinski AT, Pestka JJ. Modulation of lipopolysaccharide-induced proinflammatory cytokine production in vitro and in vivo by the herbal constituents apigenin (chamomile), ginsenoside Rb(1) (ginseng) and parthenolide (feverfew). Food Chem Toxicol 2003;41(10):1381-1390.

Subiza J, Subiza JL, Alonso M, et al. Allergic conjunctivitis to chamomile tea. Ann Allergy 1990;65(2):127-132.

Subiza J, Subiza JL, Hinojosa M, et al. Anaphylactic reaction after the ingestion of chamomile tea: a study of cross-reactivity with other composite pollens. J Allergy Clin Immunol 1989;84(3):353-358.

Thien FC. Chamomile tea enema anaphylaxis. Med J Aust 2001;175(1):54.

van Ketel WG. Allergy to *Matricaria chamomilla*. Contact Dermatitis 1987;16(1):50-51.

Weizman Z, Alkrinawi S, Goldfarb D, et al. Efficacy of herbal tea preparation in infantile colic. J Pediatr 1993;122(4):650-652

Wilkinson S, Aldridge J, Salmon I, et al. An evaluation of aromatherapy massage in palliative care. Palliat Med 1999;13(5):409-417.

Chaparral

(Larrea tridentata [DC] Coville, Larrea divaricata Cav)

C

RELATED TERMS

- Chaparro, creosote bush, dwarf evergreen oak, el gobernadora, falsa alcaparra, geroop, greasewood, guamis, gumis, hediondilla, hideonodo, jarillo, kovanau, kreosotstrauch, *Larrea divaricata, Larrea glutiosa, Larrea mexicana* Moric, obernadora, palo ondo, shoegoi, sonora covillea, tasago, yah-temp, Zygophyllaceae.

BACKGROUND

- Chaparral and its constituent nordihydroguaiaretic acid (NDGA) have been reported to possess antioxidant/free-radical scavenging properties. Although they have been proposed as a treatment for cancer, effectiveness has not been demonstrated in clinical trials. Chaparral and NDGA have been reported to be associated with cases of hepatitis, cirrhosis, liver failure, renal cysts, and renal cell carcinoma. In response to these reports, in 1970 the U.S. Food and Drug Administration removed chaparral from its "generally recognized as safe" (GRAS) list. Chaparral and NDGA are generally considered unsafe and are not recommended for use.

USES BASED ON SCIENTIFIC EVIDENCE	Grade*
Cancer Chaparral and one of its components called nordihydroguaiaretic acid (NDGA) have antioxidant ("free-radical scavenging") properties, and have been proposed as treatment for cancer. However, both chaparral and NDGA have been reported to be associated with cases of kidney and liver failure, liver cirrhosis, kidney cysts, and kidney cancer in humans. In response to these reports, in 1970 the U.S. Food and Drug Administration (FDA) removed chaparral from its "generally recognized as safe" (GRAS) list. Chaparral and NDGA are generally considered unsafe and are not recommended for use.	C

*Key to grades: *A:* Strong scientific evidence for this use; *B:* Good scientific evidence for this use; *C:* Unclear scientific evidence for this use; *D:* Fair scientific evidence against this use (it may not work); *F:* Strong scientific evidence against this use (it likely does not work). For a more detailed explanation of efficacy criteria, see "Natural Standard Evidence-Based Validated Grading Rationale" in the Introduction.

Uses Based on Tradition, Theory, or Limited Scientific Evidence

Allergies, antibacterial, anti-inflammatory, anti-parasitic, antiviral, arthritis, blood purifier, bowel cramps, bruises, central nervous system disorders, chickenpox, colds, cough, diabetes, diarrhea, diuretic (increasing urine flow), flatulence (gas),

Continued

Uses Based on Tradition, Theory, or Limited Scientific Evidence *(cont'd)*

gastrointestinal disorders, hair tonic, hallucinations (including those due to LSD ingestion), heartburn, immune system disorders, indigestion, influenza, menstrual cramps, pain, respiratory tract infections, rheumatic diseases, skin disorders, snakebite pain, stomach ulcer, tuberculosis, urinary tract infections, venereal disease, vomiting, wound healing.

DOSING

The following doses are based on scientific research, publications, traditional use, or expert opinion. Many herbs and supplements have not been thoroughly tested, and their safety and effectiveness may not be proven. Brands may be made differently, with variable ingredients even within the same brand. The doses shown may not apply to all products. It is important to always read product labels and discuss doses with a qualified healthcare provider before therapy is started.

Standardization

- Standardization involves measuring the amounts of certain chemicals in products to try to make different preparations similar to each other. It is not always known if the chemicals being measured are the "active" ingredients. There is no widely accepted standardization for chaparral.

Adults (18 Years and Older)

- Safety has not been established for any dose. Small doses of tea have been used—for example, 1 teaspoon of chaparral leaves and flowers steeped in 1 pint of water for 15 minutes, 1 to 3 cups daily up to a maximum of several days. Tinctures have also been used—for example, 20 drops up to three times daily. These preparations may be associated with less toxicity, and possibly contain fewer allergenic compounds than capsules or tablets. Oil or powder forms of chaparral have also been applied to an affected area of skin several times daily.
- Capsules or tablets may deliver large doses leading to toxicity and are not recommended. Exposure to lignans, which may lead to toxicity, appears to be greater from capsules or tablets than from chaparral tea.

Children (Younger Than 18 Years)

- Chaparral is not recommended for use in children, because of lack of scientific data in this area and its potential toxicity.

SAFETY

The U.S. Food and Drug Administration does not strictly regulate herbs and supplements. There is no guarantee of the strength, purity, or safety of products, and effects may vary. It is important to always read product labels. People who have a medical condition, or are taking other drugs, herbs, or supplements, should consult a qualified healthcare provider before starting a new therapy. A healthcare provider should be contacted immediately about any side effects.

Allergies

- People with allergy/hypersensitivity to any of the components of chaparral, including NDGA, nor-isoguaiasin, dihydroguaiaretic acid, partially demethylated

dihydroguaiaretic acid, and demethoxyisoguaiasin, may have allergic reactions to chaparral.
- There have been case reports of allergic hypersensitivity (contact dermatitis) to chaparral and its resin.

Side Effects and Warnings

- Chaparral has been associated with multiple serious and potentially fatal adverse effects in animals and humans. Animals given the chaparral component NDGA developed kidney or gastrointestinal cysts and liver cell death. In humans, chaparral has been associated with kidney and liver failure, liver cirrhosis, kidney cysts, and kidney cancer. Case reports noted rash and fever with the use of chaparral. Exposure to lignans, which may lead to toxicity, appears to be greater from capsules and tablets than from decoctions of chaparral tea. The U.S. Food and Drug Administration removed chaparral from the "generally recognized as safe" (GRAS) list in 1970 and considers chaparral to be unsafe. Elevations of liver enzymes or kidney function tests (serum creatinine) may occur with chaparral.
- Based on a study in animals, chaparral may lower blood sugar levels. Caution is advised in people who have diabetes or hypoglycemia, and in those taking drugs, herbs, or supplements that affect blood sugar levels. Serum glucose levels should be monitored closely, and medication adjustments may be necessary.

Pregnancy and Breastfeeding

- There is insufficient scientific evidence to support the safe use of any dose of chaparral during pregnancy or breastfeeding.

INTERACTIONS

Most herbs and supplements have not been thoroughly tested for interactions with other herbs, supplements, drugs, or foods. The interactions listed here are based on reports in scientific publications, laboratory experiments, or traditional use. It is important to always read product labels. People who have a medical condition, or are taking other drugs, herbs, or supplements, should consult a qualified healthcare provider before starting a new therapy.

Interactions with Drugs

- Based on studies in animals and human case reports, chaparral has been associated with kidney damage, including cysts and cancer, and kidney failure. Theoretically, the use of chaparral with other agents known to alter kidney function or induce toxicity should be avoided, including sulfa antibiotics, aminoglycoside antibiotics, COX-2 inhibitors, and NSAIDs. People who are using other medications and considering the use of chaparral should consult a qualified healthcare provider before starting a new therapy. In studies in animals and case reports, chaparral was associated with liver damage. Theoretically, the use of chaparral with other agents known to induce liver toxicity should be avoided. Examples of such agents are amiodarone, carmustine, danazol, fluoxymesterone, isoniazid, ketoconazole, mercaptopurine, methotrexate, methyltestosterone, oxandrolone, oxymetholone, plicamycin, stanozolol, tacrine, testosterone, and valproic acid.
- Based on a study in animals, chaparral may lower blood sugar levels. Caution is advised when using medications that may also lower blood sugar levels. People who are taking drugs for diabetes by mouth or insulin should be monitored closely by a qualified healthcare provider. Medication adjustments may be necessary.

- Based on research studies in humans, chaparral may increase the risk of bleeding when taken with drugs that increase the risk of bleeding. Examples are anticoagulants (blood thinners) such as warfarin (Coumadin) and heparin, antiplatelet drugs such as clopidogrel (Plavix), aspirin, and nonsteroidal anti-inflammatory drugs such as ibuprofen (Motrin, Advil) and naproxen (Naprosyn, Aleve).
- Studies in animals suggest that chaparral may interfere with how the body uses the liver's cytochrome P450 enzyme system to process components of certain drugs. As a result, blood levels of these components may be elevated and may cause increased effects or potentially serious adverse reactions. People who are using other medications should always read the package insert and consult their healthcare provider or pharmacist about possible interactions.
- Historically, chaparral may interact with monoamine oxidase inhibitors such as isocarboxazid (Marplan), phenelzine (Nardil), and tranylcypromine (Parnate).

Interactions with Herbs and Dietary Supplements

- In studies of animals and case reports in humans, chaparral has been associated with kidney damage, cysts, cancer and kidney failure. Theoretically, the use of chaparral with other herbs or supplements known to alter kidney function or induce toxicity, such as agents with high levels of tannins, should be avoided. Chaparral has also been associated with liver damage. Theoretically, the use of chaparral with other herbs or supplements known to induce liver toxicity should be avoided. Examples of such agents are ackee, bee pollen, birch oil, blessed thistle, borage, bush tea, butterbur, coltsfoot, comfrey, DHEA, *Echinacea purpurea*, *Echium* spp., germander, *Heliotropium* spp., horse chestnut (intravenous preparations), jin-bu-huan (*Lycopodium serratum*), kava, lobelia, L-tetrahydropalmatine, mate, niacin (vitamin B_3), niacinamide, Paraguay tea, periwinkle, *Plantago lanceolata*, pride of Madeira, rue, *sassafras*, scullcap, *Senecio* spp./groundsel, tansy ragwort, turmeric/curcumin, tu-san-chi (*Gynura segetum*), uva ursi, and valerian.
- One study in animals suggested that chaparral may lower blood sugar levels. Caution is advised in people who are using herbs or supplements that may also lower blood sugar levels. Blood glucose levels may require monitoring, and doses may need adjustment. Examples of such herbs are *Aloe vera*, American ginseng, bilberry, bitter melon, burdock, fenugreek, fish oil, gymnema, horse chestnut seed extract (HCSE), marshmallow, milk thistle, *Panax ginseng*, rosemary, Siberian ginseng, stinging nettle, and white horehound. Agents that may raise blood sugar levels include arginine, cocoa, and ephedra (when combined with caffeine).
- Based on a study in humans, chaparral may increase the risk of bleeding when taken with herbs and supplements that may also increase the risk of bleeding. Multiple cases of bleeding have been reported with the use of *Ginkgo biloba*, fewer cases with garlic, and two cases with saw palmetto. Numerous other agents may theoretically increase the risk of bleeding, although this has not been proven in most cases. Examples are alfalfa, American ginseng, angelica, anise, *Arnica montana*, asafetida, aspen bark, bilberry, birch, black cohosh, bladderwrack, bogbean, boldo, borage seed oil, bromelain, capsicum, cat's claw, celery, chamomile, clove, coleus, cordyceps, danshen, devil's claw, dong quai, evening primrose, fenugreek, feverfew, flaxseed/flax powder (not a concern with flaxseed oil), ginger, grapefruit juice, grapeseed, green tea, guggul, gymnestra, horse chestnut, horseradish, licorice root, lovage root, male fern, meadowsweet, onion, *Panax ginseng*, papain, parsley, passion flower, poplar, prickly ash, propolis, quassia, red clover, reishi, Siberian ginseng, sweet birch,

sweet clover, turmeric, vitamin E, white willow, wild carrot, wild lettuce, willow, wintergreen, and yucca.

- Studies in animals suggest that chaparral may interfere with how the body uses the liver's cytochrome P450 enzyme system to process components of other herbs and supplements. As a result, blood levels of these components may be elevated. Chaparral may alter the effects of other herbs on the cytochrome P450 system. Examples of such herbs are bloodroot, cat's claw, chamomile, chasteberry, damiana, *Echinacea angustifolia*, goldenseal, grapefruit, licorice, oregano, red clover, St. John's wort, wild cherry, and yucca. People who are using other medications should always read the package insert and consult their healthcare provider or pharmacist about possible interactions.
- Based on historical use, chaparral may interact with herbs or supplements with possible monoamine oxidase inhibitor effects, such as California poppy, chromium, dehydroepiandrosterone (DHEA), 5-hydroxytryptophan (5-HTP), D,L-phenylalanine (DLPA), ephedra, evening primrose oil, fenugreek, *Ginkgo biloba*, hops, mace, *S*-adenosylmethionine (SAMe), sepia, St. John's wort, tyrosine, valerian, vitamin B_6, and yohimbe bark extract.

Selected References

Natural Standard developed the preceding evidence-based information based on a systematic review of more than 55 scientific articles. For comprehensive information about alternative and complementary therapies on the professional level, go to www.naturalstandard.com. Selected references are listed here.

Alderman S, Kailas S, Goldfarb S, et al. Cholestatic hepatitis after ingestion of chaparral leaf: confirmation by endoscopic retrograde cholangiopancreatography and liver biopsy. J Clin Gastroenterol 1994;19(3):242-247.

Anonymous. From the Centers for Disease Control and Prevention. Chaparral-induced toxic hepatitis—California and Texas, 1992. JAMA. 1992;268(23):3295, 3298.

Anonymous. Chaparral-induced toxic hepatitis—California and Texas, 1992. MMWR Morb Mortal Wkly Rep 1992;41(43):812-814.

Batchelor WB, Heathcote J, Wanless IR. Chaparral-induced hepatic injury. Am J Gastroenterol 1995;90(5):831-838.

Chitturi S, Farrell GC. Drug-induced cholestasis. Semin Gastrointest Dis 2001;12(2): 113-124.

Fleiss PM. Chaparral and liver toxicity. JAMA 1995;274(11):871; author reply 871-872. Comment on JAMA 1995;273(6):489-490.

Gordon DW, Rosenthal G, Hart J, et al. Chaparral ingestion. The broadening spectrum of liver injury caused by herbal medications. JAMA 1995;273(6):489-490. Comment in JAMA 1995;273(6):502; and JAMA 1995;274(11):871; author reply 871-872.

Heron S, Yarnell E. The safety of low-dose *Larrea tridentata* (DC) Coville (creosote bush or chaparral): a retrospective clinical study. J Altern Complement Med. 2001;7(2):175-185.

Ippen H. Chaparral and liver toxicity. JAMA 1995;274(11):871; author reply 871-872. Erratum in JAMA 1995;274(23):1838. Comment in JAMA 1995;273(6):489-490.

Katz M, Saibil F. Herbal hepatitis: subacute hepatic necrosis secondary to chaparral leaf. J Clin Gastroenterol 1990;12(2):203-206.

Luo J, Chuang T, Cheung J, et al. Masoprocol (nordihydroguaiaretic acid): a new antihyperglycemic agent isolated from the creosote bush (*Larrea tridentata*). Eur J Pharmacol 1998;346(1):77-79.

Obermeyer WR, Musser SM, Betz JM, et al. Chemical studies of phytoestrogens and related compounds in dietary supplements: flax and chaparral. Proc Soc Exp Biol Med 1995; 208(1):6-12.

Shad JA, Chinn CG, Brann OS. Acute hepatitis after ingestion of herbs. South Med J. 1999; 92(11):1095-1097.

Sheikh NM, Philen RM, Love LA. Chaparral-associated hepatotoxicity. Arch Intern Med. 1997;157(8):913-919.

Smart CR, Hogle HH, Vogel H, et al. Clinical experience with nordihydroguaiaretic acid—"chaparral tea" in the treatment of cancer. Rocky Mt Med J 1970;67(11):39-43.

Smith AY, Feddersen RM, Gardner KD, Jr., et al. Cystic renal cell carcinoma and acquired renal cystic disease associated with consumption of chaparral tea: a case report. J Urol 1994; 152(6 Pt 1):2089-2091.

Smith BC, Desmond PV. Acute hepatitis induced by ingestion of the herbal medication chaparral. Aust N Z J Med 1993;23(5):526.

Stashower ME, Torres RZ. Chaparral and liver toxicity. JAMA 1995;274(11):871; author reply 871-872. Comment in JAMA 1995;273(6):489-490.

Stickel F, Egerer G, Seitz HK. Hepatotoxicity of botanicals. Public Health Nutr 2000;3(2): 113-124. Comment in Public Health Nutr 2000;3(2):111.

Stickel F, Seitz HK, Hahn EG, Schuppan D. Liver toxicity of drugs of plant origin [in German]. Z Gastroenterol 2001;39(3):225-232, 234-237.

Zang LY, Cosma G, Gardner H, et al. Scavenging of superoxide anion radical by chaparral. Mol Cell Biochem 1999;196(1-2):157-161.

Chondroitin Sulfate

C

RELATED TERMS

- ACS4-ACS6, CDS, chondroitin sulfate A, chondroitin sulfate C, chondroitin sulphate A sodium, chondroitin-4-sulfate, chondroitin-6-sulfate, chondroitin sulfuric acid, chondroprotective agents, chonsurid, condroitin, Condrosulf CS, CSA, CSC, disease-modifying osteoarthritis drugs (DMOADs), GAG, galacotosamino-glucuronoglycan sulfate (Matrix), mesoglycan (heparan sulfate-52%, dermatan sulfate-35%, heparin-8%, chondroitin sulfate-5%), symptomatic slow-acting drug in osteoarthritis (SYSADOA).

BACKGROUND

- Chondroitin was first extracted and purified in the 1960s. It is currently manufactured from natural sources (shark/beef cartilage or bovine trachea) or by synthetic means. The consensus of expert and industry opinions support the use of chondroitin and its common partner agent, glucosamine, for improving symptoms and arresting (or possibly reversing) the degenerative process of osteoarthritis.

USES BASED ON SCIENTIFIC EVIDENCE	Grade*
Osteoarthritis Multiple controlled clinical trials since the 1980s have examined the use of oral chondroitin in patients with osteoarthritis of the knee and other locations (spine, hips, finger joints). Most of these studies have reported significant benefits in terms of symptoms (such as pain), function (such as mobility), and reduced medication requirements (such as anti-inflammatories). However, most studies have been brief (6 months' duration) with methodological weaknesses: a wide variety of patient classifications and outcome variables have been used, resulting in heterogeneity between trials; most analyses were not on an intention-to-treat basis; relationships between investigators and manufacturers were often not clarified; and blinding and randomization were frequently not well described. Despite these weaknesses and potential for bias in the available results, the weight of scientific evidence points to a beneficial effect when chondroitin is used for 6 to 24 months. Longer term effects are not clear. Preliminary studies of topical chondroitin have also been conducted. Chondroitin is frequently used with glucosamine. Glucosamine has independently been demonstrated to benefit patients with osteoarthritis (particularly of the knee). It remains unclear whether there is added benefit of using these two agents together compared to using either alone.	A

Continued

Ophthalmologic uses Chondroitin is sometimes used as a component of eye drop solutions, including prescription-only preparations such as Viscoat. These solutions should be used only under the supervision of an ophthalmologist.	B
Coronary artery disease (secondary prevention) Several studies in the early 1970s assessed the use of oral chondroitin for the prevention of subsequent coronary events in patients with a history of heart disease or myocardial infarction. Although favorable results were reported, because of methodological weaknesses in this research and the widespread current availability of more proven drug therapies for patients in this setting, a recommendation cannot be made in this area.	C
Interstitial cystitis There is preliminary research administering intravesicular chondroitin in patients diagnosed with interstitial cystitis. Additional evidence is necessary before a firm conclusion can be drawn.	C

*Key to grades: *A:* Strong scientific evidence for this use; *B:* Good scientific evidence for this use; *C:* Unclear scientific evidence for this use; *D:* Fair scientific evidence against this use (it may not work); *F:* Strong scientific evidence against this use (it likely does not work). For a more detailed explanation of efficacy criteria, see "Natural Standard Evidence-Based Validated Grading Rationale" in the Introduction.

Uses Based On Tradition, Theory, or Limited Scientific Evidence

Angina, anti-inflammatory, chronic venous ulcers, gonarthrosis, hyperlipidemia, iron deficiency anemia, kidney stones, leukemia, malaria, myocardial infarction, osteoporosis, premature labor prevention.

DOSING

The following doses are based on scientific research, publications, traditional use, or expert opinion. Many herbs and supplements have not been thoroughly tested, and their safety and effectiveness may not be proven. Brands may be made differently, with variable ingredients even within the same brand. The doses shown may not apply to all products. It is important to always read product labels and discuss doses with a qualified healthcare provider before therapy is started.

Standardization

- Standardization involves measuring the amounts of certain chemicals in products to try to make different preparations similar to each other. It is not always known if the chemicals being measured are the "active" ingredients.

Adult (18 Years and Older)

Oral (by Mouth)

- **Monotherapy:** Doses of 200 to 400 mg twice to three times daily, or 800 to 1200 mg once daily have been used. Higher doses (up to 2000 mg) appear to have similar efficacy. In the treatment of osteoarthritis, full effects may take several weeks to occur.

- **Combination with glucosamine:** It is not clear what dose is optimal when chondroitin used in combination with glucosamine or whether the combination is as effective as or more effective than either agent alone.

Intravenous/Intramuscular

- For osteoarthritis, 50 to 100 mg as a single daily injection or divided into two daily injections has been used. Medical supervision is recommended.

Children (Younger Than 18 Years)

- Because of insufficient scientific evidence, chondroitin is not recommended for use in children.

SAFETY

The U.S. Food and Drug Administration does not strictly regulate herbs and supplements. There is no guarantee of the strength, purity, or safety of products, and effects may vary. It is important to always read product labels. People who have a medical condition, or are taking other drugs, herbs, or supplements, should consult a qualified healthcare provider before starting a new therapy. A healthcare provider should be contacted immediately about any side effects.

Allergies

- Use cautiously if allergic or hypersensitive to chondroitin sulfate products.

Side Effects and Warnings

- There are limited data about the long-term safety of chondroitin, although it appears to be well tolerated in most trials.
- Adverse effects that have been rarely reported or are theoretical include bone marrow suppression, breathing difficulties, chest pain, constipation, diarrhea, elevated blood pressure, euphoria, exacerbation of previously well-controlled asthma, eyelid edema, gastrointestinal pain/dyspepsia, hair loss, headache, hives, increased risk of bleeding, lower extremity edema, motor uneasiness, nausea, photosensitivity, rash, subjective tightness in the throat or chest, and transaminitis.
- Chondroitin should be used with caution in people who have bleeding disorders or are taking anticoagulant medications.

Pregnancy and Breastfeeding

- The use of chondroitin should be avoided in pregnant or breastfeeding women because effects are unknown, and chondroitin is structurally similar to heparin, which is contraindicated during pregnancy.

INTERACTIONS

Most herbs and supplements have not been thoroughly tested for interactions with other herbs, supplements, drugs, or foods. The interactions listed here are based on reports in scientific publications, laboratory experiments, or traditional use. It is important to always read product labels. People who have a medical condition, or are taking other drugs, herbs, or supplements, should consult a qualified healthcare provider before starting a new therapy.

Interactions with Drugs

- In theory, chondroitin may increase the risk of bleeding when taken with other agents that may increase the risk of bleeding. Examples of such agents are anticoagulants (blood thinners) such as warfarin (Coumadin) and heparin, antiplatelet drugs such as clopidogrel (Plavix), aspirin, and nonsteroidal anti-inflammatory drugs such as ibuprofen (Motrin, Advil) and naproxen (Naprosyn, Aleve).

Interactions with Herbs and Dietary Supplements

- In theory, chondroitin may increase the risk of bleeding when taken with herbs and supplements that may also increase the risk of bleeding. Multiple cases of bleeding have been reported with the use of *Ginkgo biloba*, and fewer cases with garlic and saw palmetto. Numerous other agents may theoretically increase the risk of bleeding, although this has not been proven in most cases. Examples of such agents are alfalfa, American ginseng, angelica, anise, *Arnica montana*, asafetida, aspen bark, bilberry, birch, black cohosh, bladderwrack, bogbean, boldo, borage seed oil, bromelain, capsicum, cat's claw, celery, chamomile, chaparral, clove, coleus, cordyceps, dandelion, danshen, devil's claw, dong quai, eicosapentaenoic acid (EPA), evening primrose oil, fenugreek, feverfew, fish oil, flaxseed/flax powder (not a concern with flaxseed oil), ginger, grapefruit juice, grape seed, green tea, guggul, gymnestra, horse chestnut, horseradish, licorice root, lovage root, male fern, meadowsweet, melatonin, nordihydroguaiaretic acid (NDGA), omega-3 fatty acids, onion, *Panax ginseng*, papain, parsley, passion flower, poplar, prickly ash, propolis, quassia, red clover, reishi, rue, Siberian ginseng, sweet birch, sweet clover, turmeric, vitamin E, white willow, wild carrot, wild lettuce, willow, wintergreen, and yucca.

Selected References

Natural Standard developed the preceding evidence-based information based on a systematic review of more than 175 articles. For comprehensive information about alternative and complementary therapies on the professional level, go to www.naturalstandard.com. Selected references are listed here.

Blotman F, Loyau G. Clinical trial with chondroitin sulfate in gonarthrosis [abstract]. Osteoarthritis Cartilage 1993;1:68.

Bourgeois P, Chales G, Dehais J, et al. Efficacy and tolerability of chondroitin sulfate 1200 mg/day vs chondroitin sulfate 3 × 400 mg/day vs placebo. Osteoarthritis Cartilage 1998; 6(Suppl A):25-30.

Bucsi L, Poor G. Efficacy and tolerability of oral chondroitin sulfate as a symptomatic slow-acting drug for osteoarthritis (SYSADOA) in the treatment of knee osteoarthritis. Osteoarthritis Cartilage 1998;6(Suppl A)31-36.

Cohen M, Wolfe R, Mai T, et al. A randomized, double blind, placebo controlled trial of a topical cream containing glucosamine sulfate, chondroitin sulfate, and camphor for osteoarthritis of the knee. J Rheumatol 2003;30(3):523-528.

Conrozier T. [Anti-arthrosis treatments: efficacy and tolerance of chondroitin sulfates (CS 4 & 6).] Presse Med 1998;27(36):1862-1865.

Danao-Camara T. Potential side effects of treatment with glucosamine and chondroitin. Arthritis Rheum 2000;43(12):2853.

Das A Jr, Hammad TA. Efficacy of a combination of FCHG49 glucosamine hydrochloride, TRH122 low molecular weight sodium chondroitin sulfate and manganese ascorbate in the management of knee osteoarthritis. Osteoarthritis Cartilage 2000;8(5):343-350.

Du J, White N, Eddington ND. The bioavailability and pharmacokinetics of glucosamine hydrochloride and chondroitin sulfate after oral and intravenous single dose administration in the horse. Biopharm Drug Dispos 2004;25(3):109-116.

Fleish AM, Merlin C, Imhoff A, et al. A one-year randomized, double-blind, placebo-controlled study with oral chondroitin sulfate in patients with knee osteoarthritis. Osteoarthritis Cartilage 1997;5:70.

L'Hirondel JL. [Clinical double blind study with oral application of chondroitin sulfate vs. placebo for treatment of tibio femoral gonarthrosis in 125 patients.] Litera Rheumatologica 1992;14:77-84.

Leeb BF, Petera P, Neumann K. [Results of a multicenter study of chondroitin sulfate (Condrosulf) use in arthroses of the finger, knee and hip joints.] Wien Med Wochenschr 1996;146(24):609-614.

Leeb BF, Schweitzer H, Montag K, et al. A metaanalysis of chondroitin sulfate in the treatment of osteoarthritis. J Rheumatol 2000;27(1):205-211.

Leffler CT, Philippi AF, Leffler SG, et al. Glucosamine, chondroitin, and manganese ascorbate for degenerative joint disease of the knee or low back: a randomized, double-blind, placebo-controlled pilot study. Mil Med 1999;164(2):85-91.

Limberg MB, McCaa C, Kissling GE, et al. Topical application of hyaluronic acid and chondroitin sulfate in the treatment of dry eyes. Am J Ophthalmol 1987;103(2):194-197.

Malaise M, et al. Efficacy and tolerability of 800 mg oral chondroitin sulfate in the treatment of knee osteoarthritis: a randomized double-blind multicentre study versus placebo. Litera Rheumatologica 1999;24:31-42.

Mazieres B, Loyau G, Menkes CJ, et al. [Chondroitin sulfate in the treatment of gonarthrosis and coxarthrosis. 5-months result of a multicenter double-blind controlled prospective study using placebo.] Rev Rhum Mal Osteoartic 1992;59(7-8):466-472.

McAlindon TE, LaValley MP, Gulin JP, et al. Glucosamine and chondroitin for treatment of osteoarthritis: a systematic quality assessment and meta-analysis. JAMA 2000;283(11): 1469-1475.

McGee M, Wagner WD. Chondroitin sulfate anticoagulant activity is linked to water transfer: relevance to proteoglycan structure in atherosclerosis. Arterioscler Thromb Vasc Biol 2003; 23(10):1921-1927.

Morreale P, Manopulo R, Galati M, et al. Comparison of the antiinflammatory efficacy of chondroitin sulfate and diclofenac sodium in patients with knee osteoarthritis. J Rheumatol 1996;23(8):1385-1391.

Morrison LM, Branwood AW, Ershoff BH, et al. The prevention of coronary arteriosclerotic heart disease with chondroitin sulfate A: preliminary report. Exp Med Surg 1969;27(3): 278-289.

Morrison LM. Reduction of ischemic coronary heart disease by chondroitin sulfate A. Angiology 1971;22(3):165-174.

Obara M, Hirano H, Ogawa M, et al. Does chondroitin sulfate defend the human uterine cervix against ripening in threatened premature labor? Am J Obstet Gynecol 2000;182(2): 334-339.

Richy F, Bruyere O, Ethgen O, et al. Structural and symptomatic efficacy of glucosamine and chondroitin in knee osteoarthritis: a comprehensive meta-analysis. Arch Intern Med 2003; 163(13):1514-1522.

Rozenfeld V, Crain JL, Callahan AK. Possible augmentation of warfarin effect by glucosamine-chondroitin. Am J Health Syst Pharm 2004;61(3):306-307.

Shankland WE. The effects of glucosamine and chondroitin sulfate on osteoarthritis of the TMJ: a preliminary report of 50 patients. Cranio 1998;16(4):230-235.

Steinhoff G, Ittah B, Rowan S. The efficacy of chondroitin sulfate 0.2% in treating interstitial cystitis. Can J Urol 2002;9(1):1454-1458.

Tallia AF, Cardone DA. Asthma exacerbation associated with glucosamine-chondroitin supplement. J Am Board Fam Pract 2002;15(6):481-484.

Towheed TE, Anastassiades TP. Glucosamine and chondroitin for treating symptoms of osteoarthritis: evidence is widely touted but incomplete. JAMA 2000;283(11):1483-1484.

Uebelhart D, Chantraine A. Efficacite clinique du sulfate de chondroitine dans la gonarthrose: Etude randomisee en double-insu versus placebo [abstract]. Rev Rhumatisme 1994;10:692.

Uebelhart D, Knüssel O, Theiler R. Efficacy and tolerability of oral avian chondroitin sulfate in painful knee osteoarthritis [abstract]. Schweiz Med Wochenschr 1999;129(33):1174.

Uebelhart D, Thonar EJ, Zhang J, et al. Protective effect of exogenous chondroitin 4,6-sulfate in the acute degradation of articular cartilage in the rabbit. Osteoarthritis Cartilage 1998;6(Suppl A):6-13.

Uebelhart D, Malaise M, Marcolongo R, et al. Intermittent treatment of knee osteoarthritis with oral chondroitin sulfate: a one-year, randomized, double-blind, multicenter study versus placebo. Osteoarthritis Cartilage 2004;12(4):269-276.

Van Blitterswijk WJ, Van De Nes JC, Wuisman PI. Glucosamine and chondroitin sulfate supplementation to treat symptomatic disc degeneration: Biochemical rationale and case report. BMC Complement Altern Med 2003;3(1):2.

Verbruggen G, Goemaere S, Veys EM. Chondroitin sulfate: S/DMOAD (structure/disease modifying anti-osteoarthritis drug) in the treatment of finger joint OA. Osteoarthritis Cartilage 1998;6 Suppl A:37-38.

Volpi N. Oral bioavailability of chondroitin sulfate (Condrosulf) and its constituents in healthy male volunteers. Osteoarthritis Cartilage 2002;10(10):768-777.

Clay

C

RELATED TERMS

- Akipula, aluminium silicate, anhydrous aluminum silicate, askipula, beidellitic montmorillonite, benditos, bioelectrical minerals, cipula, chalk, clay dust, clay lozenges, clay suspension products, clay tablets, colloidal minerals, colloidal trace minerals, fossil farina, humic shale, Indian healing clay, kipula, mountain meal, panito del senor, phyllosilicate clay plant-derived liquid minerals, *Terra sigillata*, tirra santa, white clay, white mud.

BACKGROUND

- Clay has been used medicinally for centuries in Africa, India, and China, and by Native American groups. Uses have included gastrointestinal disorders and as an antidote for poisoning.
- The practice of eating dirt, clay, or other non-nutritious substances may be referred to as "pica" or "geophagia" and is common in early childhood and in mentally handicapped or psychotic patients. There is some evidence that mineral deficiencies such as iron deficiency may lead to pica, and prevalence is higher in developing countries and in poor communities. Chronic clay ingestion may lead to iron malabsorption and further precipitate this condition.
- There is insufficient scientific evidence to recommend for or against the use of clay for any medical condition. The potential for adverse effects with chronic oral ingestion of clay may outweigh any potential benefits.

USES BASED ON SCIENTIFIC EVIDENCE	Grade*
Fecal incontinence associated with psychiatric disorders (encopresis): clay modeling therapy in children There is not enough scientific research to support a recommendation for play with modeling clay as an effective therapeutic intervention in children with encopresis.	C
Functional gastrointestinal disorders There is not enough scientific evidence to recommend the medicinal use of clay by mouth in patients with gastrointestinal disorders. Some clay preparations have been found to be similar to Kaolin and Kaopectate, which are used to treat gastrointestinal disturbances including diarrhea. However, overall, there are significant potential risks that accompany the use of clay, including intestinal blockage and injury, as well as lead poisoning.	C
Mercuric chloride poisoning Clay lozenges have been used historically in the treatment of mercuric chloride poisoning and were officially mentioned in several European	C

Continued

pharmacopoeias, including the Royal College, until the middle nineteenth century. However, there is not enough scientific evidence to recommend the use of clay by mouth for poisoning at this time, as there is risk of clay itself containing contaminants.	
Protection from aflatoxins Aflatoxins are toxic substances from the fungus *Aspergillus flavus*, which may infect peanuts and stored grains. Ingestion of aflatoxins from peanuts and cereals (primarily in warm and humid regions) has been associated with liver cancers in humans and multiple cancers in animals. Phyllosilicate clay has been shown to adhere to aflatoxins in laboratory study, and HSACS clay in animal diets may diminish or block exposure to aflatoxins. However, the toxicity risks from chronic clay exposure do not justify the potential benefit.	C

*Key to grades: *A:* Strong scientific evidence for this use; *B:* Good scientific evidence for this use; *C:* Unclear scientific evidence for this use; *D:* Fair scientific evidence against this use (it may not work); *F:* Strong scientific evidence against this use (it likely does not work). For a more detailed explanation of efficacy criteria, see "Natural Standard Evidence-Based Validated Grading Rationale" in the Introduction.

Uses Based on Tradition, Theory, or Limited Scientific Evidence

Animal bites, cancer, constipation, diarrhea, dysentery, eye disorders, fevers, heart disorders, menstruation difficulties, nutrition, plague, poisoning, skin protection, smoking, stomach disorders, syphilis, vomiting, vomiting/nausea during pregnancy, water purification, weight loss.

DOSING

The following doses are based on scientific research, publications, traditional use, or expert opinion. Many herbs and supplements have not been thoroughly tested, and their safety and effectiveness may not be proven. Brands may be made differently, with variable ingredients even within the same brand. The doses shown may not apply to all products. It is important to always read product labels and discuss doses with a qualified healthcare provider before therapy is started.

Adults (18 Years and Older)

- There is insufficient scientific evidence to recommend the safe use of clay in adults.

Children (Younger Than 18 Years)

- There is insufficient scientific evidence to recommend the safe use of clay in children.

SAFETY

The U.S. Food and Drug Administration does not strictly regulate herbs and supplements. There is no guarantee of the strength, purity, or safety of products, and effects may vary. It is important

to always read product labels. People who have a medical condition, or are taking other drugs, herbs, or supplements, should consult a qualified healthcare provider before starting a new therapy

Allergies

- There are no reports of allergy to clay in the available scientific literature. However, in theory, allergy/hypersensitivity to clay, clay products, or constituents of clay may occur.

Side Effects and Warnings

- The practice of eating dirt, clay, or other non-nutritious substances is called *pica*, or *geophagia*, and may be seen in young children and in mentally handicapped people. Pica has been associated with lead poisoning in infants and children and with potential risks such as a low red blood cell count and brain damage. In one case report, death was related to complications of lead poisoning and brain damage after drinking from a glazed clay pitcher. Clay pots containing candy were recalled by the U.S. Food and Drug Administration because of high levels of lead in the candy, which was absorbed from the clay.
- Clay products may contain varying amounts of contaminants including aluminum, arsenic, barium, nickel, and titanium. Elevated levels of 2,3,7,8-tetracholorodibenzo-*p*-dioxin have been found in fish and eggs from chickens fed a diet containing clay. Chronic clay pica has been associated with imbalances in blood chemistry such as increased calcium and magnesium and decreased iron and potassium.
- In the 19th century, a condition called "Cachexia Africana" was reported, characterized by a swollen appearance, enlarged heart, increased urination, and death. There were also descriptions of people who chronically ate clay noting that their skin was initially dry and shiny and that, in late stages of disease, especially in children, skin ulcerations appeared on the arms and legs.
- Chronic clay eating has been associated with small gonads (testes), and muscle injury.
- Heartburn, flatulence (gas), loss of appetite, constipation, and diarrhea and vomiting after meals have been reported with ingestion of clay. Clay eating has also been associated with intestinal blockage and injury, bowel rupture (perforation), formation of stones in the intestine, and enlarged liver/spleen.
- It is reported that children with pica are more likely to develop lung infections. Chronic bronchitis, trouble breathing, and infections have been associated with dust exposure in the heavy clay industry. Hookworm infections may result from eating clay. Tetanus contracted from clay has been described in an infant who ate clay and in a newborn whose umbilical cord was wrapped in clay.
- Chronic clay eating may cause imbalances in blood chemistry such as increased calcium or magnesium, as well as decreased iron and potassium.

Pregnancy and Breastfeeding

- Use of clay during pregnancy or breastfeeding is not recommended. Eating clay during pregnancy may increase the risk of toxemia and complications at birth.

INTERACTIONS

Most herbs and supplements have not been thoroughly tested for interactions with other herbs, supplements, drugs, or foods. The interactions listed here are based on reports in scientific publications, laboratory experiments, or traditional use. It is important to always read product labels. People who have a medical condition, or are taking other drugs, herbs, or supplements, should consult a qualified healthcare provider before starting a new therapy.

Interactions with Drugs

- When taken together with drugs such as cimetidine (Tagamet), clay may inhibit their absorption.

Interactions with Herbs and Dietary Supplements

- Clay can interfere with iron absorption.

Selected References

Natural Standard developed the preceding evidence-based information based on a systematic review of more than 100 scientific articles. For comprehensive information about alternative and complementary therapies on the professional level, go to www.naturalstandard.com. Selected references are listed here.

Feldman PC, Villanueva S, Lanne V, et al. Use of play with clay to treat children with intractable encopresis. J Pediatr 1993;122(3):483-488.

Fredj G, Farinotti R, Salvadori C, et al. [Topical digestive drugs with a clay base. Influence on the absorption of cimetidine.] Therapie 1986;41(1):23-25.

Gonzalez JJ, Owens W, Ungaro PC, et al. Clay ingestion: a rare cause of hypokalemia. Ann Intern Med 1982;97(1):65-66.

Love RG, Waclawski ER, Maclaren WM, et al. Risks of respiratory disease in the heavy clay industry. Occup Environ Med 1999;56(2):124-133.

Montoya-Cabrera MA, Hernandez-Zamora A, Portilla-Aguilar J, et al. [Fatal lead poisoning caused by the ingestion of lemonade from glazed clay chinaware.] Gac Med Mex 1981; 117(4):1 54-158.

Obialo CI, Crowell AK, Wen XJ, et al. Clay pica has no hematologic or metabolic correlate in chronic hemodialysis patients. J Ren Nutr 2001;11(1):32-36.

Pariente EA, De La Garoullaye G. [A multicenter comparative study of a mucilage (Karaya gum + PVPP) versus clay in functional intestinal disorders.] Med Chir Dig 1994;23(3):193-199.

Phillips TD, Sarr AB, Grant PG. Selective chemisorption and detoxification of aflatoxins by phyllosilicate clay. Nat Toxins 1995;3(4):204-213.

Phillips TD. Dietary clay in the chemoprevention of aflatoxin-induced disease. Toxicol Sci 1999; 52(Suppl 2):118-126.

Severance HW Jr, Holt T, Patrone NA, et al. Profound muscle weakness and hypokalemia due to clay ingestion. South Med J 1988;81(2):272-274.

Clove and Clove Oil
(*Eugenia aromatica*)

C

RELATED TERMS

- 2-methoxy-4-(2-propenyl)-phenol, caryophylli, *Caryophylli atheroleum*, caryophyllum, caryophyllus, *Caryophyllus aromaticus*, chiodo di garofano, clavos, clous de girolfe, clove cigarettes, clove oil, *Eugenia caryophyllata*, *Eugenia caryophyllus*, *Flores caryophylli*, gewurznelken nagelein, kreteks, Myrtaceae, oil of clove, oleum caryophylli, pentogen, *Syzigium aromaticum*, tropical myrtle.
- **Combination products:** Dent-Zel-Ite toothache relief drops, Red Cross Toothache Medication.

BACKGROUND

- Clove is widely cultivated in Indonesia, Sri-Lanka, Madagascar, Tanzania, and Brazil. It is used in limited amounts in food products as a fragrant, flavoring agent, and antiseptic.
- Clinical trials assessing clove monotherapy are limited, although the expert panel German Commission E has approved the use of clove as a topical antiseptic and anesthetic. Other uses for clove, such as treatment for premature ejaculation, inflammation after tooth extraction (dry socket), and fever reduction, lack reliable human clinical evidence.
- Clove is sometimes added to tobacco in cigarettes. Clove cigarettes (kreteks) typically contain 60% tobacco and 40% ground cloves.

USES BASED ON SCIENTIFIC EVIDENCE	Grade*
Fever reduction Studies in animals suggest that clove can lower fever, but no reliable studies in humans are available.	C
Inflammation after tooth extraction (dry socket) Preliminary studies have reported that oil of clove combined with zinc oxide paste is effective for treatment of dry socket. The benefits of clove alone need to be studied before a recommendation can be made.	C
Premature ejaculation A small amount of human research reports that a combination cream with clove and other herbs may be helpful in the treatment of premature ejaculation. However, well-designed studies of the effectiveness of clove alone are needed before a conclusion can be drawn.	C

*Key to grades: *A:* Strong scientific evidence for this use; *B:* Good scientific evidence for this use; *C:* Unclear scientific evidence for this use; *D:* Fair scientific evidence against this use (it may not work); *F:* Strong scientific evidence against this use (it likely does not work). For a more detailed explanation of efficacy criteria, see "Natural Standard Evidence-Based Validated Grading Rationale" in the Introduction.

Uses Based on Tradition, Theory, or Limited Scientific Evidence

Abdominal pain, antifungal, antihistamine, antioxidant, antiseptic, antiviral, asthma, athlete's foot, bad breath, blood purifier, blood thinner (antiplatelet agent), cancer, dental cavities, colic, cough, counterirritant, decreased gastric transit time, diabetes, diarrhea, dust mites, expectorant, flatulence (gas), flavoring for food and cigarettes, gout, hernia, herpes simplex virus, hiccups, high blood pressure, inflammation, mouth and throat inflammation, mouthwash, muscle spasm, nausea and vomiting, pain, parasites, smooth muscle relaxant, tooth or gum pain, vasorelaxant.

DOSING

The following doses are based on scientific research, publications, traditional use, or expert opinion. Many herbs and supplements have not been thoroughly tested, and their safety and effectiveness may not be proven. Brands may be made differently, with variable ingredients even within the same brand. The doses shown may not apply to all products. It is important to always read product labels and discuss doses with a qualified healthcare provider before therapy is started.

Standardization

- Standardization involves measuring the amounts of certain chemicals in products to try to make different preparations similar to each other. It is not always known if the chemicals being measured are the "active" ingredients. Some sources recommend that clove oil should not be used in concentrations higher than 0.06%, and that the daily dose of eugenol, a component of clove, should not be higher than 2.5 milligrams for each kilogram of body weight.

Adults (18 Years and Older)

- There is insufficient scientific evidence available to recommend a specific dose of clove by mouth, on the skin, or by any other route.

Children (Younger Than 18 Years)

- There is insufficient scientific evidence available to recommend a specific dose of clove by mouth, on the skin, or by any other route.

SAFETY

The U.S. Food and Drug Administration does not strictly regulate herbs and supplements. There is no guarantee of the strength, purity, or safety of products, and effects may vary. It is important to always read product labels. People who have a medical condition, or are taking other drugs, herbs, or supplements, should consult a qualified healthcare provider before starting a new therapy. A healthcare provider should be contacted immediately about any side effects.

Allergies

- Allergic reactions to clove and its component eugenol have been reported, including severe reactions (anaphylaxis). Eugenol or clove can cause allergic rashes when applied to the skin or inside the mouth. Hives have been reported in clove cigarette smokers. People who are allergic to balsam of Peru may also be allergic to clove. Persons with known allergy to clove, its component eugenol, or to balsam of Peru should avoid the use of clove by mouth, inhaled from cigarettes, or applied to the skin.

Side Effects and Warnings

- Clove is generally regarded as safe for food use in the United States. However, when clove is taken by mouth in large doses, in its undiluted oil form, or used in clove cigarettes, side effects may occur, including vomiting, sore throat, seizure, sedation, difficulty breathing, fluid in the lungs, vomiting of blood, blood disorders, kidney failure, and liver damage. People with kidney or liver disorders or who have had seizures should avoid clove. Serious side effects are reported more often in young children. It is recommended to avoid the use of clove supplements in children and pregnant or nursing women.
- Laboratory research studies suggest that clove or clove oil may cause an increased risk of bleeding. Caution is advised in people with bleeding disorders or those taking drugs that may increase the risk of bleeding. Dosing adjustments may be necessary. It is unclear what doses or methods of using clove may contribute to this risk. One case of disseminated intravascular coagulation (DIC) (a severe reaction including bleeding and liver damage) was reported in a person taking clove by mouth.
- When applied to the skin or the inside of the mouth, clove can cause burning, loss of sensation, local tissue damage, dental pulp damage, and lip sores and can increase the risk of cavities. There is a high risk of contact dermatitis (rash) and even burns if undiluted, full-strength clove oil is applied to the skin. The application of clove combination herbal creams to the penis has been reported to cause episodes of difficulty with erection or ejaculation.
- Based on an infant case report, clove oil taken by mouth may lower blood sugar levels. Caution is advised in patients with diabetes or hypoglycemia, and in those taking drugs, herbs, or supplements that affect blood sugar levels. Serum glucose levels may need to be monitored by a healthcare provider, and medication adjustments may be necessary.
- Contamination of clove can occur if the herb is improperly stored. Fungi and aflatoxins are among the most common contaminants. Ingesting contaminated clove can result in health problems in humans as well as in animals.

Pregnancy and Breastfeeding

- Insufficient information about safety is available to recommend the use of clove supplements in pregnant or breastfeeding women.

INTERACTIONS

Most herbs and supplements have not been thoroughly tested for interactions with other herbs, supplements, drugs, or foods. The interactions listed here are based on reports in scientific publications, laboratory experiments, or traditional use. It is important to always read product labels. People who have a medical condition, or are taking other drugs, herbs, or supplements, should consult a qualified healthcare provider before starting a new therapy.

Interactions with Drugs

- Based on laboratory research, clove theoretically may increase the risk of bleeding when taken with drugs that increase the risk of bleeding. It is unclear what doses or methods of using clove may increase this risk. Examples of such drugs are

anticoagulants (blood thinners) such as warfarin (Coumadin) and heparin, antiplatelet drugs such as clopidogrel (Plavix), aspirin, and nonsteroidal anti-inflammatory drugs such as ibuprofen (Motrin, Advil) and naproxen (Naprosyn, Aleve).
- Based on an infant case report, clove oil taken by mouth may lower blood sugar levels. Caution is advised when using medications that may also lower blood sugar levels. People taking drugs for diabetes by mouth or insulin should be monitored closely by a qualified healthcare provider. Medication adjustments may be necessary.
- When applied to the skin, eugenol, a component of clove, may reduce the ability to feel and react to painful stimulation. Therefore, use of clove products on the skin with other numbing or pain-reducing products such as lidocaine/prilocaine cream (Emla) theoretically may increase effects.

Interactions with Herbs and Dietary Supplements

- Based on laboratory research studies, clove may increase the risk of bleeding when taken with herbs and supplements that may also increase the risk of bleeding. It is unclear what doses or methods of using clove may increase this risk. Multiple cases of bleeding have been reported with the use of *Ginkgo biloba*, some cases with garlic, and fewer cases with saw palmetto. Numerous other agents may theoretically increase the risk of bleeding, although this has not been proven in most cases. Examples of such agents are alfalfa, American ginseng, angelica, anise, *Arnica montana*, asafetida, aspen bark, bilberry, birch, black cohosh, bladderwrack, bogbean, boldo, borage seed oil, bromelain, capsicum, cat's claw, celery, chamomile, chaparral, coleus, cordyceps, danshen, devil's claw, dong quai, eicosapentaenoic acid (EPA), evening primrose, fenugreek, feverfew, fish oil, flaxseed/flax powder (not a concern with flaxseed oil), ginger, grapefruit juice, grape seed, green tea, guggul, gymnestra, horse chestnut, horseradish, licorice root, lovage root, male fern, meadowsweet, nordihydroguaiaretic acid (NDGA), onion, *Panax ginseng*, papain, parsley, passion flower, poplar, prickly ash, propolis, quassia, red clover, reishi, rue, Siberian ginseng, sweet birch, sweet clover, turmeric, vitamin E, white willow, wild carrot, wild lettuce, willow, wintergreen, and yucca.
- Based on an infant case report, clove may lower blood sugar levels. Caution is advised when using herbs or supplements that may also lower blood sugar levels. Blood glucose levels may require monitoring, and doses may need adjustment. Examples of such herbs are *Aloe vera*, American ginseng, bilberry, bitter melon, burdock, fenugreek, fish oil, gymnema, horse chestnut seed extract (HCSE), maitake mushroom, marshmallow, milk thistle, *Panax ginseng*, rosemary, Siberian ginseng, stinging nettle, and white horehound.
- When applied to the skin, eugenol, a component of clove, may reduce the ability to feel and react to painful stimulation. Therefore, use with other numbing or pain-reducing products such as capsaicin cream (Zostrix) may in theory cause exaggerated effects.

Selected References

Natural Standard developed the preceding evidence-based information based on a systematic review of more than 220 scientific articles. For comprehensive information about alternative and complementary therapies on the professional level, go to www.naturalstandard.com. Selected references are listed here.

Burt SA, Reinders RD. Antibacterial activity of selected plant essential oils against *Escherichia coli* O157:H7. Lett Appl Microbiol 2003;36(3):162-167.

Choi HK, Jung GW, Moon KH, et al. Clinical study of SS-cream in patients with lifelong premature ejaculation. Urology 2000;55(2):257-261.

Consolini AE, Sarubbio MG. Pharmacological effects of *Eugenia uniflora* (Myrtaceae) aqueous crude extract on rat's heart. J Ethnopharmacol 2002;81(1):57-63.

Damiani CE, Rossoni LV, Vassallo DV. Vasorelaxant effects of eugenol on rat thoracic aorta. Vascul Pharmacol 2003;40(1):59-66.

Dragland S, Senoo H, Wake K, et al. Several culinary and medicinal herbs are important sources of dietary antioxidants. J Nutr 2003;133(5):1286-1290.

Elshafie AE, Al-Rashdi TA, Al-Bahry SN, et al. Fungi and aflatoxins associated with spices in the Sultanate of Oman. Mycopathologia 2002;155(3):155-160.

Friedman M, Henika PR, Mandrell RE. Bactericidal activities of plant essential oils and some of their isolated constituents against *Campylobacter jejuni*, *Escherichia coli*, *Listeria monocytogenes*, and *Salmonella enterica*. J Food Prot 2002;65(10):1545-1560.

Grover JK, Rathi SS, Vats V. Amelioration of experimental diabetic neuropathy and gastropathy in rats following oral administration of plant (*Eugenia jambolana*, *Mucuna pruriens* and *Tinospora cordifolia*) extracts. Indian J Exp Biol 2002;40(3):273-276.

Guynot ME, Ramos AJ, Seto L, et al. Antifungal activity of volatile compounds generated by essential oils against fungi commonly causing deterioration of bakery products. J Appl Microbiol 2003;94(5):893-899.

Huss U, Ringbom T, Perera P, et al. Screening of ubiquitous plant constituents for COX-2 inhibition with a scintillation proximity based assay. J Nat Prod 2002;65(11):1517-1521.

Juglal S, Govinden R, Odhav B. Spice oils for the control of co-occurring mycotoxin-producing fungi. J Food Prot 2002;65(4):683-687.

Kalemba D, Kunicka A. Antibacterial and antifungal properties of essential oils. Curr Med Chem 2003;10(10):813-829.

Kim EH, Kim HK, Ahn YJ. Acaricidal activity of clove bud oil compounds against *Dermatophagoides farinae* and *Dermatophagoides pteronyssinus* (Acari: Pyroglyphidae). J Agric Food Chem 2003;51(4):885-889.

Pallares DE. Link between clove cigarettes and urticaria? Postgrad Med 1999;106(4):153.

Sanchez-Perez J, Garcia-Diez A. Occupational allergic contact dermatitis from eugenol, oil of cinnamon and oil of cloves in a physiotherapist. Contact Dermatitis 1999;41(6):346-347.

Soetiarto F. The relationship between habitual clove cigarette smoking and a specific pattern of dental decay in male bus drivers in Jakarta, Indonesia. Caries Res 1999;33(3):248-250.

Coenzyme Q10

(Ubiquinone)

RELATED TERMS

- Andelir, coenzyme Q, co-enzyme Q10, coenzyme Q (50), coQ, coQ10, coQ(50), co-Q10, CoQ-10, 2,3-dimethoxy-5-methyl-6-decaprenyl benzoquinone, Heartcin, idebenone (synthetic analogue), mitoquinone, Neuquinone, Q10, Taidecanone, ubidecarenone, ubiquinone, ubiquinone-10, ubiquinone-Q10, Udekinon, vitamin q10, vitamin Q10.

BACKGROUND

- Coenzyme Q10 (CoQ10) is produced by the human body and is necessary for the basic functioning of cells. CoQ10 levels are reported to decrease with age and to be low in people with chronic diseases such as heart conditions, muscular dystrophy, Parkinson's disease, cancer, diabetes, and HIV/AIDS. Some prescription drugs may also decrease CoQ10 levels. Levels of CoQ10 in the body can be increased by taking CoQ10 supplements, although it is not clear whether this is beneficial. CoQ10 has been used, recommended, or studied for numerous conditions and remains controversial as a treatment in many areas.

USES BASED ON SCIENTIFIC EVIDENCE	Grade*
High blood pressure (hypertension) Preliminary research suggests that CoQ10 causes small decreases in blood pressure (systolic and possibly diastolic). Low blood levels of CoQ10 have been found in people with hypertension, although it is not clear if CoQ10 "deficiency" is a cause of high blood pressure. It is not known what dose is safe or effective. CoQ10 is less commonly used to treat hypertension than it is for other heart conditions such as congestive heart failure. Well-designed long-term research is needed to strengthen this recommendation.	B
Alzheimer's disease Promising preliminary evidence from human research suggests that CoQ10 supplements may slow down, but not cure, dementia in people with Alzheimer's disease. Additional well-designed studies are needed to confirm this result before a firm recommendation can be made.	C
Angina (chest pain from clogged heart arteries) Preliminary small human studies suggest that CoQ10 may reduce angina and improve exercise tolerance in people with clogged heart arteries. Better studies are needed before a firm recommendation can be made.	C
Anthracycline chemotherapy heart toxicity Anthracycline chemotherapy drugs, such as doxorubicin (Adriamycin), are commonly used to treat cancers such as breast cancer or lymphoma.	C

Continued

Heart damage (cardiomyopathy) is a major concern with the use of anthracyclines, and CoQ10 has been suggested to protect the heart. However, studies in this area are small and not high quality, and the effects of CoQ10 remain unclear.	
Breast cancer Several studies in women with breast cancer report reduced levels of CoQ10 in diseased breast tissue or blood. It has been suggested by some researchers that raising CoQ10 levels with supplements might be helpful. However, it is not clear if CoQ10 is beneficial in these patients or if the low levels of CoQ10 may actually be a part of the body's natural response to cancer, helping to fight disease. Supplementation with CoQ10 has not been proven to reduce cancer and has not been compared with other forms of treatment for breast cancer.	C
Cardiomyopathy (dilated, hypertrophic) There is conflicting evidence from research on the use of CoQ10 in patients with dilated or hypertrophic cardiomyopathy. Different levels of disease severity have been studied (New York Heart Association heart failure classes I through IV). Some studies report improved heart function (ejection fraction, stroke volume, cardiac index, exercise tolerance), while others find no improvements. Most trials are small or not well designed. Better research is needed in this area before a recommendation can be made.	C
Exercise performance The effects of CoQ10 on exercise performance have been tested in athletes, normal healthy individuals, and people with chronic lung disease. Results are variable; some studies reported benefits, and others showed no effects. Most trials have not been well designed. Better research is necessary before a firm conclusion can be drawn.	C
Friedreich's ataxia Preliminary research reports promising evidence for the use of CoQ10 in the treatment of Friedreich's ataxia. Further evidence is necessary before a firm conclusion can be drawn.	C
Gum disease (periodontitis) Preliminary studies in humans suggest possible benefits of CoQ10 taken by mouth or placed on the skin or gums in the treatment of periodontitis. Improvement in bleeding, swelling, and pain were reported. However, the available studies are small and of poor quality. Better research is needed before a conclusion can be drawn.	C
Heart attack (acute myocardial infarction) There is preliminary human study of CoQ10 given to patients within 3 days after a heart attack. Reductions in deaths, abnormal heart rhythms, and second heart attacks are reported, although better research is needed before a firm conclusion can be drawn.	C

Continued

Heart failure The evidence for CoQ10 in the treatment of heart failure is controversial and remains unclear. Different levels of disease severity have been studied (New York Heart Association classes I through IV). Some studies report improved heart function (ejection fraction, stroke volume, cardiac index, exercise tolerance), while others find no improvements. Most trials are small or not well designed. In some parts of Europe, Russia, and Japan, CoQ10 is considered a part of standard therapy for congestive heart failure patients. Better research is needed in this area, studying effects on quality of life, hospitalization, and death rates, before a recommendation can be made.	C
Heart protection during surgery Several studies suggest that cardiac function may be improved following major heart surgery such as coronary artery bypass graft (CABG) or valve replacement when CoQ10 is given to patients before or during surgery. Better-designed studies that measure effects on long-term cardiac function and survival are necessary before a recommendation can be made.	C
HIV/AIDS Limited evidence suggests that natural levels of CoQ10 in the body may be reduced in people with HIV/AIDS. There is no reliable scientific research showing that CoQ10 supplements have any effect on this disease.	C
Mitochondrial diseases and Kearns-Sayre syndrome CoQ10 is often recommended for people with mitochondrial diseases such as myopathies, encephalomyopathies, and Kearns-Sayre syndrome. Several early studies reported improvement in metabolism and physical endurance in people with these conditions after treatment with CoQ10, although most available research is not of high quality or definitive. Better studies are needed before a strong recommendation can be made.	C
Muscular dystrophy Preliminary studies in people with muscular dystrophy who were given CoQ10 supplements reported improvement in exercise capacity, heart function, and overall quality of life. Additional research is needed in this area.	C
Diabetes Evidence from preliminary studies suggest that CoQ10 does not affect blood sugar levels in people with type 1 or type 2 diabetes and does not alter the need for diabetes medications.	D

*Key to grades: *A:* Strong scientific evidence for this use; *B:* Good scientific evidence for this use; *C:* Unclear scientific evidence for this use; *D:* Fair scientific evidence against this use (it may not work); *F:* Strong scientific evidence against this use (it likely does not work). For a more detailed explanation of efficacy criteria, see "Natural Standard Evidence-Based Validated Grading Rationale" in the Introduction.

Uses Based on Tradition, Theory, or Limited Scientific Evidence

Amyotrophic lateral sclerosis (ALS), antioxidant, asthma, Bell's palsy, breathing difficulties, cancer, cerebellar ataxia, chronic fatigue syndrome, chronic obstructive pulmonary disease (COPD), deafness, decreased sperm motility (idiopathic asthenozoospermia), gingivitis, hair loss (and hair loss from chemotherapy), hepatitis B, high cholesterol, Huntington's chorea/disease, immune system diseases, infertility, insomnia, irregular heart beat, kidney failure, leg swelling (edema), life extension, liver enlargement/disease, lung cancer/disease, macular degeneration, maternally inherited diabetes mellitus and deafness (MIDD), MELAS syndrome, mitral valve prolapse, obesity, Papillon-Lefevre syndrome, Parkinson's disease, physical performance enhancement, prevention of muscle damage from statin cholesterol-lowering drugs, psychiatric disorders, QT-interval shortening; reduction of phenothiazine side effects, reduction of tricyclic antidepressant (TCA) side effects, stomach ulcers.

DOSING

The following doses are based on scientific research, publications, traditional use, or expert opinion. Many herbs and supplements have not been thoroughly tested, and their safety and effectiveness may not be proven. Brands may be made differently, with variable ingredients even within the same brand. The doses shown may not apply to all products. It is important to always read product labels and discuss doses with a qualified healthcare provider before therapy is started.

Standardization

- Standardization involves measuring the amounts of certain chemicals in products to try to make different preparations similar to each other. It is not always known if the chemicals being measured are the "active" ingredients. CoQ10 products sold in stores have been found to contain variable amounts of claimed ingredients. Early studies used low doses, while more recent research suggests that higher doses may be safe and have greater effects.

Adults (18 Years and Older)

Oral Use (by Mouth)

- **High blood pressure:** 30 to 360 mg of CoQ10 per day have been used. The ideal starting dose is not established. The reason why some people seem to respond better than others is unclear.
- **Congestive heart failure/cardiomyopathy:** Studies have used 100 to 200 mg of CoQ10 per day, or 2 mg per kilogram (2.2 pounds) of body weight per day. Limited research suggests that up to 600 mg per day may be tolerated. CoQ10 has been tested alone or as an addition to prescription drugs for these conditions. People with congestive heart failure or cardiomyopathy should consult a qualified healthcare provider before starting a new therapy.
- **Heart attack:** 120 mg of CoQ10 per day started 3 days after a heart attack has been studied, but the safety and effectiveness of this therapy are not established. People should consult a qualified healthcare provider before starting a new therapy.
- **Breast cancer:** 90 mg of CoQ10 per day in combination with multivitamin/multimineral supplementation has been studied.

- **Alzheimer's disease:** Doses of CoQ10 ranging from 60 mg once daily to 120 mg three times a day have been used. A preliminary study reported that higher doses may be more beneficial, although this has not been proven.
- **Anthracycline chemotherapy heart toxicity:** Preliminary research studies have used 50 to 100 mg of CoQ10 per day in children and adults receiving doxorubicin (Adriamycin) chemotherapy.
- **Angina:** 60 mg of CoQ10 per day for up to 4 weeks has been studied.
- **Heart protection during surgery:** Several studies in the 1980s and early 1990s used 30 to 150 mg of CoQ10 per day, starting 1 to 2 weeks prior to surgery and continuing for up to 1 month after surgery. Patients should consult their surgeon before starting a new therapy.
- **Exercise performance:** 90 to 150 mg per day of CoQ10 has been studied.
- **HIV/AIDS:** A dose of CoQ10 per day has been studied, but effectiveness has not been proved.
- **Muscular dystrophy:** In one study, 100 mg of CoQ10 per day divided into three doses was used.
- **Mitochondrial diseases:** 120 to 160 mg per day, or 2 mg per kilogram of body weight, has been used.
- **Gum disease (periodontitis):** In one study, 5 ml (1 teaspoonful) per day, concentrated to 200 mg of CoQ10 per ml of corn oil, taken by mouth in divided doses has been used.

Topical (on the Skin)

- **Gum disease (periodontitis):** In one study, 85 mg of CoQ10 per ml of soybean oil suspension was applied to the surface of affected areas once weekly using a plastic syringe.

Intravenous (Through the Veins)

- **Heart protection during surgery:** Most studies of the use of CoQ10 for heart protection during bypass surgery have used CoQ10 taken by mouth. However, one study used intravenous CoQ10, 5 mg per kilogram of body weight, given 2 hours prior to surgery. Safety was not proven. People who are planning to use any therapies close to the time of surgery should discuss this with their surgeon.

Children (Younger Than 18 Years)

- There is not enough scientific information to recommend the safe use of CoQ10 in children. A qualified healthcare provider should be consulted before considering use. One small study in children used 100 mg of CoQ10 by mouth twice daily to reduce the heart toxicity of anthracycline (doxorubicin) chemotherapy. Another study used 3 to 3.4 mg per kilogram of body weight daily in children with mitral valve prolapse.

SAFETY

The U.S. Food and Drug Administration does not strictly regulate herbs and supplements. There is no guarantee of the strength, purity, or safety of products, and effects may vary. It is important to always read product labels. People who have a medical condition, or are taking other drugs, herbs, or supplements, should consult a qualified healthcare provider before starting a new therapy. A healthcare provider should be contacted immediately about any side effects.

Allergies

- In theory, allergic reactions to supplements containing CoQ10 may occur.

Side Effects and Warnings

- Few serious side effects of CoQ10 have been reported. Side effects typically are mild and brief, stopping without any treatment needed. Reactions may include diarrhea, dizziness, fatigue, flu-like symptoms, headache, heartburn, increased sensitivity to light, insomnia, irritability, itching, loss of appetite, nausea and vomiting, rash, and stomach upset.
- CoQ10 may decrease blood sugar levels. Caution is advised in people with diabetes or hypoglycemia, and in those taking drugs, herbs, or supplements that affect blood sugar levels. Serum glucose levels may need to be monitored by a healthcare provider, and medication adjustments may be necessary.
- Low blood platelet numbers were reported in one person taking CoQ10. However, other factors (viral infection, other medications) may have been responsible. A decrease in platelets may increase the risk of bruising or bleeding, although there are no known reports of bleeding caused by CoQ10. Caution is advised in people who have bleeding disorders or who are taking drugs that increase the risk of bleeding. Dosing adjustments may be necessary.
- CoQ10 may decrease blood pressure, and caution is advised in patients with low blood pressure or taking blood pressure medications. Elevations of liver enzymes have been reported rarely, and caution is advised in people with liver disease or taking medications that may harm the liver. CoQ10 may lower blood levels of cholesterol or triglycerides. In one study, thyroid hormone levels were altered.
- Organ damage due to lack of oxygen/blood flow during intense exercise was reported in a study of people with heart disease, although the specific role of CoQ10 was not clear. Vigorous exercise is often discouraged in people using CoQ10 supplements.

Pregnancy and Breastfeeding

- Scientific evidence is insufficient to recommend the safe use of CoQ10 during pregnancy or breastfeeding.

INTERACTIONS

Most herbs and supplements have not been thoroughly tested for interactions with other herbs, supplements, drugs, or foods. The interactions listed here are based on reports in scientific publications, laboratory experiments, or traditional use. It is important to always read product labels. People who have a medical condition, or are taking other drugs, herbs, or supplements, should consult a qualified healthcare provider before starting a new therapy.

Interactions with Drugs

- In theory and based on a single case report, coenzyme Q10 may reduce the effectiveness of warfarin (Coumadin), and may limit or prevent effective anticoagulation (blood thinning). CoQ10 may reduce blood pressure and may add to the effects of other blood pressure–lowering agents. In theory, CoQ10 may affect thyroid hormone levels and alter the effects of thyroid drugs such as levothyroxine (Synthroid), although this has not been proven in humans.
- In theory and based on research studies in humans, a number of drugs may deplete natural levels of CoQ10 in the body. It has not been shown that there are benefits of CoQ10 supplements in people using these agents. Examples of such agents are antipsychotic medications such as chlorpromazine, fluphenazine, haloperidol, mesoridazine, prochlorperazine, promethazine, thioridazine, trifluoperazine, and

trimipramine; beta-blocker drugs such as acebutolol, atenolol, betaxolol, bisoprolol, carvedilol, esmolol, labetalol, metoprolol, nadolol, penbutolol, pindolol, propranolol, sotalol, and timolol; clonidine; diabetes drugs such as acetohexamide, chlorpropamide, glimepiride, glipizide, glyburide, metformin, tolazamide, and tolbutamide; diuretic drugs ("water pills") such as benzthiazide, chlorothiazide, hydralazine, hydrochlorothiazide, indapamide, methyclothiazide, metolazone, and polythiazide; gemfibrozil; HMG-CoA reductase inhibitors ("statins") such as atorvastatin, cerivastatin (no longer available in U.S.), fluvastatin, lovastatin, pravastatin, and simvastatin; methyldopa; and tricyclic antidepressant drugs such as amitriptyline, clomipramine, doxepin, imipramine, and trimipramine.

Interactions with Herbs and Dietary Supplements

- CoQ10 may reduce blood pressure and may result in additive effects when taken with other herbs or supplements that also lower blood pressure. Herbs that may lower blood pressure include aconite/monkshood, arnica, baneberry, betel nut, bilberry, black cohosh, bryony, calendula, California poppy, coleus, curcumin, eucalyptol, eucalyptus oil, ginger, goldenseal, green hellebore, hawthorn, horsetail, Indian tobacco, jaborandi, licorice, mistletoe, night blooming cereus, oleander, pasque flower, periwinkle, pleurisy root, shepherd's purse, Texas milkweed, turmeric, and wild cherry.
- Based on results of studies in humans, vitamin E may reduce CoQ10 blood levels. In theory, red rice yeast may decrease CoQ10 levels. CoQ10 may add to the effects or side effects of L-carnitine.

Selected References

Natural Standard developed the preceding evidence-based information based on a systematic review of more than 600 scientific articles. For comprehensive information about alternative and complementary therapies on the professional level, go to www.naturalstandard.com. Selected references are listed here.

Albano CB, Muralikrishnan D, Ebadi M. Distribution of coenzyme Q homologues in brain. Neurochem Res 2002;27(5):359-368.

Baggio E, Gandini R, Plancher AC, et al. Italian multicenter study on the safety and efficacy of coenzyme Q10 as adjunctive therapy in heart failure. CoQ10 Drug Surveillance Investigators. Mol Aspects Med 1994;15(Suppl):s287-s294.

Baker SK, Tarnopolsky MA. Targeting cellular energy production in neurological disorders. Expert Opin Investig Drugs 2003;12(10):1655-1679.

Balercia G, Arnaldi G, Lucarelli G, et al. Effects of exogenous CoQ10 administration in patients with idiopathic asthenozoospermia. Int J Andrology 2000;23(Suppl):43.

Batino M, Ferreiro MS, Quiles JL, et al. Alterations in the oxidation products, antioxidant markers, antioxidant capacity and lipid patterns in plasma of patients affected by Papillon-Lefevre syndrome. Free Radic Res 2003;37(6):603-609.

Blasi MA, Bovina C, Carella G, et al. Does coenzyme Q10 play a role in opposing oxidative stress in patients with age-related macular degeneration? Ophthalmologica 2001;215(1):51-54.

Bleske B, Willis R, Anthony M, et al. The effect of pravastatin and atorvastatin on coenzyme Q10. Am Heart J 2001;142(2):e2.

Bonetti A, Solito F, Carmosino G, et al. Effect of ubidecarenone oral treatment on aerobic power in middle-aged trained subjects. J Sports Med Phys Fitness 2000;40(1):51-57.

Braun B, Clarkson PM, Freedson PS, et al. Effects of coenzyme Q10 supplementation on exercise performance, VO_{2max}, and lipid peroxidation in trained cyclists. Int J Sport Nutr 1991;1(4):353-365.

Bresolin N, Doriguzzi C, Ponzetto C, et al. Ubidecarenone in the treatment of mitochondrial myopathies: a multi-center double-blind trial. J Neurol Sci 1990;100(1-2):70-78.

Burke BE, Neuenschwander R, Olson RD. Randomized, double-blind, placebo-controlled trial of coenzyme Q10 in isolated systolic hypertension. South Med J 2001;94(11): 1112-1117.

Chello M, Mastroroberto P, Romano R, et al. Protection by coenzyme Q10 from myocardial reperfusion injury during coronary artery bypass grafting. Ann Thorac Surg 1994;58(5): 1427-1432.

Chen RS, Huang CC, Chu NS. Coenzyme Q10 treatment in mitochondrial encephalomyopathies. Short-term double-blind, crossover study. Eur Neurol 1997;37(4):212-218.

Chen YF, Lin YT, Wu SC. Effectiveness of coenzyme Q10 on myocardial preservation during hypothermic cardioplegic arrest. J Thorac Cardiovasc Surg 1994;107(1):242-247.

de Bustos F, Jimenez-Jimenez FJ, Molina JA, et al. Serum levels of coenzyme Q10 in patients with multiple sclerosis. Acta Neurol Scand 2000;101(3):209-211.

Digiesi V, Cantini F, Brodbeck B. Effect of coenzyme Q10 on essential arterial hypertension. Curr Ther Res 1990;47(5):841-845.

Eaton S, Skinner R, Hale JP, et al. Plasma coenzyme Q(10) in children and adolescents undergoing doxorubicin therapy. Clin Chim Acta 2000;302(1-2):1-9.

Eriksson JG, Forsen TJ, Mortensen SA, et al. The effect of coenzyme Q10 administration on metabolic control in patients with type 2 diabetes mellitus. Biofactors 1999;9(2-4):315-318.

Folkers K, Langsjoen P, Willis R, et al. Lovastatin decreases coenzyme Q levels in humans. Proc Natl Acad Sci U S A 1990;87(22):8931-8934.

Folkers K, Vadhanavikit S, Mortensen SA. Biochemical rationale and myocardial tissue data on the effective therapy of cardiomyopathy with coenzyme Q10. Proc Natl Acad Sci U S A 1985; 82(3):901-904.

Fujimoto S, Kurihara N, Hirata K, et al. Effects of coenzyme Q10 administration on pulmonary function and exercise performance in patients with chronic lung diseases. Clin Investig 1993; 71(Suppl 8):S162-S166.

Gazdikova K, Gvozdjakova A, Kucharska J, et al. Effect of coenzyme Q10 in patients with kidney diseases. Cas Lek Cesk 2000;140:307-310.

Ghirlanda G, Oradei A, Manto A, et al. Evidence of plasma CoQ10-lowering effect by HMG-CoA reductase inhibitors: a double-blind, placebo-controlled study. J Clin Pharmacol 1993; 33(3):226-229.

Gutzmann H, Hadler D. Sustained efficacy and safety of idebenone in the treatment of Alzheimer's disease: update on a 2-year double-blind multicentre study. J Neural Transm Suppl 1998;54:301-310.

Hanioka T, Tanaka M, Ojima M, et al. Effect of topical application of coenzyme Q10 on adult periodontitis. Mol Aspects Med 1994;15(Suppl):s241-s248.

Henriksen JE, Andersen CB, Hother-Nielsen O, et al. Impact of ubiquinone (coenzyme Q10) treatment on glycaemic control, insulin requirement and well-being in patients with Type 1 diabetes mellitus. Diabet Med 1999;16(4):312-318.

Ishiyama T, Morita Y, Toyama S, et al. A clinical study of the effect of coenzyme Q on congestive heart failure. Jpn Heart J 1976;17(1):32-42.

Jimenez-Jimenez FJ, Molina JA, de Bustos F, et al. Serum levels of coenzyme Q10 in patients with Parkinson's disease. J Neural Transm 2000;107(2):177-181.

Judy WV, Stogsdill WW, Folkers K. Myocardial preservation by therapy with coenzyme Q10 during heart surgery. Clin Investig 1993;71(Suppl 8):S155-S161.

Kamikawa T, Kobayashi A, Yamashita T, et al. Effects of coenzyme Q10 on exercise tolerance in chronic stable angina pectoris. Am J Cardiol 1985;56(4):247-251.

Khatta M, Alexander BS, Krichten CM, et al. The effect of coenzyme Q10 in patients with congestive heart failure. Ann Intern Med 2000;132(8):636-640.

Lampertico M, Comis S. Italian multicenter study on the efficacy and safety of coenzyme Q10 as adjuvant therapy in heart failure. Clin Investig 1993;71(8 Suppl):S129-S133.

Landbo C, Almdal TP. [Interaction between warfarin and coenzyme Q10.] Ugeskr Laeger 1998;160(22):3226-3227.

Langsjoen H, Langsjoen P, Langsjoen P, et al. Usefulness of coenzyme Q10 in clinical cardiology: a long-term study. Mol Aspects Med 1994;15(Suppl):s165-s175.

Langsjoen P, Langsjoen P, Willis R, et al. Treatment of essential hypertension with coenzyme Q10. Mol Aspects Med 1994;15(Suppl):s265-s272.

Langsjoen PH, Folkers K, Lyson K, et al. Pronounced increase of survival of patients with cardiomyopathy when treated with coenzyme Q10 and conventional therapy. Int J Tissue React 1990;12(3):163-168.

Langsjoen PH, Langsjoen PH, Folkers K. A six-year clinical study of therapy of cardiomyopathy with coenzyme Q10. Int J Tissue React 1990;12(3):169-171.

Langsjoen PH, Langsjoen PH, Folkers K. Long-term efficacy and safety of coenzyme Q10 therapy for idiopathic dilated cardiomyopathy. Am J Cardiol 1990;65(7):521-523.

Lerman-Sagie T, Rustin P, Lev D, et al. Dramatic improvement in mitochondrial cardiomyopathy following treatment with idebenone. J Inherit Metab Dis 2001;24(1):28-34.

Lockwood K, Moesgaard S, Folkers K. Partial and complete regression of breast cancer in patients in relation to dosage of coenzyme Q10. Biochem Biophys Res Commun 1994;199(3):1504-1508.

Lockwood K, Moesgaard S, Hanioka T, et al. Apparent partial remission of breast cancer in "high risk" patients supplemented with nutritional antioxidants, essential fatty acids and coenzyme Q10. Mol Aspects Med 1994;15(Suppl):s231-s240.

Lockwood K, Moesgaard S, Yamamoto T, et al. Progress on therapy of breast cancer with vitamin Q10 and the regression of metastases. Biochem Biophys Res Commun 1995;212(1):172-177.

Matsumura T, Saji S, Nakamura R, et al. Evidence for enhanced treatment of periodontal disease by therapy with coenzyme Q. Int J Vitam Nutr Res 1973;43(4):537-548.

Mazzola C, Guffanti EE, Vaccarella A, et al. Noninvasive assessment of coenzyme Q10 in patients with chronic stable effort angina and moderate heart failure. Curr Ther Res 1987; 41(6):923-932.

Miyake Y, Shouzu A, Nishikawa M, et al. Effect of treatment with 3-hydroxy-3-methylglutaryl coenzyme A reductase inhibitors on serum coenzyme Q10 in diabetic patients. Arzneimittelforschung 1999;49(4):324-329.

Morisco C, Trimarco B, Condorelli M. Effect of coenzyme Q10 therapy in patients with congestive heart failure: a long-term multicenter randomized study. Clin Investig 1993; 71(Suppl 8):S134-S136.

Mortensen SA. Coenzyme Q10 as an adjunctive therapy in patients with congestive heart failure. J Am Coll Cardiol 2000;36(1):304-305.

Mortensen SA, Leth A, Agner E, et al. Dose-related decrease of serum coenzyme Q10 during treatment with HMG-CoA reductase inhibitors. Mol Aspects Med 1997;18(Suppl): s137-s144.

Mortensen SA, Vadhanavikit S, Muratsu K, et al. Coenzyme Q10: clinical benefits with biochemical correlates suggesting a scientific breakthrough in the management of chronic heart failure. Int J Tissue React 1990;12(3):155-162.

Munkholm H, Hansen HH, Rasmussen K. Coenzyme Q10 treatment in serious heart failure. Biofactors 1999;9(2-4):285-289.

Musumeci O, Naini A, Slonim AE, et al. Familial cerebellar ataxia with muscle coenzyme Q10 deficiency. Neurology 2001;56(7):849-855.

Nielsen AN, Mizuno M, Ratkevicius A, et al. No effect of antioxidant supplementation in triathletes on maximal oxygen uptake, 31P-NMRS detected muscle energy metabolism and muscle fatigue. Int J Sports Med 1999;20(3):154-158.

Ogasahara S, Nishikawa Y, Yorifuji S, et al. Treatment of Kearns-Sayre syndrome with coenzyme Q10. Neurology 1986;36(1):45-53.

Permanetter B, Rossy W, Klein G, et al. Ubiquinone (coenzyme Q10) in the long-term treatment of idiopathic dilated cardiomyopathy. Eur Heart J 1992;13(11):1528-1533.

Pogessi L, Galanti G, Corneglio M, et al. Effect of coenzyme Q10 on left ventricular function in patients with dilative cardiomyopathy. Curr Ther Res 1991;49:878-886.

Porter DA, Costill DL, Zachwieja JJ, et al. The effect of oral coenzyme Q10 on the exercise tolerance of middle-aged, untrained men. Int J Sports Med 1995;16(7):421-427.

Shults CW, Beal MF, Fontaine D, et al. Absorption, tolerability, and effects on mitochondrial activity of oral coenzyme Q10 in parkinsonian patients. Neurology 1998;50(3):793-795.

Singh RB, Khanna HK, Niaz MA. Randomized, double-blind placebo-controlled trial of coenzyme Q10 in chronic renal failure: discovery of a new role. J Nutr Environ Med 2000;10:281-288.

Singh RB, Niaz MA, Rastogi SS, et al. Effect of hydrosoluble coenzyme Q10 on blood pressures and insulin resistance in hypertensive patients with coronary artery disease. J Hum Hypertens 1999;13(3):203-208.

Singh RB, Wander GS, Rastogi A, et al. Randomized, double-blind placebo-controlled trial of coenzyme Q10 in patients with acute myocardial infarction. Cardiovasc Drugs Ther 1998;12(4):347-353.

Soja AM, Mortensen SA. [Treatment of chronic cardiac insufficiency with coenzyme Q10, results of meta-analysis in controlled clinical trials.] Ugeskr Laeger 1997;159(49): 7302-7308.

Sunamori M, Tanaka H, Maruyama T, et al. Clinical experience of coenzyme Q10 to enhance intraoperative myocardial protection in coronary artery revascularization. Cardiovasc Drugs Ther 1991;5 Suppl 2:297-300.

Tanaka J, Tominaga R, Yoshitoshi M, et al. Coenzyme Q10: the prophylactic effect on low cardiac output following cardiac valve replacement. Ann Thorac Surg 1982;33(2):145-151.

The Huntington Study Group. A randomized, placebo-controlled trial of coenzyme Q10 and remacemide in Huntington's disease. Neurology 2001;57(3):397-404.

Tran MT, Mitchell TM, Kennedy DT, et al. Role of coenzyme Q10 in chronic heart failure, angina, and hypertension. Pharmacotherapy 2001;21(7):797-806.

Watson PS, Scalia GM, Galbraith A, et al. Lack of effect of coenzyme Q on left ventricular function in patients with congestive heart failure. J Am Coll Cardiol 1999;33(6):1549-1552.

Weston SB, Zhou S, Weatherby RP, et al. Does exogenous coenzyme Q10 affect aerobic capacity in endurance athletes? Int J Sport Nutr 1997;7(3):197-206.

Yamagami T, Takagi M, Akagami H, et al. Effect of coenzyme Q10 on essential hypertension: a double-blind controlled study. *In* Folkers K, Yamamura Y (eds): Biomedical and Clinical Aspects of Coenzyme Q. Amsterdam, Elsevier, 1986, pp 337-343.

Yikoski T, Piirainen J, Hanninen O, et al. The effect of coenzyme Q10 on the exercise performance of cross-country skiers. Molec Aspects Med 1997;18(Suppl):s283-s290.

Zhou M, Zhi Q, Tang Y, et al. Effects of coenzyme Q10 on myocardial protection during cardiac valve replacement and scavenging free radical activity in vitro. J Cardiovasc Surg (Torino) 1999;40(3):355-361.

Cranberry
(*Vaccinium macrocarpon*)

RELATED TERMS

- American cranberry, Arandano Americano, Arandano trepador, bear berry, black cranberry, bog cranberry, Ericaceae, European cranberry, grosse moosebeere, isokarpalo, kranbeere, kronsbeere, large cranberry, low cranberry, marsh apple, mountain cranberry, moosebeere, mossberry, *Oxycoccus hagerupii, Oxycoccus macrocarpus, Oxycoccus microcarpus, Oxycoccus palustris, Oxycoccus quadripetalus*, pikkukarpalo, preisselbeere, ronce d'Amerique, trailing swamp cranberry, tsuru-kokemomo, *Vaccinium edule, Vaccinium erythrocarpum, Vaccinium hageruppi, Vaccinium microcarpum, Vaccinium occycoccus, Vaccinium plaustre, Vaccinium vitis.*

BACKGROUND

- Cranberry is widely used to prevent urinary tract infection (UTI). It was initially believed to have this effect by acidifying urine. However, the mechanism is now believed to be inhibition of adhesion of bacteria to uroepithelial cells by proanthocyanadin, a compound present in cranberry.
- Preliminary clinical evidence supports the use of cranberry juice and cranberry supplements to *prevent* UTI, although most available studies are of poor methodologic quality. Most studies have focused on effects against *E. coli*, although in vitro research suggests activity against *Proteus*, *Pseudomonas* and other species. There are no clear dosing guidelines, but given the safety of cranberry, it is reasonable to recommend the use of moderate amounts of cranberry juice cocktail to prevent UTI in individuals who are not chronically ill.
- Cranberry has not been shown to be effective as a *treatment* for documented UTI. Although cranberry may be a viable adjunct therapy at a time when antimicrobial resistance is of concern, given the proven efficacy of antibiotics, cranberry should not be considered a first-line agent.
- Cranberry has been investigated for numerous other medicinal uses, and promising areas of investigation include prevention of *H. pylori* infection and dental plaque.

USES BASED ON SCIENTIFIC EVIDENCE	Grade*
Urinary tract infection (UTI) prevention There are multiple studies of cranberry (juice or capsules) for the prevention of urinary tract infections in healthy women and nursing home residents. Although no single study convincingly demonstrates the ability of cranberry to prevent UTIs, the sum total of favorable evidence combined with laboratory research tends to support this use. It is not clear what dose is best. Most research has focused on the bacteria *E. coli*, although laboratory research suggests possible effects against other bacteria such as *Proteus* or *Pseudomonas*.	B

Continued

Cranberry seems to work by preventing bacteria from sticking to cells that line the bladder. Contrary to prior belief, urine acidification does not appear to play a role. Notably, many studies have been sponsored by the cranberry product manufacturer Ocean Spray. Additional research is needed in this area before a strong recommendation can be made.	
Antioxidant Laboratory studies suggest that cranberry has antioxidant properties. However, studies in humans are needed before a recommendation can be made.	C
Antiviral and antifungal activity Limited laboratory research has examined the antiviral and antifungal activity of cranberry. There are no reliable human studies supporting the use of cranberry in this area.	C
B_{12} absorption in people using antacids Preliminary studies suggest that cranberry juice may increase vitamin B_{12} absorption in people who are taking drugs that reduce stomach acid, such as lansoprazole (Prevacid), a proton pump inhibitor. However, this effect may be due to the acidity of the juice rather than an active component of cranberry. Further study is needed before a recommendation can be made.	C
Cancer prevention Based on a small amount of laboratory research, cranberry has been proposed for cancer prevention. Studies in humans are needed before a recommendation can be made.	C
Dental plaque Because of its activity against some bacteria, cranberry juice has been proposed as helpful for mouth care. However, because many commercial cranberry juice products have a high sugar content, they may not be suitable for this purpose. Research in this area is insufficient to make a clear recommendation.	C
Kidney stones Based on preliminary research, it is not clear if drinking cranberry juice increases or decreases the risk of kidney stone formation. Cranberry juice is reported to decrease urine levels of calcium, increase levels of urine magnesium and potassium, and increase urine levels of oxalate.	C
Reduction of odor from incontinence/bladder catheterization There is preliminary evidence that cranberry juice may reduce urine odor from incontinence or bladder catheterization. Further study is needed before a recommendation can be made.	C

Continued

Stomach ulcers caused by *Helicobacter pylori* bacteria Laboratory studies indicate that cranberry may reduce the ability of *H. pylori* to live in the stomach. However, reliable human studies are needed before a recommendation can be made.	C
Urinary tract infection (UTI) treatment There are no well-designed human studies available of cranberry used for the treatment of UTI. Laboratory research suggests that cranberry may not be effective when used alone, but it may be helpful as an adjunct to antibiotic therapy.	C
Urine acidification Taken in large quantities, cranberry juice may lower urine pH. Contrary to prior opinion, urine acidification does not appear to be the mechanism by which cranberry prevents urinary tract infection.	C
Urostomy care It is proposed that skin irritation at urostomy sites may be related to urine pH. Cranberry juice can lower urine pH and has been tested for this purpose. Further study is needed before a recommendation can be made.	C
Chronic urinary tract infection prevention: children with neurogenic bladder There is preliminary evidence that cranberry is not effective in preventing urinary tract infections in children with neurogenic bladder.	D
Radiation therapy side effects (prostate cancer) Evidence from preliminary studies suggests that cranberry is not effective in preventing urinary symptoms related to pelvic radiation therapy in patients with prostate cancer.	D

*Key to grades: *A:* Strong scientific evidence for this use; *B:* Good scientific evidence for this use; *C:* Unclear scientific evidence for this use; *D:* Fair scientific evidence against this use (it may not work); *F:* Strong scientific evidence against this use (it likely does not work). For a more detailed explanation of efficacy criteria, see "Natural Standard Evidence-Based Validated Grading Rationale" in the Introduction.

Uses Based on Tradition, Theory, or Limited Scientific Evidence

Anorexia, antibacterial, blood disorders, cancer treatment, diuresis (increasing urine flow), gallbladder stones, liver disorders, rheumatoid arthritis, scurvy, stomach disorders, vomiting, wound care.

DOSING

The following doses are based on scientific research, publications, traditional use, or expert opinion. Many herbs and supplements have not been thoroughly tested, and their safety and effectiveness may not be proven. Brands may be made differently, with variable ingredients even within the same brand. The doses shown may not apply to all products. It is important to always read product labels and discuss doses with a qualified healthcare provider before therapy is started.

Standardization

- Standardization involves measuring the amounts of certain chemicals in products to try to make different preparations similar to each other. It is not always known if the chemicals being measured are the "active" ingredients. There is no widely accepted standardization for cranberry juice products, although some cranberry preparations are standardized to 11% to 12% quinic acid per dose.

Adults (18 Years and Older)

- **Urinary tract infection prevention:** Recommended doses range from 90 to 480 ml (3 to 16 ounces) of cranberry cocktail twice daily, or 15 to 30 ml of unsweetened 100% cranberry juice daily. A daily dose of 300 ml (10 ounces) of commercially available cranberry cocktail (Ocean Spray) has been used in well-designed studies.
- Other forms of cranberry used include capsules, concentrate, and tinctures. Between one and six 300 to 400-mg hard gelatin capsules of concentrated cranberry juice extract, twice daily by mouth, given with water 1 hour before meals or 2 hours after meals, has been used. Soft gelatin capsules may contain vegetable oil and smaller amounts of the cranberry component. A dose of 1.5 ounces of frozen juice concentrate twice daily by mouth has been used, as well as 4 to 5 ml of cranberry tincture three times daily by mouth.

Children (Younger Than 18 Years)

- Scientific evidence is insufficient to recommend cranberry supplementation in children (beyond amounts found in a normal, balanced diet). Cranberry has been used safely in doses of 15 ml per kilogram of body weight in one study, or 300 ml, of cranberry juice taken daily for three months.

SAFETY

The U.S. Food and Drug Administration does not strictly regulate herbs and supplements. There is no guarantee of the strength, purity, or safety of products, and effects may vary. It is important to always read product labels. People who have a medical condition, or are taking other drugs, herbs, or supplements, should consult a qualified healthcare provider before starting a new therapy. A healthcare provider should be contacted immediately about any side effects.

Allergies

- Cranberry should be avoided by people with allergy/hypersensitivity to *Vaccinium* species (cranberries and blueberries).

Side Effects and Warnings

- It is advisable for people with diabetes or glucose intolerance to drink sugar-free cranberry juice to avoid a high sugar intake. Drinking more than 3 liters of cranberry juice daily may cause stomach distress and diarrhea. Drinking more than 1 liter of cranberry juice daily may increase the risk of kidney stones in people with a history of oxalate stones. Some commercially available products are high in calories. On average, 6 ounces of cranberry juice contains approximately 100 calories.

Pregnancy and Breastfeeding

- Safety has not been determined for use of cranberry juice during pregnancy and breastfeeding, although cranberry juice is believed to be safe in amounts commonly found in foods. Many tinctures contain high levels of alcohol and should be avoided during pregnancy.

INTERACTIONS

Most herbs and supplements have not been thoroughly tested for interactions with other herbs, supplements, drugs, or foods. The interactions listed here are based on reports in scientific publications, laboratory experiments, or traditional use. It is important to always read product labels. People who have a medical condition, or are taking other drugs, herbs, or supplements, should consult a qualified healthcare provider before starting a new therapy.

Interactions with Drugs

- Because of its acidic pH, cranberry juice may counteract antacids. Cranberry juice theoretically may increase the effects of antibiotics in the urinary tract and increase the excretion of some drugs in the urine. Cranberry juice may increase absorption of vitamin B_{12} in people taking proton pump inhibitors such as esomeprazole (Nexium).
- Some cranberry tinctures have a high alcohol content and cause vomiting if they are used with disulfiram (Antabuse) or metronidazole (Flagyl).

Interactions with Herbs and Dietary Supplements

- In theory, cranberry juice may increase the excretion of some herbs or supplements in the urine.

Selected References

Natural Standard developed the preceding evidence-based information based on a systematic review of more than 200 scientific articles. For comprehensive information about alternative and complementary therapies on the professional level, go to www.naturalstandard.com. Selected references are listed here.

Avorn J, Monane M, Gurwitz J, et al. Reduction of bacteriuria and pyuria using cranberry juice. JAMA 1994;272(8):588-590.

Avorn J, Monane M, Gurwitz JH, et al. Reduction of bacteriuria and pyuria after ingestion of cranberry juice. JAMA 1994;271(10):751-754.

Burger O, Ofek I, Tabak M, et al. A high molecular mass constituent of cranberry juice inhibits *Helicobacter pylori* adhesion to human gastric mucus. FEMS Immunol Med Microbiol 2000; 29(4):295-301.

Campbell G, Pickles T, D'yachkova Y. A randomised trial of cranberry versus apple juice in the management of urinary symptoms during external beam radiation therapy for prostate cancer. Clin Oncol (R Coll Radiol) 2003;15(6):322-328.

Carson CF, Riley TV. Non-antibiotic therapies for infectious diseases. Commun Dis Intell 2003; 27(Suppl):S143-S146.

Cavanagh HM, Hipwell M, Wilkinson JM. Antibacterial activity of berry fruits used for culinary purposes. J Med Food 2003;6(1):57-61.

Dignam R, Ahmed M, Denman S, et al. The effect of cranberry juice on UTI rates in a long term care facility. J Amer Ger Soc 1997;45(9):S53.

Ebringer A, Rashid T, Wilson C. Rheumatoid arthritis: proposal for the use of anti-microbial therapy in early cases. Scand J Rheumatol 2003;32(1):2-11. Review.

Fleet JC. New support for a folk remedy: cranberry juice reduces bacteriuria and pyuria in elderly women. Nutr Rev 1994;52(5):168-170.

C

Foda M, Middlebrook PF, Gatfield CT, et al. Efficacy of cranberry in prevention of urinary tract infection in a susceptible pediatric population. Canadian J Urol 1995;2(1):98-102.
Foxman B, Geiger AM, Palin K, et al. First-time urinary tract infection and sexual behavior. Epidemiology 1995;6(2):162-168.
Gibson L, Pike L, Kilbourne J. Effectiveness of cranberry juice in preventing urinary tract infections in long-term care facility patients. J Naturopath Med 1991;2(1):45-47.
Goodfriend R. Reduction of bacteriuria and pyuria using cranberry juice. JAMA 1994;272(8): 588; author reply 588-590.
Haverkorn MJ, Mandigers J. Reduction of bacteriuria and pyuria using cranberry juice. JAMA 1994;272(8):590.
Hopkins WJ, Heisey DM, Jonler M, et al. Reduction of bacteriuria and pyuria using cranberry juice. JAMA 1994;272(8):588-589; author reply 589-590.
Howell AB, Foxman B. Cranberry juice and adhesion of antibiotic-resistant uropathogens. JAMA 2002;287(23):3082-3083.
Jepson RG, Mihaljevic L, Craig J. Cranberries for preventing urinary tract infections. Cochrane Database Syst Rev 2000;(2):CD001321.
Kontiokari T, Sundqvist K, Nuutinen M, et al. Randomised trial of cranberry-lingonberry juice and *Lactobacillus GG* drink for the prevention of urinary tract infections in women. BMJ 2001;322(7302):1571-1573.
Lee YL, Owens J, Thrupp L, et al. Does cranberry juice have antibacterial activity? JAMA 2000;283(13):1691.
Papas PN, Brusch CA, Ceresia GC. Cranberry juice in the treatment of urinary tract infections. Southwest Med 1966;47(1):17-20.
Pedersen CB, Kyle J, Jenkinson AM, et al. Effects of blueberry and cranberry juice consumption on the plasma antioxidant capacity of healthy female volunteers. Eur J Clin Nutr 2000;54(5): 405-408.
Schlager TA, Anderson S, Trudell J, et al. Effect of cranberry juice on bacteriuria in children with neurogenic bladder receiving intermittent catheterization. J Pediatr 1999;135(6):698-702.
Schmidt DR, Sobota AE. An examination of the anti-adherence activity of cranberry juice on urinary and nonurinary bacterial isolates. Microbios 1988;55(224-225):173-181.
Terris MK, Issa MM, Tacker JR. Dietary supplementation with cranberry concentrate tablets may increase the risk of nephrolithiasis. Urology 2001;57(1):26-29.
Walker EB, Barney DP, Mickelsen JN, et al. Cranberry concentrate: UTI prophylaxis. J Fam Pract 1997;45(2):167-168.

Creatine

RELATED TERMS

- *N*-amidinosarcosine, *N*-(aminoiminomethyl)-*N* methyl glycine, Athletic Series Creatine, beta-GPA, Challenge Creatine Monohydrate, Creapure, Creatine Booster, creatine citrate, creatine monohydrate powder, creatine phosphate, Creatine Powder Drink Mix, Creatine Xtreme Lemonade, Creatine Xtreme Punch, Creavescent, cyclocreatine, EAS Phosphagen HP, Hardcore Formula Creatine Powder, HPCE pure creatine monohydrate, methyl guanidine–acetic acid, Neoton, Performance Enhancer Creatine Fuel, Phosphagen, Power Creatine, Total Creatine Transport.
- **Selected combination products that contain creatine:** Creatine Xtreme Punch (6 g creatine monohydrate, 1000 mg taurine, 500 mg L-glutamine, 500 mg L-glutamicacid, 200 mg hydroxycitrate, 15 mg vanadyl nicotinate, 120 g chromium); Met-Rx Anabolic Drive Series (12.4 g micronized creatine, 400 mg alpha-lipoic acid, 10 g glutamine peptide); Muscle Link/Effervescent Creatine Elite (5 g 99.5% pure creatine monohydrate, 20 g dextrose); Optimum Nutrition Creatine Liquid Energy Tropical Punch (6 g 99% pure pharmaceutical grade creatine monohydrate, 500 mg methylsulfonylmethane); Phosphagain (64 g daily carbohydrate, 67 g daily protein, 5 g daily fat, 20 g daily creatine, yeast-derived RNA, taurine).

BACKGROUND

- Creatine is naturally synthesized in the human body from amino acids, primarily in the kidney and liver, and transported in the blood to the muscles. Approximately 95% of the body's total creatine content is located in skeletal muscle. Creatine is found in meat and fish; on average, most adults in the United States consume 1-2 g of creatine daily from dietary sources.
- Creatine was discovered in the 1800s as an organic constituent of meat. In the 1970s, Soviet scientists reported that oral creatine supplements improved athletic performance during brief, intense activities such as sprints. Creatine gained popularity in the 1990s as a "natural" way to enhance athletic performance and build lean body mass. It was reported that skeletal muscle total creatine content increased with oral creatine supplementation, although response was variable. Factors that may account for this variation are carbohydrate intake, physical activity, training status, and muscle fiber type. The finding that carbohydrate enhanced muscle creatine uptake increased the market for creatine multi-ingredient sports drinks.
- Annual consumption of creatine products is estimated to exceed four million kilograms. The use of creatine is especially popular among adolescent athletes, who are reported to take doses that are not consistent with scientific evidence and that frequently exceed recommended loading and maintenance doses.
- Published reports suggest that approximately 25% of professional baseball players and up to 50% of professional football players consume creatine supplements. According to a survey of high school athletes, creatine use is common among football players, wrestlers, hockey players, gymnasts, and lacrosse players. In 1998, the creatine market in the United States. was estimated at $200 million. Most athletic associations (including the International Olympic Committee, the International

Amateur Athletic Federation, and the National Collegiate Athletic Association) have not banned this supplement.

- Creatinine excreted in urine is derived from creatine stored in muscle.

USES BASED ON SCIENTIFIC EVIDENCE	Grade*
Congestive heart failure (chronic) It has been reported that cardiac creatine levels lowered in people with chronic heart failure. Several studies reported that creatine supplementation was associated with improved heart muscle strength and endurance in patients with heart failure. However, standards for a safe and effective dose have not been established. Creatine supplementation has also been reported to increase creatine levels in skeletal muscle in these patients, helping to increase strength and endurance. Comparisons with drugs used to treat heart failure have not been conducted. People who have symptoms of heart failure should consult a qualified healthcare provider.	C
Enhanced athletic endurance It has been suggested that creatine may help improve athletic endurance by increasing time to fatigue (possibly by shortening muscle recovery periods). However, the results of research evaluating this claim are mixed. Findings from different studies disagree with each other, and most studies do not support the use of creatine to enhance sustained aerobic activities.	C
Enhanced athletic sprinting Creatine has been suggested to enhance athletic performance and to delay onset of fatigue during short sprints. Effects have been attributed to increased creatine concentrations in muscle. Although results from different studies disagree with each other, most research reports some improvement when creatine is used as a supplement. Creatine may enhance performance when used during brief bursts of aerobic activities and when there are short recovery times between bouts of activity. Better research is necessary before a firm conclusion can be reached.	C
Enhanced muscle mass/strength Multiple studies suggest that creatine may improve muscle mass and strength in men and women, particularly when accompanied by increased physical activity. However, studies of creatine in athletes have disagreed with each other. Although many experts believe that creatine may be useful for high-intensity, short-duration exercise, it has not been demonstrated effective in endurance sports. Benefit may be greatest when levels of creatine before supplementation are low, and in specific sub-populations such as older men. Of the approximately 300 studies that have evaluated the potential ergogenic value of creatine supplementation, about 70% report	C

Continued

statistically significant results while the remaining studies generally report non-significant gains in performance. Because of methodological problems with available studies, a firm conclusion cannot be reached.	
GAMT deficiency Some individuals are born with a genetic disorder in which there is a deficiency of the enzyme guanidinoacetate methyltransferase (GAMT). A lack of this enzyme causes severe developmental delays and abnormal movement disorders. The condition is diagnosed by a lack of creatine in the brain. Although there is only limited research in this area, significant improvements were noted in two individuals who were given supplemental creatine, suggesting that this supplement may be an effective treatment for disorders caused by a lack of creatine.	**C**
Heart muscle protection during heart surgery There is early evidence that heart muscle may recover better and more rapidly after open-heart surgery if intravenous creatinine is administered during the operation. Further study is needed before a recommendation can be made.	**C**
High cholesterol There is limited research in this area, and results from different studies disagree with each other (with some trials noting reductions in total cholesterol and triglyceride levels). It remains unclear what effect creatine has on lipids. Additional studies are needed before a clear conclusion can be drawn.	**C**
Hyperornithinemia (high levels of ornithine in the blood) Ornithine is a by-product formed in the liver. Some persons are born with a genetic disorder that prevents the breakdown of ornithine, resulting in excessively high levels of ornithine in the blood. This imbalance can result in muscle weakness, reduced storage of creatine in the muscles and brain, and blindness. Although research in this area is limited, early evidence suggests that long-term, daily creatine supplements may replace the deficient creatine and may slow vision loss.	**C**
McArdle's disease McArdle's disease is characterized by a deficiency of energy compounds stored in muscle, resulting in muscle fatigue, exercise intolerance, and pain when exercising. Creatine has been proposed as a possible therapy for this condition. However, research in this area has been limited, and the results of existing studies disagree. It is unclear whether creatine offers any benefits to patients with McArdle's disease.	**C**
Mental deterioration It has been reported that use of creatine phosphate may have a favorable effect on mental deterioration in "cardio-cerebral syndrome" following heart attacks in the elderly.	**C**

Continued

Muscular dystrophy Creatine loss is suspected to cause muscle weakness and breakdown in Duchenne muscular dystrophy. Studies in animals report increased muscle formation and survival with creatine. Studies in humans have been small, although early evidence suggests that creatine may be beneficial in treating muscular dystrophies. Further research is needed.	C
Myocardial infarction (heart attack) There is early evidence that intravenous creatine following a heart attack may be beneficial to heart muscle function and may prevent ventricular arrhythmias. Further study is needed before a recommendation can be made in this area.	C
Neuromuscular disorders Numerous studies suggest that creatine may be helpful in the treatment of various neuromuscular diseases, such as amyotrophic lateral sclerosis (ALS) and myasthenia gravis, and may delay onset of symptoms when used as an adjunct to conventional treatment. However, creatine ingestion does not appear to have a significant effect on muscle creatine stores or high-intensity exercise capacity in individuals with multiple sclerosis. Although early studies were encouraging, recent research reports no beneficial effects on survival or disease progression. Additional studies are needed to provide clearer answers.	C

*Key to grades: *A:* Strong scientific evidence for this use; *B:* Good scientific evidence for this use; *C:* Unclear scientific evidence for this use; *D:* Fair scientific evidence against this use (it may not work); *F:* Strong scientific evidence against this use (it likely does not work). For a more detailed explanation of efficacy criteria, see "Natural Standard Evidence-Based Validated Grading Rationale" in the Introduction.

Uses Based on Tradition, Theory, or Limited Scientific Evidence

Alzheimer's disease, anti-arrhythmic, anti-convulsant, anti-inflammatory, antioxidant, arginine:glycine amidinotransferase (AGAT) deficiency, breast cancer, cervical cancer, circadian clock acceleration, colon cancer, diabetes and diabetic complications, disuse muscle atrophy, fibromyalgia, growth stimulation, herpes, Huntington's disease, hyperhomocysteinemia, hypoxic seizures, mitochondrial diseases, neuroprotection, Parkinson's disease, rheumatoid arthritis, wasting of brain regions.

DOSING

The following doses are based on scientific research, publications, traditional use, or expert opinion. Many herbs and supplements have not been thoroughly tested, and their safety and effectiveness may not be proven. Brands may be made differently, with variable ingredients even within the same brand. The doses shown may not apply to all products. It is important to always read product labels and discuss doses with a qualified healthcare provider before therapy is started.

Standardization

- Standardization involves measuring the amounts of certain chemicals in products to try to make different preparations similar to each other. It is not always known if the chemicals being measured are the "active" ingredients. Products contain different forms of creatine (e.g., creatine monohydrate, creatine monophosphate) in varying concentrations and may be combined with other supplements. There are no standard doses of creatine, and many different doses are used.

Adults (18 Years and Older)

- *Note*: Creatine appears to be absorbed best as a solution, although it is also readily absorbed when natural sources such as meat and fish are ingested. Elevation of muscle creatine levels may best be achieved by taking creatine with carbohydrates. Experts often recommend maintaining good hydration during creatine use.
- **Oral (powder):** A wide range of dosing has been used or studied. To enhance athletic performance, 9 to 20 g daily in divided doses for 4 to 7 days has been used, with maintenance doses of 2 to 5 g, or 0.3 mg per kilogram of body weight, daily. For cholesterol reduction, 20 to 25 g daily for 5 days, followed by 5 to 10 g thereafter, has been used. To treat hyperornithinemia, 1.5 g daily has been used. For neuromuscular diseases, including muscular dystrophy, 10 g daily has been suggested, although lower doses (5 g) and higher doses (20 g) have also been used. A dose of 400 to 670 mg per kilogram of body weight daily has been used to treat GAMT deficiency. For congestive heart failure, 20 g per day has been studied. For symptomatic therapy of ALS, 20 g daily for 7 days, and then 3 g daily for 3 to 6 months has been used. A dose of 150 mg per kilogram of body weight has been used daily for 5 days, followed by 60 mg per kilogram daily for 5 weeks, for McArdle's disease
- **Intravenous/intramuscular (IV/IM):** Numerous dosing regimens have been used in studies in humans. IV/IM dosing should be administered only under strict medical supervision.

Children (Younger Than 18 Years)

Dosing in children should be carried out under medical supervision because of potential adverse effects. A dose of 5 g daily has been used in children with muscular dystrophy, and various doses have been used in children with GAMT deficiency, including 2 g per kilogram of body weight, 4-8 g daily in an infant, and 400-670 mg per kilogram of body weight.

SAFETY

The U.S. Food and Drug Administration does not strictly regulate herbs and supplements. There is no guarantee of the strength, purity, or safety of products, and effects may vary. It is important to always read product labels. People who have a medical condition, or are taking other drugs, herbs, or supplements, should consult a qualified healthcare provider before starting a new therapy. A healthcare provider should be contacted immediately about any side effects.

Allergies

- Creatine has been associated with asthmatic symptoms. People should not take creatine if they have a known allergy to this supplement.

Side Effects and Warnings

- Systematic studies of the safety, pharmacology, and toxicology of creatine are limited. People using creatine, including athletes, should be monitored by a qualified healthcare provider.
- Some individuals may experience gastrointestinal symptoms, including loss of appetite, stomach discomfort, diarrhea, or nausea.
- Creatine may cause muscle cramps or muscle breakdown, leading to discomfort and possibly muscle tears. Weight gain and increased body mass may occur. Heat intolerance, fever, dehydration, reduced blood volume, and electrolyte imbalances (and resulting seizures) may occur.
- There is less concern today than formerly about possible kidney damage from creatine, although there have been reports of kidney damage, such as interstitial nephritis. People with kidney disease should avoid the use of creatine. Similarly, because liver function may be affected by creatine supplements, caution is advised in people with underlying liver disease.
- In theory, creatine may alter the activities of insulin. Caution is advised in people with diabetes or hypoglycemia, and in those taking drugs, herbs, or supplements that affect blood sugar levels. Serum glucose levels may need to be monitored by a healthcare provider, and medication adjustments may be necessary.
- Chronic administration of a large quantity of creatine is reported to increase the production of formaldehyde, which may cause serious side effects.
- Based on a case report, creatine may increase the risk of compartment syndrome of the lower leg, a condition characterized by pain in the lower leg associated with inflammation and ischemia (diminished blood flow), which is a potential surgical emergency.

Pregnancy and Breastfeeding

- Creatine cannot be recommended during pregnancy or breastfeeding because of the lack of scientific information in these areas.
- Pasteurized cow's milk appears to contain higher levels of creatine than human milk. The clinical significance of this is unclear.

INTERACTIONS

Most herbs and supplements have not been thoroughly tested for interactions with other herbs, supplements, drugs, or foods. The interactions listed here are based on reports in scientific publications, laboratory experiments, or traditional use. It is important to always read product labels. People who have a medical condition, or are taking other drugs, herbs, or supplements, should consult a qualified healthcare provider before starting a new therapy.

Interactions with Drugs

- In theory, creatine may alter the activities of insulin, particularly when it is taken with carbohydrates. Caution is advised in people who are using medications that may also alter blood sugar levels. People taking drugs for diabetes by mouth or insulin should be monitored closely by a qualified healthcare provider. Medication adjustments may be necessary.
- Use of creatine with probenecid may increase levels of creatine in the body, leading to increased side effects.

- Use of creatine with diuretics such as hydrochlorothiazide and furosemide (Lasix) should be avoided because of the risks of dehydration and electrolyte disturbances. The likelihood of kidney damage may be greater when creatine is used with drugs that may damage the kidneys, including amikacin, anti-inflammatory drugs such as ibuprofen (Advil, Motrin), cimetidine (Tagamet), cyclosporine (Neoral, Sandimmune), gentamicin, tobramycin, and trimethoprim.
- Creatine may increase the cholesterol-lowering effects of other drugs used to lower cholesterol levels, such as lovastatin (Mevacor).
- Studies in animals reported that the combination of creatine and nonsteroidal anti-inflammatory drugs was more effective in reducing inflammation than either agent used alone.
- Creatine and nifedipine, when used together, may enhance heart function, although research in this area is limited.

Interactions with Herbs and Dietary Supplements

- Creatine may increase the risk of adverse effects, including stroke, when used with caffeine and ephedra. In addition, caffeine may reduce the beneficial effects of creatine during intense intermittent exercise.
- Because creatine theoretically may alter the activities of insulin, caution is advised when using herbs or supplements that may also alter blood sugar levels. Blood glucose levels may require monitoring, and doses may need adjustment. Examples of herbs and supplements that may cause hypoglycemia (low blood sugar levels) are *Aloe vera*, American ginseng, bilberry, bitter melon, burdock, fenugreek, fish oil, gymnema, horse chestnut seed extract (HCSE), maitake mushroom, marshmallow, milk thistle, *Panax ginseng*, rosemary, shark cartilage, Siberian ginseng, stinging nettle, and white horehound. Agents that may raise blood sugar levels (hyperglycemia) include arginine, cocoa, and ephedra (when combined with caffeine).
- Creatine may reduce the effectiveness of vitamins A, D, E, and K.
- Creatine may affect liver function, and should be used cautiously with potentially hepatotoxic (liver-damaging) herbs and supplements. Examples are ackee, bee pollen, birch oil, blessed thistle, borage, bush tea, butterbur, chaparral, coltsfoot, comfrey, DHEA, *Echinacea purpurea*, *Echium* spp., germander, *Heliotropium* spp., horse chestnut (parenteral preparations), jin-bu-huan (*Lycopodium serratum*), kava, lobelia, mate, niacin (vitamin B_3), niacinamide, Paraguay tea, periwinkle, *Plantago lanceolata*, pride of Madeira, rue, sassafras, scullcap, *Senecio* spp./groundsel, tansy ragwort, L-tetrahydropalmatine (THP), turmeric/curcumin, tu-san-chi (*Gynura segetum*), uva ursi, valerian, and white chameleon.
- Use of creatine with diuretics should be avoided because of the risk of dehydration and electrolyte disturbances. Herbs with possible diuretic effects include artichoke, celery, corn silk, couchgrass, dandelion, elder flower, horsetail, juniper berry, kava, shepherd's purse, uva ursi, and yarrow.
- It is possible that creatine may increase the cholesterol-lowering effects of herbs and supplements that lower cholesterol levels, such as red yeast (*Monascus purpureus*).

Selected References

Natural Standard developed the preceding evidence-based information based on a systematic review of more than 3000 articles. For comprehensive information about alternative and complementary therapies on the professional level, go to www.naturalstandard.com. Selected references are listed here.

Aaserud R, Gramvik P, Olsen SR, Jensen J. Creatine supplementation delays onset of fatigue during repeated bouts of sprint running. Scand J Med Sci Sports 1998;8(5 Pt 1):247-251.

Andrews R, Greenhaff P, Curtis S, et al. The effect of dietary creatine supplementation on skeletal muscle metabolism in congestive heart failure. Eur Heart J 1998;19(4):617-622.

Balestrino M, Lensman M, Parodi M, et al. Role of creatine and phosphocreatine in neuronal protection from anoxic and ischemic damage. Amino Acids 2002;23(1-3):221-229.

Batley MA, Walton T, Scott DL, et al. Creatine supplementation in fibromyalgia. ULAR 2002 European Congress of Rheumatology, June 12-15, 2002, Stockholm.

Battini R, Leuzzi V, Carducci C, et al. Creatine depletion in a new case with AGAT deficiency: clinical and genetic study in a large pedigree. Mol Genet Metab 2002;77(4):326-331.

Becque MD, Lochmann JD, Melrose DR. Effects of oral creatine supplementation on muscular strength and body composition. Med Sci Sports Exerc 2000;32(3):654-658.

Bemben MG, Bemben DA, Loftiss DD, et al. Creatine supplementation during resistance training in college football athletes. Med Sci Sports Exerc 2001;33(10):1667-1673.

Biwer CJ, Jensen RL, Schmidt WD, Watts PB. The effect of creatine on treadmill running with high-intensity intervals. J Strength Cond Res 2003;17(3):439-445.

Branch JD. Effect of creatine supplementation on body composition and performance: a meta-analysis. Int J Sport Nutr Exerc Metab 2003;13(2):198-226.

Brose A, Parise G, Tarnopolsky MA. Creatine supplementation enhances isometric strength and body composition improvements following strength exercise training in older adults. J Gerontol A Biol Sci Med Sci 2003;58(1):11-19.

Chwalbinska-Moneta J. Effect of creatine supplementation on aerobic performance and anaerobic capacity in elite rowers in the course of endurance training. Int J Sport Nutr Exerc Metab 2003;13(2):173-183.

Delecluse C, Diels R, Goris M. Effect of creatine supplementation on intermittent sprint running performance in highly trained athletes. J Strength Cond Res 2003;17(3):446-454.

Eijnde BO, Van Leemputte M, Goris M, et al. Effects of creatine supplementation and exercise training on fitness in men 55-75 yr old. J Appl Physiol 2003;95(2):818-828.

Fagbemi O, Kane KA, Parratt JR. Creatine phosphate suppresses ventricular arrhythmias resulting from coronary artery ligation. J Cardiovasc Pharmacol 1982;4(1):53-58.

Farquhar WB, Zambraski EJ. Effects of creatine use on the athlete's kidney. Curr Sports Med Rep 2002;1(2):103-106.

Ferraro S, Codella C, Palumbo F, et al. Hemodynamic effects of creatine phosphate in patients with congestive heart failure: a double-blind comparison trial versus placebo. Clin Cardiol 1996;19(9):699-703.

Gordon A, Hultman E, Kaijser L, et al. Creatine supplementation in chronic heart failure increases skeletal muscle creatine phosphate and muscle performance. Cardiovasc Res 1995;30(3):413-418.

Gotshalk LA, Volek JS, Staron RS, et al. Creatine supplementation improves muscular performance in older men. Med Sci Sports Exerc 2002;34(3):537-543.

Green AL, Hultman E, Macdonald IA, et al. Carbohydrate ingestion augments skeletal muscle creatine accumulation during creatine supplementation in humans. Am J Physiol 1996; 271(5 Pt 1):E821-E826.

Green AL, Simpson EJ, Littlewood JJ, et al. Carbohydrate ingestion augments creatine retention during creatine feeding in humans. Acta Physiol Scand 1996;158(2):195-202.

Greenwood M, Kreider RB, Melton C, et al. Creatine supplementation during college football training does not increase the incidence of cramping or injury. Mol Cell Biochem 2003;244(1-2):83-88.

Grindstaff PD, Kreider R, Bishop R, et al. Effects of creatine supplementation on repetitive sprint performance and body composition in competitive swimmers. Int J Sport Nutr 1997; 7(4):330-346.

Groeneveld GJ, Veldink JH, van der Tweel I, et al. A randomized sequential trial of creatine in amyotrophic lateral sclerosis. Ann Neurol 2003;53(4):437-445.

Hespel P, Op't Eijnde B, Van Leemputte M. Opposite actions of caffeine and creatine on muscle relaxation time in humans. J Appl Physiol 2002;92(2):513-518.

Hulsemann J, Manz F, Wember T, Schoch G. [Administration of creatine and creatinine with breast milk and infant milk preparations.] Klin Padiatr 1987;199(4):292-295.

Izquierdo M, Ibanez J, Gonzalez-Badillo JJ, Gorostiaga EM. Effects of creatine supplementation on muscle power, endurance, and sprint performance. Med Sci Sports Exerc 2002; 34(2):332-343.

Jacobstein MD, Gerken TA, Bhat AM, Carlier PG. Myocardial protection during ischemia by prior feeding with the creatine analog: cyclocreatine. J Am Coll Cardiol 1989;14(1):246-251.

Jones AM, Atter T, Georg KP. Oral creatine supplementation improves multiple sprint performance in elite ice-hockey players. J Sports Med Phys Fitness 1999; 39(3):189-196.

Kilduff LP, Vidakovic P, Cooney G, et al. Effects of creatine on isometric bench-press performance in resistance-trained humans. Med Sci Sports Exerc 2002;34(7):1176-1183.

Klopstock T, Querner V, Schmidt F, et al. A placebo-controlled crossover trial of creatine in mitochondrial diseases. Neurology 2000;55(11):1748-1751.

Komura K, Hobbiebrunken E, Wilichowski EK, Hanefeld FA. Effectiveness of creatine monohydrate in mitochondrial encephalomyopathies. Pediatr Neurol 2003;28(1):53-58.

Koshy KM, Griswold E, Schneeberger EE. Interstitial nephritis in a patient taking creatine. N Engl J Med 1999;340(10):814-815.

Kreider RB, Ferreira M, Wilson M, et al. Effects of creatine supplementation on body composition, strength, and sprint performance. Med Sci Sports Exerc 1998;30(1):73-82.

Kreider RB, Melton C, Rasmussen CJ, et al. Long-term creatine supplementation does not significantly affect clinical markers of health in athletes. Mol Cell Biochem 2003;244(1-2):95-104.

Kuehl K, Goldberg L, Elliot D. Re: Long-term oral creatine supplementation does not impair renal function in healthy athletes. Med Sci Sports Exerc 2000;32(1):248-249.

Lawler JM, Barnes WS, Wu G, et al. Direct antioxidant properties of creatine. Biochem Biophys Res Commun 2002;290(1):47-52.

Lehmkuhl M, Malone M, Justice B, et al. The effects of 8 weeks of creatine monohydrate and glutamine supplementation on body composition and performance measures. J Strength Cond Res 2003;17(3):425-438.

Mayhew DL, Mayhew JL, Ware JS. Effects of long-term creatine supplementation on liver and kidney functions in American college football players. Int J Sport Nutr Exerc Metab 2002; 12(4):453-460.

Mazzini L, Balzarini C, Colombo R, et al. Effects of creatine supplementation on exercise performance and muscular strength in amyotrophic lateral sclerosis: preliminary results. J Neurol Sci 2001;191(1-2):139-144.

McNaughton LR, Dalton B, Tarr J. The effects of creatine supplementation on high-intensity exercise performance in elite performers. Eur J Appl Physiol Occup Physiol 1998;78(3): 236-240.

Mujika I, Chatard JC, Lacoste L, et al. Creatine supplementation does not improve sprint performance in competitive swimmers. Med Sci Sports Exerc 1996;28(11):1435-1441.

Mujika I, Padilla S, Ibanez J, et al. Creatine supplementation and sprint performance in soccer players. Med Sci Sports Exerc 2000;32(2):518-525.

Newman JE, Hargreaves M, Garnham A, Snow RJ. Effect of creatine ingestion on glucose tolerance and insulin sensitivity in men. Med Sci Sports Exerc 2003;35(1):69-74.

O'Reilly DS, Carter R, Bell E, et al. Exercise to exhaustion in the second-wind phase of exercise in a case of McArdle's disease with and without creatine supplementation. Scott Med J 2003; 48(2):46-48.

Peyrebrune MC, Nevill ME, Donaldson FJ, Cosford DJ. The effects of oral creatine supplementation on performance in single and repeated sprint swimming. J Sports Sci 1998;16(3): 271-279.

Potteiger JA, Randall JC, Schroeder C, et al. Elevated anterior compartment pressure in the leg after creatine supplementation: A controlled case report. J Athl Train 2001;36(1):85-88.

Preen D, Dawson B, Goodman C, et al. Effect of creatine loading on long-term sprint exercise performance and metabolism. Med Sci Sports Exerc 2001;33(5):814-821.

Robinson TM, Sewell DA, Casey A, et al. Dietary creatine supplementation does not affect some haematological indices, or indices of muscle damage and hepatic and renal function. Br J Sports Med 2000;34(4):284-288.

Romer LM, Barrington JP, Jeukendrup AE. Effects of oral creatine supplementation on high intensity, intermittent exercise performance in competitive squash players. Int J Sports Med 2001;22(8):546-552.

Rooney KB, Bryson JM, Digney AL, et al. Creatine supplementation affects glucose homeostasis but not insulin secretion in humans. Ann Nutr Metab 2003;47(1):11-15.

Schneider-Gold C, Beck M, Wessig C, et al. Creatine monohydrate in DM2/PROMM: a double-blind placebo-controlled clinical study. Proximal myotonic myopathy. Neurology 2003;60(3):500-502.

Schroeder C, Potteiger J, Randall J, et al. The effects of creatine dietary supplementation on anterior compartment pressure in the lower leg during rest and following exercise. Clin J Sport Med 2001;11(2):87-95.

Skare OC, Skadberg, Wisnes AR. Creatine supplementation improves sprint performance in male sprinters. Scand J Med Sci Sports 2001;11(2):96-102.

Tarnopolsky MA, MacLennan DP. Creatine monohydrate supplementation enhances high-intensity exercise performance in males and females. Int J Sport Nutr Exerc Metab 2000; 10(4):452-463.

Vandenberghe K, Gillis N, Van Leemputte M, et al. Caffeine counteracts the ergogenic action of muscle creatine loading. J Appl Physiol 1996;80(2):452-457.

Vorgerd M, Zange J, Kley R, et al. Effect of high-dose creatine therapy on symptoms of exercise intolerance in McArdle disease: double-blind, placebo-controlled crossover study. Arch Neurol 2002;59(1):97-101.

Dandelion

(*Taraxacum officinale*)

RELATED TERMS

- Asteraceae/Compositae, blowball, cankerwort, Cichoroideae, clock flower, common dandelion, dandelion herb, dent de lion, diente de lion, dudhal, dumble-dor, fairy clock, fortune teller, hokouei-kon, huang hua di ding, Irish daisy, *Leontodon taraxacum*, lion's teeth (lion's tooth), lowenzahn, lowenzahnwurzel, maelkebotte, milk gowan, min-deul-rre, mok's head, mongoloid dandelion, pee in the bed, pissenlit, piss-in-bed, pries' crown (priest's crown), puffball, pu gong ying, pu kung ying, radix taraxaci, swine snout, taraxaci herba, taraxacum, *Taraxacum mongolicum*, *Taraxacum palustre*, *Taraxacum vulgare*, telltime, white endive, wild endive, witch gowan, witches' milk, yellow flower earth nail.

BACKGROUND

- Dandelion is a member of the Asteraceae/Compositae family and is closely related to chicory. It is a perennial herb, native throughout the Northern hemisphere and found growing wild in meadows, pastures, and waste grounds of the temperate zones. Most commercial dandelion is cultivated in Bulgaria, Hungary, Poland, Romania, and the United Kingdom.
- Dandelion was commonly used in Native American medicine. The Iroquois, Ojibwe, and Rappahannock prepared infusions and decoctions of the root and herb to treat kidney disease, dyspepsia, and heartburn. In traditional Arabian medicine, dandelion has been used to treat liver and spleen ailments. In traditional Chinese medicine (TCM), dandelion is combined with other herbs to treat hepatitis; to enhance immune response to upper respiratory tract infections, bronchitis, and pneumonia; and as a topical compress for mastitis (breast inflammation).
- Dandelion root and leaf are used throughout Europe for gastrointestinal ailments. The European Scientific Cooperative on Phytotherapy (ESCOP) recommends dandelion root for "restoration of hepatic and biliary function, dyspepsia [indigestion], and loss of appetite." The German Commission E authorizes the use of combination products containing dandelion root and herb for biliary abnormalities, appetite loss, dyspepsia, and for stimulation of diuresis (urine flow). Some modern naturopathic physicians assert that dandelion can detoxify the liver and gallbladder, reduce side effects of medications metabolized by the liver, and relieve symptoms associated with liver disease.
- Dandelion is generally regarded as safe, with rare side effects including contact dermatitis, diarrhea, and gastrointestinal upset. Traditionally, the herb is not recommended in patients with liver or gallbladder disease, based on the belief that dandelion stimulates bile secretion (an assertion not demonstrated in studies in animals or humans).
- Dandelion is used as a salad ingredient, and the roasted root and its extracts are sometimes used as a coffee substitute.

USES BASED ON SCIENTIFIC EVIDENCE	Grade*
Anti-inflammatory Research in laboratory animals suggests that dandelion root may possess anti-inflammatory properties. There have been no well-conducted studies in humans in this area.	C
Antioxidant Several laboratory studies report antioxidant properties of dandelion flower extract, although this research is preliminary, and effects in humans are not known.	C
Cancer Limited animal research does not provide a clear assessment of the effects of dandelion on tumor growth. There have been no well-conducted human studies in this area.	C
Colitis There is a report that a combination herbal preparation containing dandelion improved chronic pain associated with colitis in several patients. Because multiple herbs were used and this study was not well designed or reported, the effects of dandelion are unclear.	C
Diabetes There has been limited research on the effects of dandelion on blood sugar levels in animals. One study reported decreases in glucose levels in non-diabetic rabbits, whereas another noted no changes in mice. Effects in humans are not known.	C
Diuretic (increasing urine flow) Dandelion leaves have traditionally been used to increase urine production and excretion. Studies in animals reported mixed results, and there has been no reliable research in humans in this area.	C
Hepatitis B One study reported improved liver function in people with hepatitis B after they took a combination herbal preparation containing dandelion root, called jiedu yanggan gao (the combination also included *Artemisia capillaris, Astragalus membranaceus, Cephalanoplos segetum, flos chrysanthemi indici, fructus polygonii orientalis, Hedyotis diffusa,* plantago seed, *Polygonatum sibiricum, radix paeoniae albae, Salviae miltiorrhizae, smilax glabra,* and *Taraxacum mongolicum*). Because multiple herbs were used and this study was not well designed or reported, the effects of dandelion are unclear.	C

*Key to grades: *A:* Strong scientific evidence for this use; *B:* Good scientific evidence for this use; *C:* Unclear scientific evidence for this use; *D:* Fair scientific evidence against this use (it may not work); *F:* Strong scientific evidence against this use (it likely does not work). For a more detailed explanation of efficacy criteria, see "Natural Standard Evidence-Based Validated Grading Rationale" in the Introduction.

Uses Based on Tradition, Theory, or Limited Scientific Evidence

Abscess, acne, age spots, AIDS, alcohol withdrawal, allergies, analgesia, anemia, antibacterial, antifungal, antioxidant, antiviral, aphthous ulcers, appendicitis, appetite stimulant, arthritis, benign prostate hypertrophy, bile flow stimulation, bladder irritation, blood purifier, boils, breast augmentation, breast cancer, breast infection, breast inflammation, breast milk stimulation, bruises, cardiovascular disorders, chronic fatigue syndrome, circulation, clogged arteries, CNS stimulant, coffee substitute, congestive heart failure, dandruff, diarrhea, dropsy, eye problems, fertility, fever reduction, flatulence (gas), food uses, frequent urination, gallbladder disease, gallstones, gout, headache, heartburn, high blood pressure, high cholesterol, immune stimulation, increased sweating, jaundice, kidney disease, kidney stones, leukemia, liver cleansing, liver disease, menopause, menstrual period stimulation, muscle aches, nutrition, osteoarthritis, postpartum support, pregnancy, premenstrual syndrome, psoriasis, rheumatoid arthritis, skin conditions, skin toner, smoking cessation, stiff joints, stomachache, urinary stimulant, urinary tract inflammation, warts, weight loss.

DOSING

The following doses are based on scientific research, publications, traditional use, or expert opinion. Many herbs and supplements have not been thoroughly tested, and their safety and effectiveness may not be proven. Brands may be made differently, with variable ingredients even within the same brand. The doses shown may not apply to all products. It is important to always read product labels and discuss doses with a qualified healthcare provider before therapy is started.

Standardization

- Standardization involves measuring the amounts of certain chemicals in products to try to make different preparations similar to each other. It is not always known if the chemicals being measured are the "active" ingredients. There are no standard or well-studied doses of dandelion, and many different doses are used traditionally. Safety of use beyond 4 months has not been evaluated.
- Dandelion leaves are a source of vitamin A, containing up to 1400 IU per 100 g.

Adults (18 Years and Older)

- **Dried root:** Doses of 2 to 8 g taken as an infusion or decoction have been used.
- **Leaf fluid extract:** Doses of 4 to 8 mg of a 1:1 extract in 25% alcohol have been used.
- **Root tincture:** Doses of 1 or 2 teaspoons of a 1:5 tincture in 45% alcohol have been used.

Children (Younger Than 18 Years)

- There is insufficient scientific research to recommend dandelion for use in children in amounts greater than found in food.

SAFETY

The U.S. Food and Drug Administration does not strictly regulate herbs and supplements. There is no guarantee of the strength, purity, or safety of products, and effects may vary. It is important

to always read product labels. People who have a medical condition, or are taking other drugs, herbs, or supplements, should consult a qualified healthcare provider before starting a new therapy. A healthcare provider should be contacted immediately about any side effects.

Allergies

- Dandelion should be avoided by people with known allergy to dandelion, honey, chamomile, chrysanthemums, yarrow, feverfew, or any members of the Asteraceae/Compositae plant families (e.g., ragweed, sunflower, daisies).
- The most common type of allergy is dermatitis (skin inflammation) after direct skin contact with dandelion, which may include itching, rash, and red, swollen, or eczematous areas on the skin. Skin reactions have also been reported in dogs. The main chemicals in dandelion responsible for allergic reactions are believed to be sesquiterpene lactones. Patch tests have been developed to assess for dandelion allergy.
- Rhinoconjunctivitis and asthma have been reported in people who have handled products containing dandelion and other herbs (such as birdfeed), with reported positive skin tests for dandelion hypersensitivity.

Side Effects and Warnings

- Dandelion was well tolerated in a small number of studies in humans. Safety of use beyond 4 months has not been evaluated.
- The most common reported adverse effects are skin allergy, eczema, and increased sun sensitivity following direct contact with dandelion.
- According to traditional accounts, gastrointestinal symptoms may occur, including stomach discomfort, diarrhea, and heartburn. There is a case report of a patient who developed intestinal blockage from ingesting a large amount of dandelion greens 3 weeks after undergoing a stomach operation.
- Parasitic infection due to ingestion of contaminated dandelion has been reported, affecting the liver and bile ducts and characterized by fever, stomach upset, vomiting, loss of appetite, coughing, and liver damage.
- Dandelion may lower blood sugar levels, based on one study in animals; however, another study noted no changes. Effects in humans are unknown. Caution is advised in people with diabetes or hypoglycemia, and in those taking drugs, herbs, or supplements that affect blood sugar levels. Serum glucose levels may need to be monitored by a healthcare provider, and medication adjustments may be necessary.
- In theory, because of the chemical coumarin that is found in dandelion leaf extracts, dandelion may increase the risk of bleeding when taken with drugs that increase the risk of bleeding. Examples of such drugs are anticoagulants (blood thinners) such as warfarin (Coumadin) and heparin, antiplatelet drugs such as clopidogrel (Plavix), aspirin, and nonsteroidal anti-inflammatory drugs such as ibuprofen (Motrin, Advil) and naproxen (Naprosyn, Aleve).
- Historically, dandelion is believed to possess diuretic (increasing urine flow) properties and to lower blood potassium levels.
- Dandelion may be prepared as a tincture containing high levels of alcohol. Tinctures should therefore be avoided during pregnancy or by persons who are driving or operating heavy machinery.

Pregnancy and Breastfeeding

- Dandelion cannot be recommended during pregnancy and breast-feeding in amounts greater than found in foods, because of lack of scientific information.

Many tinctures contain high levels of alcohol and their use should be avoided during pregnancy.

INTERACTIONS

Most herbs and supplements have not been thoroughly tested for interactions with other herbs, supplements, drugs, or foods. The interactions listed here are based on reports in scientific publications, laboratory experiments, or traditional use. It is important to always read product labels. People who have a medical condition, or are taking other drugs, herbs, or supplements, should consult a qualified healthcare provider before starting a new therapy.

Interactions with Drugs

- Drug interactions with dandelion have rarely been identified, although studies in this area have been limited.
- Based on research studies in animals, dandelion, when taken at the same time as the antibiotic ciprofloxacin (Cipro), may reduce absorption of the drug. In theory, dandelion may have a similar effect on other drugs taken at the same time.
- In one study in animals, it was suggested that dandelion may lower blood sugar levels, although another study noted no changes. Although effects in humans are unknown, caution is advised in people taking prescription drugs that may also lower blood sugar levels. Persons taking oral drugs for diabetes or insulin at the same time that they are using dandelion should be monitored closely by a qualified healthcare provider. Dosing adjustments may be necessary.
- Historically, dandelion is believed to possess diuretic (increasing urine flow) properties and to lower blood potassium levels. In theory, the effects or side effects of other drugs may be increased, including corticosteroids such as prednisone, digoxin (Lanoxin), other diuretics, and lithium. The effects or side effects of niacin or nicotinic acid may be increased (such as flushing and gastrointestinal upset), because of small amounts of nicotinic acid present in dandelion.
- In theory, because of the presence of the chemical coumarin in dandelion leaf extracts, dandelion may increase the risk of bleeding when used with anticoagulants (blood thinners) or antiplatelet drugs. Examples of such drugs are clopidogrel (Plavix), heparin, and warfarin (Coumadin). Some pain relievers may also increase the risk of bleeding if used with dandelion. Examples are aspirin, ibuprofen (Motrin, Advil), and naproxen (Naprosyn, Aleve, Anaprox). It is possible that dandelion may reduce the effectiveness of antacids or drugs commonly used to treat peptic ulcer disease, such as esomeprazole (Nexium) and famotidine (Pepcid).
- Studies in animals suggest that dandelion may interfere with how the body uses the liver's cytochrome P450 enzyme system to process components of some drugs. As a result, blood levels of these components may be elevated and may cause increased effects or potentially serious adverse reactions. People using any medications should always read the package insert and consult with their healthcare provider or pharmacist about possible interactions.
- One study reported improved liver function in people with hepatitis B after they took a combination herbal preparation containing dandelion root, called jiedu yanggan gao (the combination also included *Artemisia capillaris, Astragalus membranaceus, Cephalanoplos segetum, flos chrysanthemi indici, fructus polygonii orientalis, Hedyotis diffusa*, plantago seed, *Polygonatum sibiricum, radix paeoniae albae, Salviae miltiorrhizae, smilax glabra,* and *Taraxacum mongolicum*). Because multiple herbs were used and this study was not well designed or reported, the effects of dandelion are unclear.

- *Note:* Many tinctures contain high levels of alcohol and may cause nausea or vomiting when taken with metronidazole (Flagyl) or disulfiram (Antabuse).

Interactions with Herbs and Dietary Supplements

- Reports of interactions of dietary supplements with dandelion have rarely been published, although there have been limited studies in this area.
- One study in animals suggested that dandelion may lower blood sugar levels, although another study noted no changes. Although effects in humans are unknown, caution is advised in people who are using herbs or supplements that may also lower blood sugar. Blood glucose levels may require monitoring, and doses may need adjustment. Examples of such agents are *Aloe vera*, American ginseng, bilberry, bitter melon, burdock, fenugreek, fish oil, gymnema, horse chestnut seed extract (HCSE), maitake mushroom, marshmallow, milk thistle, *Panax ginseng*, rosemary, shark cartilage, Siberian ginseng, stinging nettle, and white horehound.
- Historically, dandelion is believed to possess diuretic (increased urination) properties and may increase the effects of other herbs with potential diuretic effects, such as artichoke, celery, corn silk, couchgrass, elder flower, horsetail, juniper berry, kava, shepherd's purse, uva ursi, and yarrow.
- In theory, because of the presence of the chemical coumarin in dandelion leaf extracts, dandelion may increase the risk of bleeding when taken with other herbs and supplements that may increase the risk of bleeding. Multiple cases of bleeding have been reported with the use of *Ginkgo biloba*, and fewer cases with garlic and saw palmetto. Numerous other agents may theoretically increase the risk of bleeding, although this has not been proven in most cases. Examples are alfalfa, American ginseng, angelica, anise, *Arnica montana*, asafetida, aspen bark, bilberry, birch, black cohosh, bladderwrack, bogbean, boldo, borage seed oil, bromelain, capsicum, cat's claw, celery, chamomile, chaparral, clove, coleus, cordyceps, danshen, devil's claw, dong quai, eicosapentaenoic acid (EPA), evening primrose oil, fenugreek, feverfew, fish oil, flaxseed/flax powder (not a concern with flaxseed oil), ginger, grapefruit juice, grape seed, green tea, guggul, gymnestra, horse chestnut, horseradish, licorice root, lovage root, male fern, meadowsweet, nordihydroguaiaretic acid (NDGA), omega-3 fatty acids, onion, *Panax ginseng*, papain, parsley, passion flower, poplar, prickly ash, propolis, quassia, red clover, reishi, rue, Siberian ginseng, sweet birch, sweet clover, turmeric, vitamin E, white willow, wild carrot, wild lettuce, willow, wintergreen, and yucca.
- Studies in animals suggest that dandelion may interfere with how the body uses the liver's cytochrome P450 enzyme system to process components of certain drugs. As a result, the blood levels of other herbs or supplements may be too high. Dandelion may alter the effects of other herbs on the cytochrome P450 enzyme system. Examples of such herbs are bloodroot, cat's claw, chamomile, chaparral, chasteberry, damiana, *Echinacea angustifolia*, goldenseal, grapefruit juice, licorice, oregano, red clover, St. John's wort, wild cherry, and yucca.
- Because dandelion leaves contain vitamin A, lutein, and beta-carotene, supplemental doses of these agents may have additive effects or side effects.

Selected References

Natural Standard developed the preceding evidence-based information based on a systematic review of more than 95 scientific articles. For comprehensive information about alternative and complementary therapies on the professional level, go to www.naturalstandard.com. Selected references are listed here.

Chakurski I, Matev M, Koichev A, et al. [Treatment of chronic colitis with an herbal combination of *Taraxacum officinale, Hipericum perforatum, Melissa officinalis, Calendula officinalis* and *Foeniculum vulgare.*] Vutreshni bolesti 1981;20(6):51-54.

Chen Z. [Clinical study of 96 cases with chronic hepatitis B treated with jiedu yanggan gao by a double-blind method.] Zhong Xi Yi Jie He Za Zhi 1990;10(2):71-74, 67.

Davies MG, Kersey PJ. Contact allergy to yarrow and dandelion. Contact Dermatitis 1986; 14(4):256-257.

Grases F, Melero G, Costa-Bauza A, et al. Urolithiasis and phytotherapy. Int Urol Nephrol 1994;26(5):507-511.

Danshen
(*Salvia miltiorrhiza*)

D

RELATED TERMS

- Ch'ih shen, dan-shen, dan shen, danshen root, hang ken, hung ken, pin-ma ts'ao (horse-racing grass), radix salvia miltiorrhiza, red-rooted sage, red roots, red sage root, *Salvia bowelyana, Salvia miltiorrhiza* Bunge, *Salviae miltiorrhizae, Salvia przewalskii, Salvia przewalskii* mandarinorum, *Salvia yunnanensis,* salvia root, scarlet sage, sh'ih shen, shu-wei ts'ao (rat-tail grass), tan seng, tan-shen, tzu tan-ken (roots of purple sage).

BACKGROUND

- Danshen (*Salvia miltiorrhiza*) is widely used in traditional Chinese medicine (TCM), often in combination with other herbs. Remedies containing danshen are used traditionally to treat a diversity of ailments, particularly cardiac (heart) and vascular (blood vessel) disorders such as atherosclerosis (hardening of the arteries with cholesterol plaques) and blood clotting abnormalities.
- The ability of danshen to thin the blood and reduce blood clotting is well documented, although the herb's purported ability to "invigorate" the blood or improve circulation has not been demonstrated in high-quality trials in humans. Constituents of the danshen root, particularly protocatechualdehyde and 3,4-dihydroxyphenyl-lactic acid, are believed to be responsible for its vascular effects. Because danshen can inhibit platelet aggregation and has been reported to potentiate (increase) the blood-thinning effects of warfarin, it should be avoided in persons with bleeding disorders, prior to some surgical procedures, or in those taking anticoagulant (blood-thinning) drugs, herbs, or supplements.
- In the mid-1980s, scientific interest was shown in danshen's possible cardiovascular benefits, particularly in patients with ischemic stroke or coronary artery disease/angina. More recent studies have focused on danshen's possible role in the treatment of liver disease (hepatitis and cirrhosis), and as an antioxidant. However, most research in these areas has been in studies in animals and small trials of poor methodological quality in humans. Therefore, firm evidence-based conclusions are not possible at this time about the effects of danshen for any medical condition.

USES BASED ON SCIENTIFIC EVIDENCE	Grade*
Asthmatic bronchitis A small amount of research studies in humans suggest that danshen may improve breathing and lessen cough and wheeze in persons with chronic asthmatic bronchitis. Better studies are needed that compare danshen with established treatments for this condition before a clear conclusion can be drawn.	C

Continued

Burn healing Although studies in animals suggest that danshen may speed healing of burns and wounds, there are no reliable studies in humans available that evaluate this claim.	C
Cardiovascular disease/angina A small number of poor-quality studies in animals and humans report that danshen may provide benefits for treating disorders of the heart and blood vessels, including heart attacks, cardiac chest pain (angina), or myocarditis. Traditionally, danshen is most frequently used for these problems in combination with other herbs. Because most studies have been small and brief with flaws in their designs, and the results of different trials have disagreed with each other, it is not clear whether there is any benefit from danshen for these conditions. No specific dose or standardized preparation is widely accepted for these disorders. Danshen may have effects on blood clotting and therefore may be unsafe when combined with other drugs used in patients with cardiovascular disease. Patients should check with a physician and pharmacist before combining danshen with prescription drugs.	C
Glaucoma Danshen has been proposed as a possible glaucoma therapy, but further studies are needed in humans before a clear conclusion can be drawn. Danshen should not be used in place of established therapies, and patients with glaucoma should be evaluated by a qualified eye care specialist.	C
Increased rate of peritoneal dialysis One study suggested that danshen may speed peritoneal dialysis and ultrafiltration rates when added to dialysate solution. Although this evidence is promising, it is not known whether danshen is safe for this use.	C
Ischemic stroke In limited research from the 1970s, danshen was administered intravenously (through the veins) for up to 4 weeks in patients with ischemic stroke. Due to poor quality of this evidence, unclear safety, and the existence of more proven treatments for ischemic stroke, this use of danshen cannot be recommended.	C
Liver disease (cirrhosis/chronic hepatitis B) Some studies suggest that danshen may provide benefits for treating liver diseases such as cirrhosis and chronic hepatitis B. Traditionally, danshen is most frequently used for these problems in combination with other herbs. Although early research in humans suggests a possible reduction in liver fibrosis in people with cirrhosis, as well as some improvements in liver function in chronic hepatitis, these studies have been small with flaws in their designs. Therefore it is unclear whether there are any clinically significant effects of danshen in patients with liver disease.	C

*Key to grades: *A:* Strong scientific evidence for this use; *B:* Good scientific evidence for this use; *C:* Unclear scientific evidence for this use; *D:* Fair scientific evidence against this use (it may not work); *F:* Strong scientific evidence against this use (it likely does not work). For a more detailed explanation of efficacy criteria, see "Natural Standard Evidence-Based Validated Grading Rationale" in the Introduction.

Uses Based on Tradition, Theory, or Limited Scientific Evidence

Acne, anoxic brain injury, antioxidant, antiphospholipid syndrome, anxiety, bleomycin-induced lung fibrosis, blood-clotting disorders, bruising, cancer, cataracts, circulation, clogged arteries, diabetic nerve pain, ectopic pregnancy, eczema, gastric ulcers, gentamicin toxicity, hearing loss, heart palpitations, high cholesterol, HIV, hypercoagulability, intrauterine growth retardation, kidney failure, left ventricular hypertrophy, leukemia, liver cancer, lung fibrosis, menstrual problems, preeclampsia, psoriasis, pulmonary hypertension, radiation-induced lung damage, restlessness, sleep difficulties, stimulation of gamma-aminobutyric acid (GABA) release, stomach ulcers, wound healing.

DOSING

The following doses are based on scientific research, publications, traditional use, or expert opinion. Many herbs and supplements have not been thoroughly tested, and their safety and effectiveness may not be proven. Brands may be made differently, with variable ingredients even within the same brand. The doses shown may not apply to all products. It is important to always read product labels and discuss doses with a qualified healthcare provider before therapy is started.

Standardization

- Standardization involves measuring the amounts of certain chemicals in products to try to make different preparations similar to each other. It is not always known if the chemicals being measured are the "active" ingredients. There is no widely accepted standardization or well-studied dosing of danshen, and many different doses are used traditionally. Danshen is frequently used in combination with other herbs.

Adults (18 Years and Older)

- **By mouth:** Oral dosing has not been studied in well-conducted trials in humans, and therefore no specific dose can be recommended.
- **By intravenous injection:** In research from the 1970s, an 8-ml injection of danshen (16 g of the herb) was given intravenously (diluted in 500 ml of a 10% glucose solution) for up to 4 weeks for ischemic stroke. Safety and effectiveness have not been established for this route of administration and it cannot be recommended at this time.

Children (Younger Than 18 Years)

- There is insufficient scientific evidence to recommend the safe use of danshen in children, and its use should be avoided because of potentially serious side effects.

SAFETY

The U.S. Food and Drug Administration does not strictly regulate herbs and supplements. There is no guarantee of the strength, purity, or safety of products, and effects may vary. It is important to always read product labels. People who have a medical condition, or are taking other drugs, herbs, or supplements, should consult a qualified healthcare provider before starting a new therapy. A healthcare provider should be contacted immediately about any side effects.

Allergies

- People with known allergy to danshen or its constituents (i.e., protocatechualdehyde, 3,4-dihydroxyphenyl-lactic acid, tanshinone I, dihydrotanshinone, cryptotanshione, miltirone, salvianolic acid B) should avoid this herb. Danshen is often found in combination with other herbs in various formulations, and patients should read product labels carefully and consult their healthcare provider and pharmacist about possible interactions.

Side Effects and Warnings

- Although danshen has been well tolerated in most studies, there is limited research using preparations consisting of danshen only for extended periods of time, and safety has not been studied systematically.
- Danshen may increase the risk of bleeding. This herb has been reported to inhibit platelet aggregation and increase the blood-thinning effects of warfarin in humans. Caution is advised in people with bleeding disorders who are taking drugs that may increase the risk of bleeding, or prior to some surgical procedures. Dosing adjustments may be necessary.
- Some people may experience stomach discomfort, reduced appetite, or itching.
- In theory, danshen may lower blood pressure and therefore it should be used cautiously by patients with blood pressure abnormalities or taking drugs that alter blood pressure.
- In theory, the chemical miltirone, which is present in danshen, may increase drowsiness. Caution is advised in people who are driving or operating machinery.

Pregnancy and Breastfeeding

- Danshen should be avoided during pregnancy and breastfeeding. In theory, the blood-thinning properties of danshen may increase the risk of miscarriage, and effects on the fetus or nursing infants are unknown.

INTERACTIONS

Most herbs and supplements have not been thoroughly tested for interactions with other herbs, supplements, drugs, or foods. The interactions listed here are based on reports in scientific publications, laboratory experiments, or traditional use. It is important to always read product labels. People who have a medical condition, or are taking other drugs, herbs, or supplements, should consult a qualified healthcare provider before starting a new therapy.

Interactions with Drugs

- Danshen may increase the risk of bleeding when it is taken with drugs that increase the risk of bleeding. This herb has been reported to inhibit platelet aggregation and to cause excessive anticoagulation (blood-thinning effects) in persons taking the blood thinner warfarin (Coumadin). Examples of drugs that increase the risk of bleeding are anticoagulants such as warfarin (Coumadin) and heparin, antiplatelet drugs such as clopidogrel (Plavix), aspirin, and nonsteroidal anti-inflammatory drugs such as ibuprofen (Motrin, Advil) and naproxen (Naprosyn, Aleve).
- In theory, the risk of side effects or toxicity from digoxin (Lanoxin) may be increased if this agent is taken with danshen. In addition, danshen may cause inaccurate (too high or too low) laboratory measurements of digoxin blood levels.
- Danshen may cause hypotension (dangerously low blood pressure) if it is taken with drugs that also lower blood pressure. Examples of such drugs are ACE inhibitors

such as captopril (Capoten) and lisinopril (Prinivil) and beta-blockers such as atenolol (Tenormin) and propranolol (Inderal). In addition, the use of danshen with beta-blockers may cause bradycardia (dangerously slow heart rate).

- In theory, the chemical miltirone, which is present in danshen, may increase sleepiness or other side effects associated with some drugs taken for anxiety or insomnia, such as lorazepam (Ativan), alprazolam (Xanax), and diazepam (Valium), and alcohol. In addition, based on studies in animals, danshen may affect the absorption of alcohol in the blood.

Interactions with Herbs and Dietary Supplements

- Danshen may increase the risk of bleeding when taken with herbs and supplements that may also increase the risk of bleeding. Multiple cases of bleeding have been reported with the use of *Ginkgo biloba*, and fewer cases with garlic and saw palmetto. Numerous other agents may theoretically increase the risk of bleeding, although this has not been proven in most cases. Examples are alfalfa, American ginseng, angelica, anise, *Arnica montana*, asafetida, aspen bark, bilberry, birch, black cohosh, bladderwrack, bogbean, boldo, borage seed oil, bromelain, capsicum, cat's claw, celery, chamomile, chaparral, clove, coleus, cordyceps, devil's claw, dong quai, eicosapentaenoic acid (EPA), evening primrose oil, fenugreek, feverfew, fish oil, flaxseed/flax powder (not a concern with flaxseed oil), ginger, grapefruit juice, grape seed, green tea, guggul, gymnestra, horse chestnut, horseradish, licorice root, lovage root, male fern, meadowsweet, nordihydroguaiaretic acid (NDGA), omega-3 fatty acids, onion, *Panax ginseng*, papain, parsley, passion flower, poplar, prickly ash, propolis, quassia, red clover, reishi, rue, Siberian ginseng, sweet birch, sweet clover, turmeric, vitamin E, white willow, wild carrot, wild lettuce, willow, wintergreen, and yucca.
- In theory, danshen may add to the effects of other herbs with potential cardiac glycoside properties, potentially resulting in slow heart rate or toxicity. Examples of such agents are adonis, balloon cotton, black hellebore root/melampode, black Indian hemp, bushman's poison, cactus grandifloris, convallaria, eyebright, figwort, foxglove/digitalis, frangipani, hedge mustard, hemp root/Canadian hemp root, king's crown, lily-of-the-valley, motherwort, oleander leaf, pheasant's eye plant, plantain leaf, pleurisy root, psyllium husks, redheaded cotton-bush, rhubarb root, rubber vine, sea-mango, senna fruit, squill, strophanthus, uzara, wallflower, wintersweet, yellow dock root, and yellow oleander. Notably, bufalin/chan suis is a Chinese herbal formula that has been reported as toxic or fatal when taken with cardiac glycosides.
- Danshen should be used cautiously with herbs/supplements that may also lower blood pressure, such as aconite/monkshood, arnica, baneberry, betel nut, bilberry, black cohosh, bryony, calendula, California poppy, coleus, curcumin, eucalyptol, eucalyptus oil, flaxseed/flaxseed oil, garlic, ginger, ginkgo, goldenseal, green hellebore, hawthorn, Indian tobacco, jaborandi, mistletoe, night-blooming cereus, oleander, pasque flower, periwinkle, pleurisy root, *Polypodium vulgare*, shepherd's purse, Texas milkweed, turmeric, and wild cherry.
- In theory, the chemical miltirone, which is present in danshen, can increase the amount of drowsiness that may be caused by other herbs or supplements, including calamus, calendula, California poppy, capsicum, catnip, celery, couch grass, dogwood, elecampane, German chamomile, goldenseal, gotu kola, hops, kava (may help sleep without drowsiness), lavender aromatherapy, lemon balm, sage, sassafras, scullcap,

shepherd's purse, Siberian ginseng, St. John's wort, stinging nettle, valerian, wild carrot, wild lettuce, withania root, and yerba mansa.

Selected References

Natural Standard developed the preceding evidence-based information based on a systematic review of more than 225 articles. For comprehensive information about alternative and complementary therapies on the professional level, go to www.naturalstandard.com. Selected references are listed here.

Brunetti G, Serra S, Vacca G, et al. IDN 5082, a standardized extract of *Salvia miltiorrhiza*, delays acquisition of alcohol drinking behavior in rats. J Ethnopharmacol 2003;85(1):93-97.

Cao CM, Xia Q, Zhang X, et al. *Salvia miltiorrhiza* attenuates the changes in contraction and intracellular calcium induced by anoxia and reoxygenation in rat cardiomyocytes. Life Sci 2003;72(22):2451-2463.

Chan TY. Interaction between warfarin and danshen (*Salvia miltiorrhiza*). Ann Pharmacother 2001;35(4):501-504.

Chen Y, Ruan Y, Li L, et al. Effects of *Salvia miltiorrhiza* extracts on rat hypoxic pulmonary hypertension, heme oxygenase-1 and nitric oxide synthase. Chin Med J (Engl) 2003;116(5): 757-760.

Cheng TO. Warfarin danshen interaction. Ann Thorac Surg 1999;67(3):894.

Ji X, Tan BK, Zhu YC, et al. Comparison of cardioprotective effects using ramipril and DanShen for the treatment of acute myocardial infarction in rats. Life Sci 2003;73(11):1413-1426.

Kang HS, Chung HY, Byun DS, et al. Further isolation of antioxidative (+)-1-hydroxypinoresinol-1-*O*-beta-D-glucoside from the rhizome of *Salvia miltiorrhiza* that acts on peroxynitrite, total ROS and 1,1-diphenyl-2-picrylhydrazyl radical. Arch Pharm Res 2003; 26(1):24-27.

Lay IS, Chiu JH, Shiao MS, et al. Crude extract of *Salvia miltiorrhiza* and salvianolic acid B enhance in vitro angiogenesis in murine SVR endothelial cell line. Planta Med 2003;69(1): 26-32.

Lee TY, Mai LM, Wang GJ, et al. Protective mechanism of *Salvia miltiorrhiza* on carbon tetrachloride–induced acute hepatotoxicity in rats. J Pharmacol Sci 2003;91(3):202-210.

Liu GY. Analysis of effect of composite danshen droplet pills in treatment of chronic stable angina. Hubei J Trad Chin Med 1997;19(2):33-34.

Liu F, Liu Y, Li J. [Effects of danshen on solute transport by peritoneal dialysis.] Hunan Yi Ke Da Xue Xue Bao 1997;22(3):237-239.

Lo CJ, Lin JG, Kuo JS, et al. Effect of *Salvia miltiorrhiza* Bunge on cerebral infarct in ischemia-reperfusion injured rats. Am J Chin Med 2003;31(2):191-200.

Mashour NH, Lin GI, Frishman WH. Herbal medicine for the treatment of cardiovascular disease: clinical considerations. Arch Intern Med 1998;158(20):2225-2234.

Sha Q, Cheng HZ, Xie XY. *Salviae miltiorrhizae* composita pill for treating 47 cases of active liver cirrhosis. Chin J Integrat Trad West Med Liver Dis 1999;9(6):50.

Vacca G, Colombo G, Brunetti G, et al. Reducing effect of *Salvia miltiorrhiza* extracts on alcohol intake: influence of vehicle. Phytother Res 2003;17(5):537-541.

Wu CT, Mulabagal V, Nalawade SM, et al. Isolation and quantitative analysis of cryptotanshinone, an active quinoid diterpene formed in callus of *Salvia miltiorrhiza* BUNGE. Biol Pharm Bull 2003;26(6):845-848.

Yagi A, Takeo S. [Anti-inflammatory constituents, aloesin and aloemannan in Aloe species and effects of tanshinon VI in Salvia miltiorrhiza on heart.] Yakugaku Zasshi 2003;123(7): 517-532.

Devil's Claw

(*Harpagophytum procumbens*)

D

RELATED TERMS

- Algophytum, Arthrosetten H, Arthrotabs, Artigel, Artosan, Defencid, Devil's Claw Capsule, Devil's Claw Secondary Root, Devil's Claw Vegicaps, Doloteffin, duiwelsklou, Fitokey Harpagophytum, grapple plant, *griffe du diable*, Harpadol, Hariosen, HarpagoMega, Harpagon, harpagophyti radix, *Harpagophytum zeyheri*, Jucurba N, Pedaliaceae, Rheuma-Sern, Rheuma-Tee, Salus, sengaparile, sudafrikanische, teufelskralle, trampelklette, venustorn, Windhoek's root, wood spider.
- **Multi-ingredient preparations containing devil's claw root:** Arktophytum, Arthritic Pain Herbal Formula, Devil's Claw Plus, Lifesystem Herbal Formula 1 Arthritic Aid, Lifesystem Herbal Formula 12 Willowbark, Prost-1, green-lipped mussel (FM).

BACKGROUND

- The medicinal ingredient of devil's claw (*Harpagophytum procumbens*) is extracted from the dried tuberous roots of the plant, which originated in the Kalahari and savannah desert regions of South and Southeast Africa, where it has historically been used to treat a wide range of conditions including fever, malaria, and indigestion.
- Currently, the major clinical uses of devil's claw are as an anti-inflammatory and analgesic (pain reliever) for joint diseases, back pain, and headache. Initial evidence from scientific studies in animals and humans has been popularized and has resulted in widespread use of standardized devil's claw as a mild analgesic for joint pain in Europe. Scientific evaluation is lacking regarding its effectiveness as an appetite stimulant or liver tonic, but it is widely used for these purposes as well.
- Potential side effects include gastrointestinal upset, hypotension (low blood pressure) and arrhythmic (abnormal) heartbeat. Devil's claw may have chronotropic (increased heart rate) and inotropic (increased heart squeezing) effects.
- Traditionally, it has been recommended to avoid using devil's claw in people with gastric or duodenal ulcers and in those using anticoagulants (blood thinners). Clinical data to substantiate these recommendations are insufficient.

USES BASED ON SCIENTIFIC EVIDENCE	Grade*
Osteoarthritis A small amount of research reports that devil's claw may be effective for treating pain and for improving mobility in individuals with osteoarthritis (particularly affecting the hip or knee). These studies suggest that the use of devil's claw may allow the dose of pain medications to be reduced. However, there are problems with the design and reporting of these trials, and better research is needed before a firm conclusion can be drawn.	B

Continued

Low back pain The results of several studies in humans of devil's claw for low back pain are conflicting. Additional research is needed to provide clearer answers.	**C**

*Key to grades: *A:* Strong scientific evidence for this use; *B:* Good scientific evidence for this use; *C:* Unclear scientific evidence for this use; *D:* Fair scientific evidence against this use (it may not work); *F:* Strong scientific evidence against this use (it likely does not work). For a more detailed explanation of efficacy criteria, see "Natural Standard Evidence-Based Validated Grading Rationale" in the Introduction.

Uses Based on Tradition, Theory, or Limited Scientific Evidence

Allergies, anti-inflammatory, antioxidant, appetite stimulant, arrhythmias, atherosclerosis (clogged arteries), bitter tonic, blood diseases, boils (used topically), childbirth difficulties, choleretic (bile secretion), constipation, diabetes, diarrhea, diuretic, dyspepsia, edema, fever, fibromyalgia, flatulence (gas), gastrointestinal disorders, gout, headache, heartburn, high cholesterol, hip pain, indigestion, irregular heartbeat, knee pain, liver and gallbladder tonic, loss of appetite, malaria, menopausal symptoms, menstrual cramps, migraines, muscle pain, nerve pain, nicotine poisoning, pain, rheumatoid arthritis, sedative, skin cancer (used topically), skin ulcers (used topically), sores (used topically), spasmolytic, tendonitis, urinary tract infections, wound healing for skin injuries (used topically).

DOSING

The following doses are based on scientific research, publications, traditional use, or expert opinion. Many herbs and supplements have not been thoroughly tested, and their safety and effectiveness may not be proven. Brands may be made differently, with variable ingredients even within the same brand. The doses shown may not apply to all products. It is important to always read product labels and discuss doses with a qualified healthcare provider before therapy is started.

Standardization

- Standardization involves measuring the amounts of certain chemicals in products to try to make different products similar to each other. It is not always known if the chemicals being measured are the "active" ingredients. Devil's claw products may be standardized to contain a specific amount of harpagoside and often contain greater than 1% to 2% harpagoside. Some studies have used a special preparation called WS 1531, which contains 8.5% harpagoside.

Adults (18 Years and Older)

- **Tablets:** A dose of 600 to 1200 mg (standardized to contain 50 to 100 mg of harpagoside) by mouth three times daily has been used in studies of therapy for joint and muscle problems.
- **Dried root:** A dose of 0.5 to 1.5 g by mouth three times daily in an aqueous (water-based) solution has been used traditionally for appetite loss and stomach discomfort.

- **Tincture:** A dose of 0.2 to 1 ml (1:5 in 25% alcohol) by mouth three times daily has been used traditionally. A dose of 3 ml (1:10 in 25% alcohol) by mouth three times daily has also been used traditionally.
- **Fluid extract:** A dose of 0.25 to 1.5 ml (1:1 in 25% alcohol) by mouth three times daily has been used traditionally.

Children (Younger Than 18 Years)

- The dosing and safety of devil's claw have not been studied thoroughly in children, and safety is not established.

SAFETY

The U.S. Food and Drug Administration does not strictly regulate herbs and supplements. There is no guarantee of the strength, purity, or safety of products, and effects may vary. It is important to always read product labels. People who have a medical condition, or are taking other drugs, herbs, or supplements, should consult a qualified healthcare provider before starting a new therapy. A healthcare provider should be contacted immediately about any side effects.

Allergies

- People with allergies to *Harpagophytum procumbens* should avoid devil's claw products.

Side Effects and Warnings

- At recommended doses, devil's claw traditionally is believed to be well tolerated. However, there are published reports of headache, ringing in the ears, loss of taste and appetite, and diarrhea in those taking this herb. Whether the use of devil's claw for longer than 3 to 4 months is safe or effective is unknown.
- Devil's claw may change the rate and force of heartbeats (chronotropic and inotropic effects). People with heart disease or arrhythmias (abnormal heart rhythms) should consult their cardiologist or other qualified healthcare provider before taking devil's claw. Devil's claw may affect levels of acid in the gastrointestinal tract and should be avoided by people with gastric (stomach) or duodenal (intestinal) ulcers. Devil's claw should be used cautiously in people with gallstones.
- In theory, devil's claw may lower blood sugar levels. Caution is advised in people with diabetes or hypoglycemia and in those taking drugs, other herbs, or supplements that affect blood sugar levels. Serum glucose levels may need to be monitored by a qualified healthcare provider, and medication adjustments may be necessary.
- In theory, devil's claw may increase the risk of bleeding. Caution is advised in people with bleeding disorders or those taking drugs that may increase the risk of bleeding. Dosing adjustments may be necessary. People may need to stop taking devil's claw before some surgeries and should discuss this with their primary healthcare provider.
- Devil's claw products may be contaminated with other herbs or with pesticides, herbicides, heavy metals, or drugs.

Pregnancy and Breastfeeding

- Devil's claw may stimulate contractions of the uterus and cannot be recommended during pregnancy and breastfeeding. People should be aware that many tinctures contain high levels of alcohol and should be avoided during pregnancy.

INTERACTIONS

Most herbs and supplements have not been thoroughly tested for interactions with other herbs, supplements, drugs, or foods. The interactions listed here are based on reports in scientific publications, laboratory experiments, or traditional use. It is important to always read product labels. People who have a medical condition, or are taking other drugs, herbs, or supplements, should consult a qualified healthcare provider before starting a new therapy.

Interactions with Drugs

- Devil's claw may lower blood sugar levels. Caution is advised in people who are using medications that may also lower blood sugar levels. Persons taking drugs for diabetes by mouth or insulin closely should be monitored by a qualified healthcare provider, and medication adjustments may be necessary.
- In theory, devil's claw may have an additive effect when taken with drugs used for pain, inflammation, high cholesterol, and gout. Devil's claw may add to the effects of drugs that reduce cholesterol levels. Devil's claw may also increase stomach acidity and therefore may affect drugs used to decrease the amount of acid in the stomach, such as antacids, esomeprazole (Nexium), ranitidine (Zantac), and sucralfate. People who are taking any of these drugs should consult their healthcare provider and pharmacist before taking devil's claw.
- Because devil's claw may affect heart rhythm, heart rate, and the force of heartbeats, individuals taking prescription drugs such as antiarrhythmics and digoxin (Lanoxin) should consult their healthcare provider before taking devil's claw.
- In theory, devil's claw may increase the risk of bleeding when taken with drugs that increase the risk of bleeding. Examples are anticoagulants (blood thinners) such as warfarin (Coumadin) and heparin, antiplatelet drugs such as clopidogrel (Plavix), aspirin, and nonsteroidal anti-inflammatory drugs such as ibuprofen (Motrin, Advil) and naproxen (Naprosyn, Aleve).

Interactions with Herbs and Dietary Supplements

- In theory, devil's claw may lower blood sugar levels. Caution is advised in people who are using herbs or supplements that may also lower blood sugar levels. Blood glucose levels may require monitoring, and doses may need adjustment. Examples of herbs that may lower blood sugar levels are *Aloe vera*, American ginseng, bilberry, bitter melon, burdock, fenugreek, fish oil, gymnema, horse chestnut seed extract (HCSE), maitake mushroom, marshmallow, milk thistle, *Panax ginseng*, rosemary, shark cartilage, Siberian ginseng, stinging nettle, and white horehound. Agents that may raise blood sugar levels include arginine, cocoa, and ephedra (when combined with caffeine).In theory, devil's claw may interfere with other herbs and dietary supplements that affect heart rhythm, heart rate, and the force of heartbeats. Potential cardiac glycoside herbs and supplements include adonis, balloon cotton, black hellebore root/melampode, black Indian hemp, bushman's poison, cactus grandifloris, convallaria, eyebright, figwort, foxglove/digitalis, frangipani, hedge mustard, hemp root/Canadian hemp root, king's crown, lily-of-the-valley, motherwort, oleander leaf, pheasant's eye plant, plantain leaf, pleurisy root; psyllium husks, redheaded cotton-bush, rhubarb root, rubber vine, sea-mango, senna fruit, squill, strophanthus, uzara, wallflower, wintersweet, yellow dock root, and yellow oleander. Notably, bufalin/chan suis is a Chinese herbal formula that has been reported as toxic or fatal when taken with cardiac glycosides.

- Devil's claw may affect herbs and dietary supplements that are used for pain, inflammation, high cholesterol, and gout. Because devil's claw may increase stomach acidity, it may affect herbs and supplements used to decrease the amount of acid in the stomach.
- Devil's claw may increase the risk of bleeding when taken with herbs and supplements that may also increase the risk of bleeding. Multiple cases of bleeding have been reported with the use of *Ginkgo biloba*, and fewer cases with garlic and saw palmetto. Numerous other agents may theoretically increase the risk of bleeding, although this has not been proven in most cases. Examples are alfalfa, American ginseng, angelica, anise, *Arnica montana*, asafetida, aspen bark, bilberry, birch, black cohosh, bladderwrack, bogbean, boldo, borage seed oil, bromelain, capsicum, cat's claw, celery, chamomile, chaparral, clove, coleus, cordyceps, danshen, dong quai, eicosapentaenoic acid (EPA), evening primrose oil, fenugreek, feverfew, fish oil, flaxseed/flax powder (not a concern with flaxseed oil), ginger, grapefruit juice, grape seed, green tea, guggul, gymnestra, horse chestnut, horseradish, licorice root, lovage root, male fern, meadowsweet, nordihydroguaiaretic acid (NDGA), omega-3 fatty acids, onion, *Panax ginseng*, papain, parsley, passion flower, poplar, prickly ash, propolis, quassia, red clover, reishi, rue, Siberian ginseng, sweet birch, sweet clover, turmeric, vitamin E, white willow, wild carrot, wild lettuce, willow, wintergreen, and yucca.

Selected References

Natural Standard developed the preceding evidence-based information based on a systematic review of more than 75 articles. For comprehensive information about alternative and complementary therapies on the professional level, go to www.naturalstandard.com. Selected references are listed here.

Chantre P, Cappelaere A, Leblan D, et al. Efficacy and tolerance of *Harpagophytum procumbens* versus diacerhein in treatment of osteoarthritis. Phytomedicine 2000;7(3):177-183.

Chrubasik S, Zimpfer C, Schutt U, et al. Effectiveness of *Harpagophytum procumbens* in treatment of acute low back pain. Phytomedicine 1996;3(1):1-10.

Chrubasik S, Junck H, Conradt C, et al. Effectiveness of oral *Harpagophytum* extract WS 1531 in treating low back pain [abstract]. Arthr Rheum 1998;41(Suppl 9):S261.

Chrubasik S, Junck H, Breitschwerdt H, et al. Effectiveness of *Harpagophytum* extract WS 1531 in the treatment of exacerbation of low back pain: a randomized, placebo-controlled, double-blind study. Eur J Anaesthesiol 1999;16(2):118-129.

Chrubasik S, Junck H, Breitschwerdt H, et al. Effectiveness of *Harpagophytum* extract WS 1531 in the treatment of exacerbation of low back pain: a randomized, placebo-controlled, double-blind study. Eur J Anaesthesiol 1999;16(2):118-129.

Chrubasik S, Sporer F, Dillmann-Marschner R, et al. Physicochemical properties of harpagoside and its in vitro release from *Harpagophytum procumbens* extract tablets. Phytomedicine 2000; 6(6):469-473.

Chrubasik S, Künzel O, Thanner J, et al. A short-term follow-up after a randomised double-blind pilot study comparing Doloteffin vs Rofecoxib for low back pain. 9th Annual Symposium on Complementary Health Care, Exeter, UK, 2002.

Chrubasik S, Model A, Ullmann H, et al. Doloteffin vs Vioxx for low back pain—a randomized, double-blind pilot study. Focus Altern Complement Ther 2002;7:90.

Chrubasik S, Fiebich B, Black A, et al. Treating low back pain with an extract of *Harpagophytum procumbens* that inhibits cytokine release. Eur J Anaesthesiol 2002;19:209.

Chrubasik S, Pollak S, Black A. Effectiveness of devil's claw for osteoarthritis. Rheumatology (Oxford) 2002;41(11):1332-1333.

Chrubasik S, Thanner J, Kunzel O, et al. Comparison of outcome measures during treatment with the proprietary *Harpagophytum* extract doloteffin in patients with pain in the lower back, knee or hip. Phytomedicine 2002;9(3):181-194.
Chrubasik S, Pollak S. [In Process Citation.] Wien Med Wochenschr 2002;152(7-8):198-203.
Ernst E, Chrubasik S. Phyto-anti-inflammatories: a systematic review of randomized, placebo-controlled, double-blind trials. Rheum Dis Clin North Am 2000;26(1):13-27.
Grahame R, Robinson BV. Devil's claw (*Harpagophytum procumbens*): pharmacological and clinical studies. Ann Rheum Dis 1981;40(6):632.
Guyader M. Les plantes antirhumatismales. Etude historique et pharmacologique, et etude clinique du nebulisat d'*Harpagophytum procumbens* DC chez 50 patients arthrosiques suivis en service hospitalier [Dissertation]. Paris, Universite Pierre et Marie Curie, 1984.
Leblan D, Chantre P, Fournie B. *Harpagophytum procumbens* in the treatment of knee and hip osteoarthritis: four-month results of a prospective, multicenter, double-blind trial versus diacerhein. Joint Bone Spine 2000;67(5):462-467.
Lecomte A, Costa JP. *Harpagophytum* dans l'arthrose: Etude en double insu contre placebo. Le Magazine 1992;15:27-30.
Munkombwe NM. Acetylated phenolic glycosides from *Harpagophytum procumbens.* Phytochemistry 2003;62(8):1231-1234.

DHEA

(Dehydroepiandrosterone)

D

RELATED TERMS

- 5-androsten-3-β-ol-17-one Atlantic yam, barbasco, China root, colic root, dehydroepiandrosterone sulfate, devil's bones, DHEA-S, dioscorea, *Dioscorea composita, Dioscorea floribunda, Dioscorea macrostachya, Dioscorea mexicana, Dioscorea villosa*, Mexican yam, natural DHEA, phytoestrogen, Prasterone, rheumatism root, wild Mexican yam, yam, yuma.
- **Combination products/trade names:** Born Again's DHEA Eyelift Serum, DHEA Men's Formula, DHEA with Antioxidants 25 mg, DHEA with Bioperine 50 mg.
- *Note*: DHEA can be synthesized in the laboratory using wild yam extract. However, it is believed that wild yam cannot be converted by the body into DHEA. Therefore, information citing wild yam as "natural DHEA" may be inaccurate.

BACKGROUND

- DHEA (dehydroepiandrosterone) is an endogenous hormone (made in the human body), and secreted by the adrenal glands. DHEA serves as a precursor to male and female sex hormones (androgens and estrogens). DHEA levels in the body begin to decrease after age 30, and are reported to be low in some people with anorexia, end-stage kidney disease, type 2 diabetes (non-insulin dependent diabetes), AIDS, adrenal insufficiency, and in the critically ill. DHEA levels may also be depleted by a number of drugs, including insulin, corticosteroids, opiates, and danazol.
- No studies of the long-term effects of DHEA have been conducted. DHEA can cause higher than normal levels of androgens and estrogens in the body and theoretically may increase the risk of prostate, breast, ovarian, and other hormone-sensitive cancers. Therefore, it is not recommended for regular use without supervision by a qualified healthcare provider.

USES BASED ON SCIENTIFIC EVIDENCE	Grade*
Adrenal insufficiency Several studies suggest that DHEA may improve well-being, quality of life, exercise capacity, sex drive, and hormone levels in people with insufficient adrenal function (Addison's disease). These studies have been small, and better research is needed to provide more definitive answers. Adrenal insufficiency is a serious medical condition and should be treated under the supervision of a qualified healthcare provider.	C
Atherosclerosis (cholesterol plaques in the arteries) Initial studies report possible benefits of DHEA supplementation in patients with cholesterol plaques in the arteries (hardening of the arteries). However, other, more proven therapies are available, and people with high cholesterol, atherosclerosis, or heart disease should discuss treatment options with their primary healthcare provider.	C

Continued

Bone density The ability of DHEA to increase bone density is under investigation. Effects are unclear at this time.	C
Cervical dysplasia Initial research studies suggest that the use of intravaginal DHEA is safe and promotes regression of low-grade cervical lesions. However, further study is necessary in this area before a firm conclusion can be drawn. Patients should not substitute the use of DHEA for better-established therapies, and should discuss management options and follow-up with their primary healthcare provider or a gynecologist.	C
Chronic fatigue syndrome Scientific evidence is unclear regarding the effects of DHEA supplementation in patients with chronic fatigue syndrome. Better-quality research is necessary before a clear conclusion can be drawn.	C
Critical illness Scientific evidence is unclear regarding the safety and effectiveness of DHEA supplementation in critically ill patients. At this time, it is recommended that severe illness in the intensive care unit be treated with better-established therapies.	C
Crohn's disease Initial research studies suggested that DHEA supplements are safe for short-term use in patients with Crohn's disease. Preliminary trials suggest possible beneficial effects, but additional research is necessary before a clear conclusion can be drawn.	C
Depression Results of studies on the use of DHEA supplements for depression are conflicting, with some results suggesting benefits, and others reporting no effects. Better-quality research is necessary before a clear conclusion can be drawn.	C
Heart failure There is conflicting scientific evidence regarding the use of DHEA supplements in patients with heart failure or diminished ejection fraction. Other, more proven therapies are available in this area, and people with heart failure or other types of heart disease should discuss treatment options with their primary healthcare provider or a cardiologist.	C
HIV/AIDS Although some studies suggest that DHEA supplementation may be beneficial in patents with HIV, results from different studies do not agree. Most research in this area was not well designed or reported. There is currently not enough scientific evidence to recommend DHEA for this condition, and other, more proven therapies are available in this area.	C

Menopausal disorders C

Many different aspects of menopause have been studied using DHEA as a treatment. When DHEA is applied topically (on the skin) as a cream, it may lessen vaginal pain and discomfort associated with menopause. However, it is not clear whether DHEA cream has any benefits in treating osteoporosis after menopause.

Early evidence suggests that DHEA is not an effective treatment for hot flashes or emotional disturbances such as fatigue, irritability, anxiety, depression, insomnia, difficulties with concentration, memory, or decreased sex drive (which may occur at the time of menopause).

Muscle mass/body C

DHEA has been studied for improving body mass index, decreasing body fat, and increasing muscle mass. Early research reports that muscle mass is not increased when adding DHEA supplements to compensate for the natural decrease in dehydroepiandrosterone levels that occurs with aging (in otherwise healthy adults). It is not known if there are medical conditions in which DHEA supplementation might contribute to the preservation or improvement of muscle mass.

Myotonic dystrophy C

There is conflicting scientific evidence regarding the use of DHEA supplements for myotonic dystrophy. Better-quality research is necessary before a clear conclusion can be drawn.

Ovulation disorders C

Low-quality studies suggest that DHEA supplementation may be beneficial in women with ovulation disorders. However, results of research in this area are conflicting, and safety is not established. Currently, there is insufficient scientific evidence to form a clear conclusion about the use of DHEA for this condition.

Schizophrenia C

Initial research studies suggest benefits of DHEA supplementation in the management of negative, depressive, and anxiety symptoms of schizophrenia. Further study is needed to confirm these results before a firm conclusion can be drawn.

Septicemia (serious bacterial infections in the blood) C

Scientific evidence is unclear concerning the safety and effectiveness of DHEA supplementation in patients with septicemia. Other, more proven therapies are available.

Sexual function/libido/erectile dysfunction C

The results of studies vary on the benefits of use of DHEA in erectile dysfunction and sexual function in both men and women. Better-quality research is necessary before a clear conclusion can be drawn.

Continued

Systemic lupus erythematosus (SLE) Most studies on DHEA supplementation in people with SLE have not been well designed or reported. The results of various studies do not agree, with some results suggesting benefits, and others reporting no effects. Better-quality research is necessary before a clear conclusion can be drawn.	**C**
Alzheimer's disease Initial studies suggest that DHEA does not significantly improve cognitive performance or change symptom severity in people with Alzheimer's disease. Additional research is warranted in this area.	**D**
Brain function and well-being in the elderly Some textbooks and review articles suggest that DHEA supplements may improve brain function, memory, and overall feelings of well-being in the elderly. However, most studies reported no benefits. Additional study is warranted in this area.	**D**
Immune system stimulant It is suggested in some textbooks and review articles that DHEA may stimulate the immune system. However, current scientific evidence does not support this claim.	**D**

*Key to grades: *A:* Strong scientific evidence for this use; *B:* Good scientific evidence for this use; *C:* Unclear scientific evidence for this use; *D:* Fair scientific evidence against this use (it may not work); *F:* Strong scientific evidence against this use (it likely does not work). For a more detailed explanation of efficacy criteria, see "Natural Standard Evidence-Based Validated Grading Rationale" in the Introduction.

Uses Based on Tradition, Theory, or Limited Scientific Evidence

Aging, allergic disorders, amenorrhea associated with anorexia, andropause/adrenopause, angioedema, anxiety, asthma, bone diseases, bone loss associated with anorexia, bladder cancer, breast cancer, burns, colon cancer, dementia, diabetes, heart attack, high cholesterol, Huntington's disease, influenza, joint diseases, lipodystrophy in HIV, liver protection, malaria, malnutrition, movement disorders, multiple sclerosis, obesity, osteoporosis, pancreatic cancer, Parkinson's disease, performance enhancement, polycystic ovarian syndrome, post-traumatic stress disorder (PTSD), premenstrual syndrome, prostate cancer, psoriasis, Raynaud's phenomenon, rheumatic diseases, skin graft healing, sleep disorders, stress, tetanus, ulcerative colitis, viral encephalitis, weight loss.

DOSING

The following doses are based on scientific research, publications, traditional use, or expert opinion. Many herbs and supplements have not been thoroughly tested, and their safety and effectiveness may not be proven. Brands may be made differently, with variable ingredients even within the same brand. The doses shown may not apply to all products. It is important to always read product labels and discuss doses with a qualified healthcare provider before therapy is started.

Standardization

- Standardization involves measuring the amounts of certain chemicals in products to try to make different preparations similar to each other. It is not always known if the chemicals being measured are the "active" ingredients.
- *Note:* Some products are micronized and compounded with polyunsaturates. Information on the safety of long-term use of DHEA supplements is not available.

Adults (18 Years and Older)

Oral (Capsules/Tablets)

- **Addison's disease:** A dose of 50 mg taken daily has been used for Addison's disease/adrenal insufficiency. Adrenal insufficiency is a serious medical condition and should be treated under the supervision of a qualified healthcare provider.
- **Depression:** A dose of 30 to 90 mg taken daily has been used for depression. Higher doses of 200 to 500 mg per day have been studied for depression in HIV/AIDS.
- **Crohn's disease/ulcerative colitis:** A dose of 200 mg taken daily has been used in a small pilot study of therapy for Crohn's disease and ulcerative colitis.
- **Systemic lupus erythematosus (SLE):** Doses of 50 to 200 mg taken daily have been used in multiple studies for treatment of SLE.

Intravenous Administration

- **Dementia (multi-infarct):** A dose of 200 mg taken daily has been studied for multi-infarct dementia given intravenously. Safety is not established.

Topical (Cream)

- **Menopausal symptoms:** A cream containing 10% DHEA was applied on an area 20 cm by 20 cm on both thighs once daily for vaginal discomfort associated with menopause.

Children (Younger Than 18 Years)

- The dosing and safety of DHEA have not been well studied in children. In theory, DHEA may interfere with normal hormone balance and growth in children.

SAFETY

The U.S. Food and Drug Administration does not strictly regulate herbs and supplements. There is no guarantee of the strength, purity, or safety of products, and effects may vary. It is important to always read product labels. People who have a medical condition, or are taking other drugs, herbs, or supplements, should consult a qualified healthcare provider before starting a new therapy. A healthcare provider should be contacted immediately about any side effects.

Allergies

- People who are allergic to any DHEA product should avoid the use of all DHEA products.

Side Effects and Warnings

- Few side effects have been reported when DHEA supplements have been taken by mouth in recommended doses. The most common complaints include fatigue, nasal congestion, and headache. Rarely, rapid/irregular heartbeats or palpitations have been reported. People taking DHEA supplements may have a higher risk of developing blood clots or liver damage, although these effects have not been widely studied in humans. Individuals with a history of abnormal heart rhythms, blood clots, or hypercoagulability, and those with a history of liver disease, should avoid DHEA supplements.

- Because DHEA is a hormone related to other male and female hormones, there may be side effects related to its hormonal activities. For example, masculinization may occur in women, including acne, increased facial hair, hair loss, increased sweating, weight gain around the waist, and development of a deeper voice. Likewise, men may develop more prominent breasts (gynecomastia) and breast tenderness. Men may also experience increased blood pressure, testicular wasting, and increased aggressiveness.
- DHEA supplementation may alter the production or balance of various other hormones in the body. Possible hormone-related side effects include increased blood sugar levels, insulin resistance, altered cholesterol levels, altered thyroid hormone levels, and altered adrenal function. Caution is advised in persons with diabetes or hyperglycemia, high cholesterol, thyroid disorders, and other endocrine (hormonal) abnormalities. Serum glucose, cholesterol, and thyroid levels may need to be monitored by a healthcare provider, and medication adjustments may be necessary.
- In theory, DHEA may increase the risk of developing prostate, breast, and ovarian cancer. Based on laboratory research, DHEA may contribute to tamoxifen resistance in persons with breast cancer. Other possible side effects include insomnia, agitation, delusions, mania, nervousness, irritability, and psychosis.
- High DHEA levels have been correlated with Cushing's syndrome, which may be caused by excessive supplementation.

Pregnancy and Breastfeeding

- DHEA is not recommended during pregnancy or breastfeeding. Because DHEA is a hormone, it may be unsafe for the fetus or nursing infant. DHEA has caused abortions in studies of rats.

INTERACTIONS

Most herbs and supplements have not been thoroughly tested for interactions with other herbs, supplements, drugs, or foods. The interactions listed here are based on reports in scientific publications, laboratory experiments, or traditional use. It is important to always read product labels. People who have a medical condition, or are taking other drugs, herbs, or supplements, should consult a qualified healthcare provider before starting a new therapy.

Interactions with Drugs

- Laboratory research and studies in animals suggest that DHEA may interfere with how the body uses the liver's cytochrome P450 enzyme system to process components of some drugs. As a result, blood levels of these components may be elevated and may cause increased effects or potentially serious adverse reactions. Central nervous system agents, including carbamazepine and phenytoin, induce the P450 enzymes that metabolize DHEA and DHEA-S and therefore can decrease circulating concentrations of these hormones. People who are using any medications should always read the package insert and consult their healthcare provider and pharmacist about possible interactions.

- Based on data from studies in humans, DHEA may increase blood sugar levels. Caution is advised in people who are using medications that may also lower blood sugar levels such as metformin (Glucophage). In postmenopausal women, DHEA (1600 mg daily by mouth for 28 days) has been shown to cause insulin resistance. People who are taking drugs for diabetes by mouth or insulin should be closely monitored by a qualified healthcare provider. Medication adjustments may be necessary.
- In theory, DHEA may increase the risk of blood clotting. Persons who are taking anticoagulants (blood thinners) or antiplatelet drugs (such as aspirin) to prevent blood clots should discuss the use of DHEA with their healthcare provider. Examples of blood-thinning drugs are clopidogrel (Plavix), heparin, and warfarin (Coumadin). The risk of blood clots is also increased by smoking and by taking other hormones (such as oral contraceptives or hormone replacement therapy), and these hormones should not be combined with DHEA except under medical supervision.
- DHEA may alter heart rates or rhythm, and should be used cautiously with heart medications or drugs that may also affect heart rhythm.
- Although studies in this area have been limited, there are some reports that drugs such as amlodipine, nicardipine and other calcium channel blockers (e.g., diltiazem [Cardizem] and alprazolam [Xanax]) may increase DHEA levels in the body, which may lead to increased side effects when taken with DHEA supplements. In theory, increased hormone levels may occur if DHEA is used with estrogen or androgen hormonal therapies. DHEA may interact with psychiatric drugs such as clozapine (Clozaril).
- DHEA may interact with GABA-receptor drugs used for seizures or pain. Studies in animals suggest that DHEA may decrease the effectiveness of methadone and may add to the effects of clofibrate. Laboratory research studies reported that DHEA may contribute to tamoxifen resistance in breast cancer.
- Drugs that reduce the normal levels of DHEA produced by the body include dopamine, insulin, corticosteroids such as dexamethasone, drugs used to treat endometriosis such as danazol, opiate pain-killers, and estrogen-containing drugs. Metopirone and benfluorex may increase blood DHEA levels.

Interactions with Herbs and Dietary Supplements

- Laboratory research and studies in animals suggest that DHEA may interfere with how the body uses the liver's cytochrome P450 enzyme system to process components of other herbs and supplements. As a result, blood levels of these components may be elevated. DHEA may alter the effects that other herbs have on the cytochrome P450 system. Examples of such herbs are bloodroot, cat's claw, chamomile, chaparral, chasteberry, damiana, *Echinacea angustifolia*, goldenseal, grapefruit juice, licorice, oregano, red clover, St. John's wort, wild cherry, and yucca. People who are using any medications should always read the package insert and consult their healthcare provider and pharmacist about possible interactions.
- DHEA may raise blood sugar levels or cause insulin resistance, and may add to the effects of herbs/supplements that may also increase blood sugar levels, such as arginine, cocoa, ephedra (when combined with caffeine), and melatonin. DHEA may work against the effects of herbs/supplements that may decrease blood sugar levels, such as *Aloe vera*, American ginseng, bilberry, bitter melon, burdock, fenugreek, fish oil, gymnema, horse chestnut seed extract (HCSE), maitake

mushroom, marshmallow, milk thistle, *Panax ginseng*, rosemary, shark cartilage, Siberian ginseng, stinging nettle, and white horehound. Serum glucose levels in people with diabetes who are using DHEA should be monitored closely by a qualified healthcare provider. Dosing adjustments may be necessary.

- In theory, DHEA may increase the risk of blood clotting and may add to the effects of herbs and supplements that may also increase the risk of clotting, such as coenzyme Q10 and *Panax ginseng*. DHEA may work against the effects of herbs and supplements that may have blood-thinning effects and may reduce the risk of clotting, Examples of such herbs are alfalfa, American ginseng, angelica, anise, *Arnica montana*, asafetida, aspen bark, bilberry, birch, black cohosh, bladderwrack, bogbean, boldo, borage seed oil, bromelain, capsicum, cat's claw, celery, chamomile, chaparral, coleus, clove, cordyceps, danshen, devil's claw, dong quai, eicosapentaenoic acid (EPA), evening primrose oil, fenugreek, feverfew, fish oil, flaxseed/flax powder (not a concern with flaxseed oil), garlic, ginger, *Ginkgo biloba*, grapefruit juice, grape seed, green tea, guggul, gymnestra, horse chestnut, horseradish, licorice root, lovage root, male fern, meadowsweet, nordihydroguaiaretic acid (NDGA), omega-3 fatty acids, onion, *Panax ginseng*, papain, parsley, passion flower, poplar, prickly ash, propolis, quassia, red clover, reishi, rue, saw palmetto, Siberian ginseng, sweet birch, sweet clover, turmeric, vitamin E, white willow, wild carrot, wild lettuce, willow, wintergreen, and yucca.
- It is not known what effects occur when DHEA is used with herbs that may have hormonal effects in the body. Examples of agents with possible estrogen-like (phytoestrogenic) effects in the body are alfalfa, black cohosh, bloodroot, burdock, hops, kudzu, licorice, pomegranate, red clover, soy, thyme, white horehound, and yucca. Agents with possible progestin-like (phytoprogestational) effects in the body include bloodroot, chasteberry, damiana, oregano, and yucca.
- DHEA may alter heart rates and rhythms. Caution is advised in people who are taking herbs or supplements that may alter heart function or that contain cardiac glycosides. Examples are adonis, balloon cotton, black hellebore root/melampode, black Indian hemp, bushman's poison, cactus grandifloris, convallaria, eyebright, figwort, foxglove/digitalis, frangipani, hedge mustard, hemp root/Canadian hemp root, king's crown, lily-of-the-valley, motherwort, oleander leaf, pheasant's eye plant, plantain leaf, pleurisy root, psyllium husks, redheaded cotton-bush, rhubarb root, rubber vine, sea-mango, senna fruit, squill, strophanthus, uzara, wallflower, wintersweet, yellow dock root, and yellow oleander. Notably, bufalin/chan suis is a Chinese herbal formula that has been reported as toxic or fatal when taken with other agents that may alter conduction properties of the heart.
- Chromium picolinate may increase blood DHEA levels. Carnitine combined with DHEA may have additive effects. Studies in animals suggest that DHEA may increase melatonin secretion and prevent breakdown of vitamin E in the body.

Selected References

Natural Standard developed the preceding evidence-based information based on a systematic review of more than 800 articles. For comprehensive information about alternative and complementary therapies on the professional level, go to www.naturalstandard.com. Selected references are listed here.

Achermann JC, Silverman BL. Dehydroepiandrosterone replacement for patients with adrenal insufficiency. Lancet 2001;357(9266):1381-1382.

Andus T, Klebl F, Rogler G, et al. Patients with refractory Crohn's disease or ulcerative colitis respond to dehydroepiandrosterone: a pilot study. Aliment Pharmacol Ther 2003;17(3): 409-414.

Angold A. Adolescent depression, cortisol and DHEA. Psychol Med 2003;33(4):573-581.

Arlt W, Callies F, Allolio B. DHEA replacement in women with adrenal insufficiency—pharmacokinetics, bioconversion and clinical effects on well-being, sexuality and cognition. Endocr Res 2000;26(4):505-511.

Arlt W, Callies F, Koehler I, et al. Dehydroepiandrosterone supplementation in healthy men with an age-related decline of dehydroepiandrosterone secretion. J Clin Endocrinol Metab 2001;86(10):4686-4692.

Arlt W, Callies F, van Vlijmen JC, et al. Dehydroepiandrosterone replacement in women with adrenal insufficiency. N Engl J Med 1999;341(14):1013-1020.

Arlt W, Haas J, Callies F, et al. Biotransformation of oral dehydroepiandrosterone in elderly men: significant increase in circulating estrogens. J Clin Endocrinol Metab 1999;84(6):2170-2176.

Arlt W, Justl HG, Callies F, et al. Oral dehydroepiandrosterone for adrenal androgen replacement: pharmacokinetics and peripheral conversion to androgens and estrogens in young healthy females after dexamethasone suppression. J Clin Endocrinol Metab 1998;83(6): 1928-1934.

Azuma T, Nagai Y, Saito T, et al. The effect of dehydroepiandrosterone sulfate administration to patients with multi-infarct dementia. J Neurol Sci 1999;162(1):69-73.

Barry NN, McGuire JL, van Vollenhoven RF. Dehydroepiandrosterone in systemic lupus erythematosus: relationship between dosage, serum levels, and clinical response. J Rheumatol 1998;25(12):2352-2356.

Baulieu EE, Thomas G, Legrain S, et al. Dehydroepiandrosterone (DHEA), DHEA sulfate, and aging: contribution of the DHEAge study to a sociobiomedical issue. Proc Natl Acad Sci U S A 2000;97(8):4279-4284.

Bloch E, Newman E. Comparative placental steroid synthesis. I. Conversion of (7-3-H) dehydroepiandrosterone to (3-H)-androst-4-ene-3,17-dione. Endocrinology 1966;79(3): 524-530.

Bloch M, Schmidt PJ, Danaceau MA, et al. Dehydroepiandrosterone treatment of midlife dysthymia. Biol Psychiatry 1999;45(12):1533-1541.

Brown RC, Han Z, Cascio C, et al. Oxidative stress-mediated DHEA formation in Alzheimer's disease pathology. Neurobiol Aging 2003;24(1):57-65.

Buffington CK, Givens JR, Kitabchi AE. Opposing actions of dehydroepiandrosterone and testosterone on insulin sensitivity. In vivo and in vitro studies of hyperandrogenic females. Diabetes 1991;40(6):693-700.

Buffington CK, Pourmotabbed G, Kitabchi AE. Case report: amelioration of insulin resistance in diabetes with dehydroepiandrosterone. Am J Med Sci 1993;306(5):320-324.

Calhoun K, Pommier R, Cheek J, et al. The effect of high dehydroepiandrosterone sulfate levels on tamoxifen blockade and breast cancer progression. Am J Surg 2003;185(5):411-415.

Callies F, Fassnacht M, van Vlijmen JC, et al. Dehydroepiandrosterone replacement in women with adrenal insufficiency: effects on body composition, serum leptin, bone turnover, and exercise capacity. J Clin Endocrinol Metab 2001;86(5):1968-1972.

Casson PR, Andersen RN, Herrod HG, et al. Oral dehydroepiandrosterone in physiologic doses modulates immune function in postmenopausal women. Am J Obstet Gynecol 1993;169(6): 1536-1539.

Casson PR, Buster JE, Lindsay MS, et al. Dehydroepiandrosterone (DHEA) supplementation augments ovulation induction (OI) in poor responders: a case series [abstract]. Fertil Steril 1998;70(2S)(Suppl 1):475S-476S.

Casson PR, Buster JE. DHEA administration to humans: panacea or palaver? Semin Reprod Endocrinol 1995;13:247-256.

Casson PR, Carson SA, Buster JE, et al. Replacement dehydroepiandrosterone in elderly: rationale and prospects for the future. Endocrinologist 1998;8:187-194.

Casson PR, et al. Dehydroepiandrosterone (DHEA) replacement in postmenopausal women: present status and future promise. J North Am Menopause Soc 1997;4:225.

Casson PR, Faquin LC, Stentz FB, et al. Replacement of dehydroepiandrosterone enhances T-lymphocyte insulin binding in postmenopausal women. Fertil Steril 1995;63(5): 1027-1031.

Casson PR, Fisher J, Umstot ES, et al. Vaginal dehydroepiandrosterone (DHEA) bioavailability in a hypopituitary woman with induction of adrenarche [Abstract P17]. Society for Gynecologic Investigation 1994.

Casson PR, Lindsay MS, Pisarska MD, et al. Dehydroepiandrosterone supplementation augments ovarian stimulation in poor responders: a case series. Hum Reprod 2000;15(10): 2129-2132.

Casson PR, Santoro N, Elkind-Hirsch K, et al. Postmenopausal dehydroepiandrosterone administration increases free insulin-like growth factor-I and decreases high-density lipoprotein: a six-month trial. Fertil Steril 1998;70(1):107-110.

Casson PR, Straughn AB, Umstot ES, et al. Delivery of dehydroepiandrosterone to premenopausal women: effects of micronization and nonoral administration. Am J Obstet Gynecol 1996;174(2):649-653.

Centurelli MA, Abate MA. The role of dehydroepiandrosterone in AIDS. Ann Pharmacother 1997;31(5):639-642.

Chang DM, Lan H, Lan HY, et al. GL701 (Prasterone, DHEA) significantly reduces flares in female patients with mild to moderate systemic lupus erythematosus. Arthritis Rheum 2000;43(Suppl):S241.

Chassany O. [Does dehydroepiandrosterone improve well-being?] Presse Med 2000;29(24): 1354-1355.

Colker C, Torina G, Swain M, et al. Double-blind, placebo-controlled, randomized clinical trial evaluating the effects of exercise plus 3-acetyl-7-oxo-dehydroepiandrosterone on body composition and the endocrine system in overweight adults [abstract]. J Exercise Physiol 1999;2(4).

Derksen RH. Dehydroepiandrosterone (DHEA) and systemic lupus erythematosus. Semin Arthritis Rheum 1998;27(6):335-347.

Dockhorn R, Wanger J, McKay L, et al. Safety and efficacy of DHEA in asthmatics undergoing a cat room challenge [abstract]. Ann Allergy Asthma Immunol 1999;82(1):111.

Dyner T, Lang W, Geaga JV, et al. Phase I study of dehydroepiandrosterone (EL-10) therapy in symptomatic HIV disease [abstract]. 6th Intl Conf on AIDS 1990;3:208.

Dyner TS, Lang W, Geaga J, et al. An open-label dose-escalation trial of oral dehydroepiandrosterone tolerance and pharmacokinetics in patients with HIV disease. J Acquir Immune Defic Syndr 1993;6(5):459-465.

Fassati P, Fassati M, Sonka J, et al. [New approach to the treatment of angina pectoris by dehydroepiandrosterone-sulfate.] Cas Lek Cesk 1971;110(26):606-609.

Fassati P, Fassati M, Sonka J, et al. Dehydroepiandrosterone sulphate—a new approach to some cases of angina pectoris therapy. Agressologie 1970;11(5):445-448.

Forrest AD, Drewery J, Fotherby K, et al. A clinical trial of dehydroepiandrosterone (Diandrone). J Neurol Neurosurg Psychiat 1960;23:52-55.

Furie R. Dehydroepiandrosterone and biologics in the treatment of systemic lupus erythematosus. Curr Rheumatol Rep 2000;2(1):44-50.

Gebre-Medhin G, Husebye ES, Mallmin H, et al. Oral dehydroepiandrosterone (DHEA) replacement therapy in women with Addison's disease. Clin Endocrinol (Oxf) 2000;52(6): 775-780.

Giltay EJ, van Schaardenburg D, Gooren LJ, et al. Dehydroepiandrosterone sulfate in patients with rheumatoid arthritis. Ann N Y Acad Sci 1999;876:152-154.

Giltay EJ, van Schaardenburg D, Gooren LJ, et al. Effects of dehydroepiandrosterone administration on disease activity in patients with rheumatoid arthritis. Br J Rheumatol 1998;37(6): 705-706.

Gordon CM, Grace E, Emans SJ, et al. Changes in bone turnover markers and menstrual function after short- term oral DHEA in young women with anorexia nervosa. J Bone Miner Res 1999;14(1):136-145.

Gordon GB, Bush DE, Weisman HF. Reduction of atherosclerosis by administration of dehydroepiandrosterone. A study in the hypercholesterolemic New Zealand white rabbit with aortic intimal injury. J Clin Invest 1988;82(2):712-720.

Gordon GB, Bush TL, Helzlsouer KJ, et al. Relationship of serum levels of dehydroepiandrosterone and dehydroepiandrosterone sulfate to the risk of developing postmenopausal breast cancer. Cancer Res 1990;50(13):3859-3862.

Gordon GB, Helzlsouer KJ, Alberg AJ, et al. Serum levels of dehydroepiandrosterone and dehydroepiandrosterone sulfate and the risk of developing gastric cancer. Cancer Epidemiol Biomarkers Prev 1993;2(1):33-35.

Gordon GB, Helzlsouer KJ, Comstock GW. Serum levels of dehydroepiandrosterone and its sulfate and the risk of developing bladder cancer. Cancer Res 1991;51(5):1366-1369.

Gordon GB, Shantz LM, Talalay P. Inhibitory effects of dehydroepiandrosterone on cell proliferation, differentiation, and carcinogenesis: role of glucose-6-phosphate dehydrogenase. *In* Hardy HA, Stratman F (eds): Proceedings of the Eighteenth Steenbock Symposium. Hormones, Thermogenesis, and Obesity. New York, Elsevier Science, 1989, pp 339-354.

Gordon GB, Shantz LM, Talalay P. Modulation of growth, differentiation and carcinogenesis by dehydroepiandrosterone. Adv Enzyme Regul 1987;26:355-382.

Guay AT. Decreased testosterone in regularly menstruating women with decreased libido: a clinical observation. J Sex Marital Ther 2001;27(5):513-519.

Himmel P, Seligman TM. A pilot study employing dehydroepiandrosterone (DHEA) in the treatment of chronic fatigue syndrome. J Clin Rheumatol 1999;5(2):56-59.

Holzmann H, Krapp R, Morsches B, et al. [Therapy of psoriasis using dehydroepiandrosterone-sulfate.] Arztl Forsch 1971;25(11):345-353.

Holzmann H, Morsches B, Krapp R, et al. [Therapy of psoriasis using dehydroepiandrosterone-enanthate.] Z Haut Geschlechtskr 1972;47(3):99-110.

Holzmann H, Morsches B, Krapp R, et al. [Therapy of psoriasis with dehydroepiandrosterone-enanthate. II. Intramuscular depot application of 300 mg weekly (author's transl).] Archiv fur Dermatol Forsch 1973;247(1):23-28.

Hunt PJ, Gurnell EM, Huppert FA, et al. Improvement in mood and fatigue after dehydroepiandrosterone replacement in Addison's disease in a randomized, double blind trial. J Clin Endocrinol Metab 2000;85(12):4650-4656.

Huppert FA, Van Niekerk JK. Dehydroepiandrosterone (DHEA) supplementation for cognitive function (Cochrane Review). Cochrane Database (Issue 2) 2001;2:CD000304.

Ishikawa M, Shimizu T. Dehydroepiandrosterone sulfate and induction of labor. Am J Perinatol 1989;6(2):173-175.

Johannsson G, Burman P, Wiren L, et al. Low dose dehydroepiandrosterone affects behavior in hypopituitary androgen–deficient women: a placebo-controlled trial. J Clin Endocrinol Metab 2002;87(5):2046-2052.

Jones DL, James VH. Determination of dehydroepiandrosterone and dehydroepiandrosterone sulphate in blood and tissue. Studies of normal women and women with breast or endometrial cancer. J Steroid Biochem 1987;26(1):151-159.

Jones JA, Nguyen A, Straub M, et al. Use of DHEA in a patient with advanced prostate cancer: a case report and review. Urology 1997;50(5):784-788.

Kalman DS, Colker CM, Swain MA, et al. A randomized, double-blind, placebo-controlled study of 3-acetyl-7-oxo-dehydroepiandrosterone in healthy overweight adults. Current Therapeutic Research 2000;61(7):435-442.

Kim SS, Brody KH. Dehydroepiandrosterone replacement in Addison's disease. Eur J Obstet Gynecol Reprod Biol 2001;97(1):96-97.

Knopman D, Henderson VW. DHEA for Alzheimer's disease: a modest showing by a superhormone. Neurology 2003;60(7):1060-1061.

Kodama M, Kodama T, Murakami M. The value of the dehydroepiandrosterone-annexed vitamin C infusion treatment in the clinical control of chronic fatigue syndrome (CFS). I. A Pilot study of the new vitamin C infusion treatment with a volunteer CFS patient. In Vivo 1996;10(6):575-584.

Kodama M, Kodama T, Murakami M. The value of the dehydroepiandrosterone-annexed vitamin C infusion treatment in the clinical control of chronic fatigue syndrome (CFS). II. Characterization of CFS patients with special reference to their response to a new vitamin C infusion treatment. In Vivo 1996;10(6):585-596.

Koo E, Feher KG, Feher T, et al. Effect of dehydroepiandrosterone on hereditary angioedema. Klin Wochenschr 1983;61(14):715-717.

Lahita RG. Dehydroepiandrosterone (DHEA) and lupus erythematosus: an update. Lupus 1997;6(6):491-493.

Lahita RG. Dehydroepiandrosterone (DHEA) for serious disease, a possibility? Lupus 1999; 8(3):169-170.

Lauritzen C. [Therapeutic attempts with dehydroepiandrosterone sulfate in threatened pregnancies.] Arch Gynakol 1971;211(1):247-249.

Lauritzen C. Conversion of DHEA-sulfate to estrogens as a test of placental function. Horm Metab Res 1969;1(2):96.

Leenstra T, Ter Kuile FO, Kariuki SK, et al. Dehydroepiandrosterone sulfate levels associated with decreased malaria parasite density and increased hemoglobin concentration in pubertal girls from Western Kenya. J Infect Dis 2003;188(2):297-304.

Marcelli C. Can DHEA be used to prevent bone loss and osteoporosis? Joint Bone Spine 2003; 70(1):1-2.

Marx C, Petros S, Bornstein SR, et al. Adrenocortical hormones in survivors and nonsurvivors of severe sepsis: diverse time course of dehydroepiandrosterone, dehydroepiandrosterone-sulfate, and cortisol. Crit Care Med 2003;31(5):1382-1388.

Mease PJ, Merrill JT, Lahita R, et al. GL701 (prasterone, dehydroepiandrosterone) improves or stabilizes disease activity in systemic lupus erythematosus. The Endocrine Society's 82nd Annual Meeting, 2000.

Mease PJ, Merrill JT, Lahita RG, et al. GL701 (Prasterone, DHEA) improves systemic lupus erythematosus. Arthritis Rheum 2000;43(Suppl):S271.

Mease PL, Ginzler EM, Gluck OS, et al. Improvement in bone mineral density in steroid-treated patients during treatment with GL701 (Prasterone, DHEA). Arthritis Rheum 2000; 43(Suppl):S230.

Munarriz R, Talakoub L, Flaherty E, et al. Androgen replacement therapy with dehydroepiandrosterone for androgen insufficiency and female sexual dysfunction: androgen and questionnaire results. J Sex Marital Ther 2002;28(Suppl 1):165-173.

Munarriz RM, Talakoub L, Flaherty E, et al. Hormone, sexual function and personal sexual distress outcomes following dehydroepiandrosterone (DHEA) treatment for multi-dimensional female sexual dysfunction and androgen deficiency syndrome [abstract]. American Urological Association Annual Meeting, June 2-7, 2001.

Oelkers W. Dehydroepiandrosterone for adrenal insufficiency. N Engl J Med 1999;341(14): 1073-1074.

Patavino T, Brady DM. Natural medicine and nutritional therapy as an alternative treatment in systemic lupus erythematosus. Altern Med Rev 2001;6(5):460-471.

Percheron G, Hogrel JY, Denot-Ledunois S, et al. Effect of 1-year oral administration of dehydroepiandrosterone to 60- to 80-year-old individuals on muscle function and cross-sectional area: a double-blind placebo-controlled trial. Arch Intern Med 2003; 163(6):720-727.

Petri M, Lahita RG, McGuire J, et al. Results of the GL701 (DHEA) multicenter steroid-sparing SLE study. Arthritis Rheum 1997;40(Suppl):S327.

Rabkin JG, Ferrando SJ, Wagner GJ, et al. DHEA treatment for HIV+ patients: effects on mood, androgenic and anabolic parameters. Psychoneuroendocrinology 2000;25(1):53-68.

Rommler A. [Adrenopause and dehydroepiandrosterone: pharmacological therapy versus replacement therapy.] Gynakol Geburtshilfliche Rundsch 2003;43(2):79-90.

Sasaki K, Nakano R, Kadoya Y, et al. Cervical ripening with dehydroepiandrosterone sulphate. Br J Obstet Gynaecol 1982;89(3):195-198.

Shun YP, Shun LH, Feng YY, et al. [The effect of DHEA on body fat distribution and serum lipids in elderly overweight males.] Pract Geriatr 1999;13(1):31-33.

Stomati M, Monteleone P, Casarosa E, et al. Six-month oral dehydroepiandrosterone supplementation in early and late postmenopause. Gynecol Endocrinol 2000;14(5):342-363.

Strous RD, Maayan R, Lapidus R, et al. Dehydroepiandrosterone augmentation in the management of negative, depressive, and anxiety symptoms in schizophrenia. Arch Gen Psychiatry 2003;60(2):133-141.

Strous RD, Maayan R, Lapidus R, et al. Dehydroepiandrosterone augmentation in the management of negative, depressive, and anxiety symptoms in schizophrenia. Arch Gen Psychiatry 2003;60(2):133-141.

Sugino M, Ohsawa N, Ito T, et al. A pilot study of dehydroepiandrosterone sulfate in myotonic dystrophy. Neurology 1998;51(2):586-589.

Suh-Burgmann E, Sivret J, Duska LR, et al. Long-term administration of intravaginal dehydroepiandrosterone on regression of low-grade cervical dysplasia—a pilot study. Gynecol Obstet Invest 2003;55(1):25-31.

Trichopoulou A, Bamia C, Kalapothaki V, et al. Dehydroepiandrosterone relations to dietary and lifestyle variables in a general population sample. Ann Nutr Metab 2003;47(3-4): 158-164.

Usiskin KS, Butterworth S, Clore JN, et al. Lack of effect of dehydroepiandrosterone in obese men. Int J Obes 1990;14(5):457-463.

Vakina TN, Shutov AM, Shalina SV, et al. [Dehydroepiandrosterone and sexual function in men with chronic prostatitis]. Urologiia 2003;Jan-Feb(1):49-52.

Van Vollenhoven RF, Engleman EG, McGuire JL. An open study of dehydroepiandrosterone in systemic lupus erythematosus. Arthritis Rheum 1994;37(9):1305-1310.

Van Vollenhoven RF, Engleman EG, McGuire JL. Dehydroepiandrosterone in systemic lupus erythematosus. Results of a double-blind, placebo-controlled, randomized clinical trial. Arthritis Rheum 1995;38(12):1826-1831.

Van Vollenhoven RF, McDevitt H. Studies of the treatment of nephritis in NZB/NZW mice with dehydroepiandrosterone [abstract]. Arthritis Rheum 1992;35(Suppl):S207.

Van Vollenhoven RF, McGuire JL. Studies of dehydroepiandrosterone (DHEA) as a therapeutic agent in systemic lupus erythematosus. Ann Med Interne (Paris) 1996; 147(4):290-296.

Van Vollenhoven RF, Morabito LM, Engleman EG, et al. Treatment of systemic lupus erythematosus with dehydroepiandrosterone. Two-year follow-up from an open-label clinical trial [abstract]. Arthritis Rheum 1994;37:S407.

Van Vollenhoven RF, Morabito LM, Engleman EG, et al. Treatment of systemic lupus erythematosus with dehydroepiandrosterone: 50 patients treated up to 12 months. J Rheumatol 1998;25(2):285-289.

Van Vollenhoven RF, Morales A, Yen S, et al. In patients with systemic lupus erythematosus, treatment with oral dehydroepiandrosterone restores abnormally low in vitro production of IL-2, IL-6 and TNF-alpha [abstract]. Arthritis Rheum 1994;37:S407.

Van Vollenhoven RF, Park JL, Genovese MC, et al. A double-blind, placebo-controlled, clinical trial of dehydroepiandrosterone in severe systemic lupus erythematosus. Lupus 1999;8(3): 181-187.

Van Vollenhoven RF. Dehydroepiandrosterone for the treatment of systemic lupus erythematosus. Expert Opin Pharmacother 2002;3(1):23-31.

Van Vollenhoven RF. Dehydroepiandrosterone in systemic lupus erythematosus. Rheum Dis Clin North Am 2000;26(2):349-362.

Van Vollenhoven RF. Dehydroepiandrosterone in the treatment of systemic lupus erythematosus. Rheumatology (Oxford) 2000;39(8):929-930.

Van Weering HG, Gutknecht DR, Schats R. Augmentation of ovarian response by dehydroepiandrosterone. Hum Reprod 2001;16(7):1537-1539.

Villareal DT, Holloszy JO, Kohrt WM. Effects of DHEA replacement on bone mineral density and body composition in elderly women and men. Clin Endocrinol (Oxf) 2000;53(5): 561-568.

Wallace D. Current and emerging lupus treatments. Am J Manag Care 2001;7(16 Suppl): S490-S495.

Wallace MB, Lim J, Cutler A, et al. Effects of dehydroepiandrosterone vs androstenedione supplementation in men. Med Sci Sports Exerc 1999;31(12):1788-1792.

Wolkowitz OM, Kramer JH, Reus VI, et al. DHEA treatment of Alzheimer's disease: a randomized, double-blind, placebo-controlled study. Neurology 2003;60(7):1071-1076.

Wolkowitz OM, Reus VI, Keebler A, et al. Double-blind treatment of major depression with dehydroepiandrosterone. Am J Psychiatry 1999;156(4):646-649.

Wolkowitz OM, Reus VI, Roberts E, et al. Antidepressant and cognition-enhancing effects of DHEA in major depression. Ann N Y Acad Sci 1995;774:337-339.

Wolkowitz OM, Reus VI, Roberts E, et al. Dehydroepiandrosterone (DHEA) treatment of depression. Biol Psychiatry 1997;41(3):311-318.

Wren BG, Day RO, McLachlan AJ, et al. Pharmacokinetics of estradiol, progesterone, testosterone and dehydroepiandrosterone after transbuccal administration to postmenopausal women. Climacteric 2003;6(2):104-111.

Zelissen PM, Thijssen JH. [Role of prasterone (dehydroepiandrosterone) in substitution therapy for adrenocortical insufficiency]. Ned Tijdschr Geneeskd 2001;145(42):2018-2022.
Zumoff B, Levin J, Rosenfeld RS, et al. Abnormal 24-hr mean plasma concentrations of dehydroisoandrosterone and dehydroisoandrosterone sulfate in women with primary operable breast cancer. Cancer Res 1981;41(9 Pt 1):3360-3363.
Zumoff B, Troxler RG, O'Connor J, et al. Abnormal hormone levels in men with coronary artery disease. Arteriosclerosis 1982;2(1):58-67.
Zumoff B, Walsh BT, Katz JL, et al. Subnormal plasma dehydroisoandrosterone to cortisol ratio in anorexia nervosa: a second hormonal parameter of ontogenic regression. J Clin Endocrinol Metab 1983;56(4):668-672.
Zumoff BV, Bradlow HL. Sex difference in the metabolism of dehydroisoandrosterone sulfate. J Clin Endocrinol Metab 1980;51(2):334-336.

Dong Quai

(*Angelica sinensis* [Oliv.] Diels)

RELATED TERMS

- American angelica, *Angelica acutiloba* (Japanese), *Angelica archangelica, Angelica atropurpurea, Angelica dahurica, Angelica edulis, Angelica gigas, Angelica keiskei, Angelica koreana, Angelica polymorpha* var. sinensis Oliv., *Angelica pubescens*, angelica radix, angelica root, *Angelica sylvestris*, angelique, Apiaceae/Umbellifera, *Archangelica officinalis* Moench or Hoff, beta-sitosterol, Chinese angelica, Chinese danggui, danggui, Dang Gui, danggui-nian-tong-tang (DGNTT), dang quai, dong kwai, dong qua, dong quai extract, dong quai root, dong qui, dry-kuei, engelwurzel, European angelica, European dong quai, female ginseng, FP3340010, FP334015, FT334010, garden angelica, heiligenwurzel, Japanese angelica, kinesisk kvan, kinesisk kvanurt, ligusticum glaucescens franch, ligusticum officinale Koch, ligustilides, phytoestrogen, qingui, radix angelica sinensis, root of the holy ghost, tan kue bai zhi, tang kuei, tang kuei root, tang kwei, tanggui (Korean), tanggwi (Korean), tang quai, toki (Japanese), wild angelica, wild chin quai, women's ginseng, yuan nan wild dong quai, yungui.
- **Combination herbal formulations:** Angelica-Alunite Solution, Angelica-Paeonia Powder, Bloussant Breast Enhancement Tablets, Bust Plus, Dong Quai and Royal Jelly, Dong Quai 4, Dong Quai 4, Danggui Buxue Tang, Danggui Huoxue Tang, Female Corrective Combination Containing Dong Quai, Four Things Soup, Shenyan Huayu Tang, Shimotus To, Shou Wu Chih, Sini Decoction, Siwu tang, tokishakuyakusan, Xiao Yao Powder, Yishen Tang.
- *Note:* The related species *Angelica acutiloba* appears to have properties similar to those of dong quai (*Angelica sinensis*) in laboratory experiments.

BACKGROUND

- Dong quai (*Angelica sinensis*), also known as Chinese angelica, has been used for thousands of years in traditional Chinese, Korean, and Japanese medicine. It remains one of the most popular plants in Chinese medicine and is used primarily for health conditions in women. Dong quai has been called "female ginseng," based on its use for gynecologic disorders such as painful menstruation (dysmenorrhea), pelvic pain, recovery from childbirth or illness, and fatigue/low vitality. It is also given for strengthening *xue* (loosely translated as "the blood") and for cardiovascular conditions, high blood pressure, inflammation, headache, infections, and neuropathic (nerve) pain.
- In the late 1800s, an extract of dong quai called *Eumenol* became popular in Europe as a treatment for gynecologic complaints. Recently, interest in dong quai has resurged because of its proposed weak estrogen-like properties. However, it remains unclear whether dong quai has the same effects on the body as estrogens, blocks the activity of estrogens, or has no significant hormonal effects. Results of animal studies are conflicting, and one trial in humans found no short-term estrogen-like effects on the body. Additional research is necessary in this area before a firm conclusion can be drawn.

- In Chinese medicine, dong quai is most often used in combination with other herbs. Within the Chinese medical framework, dong quai is used as a component of formulas for liver *qi* stasis and spleen deficiency. It is believed to work best in persons with a *yin* profile and is considered to be a mildly warming herb. Dong quai is thought to return the body to proper order by nourishing the blood and harmonizing vital energy. The name *dong quai* translates as "return to order," based on its alleged restorative properties.
- The part of the plant most often cultivated for medicinal use is the root, which is divided into three parts (head, body, tail). Each section is believed to have different actions within the body. For example, the tail is proposed to be best for promoting blood circulation, while the head is considered the worst.
- Although dong quai has many historical and theoretical uses based on studies in animals, there is little evidence from studies in humans supporting the effects of dong quai for any condition. Clinical studies have been limited, and in general have been either poorly designed or have reported insignificant results. Most of these studies have examined combination formulas containing multiple ingredients, making it difficult to determine which ingredient causes certain effects.

USES BASED ON SCIENTIFIC EVIDENCE	Grade*
Amenorrhea (lack of menstrual period) There have been limited poor-quality studies of dong quai as a component of herbal combinations given for amenorrhea. It is unclear from laboratory studies whether dong quai has the same effects on the body as estrogens or blocks the activity of estrogens (or neither), and how this may affect women with amenorrhea. One study in humans suggested that dong quai may not have significant short-term estrogen-like effects on the body. Additional research is necessary before a firm conclusion can be drawn.	C
Angina pectoris/coronary artery disease There is insufficient evidence to support the use of dong quai for the treatment of heart disease.	C
Arthritis Dong quai is traditionally used in the treatment of arthritis. However, there is insufficient reliable scientific evidence from studies in humans to recommend the use of dong quai alone or in combination with other herbs for osteoarthritis or rheumatoid arthritis.	C
Dysmenorrhea (painful menstruation) Results were inconclusive in preliminary, poor-quality research studies in humans of the use of dong quai in combination with other herbs for dysmenorrhea. Studies in animals reported conflicting results, with both relaxing and stimulatory effects of dong quai on the uterus. Reliable scientific evidence concerning the effects of dong quai alone in women with dysmenorrhea is not available. It is traditionally believed that therapy should begin on day 14 of the menstrual cycle and continue until menstruation has ceased.	C

Continued

Glomerulonephritis There is insufficient evidence to support the use of dong quai as a treatment for kidney diseases such as glomerulonephritis. Results were unclear in preliminary poor-quality studies of dong quai used in combination with other herbs.	C
Idiopathic thrombocytopenic purpura (ITP) One poor-quality study reported that dong quai was beneficial in patients diagnosed with ITP. However, these patients were not compared to individuals who were not receiving dong quai, and therefore the results can only be considered preliminary.	C
Menstrual migraine headache One small study reported a reduced average number of menstruation-associated migraine attacks during prophylactic treatment with a daily combination of 60 mg of soy isoflavones, 100 mg of dong quai, and 50 mg of black cohosh, with each component standardized to its primary alkaloid. Subjects in the study received medication for 24 weeks. The effects of dong quai alone for this condition are unclear, and further research is necessary before a clear conclusion can be reached.	C
Nerve pain There is insufficient evidence to support the use of dong quai as a treatment for neuropathic pain. High-quality human research is lacking.	C
Pulmonary hypertension A preliminary controlled trial reports that the combination of dong quai with the drug nifedipine may be better than either agent alone to improve pulmonary hypertension in individuals with chronic obstructive pulmonary disease (COPD). A second study of dong quai alone also noted benefits. These studies were small, not well reported, and cannot be considered conclusive. It remains unclear if dong quai is beneficial for other causes of pulmonary hypertension. Further research is needed before a recommendation can be made.	C
Menopausal symptoms Dong quai is used in traditional Chinese formulas for menopausal symptoms. It has been proposed that dong quai may contain "phytoestrogens" (chemicals with estrogen-like effects in the body). However, it remains unclear from laboratory studies whether dong quai has the same effects on the body as estrogens, blocks the activity of estrogens, or has no significant effect on estrogens. A well-designed 24-week human trial compared the effects of dong quai to a placebo in 71 women with menopausal symptoms. This study found no differences in hot flashes or in the Kupperman Index (a commonly used measure of menopausal symptoms) between dong quai and placebo groups. No changes occurred in blood estrogen levels, thickness of the uterus lining, or vaginal dryness. This study suggests that dong quai may not have short-term estrogen-like effects on the	D

Continued

body. However, there may have been too few patients enrolled in the study to accurately measure effects. In addition, the dong quai extract used, prepared by East Earth herbs, Inc. (4.5 mg per day, standardized to 0.5 mg per kg of ferulic acid), may not be manufactured in the same way as other dong quai products and may yield different results. Additional research is necessary before a strong recommendation can be made.

*Key to grades: *A:* Strong scientific evidence for this use; *B:* Good scientific evidence for this use; *C:* Unclear scientific evidence for this use; *D:* Fair scientific evidence against this use (it may not work); *F:* Strong scientific evidence against this use (it likely does not work). For a more detailed explanation of efficacy criteria, see "Natural Standard Evidence-Based Validated Grading Rationale" in the Introduction.

Uses Based on Tradition, Theory, or Limited Scientific Evidence

Abscesses, abdominal pain, abnormal fetal movement, abnormal heart rhythms, age-related nerve damage, allergy, anemia, anorexia nervosa, antibacterial, anti-aging, antifungal, antiseptic, antispasmodic, anti-tumor, antiviral, anxiety, aortitis, asthma, atherosclerosis, back pain, bleeding hemorrhoids, bleomycin-induced lung damage, blood clots, blood flow disorders, blood purifier, blood stagnation, blood vessel disorders, blurred vision, body pain, boils, bone growth, breast enlargement, bronchitis, Buerger's disease, cancer, central nervous system disorders, cervicitis, chilblains, cholagogue, chronic hepatitis, chronic obstructive pulmonary disease (COPD), chronic rhinitis, cirrhosis, colchicine-induced learning impairment, congestive heart failure (CHF), constipation, cough, cramps, dermatitis, diabetes, digestion disorders, diuretic (increasing urine flow), dysentery, eczema, emotional instability, endometritis, expectorant, fatigue, fibrocystic breast disease, fibroids, flatulence (gas), fluid retention, gastric ulcer, glaucoma, hay fever, headache, heartburn, hematopoiesis (stimulation of blood cell production), hemolytic disease of the newborn, hernia, high blood pressure, high cholesterol, hormonal abnormalities, immune cytopenias, immunosuppressant, infections, infertility, irritable bowel syndrome, joint pain, kidney disease, labor aid, laxative, leukorrhea (vaginal discharge), liver protection, lung disease, malaria, menorrhagia (heavy menstrual bleeding), menstrual cramping, migraine, miscarriage prevention, morning sickness, muscle relaxant, osteoporosis, ovulation abnormalities, pain, pain from bruises, palpitations, pelvic congestion syndrome, pelvic inflammatory disease, peritoneal dialysis, pleurisy, postpartum weakness, pregnancy support, premenstrual syndrome (PMS), prolapsed uterus, psoriasis, pulmonary fibrosis, Raynaud's disease, reperfusion injury, respiratory tract infection, retained placenta, Rhesus (Rh) factor incompatibility, rheumatic diseases, sciatica, sedative, sepsis, shingles (herpes zoster), skin pigmentation disorders, skin ulcers, stiffness, stomach cancer, stress, stroke, tinnitus (ringing in the ear), toothache, vaginal atrophy, vitamin E deficiency, wound healing.

DOSING

The following doses are based on scientific research, publications, traditional use, or expert opinion. Many herbs and supplements have not been thoroughly tested, and their safety and effectiveness may not be proven. Brands may be made differently, with variable ingredients even within the same brand. The doses shown may not apply to all products. It is important to always read product labels and discuss doses with a qualified healthcare provider before therapy is started.

Standardization

- Standardization involves measuring amounts of certain chemicals in products to try to make different preparations similar to each other. It is not always known if the chemicals being measured are the "active" ingredients.
- There are no standard or well-studied doses of dong quai, and many different doses are used traditionally. Some products standardize dong quai to 0.8% to 1.1% ligustilide per dose, or to 0.5 mg per kg of ferulic acid. One gram of 100% dong quai extract has been reported to be equivalent to approximately 4 g of raw dong quai root. Safety and effectiveness are not established for any dose.
- In Asia, dong quai is primarily used medicinally, whereas in the United States and Europe it is more common as a flavoring agent in food products (e.g., in liqueurs, vermouth, ice cream, candy, gelatins, puddings). A related species, *Angelica acutiloba*, appears to have similar properties to dong quai in laboratory experiments.

Adults (18 Years and Older)

Root Preparations

- **Combination preparations:** Dong quai is used in numerous herbal combinations, and various doses have been used traditionally and in Chinese research. Because of this variation and lack of high-quality studies, no specific recommendations can be made. Safety and effectiveness are not established for most herbal combinations, and the amounts of dong quai present may vary from batch to batch.
- **Powdered/dried root/root slices:** A dose of 1 to 5 g of root taken by mouth three times daily has been used traditionally, although more common doses range from 1 to 2 g taken three times daily. Weight-based dosing has been proposed, although there is no scientific evidence to support this practice.
- **Fluid extract/tincture:** Doses of 3 to 8 ml of a fluid extract (1:2) or 10 to 40 drops of tincture (1:5 in 50% to 70% alcohol) taken by mouth three times daily have been used.
- **Decoction:** To prepare, 1 teaspoon to 1 tablespoon of cut root is simmered for 2 to 5 minutes in 1 cup of water that has been brought to a boil; it is then removed from the heat and left to stand for 5 to 10 minutes. One to three cups have been consumed by mouth daily.
- **Intravenous injection:** Safety of intravenous use is not established, although it has been reported in research.
- **Topical (on the skin):** Ten to 15 drops of diluted essential oil has been used for skin irritation (anecdotal).

Leaf Preparations (Less Common Than Root Preparations)

- **Dried leaf:** A dose of 2 to 5 g taken by mouth three times daily has been used.
- **Leaf tincture:** A dose of 2 to 5 ml (1:5 in 45% alcohol) taken by mouth three times daily has been used.
- **Leaf fluid extract:** A dose of 0.5 to 2 ml (1:1) taken 3 times daily has been used.

Children (Younger Than 18 Years)

- There are insufficient scientific data to recommend dong quai for use in children, and it is not recommended because of potential side effects.

SAFETY

The U.S. Food and Drug Administration does not strictly regulate herbs and supplements. There is no guarantee of the strength, purity, or safety of products, and effects may vary. It is important to always read product labels. People who have a medical condition, or are taking other drugs, herbs, or supplements, should consult a qualified healthcare provider before starting a new therapy. A healthcare provider should be contacted immediately about any side effects.

Allergies

- People with known allergy/hypersensitivity to *Angelica radix* or members of the Apiaceae/Umbelliferae family (anise, caraway, carrot, celery, dill, parsley) should avoid dong quai products. Skin rash has been reported with the use of dong quai, although it is unclear whether this was an allergic response. An asthma response occurred after a person breathed in dong quai powder.

Side Effects and Warnings

- Although the safety of dong quai is accepted as a food additive in the United States and Europe, its safety in medicinal doses is not known. There are no reliable long-term studies of side effects. Most precautions are based on theory, laboratory research, tradition, or isolated case reports.
- Components of dong quai may increase the risk of bleeding due to anticoagulant and anti-platelet effects, although there are no reliable reports of clinically significant bleeding in humans. Caution is advised in people with bleeding disorders or those who are taking drugs that may increase the risk of bleeding. Dosing adjustments may be necessary. Use of dong quai products should be discontinued in persons who are going to have surgical or major dental procedures.
- It is unclear whether dong quai has the same effects on the body as estrogens, blocks the activity of estrogens, or has no significant hormonal effects. Results of studies in animals are conflicting, and one trial in human subjects reported that there were no short-term estrogen-like effects (including no hormonal changes or increases in uterus-wall thickness after 24 weeks of treatment). It is unclear whether dong quai is safe in individuals with hormone-sensitive conditions such as breast cancer, uterine cancer, ovarian cancer, or endometriosis. It is not known if dong quai possesses the beneficial effects that estrogen is believed to have on bone mass, or the potential harmful effects such as increased risk of stroke or hormone-sensitive cancers.
- Increased sun sensitivity with a risk of severe skin reactions (photosensitivity) may occur because of certain chemicals in dong quai (i.e., furocoumarins, psoralen, and bergapten). Prolonged exposure to sunlight or ultraviolet light should be avoided in people who are using dong quai. It has been reported that steam-distilled oils of the root and seed may not possess these phototoxic chemicals.
- Safrole, a volatile oil in dong quai, may be carcinogenic (cancer-causing). Long-term use should therefore be avoided, and suntan lotions that contain dong quai often limit the amount of dong quai to less than 1%.
- Dong quai has traditionally been associated with gastrointestinal symptoms (particularly with prolonged use), including laxative effects/diarrhea, upset stomach,

nausea, vomiting, loss of appetite, burping, and bloating. Published literature is limited in this area.

- Dong quai preparations may contain high levels of sucrose and should be used cautiously by patients with diabetes or glucose intolerance.
- Various other side effects have rarely been reported with dong quai taken alone or in combination with other herbs, including abnormal heart rhythms, blood pressure abnormalities, fever, gynecomastia (increased male breast size), headache, hot flashes, insomnia, irritability, kidney problems (nephrosis), lightheadedness/dizziness, reduced menstrual flow, sedation/drowsiness, skin rash, sweating, weakness, wheezing/asthma, and worsening premenstrual symptoms. However, side effects have not been evaluated in well-designed studies.
- The safety of dong quai injected into the skin, muscles, or veins is unknown, and this method of administration should be avoided. In one study, dogs stopped breathing after essential oil of dong quai was injected under their skin.

Pregnancy and Breastfeeding

- Dong quai is not recommended during pregnancy because of possible hormonal and anticoagulant/anti-platelet properties. Results of studies in animals of the effects of dong quai on the uterus were conflicting, with reports of both stimulation and relaxation. There is a published report of miscarriage in a woman taking dong quai, although it is not clear whether dong quai was the cause. Dong quai is traditionally viewed as increasing the risk of abortion. Women who are breastfeeding should avoid the use of dong quai because there is insufficient evidence regarding its safety.

INTERACTIONS

Most herbs and supplements have not been thoroughly tested for interactions with other herbs, supplements, drugs, or foods. The interactions listed here are based on reports in scientific publications, laboratory experiments, or traditional use. It is important to always read product labels. People who have a medical condition, or are taking other drugs, herbs, or supplements, should consult a qualified healthcare provider before starting a new therapy.

Interactions with Drugs

- Dong quai when taken alone may increase the risk of bleeding because of its anticoagulant and antiplatelet effects and may increase the risk of bleeding when taken with drugs that increase the risk of bleeding. Examples are anticoagulants (blood thinners) such as warfarin (Coumadin) and heparin, antiplatelet drugs such as clopidogrel (Plavix), aspirin, and nonsteroidal anti-inflammatory drugs such as ibuprofen (Motrin, Advil) and naproxen (Naprosyn, Aleve). In one review, it was reported that the effects of warfarin (Coumadin) were increased in a woman taking 565 mg of dong quai one to two times daily, as measured by 2.5-fold increases in values of blood tests for prothrombin time (PT) and international normalized ratio (INR).
- It remains unclear whether dong quai has the same effects on the body as estrogens, blocks the activity of estrogens, or has no significant hormonal effects. It has not been shown whether taking dong quai increases or decreases the effects of oral contraceptives, of hormone replacement therapies (such as Premarin) that contain estrogen, or of the anti-tumor properties of selective estrogen receptor modulators (SERMs) such as tamoxifen.

- Chemicals in dong quai may cause increased sun sensitivity, with a risk of severe skin reactions (photosensitivity). Dong quai should be avoided in people who are taking other drugs that cause photosensitivity, such as tretinoin (Retin-A, Renova), and some types of antidepressants, cancer drugs, antibiotics, and antipsychotic medications. People who are considering the use of dong quai and who are taking other medications should always read the package insert and consult their healthcare provider and pharmacist about possible interactions.
- Based on laboratory research, dong quai may increase the effects of drugs that affect heart rhythms, Examples of such drugs are beta-blockers such as metoprolol (Lopressor, Toprol), calcium channel blockers such as nifedipine (Procardia), and digoxin. Studies in animals and one report in humans noted reduced blood pressure after administration of dong quai; dong quai should be used cautiously in individuals taking blood pressure–lowering medications.

Interactions with Herbs and Dietary Supplements

- In theory, because of their anticoagulant and antiplatelet effects, components of dong quai may increase the risk of bleeding when taken with herbs and supplements that may increase the risk of bleeding. Multiple cases of bleeding have been reported with the use of *Ginkgo biloba*, and fewer cases with garlic and saw palmetto. Numerous other agents may theoretically increase the risk of bleeding, although this has not been proven in most cases. Examples are alfalfa, American ginseng, angelica, anise, *Arnica montana*, asafetida, aspen bark, bilberry, birch, black cohosh, bladderwrack, bogbean, boldo, borage seed oil, bromelain, capsicum, cat's claw, celery, chamomile, chaparral, clove, coleus, cordyceps, danshen, devil's claw, eicosapentaenoic acid (EPA), evening primrose oil, fenugreek, feverfew, fish oil, flaxseed/flax powder (not a concern with flaxseed oil), ginger, grapefruit juice, grape seed, green tea, guggul, gymnestra, horse chestnut, horseradish, licorice root, lovage root, male fern, meadowsweet, nordihydroguaiaretic acid (NDGA), onion, *Panax ginseng*, papain, parsley, passion flower, poplar, prickly ash, propolis, quassia, red clover, reishi, rue, Siberian ginseng, sweet birch, sweet clover, turmeric, vitamin E, white willow, wild carrot, wild lettuce, willow, wintergreen, and yucca.
- It is unclear whether dong quai has the same effects on the body as estrogens, blocks the activity of estrogens, or has no significant hormonal effects. Dong quai may alter the effects of agents that may have estrogen-like properties, such as alfalfa, black cohosh, bloodroot, burdock, hops, kudzu, licorice, pomegranate, red clover, soy, thyme, white horehound, and yucca.
- Chemicals in dong quai may cause increased sun sensitivity, with a risk of severe skin reactions (photosensitivity). Dong quai should not be taken with products containing *Hypericum perforatum* (St. John's wort) or capsaicin, which are also reported to cause photosensitivity.

Selected References

Natural Standard developed the preceding evidence-based information based on a systematic review of more than 200 articles. For comprehensive information about alternative and complementary therapies on the professional level, go to www.naturalstandard.com. Selected references are listed here.

Abebe W. An overview of herbal supplement utilization with particular emphasis on possible interactions with dental drugs and oral manifestations. J Dent Hyg 2003;77(1):37-46

D

Bian X, Xu Y, Zhu L, et al. Prevention of maternal-fetal blood group incompatibility with traditional Chinese herbal medicine. Chin Med J (Engl) 1998;111(7):585-587.

Burke BE, Olson RD, Cusack BJ. Randomized, controlled trial of phytoestrogen in the prophylactic treatment of menstrual migraine. Biomed Pharmacother 2002;56(6):283-288.

Bradley RR, Cunniff PJ, Pereira BJ, et al. Hematopoietic effect of Radix Angelicae sinensis in a hemodialysis patient. Am J Kidney Dis 1999;34(2):349-354.

Chou CT, Kuo SC. The anti-inflammatory and anti-hyperuricemic effects of Chinese herbal formula danggui-nian-tong-tang on acute gouty arthritis: a comparative study with indomethacin and allopurinol. Am J Chin Med 1995;23(3-4):261-271.

Dai L, Hou J, Cai H. [Using ligustrazini and angelica sinensis to treat the bleomycin-induced pulmonary fibrosis in rats.] Zhonghua Jie He He Hu Xi Za Zhi 1996;19(1):26-28.

Day C, Bailey CJ. Hypoglycaemic agents from traditional plant treatments for diabetes. Internat Industrial Biotech 1998;8(3):5-8.

Deng Y, Yang L. Effect of *Angelica sinensis* (Oliv.) on melanocytic proliferation, melanin synthesis and tyrosinase activity in vitro. Di Yi Jun Yi Da Xue Xue Bao 2003;23(3):239-241.

Ding H, Shi GG, Yu X, et al. Modulation of GdCl3 and *Angelica sinensis* polysaccharides on differentially expressed genes in liver of hepatic immunological injury mice by cDNA microarray. World J Gastroenterol 2003;9(5):1072-1076.

Fu YF. Treatment of 34 cases of infertility due to tubal occlusion with compound Danggui injection by irrigation. Jiangsu J Trad Chin Med 1988;9:15-16.

Fugh-Berman A. "Bust enhancing" herbal products. Obstet Gynecol 2003;101(6):1345-1349.

Goy SY, Loh KC. Gynaecomastia and the herbal tonic "Dong quai." Singapore Med J 2001; 42(3):115-116.

Hann SK, Park YK, Im S, et al. Angelica-induced phytophotodermatitis. Photodermatol Photoimmunol Photomed 1991;8(2):84-85.

Harada M, Suzuki M, Ozaki Y. Effect of Japanese Angelica root and peony root on uterine contraction in the rabbit in situ. J Pharmacobiodyn 1984;7(5):304-311.

He ZP, Wang DZ, Shi LY, et al. Treating amenorrhea in vital energy–deficient patients with angelica sinensis–astragalus membranaceus menstruation-regulating decoction. J Trad Chin Med 1986;6(3):187-190.

Hirata JD, Swiersz LM, Zell B, et al. Does Dong Quai have estrogenic effects in post-menopausal women? A double-blind, placebo-controlled trial. Fertil Steril 1997; 68(6): 981-986.

Huang LN, Yang BZ, Wang ZS. Treating 150 cases of postnatal lack of lactation by medicinal extract of "Zeng-Ru-Bao-Yu." Shan Xi J Trad Chin Med (Chiang-Su I Tsa Chih) 1997; 18(6):251.

Huang Z, Guo B, Liang K. [Effects of Radix Angelicae sinensis on systemic and portal hemodynamics in cirrhotics with portal hypertension.] Zhonghua Nei Ke Za Zhi 1996;35(1): 15-18.

Hudson TS, Standish L, Breed C, et al. Clinical and endocrinological effects of a menopausal botanical formula. J Naturopath Med 1998;7(1):73-77.

Huntley AL, Ernst E. A systematic review of herbal medicinal products for the treatment of menopausal symptoms. Menopause 2003;10(5):465-476.

Jujie T, Huaijun H. Effects of Radix Angelicae sinensis on hemorrheology in patients with acute ischemic stroke. J Trad Chin Med 1984;4:225-228.

Kiong HN. Gynaecomastia and the herbal tonic "Dong Quai." Singapore Med J 2001;42(6): 286-287.

Kotani N, Oyama T, Sakai I, et al. Analgesic effect of a herbal medicine for treatment of primary dysmenorrhea—a double-blind study. Am J Chin Med 1997;25(2):205-212.

Kronenberg F, Fugh-Berman A. Complementary and alternative medicine for menopausal symptoms: a review of randomized, controlled trials. Ann Intern Med 2002;137(10): 805-813.

Lee SK, Cho HK, Cho SH, et al. Occupational asthma and rhinitis caused by multiple herbal agents in a pharmacist. Ann Allergy Asthma Immunol 2001;86(4):469-474.

Li JC, Yang ZR, Zhang K. [The intervention effects of *Angelica sinensis, Salvia miltiorrhiza* and ligustrazine on peritoneal macrophages during peritoneal dialysis.] Zhongguo Zhong Xi Yi Jie He Za Zhi 2002;22(3):190-192.

Li KX, You ZL, Zhang H, et al. Clinical study on "Yi-Qi-Hua-Yu" method in treatment of pelvis congestion syndrome. J Hunan Coll Trad Chin Med 1997;17(2):11-13, 28.

Li YH. [Local injection of angelica sinensis solution for the treatment of sclerosis and atrophic lichen of the vulva.] Zhonghua Hu Li Za Zhi 1983;18(2):98-99.

Liao JZ, Chen JJ, Wu ZM, et al. Clinical and experimental studies of coronary heart disease treated with yi-qi huo-xue injection. J Tradit Chin Med 1989;9(3):193-198.

Lo AC, Chan K, Yeung JH, et al. Danggui (*Angelica sinensis*) affects the pharmacodynamics but not the pharmacokinetics of warfarin in rabbits. Eur J Drug Metab Pharmacokinet 1995;20(1):55-60.

Lu MC. Danggui shaoyao can improve colchichine-induced learning acquisition impairment in rats. Acta Pharmacol Sin 2001;22(12):1149-1153.

Mei QB, Tao JY, Cui B. Advances in the pharmacological studies of radix Angelica sinensis (Oliv) Diels (Chinese Danggui). Chin Med J (Engl) 1991;104(9):776-781.

Nambiar S, Schwartz RH, Constantino A. Hypertension in mother and baby linked to ingestion of Chinese herbal medicine. West J Med 1999;171(3):152.

Oerter Klein K, Janfaza M, Wong JA, et al. Estrogen bioactivity in fo-ti and other herbs used for their estrogen-like effects as determined by a recombinant cell bioassay J Clin Endocrinol Metab 2003;88(9):4077-4079.

Ozaki Y, Ma JP. Inhibitory effects of tetramethylpyrazine and ferulic acid on spontaneous movement of rat uterus in situ. Chem Pharm Bull (Tokyo) 1990;38(6):1620-1623.

Page RL, Lawrence JD. Potentiation of warfarin by Dong quai. Pharmacotherapy 1999;19(7): 870-876.

Pan SQ, Zhang ZD, Zhang SX, et al. Clinical observation on 121 cases of primary thrombocytopenic purpura treated by SHEN-XUE-LING powder. Hunan J Chin Trad Med 1997; 13(4):3-4.

Seibel MM. Treating hot flushes without hormone replacement therapy. J Fam Pract 2003; 52(4):291-296.

Sha H, Chou Y. The modified Dan-Guei-Nein-Tong-Tang to treat gouty arthritis with tophi. J Trad Chinese Med 1987;2:60.

Shang P, Qian AR, Yang TH, et al. Experimental study of anti-tumor effects of polysaccharides from *Angelica sinensis.* World J Gastroenterol 2003;9(9):1963-1967

Shimuzu M, Matsuzawa T, Suzuki S, et al. Evaluation of Angelicae radix (Touki) by the inhibitory effect on platelet aggregation. Chem Pharm Bull 1991;39(8):2046-2048.

Sun SW, Wang JF. [Efficacy of danggui funing pill in treating 162 cases of abdominal pain.] Zhongguo Zhong Xi Yi Jie He Za Zhi 1992;12(9):531-532, 517.

Tao JY, Ruan YP, Mei QB, et al. [Studies on the antiasthmatic action of ligustilide of dang-gui, Angelica sinensis (Oliv.) Diels.] Yao Xue Xue Bao 1984;19(8):561-565.

Tu JJ. Effects of radix Angelicae sinensis on hemorrheology in patients with acute ischemic stroke. J Tradit Chin Med 1984;4(3):225-228.

Usuki S. Effects of herbal components of Tokishakuyakusan on progesterone secretion by corpus luteum in vitro. Am J Chin Med 1991;19(1):57-60.

Wang CH, Zhang ZH, Wang Q. Therapeutic effect on 106 acute urticaria patients with the added ingredient of radix angelicae sinesis. Journal Shanxi Coll Trad Chin Med 1997; 20(3):25.

Wang X, Wei L, Ouyang JP, et al. Effects of an angelica extract on human erythrocyte aggregation, deformation and osmotic fragility. Clin Hemorheol Microcirc 2001;24(3): 201-205.

Wang Y, Zhu B. [The effect of angelica polysaccharide on proliferation and differentiation of hematopoietic progenitor cell.] Zhonghua Yi Xue Za Zhi 1996;76(5):363-366.

Wang ZH, Wang XP, Ma L. 103 cases of neonatal hemolytic disease due to ABO blood group incompatibility prevented and treated by Huo Xue Xiao Yu decoction. Forum Trad Chin Med 1997;12(2):26.

Wilasrusmee C, Siddiqui J, Bruch D, et al. In vitro immunomodulatory effects of herbal products. Am Surg. 2002;68(10):860-864.

Wilasrusmee C, Kittur S, Siddiqui J, et al. In vitro immunomodulatory effects of ten commonly used herbs on murine lymphocytes. J Altern Complement Med 2002;8(4):467-475.

Wu Y, Zhu B. [Effect of danggui buxue decoction on proliferation and expression of intercellular adhesion molecule-1 in human umbilical vein endothelial cells.] Hua Xi Yi Ke Da Xue Xue Bao 2001;32(4):593-595.

Xu JY, Li BX, Cheng SY. [Short-term effects of *Angelica sinensis* and nifedipine on chronic obstructive pulmonary disease in patients with pulmonary hypertension.] Zhongguo Zhong Xi Yi Jie He Za Zhi 1992;12(12):716-718, 707.

Xuan GC, Feng QF, Xue FM. Clinical observation on treating 400 cases of cerebral infarction with traditional Chinese herb powder. Henan J Trad Chin Med Pharmacy 1997;12(4): 28-29.

Yan TY, Hou AC, Sun BT. [Injection of *Angelica sinensis* in treating infantile pneumonia and its experimental study in rabbits]. Zhong Xi Yi Jie He Za Zhi 1987;7(3):161-162, 133.

Yang Q, Populo SM, Zhang J, et al. Effect of *Angelica sinensis* on the proliferation of human bone cells. Clin Chim Acta 2002;324(1-2):89-97.

Ye YN, Koo MW, Li Y, et al. *Angelica sinensis* modulates migration and proliferation of gastric epithelial cells. Life Sci 2001;68(8):961-968.

Ye YN, Liu ES, Li Y, et al. Protective effect of polysaccharides-enriched fraction from *Angelica sinensis* on hepatic injury. Life Sci 2001;69(6):637-646.

Ye YN, Liu ES, Shin VY, et al. A mechanistic study of proliferation induced by *Angelica sinensis* in a normal gastric epithelial cell line. Biochem Pharmacol 2001;61(11):1439-1448.

Ye YN, So HL, Liu ES, et al. Effect of polysaccharides from *Angelica sinensis* on gastric ulcer healing. Life Sci 2003;72(8):925-932.

Yim TK, Wu WK, Pak WF, et al. Myocardial protection against ischaemia-reperfusion injury by a *Polygonum multiflorum* extract supplemented 'Dang-Gui decoction for enriching blood', a compound formulation, ex vivo. Phytother Res 2000;14(3):195-199.

Zheng L. [Short-term effect and the mechanism of radix Angelicae on pulmonary hypertension in chronic obstructive pulmonary disease. Zhonghua Jie He He Hu Xi Za Zhi 1992;15(2): 95-97, 127.

Zheng M, Wang YP. Experimental study on effect of Angelica polysaccharide in inhibitory proliferation and inducing differentiation of K562 cells. Zhongguo Zhong Xi Yi Jie He Za Zhi 2002;22(1):54-57.

Zhiping H, Dazeng W, Lingyi S, et al. Treating amenorrhea in vital energy-deficient patients with *Angelica sinensis–Astragalus membranaceus* menstruation-regulating decoction. J Trad Chin Med 2002;6(3):187-190.

Zschocke S, Liu J, Stuppner H, et al. Comparative study of roots of *Angelica sinensis* and related Umbelliferous drugs by thin layer chromatography, high-performance liquid chromatography, and liquid chromatography–mass spectrometry. Phytochem Anal 1998;9(6):283-290.

D

Echinacea

(*E. angustifolia* DC, *E. pallida, E. purpurea*)

RELATED TERMS

- American coneflower, echinacin, Echinaforce, Echinaguard, black Sampson, black Susan, cock-up-hat, combflower, coneflower, hedgehog, igelkopf, Indian head, Kansas snake root, kegelblume, narrow-leaved purple coneflower, purple coneflower, red sunflower, rudbeckia, scurvy root, snakeroot, solhat, sun hat.

BACKGROUND

- Echinacea species are perennials that belong to the Aster family and that originated in eastern North America. Traditionally used for a range of infections and malignancies, the roots and herb (above-ground parts) of echinacea species have attracted recent scientific interest because of their purported "immunostimulant" properties. Oral preparations are popular in Europe and the United States for prevention and treatment of upper respiratory tract infections (URIs), and *Echinacea purpurea* herb is believed to be the most potent echinacea species used for this indication. In the United States, sales of echinacea are believed to represent approximately 10% of the dietary supplement market.
- In studies of echinacea as URI *treatment*, numerous trials in humans have reported that echinacea reduced the duration and severity of symptoms, particularly when therapy was initiated at the earliest onset of symptoms. However, the majority of trials, largely conducted in Europe, have been small or methodologically flawed. Although highly suggestive, the evidence cannot be considered definitive in favor of this use. Lack of benefit in children ages 2 to 11 has been reported. In a trial in the United states, negative results were reported on the use of echinacea in adults; however, this study used a whole-plant echinacea preparation containing both *E. purpurea* and *E. angustifolia*. Additional research is merited in this area.
- For URI *prevention* (prophylaxis), daily ingestion of echinacea was not shown to be effective in trials in humans.
- Preliminary studies of oral echinacea for genital herpes and radiation-associated toxicity were inconclusive. Topical *E. purpurea* juice has been suggested for skin and oral wound healing, and oral/injectable echinacea for vaginal *Candida albicans* infections, but evidence is lacking in these areas.
- The German Commission E discourages the use of echinacea in patients with autoimmune diseases, but this warning is based on theoretical considerations rather than human data.

USES BASED ON SCIENTIFIC EVIDENCE	Grade*
Treatment of upper respiratory tract infections Multiple studies suggest that taking echinacea by mouth when cold symptoms begin may reduce the length and severity of symptoms. However, additional studies are needed before a strong recommendation can be made.	**B**

Continued

Cancer There is no clear human evidence of the effects of echinacea on any type of cancer.	**C**
Immune system stimulation Echinacea has been studied alone and in combination preparations for immune system stimulation (including in patients receiving cancer chemotherapy). It remains unclear if there are clinically significant benefits. Additional studies are needed in this area before conclusions can be drawn regarding safety or effectiveness.	**C**
Low white blood cell counts after x-ray treatment Studies have reported mixed results, and it is not clear whether echinacea has benefits for this use.	**C**
Prevention of upper respiratory tract infections Preliminary studies in humans have found that echinacea is not helpful in preventing the common cold. However, this research was not well designed, and additional trials are needed in this area.	**C**
Genital herpes Initial studies in humans suggest that echinacea is not helpful in the treatment of genital herpes.	**D**

*Key to grades: *A:* Strong scientific evidence for this use; *B:* Good scientific evidence for this use; *C:* Unclear scientific evidence for this use; *D:* Fair scientific evidence against this use (it may not work); *F:* Strong scientific evidence against this use (it likely does not work). For a more detailed explanation of efficacy criteria, see "Natural Standard Evidence-Based Validated Grading Rationale" in the Introduction.

Uses Based on Tradition, Theory, or Limited Scientific Research

Abscesses, acne, attention deficit hyperactivity disorder (ADHD), bacterial infections, bee stings, boils, burns, cancer, cold sores, diphtheria, dizziness, eczema, gingivitis, hemorrhoids, HIV/AIDS, malaria, menopause, migraine headache, nasal congestion/runny nose, pain, psoriasis, rheumatism, skin ulcers, snake bites, stomach upset, syphilis, tonsillitis, typhoid, urinary tract infections, whooping cough (pertussis), wounds, yeast infections.

DOSING

The following doses are based on scientific research, publications, traditional use, or expert opinion. Many herbs and supplements have not been thoroughly tested, and their safety and effectiveness may not be proven. Brands may be made differently, with variable ingredients even within the same brand. The doses shown may not apply to all products. It is important to always read product labels and discuss doses with a qualified healthcare provider before therapy is started.

Standardization

- Standardization involves measuring the amounts of certain chemicals in products to try to make different preparations similar to each other. It is not always known if the chemicals being measured are the "active" ingredients. Some manufacturers standardize echinacea extracts to 4.0% to 5.0% echinacoside, whereas others standardize them to cichoric acid. Because the active ingredient(s) has not been identified, standardization may not predict effectiveness.

Adults (18 Years and Older)

- **Capsules (of powdered herb):** For treatment of upper respiratory tract infections, 500 to 1000 mg by mouth three times daily for 5 to 7 days has been used.
- **Expressed juice:** A dose of 6 to 9 ml by mouth daily, divided into two or three doses, for 5 to 7 days has been used.
- **Tincture:** 0.75 to 1.5 ml (1:5), gargled and then swallowed, has been taken two to five times daily for 5 to 7 days (daily dose equivalent to 900 mg dried echinacea root). Some herbalists prefer tinctures because of the theoretical immunostimulation of the tonsils that occurs with gargling.
- **Tea:** An infusion made from 2 teaspoons of coarsely powdered herb (4 g of echinacea), steeped in 1 cup of boiling water for 10 minutes and then strained, taken daily for 5 to 7 days has been used. There is early evidence that echinacea tea may reduce the symptoms of upper respiratory tract infection. A total of 5 to 6 cups (1.275 mg of dried herb and root per tea bag per cup or the equivalent) are taken on the first day, decreased by 1 cup each day for the next 5 days.
- **Topical (applied to the skin):** A semisolid preparation of 15% pressed herb (non-root) juice has been applied daily for wounds and skin ulcers.
- **Intravenous administration:** Preparations of echinacea to be injected into the veins are not available commercially. Severe reactions to injected echinacea have been reported, and echinacea injections are not recommended.

Children (Younger Than 18 Years)

- The dosing and safety of echinacea have not been studied thoroughly in children. Doses should be discussed with the child's healthcare provider before therapy is started. Some natural medicine practitioners recommend basing children's doses on their body weight. A child's dose is calculated by dividing the child's weight (in pounds) by 150 and then multiplying the number obtained by the recommended adult dose. However, there is no scientific support for or safety data concerning this formula.

SAFETY

The U.S. Food and Drug Administration does not strictly regulate herbs and supplements. There is no guarantee of the strength, purity, or safety of products, and effects may vary. It is important to always read product labels. People who have a medical condition, or are taking other drugs, herbs, or supplements, should consult a qualified healthcare provider before starting a new therapy. A healthcare provider should be contacted immediately about any side effects.

Allergies

- People with allergies to plants in the Asteraceae/Compositae family (ragweed, chrysanthemums, marigolds, daisies) are theoretically more likely to have allergic reactions to echinacea. Multiple cases of anaphylactic shock (severe allergic reactions) and allergic rash have been reported in people who had taken echinacea by mouth. Allergic reactions, including itching, rash, wheezing, facial swelling, and anaphylaxis may occur more commonly in people with asthma or other allergies. Echinacea intravenous injections have caused severe reactions and are not recommended.

Side Effects and Warnings

- Few side effects from echinacea have been reported when it has been used at recommended doses. Reported complaints include dizziness, drowsiness, headache, muscle aches, nausea, sore throat, stomach discomfort, rash (allergic, hives, or painful lumps called *erythema nodosum*). Rare cases of hepatitis (liver inflammation), irregular heart rate (atrial fibrillation), and kidney failure have been reported in people taking echinacea, although it is unclear whether these were due to echinacea itself. Injected echinacea may alter blood sugar levels and cause severe reactions and should be avoided.
- Some natural medicine experts discourage the use of echinacea by people with conditions affecting the immune system, such as HIV/AIDS, some types of cancer, multiple sclerosis, tuberculosis, and rheumatologic diseases (such as rheumatoid arthritis or lupus). However, there are no specific studies or reports in this area, and the risks of echinacea use with these conditions are unclear. Long-term use of echinacea may cause low white blood cell counts (leukopenia).

Pregnancy and Breastfeeding

- At this time, echinacea cannot be recommended during pregnancy or breastfeeding. Although early studies show no effect of echinacea on pregnancy, there is not enough research in this area to confirm this finding. Pregnant women should avoid tinctures because of their high alcohol content (15% to 90%).

INTERACTIONS

Most herbs and supplements have not been thoroughly tested for interactions with other herbs, supplements, drugs, or foods. The interactions listed here are based on reports in scientific publications, laboratory experiments, or traditional use. It is important to always read product labels. People who have a medical condition, or are taking other drugs, herbs, or supplements, should consult a qualified healthcare provider before starting a new therapy.

Interactions with Drugs

- Natural medicine practitioners sometimes caution that echinacea may lead to liver inflammation. There is no clear information from laboratory or human studies in this area. Nonetheless, caution should be used when combining echinacea taken by mouth with other medications that may harm the liver. Examples of such agents are acetaminophen (Tylenol), amiodarone, anabolic steroids, antifungal medications taken by mouth (such as ketoconazole), and methotrexate.
- In theory, echinacea's ability to stimulate the immune system may interfere with drugs that are taken to suppress the immune system (including azathioprine, cyclosporine, and steroids such as prednisone). No clear human studies are available.
- In one vague report, a person taking the antibiotic amoxicillin and an unspecified echinacea preparation developed muscle damage, shock, and death.
- Early research data suggest that the use of echinacea with econazole nitrate cream (Spectazole) on the skin may lower the frequency of vaginal yeast infections.

- *Note*: Many tinctures contain high levels of alcohol and may cause nausea or vomiting when taken with metronidazole (Flagyl) or disulfiram (Antabuse).

Interactions with Herbs and Dietary Supplements

- Natural medicine practitioners sometimes caution that echinacea may lead to liver inflammation. Although evidence from laboratory studies and research in humans is inconclusive in this area, in theory echinacea may add to liver toxicity caused by other agents. Herbs and supplements that have been proposed to cause possible liver damage include ackee, bee pollen, birch oil, blessed thistle, borage, bush tea, butterbur, chaparral, coltsfoot, comfrey, DHEA, *Echinacea purpurea*, *Echium* spp., germander, *Heliotropium* spp., horse chestnut (injections), jin-bu-huan (*Lycopodium serratum*), kava, lobelia, mate, niacin (vitamin B_3), niacinamide, Paraguay tea, periwinkle, *Plantago lanceolata*, pride of Madeira, rue, sassafras, scullcap, *Senecio* spp./groundsel, tansy ragwort, L-tetrahydropalmatine (L-THP), turmeric/curcumin, tu-san-chi (gynura segetum), uva ursi, and valerian.
- Echinacea is sometimes used in combination products that are believed to stimulate the immune system. For example, Esberitox (PhytoPharmica, Germany) contains *Echinacea purpurea*, *Echinacea pallida*, wild indigo root (*Baptisia tinctoria*), and thuja (white cedar). Echinacea may be combined with goldenseal and other herbs in some cold relief preparations. No high-quality studies in humans have shown added benefits or interactions of these combinations.

Interactions with Foods

- There are no available published reports of interactions with food.

Selected References

Natural Standard developed the preceding evidence-based information based on a systematic review of more than 500 scientific articles. For comprehensive information about alternative and complementary therapies on the professional level, go to www.naturalstandard.com. Selected references are listed here.

Barak V, Birkenfeld S, Halperin T, et al. The effect of herbal remedies on the production of human inflammatory and anti-inflammatory cytokines. Isr Med Assoc J 2002;4(Suppl 11): 919-922. Comment in: Isr Med Assoc J 2002;4(Suppl 11):944-946.

Barrett B. Medicinal properties of Echinacea: a critical review. Phytomedicine 2003;10(1): 66-86.

Barrett BP, Brown RL, Locken K, et al. Treatment of the common cold with unrefined echinacea. A randomized, double-blind, placebo-controlled trial. Ann Intern Med 2002; 137(12):939-946. Comment in: Ann Intern Med. 2002;137(12):1001-1002. Thorax 2003; 58(3):230. Summary for patients in: Ann Intern Med. 2002 Dec 17;137(12):I18.

Barrett B, Vohmann M, Calabrese C. Echinacea for upper respiratory tract infection. J Fam Pract 1999; 48(8):628-635.

Bielory L. Adverse reactions to complementary and alternative medicine: ragweed's cousin, the coneflower (echinacea), is "a problem more than a sneeze." Ann Allergy Asthma Immunol. 2002;88(1):7-9. Comment in: Ann Allergy Asthma Immunol 2002;88(1):42-51.

Binns SE, Hudson J, Merali S, Arnason JT. Antiviral activity of characterized extracts from echinacea spp. (Heliantheae: Asteraceae) against herpes simplex virus (HSV-I). Planta Med 2002;68(9):780-783.

Brinkeborn RM, Shah DV, Degenring FH. Echinaforce and other Echinacea fresh plant preparations in the treatment of the common cold: a randomized, placebo controlled, double-blind clinical trial. Phytomed 1999;6(1):1-6.

Cala S, Crismon ML, Baumgartner J. A survey of herbal use in children with attention-deficit-hyperactivity disorder or depression. Pharmacotherapy 2003;23(2):222-230.

Chua D. Chronic use of echinacea should be discouraged. Am Fam Physician. 2003;68(4):617; author reply, 617. Comment in: Am Fam Physician 2003;67(1):77-80.

Del Mar CB, Glasziou P; BMJ Publishing Group. Upper respiratory tract infection. Am Fam Physician 2002;66(11):2143-2144.

Dergal JM, Gold JL, Laxer DA, et al. Potential interactions between herbal medicines and conventional drug therapies used by older adults attending a memory clinic. Drugs Aging 2002;19(11):879-886.

Dorn M, Knick E, Lewith G. Placebo-controlled, double blind study of *Echinaceae pallidae* radix in upper respiratory tract infections.Complement Ther Med 1997;5:40-42.

Gaby AR. Comments on the common cold. Lancet 2003;361(9359):782; author reply, 782. Comment in: Lancet 2003;361(9351):51-59.

Gallo M, Sarkar M, Au W, Pietrzak K, et al. Pregnancy outcome following gestational exposure to echinacea: a prospective controlled study. Arch Intern Med 2000;160(20):3141-3143.

Giles JT, Palat CT, III, Chien SH, et al. Evaluation of echinacea for treatment of the common cold. Pharmacother 2000;20(6):690-697.

Grimm W, Muller HH. A randomized controlled trial of the effect of fluid extract of *Echinacea purpurea* on the incidence and severity of colds and respiratory infections. Am J Med 1999;106(2):138-143.

Henneicke-von Zepelin H, Hentschel C, et al. Efficacy and safety of a fixed combination phytomedicine in the treatment of the common cold (acute viral respiratory tract infection): results of a randomised, double blind, placebo controlled, multicentre study. Curr Med Res Opin 1999;15(3):214-227.

Hoheisel O, Sandberg M, Bertram S, et al. Echinagard treatment shortens the course of the common cold: a double blind, placebo controlled clinical trial. Eur J Clin Res 1997; 9:261-269.

Jaber R. Respiratory and allergic diseases: from upper respiratory tract infections to asthma. Prim Care 2002;29(2):231-261.

Kemp DE, Franco KN. Possible leukopenia associated with long-term use of echinacea. J Am Board Fam Pract 2002;15(5):417-419.

Kim LS, Waters RF, Burkholder PM. Immunological activity of larch arabinogalactan and Echinacea: a preliminary, randomized, double-blind, placebo-controlled trial. Altern Med Rev 2002;7(2):138-449.

Kligler B. Echinacea. Am Fam Physician. 2003 Jan 1;67(1):77-80. Comment in: Am Fam Physician. 2003 Aug 15;68(4):617; author reply, 617. Am Fam Physician. 2003;67(1):36, 38. Am Fam Physician 2003;67(1):83.

Lindenmuth GF, Lindenmuth EB. The efficacy of echinacea compound herbal tea preparation on the severity and duration of upper respiratory and flu symptoms: a randomized, double-blind placebo-controlled study. J Altern Complement Med 2000;6(4):327-334.

Mahady GB, Parrot J, Lee C, Yun GS, Dan A. Botanical dietary supplement use in peri- and postmenopausal women. Menopause 2003;10(1):65-72.

Melchart D, Clemm C, Weber B, et al. Polysaccharides isolated from *Echinacea purpurea* herba cell cultures to counteract undesired effects of chemotherapy—a pilot study. Phytother Res 2002;16(2):138-142.

Melchart D, Linde K, Fischer P, et al. Echinacea for preventing and treating the common cold. Cochrane Database Syst Rev 2000;(2):CD000530.

Melchart D, Walther E, Linde K, et al. Echinacea root extracts for the prevention of upper respiratory tract infections: a double-blind, placebo-controlled randomized trial. Arch Fam Med 1998;7(6):541-545.

Mullins R. Allergic reactions to echinacea. J Allergy Clin Immunol 2000;105(1 part 2): s268-s269.

Mullins RJ, Heddle R. Adverse reactions associated with echinacea: the Australian experience. Ann Allergy Asthma Immunol. 2002 Jan;88(1):42-51. Comment in: Ann Allergy Asthma Immunol 2002;88(1):7-9.

Paulsen E. Contact sensitization from Compositae-containing herbal remedies and cosmetics. Contact Dermatitis 2002;47(4):189-198.

Scaglione F, Lund B. Efficacy in the treatment of the common cold of a preparation containing an echinacea extract. Internat J Immunother 1995;11(4):163-166.

Soon SL, Crawford RI. Recurrent erythema nodosum associated with Echinacea herbal therapy. J Am Acad Dermatol 2001;44(2):298-299.
Turner RB, Riker DK, Gangemi JD. Ineffectiveness of echinacea for prevention of experimental rhinovirus colds. Antimicrob Agents Chemother 2000; 44(6):1708-1709.
Vonau B, Chard S, Mandalia S, et al. Does the extract of the plant *Echinacea purpurea* influence the clinical course of recurrent genital herpes? Int J STD AIDS 2001;12(3):154-158.

Elderberry and Elder Flower

(*Sambucas nigra* L.)

E

RELATED TERMS

- Almindelig hyld, baccae, baises de sureau, battree, black berried alder, black elder, black elderberry, boor tree, bountry, boure tree, Busine (Russian), Caprifoliaceae, devil's eye, elderberry, ellanwood, ellhorn, European alder, European elder, European elderberry, European elder flower, European elder fruit, frau holloe, German elder, holunderblüten, holunderbeeren, lady elder, old gal, old lady, pipe tree, rubini (elderberry extract), sambreo, sambuco, sambucus sieboldiana, sambucipunct sambucus, sambuci flos, sauco, shwarzer holunder, stinking elder, sureau noir, sweet elder, tree of doom, yakori bengestro.
- **Selected combination products that contain *Sambucus nigra*:** Sinupret (contains *Sambucus nigra* flowers, gentian root, verbena, cowslip flower, and sorrel), Sambucol Active Defense (contains elderberry extract, vitamin C, zinc, *Echinacea angustifolia*, *Echinacea purpurea*, and propolis).

BACKGROUND

- Several species of *Sambucus* produce elderberries. Most research and other publications refer to *Sambucus nigra*. Other species with similar chemical components include the American elder or common elder (*Sambucus canadensis*), antelope brush (*Sambucus tridentata*), blue elderberry (*Sambucus caerulea*), danewort (*Sambucus ebulus*), dwarf elder (*Sambucus ebulus*), red-fruited elder (*Sambucus pubens, Sambucus racemosa*), and *Sambucus formosana*. American elder (*S. canadensis*) and European elder (*S. nigra*) are often discussed simultaneously in the literature since they have many of the same uses and contain common constituents.
- European elder grows up to 30 feet tall, is native to Europe, but has been naturalized to the Americas. Historically, the flowers and leaves have been used for pain relief, swelling/inflammation, diuresis (increased urine flow), and as a diaphoretic or expectorant. The leaves have been used externally for sitz baths. The bark, when aged, has been used as a diuretic, laxative, and emetic (to induce vomiting). The berries have been used traditionally in food as flavoring and to make elderberry wine and pies.
- The flowers and berries (blue/black only) are used most often medicinally. They contain flavonoids, which possess a variety of biochemical and pharmacologic actions, including antioxidant and immunologic properties. Although hypothesized to be beneficial, there is no definitive evidence from well-conducted clinical trials in humans regarding the use of elder.
- The bark, leaves, seeds, and raw/unripe fruit contain the cyanogenic glycoside *sambunigrin*, which is potentially toxic.

USES BASED ON SCIENTIFIC EVIDENCE	Grade*
Bacterial sinusitis Elder has been observed to reduce excessive sinus mucus secretion in laboratory studies. There is only limited research specifically using elder to treat sinusitis in humans. Combination products containing elder and other herbs (such as Sinupret) have been reported to have beneficial effects when used with antibiotics to treat sinus infections, although the majority of this evidence is of poor quality and requires confirmation from better-quality research. Some studies suggest that herbal preparations containing elder result in less swelling of mucous membranes, better drainage, milder headache symptoms, and decreased nasal congestion. There is no evidence regarding the effects of elder when used alone for treatment of this condition.	C
Bronchitis There has been a small amount of research on the combination herbal product Sinupret in patients with bronchitis. This formula contains elder flowers (*Sambucus nigra*) as well as gentian root, verbena, cowslip flower, and sorrel. Although benefits have been suggested, because of design flaws in this research, no clear conclusion can be drawn either for Sinupret or elder in the management of bronchitis.	C
Influenza Some laboratory studies suggest that elder may possess anti-inflammatory and antiviral effects. One study reported that elderberry juice may improve flu-like symptoms, such as aches, cough, fever, fatigue, headache, and sore throat, in less than half the time that it normally takes to recover from the flu. However, this study was small with design flaws, and it should be noted that the berries must be cooked to prevent nausea or cyanide toxicity. It remains unclear whether there is any benefit from elder for this condition. Additional research is needed in this area before a firm conclusion can be reached. Elder should not be used in the place of other, more proven therapies, and patients are advised to discuss influenza vaccination with their primary healthcare provider.	C

*Key to grades: *A:* Strong scientific evidence for this use; *B:* Good scientific evidence for this use; *C:* Unclear scientific evidence for this use; *D:* Fair scientific evidence against this use (it may not work); *F:* Strong scientific evidence against this use (it likely does not work). For a more detailed explanation of efficacy criteria, see "Natural Standard Evidence-Based Validated Grading Rationale" in the Introduction.

Uses Based on Tradition, Theory, or Limited Scientific Evidence

Alzheimer's disease, anti-inflammatory, antioxidant, antispasmodic, asthma, astringent, blood vessel disorders, burns, cancer, chafing, circulatory stimulant, cold sores, colds, colic, cough suppressant, diabetes, diuresis (increased urine flow),

Continued

Uses Based on Tradition, Theory, or Limited Scientific Evidence *(cont'd)*

edema, epilepsy, fever, flavoring, gut disorders, hair dye, hay fever, headache, herpes, HIV, immunostimulant, increased sweating, insomnia, joint swelling, kidney disease, laryngitis, laxative, liver disease, measles, migraine, mosquito repellent, nerve pain, psoriasis, respiratory distress, sedative, stress reduction, syphilis, toothache, ulcerative colitis, vomiting, weight loss.

DOSING

The following doses are based on scientific research, publications, traditional use, or expert opinion. Many herbs and supplements have not been thoroughly tested, and their safety and effectiveness may not be proven. Brands may be made differently, with variable ingredients even within the same brand. The doses shown may not apply to all products. It is important to always read product labels and discuss doses with a qualified healthcare provider before therapy is started.

Standardization

Standardization involves measuring the amounts of certain chemicals in products to try to make different products similar to each other. It is not always known if the chemicals being measured are the "active" ingredients. There are no standard or well-studied doses of elder, and many different doses are used traditionally.

- **Berries:** The berries must be cooked to prevent nausea or cyanide toxicity.
- **Dried elder flower:** Dried elder flower may be standardized to contain at least 0.8% total flavonoids calculated as isoquercitin. The dried flower may contain at least 25% water-soluble extract.
- **Sambucol:** Sambucol Active Defense consists of a 38% standardized black elderberry extract plus vitamin C, zinc, *Echinacea angustifolia*, *Echinacea purpurea*, and propolis.
- **Sinupret:** The combination product Sinupret (formerly marketed in the United States as *Quantera Sinus Defense*), is an herbal mixture containing elder flowers as well as gentian root (radix gentianae luteae), verbena, cowslip flower (flos primulae veris cum calycibus), and sorrel (*Rumex acetosa*).
- **Rubini:** Rubini, an elderberry extract of bioflavonoids, is produced solely from elderberries, with no additives from animals, no colorings, and no preservatives. The product Rubini BioFlavonoides is produced with "organic certified fruits".

Adults (18 Years and Older)

- **Tea:** An infusion made from 3 to 5 g of dried elder flowers steeped in 1 cup of boiling water for 10 to 15 minutes and taken by mouth three times daily has been used. Be aware of possible toxicity.
- **Sinupret tablets:** For bacterial sinusitis, a dose of 2 tablets of Sinupret taken by mouth three times daily with antibiotics has been used. Sinupret contains elder and several other herbs.
- **Extract:** For treating influenza or flu-like symptoms, a dose of 4 tablespoons of elderberry extract taken daily by mouth for 3 days has been used.
- **Topical (on the skin):** A cream has been prepared by mixing several handfuls of fresh elder flowers in liquefied petroleum jelly. After simmering this mixture for 40 minutes, it is filtered and allowed to solidify. This has been applied to the hands at bedtime.

Children (Younger Than 18 Years)

- For influenza or flu-like symptoms, a dose of 1 teaspoon of elderberry juice containing extract syrup taken twice daily has been suggested. However, there is not enough scientific information available to recommend the safe use of elder in children. Toxicity has been reported, and caution is recommended.

SAFETY

The U.S. Food and Drug Administration does not strictly regulate herbs and supplements. There is no guarantee of the strength, purity, or safety of products, and effects may vary. It is important to always read product labels. People who have a medical condition, or are taking other drugs, herbs, or supplements, should consult a qualified healthcare provider before starting a new therapy. A healthcare provider should be contacted immediately about any side effects.

Allergies

- Elder should be avoided in people with known allergy to plants in the Caprifoliaceae (honeysuckle) family. There are some reports of allergies in children playing with toys made from fresh elder stems.

Side Effects and Warnings

- Elderberry products should be used under the direction of a qualified healthcare provider because of the possible risk of cyanide toxicity, especially from elder bark, root, and leaves.
- There are reports of abdominal cramps, diarrhea, gastrointestinal distress, vomiting, and weakness after drinking elderberry juice made from crushed leaves, stems and uncooked elderberries
- Allergies are possible from fresh elder stems and may include rash, skin irritation, and difficulty in breathing.
- In theory, high doses or long-term use of elder flowers may have diuretic (increasing urine flow) effects. People taking diuretics or drugs that interact with diuretics should use caution when taking products containing elder.
- *Note:* Elderberries must be cooked to prevent nausea or cyanide toxicity.

Pregnancy and Breastfeeding

- Elder cannot be recommended during pregnancy because of the theoretical risk of birth defects and spontaneous abortion. Its use is not advised in women who are breastfeeding because of the lack of sufficient scientific data about its safety.

INTERACTIONS

Most herbs and supplements have not been thoroughly tested for interactions with other herbs, supplements, drugs, or foods. The interactions listed here are based on reports in scientific publications, laboratory experiments, or traditional use. It is important to always read product labels. People who have a medical condition, or are taking other drugs, herbs, or supplements, should consult a qualified healthcare provider before starting a new therapy.

Interactions with Drugs

- Elder may possess diuretic (increasing urine flow) effects and should be used cautiously with drugs that increase urination. Elder may possess laxative effects and should be used cautiously with other laxatives.

- Based on laboratory studies, elder may lower blood sugar levels. Caution is advised in people who are using medications that may also lower blood sugar levels. Persons who are taking drugs for diabetes by mouth or insulin should be monitored by a qualified healthcare provider. Medication adjustments may be necessary.
- The flavonoid quercitin, which is present in elder, has been reported to inhibit xanthine oxidase and may affect caffeine and theophylline levels. People who are using theophylline should consult their healthcare provider before using elder.
- Animal studies suggest that elder may increase the effects and possible side effects of some cancer chemotherapies.
- Based on preliminary research, increased benefits may result when elder is used in combination with antibiotics and decongestants such as oxymetazoline (Afrin). Studies in animals suggest that elder flowers may possess anti-inflammatory properties and may add to the effects of some drugs that also decrease inflammation.

Interactions with Herbs and Dietary Supplements

- Elder may possess diuretic (increasing urine flow) effects, and should be used cautiously with other herbs or supplements that may increase urination, such as artichoke, celery, corn silk, couchgrass, dandelion, horsetail, juniper berry, kava, shepherd's purse, uva ursi, and yarrow.
- Elder may possess laxative effects, and should be used cautiously with other herbs or supplements that may have laxative effects, such as alder buckthorn, aloe dried leaf sap, black root, blue flag rhizome, butternut bark, dong quai, European buckthorn, eyebright, cascara bark, castor oil, chasteberry, colocynth fruit pulp, dandelion, gamboges bark, horsetail, jalap root, manna bark, plantain leaf, podophyllum root, psyllium, rhubarb, senna, wild cucumber fruit, and yellow dock root.
- Based on laboratory studies, elder may lower blood sugar levels. Caution is advised in people who are using other herbs or supplements that may lower blood sugar such as *Aloe vera*, American ginseng, bilberry, bitter melon, burdock, fenugreek, fish oil, gymnema, horse chestnut seed extract (HCSE), maitake mushroom, marshmallow, milk thistle, *Panax ginseng*, rosemary, shark cartilage, Siberian ginseng, stinging nettle and, white horehound. Blood glucose levels may require monitoring, and doses may need adjustment.
- Increased effects may be seen when elder is used in combination with other antioxidants, such as vitamin C, or flavonoids such as quercetin.

Selected References

Natural Standard developed the preceding evidence-based information based on a systematic review of more than 75 articles. For comprehensive information about alternative and complementary therapies on the professional level, go to www.naturalstandard.com. Selected references are listed here.

Dellagreca M, Fiorentino A, Monaco P, et al. Synthesis of degraded cyanogenic glycosides from *Sambucus nigra*. Nat Prod Res. 2003 Jun;17(3):177-181.

Ernst E, Marz RW, Sieder C. [Acute bronchitis: effectiveness of Sinupret. Comparative study with common expectorants in 3,187 patients.] Fortschr Med. 1997;115(11):52-53.

Gray AM, Abdel-Wahab YH, Flatt PR. The traditional plant treatment, *Sambucus nigra* (elder), exhibits insulin-like and insulin-releasing actions in vitro. J Nutr. 2000 Jan;130(1): 15-20.

Kunitz S, Melton RJ, Updyke T, et al. Poisoning from elderberry juice. MMWR Morb Mortal Wkly Rep1984;33(13):173-174.

Neubauer N, März RW. Placebo-controlled, randomized double-blind clinical trial with Sinupret sugar coated tablets on the basis of a therapy with antibiotics and decongestant nasal drops in acute sinusitis. Phytomed 1994;1:177-181.

Richstein A, Mann W. [Treatment of chronic sinusitis with Sinupret.] Ther Ggw 1980;119(9): 1055-1060.

Zakay-Rones Z, Varsano N, Zlotnik M, et al. Inhibition of several strains of influenza virus in vitro and reduction of symptoms by an elderberry extract (*Sambucus nigra* L.) during an outbreak of influenza B in Panama. J Altern Complement Med 1995;1(4):361-369.

Ephedra/Ma Huang

(*Ephedra sinica*)

E

RELATED TERMS

- Amsania, Brigham tea, budshur, cao ma huang, chewa, Chinese ephedra, Chinese joint fir, desert herb, *Ephedra altissima, Ephedra americana, Ephedra anti-syphilitica, Ephedra distacha* (*Ephedra distachya*), *Ephedra equisetina* (Mongolian ephedra), *Ephedra geradiana, Ephedra helvetica, Ephedra intermedia* (intermediate ephedra), *Ephedra major, Ephedra nevadensis, Ephedra shennungiana, Ephedra trifurca, Ephedra viridis, Ephedra vulgaris,* Ephedraceae, ephedrae herba, epitonin, European ephedra, herba ephedrae, horsetail, hum, huma, Indian joint fir, intermediate ephedra, joint fir, khama, mahoàng, máhuáng, mao, mao-kon, mahuuanggen, Mexican tea, môc tac ma hoàng, Mongolian ephedra, Mormon tea, mu-tsei-ma-huang, muzei mu huang, natural ecstasy, phok, popotillo, san-ma-huang, sea grape, shrubby, soma, song tuê ma hoàng, squaw tea, teamster's tea, trun aa hoàng, tsao-ma-huang, tutgantha, yellow astringent, yellow horse, zhong Ma huang.
- *Note:* There are approximately 40 species of ephedra.
- **Multi-ingredient preparations containing ephedra:** Acceleration, AllerClear, AllerPlus, Andro Heat, Better BodyEnergy for Life, Bio Trim, Biovital Plus, Bladderwrack-Dandelion Virtue, Breathe-Aid Formula, Breath Easy, Cordephrine XC, Diet Fuel, Dymetadrine Xtrem, EPH-833, Ephedra Plus, Thermogen, Guarana-Gotu Kola Virtue, Herba Fuel, Herbal Decongestant Expectorant Capsules, Herbalife–Thermojetics Original Green, Metabolife 356, Metabolift, Metaboloss, MetaboTRIM, Naturafed, Naturally Ripped, Naturatussin 1, Nettle-Reishi Virtue, Power Thin, ProLab Stoked, Pro-Ripped Ephedra, Respa-Herb, Respiratory Support Formula, Ripped Fuel, SinuCheck, SinuClear, SnoreStop, Thermadrene, Thermic Blast, Thermicore, Thermo Cuts, ThermoDiet, Ultra Diet Pep, Xenadrine RFA-1.

BACKGROUND

- On February 6, 2004 the U.S. Food and Drug Administration (FDA) issued a final rule prohibiting the sale of dietary supplements containing ephedrine alkaloids (ephedra) because such supplements present an unreasonable risk of illness or injury. The rule became effective 60 days from the date of publication.
- *Ephedra sinica*, a species of ephedra (ma huang), contains the alkaloids ephedrine and pseudoephedrine, which have been found to induce central nervous system (CNS) stimulation, bronchodilation, and vasoconstriction. In combination with caffeine, ephedrine appears to elicit weight loss (in trials of 1 to 12 months' duration). However, studies of ephedra or ephedrine monotherapy have been equivocal. The majority of trials of weight loss in humans have been small with methodological weaknesses, including large dropout rates due to adverse effects and incomplete reporting of blinding or randomization. Numerous trials have documented the efficacy of ephedrine in the management of asthmatic broncho-constriction and hypotension. However, commercial preparations of non-prescription

supplements containing ephedra have not been systematically studied for these indications.

- Major safety concerns have been associated with ephedra or ephedrine use, including arrhythmia, CNS excitation, hypertension, myocardial infarction, tachycardia, and stroke. In 1997, as the result of more than 800 reports of serious toxicity in this country (and many more worldwide), including at least 22 deaths in adolescents and young adults, the FDA adopted the following policy: Ephedra-containing products must (1) be labeled with all possible adverse effects, including death; (2) contain no more than 8 mg of ephedrine per dose; and (3) be used for no more than 7 days. The FDA also proposed a maximum daily dose of 24 mg, and a ban on ephedra-caffeine combination products (these proposed limits were subsequently withdrawn).
- In 2002, Samenuk et al. identified 926 cases of possible ephedra toxicity reported to the Adverse Reaction Monitoring System of the FDA between 1995 and 1997. In 37 patients, the use of ephedra was temporally related to stroke (16 patients), myocardial infarction (10), or sudden death (11). Autopsies performed in patients who experienced sudden death showed a normal heart in one, coronary atherosclerosis in three, and cardiomyopathies in three. In 36 of the 37 patients, use of ephedra was reported to be within the manufacturers' dosing guidelines.
- In 2003, a report was prepared by Shekelle and colleagues on behalf of the RAND Southern California Evidence-based Practice Center for the Agency for Healthcare Research and Quality, U.S. Department of Health and Human Services. This study reviewed available clinical trials, as well as more than 1500 adverse event reports to the FDA and adverse event reports to the manufacturer Metabolife. Although most prospective trials were not sufficiently large and most adverse event reports were not sufficiently detailed, the authors identified three deaths, two myocardial infarctions, two cerebrovascular accidents, one seizure, and three psychiatric cases that were considered to be "sentinel events" (i.e., strongly tied to ephedra use within 24 hours without other plausible explanations). In addition, 50 other possible sentinel events were identified.
- A 2003 analysis by Bent et al. in *Annals of Internal Medicine* found that products containing ephedra accounted for 64% of all adverse reactions to herbs in the United States, but represented only 0.82% of herbal product sales. The relative risk for an adverse reaction in a person using ephedra compared with other herbs was extremely high, ranging from 100 (95% CI, 83 to 140) for kava to 720 (95% CI, 520 to 1100) for *Ginkgo biloba*. It was concluded that ephedra use poses a greatly increased risk of adverse reactions compared with the use of other herbs. An analysis published in *Neurology* in 2003 also found increased risk of stroke associated with ephedra-containing products.
- Despite widely publicized safety concerns and the highly publicized death in 2003 of an American major league baseball pitcher thought to be related to use of ephedra, before the ban on ephedra, 14% of individuals using non-prescription weight-loss products in the U.S. continue to take ephedra or ephedrine-containing products.

USES BASED ON SCIENTIFIC EVIDENCE	Grade*
Weight loss Ephedra contains the chemical ephedrine, which appears to cause weight loss when used in combination with caffeine, based on the available scientific evidence. The results of research on ephedrine used alone without caffeine are unclear. The amount of ephedrine in commercially available products varies widely.	A
Bronchodilator (asthma) Ephedra contains the chemicals ephedrine and pseudoephedrine, which are bronchodilators (expand the airways to assist in easier breathing). It has been used and studied to treat asthma and chronic obstructive pulmonary disease in both children and adults. Other treatments such as beta-agonist inhalers (for example, albuterol) are more commonly recommended because of safety concerns with ephedra or ephedrine.	B
Allergic nasal symptoms (used as a nose wash) One study suggested that ephedrine nasal spray, a chemical in ephedra, may help treat symptoms of nasal allergies. Additional research is needed before a recommendation can be made.	C
Low blood pressure Chemicals in ephedra can stimulate the heart, increase heart rate, and raise blood pressure. Ephedrine, a component of ephedra, is sometimes used in hospitals to help control blood pressure. However, the effects of over-the-counter ephedra supplements taken by mouth have not been well described in this area.	C
Sexual arousal A small study reported that ephedra may increase sexual arousal in women. Further, well-designed research is needed to confirm these results.	C

*Key to grades: *A:* Strong scientific evidence for this use; *B:* Good scientific evidence for this use; *C:* Unclear scientific evidence for this use; *D:* Fair scientific evidence against this use (it may not work); *F:* Strong scientific evidence against this use (it likely does not work). For a more detailed explanation of efficacy criteria, see "Natural Standard Evidence-Based Validated Grading Rationale" in the Introduction.

Uses Based on Tradition, Theory, or Limited Scientific Evidence

Acute coryza (rhinitis), anaphylaxis (a severe allergic reaction), anti-inflammatory, appetite suppressant, athletic performance enhancement, bed-wetting, body-building, chills, colds, congenital myasthenic syndrome, cough, decongestant, depression, diuretic, dyspnea (shortness of breath), edema, energy enhancer, euphoria, fevers, flu, gonorrhea, gout, hay fever, hives, increased sweating, joint pain, kidney disease, lack of perspiration, metabolic enhancement, myasthenia gravis, narcolepsy, nasal congestion, nephritis, obesity, runny nose, shortness of breath, stimulation of energy, syphilis, stimulant, upper respiratory tract infections, urticaria (rash), uterine stimulant, water retention.

DOSING

The following doses are based on scientific research, publications, traditional use, or expert opinion. Many herbs and supplements have not been thoroughly tested, and their safety and effectiveness may not be proven. Brands may be made differently, with variable ingredients even within the same brand. The doses shown may not apply to all products. It is important to always read product labels and discuss doses with a qualified healthcare provider before therapy is started.

Standardization

- Standardization involves measuring the amounts of certain chemicals in products to try to make different preparations similar to each other. It is not always known if the chemicals being measured are the "active" ingredients.
- There is wide variability in the alkaloid content of different preparations of ephedra. A study in 1998 by Gurley and associates examined the pseudoephedrine and ephedrine content of nine commercially available nutritional supplements containing *Ephedra sinica*. Significant variations in content were found for pseudoephedrine, ranging from 0.52 to 9.46 mg, and for ephedrine, ranging from 1.08 to 13.54 mg per recommended dose. An earlier study by Liu and colleagues collected and evaluated 22 different ephedra products from herbal shops throughout Taiwan. A fourfold difference was found in the amounts of the various alkaloids, ranging from 0.536% to 2.308%. The average ephedra supplement content is 1% of the crude plant.
- Different ephedra species, yielding markedly different quantities of active alkaloids, are all sold as ma huang in China, making it difficult for consumers to find standardized products. *Ephedra sinica* plants grown in northern China often have a morphology and alkaloid content different from the same species grown in southern China.

Adults (18 Years and Older)

- *Note:* On February 6, 2004 the U.S. Food and Drug Administration (FDA) issued a final rule prohibiting the sale of dietary supplements containing ephedrine alkaloids (ephedra) because such supplements present an unreasonable risk of illness or injury. The rule became effective 60 days from the date of publication.
- **Controversy regarding dosing:** There is disagreement regarding the optimal form and dose of ephedra. Traditionally, herbalists have recommended a wide range of doses, which are typically higher than FDA recommendations. In the past, the FDA recommended a maximum of 8 mg up to every 6 hours (total daily dose of 24 mg) for up to 7 days. However, doses up to 25 mg of total ephedra alkaloids taken four times daily have been recommended by some experts, and doses in some studies have been as high as 50 to 100 mg of ephedra taken three times daily. Over-the-counter drugs containing ephedra generally contain warning labels advising adults not to take 12.5 to 25 mg every 4 to 6 hours and not to exceed 150 mg in 24 hours.
- **Weight loss:** In the past, the FDA has recommended a dose of not more than 8 mg every 6 hours for up to 7 days. However, doses used in some clinical trials were as high as 25 to 50 mg taken three times daily.

Children (Younger Than 18 Years)

- Ephedrine is not recommended in children because of the risk of toxicity and death. Purified ephedrine has been given in hospital settings to children older than

2 years of age in doses of 2 to 3 mg per kilogram of body weight, divided into 4 to 6 daily doses

SAFETY

The U.S. Food and Drug Administration does not strictly regulate herbs and supplements. There is no guarantee of the strength, purity, or safety of products, and effects may vary. It is important to always read product labels. People who have a medical condition, or are taking other drugs, herbs, or supplements, should consult a qualified healthcare provider before starting a new therapy. A healthcare provider should be contacted immediately about any side effects.

Allergies

- Persons with a known allergy to ephedra, ephedrine or pseudoephedrine (Sudafed) should avoid the use of products containing ephedra.

Side Effects and Warnings

- The FDA has collected thousands of reports of serious toxicity (including over 100 deaths). On December 30, 2003, U.S. federal officials announced plans to ban the sale of dietary supplements containing ephedra because of continued and growing health concerns. The FDA notified more than 60 companies that market ephedra products, and issued a consumer warning. On February 6, 2004 the U.S. Food and Drug Administration (FDA) issued a final rule prohibiting the sale of dietary supplements containing ephedrine alkaloids (ephedra) because such supplements present an unreasonable risk of illness or injury. The rule became effective 60 days from the date of publication.
- Some people may experience abdominal discomfort (constipation, diarrhea, loss of appetite, nausea and vomiting), anxiety, delirium, dizziness, dry mouth, fainting, headache, insomnia, or tremors. Ephedra may also cause euphoria, exaggerated reflexes, hallucinations, irritability, low potassium levels in the blood, muscle aches, muscle damage, Parkinson's disease–like symptoms, seizures, stroke, and weakness. Persons who have had strokes or transient ischemic attacks (TIAs; "mini-strokes"), tremors, or insomnia should avoid the use of ephedra. People with a history of psychiatric illness, especially if they were treated with monoamine oxidase inhibitors (MAOIs), should consult a qualified healthcare provider before taking supplements. Examples of MAOIs are isocarboxazid (Marplan), phenelzine (Nardil), and tranylcypromine (Parnate).
- Ephedra can cause breathing difficulties, cardiac arrest, chest tightness, fluid retention in the lungs, heart muscle damage, heart rhythm irregularity, high blood pressure, and inflammation of the heart. Ephedra should be used with extreme caution in persons with a history of heart disease, heart rate disorders, or high blood pressure. Other possible side effects include liver damage, kidney stones, difficulty passing urine or pain when urinating, increased urine production, and contractions of the uterus. These effects may limit the use of ephedra by people with kidney disease or enlarged prostate. Caution is advised in persons with thyroid gland disorders or glaucoma.
- In theory, ephedra may lower blood sugar levels. Caution is advised in patients with diabetes or hypoglycemia, and in those taking drugs, other herbs and supplements that affect blood sugar levels. Serum glucose levels may need to be monitored by a qualified healthcare provider, and medication adjustments may be necessary.

- When used for prolonged periods, even at recommended doses, ephedra may lead to anxiety, difficulty in sleeping, dry mouth, heart damage, high blood pressure, irregular heart rhythms, and weight loss.

Pregnancy and Breastfeeding

- Ephedra should not be used during pregnancy, because of risks to the mother and fetus. Ephedrine crosses the placenta, and has been found to increase fetal heart rate. Ephedra may induce uterine contractions.
- Ephedra should not be used by women who are breastfeeding, because of risks to the mother and nursing infant. Ephedrine crosses into breast milk and has been associated with irritability, crying, and insomnia in infants.

INTERACTIONS

Most herbs and supplements have not been thoroughly tested for interactions with other herbs, supplements, drugs, or foods. The interactions listed here are based on reports in scientific publications, laboratory experiments, or traditional use. It is important to always read product labels. People who have a medical condition, or are taking other drugs, herbs, or supplements, should consult a qualified healthcare provider before starting a new therapy.

Interactions with Drugs

- Many drugs can cause increased stimulation when used with ephedra or ephedrine. Examples are caffeine and theophylline. When combined with ephedra, these drugs may cause difficulty in sleeping, nervousness, and stomach upset. The combination of ephedrine and caffeine may be fatal. Many products contain both ephedrine and caffeine and should be used with caution, if at all.
- Bronchodilators used for asthma or the decongestant pseudoephedrine (Sudafed) may have increased bronchodilating effects when used with ephedra.
- If ephedra is taken with monoamine oxidase inhibitor (MOAI) antidepressants, such as isocarboxazid (Marplan), phenelzine (Nardil), and tranylcypromine (Parnate), severe side effects may develop, including dangerously high blood pressure, muscle damage, fever, and irregular heart rate. Other antidepressants and medications for psychiatric disorders (phenothiazines, tricyclics) may reduce the effects of ephedra and cause low blood pressure and rapid heartbeat.
- Because ephedra affects blood pressure and heart rate, it may alter the effectiveness of medications given to control blood pressure or heart rhythm, including alpha-blockers, angiotensin converting enzyme (ACE) inhibitors, beta-blockers, calcium-channel blockers, digoxin, and diuretics. The side effects of ephedra may be worsened by anesthetic drugs (cyclopropane, halothane, propofol), diuretics, ergot alkaloids (bromocriptine, dihydroergotamine, ergotamine), guanethidine, morphine, and oxytocin (Ptosin).
- *Note:* Use of ephedra products should be stopped 24 hours prior to surgery.
- Ephedra may lower blood sugar levels, although ephedra-caffeine combinations may increase them. Caution is advised in people who are using medications that may also lower blood sugar levels. Persons taking drugs for diabetes by mouth or insulin who are also taking ephedra products should be monitored closely by a qualified healthcare provider. Medication adjustments may be necessary.
- Ephedra may reduce the effects of steroids such as dexamethasone. Ephedra may increase serum levels of thyroid hormones and may alter the results of thyroid hormone treatments. Medications that alter the acidity of urine may reduce the effectiveness of ephedra.

- Effects of cholesterol-lowering medications may be altered by ephedra, although this has not been proven. In one study, Metabolife 356, a product containing ephedra and multiple other ingredients, was associated with heart rhythm abnormalities (arrhythmias, QT prolongation) and may therefore interact with other agents with similar effects, such as haloperidol (Haldol) and metoclopramide (Reglan).
- Phenylpropanolamine, which has been removed from the United States market, may lead to additive effects when taken with ephedra.

Interactions with Herbs and Dietary Supplements

- The stimulant effects of ephedra may be increased when combined with herbs and supplements that have stimulant properties or with supplements that contain caffeine, such as cola nut, guarana, and yerba mate. Commercially available products may contain combinations of ephedrine and caffeine or guarana. Ephedra may alter thyroid hormones and should be used cautiously with other herbs or supplements that affect thyroid hormones, such as bladderwrack (seaweed, kelp).
- Ephedra may decrease the effectiveness of herbs that contain cardiac glycosides. Examples of such drugs are adonis, balloon cotton, black hellebore root/melampode, black Indian hemp, bushman's poison, cactus grandifloris, convallaria, eyebright, figwort, foxglove/digitalis, frangipani, hedge mustard, hemp root/Canadian hemp root, king's crown, lily-of-the-valley, motherwort, oleander leaf, pheasant's eye plant, plantain leaf, pleurisy root, psyllium husks, redheaded cottonbush, rhubarb root, rubber vine, sea-mango, senna fruit, squill, strophanthus, uzara, wallflower, wintersweet, yellow dock root, and yellow oleander.
- Ephedra may raise blood pressure and may increase the blood pressure-raising effects of herbs such as American ginseng, arnica, bayberry, betel nut, blue cohosh, cayenne, cola, coltsfoot, ginger, licorice, *Polypodium vulgare*, and yerba mate. Similarly, ephedra may lessen the effects of blood pressure-lowering herbs such as aconite/monkshood, arnica, baneberry, betel nut, bilberry, black cohosh, bryony, calendula, California poppy, coleus, curcumin, eucalyptol, eucalyptus oil, evening primrose oil, flaxseed, garlic, ginger, ginkgo, goldenseal, green hellebore, hawthorn, Indian tobacco, jaborandi, mistletoe, night-blooming cereus, oleander, pasque flower, periwinkle, pleurisy root, shepherd's purse, Texas milkweed, turmeric, and wild cherry.
- Ephedra may lower blood sugar levels. Caution is advised in people who are also using other herbs or supplements that may lower blood sugar levels. Blood glucose levels may require monitoring, and doses may need adjustment. Examples include *Aloe vera*, American ginseng, bilberry, bitter melon, burdock, fenugreek, fish oil, gymnema, horse chestnut seed extract (HCSE), marshmallow, milk thistle, *Panax ginseng*, rosemary, Siberian ginseng, stinging nettle, and white horehound.
- Ephedra may increase the diuretic effects of herbs such as artichoke, celery, corn silk, couchgrass, dandelion, elder flower, horsetail, juniper berry, kava, shepherd's purse, uva ursi, and yarrow.
- Combining ephedra with herbs that have possible monoamine oxidase inhibitor (MAOI) antidepressant activity may cause severe side effects, including dangerously high blood pressure, muscle breakdown, fever, and irregular heartbeats. Other herbs and supplements with possible MAOI effects include California poppy, chromium, dihydroepiandrosterone (DHEA), DL-phenylalanine (DLPA), evening primrose oil, fenugreek, *Ginkgo biloba*, hops, 5-hydroxytryptophan (5-HTP), mace, *S*-adenosylmethionine (SAMe), sepia, St. John's wort, tyrosine, valerian, vitamin B_6, and yohimbe bark extract.

- Effects of cholesterol-lowering herbs and supplements may be altered by ephedra, although this has not been proven. One study of Metabolife 356, a product containing ephedra, showed that it may cause heart rhythm abnormalities (arrhythmias, QT prolongation) and may therefore interact with other agents with similar effects.

Interactions with Foods

- Caffeine-containing foods ingested in combination with ephedra may increase the risk of negative effects on the heart or the nervous system and may cause psychiatric changes. In several cases, the use of caffeine and ephedrine was reported to result in death.

Selected References

Natural Standard developed the preceding evidence-based information based on a systematic review of more than 225 scientific articles. For comprehensive information about alternative and complementary therapies on the professional level, go to www.naturalstandard.com. Selected references are listed here.

Abourashed EA, El Alfy AT, Khan IA, et al. Ephedra in perspective—a current review. Phytother Res 2003;17(7):703-712.

Anon. Working to get ephedra banned. Consum Rep 2003;68(2):6.

Anon. Summaries for patients. Ephedra is associated with more adverse effects than other herbs. Ann Intern Med 2003;138(6):I56.

Ashar BH, Miller RG, Getz KJ, et al. A critical evaluation of Internet marketing of products that contain ephedra. Mayo Clin Proc 2003;78(8):944-946.

Astrup A, Breum L, Toubro S, et al. The effect and safety of an ephedrine/caffeine compound compared to ephedrine, caffeine and placebo in obese subjects on an energy restricted diet. A double blind trial. Int J Obes Relat Metab Disord 1992;16(4):269-277.

Astrup A, Buemann B, Christensen NJ, et al. The effect of ephedrine/caffeine mixture on energy expenditure and body composition in obese women. Metabolism 1992;41(7): 686-688.

Backer R, Tautman D, Lowry S, et al. Fatal ephedrine intoxication. J Forensic Sci 1997;42(1): 157-159.

Bent S, Tiedt TN, Odden MC, et al. The relative safety of ephedra compared with other herbal products. Ann Intern Med 2003;138(6):468-471.

Boozer CN, Nasser JA, Heymsfield SB, et al. An herbal supplement containing Ma Huang-Guarana for weight loss: a randomized, double-blind trial. Int J Obes Relat Metab Disord 2001;25(3):316-324.

Boozer CN, Daly PA, Homel P, et al. Herbal ephedra/caffeine for weight loss: a 6-month randomized safety and efficacy trial. Int J Obes Relat Metab Disord 2002;26(5):593-604.

Borum ML. Fulminant exacerbation of autoimmune hepatitis after the use of ma huang. Am J Gastroenterol 2001;96(5):1654-1655.

Breum L, Pedersen JK, Ahlstrom F, et al. Comparison of an ephedrine/caffeine combination and dexfenfluramine in the treatment of obesity. A double-blind multi-centre trial in general practice. Int J Obes Relat Metab Disord 1994;18(2):99-103.

Bruno A, Nolte KB, Chapin J. Stroke associated with ephedrine use. Neurology 1993;43(7): 1313-1316.

Charatan F. Ephedra supplement may have contributed to sportsman's death. BMJ 2003; 326(7387):464.

Cockings JG, Brown M. Ephedrine abuse causing acute myocardial infarction. Med J Aust 1997; 167(4):199-200.

Daly PA, Krieger DR, Dulloo AG, et al. Ephedrine, caffeine and aspirin: safety and efficacy for treatment of human obesity. Int J Obes Relat Metab Disord 1993;17 Suppl 1:S73-S78.

Dickinson A. The relative safety of ephedra compared with other herbal products. Ann Intern Med 2003;139(5 Pt 1):385-387.

Fontanarosa PB, Rennie D, DeAngelis CD. The need for regulation of dietary supplements—lessons from ephedra. JAMA 2003;289(12):1568-1570.

Food & Drug Administration. Press Release, February 28, 2003: HHS Acts to Reduce Potential Risks of Dietary Supplements Containing Ephedra.

Gardner SF, Franks AM, Gurley BJ, et al. Effect of a multicomponent, ephedra-containing dietary supplement (Metabolife 356) on Holter monitoring and hemostatic parameters in healthy volunteers. Am J Cardiol 2003;91(12):1510-3, A9.

Guharoy R, Noviasky JA. Time to ban ephedra—now. Am J Health Syst Pharm 2003;60(15): 1580-1582.

Karch SB. Use of Ephedra-containing products and risk for hemorrhagic stroke. Neurology 2003;61(5):724-725.

Meadows M. Public health officials caution against ephedra use. Health officials caution consumers against using dietary supplements containing ephedra. The stimulant can have dangerous effects on the nervous system and heart. FDA Consum 2003;37(3):8-9.

Molnar D, Torok K, Erhardt E, et al. Safety and efficacy of treatment with an ephedrine/caffeine mixture. The first double-blind placebo-controlled pilot study in adolescents. Int J Obes Relat Metab Disord 2000;24(12):1573-1578.

Morgenstern LB, Viscoli CM, Kernan WN, et al. Use of Ephedra-containing products and risk for hemorrhagic stroke. Neurology 2003;60(1):132-135.

Oh RC, Henning JS. Exertional heatstroke in an infantry soldier taking ephedra-containing dietary supplements. Mil Med 2003;168(6):429-430.

Pasquali R, Baraldi G, Cesari MP, et al. A controlled trial using ephedrine in the treatment of obesity. Int J Obes 1985;9(2):93-98.

Pasquali R, Casimirri F, Melchionda N, et al. Effects of chronic administration of ephedrine during very-low-calorie diets on energy expenditure, protein metabolism and hormone levels in obese subjects. Clin Sci (Colch) 1992;82(1):85-92.

Perrotta DM. From the Centers for Disease Control and Prevention. Adverse events associated with ephedrine-containing products—Texas, December 1993–September 1995. JAMA 1996; 276(21):1711-1712.

Samenuk D, Link MS, Homoud MK, et al. Adverse cardiovascular events temporally associated with ma huang, an herbal source of ephedrine. Mayo Clin Proc 2002;77(1):12-16.

Schulman S. Addressing the potential risks associated with ephedra use: a review of recent efforts. Public Health Rep 2003;118(6):487-492.

Schweinfurth J, Pribitkin E. Sudden hearing loss associated with ephedra use. Am J Health Syst Pharm 2003;60(4):375-377.

Shekelle P, Hardy M. Safety and efficacy of ephedra and ephedrine for enhancement of athletic performance, thermogenesis and the treatment of obesity. Phytomedicine 2002;9(1):78.

Shekelle PG, Hardy ML, Morton SC, et al. Efficacy and safety of ephedra and ephedrine for weight loss and athletic performance: a meta-analysis. JAMA 2003;289(12):1537-1545.

Torpy JM, Lynm C, Glass RM. JAMA patient page. Ephedra and ephedrine. JAMA 2003; 289(12):1590.

Toubro S, Astrup AV, Breum L, et al. Safety and efficacy of long-term treatment with ephedrine, caffeine and an ephedrine/caffeine mixture. Int J Obes Relat Metab Disord 1993;17 Suppl 1:S69-S72.

Essiac

RELATED TERMS

- **Burdock root *(Arctium lappa)* synonyms/related terms:** Akujitsu, anthraxivore, arctii, *Arctium minus*, *Arctium tomentosa*, bardana, bardanae radix, bardane, bardane grande, beggar's buttons, burr, burr seed, chin, clot-burr, clotbur, cocklebur, cockle button (cocklebutton), cuckold, daiki kishi, edible burdock, fox's clote, grass burdock, great bur, great burdock, gobo, grosse klette, happy major, hardock, hare burr, hurrburr, kletterwurzel, lampazo, lappola, love leaves, niu bang zi, oil of lappa, personata, philanthropium, thorny burr, turkey burrseed, woo-bang-ja, wild gobo.
- **Sheep sorrel (*Rumex acetosella*) synonyms/related terms:** Acedera, acid sorrel, azeda-brava, buckler leaf, cigreto, common sorrel, cuckoo sorrow, cuckoo's meate, dock, dog-eared sorrel, field sorrel, French sorrel, garden sorrel, gowke-meat, greensauce, green sorrel, herba acetosa, kemekulagi, Polygonaceae, red sorrel, red top sorrel, round leaf sorrel, *Rumex scutatus*, *Rumex acetosa* L., sheephead sorrel, sheep's sorrel, sorrel, sorrel dock, sour dock, sour grass, sour sabs, sour suds, sour sauce, wiesensauerampfer, wild sorrel.
- **Slippery elm inner bark (*Ulmus fulva*) synonyms/related terms:** Indian elm, moose elm, red elm, rock elm, slippery elm, sweet elm, Ulmaceae, ulmi rubrae cortex, *Ulmus fulva* Michaux, ulmus rubra, winged elm.
- **Turkish rhubarb (*Rheum palmatum*) synonyms/related terms:** Baoshen pill, Canton rhubarb, Chinesischer rhabarber, Chinese rhubarb, chong-gi-huang, common rhubarb, da huang, daio, da huang liujingao, English rhubarb, extractum rhei liquidum, Himalayan rhubarb, Indian rhubarb, Japanese rhubarb, jiang-zhi jian-fel yao (JZJFY), jinghuang tablet, medicinal rhubarb, pie rhubarb, Polygonaceae, pyralvex, pyralvex berna, racine de rhubarbee, RET (rhubarb extract tablet), rhabarber, rhei radix, rhei rhizoma, rheum, rheum australe, *Rheum emodi* Wall., *Rheum officinale* Baill., *Rheum rhabarbarum*, *Rheum rhaponticum* L., *Rheum tanguticum* Maxim., *Rheum tanguticum* Maxim. ex. Balf., *Rheum tanguticum* Maxim. L., Rheum *undulatum*, *Rheum* x *cultorum*, *Rheum webbianum* (Indian or Himalayan rhubarb), rhizoma, rheirhubarbe de Chine, rhubarb, rubarbo, ruibarbo, shenshi rhubarb, tai huang, Turkey rhubarb.

BACKGROUND

- Essiac is a combination of herbs, including burdock root (*Arctium lappa*), sheep sorrel (*Rumex acetosella*), slippery elm inner bark (*Ulmus fulva*), and Turkish rhubarb (*Rheum palmatum*). The original formula was developed by the Canadian nurse Rene Caisse (1888-1978) in the 1920s ("Essiac" is Caisse spelled backward). The recipe is said to be based on a traditional Ojibwa (Native American) remedy, and Caisse administered the formula by mouth and injection to numerous cancer patients during the 1920s and 1930s. The exact ingredients and amounts in the original formulation remain a secret.
- During investigations by the Canadian government and public hearings in the late 1930s, it remained unclear if Essiac was an effective cancer treatment. Amidst controversy, Caisse closed her clinic in 1942. In the 1950s, Caisse provided samples

of Essiac to Dr. Charles Brusch, founder of the Brusch Medical Center in Cambridge, Massachusetts, who administered Essiac to patients (it is unclear if Brusch was given access to the secret formula). According to some accounts, additional herbs were added to these later formulations, including blessed thistle (*Cnicus benedictus*), red clover (*Trifolium pratense*), kelp (*Laminaria digitata*), and watercress (*Nasturtium officinale*).

- A laboratory at Memorial Sloan-Kettering Cancer Center tested Essiac samples (provided by Caisse) on mice during the 1970s. This research was never formally published, and there is controversy regarding the results, with some accounts noting no benefits, and others reporting significant effects (including an account by Dr. Brusch). Questions were later raised about improper preparation of the formula. Caisse subsequently refused requests by researchers at Memorial Sloan-Kettering and the U.S. National Cancer Institute for access to the recipe.
- In the 1970s, Caisse provided the formula to Resperin Corporation Ltd., with the understanding that Resperin would coordinate a scientific trial in humans. Although a study was initiated, it was stopped early because of questions about improper preparation of the formula and inadequate study design. This research was never completed. Resperin, which owned the Essiac name, formally went out of business after transferring rights to the Essiac name and selling the secret formula to Essiac Products Ltd., which currently distributes products through Essiac International.
- Despite the lack of available scientific evidence, Essiac and Essiac-like products (with similar ingredients) remain popular, particularly among people with cancer.
- Essiac is most commonly taken as a tea. A survey conducted in 2000 found that almost 15% of Canadian women with breast cancer were using Essiac. Essiac also has become popular in people with HIV and diabetes and in healthy individuals for its purported immune-enhancing properties, although there has been no reliable scientific research in these areas.
- More than 40 Essiac-like products are available in North America, Europe, and Australia. Flor-essence includes the original four herbs (burdock root, sheep sorrel, slippery elm bark, Turkish rhubarb) as well as herbs that were later added as "potentiators" (blessed thistle, red clover, kelp, watercress). Virginias Herbal E contains the four original herbs along with echinacea and black walnut. Other commercial formulations may include additional ingredients, such as cat's claw (*Uncaria tomentosa*).

USES BASED ON SCIENTIFIC EVIDENCE	Grade*
Cancer There are no properly conducted published human studies of Essiac for the treatment of cancer. A laboratory at Memorial Sloan-Kettering Cancer Center tested Essiac on mice during the 1970s, although the results were never formally published and remain controversial. Questions were raised about improper preparation of the formula. A study in humans was begun in Canada in the late 1970s but was stopped early because of concerns about inconsistent preparation of the formula and inadequate study design. In the 1980s, the Canadian Department of National Health and Welfare collected information about 86 cancer	C

Continued

patients treated with Essiac. Results were inconclusive (17 patients had died at the time of the study, inadequate information was available for 8 patients, "no benefits" were found in 47 patients, 5 patients reported reduced need for pain medications, and 1 noted subjective improvement). Most patients had also received other cancer treatments such as chemotherapy, making the effects of Essiac impossible to isolate.
Currently, there is not enough evidence to recommend for or against the use of this herbal mixture as a therapy for cancer. Different brands may contain variable ingredients, and the comparative effectiveness of these formulas is not known. None of the individual herbs used in Essiac has been tested in rigorous human cancer trials (rhubarb has shown some anti-tumor properties in experiments in animals; slippery elm inner bark has not; sheep sorrel and burdock have been used traditionally in other cancer remedies). Numerous individual patient testimonials and reports from manufacturers are available on the Internet, although these cannot be considered scientifically viable as evidence. Individuals with cancer are advised not to delay treatment with more proven therapies.

*Key to grades: *A:* Strong scientific evidence for this use; *B:* Good scientific evidence for this use; *C:* Unclear scientific evidence for this use; *D:* Fair scientific evidence against this use (it may not work); *F:* Strong scientific evidence against this use (it likely does not work). For a more detailed explanation of efficacy criteria, see "Natural Standard Evidence-Based Validated Grading Rationale" in the Introduction.

Uses Based on Tradition, Theory, or Limited Scientific Evidence

AIDS/HIV, appetite stimulant, arthritis, asthma, bladder cancer, blood cleanser, breast cancer, chelating agent (heavy metals), chronic fatigue syndrome, colon cancer, "detoxification," diabetes, endometrial cancer, energy enhancement, head/neck cancers, Hodgkin's disease, immune system enhancement, kidney diseases, leukemia, lip cancer, liver cancer (hepatocellular carcinoma), longevity, lung cancer, Lyme disease, lymphoma, multiple myeloma, non-Hodgkin's lymphoma, nutritional supplement, ovarian cancer, supportive care in advanced cancer patients, pancreatic cancer, paralysis, prostate cancer, reduction of chemotherapy side effects, stomach cancer, systemic lupus erythematosus (SLE), throat cancer, thyroid disorders, tongue cancer, well-being.

DOSING

The following doses are based on scientific research, publications, traditional use, or expert opinion. Many herbs and supplements have not been thoroughly tested, and their safety and effectiveness may not be proven. Brands may be made differently, with variable ingredients even within the same brand. The doses shown may not apply to all products. It is important to always read product labels and discuss doses with a qualified healthcare provider before therapy is started.

Standardization

- Standardization involves measuring the amounts of certain chemicals in products to try to make different preparations similar to each other. It is not always known if the chemicals being measured are the "active" ingredients. Because the formula for Essiac remains a secret, it is not clear what standards for manufacturing are followed. Some brands of Essiac-like products publish the amounts of herbal constituents, although the basis for standardization of these individual ingredients is not always clear.

Adults (18 Years and Older)

- Historically, Essiac has been administered by mouth or injection. The most common current use is as a tea. There are no reliable published human studies of Essiac or Essiac-like products, and safety or effectiveness has not been established scientifically for any dose. Instructions for tea preparation and dosing vary from product to product. People are advised to read product labels and consult their cancer healthcare provider before starting any new therapy, such as the use of Essiac or Essiac-like products.

Children (Younger Than 18 Years)

- There are insufficient scientific data available to recommend the safe use of Essiac or Essiac-like products in children.

SAFETY

The U.S. Food and Drug Administration does not strictly regulate herbs and supplements. There is no guarantee of the strength, purity, or safety of products, and effects may vary. It is important to always read product labels. People who have a medical condition, or are taking other drugs, herbs, or supplements, should consult a qualified healthcare provider before starting a new therapy. A healthcare provider should be contacted immediately about any side effects.

Allergies

- There are no reports of allergy to Essiac in published scientific literature, although reactions potentially can occur due to any of the included herbs. Anaphylaxis (severe allergic reaction) has been reported after rhubarb leaf ingestion, and allergic reactions to sorrel products taken by mouth have been reported. Contact dermatitis (skin rash after direct contact) has been reported with exposure to burdock, slippery elm bark, and rhubarb leaves. Cross-sensitivity to burdock may occur in individuals with allergy to members of the Asteraceae/Compositae family, such as ragweed, chrysanthemums, marigolds, and daisies.

Side Effects and Warnings

- The safety of Essiac has not been well studied scientifically. Safety concerns are based on theoretical and known reactions associated with herbal components of Essiac: burdock root (*Arctium lappa*), sheep sorrel (*Rumex acetosella*), slippery elm bark (*Ulmus fulva*), and Turkish rhubarb (*Rheum palmatum*). However, the safety and toxicities of these individual herbs also have not been well studied. Essiac-like products may contain different or additional ingredients, and people who plan to use such products should always read the product labels.

- Potentially toxic compounds present in Essiac include tannins, oxalic acid, and anthraquinones. Tannins, which are present in burdock, sorrel, rhubarb, and slippery elm, may cause stomach upset and, in high concentrations, may lead to kidney or liver damage. In theory, long-term use of tannins may increase the risk of head and neck cancers, although there are no documented cases in humans.
- Oxalic acid, which is present in rhubarb, slippery elm, and sorrel, can cause serious adverse effects when taken in high doses (particularly in children). Signs and symptoms of oxalic acid toxicity/poisoning include nausea and vomiting, mouth/throat burning, dangerously low blood pressure, blood electrolyte imbalances, seizures, throat swelling that interferes with breathing, and liver and kidney damage. Death from oxalic acid poisoning was reported in an adult man who had eaten soup containing sorrel and in a 4-year-old child who had eaten rhubarb leaves. The lethal dose of oxalic acid for adults has been estimated as 15 to 30 g, although doses as low as 5 g may be fatal. The amount of oxalic acid in Essiac preparations is not known. In cases of suspected oxalic acid poisoning, medical attention should be sought immediately. Regular intake of oxalic acid may increase the risk of kidney stones.
- Anthraquinones in rhubarb root and sheep sorrel may cause diarrhea, intestinal cramping, and loss of fluid and electrolytes (such as potassium). Use of rhubarb may result in discoloration of the urine (bright yellow or red) or of the inner mucosal surface of the intestine (a condition called melanosis coli). Fluoride poisoning has been reported in persons taking rhubarb fruit juice. Rhubarb products manufactured in China have been found to be contaminated with heavy metals. Chronic use of rhubarb products may lead to dependence.
- Based on research in animals and limited studies in humans, burdock may increase or decrease blood sugar levels. Caution is advised in patients with diabetes or hypoglycemia, and in those taking drugs, herbs, or supplements that affect blood sugar levels. Serum glucose levels may need to be monitored by a healthcare provider, and medication adjustments may be necessary. Diuretic effects (increasing urine flow) and estrogen-like effects have been reported in persons with HIV who were taking oral burdock supplements.
- Reports of anticholinergic reactions (such as slow heart rate and dry mouth) with the use of burdock products, reported in studies made in the 1970s, are believed to have been due to contamination with belladonna alkaloids, which resemble burdock and can be introduced during harvesting. Burdock itself has not been found to contain constituents that would be responsible for these reactions.

Pregnancy and Breastfeeding

- There is insufficient scientific evidence to recommend the safe use of Essiac or Essiac-like products in women who are pregnant or are breastfeeding, and there are potential risks from the herbal constituents. Oxalic acid and anthraquinone glycosides, which are present in the included herbs, may be unsafe during pregnancy. Rhubarb and burdock may cause contractions of the uterus; some publications note that whole slippery elm bark can lead to abortion, although there is limited supporting scientific evidence.

INTERACTIONS

Most herbs and supplements have not been thoroughly tested for interactions with other herbs, supplements, drugs, or foods. The interactions listed here are based on reports in scientific publications, laboratory experiments, or traditional use. It is important to always read product labels. People who have a medical condition, or are taking other drugs, herbs, or supplements, should consult a qualified healthcare provider before starting a new therapy.

Interactions with Drugs

- Essiac interactions have not been well studied scientifically. Most potential interactions are based on theoretical and known reactions associated with the herbal components of Essiac: burdock root (*Arctium lappa*), sheep sorrel (*Rumex acetosella*), slippery elm bark (*Ulmus fulva*), and Turkish rhubarb (*Rheum palmatum*). However, the interactions of these individual herbs also have not been well studied. Essiac-like products may contain different or additional ingredients, and people who plan to use such products should always read the product labels.
- Essiac may interfere with how the body uses the liver's cytochrome P450 enzyme system to process components of some drugs. As a result, blood levels of these components may be altered and may cause increased effects or potentially serious adverse reactions. This study reported that a patient who was taking the experimental drug DX-8951f (metabolized by CYP3A4 and CYP1A2) experienced toxic side effects and drug clearance that was 4 to 5 times slower than in other patients. This patient was also taking "Essiac tea"; however, further details are lacking, and it is unclear whether the patient was taking Essiac or an Essiac-like product. People who are using any medications should always read the package insert and consult with their healthcare provider and pharmacist about possible interactions.
- Anthraquinones in rhubarb root and sheep sorrel may lead to diarrhea, dehydration, or loss of electrolytes (such as potassium) and may increase the effects of other laxative agents. In one study in humans, burdock was associated with diuretic effects (increasing urine flow), and in theory burdock may cause excess fluid loss (dehydration) and electrolyte imbalances (such as changes in blood potassium or sodium levels). These effects may be increased when burdock is taken at the same time as diuretic drugs such as chlorothiazide (Diuril), furosemide (Lasix), hydrochlorothiazide (HCTZ), and spironolactone (Aldactone). The laxative and diuretic properties of the herbs in Essiac may lead to low potassium blood levels that are potentially dangerous in people taking digoxin or digitoxin.
- Based on animal research and limited human study, burdock may decrease or increase blood sugar levels. Caution is advised in people who are using medications that may also affect blood sugar levels. Persons who are taking drugs for diabetes by mouth or insulin should be monitored closely by a qualified healthcare provider. Medication adjustments may be necessary.
- Based on limited human evidence that is not entirely clear, burdock may have estrogen-like properties, and may act to increase the effects of estrogenic agents, including hormone replacement therapies (e.g., Premarin) and birth control pills.

Interactions with Herbs and Dietary Supplements

- One human report suggests that Essiac may interfere with how the body uses the liver's cytochrome P450 enzyme system to process components of other herbs and supplements. As a result, blood levels of these components may be elevated. Essiac may alter the effects of other herbs on the cytochrome P450 system. Examples of such herbs are bloodroot, cat's claw, chamomile, chaparral, chasteberry, damiana, *Echinacea angustifolia*, goldenseal, grapefruit juice, licorice, oregano, red clover, St. John's wort, wild cherry, and yucca.

- Anthraquinones in rhubarb root and sheep sorrel may cause diarrhea, dehydration, or loss of electrolytes (such as potassium) and may increase the effects of other agents with possible laxative properties, such as alder buckthorn, aloe dried leaf sap, black root, blue flag rhizome, butternut bark, cascara bark, castor oil, chasteberry, colocynth fruit pulp, dandelion, dong quai, European buckthorn, eyebright, gamboges bark, horsetail, jalap root, manna bark, plantain leaf, podophyllum root, psyllium, rhubarb, senna, wild cucumber fruit, and yellow dock root.
- Burdock has been associated with diuretic effects (increasing urine flow) in one study in humans and, in theory, may cause excessive fluid loss (dehydration) or electrolyte imbalances (such as changes in blood potassium and sodium levels) when used with other diuretic herbs or supplements, such as artichoke, celery, corn silk, couchgrass, dandelion, elder flower, horsetail, juniper berry, kava, shepherd's purse, uva ursi, and yarrow.
- The laxative and diuretic properties of herbs in Essiac may result in low potassium blood levels that are potentially dangerous in people taking cardiac glycoside-containing herbs such as adonis, balloon cotton, black hellebore root/melampode, black Indian hemp, bushman's poison, cactus grandifloris, convallaria, eyebright, figwort, foxglove/digitalis, frangipani, hedge mustard, hemp root/Canadian hemp root, king's crown, lily-of-the-valley, motherwort, oleander leaf, pheasant's eye plant, plantain leaf, pleurisy root, psyllium husks, redheaded cotton-bush, rhubarb root, rubber vine, sea-mango, senna fruit, squill, strophanthus, uzara, wallflower, wintersweet, yellow dock root, and yellow oleander.
- Based on research in animals and limited studies in humans, burdock may decrease or increase blood sugar levels. Caution is advised in people who are using other herbs or supplements that may also alter blood sugar levels. Blood glucose levels may require monitoring, and doses may need adjustment. Examples of herbs that may lower blood sugar levels are *Aloe vera*, American ginseng, bilberry, bitter melon, fenugreek, fish oil, gymnema, horse chestnut seed extract (HCSE), marshmallow, milk thistle, *Panax ginseng*, rosemary, Siberian ginseng, stinging nettle, and white horehound.
- Because burdock may contain estrogen-like chemicals, the effects of other agents believed to have estrogen-like properties may be altered. Examples of such agents are alfalfa, black cohosh, bloodroot, hops, kudzu, licorice, pomegranate, red clover, soy, thyme, white horehound, and yucca. These possible interactions are based on initial and unclear evidence.
- In theory, use of rhubarb and sheep sorrel may decrease the absorption of minerals such as calcium, iron, and zinc.

Selected References

Natural Standard developed the preceding evidence-based information based on a systematic review of more than 75 articles. For comprehensive information about alternative and complementary therapies on the professional level, go to www.naturalstandard.com. Selected references are listed here.

Bever BO, Zahnd GR. Plants with oral hypoglycaemic action. Quart J Crude Drug Res 1979; 17:139-196.

Boon H, Stewart M, Kennard MA, et al. Use of complementary/alternative medicine by breast cancer survivors in Ontario: prevalence and perceptions. J Clin Oncol 2000;18(13):2515-2521.

Bryson PD, Watanabe AS, Rumack BH, et al. Burdock root tea poisoning. Case report involving a commercial preparation. JAMA 1978;239(20):2157.

Bryson PD. Burdock root tea poisoning. JAMA 1978;240(15):1586.

De Jager R, Cheverton P, Tamanoi K, et al. (DX-8931f Investigators). DX-8951f: summary of phase I clinical trials. Ann N Y Acad Sci 2000;922:260-273.

Dog TL. Author of CME article offers clarification about Essiac. Altern Ther Health Med 2001;7(4):20.

Fraser SS, Allen C. Could Essiac halt cancer? Homemaker's 1977 (August issue).

Geyer C, Hammond L, Johnson T, et al. Dose-schedule optimization of the hexacyclic camptothecin (CPT) analog DX-8951f: a phase I and pharmacokinetic study with escalation of both treatment duration and dose [meeting abstract]. Proc Ann Meet Amer Soc Clin Oncol 1999:A813.

Kaegi E. Unconventional therapies for cancer: 1. Essiac. The Task Force on Alternative Therapies of the Canadian Breast Cancer Research Initiative. CMAJ 1998;158(7):897-902.

Karn H, Moore MJ. The use of the herbal remedy Essiac in an outpatient cancer population [meeting abstract]. Proc Ann Meet Amer Soc Clin Oncol 1997:A245.

LeMoine L. Essiac: an historical perspective. Can Oncol Nurs J 1997;7(4):216-221.

Rhoads PM, Tong TG, Banner W, Jr., et al. Anticholinergic poisonings associated with commercial burdock root tea. J Toxicol Clin Toxicol 1984;22(6):581-584.

Silver AA, Krantz JC. The effect of the ingestion of burdock root on normal and diabetic individuals: a preliminary report. Ann Int Med 1931;5:274-284.

Tamayo C, Richardson MA, Diamond S, et al. The chemistry and biological activity of herbs used in Flor-Essence herbal tonic and Essiac. Phytother Res 2000;14(1):1-14.

Thomas R. The Essiac report: the true story of a Canadian herbal cancer remedy and of the thousands of lives it continues to save. Los Angeles: Altern Treat Inform Network, 1993.

U.S. Congressional Office of Technology Assessment. Essiac. Washington, DC: U.S. Government Printing Office, 1990.

Zarembski PM, Hodgkinson A. Plasma oxalic acid and calcium levels in oxalate poisoning. J Clin Path 1967;20:283-285.

E

Eucalyptus Oil

(*E. globulus Labillardiere, E. fruticetorum* F. Von Mueller, *E. smithii* R.T. Baker)

RELATED TERMS

- Australian fever tree leaf, blauer gommibaum, blue gum, catheter oil, cineole, 1,8-cineole, essence of eucalyptus rectifiee, essencia de eucalipto, eucalypti aetheroleum, eucalypti folium, eucalyptol, *Eucalyptus polybractea*, eucalytpo setma ag, fevertree, gommier bleu, gum tree, kafur ag, malee, Myrtaceae, oleum eucalypti, schonmutz, southern blue gum, Tasmanian blue gum.

BACKGROUND

- Eucalyptus oil is used commonly as a decongestant and expectorant for upper respiratory tract infections or inflammation, as well as for various musculoskeletal conditions. The oil is found in numerous over-the-counter cough and cold lozenges as well as in inhalation vapors and topical ointments. Veterinarians use the oil topically for its reported antimicrobial activity, which is supported by in vitro and in vivo study. Numerous applications are suggested in the sparse literature on this topic; however, there are insufficient controlled studies supporting use in humans. Other applications include use as an aromatic in soaps or perfumes, as a flavoring agent in foodstuffs and beverages, and as a dental or industrial solvent.
- Eucalyptus oil contains 70% to 85% 1,8-cineole (eucalyptol), which is also present in other plant oils. Eucalyptol is used as an ingredient in some mouthwash and dental preparations as an endodontic solvent and may possess antimicrobial properties. Listerine mouthrinse is a combination of essential oils (eucalyptol, menthol, thymol, and methyl salicylate) that has been shown to be efficacious for the reduction of dental plaque and gingivitis.
- Topical use or inhalation of eucalyptus oil at low concentrations may be safe, although significant and potentially lethal toxicity has been consistently reported with oral use, and may occur with inhalation as well. Use of eucalyptus oil, by all routes of administration, should be avoided in children.

USES BASED ON SCIENTIFIC EVIDENCE	Grade*
Asthma Initial research suggests that long-term systemic therapy with eucalyptol (1,8-cineol, a main chemical constituent of eucalyptus oil) may decrease the amount of steroids needed in people with steroid-dependent asthma. Further research is needed to confirm eucalyptol's anti-inflammatory and mucolytic activity before this agent can be recommended in therapy for upper and lower airway diseases.	C

Continued

Decongestant/expectorant Although eucalyptus oil is commonly used in non-prescription products, results have been inconclusive in scientific studies of eucalyptus oil or eucalyptol (1,8-cineole, a main chemical constituent of eucalyptus oil) taken by mouth or inhaled as a decongestant/expectorant in people with colds or upper respiratory tract infections. Better research is necessary before a recommendation can be made.	C
Dental plaque/gingivitis (mouthwash) Results have been promising in studies in people who have used mouthwashes containing several potentially active ingredients, including eucalyptus extract or eucalyptol (1,8-cineole, a main chemical constituent of eucalyptus oil) for therapy of dental plaque/gingivitis. Although these combination mouthwashes (such as Listerine) were effective, it is unclear whether eucalyptus oil by itself is effective or safe for this purpose.	C
Headache Eucalyptus has been shown to reduce pain in studies in animals. However, the effectiveness of eucalyptus oil applied to the skin for headache relief in humans has not been supported by reliable research.	C

*Key to grades: *A*: Strong scientific evidence for this use; *B*: Good scientific evidence for this use; *C*: Unclear scientific evidence for this use; D: Fair scientific evidence against this use (it may not work); F: Strong scientific evidence against this use (it likely does not work). For a more detailed explanation of efficacy criteria, see "Natural Standard Evidence-Based Validated Grading Rationale" in the Introduction.

Uses Based on Tradition, Theory, or Limited Scientific Evidence

AIDS, alertness, antibacterial, antifungal, antiviral, aromatherapy, arthritis, astringent, back pain, bronchitis, burns, cancer prevention, chronic obstructive pulmonary disease (COPD), cleaning solvent, colds, cough, croup, deodorant, diabetes, diarrhea, ear infections, emphysema, fever, flavoring, fragrance, herpes, hookworm, inflammation, inflammatory bowel disease, influenza, insect repellent, liver protection, muscle/joint pain, muscle spasm, nerve pain, parasitic infection, rheumatoid arthritis, ringworm, runny nose, shingles, sinusitis, skin infections in children, skin ulcers, snoring, stimulant, strains/sprains, tuberculosis, urinary difficulties, urinary tract infection, whooping cough, wound healing.

DOSING

The following doses are based on scientific research, publications, traditional use, or expert opinion. Many herbs and supplements have not been thoroughly tested, and their safety and effectiveness may not be proven. Brands may be made differently, with variable ingredients even within the same brand. The doses shown may not apply to all products. It is important to always read product labels and discuss doses with a qualified healthcare provider before therapy is started.

Standardization

- Standardization involves measuring the amounts of certain chemicals in products to try to make different preparations similar to each other. It is not always known if the chemicals being measured are the "active" ingredients Standardization data for eucalyptus is limited. It has been suggested that in order to be effective medicinally, eucalyptus leaf oil must contain 70% to 85% eucalyptol (1,8-cineole).

Adults (18 Years and Older)

- **Topical (applied to the skin):** Application of 5% to 20% in an oil-based formulation or 5% to 10% in an alcohol-based formulation has been used.
- **Inhaled:** Tincture containing 5% to 10% eucalyptus oil or a few drops placed in a vaporizer as an inhalant have been used.
- **By mouth:** Caution is advised in people who are taking eucalyptus oil by mouth, because small amounts of oil taken by mouth have resulted in severe and deadly reactions. Doses of 0.05 to 0.2 ml or 0.3 to 0.6 g of eucalyptus oil taken daily have been used traditionally but may cause toxic side effects. For infusions prepared with eucalyptus leaf, a quantity of 2 to 3 g of eucalyptus leaf in 150 ml of water, three times a day, has been used traditionally but may result in toxic side effects.
- **Mouthwash:** Eucalyptol (1,8-cineole, a major chemical in eucalyptus oil) is used in some commercially sold mouthwashes.

Children (Younger Than 18 Years)

- Severe side effects have been reported in children after they were given small doses of eucalyptus by mouth or applied to the skin. Eucalyptus preparations are not recommended for use by infants and young children, especially on or near the face.

SAFETY

The U.S. Food and Drug Administration does not strictly regulate herbs and supplements. There is no guarantee of the strength, purity, or safety of products, and effects may vary. It is important to always read product labels. People who have a medical condition, or are taking other drugs, herbs, or supplements, should consult a qualified healthcare provider before starting a new therapy. A healthcare provider should be contacted immediately about any side effects.

Allergies

- Case reports describe allergic rash after exposure to eucalyptus oil, either alone or as an ingredient in creams. One child developed a rash after taking eucalyptus oil by mouth. Reports also describe hives after exposure to eucalyptus pollen.

Side Effects and Warnings

- Severe and potentially deadly side effects have been reported in children and adults who have taken eucalyptus oil by mouth, including slowing of the brain and central nervous system, drowsiness, seizures, and coma. Caution is advised in people who are driving or operating heavy machinery. Anecdotal reports suggest that serious side effects can develop after taking as little as 1 teaspoon by mouth. Reports also suggest that inhaled eucalyptus products or bathtub exposure can cause symptoms.
- Eucalyptus products should be avoided in infants and young children, because severe reactions have been reported in children after exposure to eucalyptus by mouth or by application to the skin. Ingestion by children of vaporizer formulas containing eucalyptus has been reported.

- Symptoms of adverse effects in people who ingested eucalyptus oil include abdominal pain, blue discoloration of the lips or skin, constricted pupils, convulsions, cough, delirium, diarrhea, difficulty in breathing (including sensation of suffocating), difficulty in walking, dizziness, drowsiness, fever, headache, hyperactivity, muscle weakness, nausea and vomiting, pneumonia, slurred speech, and wheezing. Case reports describe several abnormalities in heart function in people after eucalyptus oil was taken by mouth, including abnormal rhythms, loss of heartbeat, low blood pressure, and complete disruption of the heart and circulation. Caution is advised in people with seizure disorder, heart disease, disorders of the stomach or intestines, or lung disease.
- Published reports describe "attacks" following ingestion of eucalyptus oil in people with acute intermittent porphyria (AIP), an inherited disorder affecting the liver and blood. Individuals with AIP should avoid the use of eucalyptus products. Other case studies report symptoms following ingestion of eucalyptus oil in persons who have kidney or liver disease or who are taking other medications that are processed by the liver. Eucalyptus is reported to lower blood sugar levels in diabetic animals, although reliable studies in humans are lacking in this area. Nonetheless, caution is advised in persons with diabetes or hypoglycemia and in those taking drugs, herbs, or supplements that affect blood sugar levels. Serum glucose levels may need to be monitored by a healthcare provider, and medication adjustments may be necessary.

Pregnancy and Breastfeeding

- Because of the known side effects of eucalyptus and the lack of scientific data in this area, eucalyptus should be avoided by pregnant and breastfeeding women.

INTERACTIONS

Most herbs and supplements have not been thoroughly tested for interactions with other herbs, supplements, drugs, or foods. The interactions listed here are based on reports in scientific publications, laboratory experiments, or traditional use. It is important to always read product labels. People who have a medical condition, or are taking other drugs, herbs, or supplements, should consult a qualified healthcare provider before starting a new therapy.

Interactions with Drugs

- Multiple case reports associate eucalyptus oil taken by mouth with slowing of the brain and nervous system. These symptoms may be worsened when eucalyptus is taken with sedating agents. Examples are alcohol, some antidepressants, barbiturates such as phenobarbital, benzodiazepines such as lorazepam (Ativan) and diazepam (Valium), and narcotics such as codeine. Caution is advised in people who are driving or operating machinery.
- Eucalyptus has been reported to lower blood sugar levels in diabetic animals. Although studies in humans are lacking, the theoretical risk suggests that eucalyptus should be taken with caution when combined with medications that lower blood sugar levels. People who are taking drugs for diabetes by mouth or insulin should be monitored closely by a qualified healthcare provider. Medication adjustments may be necessary.
- In animals, several components of eucalyptus interfere with how the body uses the liver's cytochrome P450 enzyme system. As a result, the levels of these drugs may be decreased in the blood, with reduced intended effects. People who are

using any medications should always read the package insert and consult with their healthcare provider and pharmacist about possible interactions.
- When applied to the skin with 5-fluorouracil (5-FU) lotion (Efudex, Carac), eucalyptus may increase the absorption of 5-FU.
- *Note:* Many tinctures contain high levels of alcohol and may cause nausea or vomiting when taken with metronidazole (Flagyl) or disulfiram (Antabuse).

Interactions with Herbs and Dietary Supplements

- Eucalyptus may increase the drowsiness caused by other herbs or supplements. Examples of such agents are calamus, calendula, California poppy, capsicum, catnip, celery, couchgrass, dogwood, elecampane, German chamomile, goldenseal, gotu kola, hops, kava, lavender aromatherapy, lemon balm, sage, sassafras, skullcap, shepherd's purse, Siberian ginseng, stinging nettle, St. John's wort, valerian, wild carrot, wild lettuce, withania root, and yerba mansa. Caution is advised in people who are driving or operating machinery.
- Based on animal studies, eucalyptus may lower blood sugar levels. Caution is advised in people who are using other herbs or supplements that also may lower blood sugar levels. Blood glucose levels may require monitoring, and doses may need adjustment. Examples of such agents are *Aloe vera*, American ginseng, bilberry, bitter melon, burdock, fenugreek, fish oil, gymnema, horse chestnut seed extract (HCSE), marshmallow, milk thistle, *Panax ginseng*, rosemary, Siberian ginseng, stinging nettle, and white horehound.
- Studies in animals suggest that eucalyptus may interfere with how the body uses the liver's cytochrome P450 enzyme system to processes components of other herbs and supplements. As a result, blood levels of these components may be elevated. Eucalyptus may alter the effects of other herbs on the cytochrome P450 system. Examples of such agents are bloodroot, cat's claw, chamomile, chaparral, chasteberry, damiana, *Echinacea angustifolia*, goldenseal, grapefruit juice, licorice, oregano, red clover, St. John's wort, wild cherry, and yucca. People who are using any medications should always read the package insert and consult their healthcare provider or pharmacist about possible interactions.
- Eucalyptus has been reported to worsen the adverse effects of borage, coltsfoot, comfrey, hound's tooth, and *Senecio* species, although there have been no reliable research studies in this area.

Interactions with Foods

- **Milk and fatty foods:** In theory, the absorption of eucalyptus may be increased in the presence of milk or fat in the gastrointestinal system.

Selected References

Natural Standard developed the preceding evidence-based information based on a systematic review of more than 265 scientific articles. For comprehensive information about alternative and complementary therapies on the professional level, go to www.naturalstandard.com. Selected references are listed here.

Darben T, Cominos B, Lee CT. Topical eucalyptus oil poisoning. Australas J Dermatol 1998; 39(4):265-267.

Hindle RC. Eucalyptus oil ingestion. N Z Med J 1994;107(977):185-186.

Juergens UR, Dethlefsen U, Steinkamp G, et al. Anti-inflammatory activity of 1.8-cineol (eucalyptol) in bronchial asthma: a double-blind placebo-controlled trial. Respir Med 2003; 97(3):250-256.

Schaller M, Korting HC. Allergic airborne contact dermatitis from essential oils used in aromatherapy. Clin Exp Dermatol 1995;20(2):143-145.

Tascini C, Ferranti S, Gemignani G, et al. Clinical microbiological case: fever and headache in a heavy consumer of eucalyptus extract. Clin Microbiol Infect 2002;8(7):437,445-446.

Tibballs J. Clinical effects and management of eucalyptus oil ingestion in infants and young children. Med J Aust 1995;163(4):177-180.

Tovey ER, McDonald LG. A simple washing procedure with eucalyptus oil for controlling house dust mites and their allergens in clothing and bedding. J Allergy Clin Immunol 1997;100(4):464-466.

Webb NJ, Pitt WR. Eucalyptus oil poisoning in childhood: 41 cases in south-east Queensland. J Paediatr Child Health 1993;29(5):368-371.

Evening Primrose Oil

(*Oenothera biennis* L.)

RELATED TERMS

- Echte nachtkerze, EPO, fever plant, gamma-linolenic acid (GLA), herbe aux anes, huile d'onagre, kaempe natlys, king's cureall, la belle de nuit, nachtkerzenol, night willow-herb, *Oenothera communis* Leveill, *Oenothera graveolens* Gilib, omega-6 essential fatty acid, *Onagra biennis* Scop, *Onogra vulgaris*, onagre bisannuelle, scabish, spach, stella di sera, sun drop, teunisbloem.

BACKGROUND

- The omega-6 essential fatty acid, gamma-linolenic acid (GLA), is believed to be the active ingredient of evening primrose oil (EPO). EPO has been studied in a wide variety of disorders, particularly those affected by metabolic products of essential fatty acids. However, evidence from high-quality research for its use in most conditions is lacking.

USES BASED ON SCIENTIFIC EVIDENCE	Grade*
Eczema Several small studies suggest benefits of evening primrose oil taken by mouth in people with eczema. Large, well-designed studies are needed before a strong recommendation can be made. Evening primrose oil is approved for eczema in several countries outside of the United States.	B
Skin irritation Several small studies of people with atopic dermatitis suggest benefits of taking evening primrose oil by mouth. Large, well-designed studies are needed before a strong recommendation can be made. Evening primrose oil is approved for atopic dermatitis in several countries outside of the United States.	B
Breast cancer Insufficient data are available to advise the use of evening primrose oil for breast cancer. People with known or suspected breast cancer should consult a qualified healthcare provider about possible treatments.	C
Breast cysts Limited available research does not demonstrate that evening primrose oil has a significant effect in treatment of breast cysts.	C
Breast pain (mastalgia) Although primrose oil is used for breast pain in several European countries, no high-quality human studies have been published in this area. Therefore, the available information does not allow recommendation for or against the use of primrose oil for this condition.	C

Continued

E

Chronic fatigue syndrome/post-viral infection symptoms Insufficient scientific information is available to advise the use of evening primrose oil for symptoms of chronic fatigue syndrome or fatigue following a viral infection.	**C**
Diabetes A small number of laboratory studies and theory suggests that evening primrose oil may be helpful in diabetes, but more scientific data are needed before a recommendation can be made.	**C**
Diabetic neuropathy (nerve damage) Gamma-linolenic acid (GLA), one of the components of evening primrose oil, may be helpful in people with diabetic neuropathy. Additional studies are needed before a recommendation can be made.	**C**
Ichthyosis vulgaris (scale-like dry skin) Early studies have not shown any benefit from evening primrose oil in the treatment of ichthyosis vulgaris. Larger studies are needed to confirm these results.	**C**
Multiple sclerosis (MS) It is theorized that primrose oil may be helpful in patients with MS, based on the results of laboratory studies. Limited evidence is available from studies in humans, and a firm conclusion is not possible at this time.	**C**
Obesity/weight loss Initial studies in humans suggest that evening primrose oil may have no effects on weight loss.	**C**
Pre-eclampsia (high blood pressure during pregnancy) Evening primrose oil has been proposed to have effects on chemicals in the blood called prostaglandins, which may play a role in pre-eclampsia. However, more studies are needed before a firm conclusion can be drawn.	**C**
Raynaud's phenomenon Insufficient scientific information is available to advise the use of evening primrose oil for Raynaud's phenomenon.	**C**
Rheumatoid arthritis The benefits of evening primrose oil in the treatment of arthritis have not been clearly shown. More scientific information is needed before a recommendation can be made.	**C**
Asthma Small studies have not shown evening primrose oil to be useful in the treatment of asthma.	**D**

Continued

Attention deficit hyperactivity disorder (ADHD) Small human studies did not show any benefit from evening primrose oil in therapy for ADHD.	**D**
Menopause (flushing/bone metabolism) Available studies do not show evening primrose oil to be helpful in treatment of potential complications of menopause, such as flushing and bone loss.	**D**
Pre-menstrual syndrome (PMS) Small studies in humans did not report that evening primrose oil was helpful for the symptoms of PMS. A large, well-designed study is needed before any recommendation can be made.	**D**
Psoriasis Initial research studies have not shown any benefit from evening primrose oil in the treatment of psoriasis. However, studies have been small with design flaws, and many have combined primrose oil with other agents such as fish oil.	**D**
Schizophrenia Results from studies of mixed quality do not support the use of evening primrose oil for schizophrenia.	**D**

*Key to grades: *A:* Strong scientific evidence for this use; *B:* Good scientific evidence for this use; *C:* Unclear scientific evidence for this use; *D:* Fair scientific evidence against this use (it may not work); *F:* Strong scientific evidence against this use (it likely does not work). For a more detailed explanation of efficacy criteria, see "Natural Standard Evidence-Based Validated Grading Rationale" in the Introduction.

Uses Based on Tradition, Theory, or Limited Scientific Evidence

Alcoholism, antioxidant, atherosclerosis, bruises, cancer, cancer prevention, Crohn's disease, cystic fibrosis, diabetes, disorders of the stomach and intestines, hangover remedy, heart disease, hepatitis B, high cholesterol, inflammation, irritable bowel syndrome, kidney stones, melanoma, multiple sclerosis, pain, Sjögren's syndrome, skin conditions due to kidney failure in dialysis patients, systemic lupus erythematosus (SLE), ulcerative colitis, weight loss, whooping cough, wound healing.

DOSING

The following doses are based on scientific research, publications, traditional use, or expert opinion. Many herbs and supplements have not been thoroughly tested, and their safety and effectiveness may not be proven. Brands may be made differently, with variable ingredients even within the same brand. The doses shown may not apply to all products. It is important to always read product labels and discuss doses with a qualified healthcare provider before therapy is started.

Standardization

- Standardization involves measuring the amounts of certain chemicals in products to try to make different preparations similar to each other. It is not always known if the chemicals being measured are the "active" ingredients.
- Standardized capsules of evening primrose oil (EPO) may contain about 320 mg of linoleic acid (LA), 40 mg of gamma-linolenic acid (GLA), and 10 international units (IU) of vitamin E. Some preparations are labeled with percent content (e.g., 70% LA, 9% GLA). LA from normal daily food intake provides approximately 250 to 1000 mg of GLA daily.

Adults (18 Years and Older)

- Studies on the treatment of eczema or atopic dermatitis have used doses of 4 to 8 g of EPO daily, taken by mouth, divided into several smaller doses throughout the day. Studies of breast pain have used doses of 3 g EPO daily, taken by mouth, divided into several smaller doses throughout the day.

Children (Younger Than 18 Years)

- Studies in children treated for skin conditions have used 3 g of evening primrose oil daily, taken by mouth, divided into several smaller doses throughout the day. It is reported that the maximum dose should not be greater than 0.5 g per kilogram of body weight daily.

SAFETY

The U.S. Food and Drug Administration does not strictly regulate herbs and supplements. There is no guarantee of the strength, purity, or safety of products, and effects may vary. It is important to always read product labels. People who have a medical condition, or are taking other drugs, herbs, or supplements, should consult a qualified healthcare provider before starting a new therapy. A healthcare provider should be contacted immediately about any side effects.

Allergies

- Allergy or hypersensitivity to evening primrose oil has not been widely reported. People with allergy or adverse reactions to plants in the Onagraceae family, to gamma-linolenic acid, or to other ingredients in evening primrose oil should avoid its use.

Side Effects and Warnings

- Several reports describe seizures in individuals taking evening primrose oil (EPO). Some of these seizures developed in people with a previous seizure disorder or in individuals taking EPO in combination with anesthetics. Based on these reports, people with seizure disorders should not take EPO. EPO should be used cautiously with drugs used to treat mental illness such as chlorpromazine (Thorazine), thioridazine (Mellaril), trifluoperazine (Stelazine), or fluphenazine (Prolixin), because of an increased risk of seizures. Persons who plan to undergo surgery requiring anesthesia should stop taking EPO 2 weeks before surgery is scheduled because of the possibility of seizures.
- Other reports describe occasional abdominal pain, headache, nausea, and loose stools in people taking EPO. In studies in animals, gamma-linolenic acid (GLA) (an ingredient of evening primrose oil) was reported to decrease blood pressure. Early results in studies in humans do not show consistent changes in blood pressure.

Pregnancy and Breastfeeding

- There is insufficient scientific information to recommend the safe use of evening primrose oil during pregnancy or in women who are breastfeeding.

INTERACTIONS

Most herbs and supplements have not been thoroughly tested for interactions with other herbs, supplements, drugs, or foods. The interactions listed here are based on reports in scientific publications, laboratory experiments, or traditional use. It is important to always read product labels. People who have a medical condition, or are taking other drugs, herbs, or supplements, should consult a qualified healthcare provider before starting a new therapy.

Interactions with Drugs

- Because seizures have been reported in people taking evening primrose oil alone or in combination with certain medications used to treat mental illness, caution is advised in people who are taking evening primrose oil with medications such as chlorpromazine (Thorazine), thioridazine (Mellaril), trifluoperazine (Stelazine), and fluphenazine (Prolixin). Persons who are undergoing surgery requiring general anesthesia may be at a higher risk for developing seizures and should stop taking evening primrose oil 2 weeks before surgery is scheduled. In people with a history of seizures, doses of anti-seizure medications may require adjustment because evening primrose oil may increase the risk of seizures.
- An ingredient of evening primrose oil, gamma-linolenic acid (GLA), is reported to lower blood pressure in studies in animals. Although studies in humans do not show clear changes in blood pressure, people taking certain blood pressure medications should consult with a healthcare provider before beginning to take evening primrose oil.

Interactions with Herbs and Dietary Supplements

- In studies in animals, gamma-linolenic acid (GLA), an ingredient of evening primrose oil, has been reported to lower blood pressure. Therefore, in theory, evening primrose oil may have effects on blood pressure and should be used cautiously when combined with other agents that may lower blood pressure. Examples are aconite/monkshood, arnica, baneberry, betel nut, bilberry, black cohosh, bryony, calendula, California poppy, coleus, curcumin, eucalyptol, eucalyptus oil, flaxseed, ginger, goldenseal, green hellebore, hawthorn, Indian tobacco, jaborandi, mistletoe, night-blooming cereus, oleander, pasque flower, periwinkle, pleurisy root, shepherd's purse, Texas milkweed, turmeric, and wild cherry.

Interactions with Foods

- There are no reliable published reports available of interactions of evening primrose oil with food.

Selected References

Natural Standard developed the preceding evidence-based information based on a systematic review of more than 220 scientific articles. For comprehensive information about alternative and complementary therapies on the professional level, go to www.naturalstandard.com. Selected references are listed here.

Arimura T, Kojima-Yuasa A, Watanabe S, et al. Role of intracellular reactive oxygen species and mitochondrial dysfunction in evening primrose extract-induced apoptosis in *Ehrlichia* ascites tumor cells. Chem Biol Interact 2003;145(3):337-347.

Blommers J, de Lange-De Klerk ES, Kuik DJ, et al. Evening primrose oil and fish oil for severe chronic mastalgia: a randomized, double-blind, controlled trial. Am J Obstet Gynecol 2002; 187(5):1389-1394.

Budeiri D, Li Wan PA, Dornan JC. Is evening primrose oil of value in the treatment of premenstrual syndrome? Controlled Clin Trials 1996;17(1):60-68.

Dickerson LM, Mazyck PJ, Hunter MH. Premenstrual syndrome. Am Fam Physician 2003; 67(8):1743-1752.

Gateley CA, Pye JK, Harrison BJ, et al. Evening primrose oil (Efamol), a safe treatment option for breast disease. Breast Cancer Res Treat 2001;(14):161.

Gokhale L, Sturdee DW, Parsons AD. The use of food supplements among women attending menopause clinics in the West Midlands. J Br Menopause Soc 2003;9(1):32-35.

Halat KM, Dennehy CE. Botanicals and dietary supplements in diabetic peripheral neuropathy. J Am Board Fam Pract 2003;16(1):47-57.

Hamburger M, Riese U, Graf H, et al. Constituents in evening primrose oil with radical scavenging, cyclooxygenase, and neutrophil elastase inhibitory activities. J Agric Food Chem 2002;50(20):5533-5538.

Hederos CA, Berg A. Epogam evening primrose oil treatment in atopic dermatitis and asthma. Arch Dis Child 1996; 75(6):494-497.

Humphreys F, Symons J, Brown H, et al. The effects of gamolenic acid on adult atopic eczema and premenstrual exacerbation of eczema. Eur J Dermatol 1994;4(598):603.

Huntley AL, Ernst E. Systematic review of herbal medicinal products for the treatment of menopausal symptoms. Menopause 2003;10(5):465-476.

Jack AM, Keegan A, Cotter MA, et al. Effects of diabetes and evening primrose oil treatment on responses of aorta, corpus cavernosum and mesenteric vasculature in rats. Life Sci 2002; 71(16):1863-1877.

Joe LA, Hart LL. Evening primrose oil in rheumatoid arthritis. Ann Pharmacother 1993; 27(12):1475-1477.

Joy CB, Mumby-Croft R, Joy LA. Polyunsaturated fatty acid (fish or evening primrose oil) for schizophrenia. Cochrane Database Syst Rev 2000;(2):CD001257. Review. Update in: Cochrane Database Syst Rev 2003;(2):CD001257.

Morse PF, Horrobin DF, Manku MS, et al. Meta-analysis of placebo-controlled studies of the efficacy of Epogam in the treatment of atopic eczema: relationship between plasma essential fatty acid changes and clinical response. Br J Dermatol 1989;121(1):75-90.

Strid J, Jepson R, Moore V et al. Evening Primrose oil or other essential fatty acids for premenstrual syndrome [protocol]. Cochrane Database Syst Rev 2000;(2):CD.

van der Merwe CF, Booyens J, Joubert HF, et al. The effect of gamma-linolenic acid, an in vitro cytostatic substance contained in evening primrose oil, on primary liver cancer: a double-blind placebo controlled trial. Prostaglandins Leukot Essent Fatty Acids 1990;40(3):199-202.

Whitaker DK, Cilliers J, de Beer C. Evening primrose oil (Epogam) in the treatment of chronic hand dermatitis: disappointing therapeutic results. Dermatology 1996;193(2):115-120.

Yoshimoto-Furuie K, Yoshimoto K, Tanaka T et al. Effects of oral supplementation with evening primrose oil for six weeks on plasma essential fatty acids and uremic skin symptoms in hemodialysis patients. Nephron 1999;81(2):151-159.

Fenugreek

(*Trigonella foenum-graecum* L. Leguminosae)

RELATED TERMS

- Abish, alholva, bird's foot, bockhornsklover, bockshornsamen, bockshornklee, cemen, chilbe, fenegriek, fenogrego, fenugree, fenugreek seed, fenogreco, fenigreko, fenu-thyme, foenugraeci semen, gorogszena, graine de fenugrec, gray hay, Greek hay seed, griechische heusamen, fieno greco, halba, hilbeh, hulba, hu lu ba, kasoori methi, kozieradka pospolita, kreeka lambalaats, mente, mentikura, mentula, methi, methika, methini, methri, methro, mithiguti, pazhitnik grecheskiy, penantazi, sag methi, sambala, sarviapila, shabaliidag, shambelile, trigonella, trigonella semen, trigonella, trigonelline, uluhaal, uwatu, vendayam, venthiam.

BACKGROUND

- Fenugreek has a long history of medical uses in Indian and Chinese medicine and has been used for numerous indications, including labor induction, aiding digestion, and as a general tonic to improve metabolism and health.
- Preliminary studies in animals and methodologically weak trials in humans have suggested possible hypoglycemic and antihyperlipidemic properties of oral fenugreek seed powder. However, at this time, the evidence is insufficient to recommend either for or against fenugreek for treatment of diabetes or hyperlipidemia. Nonetheless, caution is warranted in people taking hypoglycemic agents, and their blood glucose levels should be monitored. Hypokalemia has been reported as an effect of fenugreek supplementation, and potassium levels should be monitored in people taking concomitant hypokalemic agents or with underlying cardiac disease.

USES BASED ON SCIENTIFIC EVIDENCE	Grade*
Diabetes mellitus type 1 In animal studies and in several small, methodologically weak human trials, fenugreek has been found to lower serum glucose levels both acutely and chronically. Although promising, these data cannot be considered definitive, and at this time there is insufficient evidence to recommend either for or against fenugreek for type 1 diabetes. Trials have used a diversity of preparations, dosing regimens, and outcomes measures. No long-term investigations have been conducted. Additional study is warranted in this area.	C
Diabetes mellitus type 2 Review of the literature reveals animal studies and a small, methodologically weak human trial that suggest possible efficacy of fenugreek in type 2 diabetics. Although promising, these data cannot be considered definitive. At this time there is insufficient evidence to recommend either for or against the use of fenugreek for type 2 diabetes.	C

Continued

Hyperlipidemia

C

There is insufficient evidence to support the use of fenugreek as an anti-hyperlipidemic agent. Most available studies are case reports without proper controls, randomization, or blinding.

*Key to grades: *A:* Strong scientific evidence for this use; *B:* Good scientific evidence for this use; *C:* Unclear scientific evidence for this use; *D:* Fair scientific evidence against this use (it may not work); *F:* Strong scientific evidence against this use (it likely does not work). For a more detailed explanation of efficacy criteria, see "Natural Standard Evidence-Based Validated Grading Rationale" in the Introduction.

Uses Based on Tradition, Theory, or Limited Scientific Evidence

Abortifacient, abscesses, antioxidant, aphthous ulcers, appetite stimulant, asthenia, atherosclerosis, baldness, beriberi, boils, breast enhancement, bronchitis, burns, cancer, cellulitis, chapped lips, colic, colon cancer, constipation, convalescence, cough (chronic), dermatitis, diarrhea, digestion, dropsy, dysentery, dyspepsia, eczema, flatulence (gas), furunculosis, galactagogue (lactation stimulant), gastric ulcers, gout, hepatic disease, hepatomegaly, hernia, hypertension, immunomodulator, impotence, indigestion, infections, inflammation, inflammatory bowel disease, labor induction (uterine stimulant), leg edema, leg ulcers, leukemia, lice, low energy, lymphadenitis, menopausal symptoms, myalgia, postmenopausal vaginal dryness, protection against alcohol toxicity, rickets, splenomegaly, stomach upset, thyroxine–induced hyperglycemia, tuberculosis, vitamin deficiencies, wound healing.

DOSING

The following doses are based on scientific research, publications, traditional use, or expert opinion. Many herbs and supplements have not been thoroughly tested, and their safety and effectiveness may not be proven. Brands may be made differently, with variable ingredients even within the same brand. The doses shown may not apply to all products. It is important to always read product labels and discuss doses with a qualified healthcare provider before therapy is started.

Standardization

- Standardization involves measuring the amounts of certain chemicals in products to try to make different preparations similar to each other. It is not always known if the chemicals being measured are the "active" ingredients.
- Different clinical trials have used different doses of fenugreek preparations. Because the active ingredient(s) of fenugreek has yet to be identified, it is impossible standardize dosages of these preparations.

Adults (18 Years and Older)

- *Note:* Products rich in fenugreek fiber may interfere with the absorption of oral medications because of its mucilaginous content and high viscosity in the gut. Medications should be taken separately from such products. However, it should be noted that fenugreek is rarely used for its fiber content.

- **Type 1 diabetes:** 100 g of debitterized fenugreek seed powder divided into two equal doses has been used.
- **Type 2 diabetes:** 2.5 g of fenugreek seed powder in capsule form has been used.
- **Hyperlipidemia:** 2.5 g of fenugreek seed powder in capsule form, taken twice daily for 3 months, or 100 g of debitterized fenugreek seed powder, divided in 2 equal doses, has been used.

Children (Younger Than 18 Years)

- There is insufficient evidence about the safety of fenugreek to recommend its use in children.

SAFETY

The U.S. Food and Drug Administration does not strictly regulate herbs and supplements. There is no guarantee of the strength, purity, or safety of products, and effects may vary. It is important to always read product labels. People who have a medical condition, or are taking other drugs, herbs, or supplements, should consult a qualified healthcare provider before starting a new therapy. A healthcare provider should be contacted immediately about any side effects.

Allergies

- Caution is warranted in people with known fenugreek allergy, or with allergy to chickpeas because of possible cross-reactivity. Inhaling fenugreek seed powder may cause allergic or asthmatic reactions, including bronchospasm.

Side Effects and Warnings

- Fenugreek has traditionally been considered safe and well tolerated. There have been rare reports of alteration of thyroid hormone levels, breathing problems (after inhalation from occupational exposure), diarrhea, dizziness, facial swelling, fainting, flatulence (gas), increased risk of bleeding, numbness, reduction of blood sugar levels, and reduction of serum potassium levels.
- Fenugreek has been reported to lower blood sugar levels. Caution is advised in people with diabetes. Serum glucose levels may need to monitored by a qualified healthcare provider, and medication adjustments may be necessary.
- Hypokalemia (low blood levels of potassium) has been reported in people taking fenugreek products, and potassium blood levels should be monitored in people who are also taking diuretics or other agents that affect potassium levels.

Pregnancy and Breastfeeding

- Reliable human data and systematic studies of fenugreek during pregnancy or lactation are lacking. Caution is warranted in women during pregnancy because of the potential hypoglycemic effects of fenugreek. In addition, in laboratory studies, both water-based and alcoholic extracts of fenugreek exerted a stimulating effect on isolated guinea pig uterus, especially during late pregnancy. Thus, fenugreek may possess abortifacient effects, and it is not recommended for use during pregnancy in amounts higher than those found in foods.

INTERACTIONS

Most herbs and supplements have not been thoroughly tested for interactions with other herbs, supplements, drugs, or foods. The interactions listed here are based on reports in scientific publications, laboratory experiments, or traditional use. It is important to always read product labels. People who have a medical condition, or are taking other drugs, herbs, or supplements, should consult a qualified healthcare provider before starting a new therapy.

Interactions with Drugs

- Products rich in fenugreek fiber may interfere with the absorption of oral medications because of its mucilaginous content and high viscosity in the gut. Medications should be taken separately from such products.
- Data from pre-clinical studies and small, methodologically weak studies in humans suggest that fenugreek possesses both acute and chronic hypoglycemic properties. Concomitant use with other hypoglycemic agents may lower serum glucose more than expected, and levels should be monitored closely.
- Based on theory and limited reports, fenugreek should be used cautiously with anticoagulants, cardiac glycosides, corticosteroids, diuretics, hormone replacement therapy (HRT), laxatives, medications that decrease blood potassium levels, mineralocorticoids, monoamine oxidase inhibitors, oral contraceptives, and thyroid medications.

Interactions with Herbs and Dietary Supplements

- Preliminary evidence suggests that fenugreek may lower or raise blood sugar levels. Caution is advised in people who are using other herbs or supplements that also lower or raise blood sugar levels. Blood glucose levels may require monitoring, and doses may need adjustment. Examples of agents that also may lower blood sugar levels are *Aloe vera*, American ginseng, bilberry, bitter melon, burdock, dandelion, devil's claw, fish oil, gymnema, horse chestnut seed extract (HCSE), maitake mushroom, marshmallow, melatonin, milk thistle, *Panax ginseng*, rosemary, shark cartilage, Siberian ginseng, stinging nettle, and white horehound. Agents that may raise blood sugar levels include arginine, cocoa, DHEA, ephedra (when combined with caffeine), and melatonin.
- Based on theory and a case report, fenugreek may increase the risk of bleeding when taken with herbs and supplements that also may increase the risk of bleeding. Multiple cases of bleeding have been reported with the use of *Ginkgo biloba*, and fewer cases with garlic and saw palmetto. Numerous other agents theoretically may increase the risk of bleeding, although this has not been proven in most cases. Examples are alfalfa, American ginseng, angelica, anise, *Arnica montana*, asafetida, aspen bark, bilberry, birch, black cohosh, bladderwrack, bogbean, boldo, borage seed oil, bromelain, capsicum, cat's claw, celery, chamomile, chaparral, clove, coleus, cordyceps, dandelion, danshen, devil's claw, dong quai, EPA (eicosapentaenoic acid), evening primrose oil, feverfew, fish oil, flaxseed/flax powder (not a concern with flaxseed oil), ginger, grapefruit juice, grape seed, green tea, guggul, gymnestra, horse chestnut, horseradish, licorice root, lovage root, male fern, meadowsweet, melatonin, nordihydroguaiaretic acid (NDGA), omega-3 fatty acids, onion, *Panax ginseng*, papain, parsley, passion flower, poplar, prickly ash, propolis, quassia, red clover, reishi, rue, Siberian ginseng, sweet birch, sweet clover, turmeric, vitamin E, white willow, wild carrot, wild lettuce, willow, wintergreen, and yucca.
- Based on theory and limited reports, fenugreek should be used cautiously with agents that decrease blood potassium levels, diuretic agents, laxatives, phytoestrogens, and herbs with monoamine oxidase inhibitor (MAOI) properties.

Selected References

Natural Standard developed the preceding evidence-based information based on a systematic review of more than 110 articles. For comprehensive information about alternative and complementary therapies on the professional level, go to www.naturalstandard.com. Selected references are listed here.

Abdel-Barry JA, Abdel-Hassan IA, Jawad AM, et al. Hypoglycaemic effect of aqueous extract of the leaves of *Trigonella foenum-graecum* in healthy volunteers. East Mediterr Health J 2000;6(1):83-88.

Abdo MS, al Kafawi AA. Experimental studies on the effect of Trigonella foenum-graecum. Planta Med 1969;17(1):14-18.

Bartley GB, Hilty MD, Andreson BD, et al. "Maple-syrup" urine odor due to fenugreek ingestion. N Engl J Med 1981;305(8):467.

Bordia A, Verma SK, Srivastava KC. Effect of ginger (Zingiber officinale Rosc.) and fenugreek (Trigonella foenumgraecum L.) on blood lipids, blood sugar and platelet aggregation in patients with coronary artery disease. Prostaglandins Leukot Essent Fatty Acids 1997;56(5):379-384.

Gupta A, Gupta R, Lal B. Effect of Trigonella foenum-graecum (fenugreek) seeds on glycaemic control and insulin resistance in type 2 diabetes mellitus: a double blind placebo controlled study. J Assoc Physicians India 2001;49:1057-1061.

Lambert JP, Cormier A. Potential interaction between warfarin and boldo-fenugreek. Pharmacotherapy 2001;21(4):509-512.

Madar Z, Abel R, Samish S, et al. Glucose-lowering effect of fenugreek in non–insulin dependent diabetics. Eur J Clin Nutr 1988;42(1):51-54.

Mishkinsky J, Joseph B, Sulman FG. Hypoglycemic effect of trigonelline. Lancet 1967;2(7529): 1311-1312.

Neeraja A, Pajyalakshmi P. Hypoglycemic effect of processed fenugreek seeds in humans. J Food Sci Technol 1996;33(5):427-430.

Panda S, Tahiliani P, Kar A. Inhibition of triiodothyronine production by fenugreek seed extract in mice and rats. Pharmacol Res 1999;40(5):405-409.

Patil SP, Niphadkar PV, Bapat MM. Allergy to fenugreek (*Trigonella foenum-graecum*). Ann Allergy Asthma Immunol 1997;78(3):297-300.

Raghuram TC, Sharma RD, Sivakumar B, et al. Effect of fenugreek seeds on intravenous glucose disposition in non–insulin dependent diabetic patients. Phytotherapy Research 1994; 8(2):83-86.

Rao PU, Sesikeran B, Rao PS, et al. Short term nutritional and safety evaluation of fenugreek. Nutr Res 1996;16(9):1495-1505.

Sharma RD, Raghuram TC, Dayasagar Rao V. Hypolipidaemic effect of fenugreek seeds. A clinical study. Phytother Res 1991;3(5):145-147.

Sharma RD, Raghuram TC, Rao NS. Effect of fenugreek seeds on blood glucose and serum lipids in type I diabetes. Eur J Clin Nutrit 1990;44(4):301-306.

Sharma RD, Raghuram TC. Hypoglycaemic effect of fenugreek seeds in non–insulin dependant diabetic subjects. Nutr Res 1990;10:731-739.

Sharma RD, Sarkar A, Hazra DK, et al. Toxicological evaluation of fenugreek seeds: a long term feeding experiment in diabetic patients. Phytother Res 1996;10(6):519-520.

Sharma RD, Sarkar A, Hazra DK, et al. Use of fenugreek seed powder in the management of non–insulin dependent diabetes mellitus. Nutrit Res 1996;16(8):1331-1339.

Sharma RD, Sarkar DK, Hazra B, et al. Hypolipidaemic effect of fenugreek seeds: a chronic study in non–insulin dependent diabetic patients. Phytother Res 1996;10:332-334.

Sharma RD. Effect of fenugreek seeds and leaves on blood glucose and serum insulin responses in human subjects. Nutr Res 1986;6:1353-1364.

Sowmya P, Rajyalakshmi P. Hypocholesterolemic effect of germinated fenugreek seeds in human subjects. Plant Foods Hum Nutr 1999;53(4):359-365.

Tahiliani P, Kar A. Mitigation of thyroxine-induced hyperglycaemia by two plant extracts. Phytother Res 2003;17(3):294-296.

Topaloglu AK, Zeller WP, Andersen BD, et al. Maternal fenugreek ingestion simulating maple syrup urine odor in the infant. Ann Med Sci 1996;5(1):41-42.

Zia T, Hasnain SN, Hasan SK. Evaluation of the oral hypoglycaemic effect of *Trigonella foenum- graecum* L. (methi) in normal mice. J Ethnopharmacol 2001;75(2-3):191-195.

Feverfew

(*Tanacetum parthenium* L. Schultz-Bip.)

RELATED TERMS

- Altamisa, bachelor's button, camomille grande, chrysanthemum parthenium, featherfew, featherfoil, febrifuge plant, federfoy, flirtwort, *Leucanthemum parthenium*, *Matricaria capensis*, *Matricaria eximia* Hort., *Matricaria parthenium* L., midsummer daisy, mother herb, mutterkraut, nosebleed, parthenolide, *Pyrethrum parthenium* L., santa maria, wild chamomile, wild quinine.

F

BACKGROUND

- Feverfew is a herb that has been used traditionally as an antipyretic, as its name denotes, although this use has not been well studied.
- Feverfew most commonly is used orally for the prevention of migraine headache. There is a biochemical basis for this use in preclinical studies reporting anti-inflammatory and vascular (inhibition of vasoconstriction) effects. Several controlled human trials have been conducted, with mixed results. Overall, these studies suggest that feverfew taken daily as dried leaf capsules may reduce the incidence of headache attacks in patients who experience chronic migraines. However, this research has been poorly designed and reported. Evidence from an adequately powered randomized trial comparing feverfew with placebo and other migraine therapies is warranted before a strong recommendation can be made.
- There is currently inconclusive evidence regarding the use of feverfew for symptoms associated with rheumatoid arthritis.
- Feverfew appears to be well tolerated in clinical trials, with mild and reversible side effects. The most common adverse effects appear to be mouth ulceration and inflammation with direct exposure to leaves. Preclinical reports of platelet aggregation inhibition suggest a theoretical increased risk of bleeding.

USES BASED ON SCIENTIFIC EVIDENCE	Grade*
Migraine headache prevention Feverfew often is taken by mouth for the prevention of migraine headaches. Laboratory studies show that feverfew can reduce inflammation and prevent blood vessel constriction, which may lead to headaches. Most of the available studies in humans are not of high quality, and reported results are mixed. However, overall they do suggest that feverfew may reduce the number of headaches that occur in people with frequent migraines. A large, well-designed study comparing feverfew with placebo and other migraine treatments is needed before a strong recommendation can be made.	**B**

Continued

Rheumatoid arthritis It is not clear if feverfew is helpful for treating rheumatoid arthritis symptoms such as joint stiffness or pain.	C

*Key to grades: *A:* Strong scientific evidence for this use; *B:* Good scientific evidence for this use; *C:* Unclear scientific evidence for this use; *D:* Fair scientific evidence against this use (it may not work); *F:* Strong scientific evidence against this use (it likely does not work). For a more detailed explanation of efficacy criteria, see "Natural Standard Evidence-Based Validated Grading Rationale" in the Introduction.

Uses Based on Tradition, Theory, or Limited Scientific Evidence

Abdominal pain, anemia, anti-inflammatory, asthma, blood vessel dilation (relaxation), cancer, central nervous system diseases, colds, constipation, diarrhea, digestion promotion, dizziness, fever, joint pain, induction of labor/abortion, heart muscle injury, insect bites, insect repellent, leukemia, menstrual cramps, menstruation induction, neurologic complications of malaria, rash, ringing in the ears, toothache, tranquilizer, uterine disorders.

DOSING

The following doses are based on scientific research, publications, traditional use, or expert opinion. Many herbs and supplements have not been thoroughly tested, and their safety and effectiveness may not be proven. Brands may be made differently, with variable ingredients even within the same brand. The doses shown may not apply to all products. It is important to always read product labels and discuss doses with a qualified healthcare provider before therapy is started.

Standardization

Standardization involves measuring the amounts of certain chemicals to try to make different preparations similar to each other. It is not always known if the chemicals being measured are the "active" ingredients.

- The active agent in feverfew is thought to be parthenolide, although this has been questioned recently. The amount of parthenolide may vary depending on the origin of the plant or the parts of the plant included in a feverfew product. Recent research reports that available feverfew products may contain very different amounts of parthenolide. In England and Canada, feverfew products are standardized to contain at least 0.2% parthenolide. In France, products contain at least 0.1% parthenolide. There are no standard or well-studied doses of feverfew, and many different doses are used traditionally.

Adults (18 Years and Older)

- **Migraine headache prevention:** Traditional doses of feverfew taken by mouth include 2 to 3 dried leaves (approximately 60 mg) daily and 50 to 250 mg of a dried leaf preparation daily, standardized to 0.2% parthenolide (a common dose is 125 mg daily). Studies in humans have used 50 to 114 mg of powdered feverfew leaves daily, packed into capsules and standardized to 0.2% parthenolide, or 0.50 mg of parthenolide daily.

- **Rheumatoid arthritis:** Doses of 70 to 86 mg of dried chopped feverfew leaves in capsules, taken once daily, have been used.

Children (Younger Than 18 Years)

- There is not enough scientific information to safely recommend feverfew for use in children.

SAFETY

The U.S. Food and Drug Administration does not strictly regulate herbs and supplements. There is no guarantee of strength, purity, or safety of products, and effects may vary. It is important to always read product labels. People who have a medical condition, or are taking other drugs, herbs, or supplements, should consult a qualified healthcare provider before starting a new therapy. A healthcare provider should be consulted immediately about any side effects.

Allergies

- Feverfew may cause allergy in people allergic to chrysanthemums, daisies, marigolds, or other members of the Compositae family, including ragweed. There are multiple reports of allergic skin rashes after contact with feverfew.

Side Effects and Warnings

- Few side effects are reported in studies of feverfew in humans. The side effects that do occur usually are mild and reversible. The most common complaints are inflammation and ulcers of the mouth and bleeding of the gums, which usually occur after direct contact of the mouth with the leaves, although some people report burning after swallowing a capsule containing dried leaf. Swelling of the lips and loss of taste also have been noted. Photosensitivity (sensitivity to sunlight or sunlamps) has been reported with other herbs in the Compositae plant family and may be possible with feverfew as well. Indigestion, nausea, flatulence, constipation, diarrhea, abdominal bloating, and heartburn have been reported rarely in studies in humans. Gardeners may develop skin irritation at sites of contact with feverfew plants. Feverfew also can cause allergic rashes. One small study reported increased heart rate in some patients.
- Long-term feverfew users who stop treatment suddenly may experience feverfew withdrawal symptoms, including rebound headaches, anxiety, difficulty sleeping, muscle stiffness, and joint pain.
- Laboratory tests suggest that feverfew affects blood platelets and in theory may increase the risk of bleeding. However, this effect has not been clearly shown in humans. Nonetheless, caution is advised regarding use of this herb in patients with bleeding disorders or those taking drugs that may increase the risk of bleeding. Dosing adjustments may be necessary. Caution is advised with use of feverfew before some surgical or dental procedures, because of a theoretical increase in bleeding risk.

Pregnancy and Breastfeeding

- There is not enough information about safety to recommend use of feverfew in women who are pregnant or breastfeeding. Traditional experience suggests that feverfew may stimulate menstrual flow and induce abortion and therefore should be avoided.

INTERACTIONS

Most herbs and supplements have not been thoroughly tested for interactions with other herbs, supplements, drugs, or foods. The interactions listed here are based on reports in scientific publications, laboratory experiments, or traditional use. It is important to always read product labels. People who have a medical condition, or are taking other drugs, herbs, or supplements, should consult a qualified healthcare provider before starting a new therapy.

Interactions with Drugs

- As indicated by laboratory research, feverfew theoretically may increase the risk of bleeding when taken with drugs that increase the risk of bleeding. However, this effect has not been clearly shown in humans. Some examples are aspirin, anticoagulants ("blood thinners") such as warfarin (Coumadin) and heparin, antiplatelet drugs such as clopidogrel (Plavix), and nonsteroidal anti-inflammatory drugs such as ibuprofen (Motrin, Advil) and naproxen (Naprosyn, Aleve).
- Sun sensitivity caused by certain drugs may be increased by feverfew.

Interactions with Herbs and Dietary Supplements

- In theory, feverfew may increase the risk of bleeding when taken with herbs and supplements that also are believed to increase the risk of bleeding. This risk is based on laboratory research and has not been reported clearly in humans. Multiple cases of bleeding have been reported with the use of *Ginkgo biloba*, fewer cases with garlic, and two cases with saw palmetto. Numerous other agents theoretically may increase the risk of bleeding, although this effect has not been proven in most cases. Some examples are alfalfa, American ginseng, angelica, anise, *Arnica montana*, asafetida, aspen bark, bilberry, birch, black cohosh, bladderwrack, bogbean, boldo, borage seed oil, bromelain, capsicum, cat's claw, celery, chamomile, chaparral, clove, coleus, cordyceps, danshen, devil's claw, dong quai, evening primrose, fenugreek, flaxseed/flax powder (but not a concern with flaxseed oil), ginger, grapefruit juice, grapeseed, green tea, guggul, gymnestra, horse chestnut, horseradish, licorice root, lovage root, male fern, meadowsweet, nordihydroguaiaretic acid (NDGA), onion, *Panax ginseng*, papain, parsley, passionflower, poplar, prickly ash, propolis, quassia, red clover, reishi, rue, Siberian ginseng, sweet birch, sweet clover, turmeric, vitamin E, white willow, wild carrot, wild lettuce, willow, wintergreen, and yucca.
- Sun sensitivity caused by certain herbs and supplements, such as St. John's wort or Capsaicin, may be increased by feverfew.

Selected References

Natural Standard developed the preceding evidence-based information based on a systematic review of more than 175 scientific articles. For comprehensive information about alternative and complementary therapies on the professional level, go to www.naturalstandard.com. Selected references are listed here.

Abebe W. An overview of herbal supplement utilization with particular emphasis on possible interactions with dental drugs and oral manifestations. J Dent Hyg 2003;77(1):37-46.

Aldieri E, Atragene D, Bergandi L, et al. Artemisinin inhibits inducible nitric oxide synthase and nuclear factor NF-κB activation. FEBS Lett 2003;552(2-3):141-144.

Beaton A, Broadhurst MK, Wilkins RJ, et al. Suppression of beta-casein gene expression by inhibition of protein synthesis in mouse mammary epithelial cells is associated with stimulation of NF-kappaB activity and blockage of prolactin-Stat5 signaling. Cell Tissue Res 2003;311(2):207-215. Epub 2003 Jan 16.

Campos M, Oropeza M, Ponce H, et al. Relaxation of uterine and aortic smooth muscle by glaucolides D and E from *Vernonia liatroides*. Biol Pharm Bull 2003;26(1):112-115.

Cory AH, Cory JG. Lactacystin, a proteasome inhibitor, potentiates the apoptotic effect of parthenolide, an inhibitor of NFkappaB activation, on drug-resistant mouse leukemia L1210 cells. Anticancer Res 2002;22(6C):3805-3809.

DeWeerdt CJ, Bootsman H, Hendricks H. Herbal medicines in migraine prevention. Randomized double-blind placebo-controlled crossover trial of a feverfew preparation. Phytomedicine 1996;3(3):225-230.

Ernst E, Pittler MH. The efficacy and safety of feverfew (*Tanacetum parthenium* L.): an update of a systematic review. Public Health Nutr 2000;3(4A):509-514.

Fan X, Subramaniam R, Weiss MF, et al. Methylglyoxal-bovine serum albumin stimulates tumor necrosis factor alpha secretion in RAW 264.7 cells through activation of mitogen-activating protein kinase, nuclear factor kappaB and intracellular reactive oxygen species formation. Arch Biochem Biophys 2003;409(2):274-286.

Fiebich BL, Lieb K, Engels S, Heinrich M. Inhibition of LPS-induced p42/44 MAP kinase activation and iNOS/NO synthesis by parthenolide in rat primary microglial cells. J Neuroimmunol 2002;132(1-2):18-24.

Gu Z, Lee RY, Skaar TC, et al. Association of interferon regulatory factor-1, nucleophosmin, nuclear factor-kappaB, and cyclic AMP response element binding with acquired resistance to Faslodex (ICI 182,780). Cancer Res 2002;62(12):3428-3437.

Hausen BM, Osmundsen PE. Contact allergy to parthenolide in *Tanacetum parthenium* (L.) Schulz-Bip. (feverfew, Asteraceae) and cross-reactions to related sesquiterpene lactone containing Compositae species. Acta Derm Venereol 1983;63(4):308-314.

Heptinstall S, Awang DV, Dawson BA, et al. Parthenolide content and bioactivity of feverfew (*Tanacetum parthenium* [L.] Schultz-Bip.). Estimation of commercial and authenticated feverfew products. J Pharm Pharmacol 1992;44(5):391-395.

Jovanovic M, Poljacki M. [Compositae dermatitis]. Med Pregl 2003 Jan-Feb;56(1-2):43-49.

Kuritzky A, Elhacham Y, Yerushalmi Z, et al. Feverfew in the treatment of migraine: its effect on serotonin uptake and platelet activity. Neurology 1994;44(Suppl 2):A201.

Loesche W, Groenewegen WA, Krause S, et al. Effects of an extract of feverfew (*Tanacetum parthenium*) on arachidonic acid metabolism in human blood platelets. Biomed Biochim Acta 1988;47(10-11):S241-S243.

Loesche W, Mazurov AV, Voyno-Yasenetskaya TA, et al. Feverfew—an antithrombotic drug? Folia Haematol Int Mag Klin Morphol Blutforsch 1988;115(1-2):181-184.

Murphy JJ, Heptinstall S, Mitchell JR. Randomised double-blind placebo-controlled trial of feverfew in migraine prevention. Lancet 1988;2(8604):189-192.

Nelson MH, Cobb SE, Shelton J. Variations in parthenolide content and daily dose of feverfew products. Am J Health Syst Pharm 2002;59(16):1527-1531.

Palevitch D, Earon G, Carasso R. Feverfew (*Tanacetum parthenium*) as a prophylactic treatment for migraine: a double-blind placebo-controlled study. Phytother Res 1997;11(7): 508-511.

Pattrick M, Heptinstall S, Doherty M. Feverfew in rheumatoid arthritis: a double blind, placebo controlled study. Ann Rheum Dis 1989;48(7):547-549.

Pfaffenrath V, Fischer M, Friede M, et al. Clinical dose-response study for the investigation of efficacy and tolerability of *Tanacetum parthenium* in migraine prophylaxis [abstract]. Presented at Deutscher Schmerzkongress, Munich, October 20-24, 1999.

Pittler MH, Vogler BK, Ernst E. Feverfew for preventing migraine. Cochrane Database Syst Rev 2000;(4):CD002286.

Prusinski A, Durko A, Niczyporuk-Turek A. [Feverfew as a prophylactic treatment of migraine]. Neurol Neurochir Pol 1999;33(Suppl 5):89-95.

Rodriguez E, Epstein WL, Mitchell JC. The role of sesquiterpene lactones in contact hypersensitivity to some North and South American species of feverfew (*Parthenium*—Compositae). Contact Dermatitis 1977;3(3):155-162.

Sriramarao P, Nagpal S, Rao BS, et al. Immediate hypersensitivity to *Parthenium hysterophorus*. II. Clinical studies on the prevalence of *Parthenium* rhinitis. Clin Exp Allergy 1991;21(1): 55-62.

Sriramarao P, Selvakumar B, Damodaran C, et al. Immediate hypersensitivity to *Parthenium hysterophorus*. I. Association of HLA antigens and *Parthenium* rhinitis. Clin Exp Allergy 1990;20(5):555-560.
Vogler BK, Pittler MH, Ernst E. Feverfew as a preventive treatment for migraine: a systematic review. Cephalalgia 1998;18(10):704-708.
Waller PC, Ramsay LE. Efficacy of feverfew as prophylactic treatment of migraine. BMJ (Clin Res Ed) 1985;291(6502):1128.

Fish Oil/Omega-3 Fatty Acids

F

RELATED TERMS

- Alpha-linolenic acid (ALA), cod liver oil, coldwater fish, docosahexaenoic acid (DHA) (C22:6n-3), eicosapentaenoic acid (EPA) (C20:5n-3), fish body oil, fish extract, fish liver oil, fish oil fatty acids, halibut oil, α-linolenic acid (C18:3n-3), long-chain polyunsaturated fatty acids, mackerel oil, marine oil, menhaden oil, n-3 fatty acids, n-3 polyunsaturated fatty acids, omega-3 oils, polyunsaturated fatty acids (PUFA), salmon oil, shark liver oil, w-3 fatty acids.
- Omega-3 fatty acids should not be confused with omega-6 fatty acids.

BACKGROUND

- Dietary sources of omega-3 fatty acids include fish oil and certain plant/nut oils. Fish oil contains both docosahexaenoic acid (DHA) and eicosapentaenoic acid (EPA), whereas some nuts (English walnuts) and vegetable oils (canola, soybean, flaxseed/linseed, olive) contain alpha-linolenic acid (ALA).
- There is evidence from multiple large-scale population (epidemiologic) studies and randomized controlled trials that intake of recommended amounts of DHA and EPA in the form of dietary fish or fish oil supplements lowers triglycerides; reduces the risk of death, heart attack, dangerous abnormal heart rhythms, and strokes in people with known cardiovascular disease; slows the buildup of atherosclerotic plaques (hardening of the arteries); and lowers blood pressure slightly. However, high doses may have harmful effects, such as an increased risk of bleeding. Although similar benefits are proposed for ALA, scientific evidence is less compelling, and beneficial effects may be less pronounced.
- Some species of fish are more likely to take up environmental contaminants, such as methylmercury. These toxins can have adverse effects in persons who eat such fish.

USES BASED ON SCIENTIFIC EVIDENCE	Grade*
High blood pressure Multiple trials in humans report small reductions in blood pressure with intake of omega-3 fatty acids. Reductions of 2 to 5 mm Hg have been observed, and benefits may be greater in persons with higher blood pressures. Effects appear to be dose dependent (higher doses have greater effects). DHA may provide greater benefits than those obtainable with EPA. However, intakes of greater than 3 g of omega-3 fatty acids per day may be necessary to obtain clinically relevant effects, and at this dose level, there is an increased risk of bleeding. Therefore, a physician should be consulted before treatment with these supplements is initiated. Other approaches are known to have a greater beneficial effect on blood pressure, such as salt reduction, weight loss, exercise, and antihypertensive	A

Continued

drug therapy. Therefore, although omega-3 fatty acids do appear to have effects in this area, their role in the management of high blood pressure is limited.

Hypertriglyceridemia (fish oil/EPA plus DHA) **A**

There is strong scientific evidence from human trials that omega-3 fatty acids from fish or fish oil supplements (EPA plus DHA) significantly reduce blood triglyceride levels. Benefits appear to be dose dependent, with effects at doses as low as 2 g of omega-3 fatty acids per day. Higher doses have greater effects, and 4 g per day can lower triglyceride levels by 25% to 40%. Effects appear to be additive with (HMG-CoA reductase) inhibitor (statin) drugs such as simvastatin, pravastatin, and atorvastatin. The effects of fish oil on hypertriglyceridemia are similar in persons with and those without diabetes, and in patients with kidney disease receiving dialysis. It is not clear how fish oil therapy compares with other agents used for hypertriglyceridemia, such as fibrates (examples are gemfibrozil and fenofibrate) and niacin/nicotinic acid.

Fish oil supplements also appear to cause small improvements (relative increases) in levels of high-density lipoprotein (HDL)—"good cholesterol"—by 1% to 3%. However, increases (worsening) in levels of low-density lipoprotein (LDL)—"bad cholesterol"—by 5% to 10% also are observed. Therefore, in patients with high blood levels of total cholesterol or LDL, significant improvements will likely not be seen, and a different treatment should be selected. Fish oil does not appear to affect C-reactive protein (CRP) levels.

It is not clear if ALA significantly affects triglyceride levels, and there is conflicting evidence in this area.

The American Heart Association, in its 2003 recommendations, reports that supplementation with 2 to 4 g of EPA plus DHA each day can lower triglycerides by 20% to 40%. Because of the risk of bleeding associated with use of omega-3 fatty acids (particularly at doses greater than 3 g per day), a physician should be consulted before treatment with supplements is instituted.

Primary cardiovascular disease prevention (fish intake) **A**

Several large studies of populations (epidemiologic studies) report a significantly lower rate of death from heart disease in men and women who regularly eat fish. Other epidemiologic research reports no such benefit. It is not clear if benefits occur only in certain groups of people, such as those at risk of developing heart disease. Overall, the evidence suggests a beneficial effect for regular consumption of fish oil. However, well-designed randomized controlled trials that classify patients by their risk of developing heart disease are necessary before a firm conclusion can be drawn.

The American Heart Association, in its 2003 recommendations, suggests that all adults eat fish at least two times per week. In particular, fatty fish are recommended, including mackerel, lake trout, herring, sardines, albacore tuna, and salmon.

Continued

Secondary cardiovascular disease prevention (fish oil/ EPA plus DHA) Several well-conducted randomized controlled trials report that in people with a history of heart attack, regular consumption of oily fish (200 to 400 g of fish each week, equal to 500 to 800 mg of daily omega-3 fatty acids) or fish oil/omega-3 supplements (containing 850 to 1800 mg of EPA plus DHA) reduces the risk of nonfatal heart attack, fatal heart attack, sudden death, and all-cause mortality (death due to any cause). Most patients in these studies also were using conventional drugs for treatment of heart problems, suggesting that the benefits of fish oils may add to the effects of other therapies. Benefits have been reported after 3 months of use, and after up to 3½ years of follow-up. Benefits of supplements may not occur in populations in which consumption of large amounts of dietary fish is usual. Multiple mechanisms have been proposed for the beneficial effects of omega-3 fatty acids. Possible mechanisms include reduced triglyceride levels, reduced inflammation, slightly lowered blood pressure, reduced blood clotting, reduced tendency of the heart to develop abnormal rhythms, and diminished buildup of atherosclerotic plaques in arteries of the heart. Experiments suggest that omega-3 fatty acids may reduce platelet-derived growth factor (PDGF), decrease platelet aggregation, inhibit the expression of vascular cell adhesion molecules, and stimulate relaxation of endothelial cells in the walls of blood vessels. The American Heart Association, in its 2003 recommendations, suggests that people with known coronary heart disease should take approximately 1 g of EPA plus DHA (combined) each day. This may be obtained from eating fish or from taking fish oil capsule supplements. Because of the risk of bleeding associated with use of omega-3 fatty acids (particularly at doses greater than 3 g daily), a physician should be consulted before treatment with these supplements is started.	A
Protection from cyclosporine toxicity in organ transplant recipients In a number of studies, patients who received heart or kidney transplants were given the potentially toxic drug cyclosporine (Neoral), either alone or with fish oil supplements. A majority of the trials reported improvements in kidney function (increased glomerular filtration rate, decreased serum creatinine) and less hypertension (high blood pressure) in patients taking these supplements compared with those not taking fish oil. Although several recent studies report no improvement in kidney function, the weight of scientific evidence favors a beneficial effect of fish oil. No changes have been found in rates of rejection or graft (transplant) survival.	B
Rheumatoid arthritis (fish oil) Multiple randomized controlled trials report decreases in morning stiffness and joint tenderness with the regular intake of fish oil supplements for up to 3 months. Benefits have been reported as additive with	B

Continued

those of anti-inflammatory medications—nonsteroidal anti-inflammatory drugs (NSAIDs) such as ibuprofen and aspirin. However, because of weaknesses in study design and reporting, better research is necessary before a strong favorable recommendation can be made. Effects beyond 3 months of treatment have not been well evaluated.	
Secondary cardiovascular disease prevention (ALA) Several randomized controlled trials have examined the effects of ALA in people with a history of heart attack. Although some studies suggest benefits, others do not. Weaknesses in some of this research make results difficult to interpret, such as the use of other foods that also may be beneficial. Additional research is necessary before a conclusion regarding a preventive effect can be drawn.	**B**
Angina pectoris Preliminary studies report reductions in angina associated with fish oil intake. Better research is necessary before a firm conclusion can be drawn.	**C**
Asthma Several studies on the use of omega-3 fatty acids for asthma do not provide enough reliable evidence to form a clear conclusion, with some studies reporting no effects and others finding benefits. Because most studies have been small without clear descriptions of design or results, the findings cannot be considered conclusive.	
Atherosclerosis Some research reports that regular intake of fish or fish oil supplements reduces the risk of developing atherosclerotic plaques in the arteries of the heart, whereas other research has found no risk reduction. Additional evidence is necessary before a firm conclusion can be drawn regarding this effect.	**C**
Bipolar disorder Several studies of fish oil supplementation for management of patients with bipolar disorder do not provide enough reliable evidence to allow a clear conclusion to be drawn.	**C**
Cancer prevention Several population (epidemiologic) studies report that dietary omega-3 fatty acids or fish oil may reduce the risk of developing breast, colon, or prostate cancer. Randomized controlled trials are necessary before a clear conclusion can be drawn.	**C**
Cardiac arrhythmias (abnormal heart rhythms) There is promising evidence that omega-3 fatty acids may decrease the risk of cardiac arrhythmias. This is one proposed mechanism behind the reduced number of heart attacks in people who regularly ingest fish oil or EPA plus DHA. Additional research in this area of investigation is needed before a firm conclusion can be reached.	**C**

Continued

Colon cancer C

Omega-3 fatty acids are commonly taken by cancer patients. Although preliminary studies report that growth of colon cancer cells may be reduced by taking fish oil, effects on survival or remission have not been measured adequately.

Crohn's disease C

It has been suggested that the effects of omega-3 fatty acids on inflammation may be beneficial in patients with Crohn's disease when these supplements are added to standard therapy. Several studies have been conducted to investigate this use. Results are conflicting, and no clear conclusion can be drawn at this time.

Cystic fibrosis C

Research on the use of fish oil for cystic fibrosis is limited and does not provide enough reliable evidence to allow a clear conclusion to be drawn.

Depression C

Several studies on the use of fish oil for depression do not provide enough reliable evidence to allow a clear conclusion to be drawn. Promising initial evidence requires confirmation with larger, well-designed trials.

Dysmenorrhea (painful menstruation) C

It has been suggested that anti-inflammatory or prostaglandin-mediated mechanisms associated with omega-3 fatty acids may play a role in the management of dysmenorrhea. Preliminary evidence suggests possible benefits of fish oil/omega-3 fatty acids in patients with dysmenorrhea. Additional research is necessary before a firm conclusion can be reached.

Eczema C

Several studies on the use of EPA for eczema do not provide enough reliable evidence to allow a clear conclusion to be drawn.

IgA nephropathy C

There are conflicting results from several poorly designed trials of fish oil for IgA nephropathy.

Infant eye/brain development C

It has been suggested that fatty acids, particularly DHA, may be important for normal neurologic development. Fatty acids are added to some infant formulas. Several studies have examined the effects of DHA on development of vision in preterm infants. Short-term benefits have been reported as compared with outcomes with use of formulas without DHA, although these benefits may not be meaningful in the long term. Well-designed research is necessary before a clear conclusion can be reached.

Continued

Lupus erythematosus There is not enough reliable evidence to allow a clear conclusion to be drawn regarding use of fish oil for systemic lupus erythematosus and lupus nephritis.	C
Nephrotic syndrome There is not enough reliable evidence to allow a clear conclusion to be drawn regarding use of fish oil for nephrotic syndrome.	C
Preeclampsia Several studies of fish oil supplementation for prevention or treatment of preeclampsia do not provide enough reliable evidence to allow a clear conclusion to be drawn regarding this use.	C
Prevention of graft failure after heart bypass surgery There is limited study of the use of fish oils in patients following coronary artery bypass grafting (CABG). Initial research suggests possible small benefits in reducing blood clot formation in vein grafts. Additional evidence is necessary before a firm conclusion regarding a protective effect can be drawn.	
Prevention of restenosis after coronary angioplasty Several randomized controlled trials have evaluated whether omega-3 fatty acid intake reduces blockage of arteries in the heart following balloon angioplasty (percutaneous transluminal coronary angioplasty [PTCA]). Some research has reported small significant benefits, whereas other studies have not found benefits. The evidence in this area of investigation remains inconclusive.	
Primary cardiovascular disease prevention (ALA) Several large studies of populations (epidemiologic studies) report a significantly reduced risk of fatal or nonfatal heart attack in men and women who regularly consume foods high in ALA. Other epidemi-ologic research reports no such benefits. Although the existing evidence is compelling, weaknesses in this research make results difficult to interpret, such as the use of other foods that may also be beneficial, or effects of risk factors for heart disease such as smoking. Additional research is necessary before a conclusion regarding a preventive effect can be drawn. The American Heart Association, in its 2003 recommendations, suggests that in addition to eating fish at least two times per week, all adults should consume plant-derived sources of omega-3 fatty acids, such as tofu/soybeans, walnuts, flaxseed oil, and canola oil.	C
Psoriasis Several studies on the use of fish oil for psoriasis do not provide enough reliable evidence to allow a clear conclusion to be drawn.	C

Continued

Schizophrenia There is promising preliminary evidence from several randomized controlled trials of fish oil for management of patients with schizophrenia. Additional research is necessary before a firm conclusion can be reached.	C
Stroke prevention Several large studies of populations (epidemiologic studies) have examined the effects of omega-3 fatty acid intake on stroke risk. Some studies suggest benefits, whereas others do not. Effects are likely on ischemic or thrombotic stroke risk, and very large intakes of omega-3 fatty acids ("Eskimo" amounts) may actually increase the risk of hemorrhagic (bleeding) stroke. At this time, it is unclear if there are benefits in people with or without a history of stroke, or if effects of fish oil are comparable with those of other treatment strategies. Several mechanisms have been proposed for the beneficial effects of omega-3 fatty acids. Possible mechanisms include reduced triglyceride levels, reduced inflammation, slightly lowered blood pressure, reduced blood clotting, and diminished buildup of atherosclerotic plaques in blood vessels. Experiments suggest that omega-3 fatty acids may reduce platelet-derived growth factor (PDGF), decrease platelet aggregation, inhibit the expression of vascular cell adhesion molecules, and stimulate relaxation of endothelial cells in the walls of blood vessels.	C
Ulcerative colitis It has been suggested that the effects of omega-3 fatty acids on inflammation may be beneficial in patients with ulcerative colitis when these supplements are added to standard therapy. Several studies have been conducted to investigate this use. Although results have been promising, a majority of the trials are small and not well designed. Therefore, better research is necessary before a clear conclusion can be drawn.	C
Appetite/weight loss in cancer patients There is preliminary evidence that fish oil supplementation does not improve appetite or prevent weight loss in cancer patients.	D
Diabetes Although slight increases in fasting blood glucose levels have been noted in patients with type 2 (adult-onset) diabetes, the available scientific evidence suggests that there are no significant long-term effects of fish oil in patients with diabetes, including no changes in progression of diabetic nephropathy (kidney disease), albuminuria (protein in the urine), or hemoglobin A_{1c} levels. Most studies to investigate this use are not well designed. The effects of fish oil on hypertriglyceridemia are similar in patients with and those without diabetes.	D

Continued

Hypercholesterolemia Although fish oil reduces triglycerides, beneficial effects on blood cholesterol levels have not been demonstrated. Fish oil supplements appear to cause small increases in high-density lipoprotein ("good cholesterol") by 1% to 3%. However, increases (worsening) in LDL levels ("bad cholesterol") by 5% to 10% also are observed (the effects are dose dependent, with increases likely to occur at daily intakes of 1 g or greater of omega-3 fatty acids). Therefore, for patients with high blood levels of total cholesterol or LDL, significant improvements probably will not be seen, and a different treatment should be selected. Fish oil does not appear to affect C-reactive protein (CRP) levels. Several randomized trials in patients with familial hypercholesterolemia have yielded conflicting results.	**D**
Transplant rejection prevention (kidney and heart) In several studies, patients who received heart or kidney transplants were given the drug cyclosporine (Neoral) (to prevent rejection of the transplant), either alone or with fish oil supplements. A majority of the trials reported improvements in kidney function (increased glomerular filtration rate, decreased serum creatinine) and less hypertension (high blood pressure) in the supplementation group compared with the group of patients not taking fish oil. However, several recent studies report no benefits on kidney function, and no changes have been found in rates of rejection or graft (transplant) survival.	**D**

*Key to grades: *A:* Strong scientific evidence for this use; *B:* Good scientific evidence for this use; *C:* Unclear scientific evidence for this use; *D:* Fair scientific evidence against this use (it may not work); *F:* Strong scientific evidence against this use (it likely does not work). For a more detailed explanation of efficacy criteria, see "Natural Standard Evidence-Based Validated Grading Rationale" in the Introduction.

Uses Based on Tradition, Theory, or Limited Scientific Evidence

Acute myocardial infarction (heart attack), acute respiratory distress syndrome (ARDS), age-related macular degeneration, aggressive behavior, agoraphobia, AIDS, allergies, Alzheimer's disease, anthracycline-induced cardiac toxicity, anticoagulation, antiphospholipid syndrome, attention-deficit hyperactivity disorder (ADHD), autoimmune nephritis, bacterial infections, Behçet's syndrome, borderline personality disorder, breast cysts, breast tenderness, cartilage destruction, chronic fatigue syndrome, chronic obstructive pulmonary disease, cirrhosis, common cold, congestive heart failure, critical illness, dementia, dermatomyositis, diabetic nephropathy, diabetic neuropathy, dyslexia, dyspraxia, exercise performance enhancement, fibromyalgia, gallstones, gingivitis, glaucoma, glomerulonephritis, glycogen storage diseases, gout, hay fever, headache, hepatorenal syndrome, hypoxia, ichthyosis, immunosuppression, isotretinoin toxicity protection, kidney disease prevention, kidney stones, leprosy, leukemia, malaria, male

Continued

Uses Based on Tradition, Theory, or Limited Scientific Evidence *(cont'd)*

infertility, mastalgia (breast pain), memory enhancement, menopausal symptoms, menstrual cramps, multiple sclerosis, myopathy, neuropathy, night vision enhancement, obesity, omega-3 fatty acid deficiency, osteoarthritis, osteoporosis, otitis media (ear infection), panic disorder, peripheral vascular disease, postviral fatigue syndrome, pregnancy nutritional supplement, premature birth prevention, premenstrual syndrome, prostate cancer prevention, Raynaud's phenomenon, Refsum's syndrome, Reye's syndrome, seizure disorder, systemic lupus erythematosus, tardive dyskinesia, tennis elbow, urolithiasis (bladder stones), vision enhancement.

DOSING

The following doses are based on scientific research, publications, traditional use, or expert opinion. Many herbs and supplements have not been thoroughly tested, and their safety and effectiveness may not be proven. Brands may be made differently, with variable ingredients even within the same brand. The doses shown may not apply to all products. It is important to read product labels and discuss doses with a qualified healthcare provider before therapy is started.

Standardization

- **General:** For fish oil supplements, dosing should be based on the amount of EPA and DHA (omega-3 fatty acids) in a product, not on the total amount of fish oil. Supplements vary in the amounts and ratios of EPA and DHA. Fish oil capsules commonly contain omega-3 fatty acids in the amounts of 0.18 g (180 mg) of EPA and 0.12 g (120 mg) of DHA. Five grams of fish oil contains approximately 0.17 to 0.56 g (170 to 560 mg) of EPA and 0.072 to 0.31 g (72 to 310 mg) of DHA. Different types of fish contain variable amounts of omega-3 fatty acids, and different types of nuts or oil contain variable amounts of ALA.
- **Amounts of seafood necessary to provide 1 g of DHA plus EPA** (based on USDA Nutrient Data Laboratory information): cod (Pacific): 23 g; haddock: 15 g; catfish: 15 to 20 g; flounder/sole: 7 g; shrimp: 11 g; lobster: 7.5 to 42.5 g; sardines: 2 to 3 g; crab: 8.5 g; cod (Atlantic): 12.5 g; clams: 12.5 g; scallops: 17.5 g; trout: 3 to 3.5 g; salmon: 1.4 to 4.5 g; herring: 1.5 to 2 g; oysters: 2.5 to 8 g; tuna (fresh): 2.5 to 12 g; tuna (canned, light): 12 g; tuna (canned, white): 4 g; halibut: 3 to 7.5 g; mackerel: 2 to 8.5 g.
- **Amounts of ALA in nuts and vegetable oils** (based on USDA Nutrient Data Laboratory information): canola oil: 1.3 g per tablespoon; flaxseed/linseed oil: 8.5 g per tablespoon; flaxseeds: 2.2 g per tablespoon; olive oil: 0.1 g per tablespoon; soybean oil: 0.9 g per tablespoon; walnut oil: 1.4 g per tablespoon; walnuts (English): 0.7 g per tablespoon.
- **Calories:** Fish oils contain approximately 9 calories per gram of oil.
- **Vitamin E:** Fish oil taken for many months may cause a deficiency of vitamin E, and therefore vitamin E is added to many commercial fish oil products.

Adults (18 Years and Older)

- **Average dietary intake of omega-3/omega-6 fatty acids:** Average Americans consume approximately 1.6 g of omega-3 fatty acids each day, of which about 1.4 g (approximately 90%) comes from ALA and only 0.1 to 0.2 g (approximately

10%) from EPA and DHA. In Western diets, people consume roughly 10 times more omega-6 fatty acids than omega-3 fatty acids. These large amounts of omega-6 fatty acids come from commonly used vegetable oils containing linoleic acid (for example, corn oil, evening primrose oil, pumpkin oil, safflower oil, sesame oil, soybean oil, sunflower oil, walnut oil, wheatgerm oil). Because omega-6 and omega-3 fatty acids compete with each other to be converted to active metabolites in the body, benefits can be achieved either by decreasing intake of omega-6 fatty acids or by increasing omega-3 fatty acids.

- **Recommended daily intake of omega-3 fatty acids (healthy adults):** For healthy adults with no history of heart disease, the American Heart Association recommends eating fish at least two times per week. In particular, fatty fish are recommended, such as anchovies, bluefish, carp, catfish, halibut, herring, lake trout, mackerel, pompano, salmon, striped sea bass, tuna (albacore), and whitefish. It is also recommended to consume plant-derived sources of ALA, such as tofu/soybeans, walnuts, flaxseed oil, and canola oil. The World Health Organization and governmental health agencies of several countries recommend consuming 0.3 to 0.5 g of daily EPA plus DHA and 0.8 to 1.1 g of daily ALA.
- **Hypertriglyceridemia:** The effects of omega-3 fatty acid intake on triglyceride lowering are dose responsive (higher doses have greater effects). Benefits are seen at daily doses less than 2 g of omega-3 fatty acids from EPA and DHA, although higher doses may be necessary in people with marked hypertriglyceridemia (triglyceride level greater than 750 mg/dl). The American Heart Association, in its 2003 recommendations, reports that supplementation with 2 to 4 g of EPA plus DHA each day can lower triglycerides by 20% to 40%. Effects appear to be additive with those of HMG-CoA reductase inhibitor (statin) drugs such as simvastatin (Zocor), pravastatin (Pravachol), and atorvastatin (Lipitor). Because of the risk of bleeding associated with use of omega-3 fatty acids (particularly at daily doses greater than 3 g), a physician should be consulted before treatment with supplements is started.
- **Heart disease (secondary prevention):** In people with a history of heart attack, regular consumption of oily fish (200 to 400 g of fish each week equal to 0.5 to 0.8 g [500 to 800 mg] of daily omega-3 fatty acids) or fish oil/omega-3 supplements (containing 0.85 to 1.8 g [850 to 1800 mg] of EPA plus DHA) appears to reduce the risk of nonfatal heart attack, fatal heart attack, sudden death, and all-cause mortality (death due to any cause). The American Heart Association, in its 2003 recommendations, suggests that people with known coronary heart disease consume approximately 1 g of EPA plus DHA (combined) each day. This may be obtained from eating fish or from fish oil capsule supplements. Because of the risk of bleeding associated with use of omega-3 fatty acids (particularly at daily doses greater than 3 g), a physician should be consulted before treatment with supplements is started.
- **High blood pressure:** The effects of omega-3 fatty acids on blood pressure appear to be dose responsive (higher doses have greater effects). However, intakes of greater than 3 g of omega-3 fatty acids per day may be necessary to obtain clinically relevant effects, and at this dose level, there is an increased risk of bleeding. Therefore, a physician should be consulted before treatment with supplements is started.
- **Rheumatoid arthritis:** Clinical trials have used a range of doses, most commonly between 3 and 5 g of EPA plus DHA daily (1.7 to 3.8 g of EPA and 1.1 to 2.0 g of DHA). Effects beyond 3 months of treatment have not been well evaluated.

- **Protection from cyclosporine toxicity in organ transplant recipients:** Studies have used 6 g of fish oil per day for up to 1 year. Some research has used doses starting at 3 g daily for 6 weeks and then increased to 6 g daily. Up to 12 g daily has been used.
- **Other:** Omega-3 fatty acids are used for numerous other indications, although effective doses are not clearly established.

Children (Younger Than 18 Years)

- Omega-3 fatty acids are used in some infant formulas, although effective doses are not clearly established. Ingestion of fresh fish should be limited in young children because of the presence of potentially harmful environmental contaminants. Fish oil capsules should not be used in children except under the direction of a physician.

SAFETY

The U.S. Food and Drug Administration does not strictly regulate herbs and supplements. There is no guarantee of strength, purity, or safety of products, and effects may vary. It is important to always read product labels. People who have a medical condition, or are taking other drugs, herbs, or supplements, should consult a qualified healthcare provider before starting a new therapy. A healthcare provider should be consulted immediately about any side effects.

Allergies

- People with allergy or hypersensitivity to fish should avoid fish oil or omega-3 fatty acid products derived from fish. Skin rash has been reported rarely. People with allergy or hypersensitivity to nuts should avoid ALA or omega-3 fatty acid products that are derived from the types of nuts to which they react.

Side Effects and Warnings

- **General:** The U.S. Food and Drug Administration classifies intake of up to 3 g per day of omega-3 fatty acids from fish as GRAS (generally regarded as safe). Caution may be warranted, however, in diabetic patients because of potential (albeit unlikely) increases in blood sugar levels, in patients at risk of bleeding, or in those with high LDL levels. Fish meat may contain methylmercury, and caution is warranted in young children and pregnant or breastfeeding women.
- **Bleeding:** Intake of 3 g or greater of omega-3 fatty acids daily may increase the risk of bleeding, although there is little evidence of significant bleeding risk at lower doses. Very large intakes of fish oil/omega-3 fatty acids ("Eskimo" amounts) may increase the risk of hemorrhagic (bleeding) stroke. High doses also have been associated with nosebleed and blood in the urine. Fish oils appear to decrease platelet aggregation and prolong bleeding time and to increase fibrinolysis (breaking down of blood clots) and may reduce levels of von Willebrand factor.
- **Environmental contamination:** Potentially harmful contaminants such as dioxins, methylmercury, and polychlorinated biphenyls (PCBs) are found in some species of fish. Methylmercury accumulates in fish flesh in greater concentrations than in fish oil, and fish oil supplements appear to contain almost no mercury. Therefore, safety concerns apply to eating fish but probably not to ingesting fish oil supplements. Heavy metals are most harmful in young children and pregnant/nursing women. For sport-caught fish, the U.S. Environmental Protection Agency recommends that intake be limited in pregnant/nursing women to a single 6-ounce meal

per week, and in young children to less than 2 ounces per week. For farm-raised, imported, or marine fish, the U.S. Food and Drug Administration recommends that pregnant/nursing women and young children avoid eating types with higher levels of methylmercury (approximately 1 part per million, such as mackerel, shark, swordfish, or tilefish), and less than 12 ounces per week of other fish types. Women who might become pregnant are advised to limit weekly consumption to 7 ounces or less of fish with higher levels of methylmercury (up to 1 part per million), or 14 ounces of fish types with lower levels (approximately 0.5 part per million), such as marlin, orange roughy, red snapper, and fresh tuna. Unrefined fish oil preparations may contain pesticides.

- **Gastrointestinal symptoms:** Gastrointestinal upset is common with the use of fish oil supplements, occurring in up to 5% of patients in clinical trials, with nausea in up to 1.5% of patients. Diarrhea also may occur, with potentially severe diarrhea at very high doses. There also are reports of increased burping, acid reflux/heartburn/indigestion, abdominal bloating, and abdominal pain. Fishy aftertaste is a common effect. Gastrointestinal side effects can be minimized if fish oils are taken with meals and if doses are started low and gradually increased.
- **Blood pressure effects:** Multiple trials in humans report small reductions in blood pressure with intake of omega-3 fatty acids. Reductions of 2 to 5 mm Hg have been observed, and effects appear to be dose dependent (higher doses have greater effects). DHA may have greater effects than those obtained with EPA. Caution is warranted in patients with low blood pressure or in those taking blood pressure–lowering medications.
- **Blood sugar levels/diabetes:** Although slight increases in fasting blood glucose levels have been noted in patients with type 2 (adult-onset) diabetes, the available scientific evidence suggests that there are no significant long-term effects of fish oil in patients with diabetes, including no changes in hemoglobin A_{1c} levels. Earlier, limited reports described increased need for insulin in diabetic patients taking long-term fish oil supplements, but this effect may have been related to other dietary changes or weight gain.
- **Vitamin levels:** Fish oil taken for many months may cause a deficiency of vitamin E; therefore, vitamin E is added to many commercial fish oil products. As a result, regular use of vitamin E–enriched products may lead to elevated levels of this fat-soluble vitamin. Fish liver oil contains the fat-soluble vitamins A and D; thus, fish liver oil products (such as cod liver oil) may increase the risk of vitamin A or D toxicity.
- **Cholesterol levels:** Increases (worsening) in LDL ("bad cholesterol") levels by 5% to 10% are observed with intake of omega-3 fatty acids. Effects are dose dependent, with increases likely to occur at daily intakes of 1 g or greater of omega-3 fatty acids.
- **Liver (hepatic) effects:** Mild elevations in liver enzymes (alanine aminotransferase), reflecting altered liver function, have been reported rarely.
- **Dermatologic effects:** Skin rashes have been reported rarely.
- **Neurologic/psychiatric effects:** There are rare reports of mania in patients with bipolar disorder or major depression who are taking fish oil supplements. Restlessness and formication (the sensation of ants crawling on the skin) also have been reported.
- **Calories:** Fish oils contain approximately 9 calories per gram of oil.

Pregnancy and Breastfeeding

- Potentially harmful contaminants such as dioxins, methylmercury, and polychlorinated biphenyls (PCBs) are found in some species of fish and may be harmful in pregnant or nursing women. Methylmercury accumulates in fish flesh more than in fish oil, and fish oil supplements appear to contain almost no mercury. Therefore, these safety concerns apply to eating fish but likely not to ingesting fish oil supplements. However, unrefined fish oil preparations may contain pesticides.
- For sport-caught fish, the U.S. Environmental Protection Agency recommends that intake be limited in pregnant or nursing women to a single 6-ounce meal per week. For farm-raised, imported, or marine fish, the U.S. Food and Drug Administration recommends that pregnant or nursing women avoid eating types with higher levels of methylmercury (approximately 1 part per million), such as mackerel, shark, swordfish, or tilefish, and limit weekly intake to less than 12 ounces of other fish types.
- Women who might become pregnant are advised to eat no more than 7 ounces per week of fish with higher levels of methylmercury (up to 1 part per million), or no more than 14 ounces per week of fish types with lower levels (approximately 0.5 part per million), such as marlin, orange roughy, red snapper, and fresh tuna.
- It is not known if maternal omega-3 fatty acid supplementation during pregnancy or the period of breastfeeding is beneficial to infants. It has been suggested that high intake of omega-3 fatty acids during pregnancy, particularly DHA, may increase birth weight and length of the gestational period. However, higher doses may not be advisable because of the potential risk of bleeding. Fatty acids are added to some infant formulas.

INTERACTIONS

Most herbs and supplements have not been thoroughly tested for interactions with other herbs, supplements, drugs, or foods. The interactions listed here are based on reports in scientific publications, laboratory experiments, or traditional use. It is important to always read product labels. People who have a medical condition, or are taking other drugs, herbs, or supplements, should consult a qualified healthcare provider before starting a new therapy.

Interactions with Drugs

- In theory, omega-3 fatty acids may increase the risk of bleeding when taken with drugs that also increase the risk of bleeding. Some examples are aspirin, anticoagulants (blood thinners) such as warfarin (Coumadin) and heparin, antiplatelet drugs such as clopidogrel (Plavix), and nonsteroidal anti-inflammatory drugs such as ibuprofen (Motrin, Advil) and naproxen (Naprosyn, Aleve).
- As indicated by studies in humans, omega-3 fatty acids may lower blood pressure and add to the effects of drugs that also may affect blood pressure.
- Fish oil supplements may lower blood sugar levels slightly. Caution is advised with use of these supplements with medications that also may lower blood sugar. Patients taking drugs for diabetes by mouth or insulin should be monitored closely by a qualified healthcare provider. Medication adjustments may be necessary.
- Omega-3 fatty acids lower triglyceride levels but can actually increase (worsen) LDL ("bad cholesterol") levels by a small amount. Therefore, omega-3 fatty acids may add to the triglyceride-lowering effects of agents such as niacin/nicotinic acid, fibrates such as gemfibrozil (Lopid), and resins such as cholestyramine (Questran).

However, omega-3 fatty acids may work against the LDL-lowering properties of statin drugs such as atorvastatin (Lipitor) and lovastatin (Mevacor).

Interactions with Herbs and Dietary Supplements

- In theory, omega-3 fatty acids may increase the risk of bleeding when taken with herbs and supplements that are believed to increase the risk of bleeding. Multiple cases of bleeding have been reported with the use of *Ginkgo biloba*, and fewer cases with garlic and saw palmetto. Numerous other agents may theoretically increase the risk of bleeding, although this effect has not been proven in most cases. Some examples are alfalfa, American ginseng, angelica, anise, *Arnica montana*, asafetida, aspen bark, bilberry, birch, black cohosh, bladderwrack, bogbean, boldo, borage seed oil, bromelain, capsicum, cat's claw, celery, chamomile, chaparral, clove, coleus, cordyceps, danshen, devil's claw, dong quai, evening primrose oil, fenugreek, feverfew, flaxseed/flaxseed powder (not a concern with flaxseed oil), ginger, grapefruit juice, grapeseed, green tea, guggul, gymnestra, horse chestnut, horseradish, licorice root, lovage root, male fern, meadowsweet, nordihydroguaiaretic acid (NDGA), onion, *Panax ginseng*, papain, parsley, passion flower, poplar, prickly ash, propolis, quassia, red clover, reishi, rue, Siberian ginseng, sweet birch, sweet clover, turmeric, vitamin E, white willow, wild carrot, wild lettuce, willow, wintergreen, and yucca.
- As suggested by studies in humans, omega-3 fatty acids may lower blood pressure and theoretically may add to the effects of agents that also may affect blood pressure. Examples are aconite/monkshood, arnica, baneberry, betel nut, bilberry, black cohosh, bryony, calendula, California poppy, coleus, curcumin, eucalyptol, eucalyptus oil, flaxseed/flaxseed oil, garlic, ginger, ginkgo, goldenseal, green hellebore, hawthorn, Indian tobacco, jaborandi, mistletoe, night-blooming cereus, oleander, pasque flower, periwinkle, pleurisy root, *Polypodium vulgare*, shepherd's purse, Texas milkweed, turmeric, and wild cherry.
- Fish oil supplements may lower blood sugar levels slightly. Caution is advised with use of herbs or supplements that also may lower blood sugar. Blood glucose levels may require monitoring, and doses may need adjustment. Possible examples are *Aloe vera*, American ginseng, bilberry, bitter melon, burdock, fenugreek, gymnema, horse chestnut seed extract (HCSE), maitake mushroom, marshmallow, milk thistle, *Panax ginseng*, rosemary, shark cartilage, Siberian ginseng, stinging nettle, and white horehound. Agents that may raise blood sugar levels include arginine, cocoa, and ephedra (when combined with caffeine).
- Omega-3 fatty acids lower triglyceride levels but can actually increase (worsen) levels of LDL ("bad cholesterol") by a small amount. Therefore, omega-3 fatty acids may add to the triglyceride-lowering effects of agents such as niacin/nicotinic acid but may work against the potential LDL-lowering properties of agents such as barley, garlic, guggul, psyllium, soy, and sweet almond.
- Fish oil taken for many months may cause a deficiency of vitamin E; therefore, vitamin E is added to many commercial fish oil products. As a result, regular use of vitamin E–enriched products may lead to elevated levels of this fat-soluble vitamin. Fish liver oil contains the fat-soluble vitamins A and D; thus, fish liver oil products (such as cod liver oil) may increase the risk of vitamin A or D toxicity. Because fat-soluble vitamins can build up in the body and cause toxicity, patients taking multiple vitamins regularly or in high doses should discuss this risk with their healthcare practitioners.

Selected References

Natural Standard developed the preceding evidence-based patient information based on a systematic review of more than 1000 articles. For comprehensive information about alternative and complementary therapies on the professional level, go to www.naturalstandard.com. Selected references are listed here.

Albert CM, Hennekens CH, O'Donnell CJ, et al. Fish consumption and risk of sudden cardiac death. JAMA 1998;279(1):23-28.

Andreassen AK, Hartmann A, Offstad J, et al. Hypertension prophylaxis with omega-3 fatty acids in heart transplant recipients. J Am Coll Cardiol 1997;29(6):1324-1331.

Anonymous. Dietary supplementation with n-3 polyunsaturated fatty acids and vitamin E after myocardial infarction: results of the GISSI-Prevenzione trial. Gruppo Italiano per lo Studio della Sopravvivenza nell'Infarto Miocardico. Lancet 1999;354(9177):447-455.

Anonymous. Dietary supplementation with n-3 polyunsaturated fatty acids and vitamin E after myocardial infarction: results of the GISSI-Prevenzione trial. Gruppo Italiano per lo Studio della Sopravvivenza nell'Infarto Miocardico. Lancet 1999;354(9177):447-455.

Appel LJ, Miller ER, III, Seidler AJ, et al. Does supplementation of diet with 'fish oil' reduce blood pressure? A meta-analysis of controlled clinical trials. Arch Intern Med 1993;153(12): 1429-1438.

Archer SL, Green D, Chamberlain M, et al. Association of dietary fish and n-3 fatty acid intake with hemostatic factors in the coronary artery risk development in young adults (CARDIA) study. Arterioscler Thromb Vasc Biol 1998;18(7):1119-1123.

Arm JP, Horton CE, Mencia-Huerta JM, et al. Effect of dietary supplementation with fish oil lipids on mild asthma. Thorax 1988;43(2):84-92.

Arm JP, Horton CE, Spur BW, et al. The effects of dietary supplementation with fish oil lipids on the airways response to inhaled allergen in bronchial asthma. Am Rev Respir Dis 1989; 139(6):1395-1400.

Ascherio A, Rimm EB, Giovannucci EL, et al. Dietary fat and risk of coronary heart disease in men: cohort follow up study in the United States. BMJ 1996;313(7049):84-90.

Aslan A, Triadafilopoulos G. Fish oil fatty acid supplementation in active ulcerative colitis: a double-blind, placebo-controlled, crossover study. Am J Gastroenterol 1992;87(4):432-437.

Aucamp AK, Schoeman HS, Coetzee JH. Pilot trial to determine the efficacy of a low dose of fish oil in the treatment of angina pectoris in the geriatric patient. Prostaglandins Leukot Essent Fatty Acids 1993;49(3):687-689.

Augustsson K, Michaud DS, Rimm EB, et al. A prospective study of intake of fish and marine fatty acids and prostate cancer. Cancer Epidemiol Biomarkers Prev 2003;12(1):64-67.

Badalamenti S, Salerno F, Lorenzano E, et al. Renal effects of dietary supplementation with fish oil in cyclosporine- treated liver transplant recipients. Hepatology 1995;22(6):1695-1770.

Bakker DJ, Haberstroh BN, Philbrick DJ, et al. Triglyceride lowering in nephrotic syndrome patients consuming a fish oil concentrate. Nutr Res 1989;9:27-34.

Balestrieri GP, Maffi V, Sleiman I, et al. Fish oil supplementation in patients with heterozygous familial hypercholesterolemia. Recent Prog Med 1996;87(3):102-105.

Barber MD, Ross JA, Preston T, et al. Fish oil–enriched nutritional supplement attenuates progression of the acute-phase response in weight-losing patients with advanced pancreatic cancer. J Nutr 1999;129(6):1120-1125.

Barber MD, Ross JA, Voss AC, et al. The effect of an oral nutritional supplement enriched with fish oil on weight-loss in patients with pancreatic cancer. Br J Cancer 1999;81(1):80-86.

Barberger-Gateau P, Letenneur L, Deschamps V, et al. Fish, meat, and risk of dementia: cohort study. BMJ 2002;325(7370):932-933.

Beckles WI, Elliott TM, Everard ML. Omega-3 fatty acids (from fish oils) for cystic fibrosis. Cochrane Database Syst Rev 2002;(3.):CD002201.

Beckles WI, Willson N, Elliott TM, Everard ML. Omega-3 fatty acids (from fish oils) for cystic fibrosis. Cochrane Database Syst Rev 2002;(3):CD002201. Review.

Belluzzi A, Brignola C, Boschi S, et al. A novel enteric coated preparation of omega-3 fatty acids in a group of steroid-dependent ulcerative colitis: an open study [abstract]. Gastroenterology 1997;112(Suppl):A930.

Belluzzi A, Brignola C, Campieri M, et al. Effects of new fish oil derivative on fatty acid phospholipid-membrane pattern in a group of Crohn's disease patients. Dig Dis Sci 1994; 39(12):2589-2594.

Bemelmans WJ, Broer J, Feskens EJ, et al. Effect of an increased intake of alpha-linolenic acid and group nutritional education on cardiovascular risk factors: the Mediterranean Alpha-Linolenic Enriched Groningen Dietary Intervention (MARGARIN) study. Am J Clin Nutr 2002;75(2):221-227.

Bennett WM, Carpenter CB, Shapiro ME, et al. Delayed omega-3 fatty acid supplements in renal transplantation. A double-blind, placebo-controlled study. Transplantation 1995;59(3): 352-356.

Berthoux FC, Guerin C, Burgard G, et al. One-year randomized controlled trial with omega-3 fatty acid-fish oil in clinical renal transplantation. Transplant Proc 1992;24(6):2578-2582.

Birch DG, Birch EE, Hoffman DR, et al. Retinal development in very-low-birth-weight infants fed diets differing in omega-3 fatty acids. Invest Ophthalmol Vis Sci 1992;33(8):2365-2376.

Birch EE, Birch DG, Hoffman DR, et al. Dietary essential fatty acid supply and visual acuity development. Invest Ophthalmol Vis Sci 1992;33(11):3242-3253.

Bittiner SB, Tucker WF, Bleehen S. Fish oil in psoriasis—a double-blind randomized placebo-controlled trial. Br J Dermatol 1987;117:25-26.

Bittiner SB, Tucker WF, Cartwright I, et al. A double-blind, randomised, placebo-controlled trial of fish oil in psoriasis. Lancet 1988;1(8582):378-380.

Bjorneboe A, Smith AK, Bjorneboe GE, et al. Effect of dietary supplementation with n-3 fatty acids on clinical manifestations of psoriasis. Br J Dermatol 1988;118(1):77-83.

Bjorneboe A, Soyland E, Bjorneboe GE, et al. Effect of dietary supplementation with eicosapentaenoic acid in the treatment of atopic dermatitis. Br J Dermatol 1987;117(4): 463-469.

Bjorneboe A, Soyland E, Bjorneboe GE, et al. Effect of n-3 fatty acid supplement to patients with atopic dermatitis. J Intern Med Suppl 1989;225(731):233-236.

Bonaa KH, Bjerve KS, Straume B, et al. Effect of eicosapentaenoic and docosahexaenoic acids on blood pressure in hypertension. A population-based intervention trial from the Tromso study. N Engl J Med 1990;322(12):795-801.

Brouwer RM, Wenting GJ, Pos B, et al. Fish oil ameliorates established cyclosporin A nephrotoxicity after heart transplantation [abstract]. Kidney Int 1991;40:347-348.

Bruera E, Strasser F, Palmer JL, et al. Effect of fish oil on appetite and other symptoms in patients with advanced cancer and anorexia/cachexia: a double-blind, placebo-controlled study. J Clin Oncol 2003;21(1):129-134.

Bucher HC, Hengstler P, Schindler C, et al. N-3 polyunsaturated fatty acids in coronary heart disease: a meta- analysis of randomized controlled trials. Am J Med 2002;112(4):298-304.

Bulstra-Ramakers MT, Huisjes HJ, Visser GH. The effects of 3 g eicosapentaenoic acid daily on recurrence of intrauterine growth retardation and pregnancy induced hypertension. Br J Obstet Gynaecol 1994;102:123-126.

Burr ML, Fehily AM, Gilbert JF, et al. Effects of changes in fat, fish, and fibre intakes on death and myocardial reinfarction: diet and reinfarction trial (DART). Lancet 1989;2(8666): 757-761.

Burr ML, Sweetham PM, Fehily AM. Diet and reinfarction. Eur Heart J 1994;15(8):1152-1153.

Cairns JA, Gill J, Morton B, et al. Fish oils and low-molecular-weight heparin for the reduction of restenosis after percutaneous transluminal coronary angioplasty. The EMPAR Study. Circulation 1996;94(7):1553-1560.

Calabrese JR, Rapport DJ, Shelton MD. Fish oils and bipolar disorder: a promising but untested treatment. Arch Gen Psychiatry 1999;56(5):413-414.

Carlson SE, Werkman SH, Rhodes PG, et al. Visual-acuity development in healthy preterm infants: effect of marine- oil supplementation. Am J Clin Nutr 1993;58(1):35-42.

Carlson SE, Werkman SH, Tolley EA. Effect of long-chain n-3 fatty acid supplementation on visual acuity and growth of preterm infants with and without bronchopulmonary dysplasia. Am J Clin Nutr 1996;63(5):687-697.

Carlson SE, Werkman SH. A randomized trial of visual attention of preterm infants fed docosahexaenoic acid until two months. Lipids 1996;31(1):85-90.

Caygill CP, Hill MJ. Fish, n-3 fatty acids and human colorectal and breast cancer mortality. Eur J Cancer Prev 1995;4(4):329-332.

Chan DC, Watts GF, Barrett PH, et al. Effect of atorvastatin and fish oil on plasma high-sensitivity C-reactive protein concentrations in individuals with visceral obesity. Clin Chem 2002;48(6 Pt 1):877-883.
Chiu CC, Huang SY, Shen WW, et al. Omega-3 fatty acids for depression in pregnancy. Am J Psychiatry 2003;160(2):385.
Christensen JH, Gustenhoff P, Ejlersen E, et al. n-3 fatty acids and ventricular extrasystoles in patients with ventricular tachyarrhythmias. Nutr Res 1995;15(1):1-8.
Christensen JH, Gustenhoff P, Korup E, et al. Effect of fish oil on heart rate variability in survivors of myocardial infarction: a double blind randomised controlled trial. BMJ 1996; 312(7032):677-678.
Clark WF, Parbtani A, Naylor CD, et al. Fish oil in lupus nephritis: clinical findings and methodological implications. Kidney Int 1993;44(1):75-86.
Clark WF, Parbtani A. Omega-3 fatty acid supplementation in clinical and experimental lupus nephritis. Am J Kidney Dis 1994;23(5):644-647.
Clarke JT, Cullen-Dean G, Regelink E, et al. Increased incidence of epistaxis in adolescents with familial hypercholesterolemia treated with fish oil. J Pediatr 1990;116(1):139-141.
Cleland LG, French JK, Betts WH, et al. Clinical and biochemical effects of dietary fish oil supplements in rheumatoid arthritis. J Rheumatol 1988;15(10):1471-1475.
Cobiac L, Nestel PJ, Wing LM, et al. A low-sodium diet supplemented with fish oil lowers blood pressure in the elderly. J Hypertens 1992;10(1):87-92.
Connor WE. Importance of n-3 fatty acids in health and disease. Am J Clin Nutr 2000; 71(1 Suppl):171S-175S.
Contacos C, Barter PJ, Sullivan DR. Effect of pravastatin and omega-3 fatty acids on plasma lipids and lipoproteins in patients with combined hyperlipidemia. Arterioscler Thromb 1993;13(12):1755-1762.
D'Almeida A, Carter JP, Anatol A, et al. Effects of a combination of evening primrose oil (gamma linolenic acid) and fish oil (eicosapentaenoic + docahexaenoic acid) versus magnesium, and versus placebo in preventing pre-eclampsia. Women Health 1992;19(2-3): 117-131.
Danno K, Sugie N. Combination therapy with low-dose etretinate and eicosapentaenoic acid for psoriasis vulgaris. J Dermatol 1998;25(11):703-705.
Daviglus ML, Stamler J, Orencia AJ, et al. Fish consumption and the 30-year risk of fatal myocardial infarction. N Engl J Med 1997;336(15):1046-1053.
de Deckere EA. Possible beneficial effect of fish and fish n-3 polyunsaturated fatty acids in breast and colorectal cancer. Eur J Cancer Prev 1999;8(3):213-221.
de Lorgeril M, Salen P, Martin JL, et al. Mediterranean diet, traditional risk factors, and the rate of cardiovascular complications after myocardial infarction: final report of the Lyon Diet Heart Study. Circulation 1999;99(6):779-785.
De Vizia B, Raia V, Spano C, et al. Effect of an 8-month treatment with omega-3 fatty acids (eicosapentaenoic and docosahexaenoic) in patients with cystic fibrosis. JPEN J Parenter Enteral Nutr 2003;27(1):52-57.
Deutch B, Jorgensen EB, Hansen JC. Menstrual discomfort in Danish women reduced by dietary supplements of omega-3 PUFA and B12 (fish oil or seal oil capsules). Nutr Res 2000; 20(5):621-631.
Deutch B. [Painful menstruation and low intake of n-3 fatty acids]. Ugeskr Laeger 1996; 158(29):4195-4198.
Dichi I, Frenhane P, Dichi JB, et al. Comparison of omega-3 fatty acids and sulfasalazine in ulcerative colitis. Nutrition 2000;16(2):87-94.
Dillon JJ. Fish oil therapy for IgA nephropathy: efficacy and interstudy variability. J Am Soc Nephrol 1997;8(11):1739-1744.
Djousse L, Pankow JS, Eckfeldt JH, et al. Relation between dietary linolenic acid and coronary artery disease in the National Heart, Lung, and Blood Institute Family Heart Study. Am J Clin Nutr 2001;74(5):612-619.
Dolecek TA. Epidemiological evidence of relationships between dietary polyunsaturated fatty acids and mortality in the multiple risk factor intervention trial. Proc Soc Exp Biol Med 1992;200(2):177-182.
Donadio JV Jr. Use of fish oil to treat patients with immunoglobulin A nephropathy. Am J Clin Nutr 2000;71(1 Suppl):373S-375S.

Donadio JV. The emerging role of omega-3 polyunsaturated fatty acids in the management of patients with IgA nephropathy. J Ren Nutr 2001;11(3):122-128.

Dry J, Vincent D. Effect of a fish oil diet on asthma: results of a 1-year double-blind study. Int Arch Allergy Appl Immunol 1991;95(2-3):156-157.

Eritsland J, Arnesen H, Gronseth K, et al. Effect of dietary supplementation with n-3 fatty acids on coronary artery bypass graft patency. Am J Cardiol 1996;77(1):31-36.

Escobar SO, Achenbach R, Iannantuono R, et al. Topical fish oil in psoriasis—a controlled and blind study. Clin Exp Dermatol 1992;17(3):159-162.

Fearon KC, Von Meyenfeldt MF, Moses AG, et al. Effect of a protein and energy dense n-3 fatty acid enriched oral supplement on loss of weight and lean tissue in cancer cachexia: a randomised double blind trial. Gut 2003;52(10):1479-1486.

Fenton WS, Dickerson F, Boronow J, et al. A placebo-controlled trial of omega-3 fatty acid (ethyl eicosapentaenoic acid) supplementation for residual symptoms and cognitive impairment in schizophrenia. Am J Psychiatry 2001;158(12):2071-2074.

Fortin PR, Lew RA, Liang MH, et al. Validation of a meta-analysis: the effects of fish oil in rheumatoid arthritis. J Clin Epidemiol 1995;48(11):1379-1390.

Friedberg CE, Janssen MJ, Heine RJ, et al. Fish oil and glycemic control in diabetes. A meta-analysis. Diabetes Care 1998;21(4):494-500.

Gapinski JP, VanRuiswyk JV, Heudebert GR, et al. Preventing restenosis with fish oils following coronary angioplasty. A meta-analysis. Arch Intern Med 1993;153(13):1595-1601.

Geusens P, Wouters C, Nijs J, et al. Long-term effect of omega-3 fatty acid supplementation in active rheumatoid arthritis. A 12-month, double-blind, controlled study. Arthritis Rheum 1994;37(6):824-829.

Gillum RF, Mussolino ME, Madans JH. The relationship between fish consumption and stroke incidence. The NHANES I Epidemiologic Follow-up Study (National Health and Nutrition Examination Survey). Arch Intern Med 1996;156(5):537-542.

Glaum M, Metzelthin E, Junker S, et al. [Comparative effect of oral fat loads with saturated, omega-6 and omega- 3 fatty acids before and after fish oil capsule therapy in healthy probands]. Klin Wochenschr 1990;68 Suppl 22:103-105.

Greenfield SM, Green AT, Teare JP, et al. A randomized controlled study of evening primrose oil and fish oil in ulcerative colitis. Aliment Pharmacol Ther 1993;7(2):159-166.

Grimminger F, Mayser P, Papavassilis C, et al. A double-blind, randomized, placebo-controlled trial of n-3 fatty acid based lipid infusion in acute, extended guttate psoriasis. Rapid improvement of clinical manifestations and changes in neutrophil leukotriene profile. Clin Invest 1993;71(8):634-643.

Grimsgaard S, Bonaa KH, Hansen JB, et al. Highly purified eicosapentaenoic acid and docosahexaenoic acid in humans have similar triacylglycerol-lowering effects but divergent effects on serum fatty acids. Am J Clin Nutr 1997;66(3):649-659.

Guallar E, Aro A, Jimenez FJ, et al. Omega-3 fatty acids in adipose tissue and risk of myocardial infarction: the EURAMIC study. Arterioscler Thromb Vasc Biol 1999;19(4):1111-1118.

Gupta AK, Ellis CN, Goldfarb MT, et al. The role of fish oil in psoriasis. A randomized, double-blind, placebo-controlled study to evaluate the effect of fish oil and topical corticosteroid therapy in psoriasis. Int J Dermatol 1990;29(8):591-595.

Gupta AK, Ellis CN, Tellner DC, et al. Double-blind, placebo-controlled study to evaluate the efficacy of fish oil and low-dose UVB in the treatment of psoriasis. Br J Dermatol 1989; 120(6):801-807.

Hansen JM, Lokkegaard H, Hoy CE, et al. No effect of dietary fish oil on renal hemodynamics, tubular function, and renal functional reserve in long-term renal transplant recipients. J Am Soc Nephrol 1995;5(7):1434-1440.

Harel Z, Biro FM, Kottenhahn RK, et al. Supplementation with omega-3 polyunsaturated fatty acids in the management of dysmenorrhea in adolescents. Am J Obstet Gynecol 1996; 174(4):1335-1338.

Harris WS. N-3 fatty acids and serum lipoproteins: human studies. Am J Clin Nutr 1997;65(5 Suppl):1645S-1654S.

Harris WS, Dujovne CA, Zucker M, et al. Effects of a low saturated fat, low cholesterol fish oil supplement in hypertriglyceridemic patients. A placebo-controlled trial. Ann Intern Med 1988;109(6):465-470.

Hawthorne AB, Daneshmend TK, Hawkey CJ, et al. Fish oil in ulcerative colitis: final results of a controlled clinical trial [abstract]. Gastroenterology 1990;98(5 pt 2):A174.
Hawthorne AB, Daneshmend TK, Hawkey CJ, et al. Treatment of ulcerative colitis with fish oil supplementation: a prospective 12 month randomised controlled trial. Gut 1992;33(7): 922-928.
Helland IB, Saugstad OD, Smith L, et al. Similar effects on infants of n-3 and n-6 fatty acids supplementation to pregnant and lactating women. Pediatrics 2001;108(5):E82.
Henderson WR. Omega-3 supplementation in CF [abstract]. In Proceedings of the 6th North American Cystic Fibrosis Conference, 1992;s21-s22.
Henderson WR Jr, Astley SJ, McCready MM, et al. Oral absorption of omega-3 fatty acids in patients with cystic fibrosis who have pancreatic insufficiency and in healthy control subjects. J Pediatr 1994;124(3):400-408.
Henderson WR Jr, Astley SJ, Ramsey BW. Liver function in patients with cystic fibrosis ingesting fish oil. J Pediatr 1994;125(3):504-505.
Henneicke-von Zepelin HH, Mrowietz U, Farber L, et al. Highly purified omega-3-polyunsaturated fatty acids for topical treatment of psoriasis. Results of a double-blind, placebo-controlled multicentre study. Br J Dermatol 1993;129(6):713-717.
Hoffman DR, Birch EE, Birch DG, et al. Effects of supplementation with omega 3 long-chain polyunsaturated fatty acids on retinal and cortical development in premature infants. Am J Clin Nutr 1993;57(5 Suppl):807S-812S.
Holm T, Andreassen AK, Aukrust P, et al. Omega-3 fatty acids improve blood pressure control and preserve renal function in hypertensive heart transplant recipients. Eur Heart J 2001; 22(5):428-436.
Homan van der Heide JJ, Bilo HJ, Donker AJ, et al. Dietary supplementation with fish oil modifies renal reserve filtration capacity in postoperative, cyclosporin A–treated renal transplant recipients. Transpl Int 1990;3(3):171-175.
Homan van der Heide JJ, Bilo HJ, Donker AJ, et al. The effects of dietary supplementation with fish oil on renal function and the course of early postoperative rejection episodes in cyclosporine-treated renal transplant recipients. Transplantation 1992;54(2):257-263.
Homan van der Heide JJ, Bilo HJ, Tegzess AM, et al. Omega-3 polyunsaturated fatty acids improve renal function in renal transplant recipients treated with cyclosporin-A [abstract]. Kidney Int 1989;35:516A.
Horrobin DF. Omega-3 Fatty acid for schizophrenia. Am J Psychiatry 2003;160(1):188-189.
Howe PR. Dietary fats and hypertension. Focus on fish oil. Ann N Y Acad Sci 1997;827:339-352.
Hu FB, Bronner L, Willett WC, et al. Fish and omega-3 fatty acid intake and risk of coronary heart disease in women. JAMA 2002;287(14):1815-1821.
Hu FB, Stampfer MJ, Manson JE, et al. Dietary intake of alpha-linolenic acid and risk of fatal ischemic heart disease among women. Am J Clin Nutr 1999;69(5):890-897.
Iso H, Rexrode KM, Stampfer MJ, et al. Intake of fish and omega-3 fatty acids and risk of stroke in women. JAMA 2001;285(3):304-312.
Johansen O, Brekke M, Seljeflot I, et al. N-3 fatty acids do not prevent restenosis after coronary angioplasty: results from the CART study. Coronary Angioplasty Restenosis Trial. J Am Coll Cardiol 1999;33(6):1619-1626.
Joy CB, Mumby-Croft R, Joy LA. Polyunsaturated fatty acid (fish or evening primrose oil) for schizophrenia. Cochrane Database Syst Rev 2000;(2):CD001257.
Katz DP, Manner T, Furst P, et al. The use of an intravenous fish oil emulsion enriched with omega-3 fatty acids in patients with cystic fibrosis. Nutrition 1996;12(5):334-339.
Keli SO, Feskens EJ, Kromhout D. Fish consumption and risk of stroke. The Zutphen Study. Stroke 1994;25(2):328-332.
Kim YI. Can fish oil maintain Crohn's disease in remission? Nutr Rev 1996;54(8):248-252.
Kinrys G. Hypomania associated with omega 3 fatty acids. Arch Gen Psychiatry 2000;57(7): 715-716.
Kjeldsen-Kragh J, Lund JA, Riise T, et al. Dietary omega-3 fatty acid supplementation and naproxen treatment in patients with rheumatoid arthritis. J Rheumatol 1992;19(10): 1531-1536.
Klein V, Chajes V, Germain E, et al. Low alpha-linolenic acid content of adipose breast tissue is associated with an increased risk of breast cancer. Eur J Cancer 2000;36(3):335-340.

Knapp HR. Dietary fatty acids in human thrombosis and hemostasis. Am J Clin Nutr 1997; 65(5 Suppl):1687S-1698S.

Knapp HR, FitzGerald GA. The antihypertensive effects of fish oil. A controlled study of polyunsaturated fatty acid supplements in essential hypertension. N Engl J Med 1989; 320(16):1037-1043.

Kooijmans-Coutinho MF, Rischen-Vos J, Hermans J, et al. Dietary fish oil in renal transplant recipients treated with cyclosporin-A: no beneficial effects shown. J Am Soc Nephrol 1996; 7(3):513-518.

Koretz RL. Maintaining remissions in Crohn's disease: a fat chance to please. Gastroenterology 1997;112(6):2155-2156.

Kremer JM, Bigauoette J, Michalek AV, et al. Effects of manipulation of dietary fatty acids on clinical manifestations of rheumatoid arthritis. Lancet 1985;1(8422):184-187.

Kremer JM, Jubiz W, Michalek A, et al. Fish-oil fatty acid supplementation in active rheumatoid arthritis. A double-blinded, controlled, crossover study. Ann Intern Med 1987;106(4):497-503.

Kremer JM, Lawrence DA, Jubiz W, et al. Dietary fish oil and olive oil supplementation in patients with rheumatoid arthritis. Clinical and immunologic effects. Arthritis Rheum 1990; 33(6):810-820.

Kremer JM, Lawrence DA, Petrillo GF, et al. Effects of high-dose fish oil on rheumatoid arthritis after stopping nonsteroidal antiinflammatory drugs. Clinical and immune correlates. Arthritis Rheum 1995;38(8):1107-1114.

Kris-Etherton PM, Harris WS, Appel LJ. Fish consumption, fish oil, omega-3 fatty acids, and cardiovascular disease. Arterioscler Thromb Vasc Biol 2003;23(2):e20-e30.

Kristensen SD, Schmidt EB, Andersen HR, et al. Fish oil in angina pectoris. Atherosclerosis 1987;64(1):13-19.

Kromann N, Green A. Epidemiological studies in the Upernavik district, Greenland. Incidence of some chronic diseases 1950-1974. Acta Med Scand 1980;208(5):401-406.

Kromhout D, Bloemberg BP, Feskens EJ, et al. Alcohol, fish, fibre and antioxidant vitamins intake do not explain population differences in coronary heart disease mortality. Int J Epidemiol 1996;25(4):753-759.

Kromhout D, Bosschieter EB, de Lezenne CC. The inverse relation between fish consumption and 20-year mortality from coronary heart disease. N Engl J Med 1985;312(19):1205-1209.

Kromhout D, Menotti A, Bloemberg B, et al. Dietary saturated and trans fatty acids and cholesterol and 25-year mortality from coronary heart disease: the Seven Countries Study. Prev Med 1995;308-315.

Kuenzel U, Bertsch S. Clinical experiences with a standardized commercial fish oil product containing 33.5% omega-3 fatty acids - field trial with 3958 hyperlipemic patients in general practitioner practice. In: Chandra RK, ed. Health Effects of Fish and Fish Oils. Newfoundland: ARTS Biomedical Publishers and Distributors, 1989: 567-579.

Kunz B, Ring J, Braun-Falco O. Eicosapentaenoic acid (EPA) treatment in atopic eczema (AE): a prospective double-blind trial [abstract]. J Allergy Clin Immunol 1989;83:196.

Kurlandsky LE, Bennink MR, Webb PM, et al. The absorption and effect of dietary supplementation with omega-3 fatty acids on serum leukotriene B4 in patients with cystic fibrosis. Pediatr Pulmonol 1994;18(4):211-217.

Lau CS, Morley KD, Belch JJ. Effects of fish oil supplementation on non-steroidal anti-inflammatory drug requirement in patients with mild rheumatoid arthritis—a double-blind placebo controlled study. Br J Rheumatol 1993;32(11):982-989.

Lawrence R, Sorrell T. Eicosapentaenoic acid in cystic fibrosis: evidence of a pathogenetic role for leukotriene B4. Lancet 1993;342(8869):465-469.

Leaf A, Jorgensen MB, Jacobs AK, et al. Do fish oils prevent restenosis after coronary angioplasty? Circulation 1994;90(5):2248-2257.

Loeschke K, Ueberschaer B, Pietsch A, et al. N-3 fatty acids only delay early relapse of ulcerative colitis in remission. Dig Dis Sci 1996;41(10):2087-2094.

Lorenz R, Loeschke K. Placebo-controlled trials of omega 3 fatty acids in chronic inflammatory bowel disease. World Rev Nutr Diet 1994;76:143-145.

Lorenz R, Weber PC, Szimnau P, et al. Supplementation with n-3 fatty acids from fish oil in chronic inflammatory bowel disease—a randomized, placebo-controlled, double- blind cross-over trial. J Intern Med Suppl 1989;225(731):225-232.

Lungershausen YK, Abbey M, Nestel PJ, et al. Reduction of blood pressure and plasma triglycerides by omega-3 fatty acids in treated hypertensives. J Hypertens 1994;12(9): 1041-1045.

Maachi K, Berthoux P, Burgard G, et al. Results of a 1-year randomized controlled trial with omega-3 fatty acid fish oil in renal transplantation under triple immunosuppressive therapy. Transplant Proc 1995;27(1):846-849.

Marchioli R, Barzi F, Bomba E, et al. Early protection against sudden death by n-3 polyunsaturated fatty acids after myocardial infarction. Time-course analysis of the results of the Gruppo Italiano per lo Studio della Sopravvivenza nell'Infarto Miocardico (GISSI)-Prevenzione. Circulation 2002;105(16):1897-1903.

Maresta A, Balducelli M, Varani E, et al. Prevention of postcoronary angioplasty restenosis by omega-3 fatty acids: main results of the Esapent for Prevention of Restenosis Italian Study (ESPRIT). Am Heart J 2002;143(6):E5.

Masuev KA. [The effect of polyunsaturated fatty acids of the omega-3 class on the late phase of the allergic reaction in bronchial asthma patients]. Terapevticheskii Arkhiv 1997;69(3):31-33.

Mayser P, Mrowietz U, Arenberger P, et al. Omega-3 fatty acid-based lipid infusion in patients with chronic plaque psoriasis: results of a double-blind, randomized, placebo-controlled, multicenter trial. J Am Acad Dermatol 1998;38(4):539-547.

McDonald CF, Vecchie L, Pierce RJ, et al. Effect of fish-oil derived omega-3 fatty acid supplements on asthma control [abstract]. Austral New Zealand J Med 1990;20:526.

Mehrotra B, Ronquillo J. Dietary supplementation in hem/onc outpatients at a tertiary care hospital. American Society of Clinical Oncology 38th Annual Meeting, Orlando, Florida, May 18-21, 2002. 1.

Mellor J, Laugharne JD, Peet M. Omega-3 fatty acid supplementation in schizophrenic patients. Human Psychopharmacol 1996;11:39-46.

Mischoulon D, Fava M. Docosahexanoic acid and omega-3 fatty acids in depression. Psychiatr Clin North Am 2000;23(4):785-794.

Mizushima S, Moriguchi EH, Ishikawa P, et al. Fish intake and cardiovascular risk among middle-aged Japanese in Japan and Brazil. J Cardiovasc Risk 1997;4(3):191-199.

Montori VM, Farmer A, Wollan PC, et al. Fish oil supplementation in type 2 diabetes: a quantitative systematic review. Diabetes Care 2000;23(9):1407-1415.

Mori TA, Bao DQ, Burke V, et al. Docosahexaenoic acid but not eicosapentaenoic acid lowers ambulatory blood pressure and heart rate in humans. Hypertension 1999;34(2):253-260.

Mori TA, Watts GF, Burke V, et al. Differential effects of eicosapentaenoic acid and docosahexaenoic acid on vascular reactivity of the forearm microcirculation in hyperlipidemic, overweight men. Circulation 2000;102(11):1264-1269.

Morris MC, Manson JE, Rosner B, et al. Fish consumption and cardiovascular disease in the Physicians' Health Study: a prospective study. Am J Epidemiol 1995;142(2):166-175.

Morris MC, Sacks F, Rosner B. Does fish oil lower blood pressure? A meta-analysis of controlled trials. Circulation 1993;88(2):523-533.

Morris MC, Taylor JO, Stampfer MJ, et al. The effect of fish oil on blood pressure in mild hypertensive subjects: a randomized crossover trial. Am J Clin Nutr 1993;57(1):59-64.

Nagakura T, Matsuda S, Shichijyo K, et al. Dietary supplementation with fish oil rich in omega-3 polyunsaturated fatty acids in children with bronchial asthma. Eur Respir J 2000;16(5): 861-865.

Nakamura N, Hamazaki T, Ohta M, et al. Joint effects of HMG-CoA reductase inhibitors and eicosapentaenoic acids on serum lipid profile and plasma fatty acid concentrations in patients with hyperlipidemia. Int J Clin Lab Res 1999;29(1):22-25.

Natvig H, Borchgrevink CF, Dedichen J, et al. A controlled trial of the effect of linolenic acid on incidence of coronary heart disease. The Norwegian vegetable oil experiment of 1965- 66. Scand J Clin Lab Invest Suppl 1968;105:1-20.

Nemets B, Stahl Z, Belmaker RH. Addition of omega-3 fatty acid to maintenance medication treatment for recurrent unipolar depressive disorder. Am J Psychiatry 2002;159(3):477-479.

Nielsen GL, Faarvang KL, Thomsen BS, et al. The effects of dietary supplementation with n-3 polyunsaturated fatty acids in patients with rheumatoid arthritis: a randomized, double blind trial. Eur J Clin Invest 1992;22(10):687-691.

Nilsen DW, Albrektsen G, Landmark K, et al. Effects of a high-dose concentrate of n-3 fatty acids or corn oil introduced early after an acute myocardial infarction on serum triacylglycerol and HDL cholesterol. Am J Clin Nutr 2001;74(1):50-56.

Nordoy A, Bonaa KH, Sandset PM, et al. Effect of omega-3 fatty acids and simvastatin on hemostatic risk factors and postprandial hyperlipemia in patients with combined hyperlipemia. Arterioscler Thromb Vasc Biol 2000;20(1):259-265.

Nordoy A, Hansen JB, Brox J, et al. Effects of atorvastatin and omega-3 fatty acids on LDL subfractions and postprandial hyperlipemia in patients with combined hyperlipemia. Nutr Metab Cardiovasc Dis 2001;11(1):7-16.

Norrish AE, Skeaff CM, Arribas GL, et al. Prostate cancer risk and consumption of fish oils: a dietary biomarker- based case-control study. Br J Cancer 1999;81(7):1238-1242.

Okamoto M, Mitsunobu F, Ashida K, et al. Effects of dietary supplementation with n-3 fatty acids compared with n-6 fatty acids on bronchial asthma. Intern Med 2000;39(2):107-111.

Olsen SF, Secher NJ, Tabor A, et al. Randomised clinical trials of fish oil supplementation in high risk pregnancies. Fish Oil Trials In Pregnancy (FOTIP) Team. BJOG 2000;107(3): 382-395.

Olsen SF, Secher NJ. Low consumption of seafood in early pregnancy as a risk factor for preterm delivery: prospective cohort study. BMJ 2002;324(7335):447.

Olsen SF, Sorensen JD, Secher NJ, et al. Randomised controlled trial of effect of fish-oil supplementation on pregnancy duration. Lancet 1992;339(8800):1003-1007.

Onwude JL, Lilford RJ, Hjartardottir H, et al. A randomised double blind placebo controlled trial of fish oil in high risk pregnancy. Br J Obstet Gynaecol 1995;102(2):95-100.

Oomen CM, Ocke MC, Feskens EJ, et al. Alpha-linolenic acid intake is not beneficially associated with 10-y risk of coronary artery disease incidence: the Zutphen Elderly Study. Am J Clin Nutr 2001;74(4):457-463.

Orencia AJ, Daviglus ML, Dyer AR, et al. Fish consumption and stroke in men. 30-year findings of the Chicago Western Electric Study. Stroke 1996;27(2):204-209.

Palat D, Rudolph D, Rothstein M. A trial of fish oil in asthma [abstract]. Am Rev Respir Dis 1988;137(Suppl 4 part 2):329.

Peet M, Mellor J. Double-blind placebo controlled trial of n-3 polyunsaturated fatty acids as an adjunct to neuroleptics [abstract]. Schizophrenia Res 1998;29(1-2):160-161.

Roche HM, Gibney MJ. Postprandial triacylglycerolaemia: the effect of low-fat dietary treatment with and without fish oil supplementation. Eur J Clin Nutr 1996;50(9):617-624.

Rose DP, Connolly JM. Omega-3 fatty acids as cancer chemopreventive agents. Pharmacol Ther 1999;83(3):217-244.

Ross E. The role of marine fish oils in the treatment of ulcerative colitis. Nutr Rev 1993; 51(2):47-49.

Roy I, Meyer F, Gingras L, et al. A double blind randomized controlled study comparing the efficacy of fish oil and low dose ASA to prevent coronary saphenous vein graft obstruction after CABG [abstract]. Circulation 1991;84:II-285.

Sacks FM, Stone PH, Gibson CM, et al. Controlled trial of fish oil for regression of human coronary atherosclerosis. HARP Research Group. J Am Coll Cardiol 1995;25(7): 1492-1498.

Salomon P, Kornbluth AA, Janowitz HD. Treatment of ulcerative colitis with fish oil–omega-3 fatty acid: an open trial. J Clin Gastroenterol 1990;12(2):157-161.

Salvi A, Di Stefano O, Sleiman I, et al. Effects of fish oil on serum lipids and lipoprotein(a) levels in heterozygous familial hypercholesterolemia. Curr Ther Res Clin Exp 1993;53(6):717-721.

Salvig JD, Olsen SF, Secher NJ. Effects of fish oil supplementation in late pregnancy on blood pressure: a randomised controlled trial. Br J Obstet Gynaecol 1996;103(6):529-533.

Sanders TA, Oakley FR, Miller GJ, et al. Influence of n-6 versus n-3 polyunsaturated fatty acids in diets low in saturated fatty acids on plasma lipoproteins and hemostatic factors. Arterioscler Thromb Vasc Biol 1997;17(12):3449-3460.

Santos J, Queiros J, Silva F, et al. Effects of fish oil in cyclosporine-treated renal transplant recipients. Transplant Proc 2000;32(8):2605-2608.

Schlanger S, Shinitzky M, Yam D. Diet enriched with omega-3 fatty acids alleviates convulsion symptoms in epilepsy patients. Epilepsia 2002;43(1):103-104.

Sellmayer A, Witzgall H, Lorenz RL, et al. Effects of dietary fish oil on ventricular premature complexes. Am J Cardiol 1995;76(12):974-977.

Shekelle RB, Missell L, Paul O, et al. Fish consumption and mortality from coronary heart disease. N Engl J Med 1985;313:820.

Simon JA, Fong J, Bernert JT Jr, et al. Serum fatty acids and the risk of stroke. Stroke 1995;26(5):778-782.

Singer P, Melzer S, Goschel M, et al. Fish oil amplifies the effect of propranolol in mild essential hypertension. Hypertension 1990;16(6):682-691.

Singh RB, Niaz MA, Sharma JP, et al. Randomized, double-blind, placebo-controlled trial of fish oil and mustard oil in patients with suspected acute myocardial infarction: the Indian Experiment of Infarct Survival—4. Cardiovasc Drugs Ther 1997;11(3):485-491.

Skoldstam L, Borjesson O, Kjallman A, et al. Effect of six months of fish oil supplementation in stable rheumatoid arthritis. A double-blind, controlled study. Scand J Rheumatol 1992; 21(4):178-185.

Soyland E, Funk J, Rajka G, et al. Effect of dietary supplementation with very-long-chain n-3 fatty acids in patients with psoriasis. N Engl J Med 1993;328(25):1812-1816.

Sperling RI, Weinblatt M, Robin JL, et al. Effects of dietary supplementation with marine fish oil on leukocyte lipid mediator generation and function in rheumatoid arthritis. Arthritis Rheum 1987;30(9):988-997.

Stacpoole PW, Alig J, Ammon L, et al. Dose-response effects of dietary marine oil on carbohydrate and lipid metabolism in normal subjects and patients with hypertriglyceridemia. Metabolism 1989;38(10):946-956.

Stacpoole PW, Alig J, Ammon L, et al. Dose-response effects of dietary fish oil on carbohydrate and lipid metabolism in hypertriglyceridemia [abstract]. Diabetes 1988;37 (Suppl 1):12A.

Stenius-Aarniala B, Aro A, Hakulinen A, et al. Evening primrose oil and fish oil are ineffective as supplementary treatment of bronchial asthma. Ann Allergy 1989;62(6):534-537.

Stenson WF, Cort D, Beeken W, et al. A trial of fish oil supplemented diet in ulcerative colitis [abstract]. Gastroenterology 1990;98(Suppl):A475.

Stenson WF, Cort D, Rodgers J, et al. Dietary supplementation with fish oil in ulcerative colitis. Ann Intern Med 1992;116(8):609-614.

Stoll AL, Severus WE, Freeman MP, et al. Omega 3 fatty acids in bipolar disorder: a preliminary double-blind, placebo-controlled trial. Arch Gen Psychiatry 1999;56(5):407-412.

Stone NJ. Fish consumption, fish oil, lipids, and coronary heart disease. Circulation 1996; 94(9):2337-2340.

Stoof TJ, Korstanje MJ, Bilo HJ, et al. Does fish oil protect renal function in cyclosporin-treated psoriasis patients? J Intern Med 1989;226(6):437-441.

Strong AM, Hamill E. The effect of combined fish oil and evening primrose oil (Efamol Marine) on the remission phase of psoriasis: a 7-month double-blind randomized placebo-controlled trial. J Derm Treatment 1993;4:33-36.

Su KP, Huang SY, Chiu CC, et al. Omega-3 fatty acids in major depressive disorder. A preliminary double-blind, placebo-controlled trial. Eur Neuropsychopharmacol 2003;13(4): 267-271.

Sweny P, Wheeler DC, Lui SF, et al. Dietary fish oil supplements preserve renal function in renal transplant recipients with chronic vascular rejection. Nephrol Dial Transplant 1989;4(12):1070-1075.

Tanskanen A, Hibbeln JR, Hintikka J, et al. Fish consumption, depression, and suicidality in a general population. Arch Gen Psychiatry 2001;58(5):512-513.

Tato F, Keller C, Wolfram G. Effects of fish oil concentrate on lipoproteins and apolipoproteins in familial combined hyperlipidemia. Clin Invest 1993;71(4):314-318.

Terry P, Lichtenstein P, Feychting M, et al. Fatty fish consumption and risk of prostate cancer. Lancet 2001;357(9270):1764-1766.

Thien FC, Mencia-Huerta JM, Lee TH. Dietary fish oil effects on seasonal hay fever and asthma in pollen-sensitive subjects. Am Rev Respir Dis 1993;147(5):1138-1143.

Tulleken JE, Limburg PC, Muskiet FA, et al. Vitamin E status during dietary fish oil supplementation in rheumatoid arthritis. Arthritis Rheum 1990;33(9):1416-1419.

Ullmann D, Connor WE, Illingworth DR, et al. Additive effects of lovastatin and fish oil in familial hypercholesterolemia [abstract]. Arteriosclerosis 1990;10(5):846a.

van der Heide JJ, Bilo HJ, Donker JM, et al. Effect of dietary fish oil on renal function and rejection in cyclosporine-treated recipients of renal transplants. N Engl J Med 1993; 329(11):769-773.

van der Temple H, Tulleken JE, Limburg PC, et al. Effects of fish oil supplementation in rheumatoid arthritis. Ann Rheum Dis 1990;49(2):76-80.

Ventura HO, Milani RV, Lavie CJ, et al. Cyclosporine-induced hypertension. Efficacy of omega-3 fatty acids in patients after cardiac transplantation. Circulation 1993;88(5 Pt 2):II281-II285.

Volker D, Fitzgerald P, Major G, et al. Efficacy of fish oil concentrate in the treatment of rheumatoid arthritis. J Rheumatol 2000;27(10):2343-2346.

von Schacky C, Angerer P, Kothny W, et al. The effect of dietary omega-3 fatty acids on coronary atherosclerosis. A randomized, double-blind, placebo-controlled trial. Ann Intern Med 1999;130(7):554-562.

Walton AJ, Snaith ML, Locniskar M, et al. Dietary fish oil and the severity of symptoms in patients with systemic lupus erythematosus. Ann Rheum Dis 1991;50(7):463-466.

Weksler BB. Omega 3 fatty acids have multiple antithrombotic effects. World Rev Nutr Diet 1994;76:47-50.

Wigmore SJ, Barber MD, Ross JA, et al. Effect of oral eicosapentaenoic acid on weight loss in patients with pancreatic cancer. Nutr Cancer 2000;36(2):177-184.

Woods RK, Thien FC, Abramson MJ. Dietary marine fatty acids (fish oil) for asthma in adults and children. Cochrane Database Syst Rev 2002;(3):CD001283.

Yamada T, Strong JP, Ishii T, et al. Atherosclerosis and omega-3 fatty acids in the populations of a fishing village and a farming village in Japan. Atherosclerosis 2000;153(2):469-481.

Zanarini MC, Frankenburg FR. Omega-3 fatty acid treatment of women with borderline personality disorder: a double-blind, placebo-controlled pilot study. Am J Psychiatry 2003;160(1):167-169.

Zhang J, Sasaki S, Amano K, et al. Fish consumption and mortality from all causes, ischemic heart disease, and stroke: an ecological study. Prev Med 1999;28(5):520-529.

Flaxseed and Flaxseed Oil

(*Linum usitatissimum*)

F

RELATED TERMS

- Alashi, alpha-linolenic acid, Barlean's Flax Oil, Barlean's Vita-Flax, brazen, common flax, eicosapentaenoic acid, flachssamen, flax, gamma-linolenic acid, graine de lin, hu-ma-esze, leinsamen, Linaceae, linen flax, lini semen, lino, lino usuale, linseed, linseed oil, lint bells, linum, *Linum catharticum*, *Linum humile* seeds, keten, omega-3 fatty acid, phytoestrogen, sufulsi, tesi-mosina, Type I flaxseed/flaxseed (51% to 55% alpha-linolenic acid), Type II flaxseed/CDC-flaxseed (2% to 3% alpha-linolenic acid), winterlien.

BACKGROUND

- Flaxseed and its derivative flaxseed oil (also called linseed oil) are rich sources of the essential fatty acid alpha-linolenic acid, which is a biologic precursor to omega-3 fatty acids such as eicosapentaenoic acid. Although omega-3 fatty acids have been associated with improved cardiovascular outcomes, evidence from trials in humans is mixed regarding the efficacy of flaxseed products for treatment of coronary artery disease or hyperlipidemia.
- The lignan constituents of flaxseed (not flaxseed oil) possess *in vitro* antioxidant and possible estrogen receptor agonist/antagonist properties, prompting theories of efficacy for the treatment of breast cancer. However, there is not sufficient evidence in humans to make a recommendation. As a source of fiber mucilage, oral flaxseed (not flaxseed oil) may possess laxative properties, although only one trial in humans has been conducted for this indication. In large doses, or when taken with inadequate water, flaxseed may precipitate bowel obstruction via a mass effect. The effects of flaxseed on blood glucose levels are not clear, although hyperglycemic effects have been reported in one case series.
- Flaxseed oil contains only the alpha-linolenic acid component of flaxseed, and not the fiber or lignan components. Therefore, flaxseed oil may share the purported lipid-lowering properties of flaxseed, but not the proposed laxative or anticancer abilities.
- Preliminary evidence suggests that alpha-linolenic acid may be associated with an increased risk of prostate cancer.

USES BASED ON SCIENTIFIC EVIDENCE	Grade*
Laxative (flaxseed, not flaxseed oil) Early studies in humans suggest that flaxseed can be used as a laxative. However, more information is needed to compare effectiveness and dosing with those for more commonly used agents.	B

Continued

Breast cancer (flaxseed, not flaxseed oil) Information from studies in humans indicating that flaxseed is effective in preventing or treating breast cancer is lacking.	C
Diabetes (flaxseed, not flaxseed oil) Studies in humans on the effect of flaxseed on blood sugar levels report mixed results. Flaxseed cannot be recommended as a treatment for diabetes at this time. More proven therapies are recommended.	C
Heart disease (flaxseed and flaxseed oil) People who have had a heart attack are reported to benefit from diets rich in alpha-linolenic acid, which is found in flaxseed. Well-designed studies that examine the effect of flaxseed on heart disease in humans are not available. It is unclear whether flaxseed supplementation alters the course of heart disease.	C
High blood pressure (flaxseed, not flaxseed oil) In animals, diets high in flaxseed have differing effects on blood pressure. One study in humans suggests that flaxseed may lower blood pressure. Further research is needed before a recommendation can be made.	C
High cholesterol or triglycerides (flaxseed and flaxseed oil) In laboratory studies and investigations in animals, flaxseed and flaxseed oil are reported to lower blood cholesterol levels. Effects on blood triglyceride levels in animals are unclear, with increased levels in some research and decreased levels in other studies. Human data results have been mixed, with decreased blood levels of total cholesterol and low-density lipoprotein ("bad cholesterol") in some studies but no effect in others. Most research in humans has not been well designed, and further research is needed before a recommendation can be made.	C
HIV/AIDS Strong evidence is unavailable regarding the use of flaxseed for the treatment of HIV infection and AIDS.	C
Kidney disease/lupus nephritis (flaxseed, not flaxseed oil) Strong evidence is unavailable regarding the use of flaxseed for the treatment of kidney disease or lupus nephritis. More research is needed before a recommendation can be made.	C
Menopausal symptoms There is preliminary evidence from randomized controlled trials that flaxseed oil may help decrease mild menopausal symptoms. Additional research is necessary before a clear conclusion can be drawn, and this remains an area of controversy. Patients should consult a physician and a pharmacist about treatment options before starting a new therapy.	C

Continued

Menstrual breast pain (flaxseed, not flaxseed oil) Early information from one study in women, the results of which have not been fully reported, suggests that flaxseed may reduce menstrual breast pain. However, further research is needed before a firm recommendation can be made.	C
Prostate cancer (flaxseed, not flaxseed oil) Several studies in humans suggest an increased risk of prostate cancer with increased intake of alpha-linolenic acid (which is present in flaxseed). On the basis of the available research, men with prostate cancer or at risk for prostate cancer should avoid flaxseed and alpha-linolenic acid supplements.	D

*Key to grades: *A:* Strong scientific evidence for this use; *B:* Good scientific evidence for this use; *C:* Unclear scientific evidence for this use; *D:* Fair scientific evidence against this use (it may not work); *F:* Strong scientific evidence against this use (it likely does not work). For a more detailed explanation of efficacy criteria, see "Natural Standard Evidence-Based Validated Grading Rationale" in the Introduction.

F

Uses Based on Tradition, Theory, or Limited Scientific Evidence

Abdominal pain, acute respiratory distress syndrome (ARDS), allergic reactions, bladder inflammation, blood thinner, bipolar disorder, boils, bronchial irritation, burns (poultice), colon cancer, cough (suppression or loosening of mucus), debris in the eye, depression, diarrhea, diverticulitis, dry skin, eczema, enlarged prostate, gonorrhea, irritable bowel syndrome, laxative-induced colon damage, liver protection, melanoma, menstrual disorders, ovarian disorders, pimples, psoriasis, rheumatoid arthritis, skin infections, sore throat, ulcerative colitis, upper respiratory tract infection, skin inflammation, stomach upset, urinary tract infection, vision improvement, vaginitis, weight loss.

DOSING

The following doses are based on scientific research, publications, traditional use, or expert opinion. Many herbs and supplements have not been thoroughly tested, and their safety and effectiveness may not be proven. Brands may be made differently, with variable ingredients even within the same brand. The doses shown may not apply to all products. It is important to always read product labels and discuss doses with a qualified healthcare provider before therapy is started.

Standardization

- Standardization involves measuring the amounts of certain chemicals in products to try to make different preparations similar to each other. It is not always known if the chemicals being measured are the "active" ingredients.
- In general, flaxseed products are not standardized with regard to specific chemical components, although products often are evaluated by manufacturers using a number of chemical tests.

Adults (18 Years and Older)

- Flaxseed oil should be kept refrigerated in an opaque (nontransparent) bottle, because its chemical parts may break down if the oil is exposed to light, oxygen, or heat. Whole flaxseed can be stored for up to 1 year in a dry location. Ground flaxseed can be kept in a refrigerator for 3 months or in a freezer for 6 months. The chemical parts of flaxseed oil and powder/flour will break down at high temperatures, such as in cooking.
- **Flaxseed oil (liquid form):** Flaxseed oil contains only the alpha-linolenic acid component of flax, not the fiber found in flaxseed. Flaxseed oil most often is used in a liquid form, which contains approximately 7 g of alpha-linolenic acid per 15-ml tablespoon (approximately 130 calories).
- **Flaxseed oil (capsule form):** Flaxseed oil is available in a capsule form, which typically contains 500 mg of alpha-linolenic acid per 1000-mg capsule (10 calories).
- **Flaxseed powder/flour/soluble fiber:** In several reported studies, adults have taken ground, raw flaxseeds by mouth in doses up to 50 g daily for up to 4 weeks. For shorter periods of time (less than 2 weeks), studies have used doses of 10 to 60 g by mouth daily. A dose of 50 g of flaxseed may be equal to 250 g of flaxseed flour. A dose of flaxseed that has been used for stomach or abdominal discomfort is 1 tablespoon of whole or bruised seed mixed with 150 ml (about ⅔ cup) of liquid, taken by mouth 2 or 3 times a day. As a laxative, 2 to 3 tablespoons of bulk seed mixed in 10 times that amount of water has been used. Studies in humans report that doses of 45 g daily have laxative effects. For lupus nephritis, 30 g of flaxseed daily has been studied. For menopausal symptoms, 40 g of flaxseed daily has been studied.
- **Flaxseed liquid:** Whole or bruised (not ground) flaxseed can be mixed with liquid and taken by mouth. Generally, 1 tablespoon in this form is mixed with 6 to 12 ounces of liquid and taken by mouth up to three times a day. Some studies use doses of soluble flaxseed mucilage/fiber as high as 60 to 80 g per kilogram (1 kg equals 2.2 lb) of the person's body weight. These liquid forms of flaxseed should not be confused with preparations of flaxseed oil.
- **Leaf:** There is not enough scientific information to recommend the use of the leaves of the flax plant for any medical condition.
- **In foods:** At high temperatures, such as in cooking, flaxseed oil and powder/flour will break down. Reports show that eating four eggs per day from chickens fed flaxseed can increase the levels of total omega-3 fatty acids in the blood. Long-term effects are not clear.
- **Applied to the skin (flaxseed poultice):** Anecdotally, 30 to 100 g of flaxseed flour can be mixed with warm or hot water to form a moist compress. Such compresses can be applied up to three times a day. It is not clear how long a flaxseed poultice should be used.
- **Applied to the eye (flaxseed):** Flaxseeds historically are used for removing debris from the eye. A single whole flaxseed is placed under the eyelid, where it collects the debris and mucus, thereby allowing removal. This process may be unsafe. The help of a healthcare professional is recommended for removal of eye debris.

Children (Younger Than 18 Years)

- Not enough information is available to recommend the use of flaxseed or flaxseed oil in children.

SAFETY

The U.S. Food and Drug Administration does not strictly regulate herbs and supplements. There is no guarantee of strength, purity, or safety of products, and effects may vary. It is important to always read product labels. People who have a medical condition, or are taking other drugs, herbs, or supplements, should consult a qualified healthcare provider before starting a new therapy. A healthcare provider should be consulted immediately about any side effects.

Allergies

- People with known allergy to flaxseed, flaxseed oil, or any other members of the Linaceae plant family or *Linum* genus plant family should avoid flaxseed products. Allergy-like reactions have developed in workers after inhaling flaxseed powder (occupational exposure). Two reports described possible allergic reactions in adults, whose symptoms included itching, hives, eye watering, nasal congestion, sneezing, nausea, abdominal pain, diarrhea, and mild shortness of breath. In these reports, multiple symptoms developed within minutes of taking a spoonful of linseed oil (from flaxseed) by mouth or eating multigrain bread. Allergy tests showed that both people were allergic to flaxseed.

Side Effects and Warnings

- There are few studies of flaxseed safety in humans. Flaxseed and flaxseed oil supplements appear to be well tolerated in the available research, and there is long-standing historical use of flaxseed products without many reports of side effects. However, unripe flaxseed pods are believed to be poisonous and should not be eaten. Raw flaxseed or flaxseed plant may increase blood levels of cyanide, a toxic chemical (this effect has not been reported when flaxseed supplements are taken at recommended doses). Flaxseed or flaxseed oil must not be applied to open wounds or broken skin.
- As indicated by studies in animals, overdose of flaxseed may cause shortness of breath, rapid breathing, weakness, or difficulty walking and may cause seizures or paralysis. Theoretically, flaxseed (*not* flaxseed oil) may increase the risk of cell damage from a reaction called oxidative stress. Studies report conflicting results in this area. Evidence from one study suggests that flaxseed or flaxseed oil taken by mouth may cause mania or hypomania in people with bipolar disorder. In theory, the laxative effects of flaxseed (*not* flaxseed oil) may cause diarrhea, increased number of bowel movements, and abdominal discomfort. Laxative effects are reported in several studies of people taking flaxseed or omega-3 acids. Large amounts of flaxseed by mouth may cause the intestines to stop moving (ileus). People with diarrhea, irritable bowel syndrome, diverticulitis, or inflammatory bowel disease (Crohn's disease or ulcerative colitis) should avoid flaxseed because of its possible laxative effects. Nausea, vomiting, and abdominal pain were reported in two people shortly after taking flaxseed products by mouth; these reactions may have been caused by allergy.
- Taking a large amount of flaxseed (*not* flaxseed oil) by mouth may cause obstruction of the intestines, especially when flaxseed is taken with too little fluid. Flaxseed should be taken with 10 times that amount of water or other liquid. People with narrowing of the esophagus or intestine, ileus, or bowel obstruction should avoid flaxseed (*not* flaxseed oil). Persons with high blood triglyceride levels should avoid flaxseed and flaxseed oil because of unclear effects on triglyceride levels in animal research. People with diabetes should use caution if taking flaxseed products by

mouth, because the omega-3 fatty acids in flaxseed and flaxseed oil may increase blood sugar levels. This increase was reported in one study of adults with type 2 diabetes who took omega-3 fatty acids for 1 month, but the effect was not reported in another study of people taking flaxseed (50 g) by mouth.

- One study reports that the menstrual period may be altered in women who take 10 g of flaxseed powder by mouth daily. Because of the possible estrogen-like effects of flaxseed (*not* flaxseed oil), it should be used cautiously in women with hormone-sensitive conditions such as endometriosis, polycystic ovary syndrome, uterine fibroids, or cancer of the breast, uterus, or ovary. Some natural medicine textbooks advise caution in patients with hypothyroidism, although little scientific information is available in this area. Flaxseed and flaxseed oil may increase the risk of bleeding, as indicated by early studies showing decreased clotting of blood. In studies in people taking alpha-linolenic acid, a substance present in flaxseed, bleeding time (time before normal clotting occurs) has been longer in laboratory tests, but dangerous bleeding problems have not been reported in the available scientific literature. Caution is advised in patients with bleeding disorders, in people taking drugs that increase the risk of bleeding, and in people planning to undergo medical, surgical, or dental procedures. Dosing of blood-thinning medications may need to be adjusted. In studies in animals, flaxseed has increased the number of red blood cells.
- Several studies in humans report an increased risk of prostate cancer in men taking alpha-linolenic acid (which is present in flaxseed) by mouth. One small study of men with prostate cancer reports that flaxseed supplements do not increase prostate-specific antigen (PSA) levels. Until more information is available, men with prostate cancer or at risk for prostate cancer should avoid flaxseed and alpha-linolenic acid supplements.

Pregnancy and Breastfeeding

- The use of flaxseed or flaxseed oil in women who are pregnant or breastfeeding is not recommended. Studies in animals show possible harmful effects, and there is little information in humans. Flaxseed may stimulate menstruation or have other hormonal effects and could be harmful to the pregnancy.

INTERACTIONS

Most herbs and supplements have not been thoroughly tested for interactions with other herbs, supplements, drugs, or foods. The interactions listed here are based on reports in scientific publications, laboratory experiments, or traditional use. It is important to always read product labels. People who have a medical condition, or are taking other drugs, herbs, or supplements, should consult a qualified healthcare provider before starting a new therapy.

Interactions with Drugs

- Taking flaxseed (*not* flaxseed oil) by mouth may reduce the absorption of other medications. Drugs used by mouth should be taken 1 hour before or 2 hours after flaxseed to prevent decreased absorption. Based on one study, flaxseed may provoke mania or hypomania in persons with bipolar disorder. People taking mood stabilizers such as lithium should use caution. Flaxseed contains alpha-linolenic acid, which theoretically may lower blood pressure. People taking medications to lower blood pressure should use caution when taking flaxseed. Laxatives and stool softeners may enhance the laxative effects of flaxseed. Flaxseed and flaxseed oil can lower cholesterol levels in animals, but studies in humans show mixed results. In theory, flaxseed may increase the effect of other medications that lower blood levels of lipids (cholesterol and triglycerides).

- Although studies report conflicting results, the omega-3 fatty acids in flaxseed and flaxseed oil may increase blood sugar, reducing the effects of drugs used to treat diabetes, including insulin and glucose-lowering medications taken by mouth. Flaxseed (*not* flaxseed oil) is a rich source of plant lignans. Lignans are sometimes referred to as phytoestrogens and may possess estrogen-like properties. It is not known if flaxseed can alter the effect of birth control pills or hormone replacement therapies. Flaxseed and flaxseed oil theoretically may increase the risk of bleeding, and caution should be used when flaxseed products are taken with drugs that increase the risk of bleeding. Some examples are aspirin, anticoagulants ("blood thinners") such as warfarin (Coumadin) and heparin, antiplatelet drugs such as clopidogrel (Plavix), and nonsteroidal anti-inflammatory drugs such as ibuprofen (Motrin, Advil) and naproxen (Naprosyn, Aleve).

Interactions with Herbs and Dietary Supplements

- Consumption of flaxseed (*not* flaxseed oil) may reduce the absorption of vitamins or supplements taken by mouth at the same time. Therefore, vitamins and supplements should be taken 1 hour before or 2 hours after a dose of flaxseed to prevent decreased absorption.
- Caution is indicated with use of flaxseed in combination with other mood-altering herbs, including St. John's wort (*Hypericum perforatum*), kava (*Piper methysticum*), and valerian (*Valeriana officinalis*). Flaxseed contains alpha-linolenic acid, which theoretically may lower blood pressure. Caution also is indicated with use of flaxseed along with other herbs or supplements that can lower blood pressure. Some examples are aconite/monkshood, arnica, baneberry, betel nut, bilberry, black cohosh, bryony, calendula, California poppy, coleus, curcumin, eucalyptol, eucalyptus oil, ginger, goldenseal, green hellebore, hawthorn, Indian tobacco, jaborandi, mistletoe, night-blooming cereus, oleander, pasque flower, periwinkle, pleurisy root, shepherd's purse, Texas milkweed, turmeric, and wild cherry.
- Because of the laxative effects of flaxseed, caution is advised with the use of flaxseed products in combination with other supplements that have laxative effects. Possible laxative herbs include alder buckthorn, aloe dried leaf sap, black root, blue flag rhizome, butternut bark, dong quai, European buckthorn, eyebright, cascara bark, castor oil, chasteberry, colocynth fruit pulp, dandelion, gamboges bark, horsetail, jalap root, manna bark, plantain leaf, podophyllum root, psyllium, rhubarb, senna, wild cucumber fruit, and yellow dock root.
- Studies on the effects of flaxseed on blood sugar in people with type 2 diabetes report mixed results. Caution is advised regarding the use of flaxseed products in combination with supplements or foods that may raise blood sugar levels. Examples are arginine, cocoa, and ephedra (when combined with caffeine). In theory, flaxseed may contain estrogen-like chemicals. Caution is indicated with use of flaxseed (*not* flaxseed oil) along with supplements believed to have estrogen-like properties. Possible examples include alfalfa, black cohosh, bloodroot, burdock, hops, kudzu, licorice, pomegranate, red clover, soy, thyme, white horehound, and yucca.
- Early studies in humans show that flaxseed and flaxseed oil theoretically may increase the risk of bleeding. Although no reports of dangerous bleeding are available, caution should be used when flaxseed products are taken with herbs

and supplements that also are believed to increase the risk of bleeding. Numerous cases of bleeding have been reported with the use of *Ginkgo biloba*, fewer cases with garlic, and two cases with saw palmetto. Numerous other agents theoretically may increase the risk of bleeding, although this effect has not been proven in most cases. Some examples are alfalfa, American ginseng, angelica, anise, *Arnica montana*, asafetida, aspen bark, bilberry, birch, black cohosh, bladderwrack, bogbean, boldo, borage seed oil, bromelain, capsicum, cat's claw, celery, chamomile, chaparral, clove, coleus, cordyceps, danshen, devil's claw, dong quai, evening primrose, fenugreek, feverfew, ginger, grapefruit juice, grapeseed, green tea, guggul, gymnestra, horse chestnut, horseradish, licorice root, lovage root, male fern, meadowsweet, nordihydroguaiaretic acid (NDGA), onion, *Panax ginseng*, papain, parsley, passion flower, poplar, prickly ash, propolis, quassia, red clover, reishi, rue, Siberian ginseng, sweet birch, sweet clover, turmeric, vitamin E, white willow, wild carrot, wild lettuce, willow, wintergreen, and yucca.

Interactions with Foods

- At high temperatures, such as in cooking, flaxseed oil and powder/flour will degrade. It is reported that eating four eggs per day from chickens fed flaxseed results in elevated serum levels of total omega-3 fatty acids. Long-term effects are not clear.

Selected References

Natural Standard developed the preceding evidence-based information based on a systematic review of more than 275 scientific articles. For comprehensive information about alternative and complementary therapies on the professional level, go to www.naturalstandard.com. Selected references are listed here.

Anonymous. Dietary supplementation with n-3 polyunsaturated fatty acids and vitamin E after myocardial infarction: results of the GISSI-Prevenzione trial. Gruppo Italiano per lo Studio della Sopravvivenza nell'Infarto Miocardico. Lancet 1999;354(9177):447-455.

Arjmandi BH, Khan DA, Juma S, et al. Whole flaxseed consumption lowers serum LDL-cholesterol and lipoprotein(a) concentrations in postmenopausal women. Nutr Res 1998;18(7):1203-1214.

Dabrosin C, Chen J, Wang L, et al. Flaxseed inhibits metastasis and decreases extracellular vascular endothelial growth factor in human breast cancer xenografts. Cancer Lett 2002; 185(1):31-37.

Demark-Wahnefried W, Price DT, Polascik TJ, et al. Pilot study of dietary fat restriction and flaxseed supplementation in men with prostate cancer before surgery: exploring the effects on hormonal levels, prostate-specific antigen, and histopathologic features. Urology 2001; 58(1):47-52.

Endoh D, Okui T, Ozawa S, et al. Protective effect of a lignan-containing flaxseed extract against CCl(4)-induced hepatic injury. J Vet Med Sci 2002;64(9):761-765.

Gross PE, Li T, Theriault M, et al. Effects of dietary flaxseed in women with cyclic mastalgia. Breast Cancer Res Treat 2000;64:49.

Hu FB, Stampfer MJ, Manson JE, et al. Dietary intake of alpha-linolenic acid and risk of fatal ischemic heart disease among women. Am J Clin Nutr 1999;69(5):890-897.

Lemay A, Dodin S, Kadri N, et al. Flaxseed dietary supplement versus hormone replacement therapy in hypercholesterolemic menopausal women. Obstet Gynecol 2002;100(3):495-504.

Lin X, Gingrich JR, Bao W, et al. Effect of flaxseed supplementation on prostatic carcinoma in transgenic mice. Urology 2002;60(5):919-924.

Lord RS, Bongiovanni B, Bralley JA. Estrogen metabolism and the diet-cancer connection: rationale for assessing the ratio of urinary hydroxylated estrogen metabolites. Altern Med Rev 2002;7(2):112-129.

Lucas EA, Wild RD, Hammond LJ, et al. Flaxseed improves lipid profile without altering biomarkers of bone metabolism in postmenopausal women. J Clin Endocrinol Metab 2002; 87(4):1527-1532.

Manthey FA, Lee RE, Hall CA 3rd. Processing and cooking effects on lipid content and stability of alpha-linolenic acid in spaghetti containing ground flaxseed. J Agric Food Chem 2002; 50(6):1668-1671.

Newton M, Combest W, Kosier JH, et al. Selected herbal dietary supplements used to manage climacteric (menopausal-type) symptoms. Urol Nurs 2002;22(4):267-272.

Ogborn MR, Nitschmann E, Bankovic-Calic N, et al. Dietary flax oil reduces renal injury, oxidized LDL content, and tissue n-6/n-3 FA ratio in experimental polycystic kidney disease. Lipids 2002;37(11):1059-1065.

Oomen CM, Ocke MC, Feskens EJ, et al. Alpha-linolenic acid intake is not beneficially associated with 10-y risk of coronary artery disease incidence: the Zutphen Elderly Study. Am J Clin Nutr 2001;74(4):457-463.

Prasad K. Dietary flax seed in prevention of hypercholesterolemic atherosclerosis. Atherosclerosis 1997;132(1):69-76.

Prasad K, Mantha SV, Muir AD, et al. Reduction of hypercholesterolemic atherosclerosis by CDC-flaxseed with very low alpha-linolenic acid. Atherosclerosis 1998;136(2):367-375.

Stoll AL, Severus WE, Freeman MP, et al. Omega 3 fatty acids in bipolar disorder: a preliminary double-blind, placebo-controlled trial. Arch Gen Psychiatry 1999;56(5):407-412.

Tarpila S, Aro A, Salminen I, et al. The effect of flaxseed supplementation in processed foods on serum fatty acids and enterolactone. Eur J Clin Nutr 2002;56(2):157-165.

von Schacky C, Angerer P, Kothny W, et al. The effect of dietary omega-3 fatty acids on coronary atherosclerosis: a randomized, double-blind, placebo-controlled trial. Ann Intern Med 1999;130(7):554-562.

Garlic

(*Allium sativum* L.)

RELATED TERMS

- Alisat, allicin, *Allii sativi* bulbus, alliinase, allium, allyl mercaptan, alubosa elewe, *Amaryllidaceae*, ayo-ishi, ayu, banlasun, camphor of the poor, clove garlic, da-suan, dai toan, dasuan, dawang, diallyl disulphide, diallyl sulfide, diallyl sulphide, dipropyl disulphide, dipropyl sulphide, dra thiam, foom, garlic clove, garlic corns, garlic extract, garlic oil, gartenlauch, hom khaao, hom kia, hom thiam, hua thiam, kesumphin, kitunguu-sumu, knoblauch, kra thiam, krathiam, krathiam cheen, krathiam khaao, Kwai, Kyolic, lai, l'ail, lahsun, la-juan, lasan, lashun, la-suan, lasun, lasuna, lauch, lay, layi, lehsun, lesun, *Liliaceae*, lobha, majo, naharu, nectar of the gods, ninniku, pa-se-waa, poor man's treacle, rason, rasonam, rasun, rustic treacle, rust treacle, *S*-allylcysteine (SAC), seer, skordo, sluon, stinking rose, sudulunu, tafanuwa, ta-suam, ta-suan, tellagada, tellagaddalu, thiam, thioallyl derivative, thiosulfinates, toi thum, tum, umbi bawang putih, vallaippundu, velluli, vellulli, verum, vinyl dithiin.

BACKGROUND

- Numerous controlled trials have examined the effects of oral garlic on serum lipids. Most studies have been small (<100 subjects), with poorly described design and results, and most have reported insignificant modest benefits. Several overlapping meta-analyses have pooled these studies, concluding that non–enteric-coated tablets containing dehydrated garlic powder (standardized to 1.3% alliin) elicit modest reductions in total cholesterol versus placebo (<20 mg/dl) in the short term (4 to 12 weeks), with unclear effects after 20 weeks. Small reductions in low-density lipoprotein (LDL) (<10 mg/dl) and triglycerides (<20 mg/dl) may also occur in the short term, although results were variable. High-density lipoprotein (HDL) levels were not significantly affected. Long-term effects on lipids or cardiovascular morbidity and mortality remain unknown. Other preparations (such as enteric-coated or raw garlic) have not been well studied.
- Small reductions in blood pressure (<10 mm Hg), inhibition of platelet aggregation, and enhancement of fibrinolytic activity have been reported, and may exert effects on cardiovascular outcomes, although evidence is preliminary in these areas.
- Numerous case-control/population-based studies suggest that regular consumption of garlic (particularly unprocessed garlic) may reduce the risk of developing several types of cancer, including gastric and colorectal malignancies. However, prospective controlled trials are lacking.
- Multiple cases of bleeding have been associated with garlic use, and caution is warranted in people at risk of bleeding. Supplemental garlic use is not advisable before some surgical/dental procedures. Garlic does not appear to significantly affect blood glucose levels.

USES BASED ON SCIENTIFIC EVIDENCE	Grade*
High cholesterol Multiple studies in humans have reported small reductions in total blood cholesterol and low-density lipoproteins ("bad cholesterol") over short periods of time (4 to 12 weeks). It is not clear if there are benefits after this amount of time. Effects on high-density lipoproteins ("good cholesterol") are not clear. This remains an area of controversy. Well-designed and longer studies are needed in this area.	B
Anti-fungal agent Several laboratory studies and historical reports describe the application of garlic to the skin to treat fungal infections, including yeast infections. However, little information on effectiveness is available. Caution should be used when using garlic topically because garlic can cause severe burns and rash when applied to the skin of sensitive individuals.	C
Anti-platelet (blood-thinning) effects Laboratory studies and trials in humans suggest that garlic may reduce blood clotting because of its effects on blood platelets. Excessive bleeding has been reported in people who take garlic supplements. The dose of garlic that can reduce blood clotting has not been established, and caution is warranted in people with bleeding problems or taking drugs that increase the risk of bleeding. Additional safety studies are needed.	C
Atherosclerosis (hardening of the arteries) Preliminary research in humans suggests that there may be relatively smaller deposits of cholesterol in blood vessels of people who take garlic. It is unclear whether this is due to the ability of garlic to lower cholesterol or to other effects of garlic.	C
Cancer prevention It is unclear whether eating garlic or taking garlic supplements regularly prevents cancer. More study is needed in this area before a conclusion can be drawn.	C
Familial hypercholesterolemia Familial hypercholesterolemia is a genetic disorder in which very high cholesterol levels occur in families. Research in children with this disorder suggests that garlic does not have a large effect in lowering their cholesterol.	C
Heart attack prevention in patients with known heart disease It is unclear whether garlic prevents future heart attacks in people who have already had a heart attack. The effects of garlic on cholesterol may be beneficial.	C
High blood pressure Numerous studies in humans report that garlic can lower blood pressure by a small amount, but larger, well-designed studies are needed to confirm this possible effect.	C

Continued

Peripheral vascular disease (blocked arteries in the legs) Some studies in humans suggest that garlic may improve circulation in the legs by a small amount, but this issue remains unclear. Better-designed studies are needed.	**C**
Tick repellent Reliable scientific information is unavailable on using garlic as a tick repellent.	**C**
Upper respiratory tract infection Preliminary reports suggest that garlic may reduce the severity of upper respiratory tract infections. However, this has not been demonstrated in well-designed studies in humans.	**C**
Diabetes Studies in animals suggest that garlic may lower blood sugar and increase the release of insulin, but studies in humans do not confirm this effect.	**D**
Stomach ulcers caused by *Helicobacter pylori* bacteria Early studies in humans show no effect of garlic on gastric or duodenal ulcers.	**D**

*Key to grades: *A:* Strong scientific evidence for this use; *B:* Good scientific evidence for this use; *C:* Unclear scientific evidence for this use; *D:* Fair scientific evidence against this use (it may not work); *F:* Strong scientific evidence against this use (it likely does not work). For a more detailed explanation of efficacy criteria, see "Natural Standard Evidence-Based Validated Grading Rationale" in the Introduction.

Uses Based on Tradition, Theory, or Limited Scientific Evidence

Abortion, age-related memory problems, AIDS, allergies, amoeba infections, antioxidant, antitoxin, anti-viral, aphrodisiac, arthritis, ascaridiasis (worms in the gut or liver), asthma, athlete's foot, bile secretion problems, bloody urine, bronchitis, cholera, claudication (leg pain due to poor blood flow), colds, cough, cryptococcal meningitis, cytomegalovirus infection, dental pain, digestive aid, diphtheria, dysentery, diuretic (increasing urine flow), earache, fatigue, fever, gallstones, hair growth stimulant, headache, heart rhythm disorders, hemorrhoids, hepatopulmonary syndrome, HIV, hormonal effects, immune system stimulation, inflammation, inflammatory bowel disease, influenza, kidney problems, kidney damage from antibiotics, leukemia, liver health, malaria, mucus thinning, muscle spasms, nephrotic syndrome, obesity, parasites and worms, perspiration, pneumonia, psoriasis, Raynaud's disease, ringworm (*Tinea corpori*, *Tinea cruris*), sedative, sinus decongestant, snake venom protection, spermicide, stomachache, stomach acid reduction, stress (anxiety), stroke, thrush, toothache, traveler's diarrhea, tuberculosis, vaginal trichomoniasis, typhus, urinary tract infections, vaginal irritation, vomiting (induction of), warts, well-being, whooping cough.

DOSING

The following doses are based on scientific research, publications, traditional use, or expert opinion. Many herbs and supplements have not been thoroughly tested, and their safety and effectiveness may not be proven. Brands may be made differently, with variable ingredients even within the same brand. The doses shown may not apply to all products. It is important to always read product labels and discuss doses with a qualified healthcare provider before therapy is started.

Standardization

- Standardization involves measuring the amounts of certain chemicals in products to try to make different preparations similar to each other. It is not always known if the chemicals being measured are the "active" ingredients.
- Although allicin was once thought to be the major active ingredient in garlic, it now appears that additional compounds may contribute to the effects of garlic. The amounts of these compounds likely vary according to the process used to manufacture the garlic product. Dried garlic powder is thought to have similar activity to that of fresh, crushed garlic. However, garlic products prepared by other methods may not have as strong effects. For example, steam-distilled oils, oils from crushed garlic, and aged-garlic in alcohol may have less blood-thinning effects. The method of processing may be as important as the ingredients reported.
- The standardized garlic powder product Kwai (Lichtwer Pharma GmbH, Berlin, Germany) has been used in numerous studies. It is standardized to contain 1.3% allicin. Other studies have used a standardized preparation containing 220 mg of garlic powder containing 2.4 mg of allicin. In the United States, pharmacy-grade garlic contains 0.3% (powdered) to 0.5% (fresh, dried) allicin, whereas in Europe, pharmacy-grade garlic must contain at least 0.45% allicin.

Adults (18 Years and Older)

- **Tablets or capsules:** 600 to 900 mg daily of non-coated, dehydrated garlic powder in three divided doses, standardized to 1.3% allicin content, has been used. The European Scientific Cooperative on Phytotherapy (ESCOP) recommends 3 to 5 mg of allicin daily (one clove or 0.5 to 1.0 g of dried powder) for prevention of atherosclerosis. The World Health Organization (WHO) recommends 2 to 5 g of fresh garlic, 0.4 to 1.2 g of dried powder, 2 to 5 mg of oil, 300 to 1000 mg of extract, or other formulations that are equal to 2 to 5 mg of allicin daily.
- **Oil:** Studies in humans have used 4 to 12.3 mg of garlic oil given by mouth daily. Steam-distilled oils, oil from crushed garlic, and aged-garlic in alcohol may be less effective in some uses, particularly as a blood thinner.
- **Tincture:** The European Scientific Cooperative on Phytotherapy recommends 2 to 4 g of dried bulb or 2 to 4 ml of tincture (1:5 dilution in 45% ethanol), by mouth three times a day for upper respiratory tract infections.

Children (Younger Than 18 Years)

- The safety and effectiveness of garlic supplements has not been proven in children. One small study involving children with a hereditary form of high cholesterol showed no benefit from 900 mg of dehydrated garlic powder tablets (Kwai) taken in three divided daily doses when compared to placebo (sugar pills). Garlic in amounts found in food is likely safe.

SAFETY

The U.S. Food and Drug Administration does not strictly regulate herbs and supplements. There is no guarantee of the strength, purity, or safety of products, and effects may vary. It is important to always read product labels. People who have a medical condition, or are taking other drugs, herbs, or supplements, should consult a qualified healthcare provider before starting a new therapy. A healthcare provider should be contacted immediately about any side effects.

Allergies

- People with a known allergy to garlic, any of its ingredients, or to other members of the Liliaceae (lily) family, which includes hyacinths, tulips, onions, leeks, and chives, should avoid the use of garlic and garlic supplements. Allergic reactions have been reported with garlic taken by mouth, inhaled, or applied to the skin. Some of these reactions were severe, including throat swelling and difficulty breathing (anaphylaxis). It has been suggested that some cases of asthma from inhaling garlic may be caused by mites on the garlic. Fresh garlic applied to the skin may be more likely than garlic extract to cause rashes.

Side Effects and Warnings

- Bad breath, body odor, and allergic reactions are the most commonly reported side effects. Fresh garlic has caused rash or skin burns, both in people taking garlic therapy and in food preparers handling garlic. Most reactions improve after stopping garlic therapy or handling garlic. Garlic products should not be applied to the skin of infants or children, because there have been multiple reports of skin burns, and should be used cautiously in adults. Other reported side effects are asthma flares, chills, dizziness, fever, increased sweating, and runny nose.
- Bleeding is a potentially serious side effect of garlic use, including bleeding after surgery and spontaneous bleeding. Several cases of bleeding have been reported that may have been due to effects of garlic on blood platelets or to increased breakdown of blood clots (fibrinolysis). There is debate about the effects of garlic in people treated with warfarin (Coumadin), but studies suggest that garlic does not alter the international normalized ratio (INR) (values that are used to measure the effect of warfarin on blood thinning). Use of garlic should be stopped prior to certain surgical or dental procedures because of the increased risk of bleeding. Caution is urged in people who have bleeding disorders or who take blood-thinning medications (anticoagulants, aspirin/antiplatelet agents, and nonsteroidal anti-inflammatory drugs such as ibuprofen and naproxen) or herbs or supplements that may increase the risk of bleeding. Dosing adjustments may be necessary.
- Studies in animals suggest that garlic or its ingredients may lower blood sugar levels and increase the release of insulin. However, studies in humans do not show changes in blood sugar levels in people either with or without diabetes. Nonetheless, caution is advised in people with diabetes or hypoglycemia, and in those taking drugs, herbs, or supplements that affect blood sugar levels. Blood glucose levels may need to be monitored by a healthcare provider, and medication adjustments may be necessary.
- Informal reports have described low iodine absorption by the thyroid and low levels of thyroid hormone (hypothyroidism) in people taking garlic supplements. A few studies have reported that ingestion of garlic and garlic-like plants may be linked to nodules or tumors of the thyroid. Reduced sperm counts have been reported in rats given garlic supplements, but not in humans.

- Dehydrated garlic preparations or raw garlic taken by mouth may cause abdominal pain or fullness, bad breath, belching, burning of the mouth, changes in the bacteria in the gut, constipation, diarrhea, flatulence (gas), heartburn, nausea and vomiting, poor appetite, and stomach lining irritation. One report describes bowel obstruction in a man who ate a whole garlic bulb. Garlic should be used cautiously by people with stomach ulcers or who are prone to stomach irritation.
- Multiple studies show a slight reduction in blood cholesterol levels after garlic supplements are taken by mouth. Slight decreases in blood pressure also have been commonly reported. One case of heart attack was reported in a healthy man after he had eaten a large amount of garlic.
- Contamination of garlic products has been reported.
- In Vancouver, British Columbia, a commercial preparation of chopped garlic was linked to botulism. One report described overdose of colchicine and even death after meadow saffron (*Colchicum autumnale*) was mistaken for wild garlic (*Allium ursinium*) and ingested.
- Garlic and pycnogenol (another popular supplement) have been shown to increase human growth hormone secretion in laboratory experiments.

G

Pregnancy and Breastfeeding

- Garlic is likely safe during pregnancy in amounts usually eaten in food, based on historical use. However, garlic supplements or large amounts of garlic should be avoided during pregnancy because of the possible increased risk of bleeding. In addition, early studies in animals suggest that garlic may cause contraction of the uterus.
- Garlic is likely safe in women who are breastfeeding in amounts usually eaten in food, based on historical use. However, some nursing mothers who were taking garlic supplements reported increased nursing time, a "garlicky" milk odor, and reduced feeding by the infant. The safety of garlic supplements in women who are breastfeeding is not known.
- *Note:* Many tinctures contain high levels of alcohol, and should be avoided during pregnancy.

INTERACTIONS

Most herbs and supplements have not been thoroughly tested for interactions with other herbs, supplements, drugs, or foods. The interactions listed here are based on reports in scientific publications, laboratory experiments, or traditional use. It is important to always read product labels. People who have a medical condition, or are taking other drugs, herbs, or supplements, should consult a qualified healthcare provider before starting a new therapy.

Interactions with Drugs

- Studies in humans suggest that garlic may increase the risk of bleeding when taken with drugs that also increase the risk of bleeding. Examples are anticoagulants (blood thinners) such as warfarin (Coumadin) and heparin, antiplatelet drugs such as clopidogrel (Plavix), aspirin, and nonsteroidal anti-inflammatory drugs such as ibuprofen (Motrin, Advil) and naproxen (Naprosyn, Aleve). Studies in animals and humans have demonstrated that garlic may lower blood pressure. Therefore, caution is advised in people taking garlic supplements in combination with other medications that lower blood pressure.

- Several studies in humans have reported lower cholesterol levels in people taking garlic. This effect may be increased if garlic is taken with medications that also lower blood cholesterol, such as lovastatin (Mevacor) and other "statins" (HMGCoA reductase inhibitors).
- Levels of the drug saquinavir, used in treatment of HIV, may be reduced if garlic is being taken at the same time, and its effectiveness may therefore be reduced. Other antiviral drugs, such as ritonavir, also may be affected.
- Based on studies in animals, garlic may lower blood sugar levels. Although this effect is theoretical in humans, caution is advised in people who are using medications that may also lower blood sugar levels. Persons who are taking drugs for diabetes by mouth or insulin should be monitored closely by a qualified healthcare provider. Medication adjustments may be necessary. People with thyroid disorders, including those who take thyroid medications, should use caution when taking garlic supplements because they may affect the thyroid.
- Limited laboratory research and studies in animals suggest that garlic may interfere with how the body uses the liver's cytochrome P450 enzyme system to process components of some drugs. As a result, blood levels of these components may be elevated and may cause increased effects or potentially serious adverse reactions. People who are using any medications should always read the package insert and consult with their healthcare provider and pharmacist about possible interactions.
- *Note:* Many tinctures contain high levels of alcohol, and may cause nausea or vomiting when taken with metronidazole (Flagyl) or disulfiram (Antabuse).

Interactions with Herbs and Dietary Supplements

- Based on human cases reports, garlic may increase the risk of bleeding. In theory, this risk may be increased when garlic is taken with other herbs or supplements that also increase the risk of bleeding. Multiple cases of bleeding have been reported with the use of *Ginkgo biloba,* and two cases with saw palmetto. Numerous other agents theoretically may increase the risk of bleeding, although this has not been proven in most cases. Examples of such agents are alfalfa, American ginseng, angelica, anise, *Arnica montana*, asafetida, aspen bark, bilberry, birch, black cohosh, bladderwrack, bogbean, boldo, borage seed oil, bromelain, capsicum, cat's claw, celery, chamomile, chaparral, clove, coleus, cordyceps, danshen, devil's claw, dong quai, EPA (eicosapentaenoic acid, found in deep-sea fish oils), evening primrose, fenugreek, feverfew, fish oil, flaxseed/flax powder (not a concern with flaxseed oil), ginger, grapefruit, grape seed, green tea, guggul, gymnestra, horse chestnut, horseradish, licorice root, lovage root, male fern, meadowsweet, nordihydroguaiaretic acid (NDGA), onion, *Panax ginseng*, papain, parsley, passion flower, poplar, prickly ash, propolis, quassia, red clover, reishi, rue, Siberian ginseng, sweet birch, sweet clover, turmeric, vitamin E, white willow, wild carrot, wild lettuce, willow, wintergreen, and yucca.
- Studies in animals and humans suggest that garlic may have a slight effect in lowering blood pressure. Caution should be used in people who are taking garlic in combination with other herbs or supplements that can lower blood pressure. Examples of such agents are aconite/monkshood, arnica, baneberry, betel nut, bilberry, black cohosh, bryony, calendula, California poppy, coleus, curcumin, eucalyptol, eucalyptus oil, flax/flaxseed oil, ginger, ginkgo, goldenseal, green hellebore, hawthorn, Indian tobacco, jaborandi, mistletoe, night-blooming cereus,

oleander, pasque flower, periwinkle, pleurisy root, shepherd's purse, Texas milkweed, turmeric, and wild cherry.

- Although studies in animals reported that garlic may lower blood sugar levels, this effect has not been shown in humans. Nonetheless, caution is advised in people who are using other herbs or supplements that also may lower blood sugar levels. Blood glucose levels may require monitoring, and doses may need adjustment. Examples of such agents are *Aloe vera*, American ginseng, bilberry, bitter melon, burdock, fenugreek, fish oil, gymnema, horse chestnut seed extract (HCSE), maitake mushroom, marshmallow, milk thistle, *Panax ginseng*, rosemary, Siberian ginseng, stinging nettle, and white horehound.
- Studies in humans have shown that garlic may cause a slight decrease in cholesterol. This effect may be larger than expected in people who are also taking other cholesterol-lowering supplements such as fish oil, EPA (eicosapentaenoic acid, found in deep-sea fish oils), guggul, red yeast, and niacin.
- Garlic may interact with herbals and dietary supplements that are metabolized by the liver's cytochrome P450 enzyme system. Speak with your doctor and pharmacist about potential interactions.
- Garlic and pycnogenol (another popular supplement) have been shown to increase human growth hormone secretion in laboratory experiments.

G

Selected References

Natural Standard developed the preceding evidence-based information based on a systematic review of more than 600 scientific articles. For comprehensive information about alternative and complementary therapies on the professional level, go to www.naturalstandard.com. Selected references are listed here.

Ackermann R, Mulrow C. Duration of the hypocholesterolemic effect of garlic supplements. Arch Intern Med 2001;161(20):2505-2506.

Ackermann RT, Mulrow CD, Ramirez G, et al. Garlic shows promise for improving some cardiovascular risk factors. Arch Intern Med 2001;161(6):813-824.

Andrianova IV, Sobenin IA, Sereda EV, et al. Effect of long-acting garlic tablets "allicor" on the incidence of acute respiratory viral infections in children. [Article in Russian.] Ter Arkh 2003;75(3):53-56.

Andrianova IV, Fomchenkov IV, Orekhov AN. Hypotensive effect of long-acting garlic tablets allicor (a double-blind placebo-controlled trial). [Article in Russian.] Ter Arkh 2002;74(3):76-78.

Anonymous. Garlic in cryptococcal meningitis: a preliminary report of 21 cases. Chin Med J 1980;93(2):123-126.

Auer W, Eiber A, Hertkorn E, et al. Hypertension and hyperlipidaemia: garlic helps in mild cases. Br J Clin Pract Suppl 1990;69:3-6.

Banerjee SK, Mukherjee PK, Maulik SK. Garlic as an antioxidant: the good, the bad and the ugly. Phytother Res 2003;17(2):97-106.

Bordia A, Verma SK, Srivastava KC. Effect of garlic (*Allium sativum*) on blood lipids, blood sugar, fibrinogen and fibrinolytic activity in patients with coronary artery disease. Prostaglandins Leukot Essent Fatty Acids 1998;58(4):257-263.

Bordia A. [Garlic and coronary heart disease. Results of a 3-year treatment with garlic extract on the reinfarction and mortality rate.] Deutsche Apotheker Zeitung 1989;129(28 suppl 15):16-17.

Bordia A. Effect of garlic on blood lipids in patients with coronary heart disease. Am J Clin Nutr 1981;34(10):2100-2103.

Borek C. Garlic supplements and saquinavir. Clin Infect Dis. 2002;35(3):343. Comment in: Clin Infect Dis 2002;34(2):234-238.

Buz'Zard AR, Peng Q, Lau BH. Kyolic and Pycnogenol increase human growth hormone secretion in genetically-engineered keratinocytes. Growth Horm IGF Res 2002;12(1):34-40.

Carden SM, Good WV, Carden PA, et al. Garlic and the strabismus surgeon. Clin Experiment Ophthalmol 2002;30(4):303-304.

Dikasso D, Lemma H, Urga K, et al. Investigation on the antibacterial properties of garlic (*Allium sativum*) on pneumonia–causing bacteria. Ethiop Med J 2002;40(3):241-249.

Dillon SA, Burmi RS, Lowe GM, et al. Antioxidant properties of aged garlic extract: an in vitro study incorporating human low density lipoprotein. Life Sci. 2003;72(14):1583-1594.

Dirsch VM, Antlsperger DS, Hentze H, et al. Ajoene, an experimental anti-leukemic drug: mechanism of cell death. Leukemia 2002;16(1):74-83.

Ernst E. Can allium vegetables prevent cancer? Phytomed 1997;4(1):79-83.

Fleischauer AT, Arab L. Garlic and cancer: a critical review of the epidemiologic literature. J Nutr 2001;131(Suppl 3):1032S-1040S.

Fleischauer AT, Poole C, Arab L. Garlic consumption and cancer prevention: meta-analyses of colorectal and stomach cancers. Am J Clin Nutr 2000;72(4):1047-1052.

Gadkari JV, Joshi VD. Effect of ingestion of raw garlic on serum cholesterol level, clotting time and fibrinolytic activity in normal subjects. J Postgrad Med 1991;37(3):128-131.

Gallicano K, Foster B, Choudhri S. Effect of short-term administration of garlic supplements on single-dose ritonavir pharmacokinetics in healthy volunteers. Br J Clin Pharmacol 2003; 55(2):199-202.

Gardner CD, Chatterjee LM, Carlson JJ. The effect of a garlic preparation on plasma lipid levels in moderately hypercholesterolemic adults. Atherosclerosis 2001;154(1):213-220.

Groppo FC, Ramacciato JC, Simoes RP, et al. Antimicrobial activity of garlic, tea tree oil, and chlorhexidine against oral microorganisms. Int Dent J 2002;52(6):433-427.

Hodge G, Hodge S, Han P. *Allium sativum* (garlic) suppresses leukocyte inflammatory cytokine production in vitro: potential therapeutic use in the treatment of inflammatory bowel disease. Cytometry 2002;48(4):209-215.

Hsing AW, Chokkalingam AP, Gao YT, et al. Allium vegetables and risk of prostate cancer: a population-based study. J Natl Cancer Inst 2002;94(21):1648-1651.

Hughes TM, Varma S, Stone NM. Occupational contact dermatitis from a garlic and herb mixture. Contact Dermatitis 2002;47(1):48.

Graham DY, Anderson SY, Lang T. Garlic or jalapeno peppers for treatment of *Helicobacter pylori* infection. Am J Gastroenterol 1999;94(5):1200-1202.

Josling P. Preventing the common cold with a garlic supplement: a double-blind, placebo-controlled survey. Adv Ther 2001;18(4):189-193.

Jung EM, Jung F, Mrowietz C, et al. Influence of garlic powder on cutaneous microcirculation. A randomized placebo-controlled double-blind cross-over study in apparently healthy subjects. Arzneimittelforschung 1991;41(6):626-630.

Kiesewetter H, Jung F, Jung EM, et al. Effects of garlic coated tablets in peripheral arterial occlusive disease. Clin Investig 1993;71(5):383-386.

Kiesewetter H, Jung F, Pindur G, et al. Effect of garlic on thrombocyte aggregation, microcirculation, and other risk factors. Int J Clin Pharmacol Ther Toxicol 1991;29(4):151-155.

Keiss HP, Dirsch VM, Hartung T, et al. Garlic (*Allium sativum* L.) modulates cytokine expression in lipopolysaccharide-activated human blood thereby inhibiting NF-kappaB activity. J Nutr 2003;133(7):2171-2175.

Ledezma E, DeSousa L, Jorquera A, et al. Efficacy of ajoene, an organosulphur derived from garlic, in the short- term therapy of tinea pedis. Mycoses 1996;39(9-10):393-395.

Ledezma E, Lopez JC, Marin P, et al. Ajoene in the topical short-term treatment of tinea cruris and tinea corporis in humans. Randomized comparative study with terbinafine. Arzneimittelforschung 1999;49(6):544-547

Lemar KM, Turner MP, Lloyd D. Garlic (*Allium sativum*) as an anti-*Candida* agent: a comparison of the efficacy of fresh garlic and freeze-dried extracts. J Appl Microbiol 2002; 93(3):398-405.

Li M, Ciu JR, Ye Y, et al. Antitumor activity of Z-ajoene, a natural compound purified from garlic: antimitotic and microtubule-interaction properties. Carcinogenesis 2002;23(4): 573-579.

Lin JG, Chen GW, Su CC, et al. Effects of garlic components diallyl sulfide and diallyl disulfide on arylamine *N*-acetyltransferase activity and 2-aminofluorene-DNA adducts in human promyelocytic leukemia cells. Am J Chin Med 2002;30(2-3):315-325.

Lohse N, Kraghede PG, Molbak K. Botulism an a 38-year-old man after ingestion of garlic in chilli oil. [Article in Danish.] Ugeskr Laeger 2003;165(30):2962-2963.

Markowitz JS, Devane CL, Chavin KD, et al. Effects of garlic (*Allium sativum* L.) supplementation on cytochrome P450 2D6 and 3A4 activity in healthy volunteers. Clin Pharmacol Ther 2003;74(2):170-177.

McCrindle BW, Helden E, Conner WT. Alternative medicine—a randomized double blind placebo-controlled clinical trial of garlic in hypercholesterolemic children. Pediatric Res 1998;43(4 Suppl 2):115.

McNulty CA, Wilson MP, Havinga W, et al. A pilot study to determine the effectiveness of garlic oil capsules in the treatment of dyspeptic patients with *Helicobacter pylori*. Helicobacter 2001;6(3):249-253.

Mulrow C, Lawrence V, Ackerman R, et al. Garlic: effects on cardiovascular risks and disease, protective effects against cancer, and clinical adverse effects. Evidence Report/Technology Assessment No. 20 (Contract 290-97-0012 to the San Antonio Evidence-based Practice Center based at The University of Texas Health Science Center at San Antonio and the Veterans Evidence-based Research, Dissemination, and Implementation Center, a Veterans Affairs Health Services Research and Development Center of Excellence). AHRQ Publication No. 01-E023. Rockville, MD: Agency for Healthcare Research and Quality. October 2000.

Neil HA, Silagy CA, Lancaster T, et al. Garlic powder in the treatment of moderate hyperlipidaemia: a controlled trial and meta-analysis. J R Coll Physicians Lond 1996;30(4): 329-334.

Siegel G. Long-term effect of garlic in preventing arteriosclerosis—results of two controlled clinical trials. Eur Phytojournal 2001; Symposium posters(1):1.

Silagy C, Neil A. Garlic as a lipid lowering agent—a meta-analysis. J R Coll Physicians Lond 1994;28(1):39-45.

Silagy CA, Neil HA. A meta-analysis of the effect of garlic on blood pressure. J Hypertension 1994;12(4):463-468.

Stevinson C, Pittler MH, Ernst E. Garlic for treating hypercholesterolemia. A meta-analysis of randomized clinical trials. Ann Intern Med 2000;133(6):420-429.

Stjernberg L, Berglund J. Garlic as an insect repellent. JAMA 2000;284(7):831.

Warshafsky S, Kamer RS, Sivak SL. Effect of garlic on total serum cholesterol. A meta-analysis. Ann Intern Med 1993;119(7 Pt 1):599-605.

Ginger

(*Zingiber officinale* Roscoe)

RELATED TERMS

- African ginger, *Amomum zingiber* L., black ginger, chayenne ginger, cochin ginger, gan jiang, gegibre, gingembre, gingerall, ginger BP, ginger powder BP, ginger root, ginger trips, ingwer, jamaica ginger, kankyo, race ginger, rhizoma zingeberis, sheng jiang, zerzero, Zingiberaceae, *Zingiber capitatum, Zingiber zerumbet* Smith, *Zingiber blancoi* Massk, *Zingiber majus* Rumph, zingiberis rhizoma.

BACKGROUND

- The rhizomes (underground stems) and stems of ginger have assumed significant roles in Chinese, Japanese and Indian medicine beginning in the 1500s. The oleoresin of ginger is often contained in digestive, antitussive, antiflatulent, laxative, and antacid compounds.
- There is supportive evidence from one randomized controlled trial and an open-label study that ginger reduces the severity and duration of chemotherapy-induced nausea/emesis. Effects appear to be additive to those of prochlorperazine (Compazine). The optimal dose remains unclear. Ginger's effects on other types of nausea/emesis, such as postoperative nausea and motion sickness, are indeterminate.
- Ginger is used orally, topically, and intramuscularly for a wide array of other conditions, without scientific evidence of benefit.
- Ginger may inhibit platelet aggregation/decrease platelet thromboxane production, thus theoretically increasing the risk of bleeding.

USES BASED ON SCIENTIFIC EVIDENCE	Grade*
Nausea and vomiting of pregnancy (hyperemesis gravidarum) Preliminary studies suggest that ginger may be safe and effective for nausea and vomiting of pregnancy when used at recommended doses for short periods of time (less than five days). Some publications discourage large doses of ginger during pregnancy due to concerns about mutations or abortion. Additional research is needed to determine the safety and effectiveness of ginger during pregnancy before it can be recommended for longer periods of time.	B
Motion sickness, seasickness There is mixed evidence in this area, with some studies reporting that ginger has no effect on motion sickness, and other research noting that ginger may reduce vomiting (but not nausea). Before a recommendation can be made, more studies are needed comparing ginger to other drugs used for this purpose.	C

Continued

Nausea (due to chemotherapy) Initial research studies in humans report that ginger may reduce the severity and length of time that a patient feels nausea after chemotherapy. Additional studies are needed to confirm these results and to determine safety and dosing. Numerous prescription drugs are highly effective at controlling nausea in cancer patients undergoing chemotherapy, and the available options should be discussed with the patient's medical oncologist.	C
Nausea and vomiting (after surgery) Some studies in humans report improvement in nausea or vomiting after surgery when patients take ginger before surgery. However, other research shows no difference. Additional studies are needed before the use of ginger before surgery to help with nausea and vomiting can be recommended.	C
Rheumatoid arthritis, osteoarthritis, joint and muscle pain Scientific evidence is limited in this area, and it is unclear whether ginger is beneficial for arthritis.	C

G

*Key to grades: *A:* Strong scientific evidence for this use; *B:* Good scientific evidence for this use; *C:* Unclear scientific evidence for this use; *D:* Fair scientific evidence against this use (it may not work); *F:* Strong scientific evidence against this use (it likely does not work). For a more detailed explanation of efficacy criteria, see "Natural Standard Evidence-Based Validated Grading Rationale" in the Introduction.

Uses Based on Tradition, Theory, or Limited Scientific Evidence

Alcohol withdrawal, antacid, antioxidant, antiseptic, antispasm, antiviral, aphrodisiac, appetite stimulant, asthma, atherosclerosis, athlete's foot, bacterial dysentery, baldness, bile secretion problems, bleeding, blood pressure control, blood thinner, body warmer, bronchitis, burns, cancer, cholera, colds, colic, cough suppressant, depression, diarrhea, digestive aid, dysmenorrhea, dyspepsia, elevated cholesterol, fungal infections, flatulence (gas), flu, headache, heart disease, *Helicobacter pylori* infection, immunostimulation, impotence, increased drug absorption, increased metabolism, insecticide, intestinal parasites, Kawasaki's disease, kidney disease, laxative, liver disease, malaria, menstruation (promotion of), migraine headache, pain relief, perspiration, poisonous snake bites, promotion of menstruation, psoriasis, dose reduction or cessation of selective serotonin reuptake inhibitor (SSRI) drugs, serotonin-induced hypothermia, stimulant, stomachache, stomach ulcers, testicular inflammation, tonic, toothache, and upper respiratory tract infections.

DOSING

The following doses are based on scientific research, publications, traditional use, or expert opinion. Many herbs and supplements have not been thoroughly tested, and their safety and effectiveness may not be proven. Brands may be made differently, with variable ingredients even within the same brand. The doses shown may not apply to all products. It is important to always read product labels and discuss doses with a qualified healthcare provider before therapy is started.

Standardization

- Standardization involves measuring the amounts of certain chemicals in products to try to make different preparations similar to each other. It is not always known if the chemicals being measured are the "active" ingredients. Although there is no universal standard, ginger products are often standardized to gingerol content.

Adults (18 Years and Older)

- *Note:* Common forms of ginger include fresh root, dried root, tablets, capsules, liquid extract, tincture, and tea. Many publications state that the maximum recommended daily dose of ginger is 4 g. It is believed that the mild stomach upset sometimes caused by ginger may be reduced by taking ginger capsules rather than powder.
- **General use:** Many experts and publications suggest that ginger powder, tablets, or capsules or fresh cut ginger can be used in doses of 1 to 4 g daily, by mouth, divided into smaller doses.
- **Nausea and vomiting:** To prevent nausea after surgery, ginger has been given as 1 g by mouth 1 hour before surgery. For nausea and vomiting of pregnancy, 1 to 2 g daily, by mouth, in divided doses has been used for 1 to 5 days. Some sources warn against higher doses in pregnancy because of concerns about mutations or abortion. Supervision by a qualified healthcare provider is recommended for pregnant women considering the use of ginger.
- **Motion sickness, seasickness:** 1 to 2 g daily, by mouth, in divided doses has been used.
- **Arthritis:** 1 to 2 g of powdered ginger daily, by mouth, in divided doses has been used. In one study, persons who mistakenly took 2 to 4 g daily reported faster and better relief, although the superiority of this dose has not been proven.

Children (Younger Than 18 Years)

- There is insufficient scientific evidence regarding safety and efficacy to recommend the use of ginger in children.

SAFETY

The U.S. Food and Drug Administration does not strictly regulate herbs and supplements. There is no guarantee of the strength, purity, or safety of products, and effects may vary. It is important to always read product labels. People who have a medical condition, or are taking other drugs, herbs, or supplements, should consult a qualified healthcare provider before starting a new therapy. A healthcare provider should be contacted immediately about any side effects.

Allergies

- Ginger supplements should be avoided by people with a known allergy to ginger or other members of the Zingiberaceae family, which includes *Alpinia formosana*, *Alpinia purpurata* (red ginger), *Alpinia zerumbet* (shell ginger), *Costus barbatus*, *Costus malortieanus*, *Costus pictus*, *Costus productus*, *Dimerocostus strobilaceus*, and *Elettaria cardamomum* (green cardamom). Allergic contact rashes have been reported, and these rashes may be more likely in people who work with ginger, who apply ginger to the skin, or who have a positive allergy test for balsam of Peru. An allergic eye reaction has also been reported.

Side Effects and Warnings

- Few side effects have been associated with ginger taken at low doses. There are no studies confirming the safety of long-term use of ginger supplements. The most commonly reported side effects of ginger involve the gastrointestinal system. A bad taste in the mouth, belching, bloating, flatulence (gas), heartburn, irritation of the mouth, and nausea have been reported, especially with powdered forms of ginger. There are several reports that fresh ginger that was swallowed before being thoroughly chewed resulted in blockage of the intestines. People who have ulcers, inflammatory bowel disease, or blocked intestines should use caution when taking ginger supplements and should avoid ingesting large quantities of fresh-cut ginger. People with gallstones should use ginger with caution.
- In theory, ginger can cause abnormal heart rhythms, although reports in humans are lacking. Some publications suggest that ginger may raise or lower blood pressure, although limited scientific information is available. In addition, ginger theoretically may prevent blood clotting by preventing the clumping of platelets. This raises a concern that people taking medications that slow blood clotting or who are planning to undergo surgery may have a high risk of excessive bleeding if they take ginger supplements. Ginger traditionally is believed to reduce blood sugar levels at high doses, but scientific evidence regarding this is lacking. In one study, two of eight participants reported an intense urge to urinate 30 minutes after ingesting ginger.

Pregnancy and Breastfeeding

- Some authors suggest that pregnant women should not take ginger in amounts greater than amounts found in food (or more than 1 g dry weight per day). Ginger has been reported to increase discharge from the uterus during menstruation and increase the risk of abortion, mutations of the fetus, and increased bleeding. However, other reports state that there is no scientific evidence that ginger is dangerous during pregnancy. Little scientific study is available in this area to support either perspective, although ginger has been studied in a small number of pregnant women (to assess effects on nausea), without reports of adverse pregnancy outcomes. Notably, this matter is sometimes confused because the use of ginger in pregnancy is discouraged in traditional Chinese medicine (TCM), in which much higher doses of ginger may be used.

INTERACTIONS

Most herbs and supplements have not been thoroughly tested for interactions with other herbs, supplements, drugs, or foods. The interactions listed here are based on reports in scientific publications, laboratory experiments, or traditional use. It is important to always read product labels. People who have a medical condition, or are taking other drugs, herbs, or supplements, should consult a qualified healthcare provider before starting a new therapy.

Interactions with Drugs

- There is evidence that the ginger rhizome (underground stem) may increase stomach acid production. As a result, theoretically it may act against the effects of antacids, sucralfate (Carafate), and antireflux medications, including H_2 blockers such as ranitidine (Zantac) and proton pump inhibitors such as lansoprazole (Prevacid). In contrast, other laboratory and animal studies report that ginger may act to protect the stomach.

- In theory, ginger may increase the risk of bleeding when taken with blood-thinning medications (although clear evidence in humans is lacking). Examples of such medications are anticoagulants such as warfarin (Coumadin) and heparin, antiplatelet drugs such as clopidogrel (Plavix), aspirin, and nonsteroidal anti-inflammatory drugs such as ibuprofen (Motrin, Advil) and naproxen (Naprosyn, Aleve).
- In theory, large doses of ginger may increase the effects of medications that slow thinking or cause drowsiness. Ginger may also interfere with medications that change the contractions of the heart, including beta-blockers, and digoxin. Because ginger theoretically can decrease blood sugar levels, it may interfere with the effects of insulin or diabetes medications taken by mouth.

Interactions with Herbs and Dietary Supplements

- In theory, ginger may increase the risk of bleeding when taken with herbs and supplements that may also increase the risk of bleeding (although clear evidence in humans is lacking). Multiple cases of bleeding have been reported with the use of *Ginkgo biloba*, fewer cases with garlic, and two cases with saw palmetto. Numerous other agents may theoretically increase the risk of bleeding, although this has not been proven in most cases. Examples of such agents are alfalfa, American ginseng, angelica, anise, *Arnica montana*, asafetida, aspen bark, bilberry, birch, black cohosh, bladderwrack, bogbean, boldo, borage seed oil, bromelain, capsicum, cat's claw, celery, chamomile, chaparral, clove, coleus, cordyceps, danshen, devil's claw, dong quai, evening primrose, fenugreek, feverfew, flaxseed/flax powder (not a concern with flaxseed oil), grapefruit juice, grape seed, green tea, guggul, gymnestra, horse chestnut, horseradish, licorice root, lovage root, male fern, meadowsweet, nordihydroguaiaretic acid (NDGA), onion, *Panax ginseng*, papain, parsley, passion flower, poplar, prickly ash, propolis, quassia, red clover, reishi, rue, Siberian ginseng, sweet birch, sweet clover, turmeric, vitamin E, white willow, wild carrot, wild lettuce, willow, wintergreen, and yucca.
- In theory, ginger in combination with large amounts of calcium may increase the risk of abnormal heart rhythms.
- Ginger theoretically may lower blood sugar levels. Caution is advised in people taking ginger who are taking other herbs or supplements that also may affect blood sugar levels, such as *Aloe vera*, American ginseng, bilberry, bitter melon, burdock, fenugreek, fish oil, gymnema, horse chestnut seed extract (HCSE), marshmallow, milk thistle, *Panax ginseng*, rosemary, Siberian ginseng, stinging nettle, and white horehound. Blood glucose levels may require monitoring, and doses may need adjustment.

Selected References

Natural Standard developed the preceding evidence-based information based on a systematic review of more than 400 scientific articles. For comprehensive information about alternative and complementary therapies on the professional level, go to www.naturalstandard.com. Selected references are listed here.

Abebe W. Herbal medication: potential for adverse interactions with analgesic drugs. J Clin Pharm Ther 2002;27(6):391-401.

Akoachere JF, Ndip RN, Chenwi EB, et al. Antibacterial effect of *Zingiber officinale* and garcinia kola on respiratory tract pathogens. East Afr Med J 2002;79(11):588-592.

Altman RD, Marcussen KC. Effects of a ginger extract on knee pain in patients with osteoarthritis. Arthritis Rheum 2001;44(11):2531-2538.

Arfeen Z, Owen H, Plummer JL, et al. A double-blind randomized controlled trial of ginger for the prevention of postoperative nausea and vomiting. Anaesth Intensive Care 1995; 23(4):449-452.

Bean P. The use of alternative medicine in the treatment of hepatitis C. Am Clin Lab 2002 May;21(4):19-21.

Bliddal H, Rosetzsky A, Schlichting P, et al. A randomized, placebo-controlled, cross-over study of ginger extracts and ibuprofen in osteoarthritis. Osteoarthritis Cartilage 2000;8(1):9-12.

Blumenthal M. Ginger as an antiemetic during pregnancy. Altern Ther Health Med. 2003 Jan-Feb;9(1):19-21; author reply, 19-21. Comment in: Altern Ther Health Med 2002; 8(5):89-91.

Bordia A, Verma SK, Srivastava KC. Effect of ginger (*Zingiber officinale* Rosc.) and fenugreek (*Trigonella foenum-graecum* L.) on blood lipids, blood sugar and platelet aggregation in patients with coronary artery disease. Prostaglandins Leukot Essent Fatty Acids 1997;56(5):379-384.

Chandra K, Einarson A, Koren G. Taking ginger for nausea and vomiting during pregnancy. Can Fam Physician 2002;48:1441-1442.

Eberhart LH, Mayer R, Betz O, et al. Ginger does not prevent postoperative nausea and vomiting after laparoscopic surgery. Anesth Analg 2003;96(4):995-998.

Ernst E, Pittler MH. Efficacy of ginger for nausea and vomiting: a systematic review of randomized clinical trials. Br J Anaesth 2000;84(3):367-371.

Handler J. Drug-induced hypertension. J Clin Hypertens (Greenwich) 2003;5(1):83-85.

Hashimoto K, Satoh K, Murata P, et al. Component of *Zingiber officinale* that improves the enhancement of small intestinal transport. Planta Med 2002;68(10):936-939.

Hodges PJ, Kam PC. The peri-operative implications of herbal medicines. Anaesthesia 2002; 57(9):889-99 Comments in: Anaesthesia 2002;57(10):947-948; Anaesthesia 2003;58(2): 184-185; Anaesthesia 2003;58(6):597-598.

Jewell D. Nausea and vomiting in early pregnancy. Clin Evid 2002;(7):1277-1283.

Jewell D, Young G. Interventions for nausea and vomiting in early pregnancy. Cochrane Database Syst Rev. 2002;(1):CD000145. Comment in: ACP J Club. 2002 Sep-Oct;137(2): 67. Update of: Cochrane Database Syst Rev. 2000;(2):CD000145.

Kalveniene Z, Savickas A, Svambaris L, et al. Development and analysis of revitalizing tincture [Article in Lithuanian]. Medicina (Kaunas) 2002;38(10):1009-1013.

Keating A, Chez RA. Ginger syrup as an antiemetic in early pregnancy. Altern Ther Health Med. 2002;8(5):89-91. Comment in: Altern Ther Health Med 2003;9(1):19-21.

Kim DS, Kim DS, Oppel MN. Shogaols from *Zingiber officinale* protect IMR32 human neuroblastoma and normal human umbilical vein endothelial cells from beta-amyloid(25-35) insult. Planta Med 2002;68(4):375-376.

Lien HC, Sun WM, Chen YH, et al Effects of ginger on motion sickness and gastric slow-wave dysrhythmias induced by circular vection. Am J Physiol Gastrointest Liver Physiol 2003;284(3):G481-G489.

Marcus DM, Suarez-Almazor ME. Is there a role for ginger in the treatment of osteoarthritis? Arthritis Rheum 2001;44(11):2461-2462.

Meyer K, Schwartz J, Crater D, et al. *Zingiber officinale* (ginger) used to prevent 8-Mop associated nausea. Dermatol Nurs 1995;7(4):242-244.

Moneret-Vautrin DA, Morisset M, Lemerdy P, et al. Food allergy and IgE sensitization caused by spices: CICBAA data (based on 589 cases of food allergy). Allerg Immunol (Paris) 2002; 34(4):135-140.

Morelli V, Naquin C, Weaver V. Alternative therapies for traditional disease states: osteoarthritis. Am Fam Physician 2003;67(2):339-344.

Murakami A, Takahashi D, Kinoshita T, et al. Zerumbone, a Southeast Asian ginger sesquiterpene, markedly suppresses free radical generation, proinflammatory protein production, and cancer cell proliferation accompanied by apoptosis: the alpha,beta unsaturated carbonyl group is a prerequisite. Carcinogenesis. 2002;23(5):795-802. [Comment in: Carcinogenesis 2002;23(11):1961; author reply, 1963.

Visalyaputra S, Petchpaisit N, Somcharoen K, et al. The efficacy of ginger root in the prevention of postoperative nausea and vomiting after outpatient gynaecological laparoscopy. Anaesthesia 1998;53(5):506-510.

Vutyavanich T, Kraisarin T, Ruangsri R. Ginger for nausea and vomiting in pregnancy: randomized, double-masked, placebo-controlled trial. Obstet Gynecol 2001;97(4):577-582.

Ginkgo

(*Ginkgo biloba* L.)

RELATED TERMS

- Arbre aux quarante écus, adiantifolia, baiguo, bai guo ye, BN-52063, duck foot tree, elefantenohr, EGb, EGb 761, eun-haeng, facherblattbaum, fossil tree, GBE, GBE 24, GBX, ginan, gin-nan, Ginkgoaceae, ginkgo balm, ginkgoblätter, ginkgo folium, *Ginkgo biloba* blätter, ginkgogink, ginkgold, ginkgopower, ginkyo, icho, ityo, japanbaum, Japanese silver apricot, kew tree, kung sun shu, LI 1370, maidenhair tree, noyer du Japon, oriental plum tree, pei kuo, pei-wen, pterophyllus, pterophyllus salisburiensis, rokan, salisburia, salisburia adiantifolia, salisburia macrophylla, silver apricot, sophium, tempeltrae, tanakan, tanakene, tebofortan, tebonin, temple balm, tramisal, valverde, vasan, vital, ya chio, yin-guo, yin-hsing.

BACKGROUND

- *Ginkgo biloba* has been used medicinally for thousands of years. Today, it is one of the top-selling herbs in the United States, accounting for $140 million in sales in 1998.
- Ginkgo is used for the treatment of numerous conditions, many of which are under scientific investigation. Available evidence demonstrates ginkgo's efficacy in the management of intermittent claudication, Alzheimer's/multi-infarct dementia, and "cerebral insufficiency" (a syndrome thought to be secondary to atherosclerotic disease, characterized by impaired concentration, confusion, decreased physical performance, fatigue, headache, dizziness, depression, and anxiety).
- Although not definitive, there is promising early evidence favoring the use of ginkgo for memory enhancement in healthy subjects, altitude (mountain) sickness, symptoms of premenstrual syndrome (PMS), and reduction of chemotherapy-induced end-organ vascular damage.
- Although the use of ginkgo for tinnitus remains controversial, a recent large trial has shifted the evidence against the use of ginkgo for this therapy.
- Ginkgo is generally well tolerated, but because of multiple case reports of bleeding, ginkgo should be used cautiously by persons with known coagulopathy or receiving anti-coagulant therapy. People should not use ginkgo before undergoing certain surgical or dental procedures.

USES BASED ON SCIENTIFIC EVIDENCE	Grade*
Claudication (painful legs from clogged arteries) Numerous studies suggest that *Ginkgo biloba* taken by mouth causes small improvements in claudication symptoms (leg pain with exercise or at rest due to clogged arteries). However, ginkgo may not be as helpful for this condition as exercise therapy or prescription drugs. Preliminary research comparing ginkgo to pentoxifylline (Trental) has not provided clear answers. Most studies have used 120 mg of ginkgo per day, divided	A

Continued

into two or three doses, for up to 6 months. Additional evidence is needed from well-designed studies comparing or combining ginkgo with drug and exercise therapies.	
Dementia (multi-infarct and Alzheimer's type) Many laboratory studies and studies in humans have examined the use of ginkgo for dementia. Most research has not been well designed. Despite these deficiencies, the scientific literature overall does suggest that ginkgo (120 to 240 mg daily) benefits people with early stage Alzheimer's disease and multi-infarct dementia, and may be as helpful as acetylcholinesterase inhibitor drugs such as donepezil (Aricept). Well-designed research comparing ginkgo to prescription drug therapies is needed.	**A**
Cerebral insufficiency Multiple clinical trials have evaluated ginkgo for a syndrome called "cerebral insufficiency." This condition, more commonly diagnosed in Europe than the United States, may include poor concentration, confusion, absent-mindedness, decreased physical performance, fatigue, headache, dizziness, depression, and anxiety. It is believed that cerebral insufficiency is caused by decreased blood flow to the brain due to clogged blood vessels. Some research reports benefits of ginkgo in patients with these symptoms, but most have been poorly designed and do not have reliable results. Better studies are needed before a strong recommendation can be made.	**B**
Age-associated memory impairment Age-associated memory impairment (AAMI) is a nonspecific syndrome that may be caused by early Alzheimer's disease or multi-infarct dementia (conditions for which ginkgo has been shown to have benefit). There is preliminary research showing small improvements in memory and other brain functions in patients with AAMI, although some studies disagree. Overall, there is currently not enough clear evidence to recommend for or against ginkgo for this condition.	**C**
Altitude (mountain) sickness A small amount of poorly designed research studies have reported benefits of ginkgo for the treatment of altitude (mountain) sickness. Additional study is needed before a recommendation can be made.	**C**
Chemotherapy side effects reduction In limited studies in humans, ginkgo has been examined in addition to 5-fluorouracil (5-FU) in the treatment of pancreatic and colorectal cancer, to measure possible benefits on side effects. At this time, there is not conclusive evidence in this area.	**C**
Decreased libido and erectile dysfunction (impotence) Ginkgo has been used and studied for the treatment of sexual dysfunction in men and women. Ginkgo may be effective in the treatment	**C**

Continued

G

of erectile dysfunction, based on studies in humans and animals that show blood vessel relaxant properties, which may improve blood flow in the penis to achieve an erection. Ginkgo has also been reported in limited human study to treat sexual dysfunction in men and women caused by antidepressant drugs, such as fluoxetine (Prozac). In general, studies are small and not well designed. Additional research is needed before a recommendation can be made.	
Depression and seasonal affective disorder Preliminary study of seasonal affective disorder (SAD) suggests that ginkgo is not effective in preventing the development of winter depression. Other research in elderly patients with depression shows possible minor benefits. Overall, there is not enough evidence to form a clear conclusion.	**C**
Glaucoma Several small human studies reported that ginkgo may be associated with mild increases in blood flow to the eyes and slight improvement in vision and intraocular pressure. However, these studies were small and poorly designed. Additional, well-designed research is needed before a recommendation can be made.	**C**
Macular degeneration Preliminary research suggests that ginkgo may improve eye blood flow, although it remains unclear if macular degeneration is significantly affected by ginkgo. More research is needed in this area before a conclusion can be drawn.	**C**
Memory enhancement (in healthy people) A recent well-designed study reported that ginkgo at a dose of 120 mg daily for 6 weeks did not improve memory or concentration in people older than 60 years. However, prior evidence from smaller, less rigorous studies suggested that ginkgo in doses greater than or equal to 240 mg daily may enhance memory in healthy individuals. Therefore, although it remains unclear whether higher doses of ginkgo are effective, it seems unlikely that 120 mg has significant benefits.	**C**
Multiple sclerosis (MS) Based on laboratory studies, ginkgo may provide benefit in therapy for MS. However, research in humans, limited to several small studies, has not found consistent benefits. Additional research is needed before a recommendation can be made.	**C**
Premenstrual syndrome (PMS) Initial study in women with premenstrual syndrome or breast discomfort suggests that ginkgo may relieve symptoms including emotional upset. Further well-designed research is needed before a recommendation can be made.	**C**

Continued

Ringing in the ears (tinnitus) There is conflicting research regarding the use of ginkgo for tinnitus. Traditional use and multiple small, poorly designed studies from the 1980s and 1990s report benefits. However, a well-designed recent study found no benefit. Additional well-designed research is needed in order to resolve this controversy.	C
Vertigo A small amount of poorly designed research reports benefits of ginkgo for the treatment of vertigo. Additional study is needed before a recommendation can be made.	C
Vitiligo One small study using oral ginkgo biloba extract 40 mg three times daily reports that ginkgo appears to arrest the progression of this disease. Better-designed studies are needed to confirm these results.	C
Stroke Laboratory studies suggest that ginkgo may be helpful immediately following strokes because of possible antioxidant or blood vessel effects. However, initial study of ginkgo in people having strokes found no benefits.	D
Cocaine dependence One small study reported no benefit in the use of ginkgo for cocaine independence.	D

*Key to grades: *A:* Strong scientific evidence for this use; *B:* Good scientific evidence for this use; *C:* Unclear scientific evidence for this use; *D:* Fair scientific evidence against this use (it may not work); *F:* Strong scientific evidence against this use (it likely does not work). For a more detailed explanation of efficacy criteria, see "Natural Standard Evidence-Based Validated Grading Rationale" in the Introduction.

Uses Based on Tradition, Theory, or Limited Scientific Evidence

Acidosis, aging, alcoholism, allergies, angina, anti-bacterial, anti-fungal, antioxidant, anti-parasitic, anxiety, atherosclerosis (clogged arteries), asthma, attention deficit hyperactivity disorder (ADHD), blood clots, blood vessel disorders, breast disease, breast tenderness, bronchitis, cancer, cardiac rhythm abnormalities, chilblains (inflammation of toes, fingers, ears, or face with exposure to cold), chronic rhinitis, congestive heart failure, cough, deafness, dermatitis, diabetes, diabetic eye disease, diabetic nerve damage (neuropathy), digestive aid, dizziness, dysentery (bloody diarrhea), eczema, fatigue, filariasis, freckle removal, gastric cancer, genitourinary disorders, headache, hearing loss, heart attack, heart disease, hepatitis B, high cholesterol, high blood pressure, hypoxia (lack of oxygen), insomnia, labor induction, menstrual pain, migraine, mood disturbances, Raynaud's phenomenon, respiratory tract illnesses, scabies, schizophrenia, sepsis, skin sores, swelling, traumatic brain injury, ulcerative colitis, varicose veins.

DOSING

The following doses are based on scientific research, publications, traditional use, or expert opinion. Many herbs and supplements have not been thoroughly tested, and their safety and effectiveness may not be proven. Brands may be made differently, with variable ingredients even within the same brand. The doses shown may not apply to all products. It is important to always read product labels and discuss doses with a qualified healthcare provider before therapy is started.

Standardization

- Standardization involves measuring the amounts of certain chemicals in products to try to make different preparations similar to each other. It is not always known if the chemicals being measured are the "active" ingredients.
- Ginkgo is available as ginkgo leaf, ginkgo leaf extract, and ginkgo seed. Ginkgo leaf extract is the most commonly used form. Products that use standardized extracts referred to as EGb 761 should contain 24% ginkgo flavone glycosides and 6% terpenoids. Products that use standardized extracts referred to as LI 1370 should contain 25% ginkgo flavone glycosides and 6% terpenoids.

Adults (18 Years and Older)

- **General:** 80 to 240 mg of a 50:1 standardized leaf extract taken daily by mouth in two to three divided doses has been used and studied (standardized to 24% to 25% ginkgo flavone glycosides and 6% terpine lactones). Other forms used include tea (bags usually contain 30 mg of extract), 3 to 6 ml of an extract of 40 mg per ml taken daily in three divided doses, and "fortified" foods. Ginkgo seeds are potentially toxic and should be avoided. The German ginkgo product Tebonin, injected in the veins (IV), was removed from the German market because of significant side effects.
- **Claudication (painful legs from clogged arteries):** 80 to 240 mg of a 50:1 standardized leaf extract taken daily by mouth in two to three divided doses has been studied. There is evidence that 240 mg daily may be more beneficial than 120 mg daily. In another study, 3 to 6 ml of an extract of 40 mg per ml taken daily by mouth in three divided doses was used, with some evidence that 6 ml may be more effective than 3 ml. The ginkgo product Tanakan has been studied at a dose of 100 mg in 500 ml of normal saline, given twice daily into a vein (IV) for blood vessel disease, although the safety of this type of dosing has not been proven.
- **Cerebral insufficiency:** In some studies, 112 to 160 mg daily, divided into three doses for up to 12 weeks, were used.
- **Dementia:** 120 to 240 mg daily in three divided doses have been studied.
- **Memory enhancement** (in healthy people): Doses of 240 to 360 mg daily in three divided doses have been studied.

Children (Younger Than 18 Years)

- There is insufficient scientific evidence to recommend the use of ginkgo in children.

SAFETY

The U.S. Food and Drug Administration does not strictly regulate herbs and supplements. There is no guarantee of the strength, purity, or safety of products, and effects may vary. It is important to always read product labels. People who have a medical condition, or are taking other drugs, herbs, or supplements, should consult a qualified healthcare provider before starting a new therapy. A healthcare provider should be contacted immediately about any side effects.

Allergies

- Allergy/hypersensitivity to *Ginkgo biloba* or members of the Ginkgoaceae family may occur. There is a case report of a severe reaction called Stevens-Johnson syndrome, including skin blistering and sloughing-off, after use of the ginkgo product One-A-Day Memory and Concentration, which contains 60 mg of ginkgo leaf extract as well as vitamins B_6, B_{12}, and choline bitartrate. There may be cross-sensitivity to ginkgo in people allergic to urusiols (mango rind, sumac, poison ivy, poison oak, cashews). If administered through a vein (IV), ginkgo may cause a skin allergy and blood vessel irritation and damage. Ginkgo fruit or pulp has caused strong allergic reactions after skin contact, and intestinal spasms have occurred after direct contact with fleshy fruit pulp.

Side Effects and Warnings

- Overall, ginkgo leaf extract (used in most commercial products) appears to be well tolerated in most healthy adults at recommended doses for up to 6 months. In several reviews, ginkgo was associated with similar rates of side effects to placebo (sugar pill). Minor symptoms including headache, nausea, and intestinal complaints have been reported.
- Bleeding has been associated with the use of ginkgo taken by mouth, and caution is advised in people who have bleeding disorders or are taking drugs, herbs, or supplements that may increase the risk of bleeding. Dosing adjustments may be necessary. Ginkgo should be stopped prior to certain surgical or dental procedures.
- Reports of bleeding range from nose bleeds to life-threatening bleeding in several case reports. In some of these reports, ginkgo had been used with other agents that also may cause bleeding. For example, spontaneous bleeding into the eye (hyphema) was reported in a 70-year-old man taking 80 mg daily of ginkgo for 1 week. This man was also taking 325 mg daily of aspirin, which can also increase the risk of bleeding. In the following cases, spontaneous bleeding into and around the brain was reported: a 33-year-old woman taking 120 mg of ginkgo daily for 2 years with no other medications; a 72-year-old woman (subdural bleeding); a 61-year-old male taking 120 to 160 mg of ginkgo daily for more than 6 months (subarachnoid hemorrhage); a 56-year-old man who regularly used an herbal preparation including ginkgo; and a 78-year-old woman taking ginkgo for 2 months in addition to the blood thinner warfarin (intracerebral bleeding). Excessive bleeding has also been reported after gallbladder surgery (laparoscopic cholecystectomy).
- Toxicity from eating ginkgo seeds is sometimes called "gin-nan food poisoning," and has been documented in at least 70 case reports between 1930 and 1970, with the worst effects seen in infants. Eating the seeds is potentially deadly because of the risk of tonic-clonic seizures and loss of consciousness. There is a case report of two persons with well-controlled seizure disorder who had seizures after taking ginkgo. However, reports of seizure activity associated with use of ginkgo leaf extract are rare.
- Based on studies in humans, ginkgo theoretically may affect insulin and blood sugar levels. Caution is advised in people with diabetes or hypoglycemia, and in those taking drugs, herbs, or supplements that also may affect blood sugar levels. Serum glucose levels may need to be monitored by a healthcare provider, and medication adjustments may be necessary.
- There have been uncommon reports of headache, dizziness, stomach upset, nausea, diarrhea, vomiting, muscle weakness, loss of muscle tone, restlessness, heart racing,

rash, and irritation around the mouth with the use of ginkgo. There is a case report of "coma" in an elderly patient with Alzheimer's disease who was taking trazodone and ginkgo, but it is not clear that ginkgo was the cause.

- Based on laboratory research and studies in humans, ginkgo may decrease blood pressure. However, an increase in blood pressure, possibly caused by ginkgo, was reported in a person taking ginkgo as well as a thiazide diuretic ("water pill"). Theoretically, high concentrations of ginkgo may reduce male and female fertility. Contamination with the drug colchicine has been found in commercial preparations of *Ginkgo biloba*.

Pregnancy and Breastfeeding

- Use of ginkgo is not recommended in women who are pregnant or breastfeeding because of the lack of reliable scientific study in this area. The risk of bleeding associated with ginkgo may be dangerous during pregnancy.

INTERACTIONS

Most herbs and supplements have not been thoroughly tested for interactions with other herbs, supplements, drugs, or foods. The interactions listed here are based on reports in scientific publications, laboratory experiments, or traditional use. It is important to always read product labels. People who have a medical condition, or are taking other drugs, herbs, or supplements, should consult a qualified healthcare provider before starting a new therapy.

Interactions with Drugs

- Overall, controlled trials of ginkgo report few adverse effects and good tolerance, with rates of complications similar to those of placebo. However, use of ginkgo with drugs that may cause bleeding may further increase the risk of bleeding, based on multiple case reports of spontaneous bleeding in patients using ginkgo alone, with warfarin (Coumadin), or with aspirin. One case report documents a possible increase in bleeding risk with combined use of ticlopidine (Ticlid) and ginkgo. Examples of drugs that may increase the risk of bleeding include anticoagulants (blood thinners) such as warfarin (Coumadin) and heparin, antiplatelet drugs such as clopidogrel (Plavix), aspirin, and nonsteroidal anti-inflammatory drugs such as ibuprofen (Motrin, Advil) and naproxen (Naprosyn, Aleve). However, not all studies agree about the existence of this risk, and it is not clear if particular types of individuals may be at greater risk.
- Based on preliminary research, ginkgo may affect insulin and blood sugar levels. Caution is advised in people who are taking ginkgo as well as medications that also may lower blood sugar levels. People who are taking drugs for diabetes by mouth or insulin should be monitored closely by a qualified healthcare provider. Medication adjustments may be necessary.
- Ginkgo has been found to decrease blood pressure in healthy volunteers, although some studies disagree. Theoretically, ginkgo may add to the effects of medications that also lower blood pressure, although increased blood pressure was reported in a person taking a thiazide diuretic ("water pill") with ginkgo.
- Monoamine oxidase (MAO) inhibition by ginkgo was reported in one study in animals but has not been confirmed in humans. In theory, if ginkgo is taken with MAO inhibitor drugs, such as isocarboxazid (Marplan), phenelzine (Nardil), and tranylcypromine (Parnate), additive effects and side effects may occur. Based on laboratory research, ginkgo may also add to the effects of selective serotonin

reuptake inhibitor (SSRI) antidepressants such as sertraline (Zoloft), with an increased risk of causing serotonin syndrome, a condition characterized by stiff muscles, rapid heart rate, hyperthermia, restlessness, and sweating.

- Case reports suggest that ginkgo may decrease side effects of antipsychotic drugs, although scientific information in this area is limited. In one report, "coma" occurred in an elderly patient with Alzheimer's disease who was taking trazodone and ginkgo, but it is not clear that this reaction was due to ginkgo. In theory, ginkgo may increase the actions of drugs used for erectile dysfunction such as sildenafil (Viagra).
- There may be a risk of seizures when taking ginkgo, particularly in people with a history of seizure disorder. Although in most reports seizures were caused by eating ginkgo seeds (not leaf extract, which is found in most products), a study in animals found that the anti-seizure properties of sodium valproate or carbamazepine were reduced by giving ginkgo. In theory, drugs such as donepezil (Aricept) and tacrine (Cognex) may have an additive effect when used at the same time as ginkgo, potentially increasing cholinergic effects, (such as salivation and urination).
- 5-fluorouracil-induced side effects and cyclosporine kidney toxicity theoretically may be lessened by ginkgo, although evidence is not conclusive in these areas. Colchicine has been found in commercial preparations of ginkgo, and may increase blood concentrations in patients using colchicine.

G

Interactions with Herbs and Dietary Supplements

- Use of ginkgo with herbs or supplements that may cause bleeding may increase the risk of bleeding, although some studies disagree. Several cases of bleeding have been reported with the use of garlic, and two cases with saw palmetto. Numerous other agents may theoretically increase the risk of bleeding, although this has not been proven in most cases. Examples are alfalfa, American ginseng, angelica, anise, *Arnica montana*, asafetida, aspen bark, bilberry, birch, black cohosh, bladderwrack, bogbean, boldo, borage seed oil, bromelain, capsicum, cat's claw, celery, chamomile, chaparral, clove, coleus, cordyceps, danshen, devil's claw, dong quai, evening primrose, fenugreek, feverfew, flaxseed/flax powder (not a concern with flaxseed oil), ginger, grapefruit juice, grape seed, green tea, guggul, gymnestra, horse chestnut, horseradish, licorice root, lovage root, male fern, meadowsweet, nordihydroguaiaretic acid (NDGA), onion, *Panax ginseng*, parsley, papain, passion flower, poplar, prickly Ash, propolis, quassia, red clover, reishi, rue, Siberian ginseng, sweet birch, sweet clover, turmeric, vitamin E, white willow, wild carrot, wild lettuce, willow, wintergreen, and yucca.
- In some studies, ginkgo has been found to decrease blood pressure in healthy volunteers, although other studies disagree. Theoretically, ginkgo may have additive effects when used with herbs or supplements that also decrease blood pressure. However, high blood pressure was reported in a patient taking a thiazide diuretic ("water pill") plus ginkgo. Although it remains unclear whether ginkgo has clinically significant effects on blood pressure, caution may be warranted when ginkgo is used with other agents that affect blood pressure. Examples of herbs and supplements that may decrease blood pressure are aconite/monkshood, arnica, baneberry, betel nut, bilberry, black cohosh, bryony, calendula, California poppy, coleus, curcumin, eucalyptol, eucalyptus oil, garlic, ginger, goldenseal, green hellebore, hawthorn, Indian tobacco, jaborandi, mistletoe, night- blooming cereus, oleander, pasque flower, periwinkle, pleurisy root, shepherd's purse, Texas milkweed,

turmeric, and wild cherry. Examples of herbs and supplements that may increase blood pressure are American ginseng, arnica, bayberry, betel nut, blue cohosh, broom, cayenne, cola, coltsfoot, ephedra/ma huang, ginger, licorice, and yerba mate.

- Based on studies in humans, ginkgo may theoretically affect insulin and lower blood sugar levels. Caution is advised when using herbs or supplements that may also affect blood sugar levels. Blood glucose levels may require monitoring, and doses may need adjustment. Examples of agents that may lower blood sugar levels are *Aloe vera*, American ginseng, bilberry, bitter melon, burdock, fenugreek, fish oil, gymnema, horse chestnut seed extract (HCSE), marshmallow, milk thistle, *Panax ginseng*, rosemary, Siberian ginseng, stinging nettle, and white horehound. Agents that may raise blood sugar levels include arginine, cocoa, and ephedra (when combined with caffeine).
- Effects on monoamine oxidase (MAO) inhibition by ginkgo have been reported in animals but not confirmed in studies in humans. In theory, ginkgo may add to the side effects of herbs or supplements that also inhibit MOA, such as 5-hydroxytryptophan (5-HTP), California poppy, chromium, dehydroepiandrosterone (DHEA), DL-phenylalanine (DLPA), ephedra, evening primrose oil, fenugreek, hops, mace, *S*-adenosylmethionine (SAMe), sepia, St. John's wort, tyrosine, valerian, vitamin B_6, and yohimbe bark extract.
- Laboratory research suggests that ginkgo may add to the effects of herbs and supplements that affect levels of serotonin in the blood or brain and may increase the risk of serotonin syndrome (a condition characterized by muscle stiffness, rapid heart rate, hyperthermia, restlessness, and sweating). Herbs and supplements that may increase levels of serotonin in the body include adrenal extract, chromium, dehydroepiandrosterone (DHEA), DL-phenylalanine (DLPA), ephedra, evening primrose oil, fenugreek, hops, 5-hydroxytryptophan (5-HTP), *S*-adenosylmethionine (SAMe), St. John's wort, tyrosine, valerian, vitamin B_6, and yohimbe bark extract.

Interactions with Foods

- Based on the possible monoamine oxidase inhibitor (MAOI) properties of ginkgo (suggested in some research in animals, but not in other studies in animals and humans), high doses of ginkgo theoretically may lead to dangerously high blood pressure when taken with tyramine-containing foods such as wine (particularly chianti) and high-protein foods that have been aged or preserved such as cheeses (particularly aged, processed, and strong varieties) and dry sausage/salami/bologna. Other examples of foods that contain tyramine/tryptophan are anchovies, avocados, bananas, bean curd, beer (alcohol-free/reduced), caffeine (large amounts), caviar, champagne, chocolate, fava beans, figs, herring (pickled), liver (particularly chicken), meat tenderizers, papaya, protein extracts/powder, raisins, shrimp paste, sour cream, soy sauce, yeast extracts, and yogurt.

Selected References

Natural Standard developed the preceding evidence-based information based on a systematic review of more than 600 scientific articles. For comprehensive information about alternative and complementary therapies on the professional level, go to www.naturalstandard.com. Selected references are listed here.

Benjamin J, Muir T, Briggs K, et al. A case of cerebral haemorrhage: can *Ginkgo biloba* be implicated? Postgrad Med J 2001;77(904):112-113.

Biber A. Pharmacokinetics of *Ginkgo biloba* extracts. Pharmacopsychiatry 2003;36(Suppl 1): S32-S37.

Birks J, Grimley EV, Van Dongen M. *Ginkgo biloba* for cognitive impairment and dementia. Cochrane Database Syst Rev 2002;(4):CD003120.

Davydov L, Stirling AL. Stevens-Johnson syndrome with *Ginkgo biloba*. J Herbal Pharmacother 2001;13:65-69.

Drew S, Davies E. Effectiveness of *Ginkgo biloba* in treating tinnitus: double blind, placebo controlled trial. BMJ 2001;322(7278):73.

Engelsen J, Nielsen JD, Hansen KF. [Effect of Coenzyme Q10 and *Ginkgo biloba* on warfarin dosage in patients on long-term warfarin treatment. A randomized, double-blind, placebo-controlled cross-over trial.] [Article in Danish.] Ugeskr Laeger 2003;165(18):1868-1871.

Ernst E, Pittler MH. *Ginkgo biloba* for dementia: a systematic review of double-blind, placebo-controlled trials. Clin Drug Invest 1999;17(4):301-308.

Evans JR. *Ginkgo biloba* extract for age-related macular degeneration. Cochrane Database Syst Rev 2000;(2):CD001775.

Kalus JS, Piotrowski AA, Fortier CR, et al. Hemodynamic and electrocardiographic effects of short-term *Ginkgo biloba*. Ann Pharmacother 2003;37(3):345-349.

Kampman K, Majewska MD, Tourian K, et al. A pilot trial of piracetam and *Ginkgo biloba* for the treatment of cocaine dependence. Addict Behav 2003;28(3):437-448.

Kennedy DO, Scholey AB, Wesnes KA. The dose-dependent cognitive effects of acute administration of *Ginkgo biloba* to healthy young volunteers. Psychopharmacology (Berl) 2000;151(4):416-423.

Le Bars PL, Katz MM, Berman N, et al. A placebo-controlled, double-blind, randomized trial of an extract of *Ginkgo biloba* for dementia. North American EGb Study Group. JAMA 1997; 278(16):1327-1332.

Le Bars PL, Kieser M, Itil KZ. A 26-week analysis of a double-blind, placebo-controlled trial of the *Ginkgo biloba* extract EGb 761 in dementia. Dement Geriatr Cogn Disord 2000;11(4): 230-237.

Le Bars PL. Response patterns of EGb 761 in Alzheimer's disease: influence of neuropsychological profiles. Pharmacopsychiatry. 2003;36(Suppl 1):S50-S55.

Mahady GB. *Ginkgo biloba*: a review of quality, safety, and efficacy. Nutr Clin Care 2001;4(3): 140-147.

Matthews MK, Jr. Association of *Ginkgo biloba* with intracerebral hemorrhage. Neurology 1998;50(6):1933-1934.

Mauro VF, Mauro LS, Kleshinski JF, et al. Impact of *Ginkgo biloba* on the pharmacokinetics of digoxin. Am J Ther 2003;10(4):247-251.

Mix JA, Crews WD Jr. An examination of the efficacy of *Ginkgo biloba* extract EGb761 on the neuropsychologic functioning of cognitively intact older adults. J Altern Complement Med 2000;6(3):219-229.

Moulton PL, Boyko LN, Fitzpatrick JL, et al. The effect of *Ginkgo biloba* on memory in healthy male volunteers. Physiol Behav 2001;73(4):659-665.

Parsad D, Pandhi R, Juneja A. Effectiveness of oral *Ginkgo biloba* in treating limited, slowly spreading vitiligo. Clin Exp Dermatol 2003;28(3):285-287.

Peters H, Kieser M, Holscher U. Demonstration of the efficacy of *Ginkgo biloba* special extract EGb 761 on intermittent claudication: a placebo-controlled, double-blind multicenter trial. Vasa 1998;27(2):106-110.

Pittler MH, Ernst E. *Ginkgo biloba* extract for the treatment of intermittent claudication: a meta-analysis of randomized trials. Am J Med 2000;108(4):276-281.

Quaranta L, Bettelli S, Uva MG, et al. Effect of *Ginkgo biloba* extract on preexisting visual field damage in normal tension glaucoma. Ophthalmology 2003;110(2):359-362; Discussion 362-364.

Rigney U, Kimber S, Hindmarch I. The effects of acute doses of standardized *Ginkgo biloba* extract on memory and psychomotor performance in volunteers. Phytother Res 1999;13(5):408-415.

Rosenblatt M, Mindel J. Spontaneous hyphema associated with ingestion of *Ginkgo biloba* extract. N Engl J Med 1997;336(15):1108.

Rowin J, Lewis SL. Spontaneous bilateral subdural hematomas associated with chronic *Ginkgo biloba* ingestion. Neurology 1996;46(6):1775-1776.

Skogh M. Extracts of *Ginkgo biloba* and bleeding or haemorrhage. Lancet 1998;352(9134): 1145-1146.

Solomon PR, Adams F, Silver A, et al. Ginkgo for memory enhancement: a randomized controlled trial. JAMA 2002;288(7):835-840.

Vale S. Subarachnoid haemorrhage associated with *Ginkgo biloba*. Lancet 1998;352(9121):36.

van Dongen M, van Rossum E, Kessels A, et al. Ginkgo for elderly people with dementia and age-associated memory impairment: a randomized clinical trial. J Clin Epidemiol 2003;56(4): 367-376.

Weber W. Ginkgo not effective for memory loss in elderly. Lancet 2000;356:1333.

Winther KA, Randlov C, Rein E, et al. Effects of *Ginkgo biloba* extract on cognitive function and blood pressure in elderly subjects. Curr Ther Res 1998;59(12):881-888.

Winther K, Randlov C, Rein E, et al. *Ginkgo biloba* (GB-8) enhances motor and intellectual function in patients with dementia when evaluated by local nurses [abstract]. International Scientific Conference on Complementary, Alternative and Integrative Medicine Research, April 12-14 2002.

Xu AH, Chen HS, Sun BC, et al. Therapeutic mechanism of ginkgo biloba exocarp polysaccharides on gastric cancer. World J Gastroenterol 2003;9(11):2424-2427.

Ginseng

(*Panax* species including *Panax ginseng* [Asian ginseng], *Panax quinquefolius* [American ginseng]; excluding *Eleutherococcus senticosus* [Siberian ginseng])

G

RELATED TERMS

- **General:** Allheilkraut, Araliaceae (family), chikusetsu ginseng, chosen ninjin, dwarf ginseng, five-fingers, five-leaf ginseng, G115, ginseng radix, ginsengwurzel, ginsenosides (Rb1, Rb2, Rc, Rd, Re, Rf, and Rg1), hakusan, hakushan, higeninjin, hongshen, hua qi shen, hungseng, hungsheng, hunseng, insam, jenseng, jenshen, jinpi, kao-li-seng, Korean ginseng, kraftwurzel, man root, minjin, nhan sam, ninjin, ninzin, niuhan, Oriental ginseng, otane ninjin, panax de chine, panax notoginseng, *Panax vietnamensis* (Vietnamese ginseng), *Panax pseudoginseng*, *Panax pseudoginseng* Wall. var. *notoginseng*, *Panax pseudoginseng* var. *major*, *Panax trifolius* L., pannag, racine de ginseng, renshen, sanchi ginseng, sang, san-pi, schinsent, sei yang sam, seng, shanshen, shen-sai-seng, shenshaishanshen, shenghaishen, siyojin, t'ang-sne, tartar root, true ginseng, tyosenninzin, Western ginseng, Western sea ginseng, xi shen, xi yang shen, yakuyo ninjin, yakuyo ninzin, yang shen, yeh-shan-seng, yuanseng, yuansheng, zhuzishen.
- **Asian ginseng (*Panax ginseng*) synonyms:** Asiatic ginseng, Chinese ginseng, ginseng asiatique, ginseng radix, ginseng root, Japanese ginseng, jintsam, Korean red, Korean red ginseng, ninjin, Oriental ginseng, *Panax schinseng,* red ginseng, ren shen, sang, shen.
- **American ginseng (*Panax quinquefolius*) synonyms:** Anchi ginseng, Canadian ginseng, North American ginseng, Ontario ginseng, red berry, ren shen, sang, tienchi ginseng, Wisconsin ginseng.
- **Siberian ginseng (*Eleutherococcus senticosus*) synonyms:** *Acanthopanax senticosus*, ci wu jia (ciwujia), devil's bush, devil's shrub, eleuthera, eleuthero, eleuthero ginseng, eleutherococ, eleutherococcus, eleutherococci radix, shigoka, touch-me-not, wild pepper, wu-jia, wu-jia-pi, ussurian thorny pepperbrush, ussuri.

BACKGROUND

- The term *ginseng* refers to several species of the genus *Panax*. For more than 2000 years, the roots of this slow-growing plant have been valued in Chinese medicine. The two most commonly used species are Asian ginseng (*Panax ginseng* C.A. Meyer), which is mostly extinct in its natural range but is still cultivated, and American ginseng (*Panax quinquefolius* L.), which is both harvested from the wild and cultivated. *Panax ginseng* should not be confused with Siberian ginseng (*Eleutherococcus senticosus*). In Russia, Siberian ginseng was promoted as a cheaper alternative to ginseng and was believed to have identical benefits. However, Siberian ginseng does not contain the ginsenosides that are present in the *Panax* species, which are believed to be active ingredients and have been studied scientifically.

USES BASED ON SCIENTIFIC EVIDENCE	Grade*
Mental performance Several studies report that ginseng can modestly improve thinking or learning at doses of 200 to 400 mg of standardized extract G115, taken by mouth daily for up to 12 weeks. Mental performance has been assessed using standardized measurements of reaction time, concentration, learning, math, and logic. Benefits have been seen both in healthy young people and in older, ill patients. Effects also have been reported for the combined use of ginseng with *Ginkgo biloba*. Although this evidence is promising, most studies have been small and not well designed or reported. There is also a small amount of negative evidence, reporting that ginseng actually may not significantly affect thinking processes. It is not clear if people with certain conditions may benefit more than others. Therefore, although the available scientific evidence does suggest some effectiveness of short-term use of ginseng for enhancing thinking or learning, better research is necessary before a strong recommendation can be made.	B
Type 2 diabetes mellitus Several studies in humans report that ginseng may lower blood sugar levels in patients with type 2 diabetes mellitus (adult-onset diabetes), both in the fasting state and after eating. Long-term effects are not clear, and it is not known what doses are safe or effective. Preliminary research suggests that ginseng may not carry a significant risk of causing dangerously low blood sugar levels (hypoglycemia). Additional studies are needed that measure long-term effects of ginseng in patients with diabetes and that also examine interactions with standard prescription drugs for diabetes. People with diabetes should seek the care of a qualified healthcare practitioner and should not use ginseng instead of more proven therapies. Effects of ginseng in type 1 diabetes mellitus (insulin-dependent diabetes) are not well studied.	B
Cancer prevention A small number of studies report that ginseng taken by mouth may lower the risk for various cancers, especially if ginger powder or extract is used. However, most of these studies have been published by the same research group and have used a type of research design (the case-control study) that limits usefulness of results, and the findings can only be considered preliminary. Results may have been affected by other lifestyle choices in people who use ginseng, such as exercise and dietary habits. Additional trials are necessary before a clear conclusion can be reached.	C
Chronic obstructive pulmonary disease (COPD) Ginseng was reported to improve pulmonary function and exercise capacity in patients with COPD in one study. Further research is needed to confirm these results.	C

Continued

Congestive heart failure Evidence from a small amount of research is unclear regarding use of ginseng in patients with congestive heart failure.	C
Coronary artery (heart) disease Several studies from China report that ginseng in combination with various other herbs may reduce symptoms of coronary artery disease such as anginal chest pain and may correct abnormalities seen on the electrocardiogram. Most studies have not been well described or reported. Without further evidence of the effects of ginseng specifically, a firm conclusion cannot be reached.	C
Erectile dysfunction Preliminary study reports that a cream containing ginseng may be helpful for men who have difficulty with erections or decreased libido. Additional research is necessary before a clear conclusion can be reached.	C
Exercise performance Ginseng is commonly used by athletes with the intention of improving stamina. However, it remains unclear if ginseng taken by mouth significantly affects exercise performance. Numerous studies of this use have been published, with mixed results. Most research has not been well designed or reported, and results cannot be considered reliable. Trials in the 1980s reported benefits, whereas more recent research found no effects. Better studies are necessary before a clear conclusion can be reached.	C
Fatigue Limited research using ginseng extract G115 (with or without multivitamins) reports improvement in patients with fatigue of various causes. However, these results are preliminary, and studies have not been of high quality. Additional research is necessary before a clear conclusion can be reached.	C
High blood pressure Preliminary research suggests that ginseng may lower blood pressure (systolic and diastolic). It is not clear what doses are safe or effective. Well-conducted studies are needed to confirm these early results.	C
Immune system enhancement A small number of studies report that ginseng may stimulate activity of immune cells in the body (T-lymphocytes and neutrophils), improve the effectiveness of antibiotics in people with acute bronchitis, and enhance the body's response to influenza vaccines. Most research in this area has been published by the same lead author. Additional studies that examine the effects of ginseng on specific types of infections are necessary before a clear conclusion can be reached.	C

Continued

Low white blood cell counts Poorly described preliminary research reports improved blood counts in patients with aplastic anemia using ginseng in combination with other herbs, and improved white blood cell counts in patients with neutropenia using high doses of ginsenosides. Reliable studies are needed before a conclusion can be reached. Of note, decreased blood cell counts after ginseng use have been reported.	C
Menopausal symptoms Evidence from a small amount of research on use of ginseng for relief of menopausal symptoms is unclear. Some studies report less depression and improved sense of well-being, without changes in hormone levels.	C
Methicillin-resistant *Staphylococcus aureus* (MRSA) In patients taking the herbal preparation hochu-ekki-to, which contains ginseng and several other herbs, urinary MRSA decreased after a 10-week treatment period. Further study of ginseng alone is necessary before firm conclusions can be drawn.	C
Multi-infarct dementia A small study conducted in patients with multi-infarct dementia reports that a herbal combination known as Fuyuan mixture, which contains ginseng, may have therapeutic benefits. The effects of ginseng alone are not clear, and no firm conclusion can be drawn.	C
Sense of well-being Several studies have examined the effects of ginseng (with or without multivitamins) on overall sense of well-being in healthy and ill patients, when taken for up to 12 weeks. Most trials are not of high quality, and results are mixed. Preliminary research suggests that benefits may occur in people with the worst baseline quality of life. However, it remains unclear if ginseng is beneficial for this purpose in any patient group.	C

*Key to grades: *A:* Strong scientific evidence for this use; *B:* Good scientific evidence for this use; *C:* Unclear scientific evidence for this use; *D:* Fair scientific evidence against this use (it may not work); *F:* Strong scientific evidence against this use (it likely does not work). For a more detailed explanation of efficacy criteria, see "Natural Standard Evidence-Based Validated Grading Rationale" in the Introduction.

Uses Based on Tradition, Theory, or Limited Scientific Evidence

Adrenal tonic, aerobic fitness, aging, aggression, Alzheimer's disease, allergy, anemia, antidepressant, anti-inflammatory, antioxidant, antiplatelet, antitumor, anxiety, aphrodisiac, aplastic anemia, appetite stimulant, asthma, atherosclerosis, athletic stamina, attention-deficit hyperactivity disorder (ADHD), bleeding disorders, breast cancer, breast enlargement, breathing difficulty, bronchodilation, burns, cancer prevention, chemotherapy support, cold limbs, colitis, convulsions,

Continued

Uses Based on Tradition, Theory, or Limited Scientific Evidence ***(cont'd)***

dementia, diabetic nephropathy (kidney disease), digestive complaints, diuretic (water pill) effect, dizziness, dysentery, estrogen-like activity, fatigue, fever, gynecologic disorders, fibromyalgia, hangover relief, headaches, heart damage, hepatitis/hepatitis B infection, herpes, high blood pressure, HIV, inflammation, influenza, insomnia, kidney disease, learning enhancement, liver diseases, liver health, long-term debility, low sperm count, male infertility, malignant tumors, memory and thinking enhancement after menopause, menopausal symptoms, migraine, morphine tolerance, neuralgia (pain due to nerve damage or inflammation), neurosis, organ prolapse, oxygen absorption, pain relief, palpitations, physical work capacity increase, premature ejaculation, prostate cancer, *Pseudomonas* infection in cystic fibrosis, psychoasthenia, prostate cancer, qi deficiency and blood stasis syndrome in heart disease (Eastern medicine), quality of life enhancement, recovery from irradiation, rehabilitation, sedative, senile dementia, sexual arousal, sexual symptoms, spontaneous sweating, stomach cancer, stomach upset, stress, strokes, surgical recovery, upper respiratory tract infection, vomiting.

DOSING

The following doses are based on scientific research, publications, traditional use, or expert opinion. Many herbs and supplements have not been thoroughly tested, and their safety and effectiveness may not be proven. Brands may be made differently, with variable ingredients even within the same brand. The doses shown may not apply to all products. It is important to always read product labels and discuss doses with a qualified healthcare provider before therapy is started.

Standardization

- Standardization involves measuring the amount of certain chemicals in products to try to make different preparations similar to each other. It is not always known if the chemicals being measured are the "active" ingredients.
- Ginseng extracts may be standardized to 4% ginsenosides content (for example, in G115) or 7% total ginsenosides content. Standardized products have been used in studies, although tests of commercially available ginseng products have found that many brands do not contain the claimed ingredients, and some include detectable pesticides.

Adults (18 Years and Older)

- **Tablets/Capsules:** 100 to 200 mg of a standardized ginseng extract (4% ginsenosides) taken by mouth once or twice daily has been used in studies for up to 12 weeks. Doses of 0.5 to 2 g of dry ginseng root, taken daily by mouth in divided doses, also have been used. Higher doses are sometimes given in studies or under the supervision of a qualified healthcare provider. Many different doses are used traditionally. Some practitioners recommend that after taking ginseng continuously for 2 to 3 weeks, the patient should stop use of this herb for 1 or 2 weeks, and that long-term dosing should not exceed 1 g of dry root daily.
- **Decoction/Fluid Extract/Tincture:** The following dosages have been used: decoction of 1 to 2 g added to 150 ml of water, taken by mouth daily; a 1:1 (grams per milliliter) fluid extract taken as 1 to 2 ml by mouth daily; 5 to 10 ml (approximately 1 to 2 teaspoons) of a 1:5 (grams per milliliter) tincture taken by mouth

daily. Some practitioners recommend that after taking ginseng continuously for 2 to 3 weeks, the patient should stop use of this herb for 1 or 2 weeks.

Children (Younger Than 18 Years)

- There is not enough scientific information available to recommend the safe use of ginseng in children.

SAFETY

The U.S. Food and Drug Administration does not strictly regulate herbs and supplements. There is no guarantee of strength, purity, or safety of products, and effects may vary. It is important to always read product labels. People who have a medical condition, or are taking other drugs, herbs, or supplements, should consult a qualified healthcare provider before starting a new therapy. A healthcare provider should be consulted immediately about any side effects.

Allergies

- People with known allergy to plants in the Araliaceae family should avoid ginseng.

Side Effects and Warnings

- Ginseng has been well tolerated by most people in scientific studies when used at recommended doses, and serious side effects appear to be rare.
- Based on limited evidence, long-term use may be associated with skin rash or spots, itching, diarrhea, sore throat, loss of appetite, excitability, anxiety, depression, or insomnia. Less common reported side effects include headache, fever, dizziness/vertigo, blood pressure abnormalities (increases or decreases), chest pain, heart palpitations, rapid heart rate, leg swelling, nausea/vomiting, and manic episodes in people with bipolar disorder.
- Research in humans indicates that ginseng may lower blood sugar levels. This effect may be greater in patients with diabetes than in nondiabetic persons. Caution is advised in patients with diabetes or hypoglycemia and in those taking drugs, herbs, or supplements that affect blood sugar. Serum glucose levels may need to be monitored by a healthcare provider, and medication adjustments may be necessary.
- There are anecdotal reports of nosebleeds and vaginal bleeding with ginseng use, although scientific study of this potential risk is limited. In one report, ginseng reduced the effectiveness of the blood-thinning medication warfarin (Coumadin). Caution is advised regarding use of ginseng in patients with bleeding disorders or taking drugs that may affect the risk of bleeding or blood clotting. Dosing adjustments may be necessary. Severe drops in white blood cell counts were reported in several people using a combination product containing ginseng in the 1970s; this effect may have been due to contamination.
- Ginseng may have estrogen-like effects. Use of ginseng has been associated with reports of breast tenderness, loss of menstrual periods, vaginal bleeding after menopause, breast enlargement (reported in men), difficulty developing or maintaining an erection, and increased sexual responsiveness. Ginseng should be avoided by patients with hormone-sensitive conditions such as breast cancer, uterine cancer, and endometriosis.
- Ginseng may produce manic symptoms. In a single case report involving a 56-year-old woman with a previously diagnosed affective disorder, a manic episode occurred during ginseng intake. Symptoms disappeared rapidly with low doses of neuroleptics and benzodiazepines.

- A severe life-threatening rash known as Stevens-Johnson syndrome occurred in one patient and may have been due to contaminants in a ginseng product. A case report describes liver damage (cholestatic hepatitis) in a patient who took a combination product containing ginseng. High doses of ginseng have been associated with rare cases of temporary inflammation of blood vessels in the brain (cerebral arteritis), abnormal dilation of the pupils of the eye, confusion, or depression.
- There is preliminary evidence that ginseng, at doses of 200 mg of extract daily, may increase the QTc interval as seen on the electrocardiogram (thus increasing the risk of abnormal heart rhythms) and decrease diastolic blood pressure 2 hours after ingestion in healthy adults.

Pregnancy and Breastfeeding

- Ginseng traditionally has been used in pregnant and breastfeeding women. Studies in animals and preliminary research in humans suggest possible safety, although safety has not been clearly established. Therefore, ginseng use cannot be recommended during pregnancy or the period of breastfeeding. There is a report of neonatal death and the development of male sex characteristics in a baby girl whose mother had taken ginseng during pregnancy.
- Many tinctures contain high levels of alcohol and should be avoided during pregnancy.

INTERACTIONS

Most herbs and supplements have not been thoroughly tested for interactions with other herbs, supplements, drugs, or foods. The interactions listed here are based on reports in scientific publications, laboratory experiments, or traditional use. It is important to always read product labels. People who have a medical condition, or are taking other drugs, herbs, or supplements, should consult a qualified healthcare provider before starting a new therapy.

Interactions with Drugs

- As suggested by research in humans, ginseng may lower blood sugar levels. This effect may be greater in patients with diabetes than in nondiabetic persons. Caution is advised with use of medications that also may lower blood sugar. Patients taking drugs for diabetes by mouth or insulin should be monitored closely by a qualified healthcare provider. Medication adjustments may be necessary.
- Headache, tremors, mania, or insomnia may occur if ginseng is combined with prescription antidepressant drugs called monoamine oxidase inhibitors (MAOIs), such as isocarboxazid (Marplan), phenelzine (Nardil), and tranylcypromine (Parnate).
- As described in case reports, ginseng may alter the effects of blood pressure or heart medications, including calcium channel blockers such as nifedipine (Procardia). There is preliminary evidence that ginseng, at doses of 200 mg of extract daily, may increase the QTc interval as seen on the electrocardiogram (thus increasing the risk of abnormal heart rhythms) and decrease diastolic blood pressure 2 hours after ingestion in healthy adults. Therefore, caution is advised with use of other medications that may alter the QTc interval. In one case report, effects of the diuretic drug furosemide (Lasix) were decreased when the drug was used with ginseng. A Chinese study reports that the effects of the cardiac glycoside drug digoxin (Lanoxin) may be increased when it is used with ginseng in patients with heart failure. Ginseng must not be combined with heart or blood pressure medications without the advice of a qualified healthcare provider.

- As suggested by limited animal research and anecdotal reports of nosebleeds and vaginal bleeding in humans, ginseng may increase the risk of bleeding when taken with drugs that also increase the risk of bleeding. Some examples are aspirin, anticoagulants (blood thinners) such as warfarin (Coumadin) and heparin, antiplatelet drugs such as clopidogrel (Plavix), and nonsteroidal anti-inflammatory drugs such as ibuprofen (Motrin, Advil) and naproxen (Naprosyn, Aleve). By contrast, in one reported case, the effectiveness of the blood thinner warfarin (Coumadin) was reduced when ginseng was taken at the same time, with a decrease in the international normalized ratio (INR), a blood test used to measure warfarin effects.
- Limited laboratory evidence indicates that ginseng may contain estrogen-like chemicals and may affect medications with estrogen-like or estrogen-blocking properties. This effect has not been demonstrated in humans.
- In theory, ginseng may interfere with how the body uses the liver's cytochrome P450 enzyme system to process components of some drugs. As a result, blood levels of these components may be elevated, causing increased effects or potentially serious adverse reactions. People who are taking any medications should always read the package insert and consult with their healthcare provider and pharmacist about possible interactions.
- The analgesic effect of opioids may be inhibited by ginseng.
- Many tinctures contain high levels of alcohol and may cause nausea or vomiting when taken with metronidazole (Flagyl) or disulfiram (Antabuse). In a preliminary study, ginseng was reported to increase the removal of alcohol from the blood, although this effect has not been substantiated.

Interactions with Herbs and Dietary Supplements

- According to research in humans, ginseng may lower blood sugar levels. This effect may be greater in patients with diabetes than in nondiabetic persons. Caution is advised with use of herbs or supplements that also may lower blood sugar. Blood glucose levels may require monitoring, and doses may need adjustment. Possible examples include *Aloe vera*, bilberry, bitter melon, burdock, fenugreek, fish oil, gymnema, horse chestnut seed extract (HCSE), marshmallow, maitake mushroom, milk thistle, rosemary, stinging nettle, and white horehound.
- Headache, tremors, mania, and insomnia may occur if ginseng is combined with supplements that have MAOI activity or that interact with MAOI drugs. Some examples are 5-hydroxytryptophan (5-HTP), California poppy, chromium, dehydroepiandrosterone (DHEA), DL-phenylalanine (DLPA), ephedra, evening primrose oil, fenugreek, *Ginkgo biloba*, hops, mace, St. John's wort, *S*-adenosylmethionine (SAMe), sepia, tyrosine, valerian, vitamin B_6, and yohimbe bark extract. In theory, ginseng can increase the stimulatory effects of caffeine, coffee, tea, cocoa, chocolate, guarana, cola nut, and yerba mate.
- As described in case reports, ginseng may raise or lower blood pressure. Caution is advised with use of ginseng in combination with other products that can affect blood pressure. Some herbs that may lower blood pressure are aconite/monkshood, arnica, baneberry, betel nut, bilberry, black cohosh, bryony, calendula, California poppy, coleus, curcumin, eucalyptol, eucalyptus oil, evening primrose oil, flaxseed, garlic, ginger, ginkgo, goldenseal, green hellebore, hawthorn, Indian tobacco, jaborandi, mistletoe, night-blooming cereus, oleander, pasque flower, periwinkle, pleurisy root, shepherd's purse, Texas milkweed, turmeric, and wild cherry. Herbs that may increase blood pressure include arnica, bayberry, betel nut,

blue cohosh, broom, cayenne, cola, coltsfoot, ephedra/ma huang, ginger, licorice, *Polypodium vulgare*, and yerba mate.

- Preliminary evidence indicates that ginseng, at doses of 200 mg of extract daily, may increase the QTc interval as seen on the electrocardiogram (thus increasing the risk of abnormal heart rhythms) and decrease diastolic blood pressure 2 hours after ingestion in healthy adults. Therefore, caution is advised with use of other agents that may cause abnormal heart rhythms.
- As suggested by limited animal research and anecdotal reports of nosebleeds and vaginal bleeding in humans, ginseng may increase the risk of bleeding when taken with herbs and supplements that are believed to increase the risk of bleeding. Multiple cases of bleeding have been reported with the use of *Ginkgo biloba*, some cases with garlic, and fewer cases with saw palmetto. Numerous other agents may theoretically increase the risk of bleeding, although this effect has not been proven in most cases. Some examples are alfalfa, angelica, anise, *Arnica montana*, asafetida, aspen bark, bilberry, birch, black cohosh, bladderwrack, bogbean, boldo, borage seed oil, bromelain, capsicum, cat's claw, celery, chamomile, chaparral, clove, coleus, cordyceps, danshen, devil's claw, dong quai, eicosapentaenoic acid (EPA), evening primrose oil, fenugreek, feverfew, fish oil, flaxseed/flaxseed powder (not a concern with flaxseed oil), ginger, grapefruit juice, grapeseed, green tea, guggul, gymnestra, horse chestnut, horseradish, licorice root, lovage root, male fern, meadowsweet, nordihydroguaiaretic acid (NDGA), onion, papain, parsley, passion flower, poplar, prickly ash, propolis, quassia, red clover, reishi, rue, sweet birch, sweet clover, turmeric, vitamin E, white willow, wild carrot, wild lettuce, willow, wintergreen, and yucca.
- In theory, ginseng may decrease the effects of diuretic herbs such as horsetail and licorice.
- In theory, ginseng may interfere with how the body uses the liver's cytochrome P450 enzyme system to process certain components of other herbs or supplements. As a result, blood levels of these components may be elevated. It also may alter the effects of other herbs or supplements on the cytochrome P450 system. Examples of such herbs are bloodroot, cat's claw, chamomile, chaparral, chasteberry, damiana, *Echinacea angustifolia*, goldenseal, grapefruit juice, licorice, oregano, red clover, St. John's wort, wild cherry, and yucca. People who are taking any herbal medications or dietary supplements should check the package insert and consult their healthcare provider or pharmacist about possible interactions.
- Limited laboratory evidence suggests that ginseng may contain estrogen-like chemicals and may affect agents with estrogen-like or estrogen-blocking properties. This effect has not been demonstrated in humans. Examples of herbs with possible estrogen-like effects are alfalfa, black cohosh, bloodroot, burdock, hops, kudzu, licorice, pomegranate, red clover, soy, thyme, white horehound, and yucca.

Selected References

Natural Standard developed the preceding evidence-based information based on a systematic review of more than 600 scientific articles. For comprehensive information about alternative and complementary therapies on the professional level, go to www.naturalstandard.com. Selected references are listed here.

Abebe W. Herbal medication: potential for adverse interactions with analgesic drugs. J Clin Pharm Ther 2002;27(6):391-401.

Allen JD, McLung J, Nelson AG, et al. Ginseng supplementation does not enhance healthy young adults' peak aerobic exercise performance. J Am Coll Nutr 1998;17(5):462-466.

Anderson GD, Rosito G, Mohustsy MA, et al. Drug interaction potential of soy extract and *Panax ginseng*. J Clin Pharmacol 2003;43(6):643-648.

Attele AS, Wu JA, Yuan CS. Ginseng pharmacology: multiple constituents and multiple actions. Biochem Pharmacol 1999;58(11):1685-1693.

Awang DV. Maternal use of ginseng and neonatal androgenization. JAMA 1991;266(3):363.

Bahrke MS, Morgan WR. Evaluation of the ergogenic properties of ginseng: an update. Sports Med 2000;29(2):113-133.

Banskota AH, Tezuka Y, Le Tran Q, et al. Chemical constituents and biological activities of Vietnamese medicinal plants. Curr Top Med Chem 2003;3(2):227-248.

Belogortseva NI, Yoon JY, Kim KH. Inhibition of *Helicobacter pylori* hemagglutination by polysaccharide fractions from roots of *Panax ginseng*. Planta Med 2000;66(3):217-220.

Cardinal BJ, Engels HJ. Ginseng does not enhance psychological well-being in healthy, young adults: results of a double-blind, placebo-controlled, randomized clinical trial. J Am Diet Assoc 2001;101(6):655-660.

Caron MF, Hotsko AL, Robertson S, et al. Electrocardiographic and hemodynamic effects of *Panax ginseng*. Ann Pharmacother 2002;36(5):758-763.

Chang TK, Chen J, Benetton SA. In vitro effect of standardized ginseng extracts and individual ginsenosides on the catalytic activity of human CYP1A1, CYP1A2, and CYP1B1. Drug Metab Dipos 2002;30(4):378-384.

Chan RY, Chen WF, Dong A, et al. Estrogen-like activity of ginsenoside Rg1 derived from Panax notoginseng. J Clin Endocrinol Metab 2002;87(8):3691-3695.

Chavez M. Treatment of diabetes mellitus with ginseng. J Herb Pharm 2001;1(2):99-113.

Cherdrungsi P, Rungroeng K. Effects of standardized ginseng extract and exercise training on aerobic and anaerobic exercise capacities in humans. Korean J Ginseng Sci 1995;19(2):93-100.

Choi CH, Kang G, Min YD. Reversal of P-glycoprotein–mediated multidrug resistance by protopanaxatriol ginsenosides from Korean red ginseng. Planta Med 2003;69(3):235-240.

Choi HK, Seong DH, Rha KH. Clinical efficacy of Korean red ginseng for erectile dysfunction. Int J Impot Res 1995;7(3):181-186.

Choi HK, Jung GW, Moon KH, et al. Clinical study of SS-cream in patients with lifelong premature ejaculation. Urology 2000;55(2):257-261.

Choi SE, Choi S, Lee JH, et al. Effects of ginsenosides on GABA(A) receptor channels expressed in *Xenopus* oocytes. Arch Pharm Res 2003;26(1):28-33.

Choi S, Lee JH, Oh S, et al. Effects of ginsenoside Rg2 on the 5-HT3a receptor–mediated ion current in *Xenopus* oocytes. Mol Cells 2003;15(1):108-113.

Choo MK, Park EK, Han MJ, et al. Antiallergic activity of ginseng and its ginsenosides. Planta Med 2003;69(6):518-522.

Chow L, Johnson M, Wells A, et al. Effect of the traditional Chinese medicines chan su, lu-shen-wan, dan shen, and Asian ginseng on serum digoxin measurement by Tina-quant (Roche) and Synchron LX system (Beckman) digoxin immunoassays. J Clin Lab Anal 2003;17(1):22-27.

Chung WY, Yow CM, Benzie IF. Assessment of membrane protection by traditional Chinese medicines using a flow cytometric technique: preliminary findings. Redox Rep 2003;8(1):31-33.

Cicero AF, Vitale G, Savino G, et al. *Panax notoginseng* (Burk.) effects on fibrinogen and lipid plasma level in rats fed on a high-fat diet. Phytother Res 2003;17(2):174-178.

Coleman CI, Hebert JH, Reddy P. The effects of *Panax ginseng* on quality of life. J Clin Pharm Ther 2003;28(1):5-15.

Cui XM, Lo CK, Yip KL, et al. Authentication of *Panax notoginseng* by 5S-rRNA spacer domain and random amplified polymorphic DNA (RAPD) analysis. Planta Med 2003; 69(6):584-586.

Dasgupta A, Wu S, Actor J, et al. Effect of Asian and Siberian ginseng on serum digoxin measurement by five digoxin immunoassays. Significant variation in digoxin-like immunoreactivity among commercial ginsengs. Am J Clin Pathol 2003;119(2):298-303.

Donovan JL, DeVane CL, Chavin KD, et al. Siberian ginseng (*Eleutherococcus senticosus*) effects on CYP2D6 and CYP3A4 activity in normal volunteers. Drug Metab Dispos 2003;31(5): 519-522.

Dragun Z, Puntaric D, Prpic-Majic D, et al. Toxic metals and metalloids in dietetic products. Croat Med J 2003;44(2):214-218.

Ellis JM, Reddy P. Effects of *Panax ginseng* on quality of life. Ann Pharmacother 2002;36: 375-379.

Engels HJ, Wirth JC. No ergogenic effects of ginseng (*Panax ginseng* C.A. Meyer) during graded maximal aerobic exercise. J Am Diet Assoc 1997;97(10):1110-1115.

Engels HJ, Kolokouri I, Cieslak TJ, et al. Effects of ginseng supplementation on supramaximal exercise performance and short-term recovery. J Strength Cond Res 2001; 15(3):290-295.

Faleni R, Soldati F. Ginseng as cause of Stevens-Johnson syndrome? Lancet 1996; 348(9022):267.

Gingrich PM, Fogel CI. Herbal therapy use by perimenopausal women. J Obstet Gynecol Neonatal Nurs 2003;32(2):181-189.

Glenn MB, Lexell J. Ginseng. J Head Trauma Rehabil 2003;18(2):196-200.

Gonzalez-Seijo JC, Ramos YM, Lastra I. Manic episode and ginseng: report of a possible case. J Clin Psychopharmacol 1995;15(6):447-448.

Gross D, Shenkman Z, Bleiberg B, et al. Ginseng improves pulmonary functions and exercise capacity in patients with COPD. Monaldi Arch Chest Dis 2002;57(5-6):242-246. Comment in: Monaldi Arch Chest Dis 2002;57(5-6):225-226.

Han KH, Choe SC, Kim HS, et al. Effect of red ginseng on blood pressure in patients with essential hypertension and white coat hypertension. Am J Chin Med 1998;26(2):199-209.

Hong B, Ji YH, Hong JH, et al. A double-blind crossover study evaluating the efficacy of Korean red ginseng in patients with erectile dysfunction: a preliminary report. J Urol 2002; 168(5):2070-2073.

Hopkins MP, Androff L, Benninghoff AS. Ginseng face cream and unexplained vaginal bleeding. Am J Obstet Gynecol 1988;159(5):1121-1122.

Janetzky K, Morreale AP. Probable interaction between warfarin and ginseng. Am J Health Syst Pharm 1997;54(6):692-693.

Jin YH, Yim H, Park JH, et al. Cdk2 activity is associated with depolarization of mitochondrial membrane potential during apoptosis. Biochem Biophys Res Commun 2003;305(4)974-980.

Kennedy D, Scholey AB, Wesnes K. A direct cognitive comparison of the acute effects of ginseng, ginkgo and their combination in healthy volunteers. J Psychopharm 2001; 15(Suppl):A56.

Kennedy D, Scholey A. A direct cognitive comparison of the acute effects of ginseng, ginkgo and their combination in healthy volunteers. Presented at Scientific Conference on Complementary, Alternative & Integrative Medicine Research, Boston, 2002.

Keum YS, Han SS, Chun KS, et al. Inhibitory effects of the ginsenoside Rg3 on phorbol ester–induced cyclooxygenase-2 expression, NF-kappaB activation and tumor promotion. Mutat Res 2003;523-524:75-85.

Kim SW, Kwon HY, Chi DW, et al. Reversal of P-glycoprotein–mediated multidrug resistance by ginsenoside Rg(3). Biochem Pharmacol 2003;65(1):75-82.

Kolokouri I, Engels H, Cieslak T, et al. Effect of chronic ginseng supplementation on short duration, supramaximal exercise test performance [abstract]. Med Sci Sports Exerc 1999; 31(5 Suppl):S117.

Ko SR, Choi KJ, Uchida K, et al. Enzymatic preparation of ginsenosides Rg2, Rh1, and F1 from protopanaxatriol-type ginseng saponin mixture. Planta Med 2003;69(3):285-286.

Kuo SC, Teng CM, Lee JC, et al. Antiplatelet components in *Panax ginseng*. Planta Med 1990;56(2):164-167.

Kwan CY. Vascular effects of selected antihypertensive drugs derived from traditional medicinal herbs. Clin Exp Pharmacol Physiol 1995;22(Suppl 1):S297-S299.

Lee EH, Cho SY, Kim SJ, et al. Ginsenoside F1 protects human HaCaT keratinocytes from ultraviolet-B–induced apoptosis by maintaining constant levels of Bcl-2. J Invest Dermatol 2003;121(3):607-613.

Lee Y, Jin Y, Lim W, et al. A ginsenoside-Rh1, a component of ginseng saponin, activates estrogen receptor in human breast carcinoma MCF-7 cells. J Steroid Biochem Mol Biol 2003;84(4):463-468.

Lee YJ, Jin YR, Lim WC, et al. Ginsenoside-Rb1 acts as a weak phytoestrogen in MCF-7 human breast cancer cells. Arch Pharm Res 2003;26(1):58-63.

Lifton B, Otto RM, Wygand J. The effect of ginseng on acute maximal aerobic exercise. Med Sci Sports Exerc 1997;29(Suppl 5):249.

Lun X, Rong L, Yang WH. Observation on efficacy of CT positioning scalp circum-needling combined with Chinese herbal medicine in treating poly-infarctional vascular dementia. Zhongguo Zhong Xi Yi Jei He Za Zhi 2003;23(6):423-425.

Mahady GB, Parrot J, Lee C, et al. Botanical dietary supplement use in peri- and postmenopausal women. Menopause 2003;10(1):65-72.

Morris CA, Avorn J. Internet marketing of herbal products. JAMA 2003;290(11):1505-1509.

Nishida S. Effect of hochu-ekki-to on asymptomatic MRSA bacteriuria. J Infect Chemother 2003;9(1):58-61.

Noh JH, Choi S, Lee JH, et al. Effects of ginsenosides on glycine receptor alpha1 channels expressed in *Xenopus* oocytes. Mol Cells 2003;15(1):34-39.

Palazon J, Mallol A, Eibl R, et al. Growth and ginsenoside production in hairy root cultures of *Panax ginseng*: a novel bioreactor. Planta Med 2003;69(4):344-349.

Pharand C, Ackman ML, Jackevicius CA, et al. Use of OTC and herbal products in patients with cardiovascular disease. Ann Pharmacother 2003;37(6):899-904.

Rosado MF. Thrombosis of a prosthetic aortic valve disclosing a hazardous interaction between warfarin and a commercial ginseng product. Cardiology 2003;99(2):111.

Rowland DL, Tai W. A review of plant-derived and herbal approaches to the treatment of sexual dysfunctions. J Sex Marital Ther 2003;29(3):185-205.

Ryu SJ, Chien YY. Ginseng-associated cerebral arteritis. Neurology 1995;45(4):829-830.

Scaglione F, Weiser K, Alessandria M. Effects of the standardised ginseng extract G115(R) in patients with chronic bronchitis: a nonblinded, randomised, comparative pilot study. Clin Drug Invest 2001;21(1):41-45.

Scholey AB, Kennedy DO. Acute, dose-dependent cognitive effects of *Ginkgo biloba*, *Panax ginseng* and their combination in healthy young volunteers: differential interactions with cognitive demand. Hum Psychopharmacol 2002;17(1):35-44.

Sievenpiper JL, Arnason JT, Leiter LA, et al. Variable effects of American ginseng: a batch of American ginseng (*Panax quinquefolius* L.) with a depressed ginsenoside profile does not affect postprandial glycemia. Eur J Clin Nutr 2003;57(2):243-248.

Sievenpiper JL, Stavro MP, Leiter LA, et al. Variable effects of ginseng: American ginseng (*Panax quinquefolius* L.) with a low ginsenoside content does not affect postprandial glycemia in normal subjects. Diabetes 2001;50:A425.

Sorensen H, Sonne J. A double-masked study of the effects of ginseng on cognitive function. Curr Ther Res 1996;57(12):959-968.

Sotaniemi EA, Haapakoski E, Rautio A. Ginseng therapy in non–insulin-dependent diabetic patients. Diabetes Care 1995;18(10):1373-1375.

Sundgot-Brogen J, Berglund B, Torstveit MK. Nutritional supplements in Norwegian elite athletes—impact of international rank and advisors. Scand J Med Sci Sports 2003;13(2): 138-144.

Taik-koo Y, Soo-Yong C. Preventive effect of ginseng intake against various human cancers: a case-control study on 1987 pairs. Cancer Epidemiol Biomarkers Prev 1995;4:401-408.

Tesch BJ. Herbs commonly used by women: an evidence-based review. Am J Obstet Gynecol 2003;188(5 Suppl):S44-S55.

Thommessen B, Laake K. No identifiable effect of ginseng (Gericomplex) as an adjuvant in the treatment of geriatric patients. Aging (Milano) 1996;8(6):417-420.

Thompson Coon J, Ernst E. *Panax ginseng*: a systematic review of adverse effects and drug interactions. Presented at the 8th Annual Symposium on Complementary Health Care, Exeter, England, December 6-8, 2001.

Vazquez I, Aguera-Ortiz LF. Herbal products and serious side effects: a case of ginseng-induced manic episode. Acta Psychiatr Scand 2002;105(1):76-77;discussion 77-78.

Vogler BK, Pittler MH, Ernst E. The efficacy of ginseng. A systematic review of randomised clinical trials. Eur J Clin Pharmacol 1999;55(8):567-575.

Vuksan V, Xu Z, Jenkins AL, et al. American ginseng (*Panax quinquefolius* L.) improves long term glycemic control in type 2 diabetes. Diabetes 2000;49:A95.

Vuksan V, Stavro MP, Sievenpiper JL, et al. Similar postprandial glycemic reductions with escalation of dose and administration time of American ginseng in type 2 diabetes. Diabetes Care 2000;23(9):1221-1226.

Vuksan V, Sievenpiper JL, Koo VY, et al. American ginseng (*Panax quinquefolius* L.) reduces postprandial glycemia in nondiabetic subjects and subjects with type 2 diabetes mellitus. Arch Intern Med 2000;160(7):1009-1013.

Vuksan V, Sievenpiper JL, Wong J, et al. American ginseng (*Panax quinquefolius* L.) attenuates postprandial glycemia in a time-dependent but not dose-dependent manner in healthy individuals. Am J Clin Nutr 2001;73(4):753-758.

Wiklund IK, Mattsson LA, Lindgren R, et al. Effects of a standardized ginseng extract on quality of life and physiological parameters in symptomatic postmenopausal women: a double-blind, placebo-controlled trial. Swedish Alternative Medicine Group. Int J Clin Pharmacol Res 1999;19(3):89-99.

Wong HC. Probable false authentication of herbal plants: ginseng. Arch Intern Med 1999; 159(10):1142-1143.

Yeh GY, Eisenberg DM, Kaptchuk TJ, et al. Systematic review of herbs and dietary supplements for glycemic control in diabetes. Diabetes Care 2003;26(4):1277-1294.

Youl Kang H, Hwan Kim S, Jun Lee W, Byrne HK. Effects of ginseng ingestion on growth hormone, testosterone, cortisol, and insulin-like growth factor 1 responses to acute resistance exercise. J Strength Cond Res 2002;16(2):179-183.

Yun TK. Experimental and epidemiological evidence of the cancer-preventive effects of *Panax ginseng* C.A. Meyer. Nutr Rev 1996;54(11 Pt 2):S71-S81.

Yun TK. Experimental and epidemiological evidence on non-organ specific cancer preventative effect of Korean ginseng and identification of active compounds. Mutat Res 2003;523-524: 63-74.

Zeilmann CA, Dole EJ, Skipper BJ, et al. Use of herbal medicine by elderly Hispanic and non-Hispanic white patients. Pharmacotherapy 2003;23(4):526-532.

Zhu M, Chan KW, Ng LS, et al. Possible influences of ginseng on the pharmacokinetics and pharmacodynamics of warfarin in rats. J Pharm Pharmacol 1999;51(2):175-180.

Ziemba AW, Chmura J, Kaciuba-Uscilko H, et al. Ginseng treatment improves psychomotor performance at rest and during graded exercise in young athletes. Int J Sport Nutr 1999; 9(4):371-377.

Glucosamine

RELATED TERMS

- 2-Acetamido-2-deoxyglucose, acetylglucosamine, Arth-X Plus, chitosamine, D-glucosamine, enhanced glucosamine sulfate, Flexi-Factors, glucosamine chlorohydrate, Glucosamine Complex, glucosamine hydrochloride, glucosamine hydroiodide, Glucosamine Mega, glucosamine *N*-acetyl, glucosamine sulfate (glucosamine sulphate), Joint Factors, *N*-acetyl-D-glucosamine, *N*-acetylglucosamine (NAG, N-A-G), Nutri-Joint, Poly-NAG, Ultra Maximum Strength Glucosamine Sulfate.

BACKGROUND

- Glucosamine is a natural compound that is found in healthy cartilage. Glucosamine sulfate is a normal constituent of glycosaminoglycans in cartilage matrix and synovial fluid.
- Available evidence from randomized controlled trials supports the use of glucosamine sulfate in the treatment of osteoarthritis, particularly of the knee. It is believed that the sulfate moiety provides clinical benefit in the synovial fluid by strengthening cartilage and aiding glycosaminoglycan synthesis. If this hypothesis is confirmed, it would mean that only the glucosamine sulfate form is effective and that nonsulfated glucosamine forms are not effective.
- Glucosamine commonly is taken in combination with chondroitin, a glycosaminoglycan derived from articular cartilage. Use of complementary therapies, including glucosamine, is common in patients with osteoarthritis and may allow reduction in doses of nonsteroidal anti-inflammatory agents.

USES BASED ON SCIENTIFIC EVIDENCE	Grade*
Knee osteoarthritis (mild to moderate) Good evidence from research in humans supports the use of glucosamine sulfate in the treatment of mild-to-moderate knee osteoarthritis. Most studies have used glucosamine sulfate supplied by one European manufacturer (Rotta Research Laboratorium), and it is not known if glucosamine preparations made by other manufacturers are equally effective. Although some studies of glucosamine have not found benefits, such studies either have included patients with severe osteoarthritis or have used products other than the sulfate form of glucosamine. Further trials are needed to confirm safety and effectiveness, and to test different formulations of glucosamine.	A

Continued

Osteoarthritis (general) Several studies in humans and experiments in animals report benefits of glucosamine in treating osteoarthritis of various joints of the body, although the evidence is less plentiful than that for knee osteoarthritis. Some of these benefits are pain relief, possibly from an anti-inflammatory effect of glucosamine, and improved joint function. Overall, these studies have not been well designed. More research is needed in this area before a conclusion can be made.	B
Chronic venous insufficiency Chronic venous insufficiency is a syndrome that includes leg swelling, varicose veins, pain, itching, skin changes, and skin ulcers. The term is more commonly used in Europe than in the United States. Currently, there is not enough reliable scientific evidence to recommend glucosamine in the treatment of this condition.	C
Inflammatory bowel disease (Crohn's disease, ulcerative colitis) Preliminary research reports improvements with *N*-acetylglucosamine as an added therapy in inflammatory bowel disease. Further scientific evidence is necessary before a recommendation can be made.	C
Rheumatoid arthritis Preliminary research in humans reports benefits of glucosamine in the treatment of joint pain and swelling in rheumatoid arthritis. However, additional research is needed before a conclusion can be drawn. The treatment of rheumatoid arthritis can be complicated, and a qualified healthcare provider should oversee the management of patients with this disease.	C
Temporomandibular joint (TMJ) disorders There is a lack of sufficient evidence to recommend for or against the use of glucosamine (or the combination of glucosamine and chondroitin) in the treatment of TMJ disorders.	C

*Key to grades: *A:* Strong scientific evidence for this use; *B:* Good scientific evidence for this use; *C:* Unclear scientific evidence for this use; *D:* Fair scientific evidence against this use (it may not work); *F:* Strong scientific evidence against this use (it likely does not work). For a more detailed explanation of efficacy criteria, see "Natural Standard Evidence-Based Validated Grading Rationale" in the Introduction.

Uses Based on Tradition, Theory, or Limited Scientific Evidence

AIDS, athletic injuries, back pain, bleeding esophageal varices (blood vessels in the esophagus), cancer, congestive heart failure, depression, diabetes, fibromyalgia, immunosuppression, joint pain, knee pain, kidney stones, migraine headache, osteoporosis, pain, psoriasis, skin rejuvenation, spondylosis deformans (growth of bony spurs on the spine), wound healing, topical hypopigmenting agent (combination product containing multiple ingredients).

DOSING

The following doses are based on scientific research, publications, traditional use, or expert opinion. Many herbs and supplements have not been thoroughly tested, and their safety and effectiveness may not be proven. Brands may be made differently, with variable ingredients even within the same brand. The doses shown may not apply to all products. It is important to always read product labels and discuss doses with a qualified healthcare provider before therapy is started.

Standardization

- Standardization involves measuring the amounts of certain chemicals in products to try to make different preparations similar to each other. It is not always known if the chemicals being measured are the "active" ingredients.
- Glucosamine is not considered a drug in the United States and is therefore not required to be tested for quality by any agency before sale. Therefore, glucosamine preparations in the United States may vary in quality among different manufacturers and from batch to batch produced by the same manufacturer. In parts of Europe, glucosamine sulfate is available as a prescription drug of defined chemical nature. Most studies of glucosamine taken by mouth have used glucosamine sulfate, although different glucosamine salts are available, including glucosamine hydrochloride and glucosamine hydroiodide.

Adults (18 Years and Older)

- **Osteoarthritis:** In most available studies, 500 mg of glucosamine sulfate has been used, taken by mouth as tablets or capsules three times daily for 30 to 90 days. Once-daily dosing as 1.5 g (1500 mg) also has been used. Limited research studies have used 1500 mg daily as a crystalline powder, dissolved in liquid to make an oral solution, or 500 mg of glucosamine *hydrochloride* three times daily. Dosing of 20 mg per kilogram of body weight daily also has been recommended. One study used a dose of 2000 mg per day for 12 weeks.
- **Other glucosamine therapies:** Other types of glucosamine therapy studied for osteoarthritis include intra-articular (joint) injections of 400 mg of glucosamine sulfate daily for 7 days, 400 mg of glucosamine sulfate given intravenously (through a vein) daily for 7 days, and muscular injections of 400 mg twice weekly. Another kind of glucosamine that has been studied is a topical form that combines glucosamine with chondroitin, used for a 4-week period. Safety and effectiveness of these formulations are not clearly proved.
- **Glucosamine hydrochloride:** The hydrochloride form provides more glucosamine than that found in glucosamine sulfate, although this difference likely does not matter when products are prepared to provide a total of 500 mg of glucosamine per tablet.

Children (Younger Than 18 Years)

- There is not enough scientific evidence to recommend the use of glucosamine in children. Preliminary research has been done using *N*-acetylglucosamine in a small number of children with inflammatory bowel disease, at a dose of 3 to 6 g daily for an average of $2^1/_2$ years.
- Research in children has shown that there could be a relationship between the ingestion of methylsulfonylmethane (MSM) and autism; whether it is beneficial or harmful is unclear. MSM often is marketed as a combination product with glucosamine as a dietary supplement and at this time should be avoided in children.

SAFETY

The U.S. Food and Drug Administration does not strictly regulate herbs and supplements. There is no guarantee of strength, purity, or safety of products, and effects may vary. It is important to always read product labels. People who have a medical condition, or are taking other drugs, herbs, or supplements, should consult a qualified healthcare provider before starting a new therapy. A healthcare provider should be consulted immediately about any side effects.

Allergies

- Because glucosamine can be made from the shells of shrimp, crab, and other shellfish, people with shellfish allergy or iodine hypersensitivity may have an allergic reaction to glucosamine products. A serious hypersensitivity reaction including throat swelling has been reported with use of glucosamine sulfate.

Side Effects and Warnings

- In most studies in humans, glucosamine sulfate at a dose of 500 mg three times daily (tablets or capsules) has been well tolerated for 30 to 90 days. In a 3-year study and several short-term trials, the number of adverse events in patients taking glucosamine was no different from that noted with placebo (sugar pill). In laboratory animals, doses as high as 5000 mg/kg taken by mouth, 3000 mg/kg injected into muscle, and 1500 mg/kg infused into a vein have not caused death.
- Side effects may include upset stomach, drowsiness, insomnia, headache, skin reactions, sun sensitivity, and nail toughening. There are rare reports of abdominal pain, loss of appetite, vomiting, nausea, flatulence (gas), constipation, heartburn, and diarrhea. As reported in several patients, temporary increases in blood pressure and heart rate, as well as palpitations, may occur with glucosamine plus chondroitin products. As suggested by animal research, glucosamine theoretically may increase the risk for eye cataract formation.
- It remains unclear if glucosamine alters blood sugar levels. Several studies in humans suggest no effects on blood sugar, whereas other research reports effects on insulin. Preliminary studies show no effect on mean hemoglobin A_{1c} concentrations in patients with type 2 diabetes mellitus. Caution is advised in patients with diabetes or hypoglycemia, and in those taking drugs, herbs, or supplements that affect blood sugar. Serum glucose levels may need to be monitored by a healthcare provider, and medication adjustments may be necessary.
- Abnormally increased amounts of protein were found in the urine of several people taking glucosamine plus chondroitin products. The clinical meaning of this abnormality is unclear. Glucosamine is removed from the body mainly in the urine, and elimination of glucosamine from the body is delayed in patients with reduced kidney function. Increased blood levels of creatine kinase may occur with glucosamine plus chondroitin, which may be due to impurities in some products. This increase may alter certain laboratory values measured by healthcare providers.
- Reported cases suggest a link between glucosamine/chondroitin products and asthma exacerbations. Until more reliable data are available, patients with a history of asthma should not use glucosamine supplements except under the strict supervision of a physician.
- Preliminary data suggest that glucosamine may modulate the immune system, although the clinical relevance of this effect is not clear.

Pregnancy and Breastfeeding

- Glucosamine is not recommended in women who are pregnant or breastfeeding because of lack of scientific evidence.

INTERACTIONS

Most herbs and supplements have not been thoroughly tested for interactions with other herbs, supplements, drugs, or foods. The interactions listed here are based on reports in scientific publications, laboratory experiments, or traditional use. It is important to always read product labels. People who have a medical condition, or are taking other drugs, herbs, or supplements, should consult a qualified healthcare provider before starting a new therapy.

Interactions with Drugs

- In theory, glucosamine may decrease the effectiveness of insulin or other drugs used to control blood sugar levels. However, limited research in humans suggests that glucosamine may not have significant effects on blood sugar. Nonetheless, caution is advised with use of insulin or drugs for diabetes taken by mouth. Patients should be monitored closely by a qualified healthcare provider, and medication adjustments may be necessary. Based on limited evidence, the combination of glucosamine with diuretics (water pills) such as furosemide (Lasix) may cause an increased risk of glucosamine side effects.
- Laboratory studies report that glucosamine may affect recombinant erythropoietin, although the clinical relevance of this is not clear.

Interactions with Herbs and Dietary Supplements

- In theory, glucosamine may decrease the effectiveness of herbs or supplements that lower blood sugar levels. Caution is advised with use of herbs or supplements that also may alter blood sugar. Possible examples include *Aloe vera*, American ginseng, bilberry, bitter melon, burdock, fenugreek, fish oil, Gymnema, horse chestnut seed extract (HCSE), marshmallow, milk thistle, *Panax ginseng*, rosemary, Siberian ginseng, stinging nettle, and white horehound. Agents that may raise blood sugar levels include arginine, cocoa, and ephedra (when combined with caffeine).
- As suggested by limited evidence from studies in humans, side effects of glucosamine may be increased when it is used at the same time as diuretic herbs or supplements such as artichoke, celery, corn silk, couchgrass, dandelion, elder flower, horsetail, juniper berry, kava, shepherd's purse, uva ursi, and yarrow. Evidence regarding such interaction is preliminary.
- Preliminary reports indicate that use of glucosamine with vitamin C, bromelain, chondroitin sulfate, or manganese may lead to increased beneficial glucosamine effects on osteoarthritis. Simultaneous use with fish oil may have additive beneficial effects in the treatment of psoriasis, as indicated by preliminary research.

Interactions with Foods

- There are no available published reports of interactions with food.

Selected References

Natural Standard developed the preceding evidence-based information based on a systematic review of more than 300 scientific articles. For comprehensive information about alternative and complementary therapies on the professional level, go to www.naturalstandard.com. Selected references are listed here.

Altman RD, Hochberg M, Moskowitz RW, Schnitzer J, for American College of Rheumatology Subcommittee on Osteoarthritis Guidelines. Recommendations for the medical management of osteoarthritis on the hip and the knee. Arthritis Rheum 2000; 43:1905-1915.

Angermann P. Glucosamine and chondroitin sulfate in the treatment of arthritis. Ugeskr Laeger 2003;165(5):451-454.

Badia Llach X. Epidemiology and economic consequences of osteoarthritis. In: Reginster JY, Pelletier JP, Martel-Pelletier J, Henrotin Y, eds. Osteoarthritis: Clinical and Experimental Aspects. New York: Springer;1999:38-52.

Barclay TS, Tsourounis C, McCart GM. Glucosamine. Ann Pharmacother 1998;32(5): 574-579.

Bellamy N, Buchanan WW, Goldsmith CH, Campbell J, Stitt LW. Validation of WOMAC: a health status instrument for measuring clinically important patient relevant outcomes to antirheumatic drug therapy in patients with osteoarthritis of the hip or knee. J Rheumatol. 1988;15:1833-1840.

Bijlsma JW. Glucosamine and chondroitin sulfate as a possible treatment for osteoarthritis. Ned Tijdschr Geneeskd 2002;146(39):1819-1823.

Braham R, Dawson B, Goodman C. The effect of glucosamine supplementation on people experiencing regular knee pain. Br J Sports Med 2003;37(1):45-49.

Brandt KD. Animal models of osteoarthritis. Biorheology 2002;39(1-2):221-235.

Brief AA, Maurer SG, Di Cesare PE. Use of glucosamine and chondroitin sulfate in the management of osteoarthritis. J Am Acad Orthop Surg 2001;9(2):71-78.

Bruyere O, Honore A, Ethgen O, et al. Correlation between radiographic severity of knee osteoarthritis and future disease progression. Results from a 3-year prospective, placebo-controlled study evaluating the effect of glucosamine sulfate. Osteoarthritis Cartilage 2003; 11(1):1-5.

Bruyere O, Honore A, Rovati LC, et al. Radiologic features poorly predict clinical outcomes in knee osteoarthritis. Scand J Rheumatol 2002;31(1):13-16.

Cecil KM, Lin A, Ross BD, Egelhoff JC. Methylsulfonylmethane observed by in vivo proton magnetic resonance spectroscopy in a 5-year-old child with developmental disorder: effects of dietary supplementation. J Comput Assist Tomogr 2002;26(5):818-820.

Cohen M, Wolfe R, Mai T, Lewis D. A randomized, double blind, placebo controlled trial of a topical cream containing glucosamine sulfate, chondroitin sulfate, and camphor for osteoarthritis of the knee. J Rheumatol 2003;30(3):523-528.

Committee for Proprietary Medicinal Products. Points to Consider on Clinical Investigation of Medicinal Products Used in the Treatment of Osteoarthritis. London: European Agency for the Evaluation of Medicinal Products; July 1998.

Consoli G, Di Matteo L, Barlafante G, Agostinone A, Frattelli V. The analgesic effect of galactosaminoglycuronoglycan in the treatment of osteoarthritis. Minerva Med 1995; 86: 171-174.

Creamer P, Hochberg MC. Osteoarthritis. Lancet 1997:350:503-509.

Creamer P, Dieppe PA. Novel drug treatment strategies for osteoarthritis. J Rheumatol 1993; 20:1461-1464.

Crolle G, D'Este E. Glucosamine sulphate for the management of arthrosis: a controlled clinical investigation. Curr Med Res Opin 1980;7:104-109.

da Camara CC, Dowless GV. Glucosamine sulfate for osteoarthritis. Ann Pharmacother 1998; 32(5):580-587.

D'Ambrosio E, Casa B, Bompani R, Ssali G, Scali M. Glucosamine sulphate: a controlled clinical investigation in arthrosis. Pharmatherapeutica 1981:2:504-508.

Das A, Jr., Hammad TA. Efficacy of a combination of FCHG49 glucosamine hydrochloride, TRH122 low molecular weight sodium chondroitin sulfate and manganese ascorbate in the management of knee osteoarthritis. Osteoarthritis Cartilage 2000;8(5):343-350.

Das AK Jr, Hammad T, Eifel J. Efficacy of a new class of agents (glucosamine and chondroitin sulfate) in the treatment of osteoarthritis of the knee: a randomized double-blind placebo-controlled clinical trial. Paper presented at: American Academy of Orthopaedic Surgeons Annual Meeting; February 7, 1999; Anaheim, Calif. Paper 180.

Denham AC, Newton WP. Are glucosamine and chondroitin effective in treating osteoarthritis? J Fam Pract 2000;49(6):571-572.

Dodge GR, Jimenez SA. Glucosamine sulfate modulates the levels of aggrecan and matrix metalloproteinase-3 synthesized by cultured human osteoarthritis articular chondrocytes. Osteoarthritis Cartilage 2003;11(6):424-432.

Drovanti A, Bignamini AA, Rovati LC. Therapeutic activity of oral glucosamine sulfate in osteoarthritis: a placebo-controlled double-blind investigation. Clin Ther 1980;3:260-272.

Fioravanti A, Franci A, Anselmi F, et al. Clinical efficacy and tolerance of galactosoaminoglucuronoglycan sulfate in the treatment of osteoarthritis. Drugs Exp Clin Res 1991:17: 41-44.

Food and Drug Administration. Guidance for Industry: Clinical Development Programs for Drugs, Devices, and Biological Products Intended for the Treatment of Osteoarthritis. Washington, DC: Food and Drug Administration; 1999. FDA document 07/1999.

Förster KK, Schmid K, Rovati LC, et al. Longer-term treatment of mild-to-moderate osteoarthritis of the knee with glucosamine sulfate: a randomized, controlled, double-blind clinical study [abstract]. Eur J Clin Pharmacol 1996;50(6):542.

Forsyth CB, Mathews HL. Lymphocyte adhesion to *Candida albicans.* Infect Immun 2002;70(2):517-527.

Fujita T, Ohue M, Fujii Y, et al. The effect of active absorbable algal calcium (AAA Ca) with collagen and other matrix components on back and joint pain and skin impedance. J Bone Miner Metab 2002;20(5):298-302.

Gottlieb MS. Conservative management of spinal osteoarthritis with glucosamine sulfate and chiropractic treatment. J Manipulative Physiol Ther 1997;20(6):400-414.

Hehne HJ, Blasius K, Ernst HU. Treatment of gonarthritis with chondroprotective substances: a prospective comparative study of glucosamine sulphate and glycosaminoglycan polysulphate. Fortschr Med 1984;102:676-682.

Hermanns JF, Petit L, Pierard-Franchimont C, et al. Assessment of topical hypopigmenting agents on solar lentigines of Asian women. Dermatology 2002;204(4):281-286.

Houpt JB, McMillan R, Wein C, et al. Effect of glucosamine hydrochloride in the treatment of pain of osteoarthritis of the knee. J Rheumatol 1999;26(11):2423-2430.

Hua J, Sakamoto, Nagaoka I. Inhibitory actions of glucosamine, a therapeutic agent for osteoarthritis, on the functions of neutrophils. J Leukoc Biol 2002;71(4):632-640.

Hughes R, Carr A. A randomized, double-blind, placebo-controlled trial of glucosamine sulphate as an analgesic in osteoarthritis of the knee. Rheumatology 2002;41:279-284.

Hughes RA, Chertsey AJ. A randomised, double-blind, placebo-controlled trial of glucosamine to control pain in osteoarthritis of the knee [abstract]. Arthritis Rheum 2000; 43(9 suppl): S384.

Kerzberg EM, Roldan EJA Castelli G, Huberman ED. Combination of glycosaminoglycans and acetylsalicylic acid in knee osteoarthritis. Scand J Rheumatol 1987;16:377-380.

Kreder HJ. Glucosamine and chondroitin were found to improve outcomes in patients with osteoarthritis. J Bone Joint Surg Am 2000;82(9):1323.

Largo R, Alvarez-Soria MA, Diez-Ortego I, et al. Glucosamine inhibits IL-1beta-induced NFkappaB activation in human osteoarthritic chondrocytes. Osteoarthritis Cartilage 2003; 11(4):290-298.

Leffler CT, Philippi AF, Leffler SG, et al. Glucosamine, chondroitin, and manganese ascorbate for degenerative joint disease of the knee or low back: a randomized, double-blind, placebo-controlled pilot study. Mil Med 1999;164(2):85-91.

Lequesne L. The algofunctional indices for hip and knee osteoarthritis. J Rheumatol 1997; 24:779-781.

Lequesne L, Lery C, Samson M, Gerard DP. Indexes of severity for osteoarthritis of the hip and the knee. Scand J Rheumatol Suppl 1987;65:85-89.

Lopes Vas A. Double-blind clinical evaluation of the relative efficacy of ibuprofen and glucosamine sulphate in the management of osteoarthritis of the knee in out-patients. Curr Med Res Opin 1982;8:145-149.

Ma L, Rudert WA, Harnaha J, et al. Immunosuppressive effects of glucosamine. J Biol Chem 2002;277(42):39343-39349.

McAlindon TE, LaValley MP, Gulin JP, et al. Glucosamine and chondroitin for treatment of osteoarthritis: a systematic quality assessment and meta-analysis. JAMA 2000;283(11): 1469-1475.

Miller DC, Richardson J. Does glucosamine relieve arthritis joint pain? J Fam Pract 2003; 52(8):645-647.
Morelli V, Naquin C, Weaver V. Alternative therapies for traditional disease states: osteoarthritis. Am Fam Physician 2003;67(2):339-344.
Muller-Fassbender H, Bach GL, Haase W, et al. Glucosamine sulfate compared to ibuprofen in osteoarthritis of the knee. Osteoarthritis Cartilage 1994;2(1):61-69.
Noack W, Fischer M, Förster KK, et al. Glucosamine sulfate in osteoarthritis of the knee. Osteoarthritis Cartilage 1994;2(1):51-59.
Parcell S. Sulfur in human nutrition and applications in medicine. Altern Med Rev 2002; 7(1):22-44.
Pavelka K, Gatterova J, Olejarova M, et al. Glucosamine sulfate decreases progression of knee osteoarthritis in a long-term randomized placebo-controlled, independent, confirmatory trial. Arthritis Rheum 2000;43(9 suppl):S384.
Pavelka K, Gatterova J, Olejarova M, et al. Glucosamine sulfate use and delay of progression of knee osteoarthritis: a 3-year, randomized, placebo-controlled, double-blind study. Arch Intern Med 2002;162(18):2113-2123.
Pendleton A, Arden N, Dougados M, et al. EULAR recommendations for the management of osteoarthritis: report of a task force of the Standing Committee for International Clinical Studies Including Therapeutic Trials (ESCISIT). Ann Rheum Dis 2000;59:936-944.
Phoon S, Manolios N. Glucosamine. A nutraceutical in osteoarthritis. Aust Fam Physician 2002;31(6):539-541.
Priebe D, McDiarmid T, Mackler L, Tudiver F. Do[es] glucosamine or chondroitin cause regeneration of cartilage in osteoarthritis? J Fam Pract 2003;52(3):237-239.
Pujalte JM, Liavore EP, Ylescupidez FR. Double-blind clinical evaluation of oral glucosamine sulphate in the basic treatment of osteoarthritis. Curr Med Res Opin 1980; 7:110-114.
Qiu GZ, Gao SN, Giacovelli G, Rovati L, Setnikar I. Efficacy and safety of glucosamine sulfate versus ibuprofen in patients with knee osteoarthritis. Arzneimittelforschung 1998;48: 469-474.
Reginster JY, Deroisy R, Rovati LC, et al. Long-term effects of glucosamine sulphate on osteoarthritis progression: a randomized, placebo-controlled clinical trial. Lancet 2001;357: 251-256.
Reginster JY, Deroisy R, Rovati LC, et al. Long-term effects of glucosamine sulphate on osteoarthritis progression: a randomised, placebo-controlled clinical trial. Lancet 2001; 357(9252):251-256.
Reginster JY, Henrotin Y, Pavelka K, et al. Glucosamine sulfate (GS) is a specific osteoarthritis modifying drug: the results of two independent 3-year, randomized, controlled clinical trials [abstract]. North American Menopause Society 12th Annual Meeting, New Orleans, October 4-6, 2001
Reichelt A, Forster KK, Fischer M, Rovati LC. Efficacy and safety of glucosamine sulfate in osteoarthritis of the knee: a randomized, placebo-controlled, double-blind study. Arzneimittelforschung 1994;44:75-80.
Richy F, Bruyere O, Ethgen O, et al. Structural and symptomatic efficacy of glucosamine and chondroitin in knee osteoarthritis: a comprehensive meta-analysis. Arch Intern Med 2003;163(13):1514-1522.
Rindone JP, Hiller D, Collacott E, et al. Randomized, controlled trial of glucosamine for treating osteoarthritis of the knee. West J Med 2000;172(2):91-94.
Rovati LC. The clinical profile of glucosamine sulfate as a selective symptom modifying drug in osteoarthritis: current data and perspectives. Osteoarthritis Cartilage 1997;5:72.
Rovati LC, Giacovelli G, Annefeld M, et al. A large, randomised, placebo controlled, double-blind study of glucosamine sulfate vs. piroxicam and vs. their association, on the kinetics of the symptomatic effect in knee osteoarthritis [abstract]. Osteoarthritis Cartilage 1994; 2(Suppl 1):56.
Rovetta G. Galactosaminoglycuronoglycan sulfate (matrix) in therapy of tibiofibular osteoarthritis of the knee. Drugs Exp Clin Res 1991;17:53-57.
Ruane R, Griffiths P. Glucosamine therapy compared to ibuprofen for joint pain. Br J Community Nurs 2002;7(3):148-152.
Sakai K, Clemmons DR. Glucosamine induces resistance to insulin-like growth factor I

(IGF-I) and insulin in Hep G2 cell cultures: biological significance of IGF-I/insulin hybrid receptors. Endocrinology 2003;144(6):2388-2395.

Salvatore S, Heuschkel R, Tomlin S, et al. A pilot study of *N*-acetyl glucosamine, a nutritional substrate for glycosaminoglycan synthesis, in paediatric chronic inflammatory bowel disease. Aliment Pharmacol Ther 2000;14(12):1567-1579.

Scott GN, Elmer GW. Update on natural product–drug interactions. Am J Health Syst Pharm 2002;59(4):339-347.

Scroggie DA, Albright A, Harris MD. The effect of glucosamine-chondroitin supplementation on glycosylated hemoglobin levels in patients with type 2 diabetes mellitus: a placebo-controlled, double-blinded, randomized clinical trial. Arch Intern Med 2003;163(13): 1587-1590.

Shankland WE. The effects of glucosamine and chondroitin sulfate on osteoarthritis of the TMJ: a preliminary report of 50 patients. J Craniomandib Pract 1998;16(4):230-235.

Tallia AF, Cardone DA. Asthma exacerbation associated with glucosamine-chondroitin supplement. J Am Board Fam Pract 2002;15(6):481-484.

Tapadinhas MJ, Rivera IC, Bignamini AA. Oral glucosamine sulphate in the management of arthrosis: report on a multi-centre open investigation in Portugal. Pharmatherapeutica 1982; 3:157-168.

Thie NM, Prasad NG, Major PW. Evaluation of glucosamine sulfate compared to ibuprofen for the treatment of temporomandibular joint osteoarthritis: a randomized double blind controlled 3 month clinical trial. J Rheumatol 2001;28(6):1347-1355.

Towheed TE, Anastassiades TP, Shea B, et al. Glucosamine therapy for treating osteoarthritis. Cochrane Database Syst Rev 2001;(1):CD002946.

Towheed TE, Anastassiades TP. Glucosamine therapy for osteoarthritis. J Rheumatol 1999; 26(11):2294-2297.

Vajaradul Y. Double-blind clinical evaluation of intra-articular glucosamine in out-patients with gonarthrosis. Clin Ther 1981;3:336-343.

Walker-Bone K. 'Natural remedies' in the treatment of osteoarthritis. Drugs Aging 2003; 20(7):517-526.

Yang M, Butler M. Effects of ammonia and glucosamine on the heterogeneity of erythropoietin glycoforms. Biotechnol Prog 2002;18(1):129-138.

Zen K, Liu Y, Cairo D, Parkos CA. CD11b/CD18-dependent interactions of neutrophils with intestinal epithelium are mediated by fucosylated proteoglycans. J Immunol 2002; 169(9): 5270-5278.

Goldenseal

(*Hydrastis canadensis* L.)

G

RELATED TERMS

- Berberine, berberine bisulfate, curcuma, eye balm, eye root, golden root, goldensiegel, goldsiegel, ground raspberry, guldsegl, hydrastidis rhizoma, hydrophyllum, Indian dye, Indian paint, Indian plant, Indian turmeric, jaundice root, kanadische gelbwurzel, kurkuma, Ohio curcuma, orange root, tumeric root, warnera, wild curcuma, wild turmeric, yellow eye, yellow Indian plant, yellow paint, yellow paint root, yellow puccoon, yellow root, yellow seal, yellow wort.
- *Note:* Goldenseal is sometimes referred to as "Indian turmeric" or "curcuma" but should not be confused with turmeric (*Curcuma longa* L.).

BACKGROUND

- Goldenseal is one of the five top-selling herbal products in the United States. However, there is little scientific evidence about its safety or effectiveness. Goldenseal can be found in dietary supplements, eardrops, feminine cleansing products, cold/flu remedies, allergy remedies, laxatives, and digestive aids.
- Goldenseal often is found in combination with echinacea in herbal preparations for treatment of upper respiratory infections and is suggested to enhance the effects of echinacea. However, this additive effect is not scientifically proven.
- A popular notion is that goldenseal can be taken to mask the presence of illegal drugs in urine, although scientific information regarding this effect is limited.
- Studies of the effectiveness of goldenseal are limited to one of its main chemical ingredients, berberine salts (there are few published studies in humans of goldenseal itself). Because of the small amount of berberine actually present in most goldenseal preparations (from 0.5% to 6%), it is difficult to extend research findings for berberine salts to goldenseal. Thus, there is not enough scientific evidence to support the use of goldenseal in humans for any medical condition.
- The popularity of goldenseal has led to a higher demand for the herb than growers can supply. This high demand has led to the substitution of other herbs containing isoquinoline alkaloids (such as berberine). These herbs, such as Chinese goldthread (*Coptis chinensis* Fransch.) and Oregon grape (*Mahonia aquifolium* [Pursh] Nutt.), do not contain exactly the same isoquinoline alkaloids and may not have the same effects as those of goldenseal.

USES BASED ON SCIENTIFIC EVIDENCE	Grade*
Chloroquine-resistant malaria A small amount of research reports that berberine, a chemical found in goldenseal, may be beneficial in the treatment of chloroquine-resistant malaria when used in combination with pyrimethamine. Because of	C

Continued

the very small amount of berberine found in most goldenseal preparations, it is unclear whether goldenseal contains enough berberine to have these effects. In addition, the available studies have not been well designed. More research is needed before a recommendation can be made.	
Common cold/upper respiratory tract infection Goldenseal has become a popular herb for treatment of the common cold and upper respiratory tract infections and often is added to echinacea in commercial herbal cold remedies. Studies in animals and laboratory research suggest that the goldenseal component berberine has effects against bacteria and inflammation. However, because of the very small amount of berberine in most goldenseal preparations, it is unclear whether goldenseal contains enough berberine to have the same effects. Currently, there are no reliable studies in humans on the effectiveness of goldenseal or berberine in the treatment of respiratory tract infections.	C
Heart failure One study suggests that berberine, when given in addition to a standard prescription drug regimen for chronic congestive heart failure (CHF), may improve quality of life and may decrease ventricular premature complexes (VPCs) and mortality rate. Further research is needed to confirm these results.	C
Immune system stimulation Goldenseal is sometimes suggested to be an immune system stimulant. However, clinical or laboratory evidence for this effect in humans is scarce. More research is needed before a firm conclusion can be drawn.	C
Infectious diarrhea In several studies in laboratory animals and in small numbers of patients, berberine has been used as a treatment for diarrhea caused by bacterial infections (including diarrhea from cholera). However, most of this research has not been well designed, and results have been unclear. Because of the very small amount of berberine in most goldenseal products, it is unclear whether goldenseal contains enough berberine to have the same effects. Therefore, there is currently not enough scientific evidence to make a recommendation in this area.	C
Narcotic concealment (in urine analysis) It has been suggested that taking goldenseal can hide the presence of illegal drugs from urine tests. However, there is limited research to support this idea. One study from the National Institute on Drug Abuse (part of the National Institutes of Health) looked at marijuana and cocaine use and found that goldenseal probably does not have this effect.	C

Continued

Trachoma (*Chlamydia trachomatis* eye infection) — **C**

Studies in animals and laboratory research suggest that the goldenseal component berberine has effects against bacteria and inflammation. Several poorly designed studies in humans report benefits of berberine used in the eye to treat trachoma. Better research is needed before a recommendation can be made.

*Key to grades: *A:* Strong scientific evidence for this use; *B:* Good scientific evidence for this use; *C:* Unclear scientific evidence for this use; *D:* Fair scientific evidence against this use (it may not work); *F:* Strong scientific evidence against this use (it likely does not work). For a more detailed explanation of efficacy criteria, see "Natural Standard Evidence-Based Validated Grading Rationale" in the Introduction.

Uses Based on Tradition, Theory, or Limited Scientific Evidence

Abnormal heart rhythms, abortion induction, acne, AIDS, alcoholic liver disease, anal fissures, anesthetic, antibacterial, anticoagulant (blood-thinning effect), antifungal, antiheparin, antihistamine, anti-inflammatory, anxiety, appetite stimulant, arthritis, asthma, astrocytoma, atherosclerosis (hardening of the arteries), athlete's foot, bile flow stimulant, blood circulation stimulant, boils, bronchitis, cancer, *Candida* yeast infections, canker sores, cervicitis, chickenpox, chronic fatigue syndrome, colitis (intestinal inflammation), conjunctivitis, constipation, Crohn's disease, croup, cystic fibrosis, cystitis, dandruff, deafness, diabetes mellitus, diarrhea, digestion problems, diphtheria, diuretic (increasing urine flow), eczema, eyewash, fever, fistula problems, flatulence (gas), gallstones, gangrene, gastroenteritis, genital disorders, *Giardia* infection, gingivitis, glioblastoma, headache, *Helicobacter pylori* infection, hemorrhage (bleeding), hemorrhoids, hepatitis, herpes, hiatal hernia, high blood pressure, high cholesterol, high tyramine levels, hypoglycemia (low blood sugar levels), impetigo, indigestion, infections, influenza, insulin effect enhancement, itching, jaundice, keratitis (inflammation of cornea of eye), leishmaniasis, liver disorders, lupus, menstruation problems, morning sickness, mouthwash, muscle pain, muscle spasm, night sweats, obesity, osteoporosis, otorrhea (fluid from the ear), pain, pneumonia, premenstrual syndrome, prostatitis, psoriasis, sciatica, seborrhea, sedative, sinusitis, stomach ulcers, stimulant, strep throat, syphilis, tetanus, thrombocytopenia (low blood platelets), thrush, tinnitus (ringing in the ears), tonsillitis, tooth disease, trichomoniasis, tuberculosis, urinary tract disorders, uterus inflammation, uterus stimulant, vaginal irritation, varicose veins.

DOSING

The following doses are based on scientific research, publications, traditional use, or expert opinion. Many herbs and supplements have not been thoroughly tested, and their safety and effectiveness may not be proven. Brands may be made differently, with variable ingredients even within the same brand. The doses shown may not apply to all products. It is important to always read product labels and discuss doses with a qualified healthcare provider before therapy is started.

Standardization

- Standardization involves measuring the amounts of certain chemicals in products to try to make different preparations similar to each other. It is not always known if the chemicals being measured are the "active" ingredients.
- An analysis of several goldenseal products found large differences in the amounts of chemicals thought to be active (berberine and hydrastine). Some sources note standardization of goldenseal to isoquinoline alkaloids (5% to 10% total alkaloids, including hydrastine, berberine, and canadine).

Adults (18 Years and Older)

- **Goldenseal dosing:** For general use, various types of goldenseal dosing have been used, each taken by mouth three times daily, including 0.5- or 1-g tablets or capsules, 0.3 to 1 ml of liquid/fluid extract (1:1 in 60% ethanol), 0.5 to 1 g as a decoction, and 2 to 4 ml as a tincture (1:10 in 60% ethanol).
- **Berberine dosing:** For infectious diarrhea, 100 to 200 mg of berberine hydrochloride taken by mouth four times daily, or a single dose of 400 mg taken by mouth, has been studied. Berberine sulfate often is used as well, and the hydrochloride and the sulfate forms generally are thought to be equivalent.

Children (Younger Than 18 Years)

- There is not enough scientific evidence to safely recommend the use of goldenseal in children. Doses of 25 to 50 mg of berberine four times daily have been studied in children for the management of diarrhea, although safety has not been established.

SAFETY

The U.S. Food and Drug Administration does not strictly regulate herbs and supplements. There is no guarantee of strength, purity, or safety of products, and effects may vary. It is important to always read product labels. People who have a medical condition, or are taking other drugs, herbs, or supplements, should consult a qualified healthcare provider before starting a new therapy. A healthcare provider should be consulted immediately about any side effects.

Allergies

- Goldenseal should be avoided by people with known allergy/hypersensitivity to goldenseal or any of its constituents, including berberine and hydrastine.

Side Effects and Warnings

- Goldenseal is rarely reported to cause nausea, vomiting, breathing failure, or a feeling of numbness in the arms or legs. Large doses of goldenseal may cause mucous membrane irritation and worsening or stomach ulcers. Goldenseal used on the skin may cause irritation or ulcers.
- Possible effects of berberine, a chemical found in small amounts in goldenseal, include headache, slow heart rate, nausea, vomiting, abdominal bloating, and low white blood cell count. It is not clear if the amount of berberine in goldenseal products is enough to cause these reactions. Toxic doses of berberine may cause seizures or irritation of the esophagus and stomach when taken by mouth. Berberine given intravenously (through a vein) may cause abnormal heart rhythms. As suggested by studies in animals and laboratory research, berberine may increase blood concentrations of bilirubin. Berberine theoretically may cause low blood

pressure, although a different chemical in goldenseal, hydrastine, may actually cause increased blood pressure. There is limited study of the blood pressure effects of these agents in humans.
- Laboratory research and studies in animals suggest that the use of goldenseal or berberine may increase the risk of bleeding. However, there are no reliable published reports of bleeding in humans. Caution is advised in patients with bleeding disorders and in those taking drugs that may increase the risk of bleeding. Dosing adjustments may be necessary.
- Laboratory research suggests that goldenseal and berberine may cause increased sun sensitivity.
- Laboratory studies indicate that berberine may lower blood sugar. Caution is advised in patients with diabetes or hypoglycemia and in those taking drugs, herbs, or supplements that affect blood sugar. Serum glucose levels may need to be monitored by a healthcare provider, and medication adjustments may be necessary.
- The popularity of goldenseal has led to the substitution of other alkaloid-containing herbs, including Chinese goldthread (*Coptis chinensis*) and Oregon grape, that do not contain the same active components and may be associated with increased risk of serious toxicity or adverse events.

G

Pregnancy and Breastfeeding

- Use of goldenseal or berberine is not recommended in women who are pregnant or breastfeeding. The chemical hydrastine (found in goldenseal) may induce labor when taken by mouth during pregnancy and could have dangerous effects.

INTERACTIONS

Most herbs and supplements have not been thoroughly tested for interactions with other herbs, supplements, drugs, or foods. The interactions listed here are based on reports in scientific publications, laboratory experiments, or traditional use. It is important to always read product labels. People who have a medical condition, or are taking other drugs, herbs, or supplements, should consult a qualified healthcare provider before starting a new therapy.

Interactions with Drugs

- Evidence from laboratory and animal research suggests that the use of goldenseal or its component berberine may increase the risk of bleeding when either is taken with drugs that increase the risk of bleeding. Some examples are aspirin, anticoagulants (blood thinners) such as warfarin (Coumadin) and heparin, antiplatelet drugs such as clopidogrel (Plavix), and nonsteroidal anti-inflammatory drugs such as ibuprofen (Motrin, Advil) and naproxen (Naprosyn, Aleve).
- As suggested by studies in animals and laboratory research, goldenseal may interfere with how the body uses the liver's cytochrome P450 enzyme system to process components of some drugs. As a result, blood levels of these drugs may be increased, causing increased effects or potentially serious adverse reactions. As indicated by animal research, chemicals in goldenseal may increase the effects of L-phenylephrine and decrease the effects of tetracycline, neostigmine, and yohimbine.
- Laboratory research suggests that berberine may reduce the gastrointestinal absorption of P-glycoprotein–mediated substrates including chemotherapeutic agents such as daunomycin.
- Evidence from laboratory studies indicates that berberine may lower blood sugar. Caution is advised with use of medications that also may lower blood sugar.

Patients taking drugs for diabetes by mouth or insulin should be monitored closely by a qualified healthcare provider. Medication adjustments may be necessary.
- People who are using any medications should always check the package insert and consult their healthcare provider and pharmacist about possible interactions with goldenseal or berberine.

Interactions with Herbs and Dietary Supplements

- As suggested by findings from laboratory and animal research, the use of goldenseal or its component berberine may increase the risk of bleeding when either is taken with herbs or supplements that also are believed to increase the risk of bleeding. Multiple cases of bleeding have been reported with the use of *Ginkgo biloba*, fewer cases with garlic, and two cases with saw palmetto. Numerous other agents may theoretically increase the risk of bleeding, although this effect has not been proven in most cases. Some examples are alfalfa, American ginseng, angelica, anise, *Arnica montana*, asafetida, aspen bark, bilberry, birch, black cohosh, bladderwrack, bogbean, boldo, borage seed oil, bromelain, capsicum, cat's claw, celery, chamomile, chaparral, clove, coleus, cordyceps, danshen, devil's claw, dong quai, evening primrose, fenugreek, feverfew, flaxseed/flax powder (not a concern with flaxseed oil), ginger, grapefruit juice, grapeseed, green tea, guggul, gymnestra, horse chestnut, horseradish, licorice root, lovage root, male fern, meadowsweet, nordihydroguaiaretic acid (NDGA), onion, *Panax ginseng*, papain, parsley, passion flower, poplar, prickly ash, propolis, quassia, red clover, reishi, rue, Siberian ginseng, sweet birch, sweet clover, turmeric, vitamin E, white willow, wild carrot, wild lettuce, willow, wintergreen, and yucca.
- Studies in animals and laboratory research suggest that goldenseal may interfere with how the body uses the liver's cytochrome P450 system to process components of certain herbs and supplements. As a result, blood levels of these components may be too high, causing increased effects or potentially serious adverse reactions. It may also alter the effects of other herbs or supplements on the cytochrome P450 system, such as bloodroot, cat's claw, chamomile, chaparral, chasteberry, damiana, *Echinacea angustifolia*, grapefruit juice, licorice, oregano, red clover, St. John's wort, wild cherry, and yucca. Laboratory research also indicates that the goldenseal component berberine may reduce the effectiveness of yohimbine, which is found in small amounts in yohimbe bark extract.
- As indicated by laboratory studies, berberine may lower blood sugar levels. Caution is advised with use of herbs or supplements that also may lower blood sugar. Blood glucose levels may require monitoring, and doses may need adjustment. Possible examples include *Aloe vera*, American ginseng, bilberry, bitter melon, burdock, fenugreek, fish oil, gymnema, horse chestnut seed extract (HCSE), maitake mushroom, marshmallow, milk thistle, *Panax ginseng*, rosemary, shark cartilage, Siberian ginseng, stinging nettle, and white horehound.
- People who are using any herbal medications or dietary supplements should always check the package insert and consult their healthcare provider and pharmacist about possible interactions with goldenseal or berberine.

Selected References

Natural Standard developed the preceding evidence-based information based on a systematic review of more than 235 scientific articles. For comprehensive information about alternative and complementary therapies on the professional level, go to www.naturalstandard.com. Selected references are listed here.

Budzinski JW, Foster BC, Vandenhoek S, Arnason JT. An *in vitro* evaluation of human cytochrome P450 3A4 inhibition by selected commercial herbal extracts and tinctures. Phytomedicine 2000;7(4):273-282.

Cone EJ, Lange R, Darwin WD. *In vivo* adulteration: excess fluid ingestion causes false-negative marijuana and cocaine urine test results. J Anal Toxicol 1998;22(6):460-473.

Foster BC, Vandenhoek S, Hana J, et al. *In vitro* inhibition of human cytochrome P450-mediated metabolism of marker substrates by natural products. Phytomedicine 2003;10(4): 334-342.

Govindan M, Govindan G. A convenient method for the determination of the quality of goldenseal. Fitoterapia 2000;71(3):232-235.

Inbaraj JJ, Kukielczak BM, Bilski P, et al. Photochemistry and photocytotoxicity of alkaloids from Goldenseal (*Hydrastis canadensis* L.) 1. Berberine. Chem Res Toxicol 2001;14(11): 1529-1534.

Khin MU, Myo K, Nyunt NW, et al. Clinical trial of berberine in acute watery diarrhoea. BMJ (Clin Res Ed) 1985;291(6509):1601-1605.

Khin-Maung U, Myo-Khin, Nyunt-Nyunt-Wai, et al. Clinical trial of high-dose berberine and tetracycline in cholera. J Diarrhoeal Dis Res 1987;5(3):184-187.

Lahiri S, Dutta NK. Berberine and chloramphenicol in the treatment of cholera and severe diarrhoea. J Indian Med Assoc 1967;48(1):1-11.

Maeng HJ, Yoo HJ, Kim IW, et al. P-glycoprotein-mediated transport of berberine across Caco-2 cell monolayers. J Pharm Sci 2002;91(12):2614-2621.

Mahady GB, Pendland SL, Stoia A, et al. *In vitro* susceptibility of *Helicobacter pylori* to isoquinoline alkaloids from *Sanguinaria canadensis* and *Hydrastis canadensis.* Phytother Res 2003;17(3):217-221.

Pan GY, Huang ZJ, Wang GJ, et al. The antihyperglycaemic activity of berberine arises from a decrease of glucose absorption. Planta Med 2003;69(7):632-636.

Pan GY, Wang GJ, Liu XD, et al. The involvement of P-glycoprotein in berberine absorption. Pharmacol Toxicol. 2002;91(4):193-197.

Pan JF, Yu C, Zhu DY, et al. Identification of three sulfate-conjugated metabolites of berberine chloride in healthy volunteers' urine after oral administration. Acta Pharmacol Sin 2002; 23(1):77-82.

Rabbani GH, Butler T, Knight J, et al. Randomized controlled trial of berberine sulfate therapy for diarrhea due to enterotoxigenic *Escherichia coli* and *Vibrio cholerae.* J Infect Dis 1987; 155(5):979-984.

Sheng WD, Jiddawi MS, Hong XQ, et al. Treatment of chloroquine-resistant malaria using pyrimethamine in combination with berberine, tetracycline or cotrimoxazole. East African Med J 1997;74(5):283-284.

Wang DY, Yeh CC, Lee JH, et al. Berberine inhibited arylamine *N*-acetyltransferase activity and gene expression and DNA adduct formation in human malignant astrocytoma (G9T/VGH) and brain glioblastoma multiforms (GBM 8401) cells. Neurochem Res 2002;27(9):883-889.

Yin, J, Hu R, Chen M, Tang J, et al. Effects of berberine on glucose metabolism in vitro. Metabolism 2002; 51(11):1439-1543.

Zeng XH, Zeng XJ, Li YY. Efficacy and safety of berberine for congestive heart failure secondary to ischemic or idiopathic dilated cardiomyopathy. Am J Cardiol 2003;92(2):173-176.

Gotu Kola

(*Centella asiatica* L.)

RELATED TERMS

- Antanan gede, Apiacea, asiaticoside, Asiatic pennywort, asiatischer wassernabel, bavilacqua, Blasteostimulina, brahmi, brahmi-buti, brahmi manduc(a) parni, calingan rambat, Centasium, Centalase, Centellase, *Centella coriacea, Centella asiatica* triterpenic fraction (CATTF), coda-gam, Emdecassol, Fo-ti-teng, gagan-gagan, gang-gagan, HU300, hydrocotyle, hydrocotyle asiatica, hydrocotyle asiatique, idrocotyle, Indian pennywort, Indian water navelwort, indischer wassernabel, kaki kuda, kaki kuta, kerok batok, kos tekosan, lui gong gen, Madecassol, marsh penny, pagaga, panegowan, papaiduh, pegagan, pepiduh, piduh, puhe beta, rending, sheep rot, talepetrako, tete kadho, tete karo, thankuni, thick-leaved pennywort, titrated extract from *Centella asiatica* (TECA), total triterpenic fraction of *Centella asiatica* (TTFCA), Trofolastin, tsubo-kusa, tungchian, tungke-tunfke, water pennyrot, white rot.

BACKGROUND

- The most popular use of gotu kola in the United States is treatment of varicose veins or cellulitis. Preliminary evidence suggests short-term efficacy (6 to 12 months) of the total triterpenic fraction of *Centella asiatica* (TTFCA) in the treatment of chronic venous insufficiency (a syndrome characterized by lower extremity edema, varicosities, pain, pruritus, atrophic skin changes, and ulcerations, possibly due to venous valvular incompetence or a post-thrombotic syndrome). Small to moderate benefits on subjective and objective endpoints have been reported. However, trials in humans have been small and methodologically flawed and have employed varying dosages. Many reports were published by the same group of investigators. Although this evidence is sufficient to suggest efficacy, further research is necessary before a strong recommendation can be made. No other uses of gotu kola are supported by scientific evidence.
- *Note:* Gotu kola is not related to the kola nut (*Cola nitida*, *Cola acuminata*). Gotu kola is not a stimulant and does not contain caffeine.

USES BASED ON SCIENTIFIC EVIDENCE	Grade*
Chronic venous insufficiency/varicose veins Chronic venous insufficiency (CVI) is a term more commonly used in Europe than the United States. It describes a syndrome characterized by lower extremity edema, varicosities, pain, pruritus, atrophic skin changes, and ulcerations. It may be due to venous valvular incompetence, or may be a component of post-thrombotic syndrome. Measurable venous hypertension of the lower extremities may accompany this syndrome. Severity may be measured by rate of blood flow, capillary permeability, venous pressure, leg volume, or the ratio of oxygen to carbon dioxide in the blood.	B

Continued

Multiple small European trials suggest that the total triterpenoid fraction of *Centella asiatica* (TTFCA) (from gotu kola) may have small to moderate benefits on objective and subjective parameters associated with CVI. However, these trials have been methodologically flawed (e.g., dosing was inconsistent) nonclinical endpoints often were used, and have been brief (1 to 12 months). The same group of investigators were the authors of much of the available research. Although this evidence is sufficient to suggest efficacy, further research is necessary before a strong recommendation can be made.

G

Anxiety C

In Ayurvedic (traditional Indian) medicine, gotu kola is said to develop the crown chakra (the energy center at the top of the head) and to balance the right and left hemispheres of the brain. It has traditionally been used by yogis as a food for meditation. Recent research in animals demonstrated anxiolytic properties of gotu kola. This anxiolytic activity may or may not apply to humans. A single, randomized trial assessing the effects of gotu kola on startle responses in healthy (non-anxious) individuals reported some benefits. These preliminary findings are promising, although further research using established endpoints in patients with anxiety is necessary before an evidence-based therapeutic recommendation can be made.

Diabetic microangiopathy C

Studies have suggested beneficial effects of the total triterpenoid fraction of *Centella asiatica* (TTFCA) on subjective and objective parameters of venous insufficiency of the lower extremities. Based on these observations, it has been postulated that there could be a role for gotu kola in the treatment of vascular disease associated with diabetes. However, diabetic patients experience vascular disease that is often different in etiology from venous insufficiency. Nonetheless, initial controlled trials have found oral gotu kola (TTFCA, 60 mg twice daily) to have statistically significant beneficial effects on microcirculatory parameters in patients with diabetic microangiopathy. These studies were brief and methodologically weak, with limited assessment of clinical outcomes. Therefore, no recommendation can be made at this time.

Wound healing C

Numerous laboratory studies and studies in animals have demonstrated the ability of *Centella asiatica* extracts to promote wound healing, possibly through the stimulation of collagen synthesis. However, there is a paucity of evidence in studies in humans regarding the use of gotu kola or *Centella asiatica* extract in the treatment of wounds, and no recommendation can be made at this time.

*Key to grades: *A:* Strong scientific evidence for this use; *B:* Good scientific evidence for this use; *C:* Unclear scientific evidence for this use; *D:* Fair scientific evidence against this use (it may not work); *F:* Strong scientific evidence against this use (it likely does not work). For a more detailed explanation of efficacy criteria, see "Natural Standard Evidence-Based Validated Grading Rationale" in the Introduction.

Uses Based on Tradition, Theory, or Limited Scientific Evidence

Abscesses, alcoholic liver disease, Alzheimer's disease, amenorrhea, anemia, antidepressant, anti-fertility agent, anti-infective, antioxidant, anxiety, aphrodisiac, asthma, bladder lesions, blood purifier, bronchitis, bruises, burns, cancer, cellulitis, cholera, colds, corneal abrasion, dehydration, diarrhea, diuretic, dysentery, eczema, elephantiasis, energy, epilepsy, eye diseases, fatigue, fever, airline flight-induced lower extremity edema, fungal infections, gastric ulcers, gastric ulcer prophylaxis, gastritis, hair growth promoter, hemorrhoids, hepatic disorders, hepatitis, herpes simplex virus-2 infection, hot flashes, hypertension, immunomodulator, inflammation, influenza, jaundice, keloid formation prevention, leprosy, leukoderma, libido stimulant, longevity, malaria, memory enhancement, menstrual disorders, mental disorders, mood disorders, pain, periodontal disease, peripheral vasodilator, physical exhaustion, psoriasis, radiation-induced behavioral changes, restless leg syndrome, rheumatism, scabies, scar healing, scleroderma, shigellosis, shingles (post-herpetic neuralgia), skin diseases, skin graft donor wounds, snake venom antidote, striae gravidarum (stretch marks), sunstroke, syphilis, systemic lupus erythematosus, tonsillitis, tuberculosis, urinary retention, urinary tract infection, vaginal discharge, vascular fragility, venous disorders.

DOSING

The following doses are based on scientific research, publications, traditional use, or expert opinion. Many herbs and supplements have not been thoroughly tested, and their safety and effectiveness may not be proven. Brands may be made differently, with variable ingredients even within the same brand. The doses shown may not apply to all products. It is important to always read product labels and discuss doses with a qualified healthcare provider before therapy is started.

Standardization

- Standardization involves measuring the amounts of certain chemicals in products to try to make different preparations similar to each other. It is not always known if the chemicals being measured are the "active" ingredients.

Adults (18 Years and Older)

- **Chronic venous insufficiency/varicose veins/venous hypertension:** Various dosing regimens have been studied, including Centellase (TTFCA; total triterpenic fraction of *Centella asiatica*), 60 to 120 mg daily and 30 mg twice daily; and TTFCA, 30 mg three times daily, 60 mg twice daily, and 60 mg three times daily. Preliminary studies have suggested a dose-dependent response, with better results using TTFCA, 60 mg three times daily. TECA (titrated extract from *Centella asiatica*) has also been studied, at a dose of 60 to 120 mg daily.
- **Diabetic microangiopathy:** TTFCA (total triterpenic fraction of *Centella asiatica*), 60 mg twice daily, has been used.

Children (Younger Than 18 Years)

- Because of insufficient scientific evidence regarding its safety and efficacy, gotu kola is not recommended for use in children.

SAFETY

The U.S. Food and Drug Administration does not strictly regulate herbs and supplements. There is no guarantee of the strength, purity, or safety of products, and effects may vary. It is important to always read product labels. People who have a medical condition, or are taking other drugs, herbs, or supplements, should consult a qualified healthcare provider before starting a new therapy. A healthcare provider should be contacted immediately about any side effects.

Allergies

- Use of gotu kola should be avoided by people with known allergy/hypersensitivity to gotu kola or any of its constituents, including asiaticoside, asiatic acid, and madecassic acid. There may be a cross-sensitivity to other members of the Apiacea family.
- There are numerous reports of allergic contact dermatitis after topical gotu kola use, including one case which occurred after the use of topical Blasteostimulina cream, and another after the application of topical Madecassol ointment (both products contain *Centella asiatica* extract).

Side Effects and Warnings

- Studies suggest that gotu kola has few side effects when taken by mouth. Reported symptoms include stomach upset and nausea. In research in animals, large doses of gotu kola caused drowsiness, increased cholesterol levels, and raised blood sugar levels. Gotu kola should be avoided in people with diabetes or high cholesterol. Persons who are driving or operating heavy machinery should avoid the use of gotu kola. One study in animals reported that asiaticoside, an ingredient of gotu kola, may have weak cancer-causing effects when applied to the skin.
- *Note:* Gotu kola is not related to the kola nut (*Cola nitida, Cola acuminata*). Gotu kola is not a stimulant and does not contain caffeine.

Pregnancy and Breastfeeding

- In studies in animals, gotu kola reduced the ability of the female to become pregnant, but it is not known if this effect occurs in humans. Gotu kola is not recommended in women who are pregnant or breastfeeding because there is little available information regarding its safety and efficacy.

INTERACTIONS

Most herbs and supplements have not been thoroughly tested for interactions with other herbs, supplements, drugs, or foods. The interactions listed here are based on reports in scientific publications, laboratory experiments, or traditional use. It is important to always read product labels. People who have a medical condition, or are taking other drugs, herbs, or supplements, should consult a qualified healthcare provider before starting a new therapy.

Interactions with Drugs

- In theory, gotu kola may increase the amount of drowsiness caused by sedatives and other agents that cause drowsiness. Examples are alcohol, barbiturates such as phenobarbital, benzodiazepines such as lorazepam (Ativan), and narcotics such as codeine. Caution is advised in people who are driving or operating heavy machinery.
- Studies in animals suggest that gotu kola raises blood sugar levels. People taking medications for diabetes or using insulin should be monitored closely by their

healthcare provider if they are also taking gotu kola. Dosing adjustments may be necessary.
- Gotu kola theoretically may increase cholesterol levels and may work against the activity of cholesterol-lowering drugs.

Interactions with Herbs and Dietary Supplements

- In theory, gotu kola may increase the amount of drowsiness caused by herbs or supplements that may also cause drowsiness. Examples are calamus, calendula, California poppy, capsicum, catnip, celery, couchgrass, dogwood, elecampane, German chamomile, goldenseal, hops, kava, lavender aromatherapy, lemon balm, sage, sassafras, skullcap, shepherd's purse, Siberian ginseng, St. John's wort, valerian, wild carrot, wild lettuce, withania root, and yerba mansa. Caution is advised in people who are driving or operating heavy machinery.
- Animal studies suggest that gotu kola may raise blood sugar levels and may therefore counteract the effects of herbs or supplements that may lower blood sugar levels. Caution is advised in people who are using such agents in combination with gotu kola. Blood glucose levels may require monitoring, and doses may need adjustment. Examples of such agents are *Aloe vera*, American ginseng, bilberry, bitter melon, burdock, fenugreek, fish oil, flaxseed, gymnema, horse chestnut seed extract (HCSE), marshmallow, milk thistle, *Panax ginseng*, rosemary, Siberian ginseng, stinging nettle, and white horehound. Other supplements that may raise blood sugar levels include arginine, cocoa, and ephedra (when combined with caffeine).
- Studies in animals suggest that gotu kola may increase cholesterol levels. It may therefore interfere with the effectiveness of lipid-lowering agents such as fish oil, garlic, and niacin.

Selected References

Natural Standard developed the preceding evidence-based information based on a systematic review of more than 140 articles. For comprehensive information about alternative and complementary therapies on the professional level, go to www.naturalstandard.com. Selected references are listed here.

Belcaro G, Laurora G, Cesarone MR, et al. Efficacy of Centellase in the treatment of venous hypertension evaluated by a combined microcirculatory model. Curr Ther Res 1989;46(6): 1015-1026.

Belcaro GV, Grimaldi R, Guidi G, et al. Treatment of diabetic microangiopathy with TTFCA. A microcirculatory study with laser-Doppler flowmetry, P02/PC02, and capillary permeability measurements. Curr Ther Res 1990;47(3):421-428.

Belcaro GV, Rulo A, Grimaldi R. Capillary filtration and ankle edema in patients with venous hypertension treated with TTFCA. Angiology 1990;41(1):12-18.

Belcaro GV, Grimaldi R, Guidi G. Improvement of capillary permeability in patients with venous hypertension after treatment with TTFCA. Angiology 1990;41(7):533-540.

Bradwejn J, Zhou Y, Koszycki D, et al. A double-blind, placebo-controlled study on the effects of Gotu Kola (*Centella asiatica*) on acoustic startle response in healthy subjects. J Clin Psychopharmacol 2000;20(6):680-684.

Cesarone MR, Belcaro G, Rulo A, et al. Microcirculatory effects of total triterpenic fraction of *Centella asiatica* in chronic venous hypertension: measurement by laser Doppler, TcPo2-co2, and leg volumetry. Angiology 2001;52(10 suppl 2):S45-S48.

Cesarone MR, Incandela L, De Sanctis MT, et al. Evaluation of treatment of diabetic microangiopathy with total triterpenic fraction of *Centella asiatica*: a clinical prospective randomized trial with a microcirculatory model. Angiology 2001;52(10 suppl 2):S49-S54.

Cesarone MR, Incandela L, De Sanctis MT, et al. Flight microangiopathy in medium- to long-distance flights: prevention of edema and microcirculation alterations with total triterpenic fraction of *Centella asiatica*. Angiology 2001;52(10 suppl 2):S33-S37.

Cesarone MR, Belcaro G, De Sanctis MT, et al. Effects of the total triterpenic fraction of *Centella asiatica* in venous hypertensive microangiopathy: a prospective, placebo-controlled, randomized trial. Angiology 2001;52(10 suppl 2):S15-S18.

Cesarone MR, Laurora G, De Sanctis MT, et al. [The microcirculatory activity of *Centella asiatica* in venous insufficiency. A double-blind study.] Minerva Cardioangiol 1994;42(6): 299-304.

De Sanctis MT, Incandela L, Cesarone MR, et al. Acute effects of TTFCA on capillary filtration in severe venous hypertension. Panminerva Medica 1994;36(2):87-90.

De Sanctis MT, Belcaro G, Incandela L, et al. Treatment of edema and increased capillary filtration in venous hypertension with total triterpenic fraction of *Centella asiatica*: a clinical, prospective, placebo-controlled, randomized, dose-ranging trial. Angiology 2001; 52(10 suppl 2):S55-S59.

Incandela L, Belcaro G, De Sanctis MT, et al. Total triterpenic fraction of *Centella asiatica* in the treatment of venous hypertension: a clinical, prospective, randomized trial using a combined microcirculatory model. Angiology 2001;52(10 suppl 2):S61-S67.

Incandela L, Cesarone MR, Cacchio M, et al. Total triterpenic fraction of *Centella asiatica* in chronic venous insufficiency and in high-perfusion microangiopathy. Angiology 2001; 52(10 suppl 2):S9-S13.

Incandela L, Belacaro G, Cesarone MR, et al. Treatment of diabetic microangiopathy and edema with total triterpenic fraction of *Centella asiatica*: a prospective, placebo-controlled randomized study. Angiology 2001;52(10 suppl 2):S27-S31.

Marastoni F, Baldo A, Redaelli G, et al. [*Centella asiatica* extract in venous pathology of the lower limbs and its evaluation as compared with tribenoside.] Minerva Cardioangiol 1982;30(4):201-207.

Pointel JP, Boccalon H, Cloarec M, et al. Titrated extract of *Centella asiatica* (TECA) in the treatment of venous insufficiency of the lower limbs. Angiology 1987;38(1 Pt 1):46-50.

Schulman RN. Gotu kola shows anxiety-reducing activity in clinical trial. HerbalGram 2002; 55:14.

Green Tea
(*Camellia sinensis*)

RELATED TERMS

- AR25, camellia, *Camellia assamica*, *Camellia sinensis*, *Camellia sinensis* L. Kuntze, camellia tea, catechins, Chinese tea, epigallocatechin-3-gallate (ECGC), Exolise, green tea extract (GTE), matsu-cha tea, *Thea bohea*, *Thea sinensis*, *Thea viridis*, theanine, theifers.

BACKGROUND

- Green tea is made from the dried leaves of *Camellia sinensis*, a perennial evergreen shrub. Green tea has a long history of use, dating back to China approximately 5000 years ago. Green tea, black tea, and oolong tea all are derived from the same plant.
- Green tea is a source of caffeine, a methylxanthine that stimulates the central nervous system, relaxes smooth muscle in the airways to the lungs (bronchioles), stimulates the heart, and acts on the kidney as a diuretic (increasing urine). One cup of tea contains approximately 50 mg of caffeine, depending on the strength of the infusion and the size of the cup; by comparison, coffee contains 65 to 175 mg of caffeine per cup. Tea also contains polyphenols (catechins, anthocyanins, phenolic acids), tannin, trace elements, and vitamins.
- The tea plant is native to Southeast Asia; it can grow up to a height of 40 feet but usually is maintained at a height of 2 to 3 feet by regular pruning. The first spring leaf buds, called the *first flush*, are considered the highest-quality leaves. When the first flush leaf bud is picked, another one grows, and this set of leaves is called the *second flush*; the harvesting continues until an *autumn flush*. The older leaves picked farther down the stems are considered to be of poorer quality.
- Tea varieties reflect the growing region (for example, Ceylon or Assam), the district (for example, Darjeeling), the form (for example, pekoe is cut, whereas gunpowder is rolled), and the processing method (for example, black, green, or oolong). India and Sri Lanka are the major producers of green tea.
- Green tea is produced by lightly steaming the freshly cut leaf, so that oxidation of the enzymes within the leaf does not take place. Green tea is produced and consumed primarily in China, Japan, and countries in North Africa and the Middle East. By contrast, allowing the leaves of *Camellia sinensis* to oxidize produces black tea (a fermentation process that alters flavor as well as enzymes present in the tea). Oolong tea is a partially oxidized tea and accounts for less than 5% of all tea produced.
- Historically, tea has been served as a part of various ceremonies and has been used to maintain alertness during long meditations. A legend in India tells the story of Prince Siddhartha Gautama, the founder of Buddhism, who tore off his eyelids in frustration at his inability to stay awake during meditation while journeying through China. A tea plant is said to have sprouted from the spot where his eyelids fell, providing him with the means to stay awake, meditate, and reach enlightenment. Turkish traders reportedly introduced tea to Western cultures in the 6th century.

USES BASED ON SCIENTIFIC EVIDENCE	Grade*
Arthritis Research indicates that green tea may benefit arthritis by reducing inflammation and slowing cartilage breakdown. Further studies are required before a recommendation can be made.	C
Asthma Research has shown caffeine to cause improvement in air flow to the lungs (bronchodilation). However, it is not clear if caffeine or tea consumption has significant clinical benefits in people with asthma. Better research regarding this effect is needed before a conclusion can be drawn.	C
Cancer prevention Several large population-based studies have been undertaken to examine the possible association between green tea consumption and cancer incidence. Cancers of the digestive system (stomach, colon, rectum, pancreas, and esophagus) have primarily been tracked. The risk of prostate cancer, cervical cancer, and breast cancer in women also has been studied. Although much of this research suggests a cancer-protective effect of habitual green tea consumption, some studies have not observed significant benefits. In studies that have shown benefits, it is not clear if other lifestyle choices of people who drink tea may actually be the beneficial factors. If there is a benefit, it may be small and require large amounts of daily consumption (several cups per day). At this time, the scientific evidence remains indeterminate in this area. Laboratory research and studies in animals report that components of tea, such as polyphenols, have antioxidant or free radical scavenging properties and may possess various effects against tumor cells (such as angiogenesis inhibition, hydrogen peroxide generation, or induction of apoptosis). Limited evidence from studies in humans includes reports of lower estrogen levels in women drinking green tea, proposed as possibly beneficial in estrogen receptor–positive breast cancers. However, other animal and laboratory research suggests that components of green tea may actually be carcinogenic, although effects in humans are not clear. Overall, the relationship of green tea consumption and human cancer remains unclear. Evidence from a controlled trial of sufficient size and duration is needed before a recommendation regarding this possible association can be made.	C
Dental caries prevention There is limited study of tea as a gargle (mouthwash) for the prevention of dental caries (tooth decay). It is not clear if this is a beneficial therapy.	C
Heart attack prevention Early suggestive evidence indicates that regular intake of green tea may reduce the risk of heart attack or atherosclerosis (clogged arteries). Tea	C

Continued

may cause a decrease in platelet aggregation or endothelial dysfunction, proposed to be beneficial against blockage of arteries in the heart. Evidence from controlled trials of sufficient size and duration is needed before a recommendation regarding this effect can be made.	
High cholesterol Laboratory evidence, studies in animals, and limited research in humans suggest possible effects of green tea on cholesterol levels. Recent research using a theaflavin-enriched GTE is promising. Better evidence from studies in humans is necessary to confirm a lipid-lowering effect.	C
Memory enhancement Several preliminary studies have examined the effects of caffeine, tea, or coffee use on short-term and long-term memory. It remains unclear if tea is beneficial for this use.	C
Menopausal symptoms A study conducted in healthy postmenopausal women showed that a morning and evening menopausal formula containing green tea was effective in relieving menopausal symptoms including hot flashes and sleep disturbance. Further studies are needed to confirm these results.	C
Mental performance/alertness Limited, low-quality research reports that the use of green tea may improve cognition and sense of alertness. Green tea contains caffeine, which is a stimulant.	C
Sun protection There is limited evidence from studies in animals and humans for a protective effect of green tea against ultraviolet light injury of the skin. Well-designed research is needed before a recommendation regarding this effect can be made. Comparisons have not been made with well-established forms of sun protection such as use of ultraviolet light–protective sunscreen.	C
Weight loss Several small studies in humans have addressed the use of green tea extract (GTE) capsules for weight loss in overweight people or in persons of average weight. Better research is needed before a recommendation regarding this effect can be made.	C

*Key to grades: *A:* Strong scientific evidence for this use; *B:* Good scientific evidence for this use; *C:* Unclear scientific evidence for this use; *D:* Fair scientific evidence against this use (it may not work); *F:* Strong scientific evidence against this use (it likely does not work). For a more detailed explanation of efficacy criteria, see "Natural Standard Evidence-Based Validated Grading Rationale" in the Introduction.

Uses Based on Tradition, Theory, or Limited Scientific Evidence

Asbestos lung injury protection, alcohol intoxication reversal, antioxidant, astringent, bleeding from gums or tooth sockets, blood flow improvement, body temperature regulation, bone density improvement, cataracts, cognitive performance enhancement, Crohn's disease, detoxification from alcohol or other toxins, diabetes, diarrhea, digestion promotion, disease resistance enhancement, diuretic (increasing urine flow), fibrosarcoma, flatulence, fungal infections, gastritis, gum swelling, headache, heart disease, *Helicobacter pylori* infection, HIV infection/AIDS, ischemia-reperfusion injury protection, joint pain, kidney stone prevention, liver cancer, longevity promotion, lung cancer, neuroprotection, oral leukoplakia, ovarian cancer, Parkinson's disease prevention, platelet aggregation inhibition, stimulant, stomach disorders, stroke prevention, sunburn, tired eyes, urine flow improvement, vomiting.

DOSING

The following doses are based on scientific research, publications, traditional use, or expert opinion. Many herbs and supplements have not been thoroughly tested, and their safety and effectiveness may not be proven. Brands may be made differently, with variable ingredients even within the same brand. The doses shown may not apply to all products. It is important to always read product labels and discuss doses with a qualified healthcare provider before therapy is started.

Adults (18 Years and Older)

- Benefits of specific doses of green tea are not established. Most studies have examined green tea taken as a brewed beverage, rather than in capsule form. One cup of tea contains approximately 50 mg of caffeine and 80 to 100 mg of polyphenols, depending on the strength of the infusion and the size of the cup. For cancer prevention, studies have examined the effects of habitually drinking anywhere from 1 to 10 cups daily (or greater). For heart disease prevention, one study reports benefits of drinking greater than 375 ml of tea daily, although evidence in this area remains unclear.
- In capsule form, there is considerable variation in the amount of green tea extract (GTE) per capsule, which may range from 100 to 750 mg per capsule. Extracts of green tea may be standardized to contain anywhere from 60% to 97% polyphenols. A recent phase I study reported that the maximum tolerated dose of oral GTE is 4.2 g/m^2 of body surface area daily, taken once or in three divided doses (equivalent to 7 or 8 Japanese cups), or 120 ml of green tea three times daily. Currently, there is no established recommended dose for GTE capsules.

SAFETY

The U.S. Food and Drug Administration does not strictly regulate herbs and supplements. There is no guarantee of strength, purity, or safety of products, and effects may vary. It is important to always read product labels. People who have a medical condition, or are taking other drugs, herbs, or supplements, should consult a qualified healthcare provider before starting a new therapy. A healthcare provider should be consulted immediately about any side effects.

Allergies

- People with known allergy/hypersensitivity to caffeine or tannin should avoid green tea. Skin rash and hives have been reported with caffeine ingestion.

Side Effects and Warnings

- Studies of the side effects of green tea specifically are limited. However, green tea is a source of caffeine, for which multiple reactions are reported.
- Caffeine is a stimulant of the central nervous system and may cause insomnia in adults, children, and infants (including nursing infants of mothers taking caffeine). Caffeine acts on the kidneys as a diuretic (increasing urine flow and urine sodium and potassium levels and potentially decreasing blood sodium and potassium levels) and may worsen urge incontinence. Caffeine-containing beverages may increase the production of stomach acid and may worsen ulcer symptoms. Tannin in tea can cause constipation. Caffeine in doses of 250 to 350 mg can increase heart rate and blood pressure, although people who consume caffeine regularly do not seem to experience these effects in the long term.
- An increase in blood sugar levels may occur after consumption of green tea containing the equivalent of 200 mg of caffeine (4 to 5 cups, depending on tea strength and cup size). Caffeine-containing beverages such as green tea should be used cautiously in patients with diabetes. By contrast, lowering of blood sugar levels from drinking green tea also has been reported in preliminary research. Additional study of the effect of green tea on blood sugar is needed.
- People with severe liver disease should use caffeine cautiously, as levels of caffeine in the blood may build up and last longer with impaired liver function. Skin rashes have been associated with caffeine ingestion. In laboratory research and studies in animals, caffeine has been found to affect blood clotting, although effects in humans are not known.
- **Caffeine toxicity/high doses:** When the equivalent of greater than 500 mg of caffeine is consumed (usually more than 8 to 10 cups per day, depending on the strength of the infusion and the size of the cup), symptoms of anxiety, delirium, agitation, psychosis, or detrusor muscle instability (unstable bladder) may occur. Conception may be delayed in women who consume large amounts of caffeine. Seizure, muscle spasm, life-threatening muscle breakdown (rhabdomyolysis), and life-threatening abnormal heart rhythms have been reported with caffeine overdose. Doses greater than 1000 mg may be fatal.
- **Caffeine withdrawal:** Chronic use can result in tolerance and psychological dependence and may be habit forming. Abrupt discontinuation may result in withdrawal symptoms such as headache, irritation, nervousness, anxiety, tremor, and dizziness. In people with psychiatric disorders such as affective disorder or schizoaffective disorder, caffeine withdrawal may worsen symptoms or cause confusion, disorientation, excitement, restlessness, violent behavior, or mania.
- **Chronic effects:** Several population studies initially suggested a possible association between caffeine use and fibrocystic breast disease, although more recent research has not found this connection. Limited research reports a possible relationship between caffeine use and multiple sclerosis, although the evidence for this association is not definitive. Studies in animals report that tannin fractions from tea plants may increase the risk of cancer, although it is not clear that the tannin present in green tea has significant carcinogenic effects in humans.

- Drinking tannin-containing beverages such as tea may contribute to iron deficiency. In infants, tea consumption has been associated with impaired iron metabolism and microcytic anemia.
- In preliminary research, green tea has been associated with decreased levels of estrogens in the body. It is not clear if significant side effects such as hot flashes may occur.

Pregnancy and Breastfeeding

- Large amounts of green tea should be used cautiously in pregnant women, because caffeine crosses the placenta and has been associated with spontaneous abortion, intrauterine growth restriction/retardation, and low birth weight. Heavy caffeine intake (400 mg or greater daily) during pregnancy may increase the risk of sudden infant death syndrome (SIDS). Very high doses of caffeine (1100 mg or greater daily) have been associated with birth defects, including limb and palate malformations.
- Caffeine is readily transferred into breast milk. Caffeine ingestion by infants can lead to sleep disturbances/insomnia. Nursing infants of mothers consuming greater than 500 mg of caffeine daily have been reported to experience tremors and heart rhythm abnormalities. Components present in breast milk may reduce infants' ability to metabolize caffeine, resulting in higher-than-expected blood levels. Tea consumption by infants has been associated with anemia, reductions in iron metabolism, and irritability.

INTERACTIONS

Most herbs and supplements have not been thoroughly tested for interactions with other herbs, supplements, drugs, or foods. The interactions listed here are based on reports in scientific publications, laboratory experiments, or traditional use. It is important to always read product labels. People who have a medical condition, or are taking other drugs, herbs, or supplements, should consult a qualified healthcare provider before starting a new therapy.

Interactions with Drugs

- Studies of the interactions of green tea with drugs are limited. However, green tea is a source of caffeine, for which multiple interactions have been documented.
- The combination of caffeine with ephedrine, an ephedra alkaloid, has been implicated in numerous severe or life-threatening cardiovascular events such as very high blood pressure, stroke, or heart attack. This combination is commonly used in over-the-counter weight loss products and also may be associated with other adverse effects, including abnormal heart rhythms, insomnia, anxiety, headache, irritability, poor concentration, blurred vision, and dizziness. Stroke also has been reported after the nasal ingestion of caffeine with amphetamine.
- Caffeine may add to the effects and side effects of other stimulants including nicotine, beta-adrenergic agonists such as albuterol (Ventolin), and other methylxanthines such as theophylline. Conversely, caffeine can counteract drowsy effects and mental slowness caused by benzodiazepines such as lorazepam (Ativan) and diazepam (Valium). Phenylpropanolamine and caffeine should not be used together, because of reports of numerous potentially serious adverse effects, although forms of phenylpropanolamine taken by mouth have been removed from the U.S. market following reports of bleeding into the head.

- When taken with caffeine, a number of drugs may increase caffeine blood levels or the length of time caffeine acts on the body, including disulfiram (Antabuse), oral contraceptives (OCPs) or agents for hormone replacement therapy (HRT), ciprofloxacin (Cipro), norfloxacin, fluvoxamine (Luvox), cimetidine (Tagamet), verapamil, and mexiletine. Caffeine levels may be lowered with simultaneous use of dexamethasone (Decadron). The metabolism of caffeine by the liver (using the cytochrome P450 isoenzyme 1A2) may be affected by numerous drugs, although the effects in humans are not clear.
- Caffeine may lengthen the effects of carbamazepine or increase the effects of clozapine (Clozaril) and dipyridamole. Caffeine may affect serum lithium levels, and abrupt cessation of caffeine use by regular caffeine users taking lithium may result in high levels of lithium or lithium toxicity. Levels of aspirin or phenobarbital may be lowered in the body, although clinical effects in humans are not clear.
- Although caffeine by itself does not appear to have pain-relieving properties, it is used in combination with ergotamine tartrate in the treatment of migraine or cluster headaches (for example, Cafergot). It has been shown to increase the headache-relieving effects of other pain relievers such as acetaminophen and aspirin (for example, Excedrin). Caffeine also may increase the pain-relieving effects of codeine and ibuprofen (Advil, Motrin).
- As a diuretic, caffeine increases urine and sodium losses through the kidney and may add to the effects of other diuretics such as furosemide (Lasix).
- Green tea may contain vitamin K, which when used in large quantities can reduce the blood-thinning effects of warfarin (Coumadin), a phenomenon that has been reported in a human case.

Interactions with Herbs and Dietary Supplements

- Studies of green tea interactions with herbs and supplements are limited. However, green tea is a source of caffeine, for which multiple interactions have been documented.
- Caffeine may add to the effects and side effects of other stimulants. The combination of caffeine with ephedrine, which is present in ephedra (ma huang), has been implicated in numerous severe or life-threatening cardiovascular events such as sudden onset of very high blood pressure, stroke, or heart attack. This combination is commonly used in over-the-counter weight loss products and also may be associated with other adverse effects, including abnormal heart rhythms, insomnia, anxiety, headache, irritability, poor concentration, blurred vision, and dizziness.
- Cola nut, guarana (*Paullina cupana*), and yerba mate (*Ilex paraguariensis*) also are sources of caffeine and may add to the effects and side effects of caffeine in green tea. A combination product containing caffeine, yerba mate, and damania (*Turnera diffusa*) has been reported to cause weight loss, slowing of the gastrointestinal transit, and a feeling of stomach fullness.
- As a diuretic, caffeine increases urine and sodium losses through the kidney and may add to the effects of other diuretic agents. Herbs with diuretic effects may include artichoke, celery, corn silk, couchgrass, dandelion, elder flower, horsetail, juniper berry, kava, shepherd's purse, uva ursi, and yarrow.

Selected References

Natural Standard developed the preceding evidence-based information based on a systematic review of more than 900 articles. For comprehensive information about alternative and complementary therapies on the professional level, go to www.naturalstandard.com. Selected references are listed here.

Adcocks C, Collin P, Buttle DJ. Catechins from green tea (*Camellia sinensis*) inhibit bovine and human cartilage proteoglycan and type II collagen degradation in vitro. J Nutr 2003; 132(3):341-346.

Adhami VM, Ahmad N, Mukhtar H. Molecular targets for green tea in prostate cancer prevention. J Nutr 2003;133(7 Suppl):2417S-2424S.

Afaq F, Adhami VM, Ahmad N, et al. Inhibition of ultraviolet B–mediated activation of nuclear factor kappa B in normal human epidermal karatinocytes by green tea constituent (−)-epigallocatechin-3-gallate. Oncogene 2003;22(7):1035-1044.

Ahmad N, Mukhtar H. Cutaneous photochemoprotection by green tea: a brief review. Skin Pharmacol Appl Skin Physiol 2001;14(2):69-76.

Ahn WS, Huh SW, Bae SM, et al. A major constituent of green tea, EGCG, inhibits the growth of a human cervical cell line, CaSki cells, through apoptosis, G(1) arrest, and regulation of gene expression. DNA Cell Biol 2003;22(3):217-224.

Alic M. Green tea for remission maintenance in Crohn's disease? Am J Gastroenterol 1999; 94(6):1710-1711.

Anonymous. Green tea and leukoplakia. The Indian-US Head and Neck Cancer Cooperative Group. Am J Surg 1997;174(5):552-555.

Arimoto-Kobayashi S, Inada N, Sato Y, et al. Inhibitory effects of (−)-epigallocatechin gallate on the mutation, DNA strand cleavage, and DNA adduct formation by heterocyclic amines. J Agric Food Chem 203;51(17):5150-5153.

Arts IC, Hollman PC, Feskens EJ, et al. Catechin intake might explain the inverse relation between tea consumption and ischemic heart disease: the Zutphen Elderly Study. Am J Clin Nutr 2001;74(2):227-232.

Birkett NJ, Logan AG. Caffeine-containing beverages and the prevalence of hypertension. J Hypertens Suppl 1988;6(4):S620-S622.

Brown SL, Salive ME, Pahor M, et al. Occult caffeine as a source of sleep problems in an older population. J Am Geriatr Soc 1995;43(8):860-864.

Cao Y, Cao R. Angiogenesis inhibited by drinking tea. Nature 1999;398(6726):381.

Cerhan JR, Putnam SD, Bianchi GD, et al. Tea consumption and risk of cancer of the colon and rectum. Nutr Cancer 2001;41(1-2):33-40.

Chai PC, Long LH, Halliwell B. Contribution of hydrogen peroxide to the cytotoxicity of green tea and red wines. Biochem Biophys Res Commun 2003;304(4):650-654.

Chang LK, Wei TT, Chiu YF, et al. Inhibition of Epstein-Barr virus lytic cycle by (−)-epigallocatechin gallate. Biochem Biophys Res Commun 2003;301(4):1062-1068.

Chantre P, Lairon D. Recent findings of green tea extract AR25 (Exolise) and its activity for the treatment of obesity. Phytomedicine 2002;9(1):3-8.

Chen C, Shen G, Hebbar V, et al. Epigallocatechin-3-gallate–induced stress signals in HT-29 human colon adenocarcinoma cells. Carcinogenesis 2003;24(8):1369-1378.

Chow HH, Cai Y, Alberts DS, et al. Phase I pharmacokinetic study of tea polyphenols following single-dose administration of epigallocatechin gallate and polyphenon E. Cancer Epidemiol Biomarkers Prev 2001;10(1):53-58.

Chow WH, Blot WJ, McLaughlin JK. Tea drinking and cancer risk: epidemiologic evidence. Proc Soc Exp Biol Med 1999;220(4):197.

Chow WH, Swanson CA, Lissowska J, et al. Risk of stomach cancer in relation to consumption of cigarettes, alcohol, tea and coffee in Warsaw, Poland. Int J Cancer 1999;81(6):871-876.

Chung WY, Yow CM, Benzie IF. Assessment of membrane protection by traditional Chinese medicines using a flow cytometric technique: preliminary findings. Redox Rep 2003;8(1): 31-33.

Clausson B, Granath F, Ekbom A, et al. Effect of caffeine exposure during pregnancy on birth weight and gestational age. Am J Epidemiol 2002;155(5):429-436.

Cnattingius S, Signorello LB, Anneren G, et al. Caffeine intake and the risk of first-trimester spontaneous abortion. N Engl J Med 2000;343(25):1839-1845.

Disler PB, Lynch SR, Charlton RW, et al. The effect of tea on iron absorption. Gut 1975; 16(3):193-200.

Dlugosz L, Belanger K, Hellenbrand K, et al. Maternal caffeine consumption and spontaneous abortion: a prospective cohort study. Epidemiology 1996;7(3):250-255.

Dona M, Dell'Aica I, Calabrese F, et al. Neutrophil restraint by green tea: inhibition of inflammation, associated angiogenesis, and pulmonary fibrosis. J Immunol 2003;170(8):4335-4341.

Duffy SJ, Vita JA, Holbrook M, et al. Effect of acute and chronic tea consumption on platelet aggregation in patients with coronary artery disease. Arterioscler Thromb Vasc Biol 2001; 21(6):1084-1089.

Durlach PJ. The effects of a low dose of caffeine on cognitive performance. Psychopharmacology (Berl) 1998;140(1):116-119.

Esimone CO, Adikwu MU, Nwafor SV, et al. Potential use of tea extract as a complementary mouthwash: comparative evaluation of two commercial samples. J Altern Complement Med 2001;7(5):523-527.

Ewertz M, Gill C. Dietary factors and breast-cancer risk in Denmark. Int J Cancer 1990; 46(5):779-784.

Fernandes O, Sabharwal M, Smiley T, et al. Moderate to heavy caffeine consumption during pregnancy and relationship to spontaneous abortion and abnormal fetal growth: a meta-analysis. Reprod Toxicol 1998;12(4):435-444.

Ford RP, Schluter PJ, Mitchell EA, et al. Heavy caffeine intake in pregnancy and sudden infant death syndrome. New Zealand Cot Death Study Group. Arch Dis Child 1998;78(1):9-13.

Fujiki H, Suganuma M, Okabe S, et al. Cancer inhibition by green tea. Mutat Res 1998; 402(1-2):307-310.

Fung KF, Zhang ZQ, Wong JW, et al. Aluminum and fluoride concentrations of three tea varieties growing at Lantau Island, Hong Kong. Environ Geochem Health 2003;25(2): 219-232.

Gao YT, McLaughlin JK, Blot WJ, et al. Reduced risk of esophageal cancer associated with green tea consumption. J Natl Cancer Inst 1994;86(11):855-858.

Geleijnse JM, Launer LJ, Hofman A, et al. Tea flavonoids may protect against atherosclerosis: the Rotterdam Study. Arch Intern Med 1999;159(18):2170-2174.

Geleijnse JM, Witteman JC, Launer LJ, et al. Tea and coronary heart disease: protection through estrogen-like activity? Arch Intern Med 2000;160(21):3328-3329.

Grosso LM, Rosenberg KD, Belanger K, et al. Maternal caffeine intake and intrauterine growth retardation. Epidemiology 2001;12(4):447-455.

Gupta S, Ahmad N, Mohan RR, et al. Prostate cancer chemoprevention by green tea: in vitro and in vivo inhibition of testosterone-mediated induction of ornithine decarboxylase. Cancer Res 1999;59(9):2115-2120.

Gupta S, Hussain T, Mukhtar H. Molecular pathway for (–)-epigallocatechin-3-gallate–induced cell cycle arrest and apoptosis of human prostate carcinoma cells. Arch Biochem Biophys 2003;410(1):177-185.

Gupta SK, Halder N, Srivastava S, et al. Green tea (*Camellia sinensis*) protects against selenite-induced oxidative stress in experimental cataractogenesis. Opthalmic Res 2003;34(4):258-263.

Hadeed A, Siegel S. Newborn cardiac arrhythmias associated with maternal caffeine use during pregnancy. Clin Pediatr (Phila) 1993;32(1):45-47.

Hartman TJ, Tangrea JA, Pietinen P, et al. Tea and coffee consumption and risk of colon and rectal cancer in middle-aged Finnish men. Nutr Cancer 1998;31(1):41-48.

Hastak K, Gupta S, Ahmad N, et al. Role of p53 and NF-kappa B in epigallocatechin-3-gallate–induced apoptosis of LNCaP cells. Oncogene 2003;22(31):4851-4859.

Hegarty VM, May HM, Khaw KT. Tea drinking and bone mineral density in older women. Am J Clin Nutr 2000;71(4):1003-1007.

Hiatt RA, Klatsky AL, Armstrong MA. Pancreatic cancer, blood glucose and beverage consumption. Int J Cancer 1988;41(6):794-797.

Hodgson JM, Puddey IB, Burke V, et al. Effects on blood pressure of drinking green and black tea. J Hypertens 1999;17(4):457-463.

Hodgson JM, Puddey IB, Croft KD, et al. Acute effects of ingestion of black and green tea on lipoprotein oxidation. Am J Clin Nutr 2000;71(5):1103-1107.

Hoshiyama Y, Kawaguchi T, Miura Y, et al. A prospective study of stomach cancer death in relation to green tea consumption in Japan. Br J Cancer 2002;87(3):309-313.

Hsu S, Bollag WB, Lewis J, et al. Green tea polyphenols induce differentiation and proliferation in epidermal keratinocytes. J Pharmacol Exp Ther 2003;306(1):29-34.
Hsu S, Lewis J, Singh B, et al. Green tea polyphenol targets the mitochondria in tumor cells inducing caspase 3-dependant apoptosis. Anticancer Res 2003;23(2B):1533-1539.
Hu J, Nyren O, Wolk A, et al. Risk factors for oesophageal cancer in northeast China. Int J Cancer 1994;57(1):38-46.
Imai K, Suga K, Nakachi K. Cancer-preventive effects of drinking green tea among a Japanese population. Prev Med 1997;26(6):769-775.
Infante-Rivard C, Fernandez A, Gauthier R, et al. Fetal loss associated with caffeine intake before and during pregnancy. JAMA 1993;270(24):2940-2943.
Iwai N, Ohshiro H, Kurozawa Y, et al. Relationship between coffee and green tea consumption and all-cause mortality in a cohort of a rural Japanese population. J Epidemiol 2002;12(3): 191-198.
James JE. Chronic effects of habitual caffeine consumption on laboratory and ambulatory blood pressure levels. J Cardiovasc Risk 1994;1(2):159-164.
Jatoi A, Ellison N, Burch PA, et al. A phase II trial of green tea in the treatment of patients with androgen independent metastatic prostate carcinoma. Cancer 2003;97(6):1442-1446.
Jensen OM, Wahrendorf J, Knudsen JB, et al. The Copenhagen case-control study of bladder cancer. II. Effect of coffee and other beverages. Int J Cancer 1986;37(5):651-657.
Ji BT, Chow WH, Hsing AW, et al. Green tea consumption and the risk of pancreatic and colorectal cancers. Int J Cancer 1997;70(3):255-258.
Joseph SL, Joseph SL, Arab L. Tea consumption and the reduced risk of colon cancer—results from a national prospective cohort study. Public Health Nutr 2002;5(3):419-426.
Kakuda T. Neuroprotective effects of the green tea components theanine and catechins. Biol Pharm Bull 2002;25(12):1513-1518.
Katiyar SK, Ahmad N, Mukhtar H. Green tea and skin. Arch Dermatol 2000;136(8):989-994.
Kaundun SS, Matsumoto S. Development of CAPS markers based on three key genes of the phenylpropanoid pathway in tea, *Camellia sinensis* (L.) O. Kuntze, and differentiation between assamica and sinensis varieties. Theor Appl Genet 2003;106(3):375-383.
Kaundun SS, Matsumoto S. Identification of processed Japanese green tea based on polymorphisms generated by STS-RFLP analysis. J Agric Food Chem 2003;51(7):1765-1770.
Kinlen LJ, McPherson K. Pancreas cancer and coffee and tea consumption: a case-control study. Br J Cancer 1984;49(1):93-96.
Kinlen LJ, Willows AN, Goldblatt P, et al. Tea consumption and cancer. Br J Cancer 1988; 58(3):397-401.
Klatsky AL, Armstrong MA, Friedman GD. Coffee, tea, and mortality. Ann Epidemiol 1993; 3(4):375-381.
Kohlmeier L, Weterings KG, Steck S, et al. Tea and cancer prevention: an evaluation of the epidemiologic literature. Nutr Cancer 1997;27(1):1-13.
Koizumi Y, Tsubono Y, Nakaya N, et al. No association between green tea and the risk of gastric cancer: pooled analysis of two prospective studies in Japan. Cancer Epidemiol Biomarkers Prev 2003;12(5):472-473.
Kono S, Shinchi K, Ikeda N, et al. Green tea consumption and serum lipid profiles: a cross-sectional study in northern Kyushu, Japan. Prev Med 1992;21(4):526-531.
Kono S. Green tea and colon cancer. Jpn J Cancer Res 1992;83(6):669.
Kono S. Green tea and gastric cancer in Japan. N Engl J Med 2001;344(24):1867-1868.
Lambert JD, Yang CS. Cancer chemopreventive activity and bioavailability of tea and tea polyphenols. Mutat Res 2003:523-524:201-208.
Lambert JD, Yang CS. Mechanisms of cancer prevention by tea constituents. J Nutr 2003; 133(10):3262S-3267S.
La Vecchia C, Negri E, Decarli A, et al. A case-control study of diet and colo-rectal cancer in northern Italy. Int J Cancer 1988;41(4):492-498.
La Vecchia C, Negri E, Franceschi S, et al. Tea consumption and cancer risk. Nutr Cancer 1992;17(1):27-31.
Lawson DH, Jick H, Rothman KJ. Coffee and tea consumption and breast disease. Surgery 1981;90(5):801-803.

Levites Y, Amit T, Mandel S, et al. Neuroprotection and neurorescue against Abetea toxicity and PKC-dependent release of nonamyloidogenic soluble precursor protein by green tea polyphenol (–)-epifallocatechin-3-gallate. FASEB J 2003;17(8):952-954.

Lee IP, Kim YH, Kang MH, et al. Chemopreventive effect of green tea (*Camellia sinensis*) against cigarette smoke–induced mutations (SCE) in humans. J Cell Biochem Suppl 1997; 27:68-75.

Levi M, Guchelaar HJ, Woerdenbag HJ, et al. Acute hepatitis in a patient using a Chinese herbal tea—a case report. Pharm World Sci 1998;20(1):43-44.

Lill G, Voit S, Schror K, et al. Complex effects of different green tea catechins on human platelets. FEBS Lett 2003;546(2-3):265-270.

Lin YS, Tsai YJ, Tsay JS, et al. Factors affecting the levels of tea polyphenols and caffeine in tea leaves. J Agric Food Chem 2003;51(7):1864-1873.

Locher R, Emmanuele L, Suter PM, et al. Green tea polyphenols inhibit human vascular smooth muscle cell proliferation stimulated by native low-density lipoprotein. Eur J Pharmacol 2002; 434(1-2):1-7.

Lu H, Meng X, Li C, et al. Glucuronides of tea catechins: enzymology of biosynthesis and biological activities. Drug Metab Dispos 2003;31(4):452-461.

Maeda K, Kusuya M, Cheng XW, et al. Green tea catechins inhibit the cultured smooth muscle cell invasion through the basement barrier. Atherosclerosis 2003;166(1):23-20.

Maeda-Yamamoto M, Suzuki N, Sawai, et al. Association of suppression of extracellular signal–regulated kinase phosphorylation by epigallocatechin gallate with the reduction of matrix metalloproteinase activities in human fibrosarcoma HT1080 cells. J Agric Food Chem 2003;51(7):1858-1863.

Mameleers PA, Van Boxtel MP, Hogervorst E. Habitual caffeine consumption and its relation to memory, attention, planning capacity and psychomotor performance across multiple age groups. Hum Psychopharmacol 2000;15(8):573-581.

Maron DJ, Lu GP, Cai NS, et al. Cholesterol-lowering effect of a theaflavin-enriched green tea extract: a randomized controlled trial. Arch Intern Med 2003;163(12):1448-1453.

Martinez-Richa A, Joseph-Nathan P. Carbon-13 CP-MAS nuclear magnetic resonance studies of teas. Solid State Nucl Magn Reson 2003;23(3):119-135.

Mei Y, Wei D, Liu J. Reversal of cancer multidrug resistance by tea polyphenol in KB cells. J Chemother 2003;15(3):260-265.

Morre DJ, Morre DM, Sun H, et al. Tea catechin synergies in inhibition of cancer cell proliferation and of a cancer specific cell surface oxidase (ECTO-NOX). Pharmacol Toxicol 2003; 92(5):234-241.

Mukamal KJ, Maclure M, Muller JE, et al. Tea consumption and mortality after acute myocardial infarction. Circulation 2002;105:2476-2481.

Nagano J, Kono S, Preston DL, et al. A prospective study of green tea consumption and cancer incidence, Hiroshima and Nagasaki (Japan). Cancer Causes Control 2001;12(6):501-508.

Nakachi K, Eguchi H, Imai K. Can teatime increase one's lifetime? Ageing Res Rev 2003; 2(1):1-10.

Nakachi K, Suemasu K, Suga K, et al. Influence of drinking green tea on breast cancer malignancy among Japanese patients. Jpn J Cancer Res 1998;89(3):254-261.

Nakagawa K, Ninomiya M, Okubo T, et al. Tea catechin supplementation increases antioxidant capacity and prevents phospholipid hydroperoxidation in plasma of humans. J Agric Food Chem 1999;47(10):3967-3973.

Nyska A, Suttie A, Bakshi S, et al. Slowing tumorigenic progression in TRAMP mice and prostatic carcinoma cell lines using natural anti-oxidant from spinach, NAO—a comparative study of three anti-oxidants. Toxicol Pathol 2003 Jan-Feb;31(1):39-51.

Ohno Y, Wakai K, Genka K, et al. Tea consumption and lung cancer risk: a case-control study in Okinawa, Japan. Jpn J Cancer Res 1995;86(11):1027-1034.

Park AM, Dong Z. Signal transduction pathways: targets for green and black tea polyphenols. J Biochem Mol Biol 2003;36(1):66-77.

Paschka AG, Butler R, Young CY. Induction of apoptosis in prostate cancer cell lines by the green tea component, (–)-epigallocatechin-3-gallate. Cancer Lett 1998;130(1-2):1-7.

Peters U, Poole C, Arab L. Does tea affect cardiovascular disease? a meta-analysis. Am J Epidemiol 2001;154(6):495-503.

Pezzato E, Dona M, Sartor L, et al. Proteinase-3 directly activates MMP-2 and degrades gelatin and Matrigel; differential inhibition by (–)epigallacatechin-3-gallate. J Leukoc Biol 2003; 74(1):88-94.
Pisters KM, Newman RA, Coldman B, et al. Phase I trial of oral green tea extract in adult patients with solid tumors. J Clin Oncol 2001;19(6):1830-1838.
Robinson R. Green tea extract may have neuroprotective effects in Parkinson's disease. Lancet 2001;358:391.
Rosenberg L. Coffee and tea consumption in relation to the risk of large bowel cancer: a review of epidemiologic studies. Cancer Lett 1990;52(3):163-171.
Roy M, Chakrabarty S, Sinha D, et al. Anticlastogenic, antigenotoxic and apoptotic activity of epigallocatechin gallate: a green tea polyphenol. Mutat Res 2003:33-41.
Sadzuka Y, Sugiyama T, Hirota S. Modulation of cancer chemotherapy by green tea. Clin Cancer Res 1998;4(1):153-156.
Saha P, Das S. Regulation of hazardous exposure by protective exposure: modulation of phase II detoxification and lipid peroxidation by *Camellia sinensis* and *Swertia chirata*. Teratog Carcinog Mutagen 2003;Suppl 1:313-322.
Sakanaka S. A novel convenient process to obtain a raw decaffeinated tea polyphenol fraction using a lignocellulose column. J Agric Food Chem 2003;51(10):3140-3143.
Sano M, Yoshida R, Degawa M, et al. Determination of peroxyl radical scavenging activity of flavonoids and plant extracts using an automatic potentiometric titrator. J Agric Food Chem 2003;51(10):2912-2918.
Sano T, Sasako M. Green tea and gastric cancer. N Engl J Med 2001;344(9):675-676.
Santos IS, Victora CG, Huttly S, et al. Caffeine intake and pregnancy outcomes: a meta-analytic review. Cad Saude Publica 1998;14(3):523-530.
Sasazuki S, Kodama H, Yoshimasu K, et al. Relation between green tea consumption and the severity of coronary atherosclerosis among Japanese men and women. Ann Epidemiol 2000;10(6):401-408.
Sato D, Matsushima M. Preventive effects of urinary bladder tumors induced by *N*-butyl-*N*-(4-hydroxybutyl)-notrosamine in rat by green tea leaves. Int J Urol 2003;10(3):160-166.
Sato Y, Nakatsuka H, Watanabe T, et al. Possible contribution of green tea drinking habits to the prevention of stroke. Tohoku J Exp Med 1989;157(4):337-343.
Sesso HD, Gaziano JM, Buring JE, et al. Coffee and tea intake and the risk of myocardial infarction. Am J Epidemiol 1999;149(2):162-167.
Setiawan VW, Zhang ZF, Yu GP, et al. Protective effect of green tea on the risks of chronic gastritis and stomach cancer. Int J Cancer 2001;92(4):600-604.
Shibata K, Moriyama M, Fukushima T, et al. Green tea consumption and chronic atrophic gastritis: a cross-sectional study in a green tea production village. J Epidemiol 2000;10(5): 310-316.
Shirlow MJ, Mathers CD. A study of caffeine consumption and symptoms; indigestion, palpitations, tremor, headache and insomnia. Int J Epidemiol 1985;14(2):239-248.
Singh R, Ahmed S, Malemud CJ, et al. Epigallocatechin-3-gallate selectivity inhibits interleukin-1beta–induced activation of mitogen activated protein kinase subgroup c-Jun N-terminal kinase in human osteoarthritis chondrocytes. J Orthop Res;21(1):102-109.
Skrzydlewska E, Ostrowska J, Stankiewicz A, et al. Green tea as a potent antioxidant in alcohol intoxication. Addict Biol 2002;7(3):307-314.
Stavchansky S, Combs A, Sagraves R, et al. Pharmacokinetics of caffeine in breast milk and plasma after single oral administration of caffeine to lactating mothers. Biopharm Drug Dispos 1988;9(3):285-299.
Stoner GD, Mukhtar H. Polyphenols as cancer chemopreventive agents. J Cell Biochem Suppl 1995;22:169-180.
Sun J. Morning/evening menopausal formula relieves menopausal symptoms: a pilot study. J Altern Complement Med 2003;9(3):403-409.
Sung H, Nah J, Chun S, et al. *In vivo* antioxidant effect of green tea. Eur J Clin Nutr 2000; 54(7):527-529.
Suzuki Y, Shioi Y. Identification of chlorophylls and carotenoids in major teas by high-performance liquid chromatography with photodiode array detection. J Agric Food Chem 2003;51(18):5307-5314.

G

Tavani A, Pregnolato A, La Vecchia C, et al. Coffee and tea intake and risk of cancers of the colon and rectum: a study of 3,530 cases and 7,057 controls. Int J Cancer 1997;73(2):193-197.
Taylor JR, Wilt VM. Probable antagonism of warfarin by green tea. Ann Pharmacother 1999;33(4):426-428.
Tedeschi E, Suzuki H, Menegazzi M. Antiinflammatory action of EGCG, the main component of green tea, through Stat-1 inhibition. Ann N Y Acad Sci 2003:435-437.
Tokunaga S, White IR, Frost C, et al. Green tea consumption and serum lipids and lipoproteins in a population of healthy workers in Japan. Ann Epidemiol 2002;12(3):157-165.
Tombola F, Campello S, De Luca L, et al. Plant polyphenols inhibit VacA, a toxin secreted by the gastric pathogen *Helicobacter pylori*. FEBS Lett 2003;543(1-3):184-189.
Tsubono Y, Nishino Y, Komatsu S, et al. Green tea and the risk of gastric cancer in Japan. N Engl J Med 2001;344(9):632-636.
Valentao P, Fernandes E, Carvalho F, et al. Hydroxyl radical and hypochlorous acid scavenging activity of small centaury (*Centaurium erythraea*) infusion. A comparative study with green tea (*Camellia sinensis*). Phytomedicine 2003;10(6-7):517-522.
Vankemmelbeke MN, Jones GC, Fowles C, et al. Selective inhibition of ADAMTS-1, -4, and -5 by catechin gallate esters. Eur J Biochem 2003;270(11):2394-2403.
Vinson J, Zhang J. Green and black tea inhibit diabetic cataracts by three mechanisms: sorbitol, lipid peroxidation and protein glycation. Diabetes 2001;50(Suppl 2):A476.
Weber JM, Ruzindana-Umunyana A, Imbeault L, et al. Inhibition of adenovirus infection and adenain by green tea catechins. Antiviral Res 2003;58(2):167-173.
Wrenn KD, Oschner I. Rhabdomyolysis induced by a caffeine overdose. Ann Emerg Med 1989;18(1):94-97.
Wu AH, Yu MC, Tseng CC, et al. Green tea and risk of breast cancer in Asian Americans. Int J Cancer 2003;106(4):574-579.
Wu CH, Yang YC, Yao WJ, et al. Epidemiological evidence of increased bone mineral density in habitual tea drinkers. Arch Intern Med 2002;162(9):1001-1006.
Xu J, Yang F, Chen L, et al. Effect of selenium on increasing the antioxidant activity of tea leaves harvested during the early spring tea producing season. J Agric Food Chem 2003; 51(4):1081-1084.
Yamamoto T, Hsu S, Lewis J, et al. Green tea polyphenol causes differential oxidative environments in tumor versus normal epithelial cells. J Pharmacol Exp Ther 2003;301(1):230-236.
Yang TT, Koo MW. Hypocholesterolemic effects of Chinese tea. Pharmacol Res 1997; 35(6):505-512.
Yee Y-K KW, Szeto ML. Effect of Chinese tea consumption on *Helicobacter pylori* infection (abstract). J Gastroenterol Hepatol 2000;15:B33-A90.
Yee YK, Koo MW, Szeto ML. Chinese tea consumption and lower risk of *Helicobacter* infection. J Gastroenterol Hepatol 2002;17(5):552-555.
Yu GP, Hsieh CC, Wang LY, et al. Green-tea consumption and risk of stomach cancer: a population-based case-control study in Shanghai, China. Cancer Causes Control 1995; 6(6):532-538.
Zhang M, Binns CW, Lee AH. Tea consumption and ovarian cancer risk: a case control study in China. Cancer Epidemiol Biomarkers Prev 2002;11(8):713-718.
Zheng W, Doyle TJ, Kushi LH, et al. Tea consumption and cancer incidence in a prospective cohort study of postmenopausal women. Am J Epidemiol 1996;144(2):175-182.
Zhong L, Goldberg MS, Gao YT, et al. A population-based case-control study of lung cancer and green tea consumption among women living in Shanghai, China. Epidemiology 2001; 12(6):695-700.
Zhou JR, Yu L, Zhong Y, et al. Soy phytochemicals and tea bioactive components synergistically inhibit androgen-sensitive human prostate tumors in mice. J Nutr 2003;133(2):516-521.

Guggul

(*Commifora mukul*)

RELATED TERMS

- African myrrh, Arabian myrrh, Burseraceae, *Commiphora myrrha*, fraction A, guggal, guggulipid C+, guggulu, guggulsterone (4,17(20)-pregnadiene-3,16-dione), Guggulu, guglip, Gugulmax, gum guggul, gum guggulu, guggulsterone, gum myrrh, myrrha, Somali myrrh, Yemen myrhh.

G

BACKGROUND

- Guggul (gum guggul) is a resin produced by the mukul myrrh tree, which is native to India. Guggulipid is extracted from guggul and contains plant sterols (guggulsterones E and Z) that are believed to be guggul's bioactive compounds.
- Until recently, the majority of scientific evidence suggested that guggulipid elicited significant reductions in serum total cholesterol, low-density lipoprotein (LDL), and triglycerides, as well as elevations in high-density lipoprotein (HDL). However, most published studies were small and not well designed or reported. In August 2003, a well-designed trial reported by Szapary and colleagues found small significant *increases* in serum LDL levels associated with the use of guggul compared to placebo. No significant changes in total cholesterol, HDL, or triglycerides were found. These results are consistent with those of two prior published case reports. This evidence provides preliminary evidence against the efficacy of guggul for hypercholesterolemia. However, because of prior research and historical use, further study is necessary before a definitive conclusion can be reached.
- Initial research reports that guggulsterones are antagonists of the farsenoid X receptor (FXR) and the bile acid receptor (BAR), nuclear hormones that are involved in cholesterol metabolism and bile acid regulation.

USES BASED ON SCIENTIFIC EVIDENCE	Grade*
Acne Guggulipid has been found to possess anti-inflammatory properties and has been suggested as an oral therapy for nodulocystic acne vulgaris. Preliminary data from small, methodologically weak studies in humans suggest possible short-term improvements in the number of acne lesions. However, further evidence is warranted before a therapeutic recommendation can be made.	C
Hypercholesterolemia Before 2003, the majority of scientific evidence suggested that guggulipid elicits significant reductions in serum total cholesterol, low-density lipoprotein (LDL), and triglycerides, as well as elevations in high-density lipoprotein (HDL). However, most published studies were small and methodologically flawed. In August 2003, a well-designed trial by	C

Continued

Szapary et al. reported small significant *increases* in serum LDL levels associated with the use of guggul compared to placebo. No significant changes in total cholesterol, high-density lipoprotein (HDL), or triglycerides were measured. These results are consistent with two prior published case reports. Although this evidence provides preliminary evidence against the efficacy of guggul for hypercholesterolemia, due to the precedent of prior research and historical use, further study is necessary before a definitive conclusion can be reached. There is no reliable research comparing guggul preparations with HMG-CoA reductase inhibitors ("statins"), or evaluating long-term effects of guggul on cardiac morbidity or mortality outcomes.	
Obesity There is insufficient evidence to support the use of guggul or guggul derivatives for the management of obesity.	C
Osteoarthritis There is insufficient evidence to support the use of guggul or guggul derivatives in the management of osteoarthritis.	C
Rheumatoid arthritis There is insufficient evidence to support the use of guggul or guggul derivatives in the management of rheumatoid arthritis.	C

*Key to grades: *A:* Strong scientific evidence for this use; *B:* Good scientific evidence for this use; *C:* Unclear scientific evidence for this use; *D:* Fair scientific evidence against this use (it may not work); *F:* Strong scientific evidence against this use (it likely does not work). For a more detailed explanation of efficacy criteria, see "Natural Standard Evidence-Based Validated Grading Rationale" in the Introduction.

Uses Based on Tradition, Theory, or Limited Scientific Evidence

Asthma, bleeding, colitis, diabetes, gingivitis, hemorrhoids, leprosy, leukorrhoea, menstrual disorders, mouth infections, neuralgia, obesity, pain, psoriasis, rhinitis, sores, sore throat, tumors, weight loss, wound healing.

DOSING

The following doses are based on scientific research, publications, traditional use, or expert opinion. Many herbs and supplements have not been thoroughly tested, and their safety and effectiveness may not be proven. Brands may be made differently, with variable ingredients even within the same brand. The doses shown may not apply to all products. It is important to always read product labels and discuss doses with a qualified healthcare provider before therapy is started.

Standardization

- Standardization involves measuring the amounts of certain chemicals in products to try to make different preparations similar to each other. It is not always known if the chemicals being measured are the "active" ingredients. Guggulipid preparations are often standardized to contain 2.5% to 5% of guggulsterones.

Adults (18 Years and Older)

- **Hyperlipidemia:** 500 to 1000 mg of guggulipid (standardized to 2.5% guggulsterones) taken twice or three times daily has been used clinically and in research. An equivalent dose of commercially prepared guggulsterone is 25 mg three times daily or 50 mg twice daily by mouth. A higher dose has been studied (2000 mg three times daily, standardized to 2.5% guggulsterones), but this dose may be associated with a greater risk of hypersensitivity skin reactions.
- **Nodulocystic acne:** A dose of guggulipid equivalent to 25 mg guggulsterone per day has been used.

Children (Younger Than 18 Years)

- There is insufficient scientific evidence regarding its safety and efficacy to recommend guggul for use in children.

SAFETY

The U.S. Food and Drug Administration does not strictly regulate herbs and supplements. There is no guarantee of the strength, purity, or safety of products, and effects may vary. It is important to always read product labels. People who have a medical condition, or are taking other drugs, herbs, or supplements, should consult a qualified healthcare provider before starting a new therapy. A healthcare provider should be contacted immediately about any side effects.

Allergies

- The use of guggul should be avoided by people with known allergy/hypersensitivity to guggul, any of its constituents or other members of the Burseraceae family.
- Hypersensitivity skin reactions have been noted in humans. In most cases, the reactions began within 48 hours of starting therapy and resolved spontaneously within 1 week of therapy discontinuation.

Side Effects and Warnings

- Standardized guggulipid is generally regarded as safe in healthy adults when taken at recommended doses for up to 6 months. Gastrointestinal upset is the most common adverse effect. Other side effects include diarrhea, nausea and vomiting, burping, and hiccough. Headache, restlessness, and anxiety have been noted in some studies. Allergic skin rash (especially at higher doses) has been reported.
- Guggulipid has been associated with inhibition of platelets and increased fibrinolysis (blood clot breakdown), and in theory the risk of bleeding may be increased.
- Weight loss has been observed in studies in animals. Based on such studies, guggulsterone may stimulate thyroid function.

Pregnancy and Breastfeeding

- Not recommended due to lack of sufficient data.

INTERACTIONS

Most herbs and supplements have not been thoroughly tested for interactions with other herbs, supplements, drugs, or foods. The interactions listed here are based on reports in scientific publications, laboratory experiments, or traditional use. It is important to always read product labels. People who have a medical condition, or are taking other drugs, herbs, or supplements, should consult a qualified healthcare provider before starting a new therapy.

Interactions with Drugs

- In studies in humans co-administration of guggulipid has been reported to decrease the bioavailability of the beta-blocker propranolol and the calcium channel blocker diltiazem.
- Guggulipid has been associated with inhibition of platelets and increased blood clot breakdown. In theory, guggul may increase the risk of bleeding when taken with drugs that increase the risk of bleeding. Examples are anticoagulants (blood thinners) such as warfarin (Coumadin) and heparin, antiplatelet drugs such as clopidogrel (Plavix), aspirin, and nonsteroidal anti-inflammatory drugs such as ibuprofen (Motrin, Advil) and naproxen (Naprosyn, Aleve).The effect of guggul on serum lipids remains controversial. Guggul may affect serum lipid levels (decreasing cholesterol, triglycerides, and low-density lipoproteins [LDLs] and increasing high-density lipoproteins [HDLs]) and thus may increase the lipid-lowering effects of lipid-lowering agents such as niacin, garlic, or fish oil (omega-3 fatty acids).
- Studies in animals suggest that the guggul constituent Z-guggulsterone may stimulate thyroid function. Therefore, additional effects may occur in patients taking thyroid drugs and guggul.

Interactions with Herbs and Dietary Supplements

- The effect of guggul on serum lipids remains controversial. Guggul may affect serum lipid levels (decreasing cholesterol, triglycerides, and LDLs and increasing HDLs), and thus may increase the lipid-lowering effects of lipid-lowering agents such as niacin, garlic, or fish oil (omega-3 fatty acids).
- Guggulipid has been associated with inhibition of platelets and increased blood clot breakdown. In theory, guggul may increase the risk of bleeding when taken with herbs and supplements that also may increase the risk of bleeding. Multiple cases of bleeding have been reported with the use of *Ginkgo biloba*, and fewer cases with garlic and saw palmetto. Numerous other agents theoretically may increase the risk of bleeding, although this has not been proven in most cases. Examples of such agents are alfalfa, American ginseng, angelica, anise, *Arnica montana*, asafetida, aspen bark, bilberry, birch, black cohosh, bladderwrack, bogbean, boldo, borage seed oil, bromelain, capsicum, cat's claw, celery, chamomile, chaparral, clove, coleus, cordyceps, danshen, devil's claw, dong quai, evening primrose, fenugreek, feverfew, flaxseed/flax powder (not a concern with flaxseed oil), ginger, grapefruit juice, grape seed, green tea, gymnestra, horse chestnut, horseradish, licorice root, lovage root, male fern, meadowsweet, nordihydroguaiaretic acid (NDGA), onion, *Panax ginseng*, papain, parsley, passion flower, poplar, prickly ash, propolis, quassia, red clover, reishi, rue, Siberian ginseng, sweet birch, sweet clover, turmeric, vitamin E, white willow, wild carrot, wild lettuce, willow, wintergreen, and yucca.

Selected References

Natural Standard developed the preceding evidence-based information based on a systematic review of more than 140 articles. For comprehensive information about alternative and complementary therapies on the professional level, go to www.naturalstandard.com. Selected references are listed here.

Agarwal RC, Singh SP, Saran RK, et al. Clinical trial of gugulipid—a new hypolipidemic agent of plant origin in primary hyperlipidemia. Indian J Med Res 1986;84:626-634.

Amma MK, Malhotra N, Suri RK, et al. Effect of oleoresin of gum guggul (*Commiphora mukul*) on the reproductive organs of female rat. Indian J Exp Biol 1978;16(9):1021-1023.

Antonio J, Colker CM, Torina GC, et al. Effects of a standardized guggulsterone phosphate supplement on body composition in overweight adults: a pilot study. Curr Ther Res 1999; 60:220-227.

Arora RB, Kapoor V, Gupta SK, et al. Isolation of a crystalline steroidal compound from *Commiphora mukul* and its anti-inflammatory activity. Indian J Exp Biol 1971;9(3):403-404.

Arora RB, Taneja V, Sharma RC, et al. Anti-inflammatory studies on a crystalline steroid isolated from *Commiphora mukul*. Indian J Med Res 1972;60(6):929-931.

Baldwa VS, Sharma RC, Ranka PC, et al. Effect of *Commiphora mukul* (guggul) on fibrinolytic activity and platelet aggregation in coronary artery disease. Rajas Med J 1980;19(2):84-86.

Beg M, Singhal KC, Afzaal S. A study of effect of guggulsterone on hyperlipidemia of secondary glomerulopathy. Indian J Physiol Pharmacol 1996;40(3):237-240.

Bhatt AD, Dalal DG, Shah SJ, et al. Conceptual and methodologic challenges of assessing the short-term efficacy of Guggulu in obesity: data emergent from a naturalistic clinical trial. J Postgrad Med 1995;41(1):5-7.

Bordia A, Chuttani SK. Effect of gum guggulu on fibrinolysis and platelet adhesiveness in coronary heart disease. Indian J Med Res 1979;70:992-996.

Cui J, Huang L, Zhao A, et al. Guggulsterone is a farnesoid X receptor antagonist in coactivator association assays but acts to enhance transcription of bile salt export pump. J Biol Chem 2003;278(12):10214-10220.

Dalvi SS, Nayak VK, Pohujani SM, et al. Effect of gugulipid on bioavailability of diltiazem and propranolol. J Assoc Physicians India 1994;42(6):454-455.

Das Gupta RD. Gugulipid: pro-lipaemic effect. J Assoc Physicians India 1990;38(8):598.

Das Gupta R. Gugulipid: pro-lipaemic effect. J Assoc Physicians India 1990;38(12):346.

Dogra J, Aneja N, Saxena VN. Oral gugulipid in acne vulgaris management. Ind J Dermatol Venereol Leprol 1990;56(1):381-383.

Duwiejua M, Zeitlin IJ, Waterman PG, et al. Anti-inflammatory activity of resins from some species of the plant family Burseraceae. Planta Med 1993;59(1):12-16.

Gaur SP, Garg RK, Kar AM, et al. Gugulipid, a new hypolipidaemic agent, in patients of acute ischaemic stroke: effect on clinical outcome, platelet function and serum lipids. Asia Pacif J Pharm 1997;12:65-69.

Ghorai M, Mandal SC, Pal M, et al. A comparative study on hypocholesterolaemic effect of allicin, whole germinated seeds of bengal gram and guggulipid of gum gugglu. Phytother Res 2000;14(3):200-202.

Gopal K, Saran RK, Nityanand S, et al. Clinical trial of ethyl acetate extract of gum gugulu (gugulipid) in primary hyperlipidemia. J Assoc Physicians India 1986;34(4):249-251.

Gujral ML, Sareen K, Reddy GS, et al. Endocrinological studies on the oleo resin of gum guggul. Indian J Med Sci 1962;16:847-851.

Jadad AR, Moore RA, Carroll D, et al. Assessing the quality of reports of randomized clinical trials: is blinding necessary? Control Clin Trials 1996;17(1):1-12.

Jain JP. Clinical assessment of the value of oleo-resin of *Commiphora mukul* (Guggul) in obesity

Kesava RG, Dhar SC. Effect of a new non-steroidal anti-inflammatory agent on lysosomal stability in adjuvant induced arthritis. Ital J Biochem 1987;36(4):205-217.

Kesava RG, Dhar SC, Singh GB. Urinary excretion of connective tissue metabolites under the influence of a new non-steroidal anti-inflammatory agent in adjuvant induced arthritis. Agents Actions 1987;22(1-2):99-105.

Kishore P, Devi Das KV, Banarjee S. Clinical studies on the treatment of Amavata-Rheumatoid arthritis with Sunthi-Guggulu. J Res Ayur Siddha 1982;3(3-4):133-146.

Kotiyal JP, Bisht DB, Singh DS. Double blind cross-over trial of gum guggulu (*Commiphora mukul*) Fraction A in hypercholesterolemia. J Res Indian Med Yoga Hom 1979;14(2): 11-16.

Kotiyal JP, Singh DS, Bisht DB. Gum guggulu (*Commiphora mukul*) fraction 'A' in obesity—a double-blind clinical trial. J Res Ayur and Siddha 1985;6(1,3,4):20-35.

Kuppurajan K, Rajagopalan SS, Koteswara Rao T, et al. Effect of guggulu (*Commiphora mukul*—Engl) on serum lipids in obese subjects. J Res Indian Med 1973;8(4):1-8.

Kuppurajan K, Rajagopalan SS, Rao TK, et al. Effect of guggulu (*Commiphora mukul*—Engl.) on serum lipids in obese, hypercholesterolemic and hyperlipemic cases. J Assoc Physicians India 1978;26(5):367-373.

Mahesh S, Pandit M, Hakala C. A study of Shuddha Guggulu on rheumatoid arthritis. Rheumatism 1981;16(2):54-67.

Majumdar KA. A clinical study of R-Arthritis with A-Compound—a herbal formulation. Rheumatism 1984;19(3):66-74.

Majumdar KA. Role of gum guggulu with gold in rheumatic and other allied disorders. Rheumatism 1984;20(1):9-15.

Malhotra SC, Ahuja MM. Comparative hypolipidaemic effectiveness of gum guggulu (*Commiphora mukul*) fraction 'A', ethyl-*p*-chlorophenoxyisobutyrate and Ciba-13437-Su. Indian J Med Res 1971;59(10):1621-1632.

Malhotra SC, Ahuja MM, Sundaram KR. Long term clinical studies on the hypolipidaemic effect of *Commiphora mukul* (Guggulu) and clofibrate. Indian J Med Res 1977;65(3): 390-395.

Mester L, Mester M, Nityanand S. Inhibition of platelet aggregation by "guggulu" steroids. Planta Med 1979;37(4):367-369.

Nityanand S, Srivastava JS, Asthana OP. Clinical trials with gugulipid. A new hypolipidaemic agent. J Assoc Physicians India 1989;37(5):323-328.

Sharma K, Puri AS, Sharma R, et al. Effect of gum guggul on serum lipids in obese subjects. J Res Indian Med Yoga Hom 1976;11(2):132.

Sharma JN, Sharma JN. Comparison of the anti-inflammatory activity of *Commiphora mukul* (an indigenous drug) with those of phenylbutazone and ibuprofen in experimental arthritis induced by mycobacterial adjuvant. Arzneimittelforschung 1977;27(7):1455-1457.

Sidhu LS, Sharma K, Puri AS, et al. Effect of gum guggul on body weight and subcutaneous tissue folds. J Res Indian Med Yoga Hom 1976;11(2):16-22.

Singh RP, Singh R, Ram P, et al. Use of Pushkar-Guggul, an indigenous antiischemic combination, in the management of ischemic heart disease. Int J Pharmacog 1993;31(2):147-160.

Singh BB, Mishra L, Aquilina N, et al. Usefulness of guggul (*Commiphora mukul*) for osteoarthritis of the knee: An experimental case study. Altern Ther Health Med 2001;7(2):120, 112-114.

Singh GB, Atal CK. Pharmacology of an extract of salai guggal ex-Boswellia serrata, a new non-steroidal anti-inflammatory agent. Agents Actions 1986;18(3-4):407-412.

Singh RB, Niaz MA, Ghosh S. Hypolipidemic and antioxidant effects of *Commiphora mukul* as an adjunct to dietary therapy in patients with hypercholesterolemia. Cardiovasc Drugs Ther 1994;8(4):659-664.

Sosa S, Tubaro R, Della Loggia R, et al. Anti-inflammatory activity of *Commiphora mukul* extracts. Pharmacol Res 1993;27(suppl 1):89-90.

Szapary PO, Wolfe ML, Bloedon LT, et al. Guggulipid for the treatment of hypercholesterolemia: a randomized controlled trial. JAMA 2003;290(6):765-772.

Thappa DM, Dogra J. Nodulocystic acne: oral gugulipid versus tetracycline. J Dermatol 1994; 21(10):729-731.

Tripathi SN, Upadhyay BN. A clinical trial of *Commiphora mukul* in the patients of ischaemic heart disease. J Mol and Cell Cardiol 1978;10(suppl 1):124.

Tripathi SN, Gupta M, Sen SP, et al. Effect of a keto-steroid of *Commifora mukul* L. on hypercholesterolemia and hyperlipidemia induced by neomercazole and cholesterol mixture in chicks. Indian J Exp Biol 1975;13(1):15-18.

Tripathi YB, Malhotra OP, Tripathi SN. Thyroid stimulating action of Z-guggulsterone obtained from *Commiphora mukul*. Planta Med 1984;(1):78-80.

Tripathi YB, Tripathi P, Malhotra OP, et al. Thyroid stimulatory action of (Z)-guggulsterone: mechanism of action. Planta Med 1988;54(4):271-277.

Upadhyaya BN, Tripathi SN, Dwivedi LD. Hypocholesterolemic and hypolipidemic action of gum guggulu in patients of coronary heart disease. J Res Indian Med Yoga Hom 1976; 11(2):1-8.

Urizar NL, Liverman AB, Dodds DT, et al. A natural product that lowers cholesterol as an antagonist ligand for the FXR. Science 2002;296(5573):1703-1706. (Epub 2002 May 02.)

Verma SK, Bordia A. Effect of *Commiphora mukul* (gum guggulu) in patients with hyperlipidemia with special reference to HDL-cholesterol. Indian J Med Res 1988;87:356-360.

Wu J, Xia C, Meier J, et al. The hypolipidemic natural product guggulsterone acts as an antagonist of the bile acid receptor. Mol Endocrinol 2002;16(7):1590-1597.

Gymnema

(*Gymnema sylvestre* R. Br.)

G

RELATED TERMS

- Asclepias geminata roxb., Asclepiadaceae, *Gemnema melicida*, GS4 (water soluble extract of the leaves), gur-mar, gurmar, gurmarbooti, *Gymnema inodum*, kogilam, mangala gymnema, merasingi, meshashingi, meshavalli, periploca of the woods, periploca sylvestris, podapatri, Proβeta, ram's horn, small indian ipecac, sarkaraikolli, sirukurinja.

BACKGROUND

- Preliminary human evidence suggests that gymnema may be effective in the management of blood sugar levels in people with type 1 and type 2 diabetes, as an adjunct to conventional drug therapy, for up to 20 months. Gymnema appears to lower serum glucose and glycosylated hemoglobin (HbA1c) levels following chronic use but may not have significant acute effects. High-quality trials in humans are lacking in this area. There is early evidence suggesting possible efficacy of gymnema as a cholesterol-lowering agent.
- *Note:* Some of the available research has been conducted by authors affiliated with manufacturers of gymnema products.

USES BASED ON SCIENTIFIC EVIDENCE	Grade*
Diabetes Studies in animals report that gymnema can lower blood sugar levels. Preliminary research in humans reports that gymnema may be beneficial in patients with type 1 or type 2 diabetes when it is added to diabetes drugs being taken by mouth or to insulin. Further studies of dosing, safety, and effectiveness are needed before a strong recommendation can be made.	B
High cholesterol Reductions in levels of serum triglycerides, total cholesterol, and low-density lipoprotein (LDL; "bad cholesterol") have been observed in studies in animals. Preliminary research in people with type 2 diabetes reported decreased cholesterol and triglyceride levels. Better evidence is needed before a clear conclusion can be drawn.	C

*Key to grades: *A:* Strong scientific evidence for this use; *B:* Good scientific evidence for this use; *C:* Unclear scientific evidence for this use; *D:* Fair scientific evidence against this use (it may not work); *F:* Strong scientific evidence against this use (it likely does not work). For a more detailed explanation of efficacy criteria, see "Natural Standard Evidence-Based Validated Grading Rationale" in the Introduction.

Uses Based on Tradition, Theory, or Limited Scientific Evidence

Aphrodisiac, cancer, cardiovascular disease, constipation, cough, digestion stimulant, diuresis, gout, high blood pressure, laxative, liver disease, liver protection, malaria, obesity, rheumatoid arthritis, snake venom antidote, stomach ailments, uterine stimulant.

DOSING

The following doses are based on scientific research, publications, traditional use, or expert opinion. Many herbs and supplements have not been thoroughly tested, and their safety and effectiveness may not be proven. Brands may be made differently, with variable ingredients even within the same brand. The doses shown may not apply to all products. It is important to always read product labels and discuss doses with a qualified healthcare provider before therapy is started.

Standardization

- Standardization involves measuring the amounts of certain chemicals in products to try to make different preparations similar to each other. It is not always known if the chemicals being measured are the "active" ingredients. At least one manufacturer offers an extract of gymnema standardized to 25% gymnemic acid, but this extract has not been thoroughly studied.
- An extract from gymnema, labeled GS4, has been used in research in humans. GS4 has since been patented as the product Proβeta. According to the PharmaTerra, the manufacturer, Proβeta is standardized to a specific biological result, as measured by a test developed by the company, that evaluates "pancreotropic" effects.

Adults (18 Years and Older)

- **Type 1 diabetes:** 200 mg of extract GS4 taken by mouth twice daily, with careful continuation of insulin, has been studied.
- **Type 2 diabetes:** 200 mg of extract GS4 taken by mouth twice daily, or 2 ml of an aqueous decoction (10 g of shade-dried powdered leaves per 100 ml) taken by mouth three times daily has been studied.
- *Note:* PharmaTerra, the manufacturer of ProBeta (GS4), recommends a dose of two 250-mg capsules taken twice daily at mealtimes, for adults weighing more than 100 pounds, or one 250-mg capsule taken twice daily at mealtimes, for adults weighing less than 100 pounds.

Children (Younger Than 18 Years)

- There is insufficient scientific evidence about the safety of gymnema to recommend its use in children.

SAFETY

The U.S. Food and Drug Administration does not strictly regulate herbs and supplements. There is no guarantee of the strength, purity, or safety of products, and effects may vary. It is important to always read product labels. People who have a medical condition, or are taking other drugs, herbs, or supplements, should consult a qualified healthcare provider before starting a new therapy. A healthcare provider should be contacted immediately about any side effects.

Allergies

- Allergy to gymnema may occur. In theory, allergic cross-reactivity may exist with members of the Asclepiadaceae (milkweed) family.

Side Effects and Warnings

- Aside from lowered blood sugar levels and increased effects of anti-diabetic drugs with chronic use of gymnema, no significant adverse effects have been reported with the herb in several studies as long as 20 months. Caution is advised in persons with diabetes or low blood sugar levels, and in those taking drugs, other herbs, or supplements that affect blood sugar levels. Serum glucose levels may need to be monitored by a qualified healthcare provider, and medication adjustments may be necessary. Based on studies in animals and humans, gymnema may lower blood cholesterol levels.
- Gymnema is reported to suppress the ability to detect sweet tastes, because of the component gurmarin. This phenomenon prompted the Hindi name *gurmar* or "sugar destroyer."

Pregnancy and Breastfeeding

- Gymnema should not be used by women who are pregnant or breastfeeding because of lack of reliable information about its safety.

INTERACTIONS

Most herbs and supplements have not been thoroughly tested for interactions with other herbs, supplements, drugs, or foods. The interactions listed here are based on reports in scientific publications, laboratory experiments, or traditional use. It is important to always read product labels. People who have a medical condition, or are taking other drugs, herbs, or supplements, should consult a qualified healthcare provider before starting a new therapy.

Interactions with Drugs

- Based on studies in animals and humans, gymnema may lower blood sugar levels. Caution is advised when using medications that may also lower blood sugar. People taking drugs for diabetes by mouth or insulin should be monitored closely by a qualified healthcare provider. Medication adjustments may be necessary. Studies also suggest that gymnema may lower blood cholesterol levels. Therefore, increased effects may occur if gymnema is taken in combination with drugs that lower cholesterol such as the "statins" (HMGCoA reductase inhibitors) lovastatin (Mevacor) and atorvastatin (Lipitor).

Interactions with Herbs and Dietary Supplements

- Studies in animals and humans suggest that gymnema may lower blood sugar levels. Caution is advised in people who are taking gymnema in combination with other herbs or supplements that may also lower blood sugar levels. Blood glucose levels may require monitoring, and doses may need adjustment. Examples of such herbs are *Aloe vera*, American ginseng, bilberry, bitter melon, burdock, fenugreek, fish oil, horse chestnut seed extract (HCSE), marshmallow, milk thistle, *Panax ginseng*, rosemary, Siberian ginseng, stinging nettle, and white horehound. Studies also suggest that gymnema may lower blood cholesterol levels. Therefore, increased effects may occur if gymnema is taken in combination with other herbs or supplements that lower cholesterol, such as fish oil, garlic, guggul, and niacin.

Interactions with Foods

- Based on studies in animals, absorption of oleic acid (a fatty acid) may be decreased by gymnema. It is unknown whether gymnema has these effects in humans or affects the absorption of other nutritionally important lipids or fat-soluble vitamins (A, D, E, and K).

Selected References

Natural Standard developed the preceding evidence-based information based on a systematic review of more than 60 scientific articles. For comprehensive information about alternative and complementary therapies on the professional level, go to www.naturalstandard.com. Selected references are listed here.

Ananthan R, Baskar C, NarmathaBai V, et al. Antidiabetic effect of *Gymnema montanum* leaves: effect on lipid peroxidation–induced oxidative stress in experimental diabetes. Pharmacol Res 2003;48(6):551-556.

Ananthan R, Latha M, Pari L, et al. Effect of *Gymnema montanum* on blood glucose, plasma insulin, and carbohydrate metabolic enzymes in alloxan-induced diabetic rats. J Med Food 2003;6(1):43-49.

Baskaran K, Ahamath B, Shanmugasundaram K, et al. Antidiabetic effect of a leaf extract from *Gymnema sylvestre* in non–insulin-dependent diabetes mellitus patients. J Ethnopharm 1990; 30:295-305.

Chattopadhyay RR. Possible mechanism of antihyperglycemic effect of *Gymnema sylvestre* leaf extract, Part I. Gen Pharm 1998;31(3):495-496.

Gholap S, Kar A. Effects of Inula racemosa root and *Gymnema sylvestre* leaf extracts in the regulation of corticosteroid-induced diabetes mellitus: involvement of thyroid hormones. Pharmazie 2003;58(6):413-415.

Jiang H. [Advances in the study on hypoglycemic constituents of *Gymnema sylvestre* (Retz.) Schult.] Zhong Yao Cai 2003;26(4):305-307.

Kamei K, Takano R, Miyasaka A, et al. Amino acid sequence of sweet-taste-suppressing peptide (gurmarin) from the leaves of *Gymnema sylvestre*. J Biochem 1992;111:109-112.

Khare AK, Tondon RN, Tewari JP. Hypoglycaemic activity of an indigenous drug (*Gymnema sylvestre*, "Gurmar") in normal and diabetic persons. Indian J Physiol Pharm 1983;27:257-258.

Kothe A, Uppal R. Antidiabetic effects of *Gymnema sylvestre* in NIDDM—a short study. Indian J Homeopath Med 1997;32(1-2):61-62, 66.

Murakami N, Murakami T, Kadoya M, et al. New hypoglycemic constituents in "gymnemic acid" from *Gymnema sylvestre*. Chem Pharm Bull 1996;44(2):469-471.

Porchezhian E, Dobriyal RM. An overview on the advances of *Gymnema sylvestre*: chemistry, pharmacology and patents. Pharmazie 2003;58(1):5-12.

Satdive RK, Abhilash P, Fulzele DP. Antimicrobial activity of *Gymnema sylvestre* leaf extract. Fitoterapia 2003;74(7-8):699-701.

Shanmugasundaram ERB, Rajeswari G, Baskaran K, et al. Use of *Gymnema sylvestre* leaf extract in the control of blood glucose in insulin-dependent diabetes mellitus. J Ethnopharm 1990; 30(3):281-294.

Shimizu K, et al. Suppression of glucose absorption by extracts from the leaves of *Gymnema inodorum*. J Vet Med Sci 1997;59:753-757.

Xie JT, Wang A, Mehendale S, et al. Anti-diabetic effects of Gymnema yunnanense extract. Pharmacol Res 2003;47(4):323-329.

Hawthorn

(*Crataegus laevigata**)

RELATED TERMS

- Aubepine, bei shanzha, bianco spino, bread and cheese tree, cardiplant, Chinese hawthorn, cockspur, cockspur thorn, crataegi flos, crataegi folium, crataegi folium cum flore, crataegi fructus, crataegi herba, crataegisan, *Crataegus azaerolus, Crataegus cuneata, Crataegus fructi, Crataegus monogyna, Crataegus nigra, Crataegus oxyacantha, Crataegus oxyacanthoides, Crataegus pentagyna, Crataegus pinnatifida, Crataegus sinaica* Boiss, crataegutt, English hawthorn, epine blanche, epine de mai, Euphytose (EUP) (combination product), fructus oxyacanthae, fructus spinae albae, gazels, haagdorn, hagedorn, hagthorn, halves, harthorne, haw, Hawthorne Berry, Hawthorne Formula, Hawthorne Heart, Hawthorne Phytosome, Hawthorne Power, hawthorn tops, hazels, hedgethorn, huath, ladies' meat, LI 132, may, mayblossoms, maybush, mayhaw, maythorn, mehlbeerbaum, meidorn, nan shanzha, northern Chinese hawthorn, oneseed, oneseed hawthorn, quickset, red haw, RN 30/9, Rosaceae, sanza, sanzashi, shanza, shan zha rou, southern Chinese hawthorn, thorn-apple tree, thorn plum, tree of chastity, Washington thorn, weissdorn, weissdornblaetter mit blueten, whitethorn, whitethorn herb, WS 1442.

H

BACKGROUND

- Hawthorn, a flowering shrub of the rose family (Rosaceae), has an extensive history of use in cardiovascular disease, dating back to the first century AD. Modern-day laboratory research and studies in animals suggest that flavonoids and other pharmacologically active compounds found in hawthorn may synergistically improve performance of the damaged myocardium and may prevent or reduce symptoms of coronary artery disease.
- Numerous well-conducted clinical trials in humans have demonstrated safety and efficacy of hawthorn leaf and flower in New York Heart Association (NYHA) Class I-II heart failure (characterized by slight or no limitation of physical activity). An international, multi-center randomized controlled trial is currently underway to investigate long-term benefits.
- Hawthorn is widely used in Europe for treating NYHA Class I-II heart failure, with standardization of dosage of its leaves and flowers. Overall, hawthorn appears to be safe and well tolerated, and in accordance with its indication, best used under the supervision of a qualified healthcare provider.
- The therapeutic equivalence of hawthorn extracts to drugs considered standard-of-care for heart failure (such as angiotensin-converting enzyme inhibitors, diuretics, and beta-adrenergic receptor blockers) remains to be established, as does the effect of concomitant use of hawthorn with these drugs. Nonetheless, hawthorn is a potentially beneficial therapy for people who cannot or will not take prescription drugs and may offer additive benefits to prescription drug therapy.

---

*See Related Terms section for names of other *Crataegus* species of hawthorn.

USES BASED ON SCIENTIFIC EVIDENCE	Grade*
Congestive heart failure (CHF) Extracts of the leaves and flowers of hawthorn at doses of 160 to 900 mg daily have been reported as efficacious in the treatment of mild-to-moderate CHF, improving exercise capacity, and alleviating symptoms of cardiac insufficiency. This assessment is based on numerous randomized placebo-controlled clinical trials. However, the therapeutic equivalence of hawthorn extracts to drugs considered standard-of-care for heart failure (such as angiotensin-converting enzyme inhibitors, diuretics, and beta-adrenergic receptor blockers) remains to be established, as does the effect of concomitant use of hawthorn with these drugs. An equivalence trial by Tauchert and colleagues found hawthorn comparable to captopril, but this study may not have been adequately powered to detect small differences in therapies. Nonetheless, hawthorn is a potentially beneficial treatment for patients who cannot or will not take prescription drugs and may offer additive benefits to established therapies. Further study of these issues is warranted.	A
Coronary artery disease (angina) Increased myocardial perfusion and performance have been observed in animals due to hawthorn, and one randomized clinical trial indicates that hawthorn may be effective in decreasing frequency or severity of anginal symptoms. However, hawthorn has not been tested in the setting of concomitant drugs such as beta-blockers or ACE-inhibitors, which are often considered to be standard-of-care. At this time, there is insufficient evidence to recommend for or against hawthorn for coronary artery disease or angina.	C
Functional cardiovascular disorders Two randomized trials reported efficacy of herbal combinations containing hawthorn in the treatment of functional cardiovascular disorders. However, due to a lack of controlled information about hawthorn monotherapy, there is insufficient evidence to recommend for or against hawthorn for treatment of functional cardiovascular disorders.	C

*Key to grades: *A:* Strong scientific evidence for this use; *B:* Good scientific evidence for this use; *C:* Unclear scientific evidence for this use; *D:* Fair scientific evidence against this use (it may not work); *F:* Strong scientific evidence against this use (it likely does not work). For a more detailed explanation of efficacy criteria, see "Natural Standard Evidence-Based Validated Grading Rationale" in the Introduction.

Uses Based on Tradition, Theory, or Limited Scientific Evidence

Abdominal colic, abdominal distention, abdominal pain, acne, amenorrhea, angina, antibacterial, antioxidant, anxiety, appetite stimulant, asthma, astringent, bladder disorders, Buerger's disease, cancer, cardiac arrhythmia, circulation, diabetes

Uses Based on Tradition, Theory, or Limited Scientific Evidence (*cont'd*)

insipidus, diabetes mellitus, diarrhea, diuresis, dysentery, dyspepsia, dyspnea, edema, frostbite, fumitory, cardiac murmurs, hemorrhoids, HIV, hyperlipidemia, hypertension, insomnia, nephrosis, orthostatic hypotension, peripheral artery disease, skin sores, sore throat, spasmolytic, stomach aches, varicose veins.

DOSING

The following doses are based on scientific research, publications, traditional use, or expert opinion. Many herbs and supplements have not been thoroughly tested, and their safety and effectiveness may not be proven. Brands may be made differently, with variable ingredients even within the same brand. The doses shown may not apply to all products. It is important to always read product labels and discuss doses with a qualified healthcare provider before therapy is started.

Standardization

- Standardization involves measuring the amount of certain chemicals in products to try to make different preparations similar to each other. It is not always known if the chemicals being measured are the "active" ingredients.
- International standardization recommendations range from 0.6% to 1.5% flavonoids, typically calculated as hyperoside. Hawthorn extract WS 1442 is standardized to 18.75% oligomeric procyanidins. Hawthorn extract LI 132 is standardized to 2.2% flavonoids.

Adults (18 Years and Older)

Oral (congestive heart failure)

- **Products containing standardized extract WS 1442 (18.75% oligomeric procyanidins):** Statistically significant trials have used doses of 60 mg three times daily 80 mg twice daily. The United States brand HeartCare (Nature's Way) is standardized in this fashion.
- **Products containing standardized extract LI 132 (2.2% flavonoids):** Statistically significant trials have used doses of 100 mg three times daily, 200 mg twice daily, and up to 300 mg three times daily.
- **Dosage range:** The dosage range recommended in review literature is 160 to 900 mg daily of hawthorn extract in two to three divided doses (corresponding to 3.5 to 19.8 mg of flavonoids or 30 to 168.8 mg of oligomeric procyanidins). Some sources recommend a range of 240 to 480 mg daily for extracts standardized to 18.75% oligomeric procyanidins.

Children (Younger Than 18 Years)

- Because of lack of scientific information about safety, hawthorn is not recommended for use in children.

SAFETY

The U.S. Food and Drug Administration does not strictly regulate herbs and supplements. There is no guarantee of the strength, purity, or safety of products, and effects may vary. It is important to always read product labels. People who have a medical condition, or are taking other drugs, herbs, or supplements, should consult a qualified healthcare provider before starting a new therapy. A healthcare provider should be contacted immediately about any side effects.

Allergies

- People with known allergies or sensitivity to hawthorn or other species of *Crataegus* should avoid the use of hawthorn products. There has been one case report of an immediate-type hypersensitivity reaction to hawthorn plants. It is not known if this applies to oral formulations.

Side Effects and Warnings

- Numerous trials in humans, observational studies including more than 4500 patients, and case studies have reported rare adverse effects, including agitation, abdominal discomfort, diaphoresis, dizziness, dyspnea, fatigue, headache, insomnia, nausea, skin rash, and tachycardia.

Pregnancy and Breastfeeding

- Because of lack of sufficient scientific information regarding its safety, hawthorn is not recommended for use in women who are pregnant or breastfeeding.

INTERACTIONS

Most herbs and supplements have not been thoroughly tested for interactions with other herbs, supplements, drugs, or foods. The interactions listed here are based on reports in scientific publications, laboratory experiments, or traditional use. It is important to always read product labels. People who have a medical condition, or are taking other drugs, herbs, or supplements, should consult a qualified healthcare provider before starting a new therapy.

Interactions with Drugs

- When hawthorn was used with cardiac glycoside drugs such as digoxin in animals, additive inotropic effects without added toxicity were noted. Hawthorn has been used in humans with the intention of decreasing digoxin doses, but data on safe and efficacious dosing in this setting are limited.
- Based on studies in animals and clinical data, hawthorn may have additive activity when co-administered with medications that lower blood pressure. Research in animals suggests that hawthorn may add to the activity of drugs that dilate blood vessels and may decrease the effects of vasoconstrictors such as phenylephrine (Neo-Synephrine), ephedrine, and norepinephrine. Based on limited laboratory research, studies in animals, and clinical data, hawthorn may have additive activity with medications that reduce cholesterol levels.

Interactions with Herbs and Dietary Supplements

- Hawthorn may add to the effects on the heart of agents containing cardiac glycosides. Potential cardiac glycoside herbs include adonis, balloon cotton, black hellebore root/melampode, black Indian hemp, bushman's poison, cactus grandifloris, convallaria, eyebright, figwort, foxglove/digitalis, frangipani, hedge mustard, hemp root/Canadian hemp root, king's crown, lily-of-the-valley, motherwort, oleander leaf, pheasant's eye plant, plantain leaf, pleurisy root, psyllium husks, redheaded cotton-bush, rhubarb root, rubber vine, sea-mango, senna fruit, squill, strophanthus, uzara, wallflower, wintersweet, yellow dock root, and yellow oleander. Notably, bufalin/chan suis, a Chinese herbal formula, has been reported as toxic or fatal when taken with cardiac glycosides.
- Hawthorn may add to the effects of agents that lower blood pressure. Herbs that theoretically may have this effect include aconite/monkshood, arnica, baneberry,

betel nut, bilberry, black cohosh, bryony, calendula, California poppy, coleus, curcumin, eucalyptol, eucalyptus oil, ginger, goldenseal, green hellebore, Indian tobacco, jaborandi, mistletoe, night-blooming cereus, oleander, pasque flower, periwinkle, pleurisy root, shepherd's purse, Texas milkweed, turmeric, and wild cherry.

- Limited laboratory research, studies in animals, and clinical data suggest that hawthorn may have additive activity when co-administered with agents that reduce cholesterol levels, such as garlic, niacin, and fish oil (omega-3 fatty acids).

Selected References

Natural Standard developed the preceding evidence-based information based on a systematic review of more than 130 articles. For comprehensive information about alternative and complementary therapies on the professional level, go to www.naturalstandard.com. Selected references are listed here.

Ammon HP, Handel M. [Crataegus, toxicology and pharmacology, Part I: Toxicity (author's transl).] Planta Med 1981;43(2):105-120.

Ammon HP, Handel M. [Crataegus, toxicology and pharmacology. Part II: Pharmacodynamics (author's transl).] Planta Med 1981;43(3):209-239.

Ammon HP, Handel M. [Crataegus, toxicology and pharmacology. Part III: Pharmacodynamics and pharmacokinetics (author's transl).] Planta Med 1981;43(4):313-322.

Beier A, Konigstein RP, Samec V. [Clinical experiences with a crataegus pentaerythrityl-tetranitrate combination drug in heart diseases due to coronary sclerosis in old age.] Wien Med Wochenschr 1974;124(24):378-381.

Bodigheimer K, Chase D. [Effectiveness of hawthorn extract at a dosage of 3x100mg per day]. Munch Med Wschr 1994;136(Suppl 1):S7-S11.

Chen ZY, Zhang ZS, Kwan KY, et al. Endothelium-dependent relaxation induced by hawthorn extract in rat mesenteric artery. Life Sci 1998;63(22):1983-1991.

Degenring FH, Suter A, Weber M, et al. A randomised double blind placebo controlled clinical trial of a standardised extract of fresh Crataegus berries (Crataegisan) in the treatment of patients with congestive heart failure NYHA II. Phytomedicine 2003;10(5):363-369.

Forster A, Forster K, Buhring M, et al. Crataegus bei massig reduzierter linksventrikularer Auswurffraktion. Ergospirometrische Verlaufsuntersuchung bei 72 Patienten in doppelblindem Vergleich mit Plazebo. [Crataegus for moderately reduced left ventricular ejection fraction. Ergospirometric monitoring study with 72 patients in a double-blind comparison with placebo.] Munch Med Wschr 1994;136(Suppl 1):S21-S26.

Hanack T, Bruckel MH. [The treatment of mild stable forms of angina pectoris using Crategutt novo.] Therapiewoche 1983;33:4331-4333.

Holubarsch CJ, Colucci WS, Meinertz T, et al. Survival and prognosis: investigation of Crataegus extract WS 1442 in congestive heart failure (SPICE)—rationale, study design and study protocol. Eur J Heart Fail 2000;2(4):431-437.

Iwamoto M, Sato T, Ishizaki T. The clinical effect of Crataegus in heart disease of ischemic or hypertensive origin. A multicenter double-blind study. Planta Med 1981;42(1):1-16.

Leuchtgens H. [Crataegus Special Extract WS 1442 in NYHA II heart failure. A placebo controlled randomized double-blind study.] Fortschr Med 1993;111(20-21):352-354.

Loew D, Albrecht M, Podzuweit H. Efficacy and tolerability of a Hawthorn preparation in patients with heart failure Stage I and II according to NYHA—a surveillance study. Phytomedicine 1996;3(Suppl 1):S92.

O'Conolly M, Bernhoft G, Bartsch G. [Treatment of stenocardia (Angina pectoris) pain in advanced age patients with multi-morbidity.] Therapiewoche 1987;37:3587-3600.

O'Conolly M, Jansen W, Bernhoft G, et al. [Treatment of decreasing cardiac performance. Therapy using standardized crataegus extract in advanced age.] Fortschr Med 1986;104(42): 805-808.

Petkov V. Plants with hypotensive, antiatheromatous and coronarodilatating action. Am J Chinese Med 1979;7(3):197-236.

Pittler MH, Schmidt K, Ernst E. Hawthorn extract for treating chronic heart failure: meta-analysis of randomized trials. Am J Med 2003;114(8):665-674.

Rajendran S, Deepalakshmi PD, Parasakthy K, et al. Effect of tincture of Crataegus on the LDL-receptor activity of hepatic plasma membrane of rats fed an atherogenic diet. Atherosclerosis 1996;123(1-2):235-241.

Schmidt U, Kuhn U, Ploch M, et al. Efficacy of hawthorn (crataegus) preparation LI 132 in 78 patients with chronic congestive heart failure defined as NYHA functional class II. Phytomedicine 1994;1:17-24.

Schmidt U, Kuhn U, Ploch M, et al. Efficacy of the hawthorn extract LI 132 (600mg/d) during eight weeks' treatment. Placebo-controlled double-blind trial with 78 NYHA stage II heart failure patients. Munch Med Wochenschr 1994;136(suppl 1):S13-S19.

Schmidt U, Albrecht M, Schmidt S. [Effects of an herbal crataegus-camphor combination on the symptoms of cardiovascular diseases.] Arzneimittelforschung 2000;50(7):613-619.

Schroder D, Weiser M, Klein P. Efficacy of a homeopathic Crataegus preparation compared with usual therapy for mild (NYHA II) cardiac insufficiency: results of an observational cohort study. Eur J Heart Fail 2003;5(3):319-326.

Steinman HK, Lovell CR, Cronin E. Immediate-type hypersensitivity to *Crataegus monogyna* (hawthorn). Contact Dermatitis 1984;11(5):321.

Tankanow R, Tamer HR, Streetman DS, et al. Interaction study between digoxin and a preparation of hawthorn (*Crataegus oxyacantha*). J Clin Pharmacol 2003;43(6):637-642.

Tauchert M, Ploch M, Hubner WD. Effectiveness of hawthorn extract LI 132 compared with the ACE inhibitor Captopril: Multicenter double-blind study with 132 NYHA Stage II. Munch Med Wochenschr 1994;136(Suppl 1):S27-S33.

Tauchert M, Gildor A, Lipinski J. [High-dose Crataegus extract WS 1442 in the treatment of NYHA stage II heart failure]. Herz 1999;24(6):465-474.

Trunzler G, Schuler E. Comparative studies on the effects of a Crataegus extract, digitoxin, digoxin, and g-Strophanthin in the isolated heart of homoiothermals. Arzneim-Forsch 1962; 12:198-202.

Ventura P, Girola M, Lattuada V. [Clinical evaluation and tolerability of a drug with garlic and hawthorn.] Acta Toxicol Ther 1990;11(4):365-372.

Von Eiff M, Brunner H, Haegeli A, et al. Hawthorn/passion flower extract and improvement in physical exercise capacity of patients with dyspnoea class II of the NYHA functional classification. Acta Therapeutica 1994;20:47-66.

Weihmayr T, Ernst E. [Therapeutic effectiveness of Crataegus.] Fortschr Med 1996;114(1-2): 27-29.

Weikl A, Noh HS. The influence of Crataegus on global cardiac insufficiency. Herz Gefabe 1993;11:516-524.

Weikl A, Assmus KD, Neukum-Schmidt A, et al. [Crataegus Special Extract WS 1442. Assessment of objective effectiveness in patients with heart failure (NYHA II)]. Fortschr Med 1996;114(24):291-296.

Weng WL, Zhang WQ, Liu FZ, et al. Therapeutic effect of *Crataegus pinnatifida* on 46 cases of angina pectoris—a double blind study. J Tradit Chin Med 1984;4(4):293-294.

Zapfe JG. Clinical efficacy of crataegus extract WS 1442 in congestive heart failure NYHA class II. Phytomedicine 2001;8(4):262-266.

Hops

(*Humulus lupulus* L.)

RELATED TERMS

- Cannabaceae, common hops, European hops, hop, hop strobile, hopfen, houblon, humulus, lupulin, lupulus, *Lupuli strobulus*, Ze 91019.
- **Selected combination products:** Avena Sativa Compound in Species Sedative Tea, HR 129 Serene, Hova-Filmtabletten, HR 133 Stress, Melatonin with Vitamin B_6, Seda-Kneipp, Snuz Plus, Stress Aid, Valverde, Zemaphyte.

BACKGROUND

- Hops are a member of the Cannabaceae family, traditionally used for relaxation and sedation and to treat insomnia. A number of methodologically weak trials in humans have investigated hops in combination with valerian (*Valeriana officinalis*) for the treatment of sleep disturbances, and several studies in animals have examined the sedative properties of hops monotherapy. However, the results of these studies were equivocal, and there is currently insufficient evidence to recommend hops alone or in combination for any medical condition.
- Hops are sometimes found in combination products with passion flower (*Passiflora incanata*), scullcap (potentially hepatotoxic), and a high percentage of alcohol (up to 70% grain alcohol), confounding the association between the possible sedative or hypnotic effects of hops and these substances.
- Hops contain phytoestrogens, with estrogen receptor agonist or antagonist properties, which have unclear effects on hormone-sensitive conditions such as breast, uterine, cervical, and prostate cancer and endometriosis.

USES BASED ON SCIENTIFIC EVIDENCE	Grade*
Insomnia/sleep quality Studies in animals report that hops may have sedative and sleep-enhancing (hypnotic) effects. However, there has been little research evaluating the effects of hops on sleep quality in humans. Some studies combine hops with valerian (*Valeriana officinalis*), and the effects of hops cannot be separated from the possible benefits of valerian. Further study is needed in this area before a recommendation can be made.	C
Sedation Hops have been used traditionally as a sedative for relaxation and reduction of anxiety. Although some studies in animals suggest possible sedative properties, there has been limited research in humans in this area. Better studies are needed before a firm conclusion can be drawn.	C

*Key to grades: *A:* Strong scientific evidence for this use; *B:* Good scientific evidence for this use; *C:* Unclear scientific evidence for this use; *D:* Fair scientific evidence against this use (it may not work); *F:* Strong scientific evidence against this use (it likely does not work). For a more detailed explanation of efficacy criteria, see "Natural Standard Evidence-Based Validated Grading Rationale" in the Introduction.

Uses Based on Tradition, Theory, or Limited Scientific Evidence

Antidepressant, antibacterial, anti-inflammatory, antispasmodic, anti-anxiety, anxiety during menopause, aphrodisiac, appetite stimulant, breast cancer, cancer (general), Crohn's disease, dermatitis, diabetes, diarrhea caused by infection, digestion stimulant, Epstein-Barr virus infection, estrogenic effects, indigestion, irritable bowel syndrome, kidney disorders, leprosy, lung disease (from inhalation of silica dust or asbestos), mood disturbances, muscle and joint disorders, muscle spasm, pain, parasites, restlessness, skin ulcers, tuberculosis.

DOSING

The following doses are based on scientific research, publications, traditional use, or expert opinion. Many herbs and supplements have not been thoroughly tested, and their safety and effectiveness may not be proven. Brands may be made differently, with variable ingredients even within the same brand. The doses shown may not apply to all products. It is important to always read product labels and discuss doses with a qualified healthcare provider before therapy is started.

Standardization

- Standardization involves measuring the amounts of certain chemicals in products to try to make different preparations similar to each other. It is not always known if the chemicals being measured are the "active" ingredients. Some hops extracts are standardized to 5.2% bitter acids and/or to 4% flavonoids per dose.

Adults (18 Years and Older)

- **Oral (by mouth):** For insomnia or sleep disturbances, doses of 300 to 400 mg of hops extract combined with 240 to 300 mg of valerian extract, taken at bedtime, have been used. Traditionally, doses of 0.5 to 1.0 g of dried hops extract or 0.5 to 1.0 ml of liquid hops extract (1:1 in 45% alcohol) have been taken up to three times daily. However, the use of hops alone has not been well studied.
- **Intravenous/intramuscular:** Administration of hops extract by injection into the veins or muscles is not recommended. In studies in animals, large injected doses resulted in a narcotic effect, followed by death, and long-term therapy resulted in weight loss and death.

Children (Younger Than 18 Years)

- **Oral (by mouth):** Hops extract traditionally is considered one of the milder sedative herbs and is regarded as safe for children. However, there is limited research in this area, and safety has not been clearly established. Some natural medicine experts suggest adjusting the dose according to body weight (multiply the usual adult dose by the child's weight in pounds and then divide by 150).

SAFETY

The U.S. Food and Drug Administration does not strictly regulate herbs and supplements. There is no guarantee of the strength, purity, or safety of products, and effects may vary. It is important to always read product labels. People who have a medical condition, or are taking other drugs, herbs, or supplements, should consult a qualified healthcare provider before starting a new therapy. A healthcare provider should be contacted immediately about any side effects.

Allergies

- Rash (contact dermatitis) and difficulty in breathing have been reported, mainly in hops harvesters. Allergy to hops pollen has also been reported. Hops allergy occurred in a patient with previous severe allergic reactions to peanut, chestnut, and banana. Therefore, people allergic to any of these agents should avoid the use of hops.

Side Effects and Warnings

- No serious side effects associated with hops have been reported in the available scientific literature. Hops may cause mild central nervous system (CNS) depression (drowsiness, slowed breathing and thinking), especially when taken with drugs or herbs/supplements that also cause CNS depression. Caution is advised in people who are driving or operating machinery.
- Studies in animals reported that eating hops in large quantities may cause seizures, hyperthermia, restlessness, vomiting, stomach pain, and increased stomach acid. Laboratory research suggests that estrogen-like substances in hops may have stimulatory or inhibitory effects on estrogen-sensitive parts of the body, and the effects of hops are unclear in hormone-sensitive conditions such as cancer (breast, uterine, cervical, prostate) and endometriosis.
- Based on preliminary studies in animals, hops may lower blood sugar levels in normal individuals but may actually increase blood sugar in persons with diabetes. Caution is advised in patients with diabetes or hypoglycemia, and in those taking drugs, herbs, or supplements that affect blood sugar levels. Serum glucose levels may need to be monitored by a healthcare provider, and medication adjustments may be necessary.
- Long-term breathing problems have been reported in brewery workers exposed to hops dust.

Pregnancy and Breastfeeding

- Hops is not recommended for use in women who are pregnant or breastfeeding because of possible hormonal and sedative effects. Limited research is available in these areas.
- *Note:* Many tinctures contain high levels of alcohol, and should be avoided during pregnancy.

INTERACTIONS

Most herbs and supplements have not been thoroughly tested for interactions with other herbs, supplements, drugs, or foods. The interactions listed here are based on reports in scientific publications, laboratory experiments, or traditional use. It is important to always read product labels. People who have a medical condition, or are taking other drugs, herbs, or supplements, should consult a qualified healthcare provider before starting a new therapy.

Interactions with Drugs

- Hops may cause mild central nervous system (CNS) depression (drowsiness, slowed breathing and thinking), and may add to the effects of drugs that also cause CNS depression or sedation. Examples include some antidepressants, barbiturates such as phenobarbital, benzodiazepines such as lorazepam (Ativan) and diazepam (Valium), narcotics such as codeine, and alcohol. Caution is advised in people who are driving or operating machinery.

- Based on preliminary studies in animals, hops may lower blood sugar levels in normal individuals but may actually increase blood sugar in those with diabetes. Caution is advised in people who are using medications that may lower blood sugar levels. People who are taking hops as well as drugs for diabetes by mouth or insulin should be monitored closely by a qualified healthcare provider. Medication adjustments may be necessary.
- Laboratory research suggests that estrogen-like substances in hops may have stimulatory or inhibitory effects on estrogen-sensitive parts of the body. It is not clear what interactions may occur when hops is used with other hormonal therapies such as birth control pills, hormone replacement therapy, tamoxifen, and aromatase inhibitors (e.g., letrozole [Femara]).
- Limited laboratory research and studies in animals suggest that hops may interfere with how the body uses the liver's cytochrome P450 enzyme system to process components of some drugs. As a result, blood levels of these components may be elevated and may cause increased effects or potentially serious adverse reactions. People who are using any medications should always read the package insert and consult with their healthcare provider or pharmacist about possible interactions.
- Taking phenothiazine anti-psychotic drugs with hops may increase the risk of hyperthermia, although there are no reliable studies in humans in this area.
- *Note:* Many tinctures contain high levels of alcohol and may cause nausea or vomiting when taken with metronidazole (Flagyl) or disulfiram (Antabuse).

Interactions with Herbs and Dietary Supplements

- Hops may cause mild central nervous system (CNS) depression (drowsiness, slowed breathing and thinking) and may add to the effects of other herbs or supplements that may cause CNS depression or sedation. Examples are calamus, calendula, California poppy, capsicum, catnip, celery, couchgrass, dogwood, elecampane, German chamomile, goldenseal, gotu kola, kava, lavender aromatherapy, lemon balm, sage, sassafras, scullcap, shepherd's purse, Siberian ginseng, stinging nettle, St. John's wort, valerian, wild carrot, wild lettuce, withania root, and yerba mansa. Caution is advised in people who are driving or operating machinery.
- Based on preliminary studies in animals, hops may lower blood sugar levels in normal individuals but may actually increase blood sugar levels in those with diabetes. Caution is advised in people who are using herbs or supplements that may affect blood sugar levels. Blood glucose levels may require monitoring, and doses may need adjustment. Examples of agents that may lower blood sugar levels are *Aloe vera*, American ginseng, bilberry, bitter melon, burdock, fenugreek, fish oil, gymnema, horse chestnut seed extract (HCSE), marshmallow, milk thistle, *Panax ginseng*, rosemary, Siberian ginseng, stinging nettle, and white horehound. Agents that may raise blood sugar levels include arginine, cocoa, and ephedra (when combined with caffeine).
- Hops may interfere with the way the body processes certain drugs using the liver's cytochrome P450 enzyme system. As a result, the levels of other herbs and supplements may be too low in the blood. It may also alter the effects that other herbs or supplements potentially may have on the cytochrome P450 system. Examples of such herbs are bloodroot, cat's claw, chamomile, chaparral, chasteberry, damiana, *Echinacea angustifolia*, goldenseal, grapefruit juice, licorice, oregano, red clover, St. John's wort, wild cherry, and yucca. People who are using any medications should always read the package insert and consult their healthcare provider and pharmacist about possible interactions.

- Because hops contains estrogen-like chemicals, when taken in combination with other agents that may have estrogen-like properties, it may alter their effects. Examples of such agents are alfalfa, black cohosh, bloodroot, burdock, kudzu, licorice, pomegranate, red clover, soy, thyme, white horehound, and yucca.

Selected References

Natural Standard developed the preceding evidence-based information based on a systematic review of more than 200 scientific articles. For comprehensive information about alternative and complementary therapies on the professional level, go to www.naturalstandard.com. Selected references are listed here.

Collie ME, Higgins JC. Hope for hops? Arch Intern Med. 2002;162(3):364-365. Comment in: Arch Intern Med 2001;161(15):1844-1848.

Duncan KL, Hare WR, Buck WB. Malignant hyperthermia-like reaction secondary to ingestion of hops in five dogs. J Am Vet Med Assoc 1997;210(1):51-54.

Estrada JL, Gozalo F, Cecchini C, Casquete E. Contact urticaria from hops (*Humulus lupulus*) in a patient with previous urticaria-angioedema from peanut, chestnut and banana. Contact Dermatitis 2002;46(2):127.

Gerhard U, Linnenbrink N, Georghiadou C, et al. [Vigilance-decreasing effects of 2 plant-derived sedatives.] Schweiz Rundsch Med Prax 1996;85(15):473-481.

Gerhauser C, Alt A, Heiss E, et al. Cancer chemopreventive activity of Xanthohumol, a natural product derived from hop. Mol Cancer Ther 2002;1(11):959-969.

Godnic-Cvar J, Zuskin E, Mustajbegovic J, et al. Respiratory and immunological findings in brewery workers. Am J Ind Med 1999;35(1):68-75.

Hänsel R, Wohlfart R, Schmidt H. The sedative-hypnotic principle of hops. 3. Communication: contents of 2-methyl-3-butene-2-ol in hops and hop preparations. Planta Med 1982;45: 224-228.

Henderson MC, Miranda CL, Stevens JF, et al. *In vitro* inhibition of human P450 enzymes by prenylated flavonoids from hops, *Humulus lupulus*. Xenobiotica 2000;30(3):235-251.

Hengel MJ, Shibamoto T. Gas chromatographic-mass spectrometric method for the analysis of dimethomorph fungicide in dried hops. J Agric Food Chem 2003;51(6):1760.

Kapadia GJ, Azuine MA, Tokuda H, et al. Inhibitory effect of herbal remedies on 12-*O*-tetradecanoylphorbol-13-acetate–promoted Epstein-Barr virus early antigen activation. Pharmacol Res 2002;45(3):213-220.

Leathwood PD, Chauffard F, Heck E, et al. Aqueous extract of valerian root (*Valeriana officinalis* L.) improves sleep quality in man. Pharmacol Biochem Behav 1982;17(1):65-71.

Milligan S, Kalita J, Pocock V, et al. Oestrogenic activity of the hop phyto-oestrogen, 8-prenylnaringenin. Reproduction 2002;123(2):235-242.

Milligan SR, Kalita JC, Heyerick A, et al. Identification of a potent phytoestrogen in hops (*Humulus lupulus* L.) and beer. J Clin Endocrinol Metab 1999;84(6):2249-2252.

Milligan SR, Kalita JC, Pocock V, et al. The endocrine activities of 8-prenylnaringenin and related hop (*Humulus lupulus* L.) flavonoids. J Clin Endocrinol Metab 2000;85(12): 4912-4915.

Muller CE, Schumacher B, Brattstrom A, et al. Interactions of valerian extracts and a fixed valerian-hop extract combination with adenosine receptors. Life Sci 2002;71(16):1939-1949.

Muller-Limmroth W, Ehrenstein W. [Experimental studies of the effects of Seda-Kneipp on the sleep of sleep disturbed subjects; implications for the treatment of different sleep disturbances.] Med Klin 1977;72(25):1119-1125.

Newmark FM. Hops allergy and terpene sensitivity: an occupational disease. Ann Allergy 1978;41(5):311-312.

O'Donovan W. Hops dermatitis. Lancet 1924;2:597.

Pradalier A, Campinos C, Trinh C. Systemic urticaria induced by hops [article in French]. Allerg Immunol (Paris) 2002;34(9):330-332.

Schaefer O, Humpel M, Fritzemeier Khet al. 8-Prenyl naringenin is a potent ERalpha selective phytoestrogen present in hops and beer. J Steroid Biochem Mol Biol 2003;84(2-3):359-360.

Schmitz M, Jackel M. [Comparative study for assessing quality of life of patients with exogenous sleep disorders (temporary sleep onset and sleep interruption disorders) treated with a hops-valarian preparation and a benzodiazepine drug.] Wien Med Wochenschr 1998;148(13): 291-298.

Spiewak R, Dutkiewicz J. Occupational airborne and hand dermatitis to hop (*Humulus lupulus*) with non-occupational relapses. Ann Agric Environ Med 2002;9(2):249-252.

Vonderheid-Guth B, Todorova A, Brattstrom A, et al. Pharmacodynamic effects of valerian and hops extract combination (Ze 91019) on the quantitative-topographical EEG in healthy volunteers. Eur J Med Res 2000;5(4):139-144.

Wohlfart R, Hansel R, Schmidt H. [The sedative-hypnotic action of hops. 4. Communication: pharmacology of the hop substance 2-methyl-3-buten-2-ol.] Planta Med 1983;48(2): 120-123.

Zenisek A, Bednar IJ. Contribution of the identification of the estrogen activity of hops. Am Perfumer Arom 1960;75:61.

Horse Chestnut
(*Aesculus hippocastanum* L.)

H

RELATED TERMS

- Aescin, aescine, aescule, buckeye, bongay, chestnut, conkers, conquerors, eschilo, escin, escine, fish poison, graine de marronier d'Inde, *Heliantheum vulgare* Gaertnhestekastanje, hippocastani folium, hippocastani semen, horsechestnut, horse chestnut seed extract (HCSE), marron eropeen, marronier, NV-101, rokastaniensamen, rosskastanie, Spanish chestnut, Venastat, Venoplant, Venostasin.

BACKGROUND

- Horse chestnut seed extract (HCSE) is widely used in Europe for chronic venous insufficiency (CVI), a syndrome that includes leg swelling, varicose veins, leg pain, itching, and skin ulcers. Although HCSE is traditionally recommended for a variety of medical conditions, CVI is the only condition for which there is strong supportive scientific evidence.
- Side effects from HCSE have been similar to those of placebo in clinical trials. However, because of an increased risk of low blood sugar levels associated with HCSE, caution is advised in children and people with diabetes.
- Horse chestnut flower, branch bark, and leaf have not been shown effective for any indication, and it is strongly advised that they be avoided because of their known toxicity.

USES BASED ON SCIENTIFIC EVIDENCE	Grade*
Chronic venous insufficiency (CVI) CVI is more commonly diagnosed in Europe than in the United States. Its symptoms include leg swelling, varicose veins, leg pain, itching, and skin ulcers. There is evidence from laboratory research and studies in animals and humans suggest that horse chestnut seed extract (HCSE) may be beneficial to patients with this condition. Studies report significant decreases in leg size, leg pain, itchiness, fatigue and "tenseness." There is preliminary evidence that HCSE may be as effective as compression stockings for this condition.	A

*Key to grades: *A:* Strong scientific evidence for this use; *B:* Good scientific evidence for this use; *C:* Unclear scientific evidence for this use; *D:* Fair scientific evidence against this use (it may not work); *F:* Strong scientific evidence against this use (it likely does not work). For a more detailed explanation of efficacy criteria, see "Natural Standard Evidence-Based Validated Grading Rationale" in the Introduction.

Uses Based on Tradition, Theory, or Limited Scientific Evidence

Benign prostatic hypertrophy (BPH), fluid in the lungs (pulmonary edema), gallbladder pain (colic), gallbladder infection (cholecystitis), gallbladder stones (cholelithiasis), bladder disorders (incontinence, cystitis), bruising, cough, vein clots (deep venous thrombosis), diarrhea, dizziness, fever, hemorrhoids, kidney diseases, leg cramps, liver congestion, lung blood clots (pulmonary embolism), menstrual pain, nerve pain, osteoarthritis, pancreatitis, rectal complaints, "rheumatism," rheumatoid arthritis, skin conditions, postoperative/post-traumatic soft tissue swelling, ringing in the ears (tinnitus), ulcers, whooping cough.

DOSING

The following doses are based on scientific research, publications, traditional use, or expert opinion. Many herbs and supplements have not been thoroughly tested, and their safety and effectiveness may not be proven. Brands may be made differently, with variable ingredients even within the same brand. The doses shown may not apply to all products. It is important to always read product labels and discuss doses with a qualified healthcare provider before therapy is started.

Standardization

- Standardization involves measuring the amounts of certain chemicals in products to try to make different preparations similar to each other. It is not always known if the chemicals being measured are the "active" ingredients. Horse chestnut seed extract (HCSE) products are often standardized to contain 16% to 20% triterpene glycosides calculated as escin (aescin) content.

Adults (18 Years and Older)

- **Oral (by mouth):** A range of doses for HCSE taken by mouth have been used. Studies suggest a standardized product containing 50 to 75 mg of escin every 12 hours taken by mouth. This often results in an HCSE product total dose of 300 mg twice daily.
- **Topical (on the skin):** A gel preparation of horse chestnut applied to the skin has been studied for bruising, without clear benefits.
- **Intravenous/intramuscular**: Severe allergic reaction (anaphylactic shock) has been reported following administration of HCSE injected in the veins. Horse chestnut leaf has been associated with liver inflammation (hepatitis) after injection into muscle.

Children (Younger Than 18 Years)

- There is insufficient scientific evidence to recommend use of horse chestnut in children. Deaths have been reported in children who ate raw horse chestnut seeds or tea made from horse chestnut leaves and twigs.

SAFETY

The U.S. Food and Drug Administration does not strictly regulate herbs and supplements. There is no guarantee of the strength, purity, or safety of products, and effects may vary. It is important

to always read product labels. People who have a medical condition, or are taking other drugs, herbs, or supplements, should consult a qualified healthcare provider before starting a new therapy. A healthcare provider should be contacted immediately about any side effects.

Allergies

- HCSE may cause an allergic reaction in patients with known allergy to horse chestnuts, esculin, or any of its ingredients (flavonoids, biosides, trisides of quertins, and oligosaccharides including 1-ketose and 2-ketose). Anaphylactic shock (severe allergic reaction) has been reported with administration of HCSE injected in the veins.

Side Effects and Warnings

- Unprocessed horse chestnut seeds, leaves, bark, and flowers contain esculin, which has been associated with significant toxicity and death. Symptoms found with horse chestnut poisoning include vomiting, diarrhea, headache, confusion, weakness, muscle twitching, poor coordination, coma, and paralysis. HCSE standardized to escin content should not contain significant levels of esculin, and should not carry the same risks.
- Standardized HCSE is generally considered to be safe in adults at recommended doses for short periods of time. Stomach upset, muscular (calf) spasms, headache, dizziness, nausea, and itching have been reported. Contact skin irritation (dermatitis) has been reported following application of HCSE to the skin.
- Based on animal studies, HCSE may decrease blood sugar levels. Caution is advised in people with diabetes or hypoglycemia, and in those taking drugs, herbs, or supplements that affect blood sugar levels. Serum glucose levels may need to be monitored by a qualified healthcare provider, and medication adjustments may be necessary.
- In theory, horse chestnut may increase the risk of bleeding because of the hydroxycoumarin content of esculin. Properly extracted HCSE should not contain esculin and therefore should not carry this risk. However, caution is advised in people with bleeding disorders or taking drugs that may increase the risk of bleeding. Monitoring by a qualified healthcare provider is recommended, and dosing adjustments may be necessary.
- There was one case report of liver toxicity with a horse chestnut leaf product that resolved after the product was discontinued. Several cases of kidney toxicity were reported after injection of high doses of escin. Aflatoxins, considered to be cancer-causing agents, have been identified in commercial skin products containing horse chestnut, but not in HCSE.

Pregnancy and Breastfeeding

- There is insufficient scientific research to recommend the safe use of HCSE or other horse chestnut products in women who are pregnant or breastfeeding. One small study of pregnant women treated with HCSE reported no serious adverse effects after 2 weeks.

INTERACTIONS

Most herbs and supplements have not been thoroughly tested for interactions with other herbs, supplements, drugs, or foods. The interactions listed here are based on reports in scientific publications, laboratory experiments, or traditional use. It is important to always read product labels. People who have a medical condition, or are taking other drugs, herbs, or supplements, should consult a qualified healthcare provider before starting a new therapy.

Interactions with Drugs

- In theory, due to its esculin constituents, horse chestnut (but not HCSE, which, when properly prepared, does not contain esculin) may increase the risk of bleeding when taken with drugs that increase the risk of bleeding. Examples are anti-coagulants (blood thinners) such as warfarin (Coumadin) and heparin, antiplatelet drugs such as clopidogrel (Plavix), aspirin, and nonsteroidal anti-inflammatory drugs such as ibuprofen (Motrin, Advil) and naproxen (Naprosyn, Aleve).
- In theory, and based on limited studies in animals, HCSE may have an additive effect when taken with drugs that cause hypoglycemia (low blood sugar levels). Caution is advised in people who are using medications that may also lower blood sugar levels. Persons taking drugs for diabetes by mouth or insulin should be monitored closely by a qualified healthcare provider. Medication adjustments may be necessary.
- Escin in HCSE may theoretically interfere with protein-bound drugs such as phenytoin (Dilantin), warfarin (Coumadin), and amiodarone (Cordarone), although no cases have been reported in the available literature.

Interactions with Herbs and Dietary Supplements

- In theory, because of its esculin constituents, horse chestnut (but not HCSE, which, when properly prepared, does not contain esculin) may increase the risk of bleeding when taken with other herbs or supplements that may increase the risk of bleeding. Multiple cases of bleeding have been reported with the use of *Ginkgo biloba*, and fewer cases with garlic and saw palmetto. Numerous other agents may theoretically increase the risk of bleeding, although this has not been proven in most cases. Examples are alfalfa, American ginseng, angelica, anise, *Arnica montana*, asafetida, aspen bark, bilberry, birch, black cohosh, bladderwrack, bogbean, boldo, borage seed oil, bromelain, capsicum, cat's claw, celery, chamomile, chaparral, clove, coleus, cordyceps, danshen, devil's claw, dong quai, evening primrose, fenugreek, feverfew, flaxseed/flax powder (not a concern with flaxseed oil), ginger, grapefruit juice, grape seed, green tea, guggul, gymnestra, horseradish, licorice root, lovage root, male fern, meadowsweet, nordihydroguaiaretic acid (NDGA), onion, *Panax ginseng*, papain, parsley, passion flower, poplar, prickly ash, propolis, quassia, red clover, reishi, rue, Siberian ginseng, sweet birch, sweet clover, turmeric, vitamin E, white willow, wild carrot, wild lettuce, willow, wintergreen, and yucca.
- In theory, and based on limited studies in animals, HCSE may have an additive effect when taken with other herbs or supplements that may lower blood sugar levels. Caution is advised in people who are taking such herbs as well as HCSE. Blood glucose levels may require monitoring, and doses may need adjustment. Examples of agents that may lower blood sugar levels are *Aloe vera*, American ginseng, bilberry, bitter melon, burdock, fenugreek, fish oil, gymnema, marshmallow, milk thistle, *Panax ginseng*, rosemary, Siberian ginseng, stinging nettle. and white horehound. Agents that may raise blood sugar levels include arginine, cocoa, and ephedra (when combined with caffeine).

Selected References

Natural Standard developed the preceding evidence-based information based on a systematic review of more than 135 scientific articles. For comprehensive information about alternative and complementary therapies on the professional level, go to www.naturalstandard.com. Selected references are listed here.

Alter H. Zur medikamentosen therapie der varikosis. Z Allg Med 1973;49(17):1301-1304.

Bisler H, Pfeifer R, Kluken N, et al. [Effects of horse-chestnut seed extract on transcapillary filtration in chronic venous insufficiency.] Dtsch Med Wochenschr 1986;111(35):1321-1329.

Diehm C, Trampisch HJ, Lange S, et al. Comparison of leg compression stocking and oral horse-chestnut seed extract therapy in patients with chronic venous insufficiency. Lancet 1996;347(8997):292-294.

Diehm C, Vollbrecht D, Amendt K, et al. Medical edema protection—clinical benefit in patients with chronic deep vein incompetence. A placebo controlled double blind study. Vasa 1992; 21(2):188-192.

Erdlen F. Klinische wirksamkeit von Venostasin retard im Doppelblindversuch. Med Welt 1989; 40:994-996.

Erler M. Rokastaniensamenextrakt bei der therapie peripherer venoser odeme: ein klinischer therapievergleich. Med Welt 1991;43:593-596.

Friederich HC, Vogelsberg H, Neiss A. [Evaluation of internally effective venous drugs.] Z Hautkr 1978;53(11):369-374.

Kalbfleisch W, Pfalzgraf H. Odemprotektiva: aquipotente dosierung: rokastaniensamenextrakt und O-beta- hydroxyethylrutoside im vergleich. Therapiewoche 1989;39:3703-3707.

Koch R. Comparative study of Venostasin and Pycnogenol in chronic venous insufficiency. Phytother Res 2002;16(Suppl)1:S1-S5.

Lohr E, Garanin P, Jesau P, et al. [Anti-edemic therapy in chronic venous insufficiency with tendency to formation of edema.] Munch Med Wochenschr 1986;128:579-581.

Neiss A, Bohm C. [Demonstration of the effectiveness of the horse-chestnut-seed extract in the varicose syndrome complex.] MMW Munch Med Wochenschr 1976;118(7):213-216.

Pilz E. Odeme bei venenerkrankungen. Med Welt 1990;40:1143-1144.

Pittler MH, Ernst E. Horse-chestnut seed extract for chronic venous insufficiency: a criteria-based systematic review. Arch Dermatol 1998;134(11):1356-1360.

Pittler MH, Ernst E. Horse chestnut seed extract for chronic venous insufficiency. Cochrane Database Syst Rev. 2002;(1):CD003230.

Rehn D, Unkauf M, Klein P, et al. Comparative clinical efficacy and tolerability of oxerutins and horse chestnut extract in patients with chronic venous insufficiency. Arzneimittelforschung 1996;46(5):483-487.

Rudofsky G, et al. Odemprotektive wirkung und klinische wirksamkeit von rokastaniensamenextrakt im doppeltblindversuch. Phleb Prokto 1986;15:47-54.

Siebert U, Brach M, Sroczynski G, et al. Efficacy, routine effectiveness, and safety of horsechestnut seed extract in the treatment of chronic venous insufficiency. A meta-analysis of randomized controlled trials and large observational studies. Int Angiol 2002;21(4):305-315.

Simini B. Horse-chestnut seed extract for chronic venous insufficiency. Lancet 1996;337(9009): 1182-1183.

Steiner M. Untersuchungen zur odemvermindernden und odemprotektiven wirking von rokastaniensamenextrakt. Phlebol Prokto 1990;19:239-242.

Tiffany N, Ulbricht C, Bent S, Basch E. Horse chestnut: a multidisciplinary clinical review. J Herbal Pharmacother 2002;2(1):71-85.

Vayssairat M, Debure C, Maurel A, et al. Horse-chestnut seed extract for chronic venous insufficiency. Lancet 1996;347(9009):1182.

Horsetail
(*Equisetum arvense* L.)

RELATED TERMS

- Bottle brush, cola de caballo, common horsetail, common scouring rush, corncob plant, corn horsetail, Dutch rush, field horsetail, horse willow, horsetail grass, horsetail rush, mokuzoku, mokchok, muzei (*Equisetum hymale*), paddock pipes, pewterwort, prele, pribes des champs, running clubmoss, schachtelhalm, scouring rush, shenjincao, shave grass, toadpipe, wenjing, zinnkraut.
- Crude drugs derived from *Equisetum arvense* include wenjing, jiejiecao, and bitoucai.
- *Note: Equisetum arvense* should not be confused with species of the genus *Laminaria*, kelp, or brown algae, for which "horsetail" has been used as a synonym.

BACKGROUND

- Horsetail (*Equisetum arvense*) has traditionally been used in Europe as an oral diuretic for the treatment of edema. The German Commission E expert panel has approved horsetail for this indication. Horsetail is also occasionally used for osteoporosis, nephrolithiasis, urinary tract inflammation, and wound healing (topical). These uses have largely been based on anecdote and clinical tradition rather than scientific evidence.
- Preliminary studies in humans support the use of horsetail as a diuretic. One poorly designed trial in humans reported that horsetail increased bone density as effectively as calcium supplements.
- In theory (based on mechanism of action), horsetail ingestion in large amounts may cause thiamine deficiency, hypokalemia, or nicotine toxicity. Reported adverse effects include dermatitis.

USES BASED ON SCIENTIFIC EVIDENCE	Grade*
Diuresis (increasing urine flow) Horsetail (*Equisetum arvense*) was used in medicine in ancient Rome and Greece. The name *Equisetum* is derived from *equus*, "horse" and *seta*, "bristle." Preliminary laboratory research and studies in humans suggest that horsetail may increase the amount of urine produced by the body. More studies are needed to determine if horsetail is safe or useful for specific health conditions.	B
Osteoporosis (reduction in the amount of bone mass) Silicon may be beneficial for bone strengthening. Because horsetail contains silicon, it has been suggested as a possible natural treatment for osteoporosis. Preliminary studies in humans have reported benefits,	C

Continued

but more detailed research is needed before a firm recommendation can be made. People with osteoporosis should consult a qualified healthcare provider about possible treatment with more proven therapies.

*Key to grades: *A:* Strong scientific evidence for this use; *B:* Good scientific evidence for this use; *C:* Unclear scientific evidence for this use; *D:* Fair scientific evidence against this use (it may not work); *F:* Strong scientific evidence against this use (it likely does not work). For a more detailed explanation of efficacy criteria, see "Natural Standard Evidence-Based Validated Grading Rationale" in the Introduction.

Uses Based on Tradition, Theory, or Limited Scientific Evidence

Antibacterial, antioxidant, astringent, bladder disturbances, bleeding, brittle fingernails, cancer, cosmetics, cystic ulcers, diabetes, dropsy, fever, fluid in the lungs, frostbite, gonorrhea, gout, hair loss, itching, kidney disease, kidney stones, leg swelling, liver protection, malaria, menstrual pain, nosebleeds, prostate inflammation, Reiter's syndrome, rheumatism, stomach upset, styptic, thyroid disorders, tuberculosis, urinary incontinence, urinary tract infection, urinary tract inflammation, wound healing.

DOSING

The following doses are based on scientific research, publications, traditional use, or expert opinion. Many herbs and supplements have not been thoroughly tested, and their safety and effectiveness may not be proven. Brands may be made differently, with variable ingredients even within the same brand. The doses shown may not apply to all products. It is important to always read product labels and discuss doses with a qualified healthcare provider before therapy is started.

Standardization

- Standardization involves measuring the amounts of certain chemicals in products to try to make different preparations similar to each other. It is not always known if the chemicals being measured are the "active" ingredients.
- There is no widely recognized standardization for horsetail products. Standardization may be difficult, because approximately 25 species of *Equisetum* exist, and it is often difficult to differentiate between species. In Europe, the silicon content of horsetail may be less than 15%. Some experts recommend that horsetail should be standardized to 10% silicon per dose.

Adults (18 Years and Older)

- Recommended doses for horsetail are based on historical use or expert opinion. There are no reliable studies in humans that show horsetail to be effective or safe at any specific dose.

Oral (by Mouth)

- **Tablets/Capsules:** Different doses have been used, ranging from 300-mg capsules taken three times daily to 6 g daily.
- **Tea:** A maximum of 6 cups of tea, made from 1.5 g of dried stems steeped in 1 cup of hot water, has been used.

- **Tincture:** 1 to 4 ml of a 1:1 tincture in 25% alcohol, taken three times daily, has been used.

Topical (Applied to the Skin)

- **External wash:** A wash prepared by mixing 10 teaspoons of horsetail in cold water and soaking for 10 to 12 hours has been used.

Children (Younger Than 18 Years)

- There is insufficient scientific information to recommend the use of horsetail in children. Poisoning has been reported in children using horsetail stems as whistles.

SAFETY

The U.S. Food and Drug Administration does not strictly regulate herbs and supplements. There is no guarantee of the strength, purity, or safety of products, and effects may vary. It is important to always read product labels. People who have a medical condition, or are taking other drugs, herbs, or supplements, should consult a qualified healthcare provider before starting a new therapy. A healthcare provider should be contacted immediately about any side effects.

Allergies

- People with allergies to *E. arvense,* related substances, or nicotine should avoid the use of horsetail. Rash was reported in a person taking horsetail who was known to be sensitive to nicotine.

Side Effects and Warnings

- There are few scientific studies or reports of side effects with horsetail. It is often used in Germany and Canada, where it is traditionally considered to be safe when taken in appropriate doses. *Equisetum palustre* (marsh horsetail) contains a poisonous ingredient. It has been reported that some batches of *E. arvense* (horsetail) have been contaminated with *E. palustre.*
- Large doses of horsetail may cause symptoms of nicotine overdose, including fever, cold hands and feet, abnormal heart rate, difficulty walking, muscle weakness, and weight loss. People who smoke or use nicotine patches or nicotine gum should avoid the use of horsetail. Studies in animals and one case report of a person allergic to nicotine described a rash that occurred after the use of white horsetail. Other studies of horsetail used in animals reported nausea, increased frequency of bowel movements, increased urination, loss of the body's potassium stores, and muscle weakness. People with kidney disorders should avoid the use of horsetail.
- Studies in mice suggest that horsetail may change the activity of the kidneys, having adverse effects on control of the amount of water and potassium release. Low blood levels of potassium, which in theory may occur with horsetail, can have negative effects on the heart. People who have heart rhythm disorders or who take digoxin should exercise caution when taking horsetail. Studies suggest that horsetail does not affect blood pressure. Other horsetail species may cause low blood sugar levels.
- Horsetail contains an ingredient that destroys thiamine (vitamin B_1), which may result in deficiency with long-term use. This may cause permanent damage to the brain and nervous system, with symptoms such as confusion, difficulty in walking, difficulty with vision and eye movement, and memory loss. People with thiamine deficiency or poor nutrition in general should avoid the use of horsetail. Alcoholics are often thiamine deficient.

- The use of horsetail should be avoided because of the lack of information about its safety. Also, there have been anecdotal reports of poisoning in children who used horsetail stems as whistles.

Pregnancy and Breastfeeding

- Horsetail is not recommended for use by women who are pregnant or breast-feeding, because little information is available about its safety. Its potential to cause thiamine (vitamin B_1) depletion, low blood levels of potassium, and nicotine-like effects are of particular concern.
- *Note:* Many tinctures contain high levels of alcohol, and their use should be avoided during pregnancy.

INTERACTIONS

Most herbs and supplements have not been thoroughly tested for interactions with other herbs, supplements, drugs, or foods. The interactions listed here are based on reports in scientific publications, laboratory experiments, or traditional use. It is important to always read product labels. People who have a medical condition, or are taking other drugs, herbs, or supplements, should consult a qualified healthcare provider before starting a new therapy.

Interactions with Drugs

- Some diuretic drugs ("water pills") can cause the body to lose water and potassium—for example, loop diuretics such as furosemide (Lasix). The use of horsetail with certain diuretics may cause dehydration or further potassium deficiency. Some steroids and laxative drugs can also lower potassium levels and should not be combined with horsetail. People with heart rhythm disorders who are being treated with digoxin (Lanoxin) or digitoxin may be especially susceptible to low potassium levels, and potassium levels should be monitored in these individuals. Because horsetail can stimulate the brain and nervous system, caution should be used when combining horsetail with stimulant drugs. Other horsetail species can cause low blood sugar levels and therefore may increase the effects of diabetes medications.
- *Note:* Many tinctures contain high levels of alcohol and may cause nausea or vomiting when taken with metronidazole (Flagyl) or disulfiram (Antabuse).

Interactions with Herbs and Dietary Supplements

- Increased urine production, dehydration, or electrolyte imbalances may theoretically occur when horsetail is used with herbs that may increase urination (diuretic herbs). Examples include artichoke, celery, corn silk, couchgrass, dandelion, elder flower, juniper berry, kava, shepherd's purse, uva ursi, and yarrow. Dehydration or low potassium levels theoretically may occur if horsetail is used with laxative agents. Possible laxative herbs include alder buckthorn, aloe dried leaf sap, black root, blue flag rhizome, butternut bark, dong quai, European buckthorn, eyebright, cascara bark, castor oil, chasteberry, colocynth fruit pulp, dandelion, gamboges bark, jalap root, manna bark, plantain leaf, podophyllum root, psyllium, rhubarb, senna, wild cucumber fruit, and yellow dock root.
- In theory, low potassium levels caused by horsetail may be dangerous in people using herbs that have cardiac glycoside activity on the heart. Herbs with possible cardiac glycoside activity include adonis, balloon cotton, black hellebore root/melampode, black Indian hemp, bushman's poison, *Cactus grandifloris*, convallaria, eyebright, figwort, foxglove/digitalis, frangipani, hedge mustard, hemp root/

Canadian hemp root, king's crown, lily-of-the-valley, motherwort, oleander leaf, pheasant's eye plant, plantain leaf, pleurisy root, psyllium husks, redheaded cottonbush, rhubarb root, rubber vine, sea-mango, senna fruit, squill, strophanthus, uzara, wallflower, wintersweet, yellow dock root, and yellow oleander.

- Horsetail may break down thiamine and may cause thiamine deficiency. This has been reported only in animals, and there are no reliable reports of this interaction in humans. Other horsetail species have caused low blood sugar and therefore may increase effects of herbs and supplements that also lower blood sugar levels.

Selected References

Natural Standard developed the above evidence-based information based on a systematic review of more than 60 scientific articles. For comprehensive information about alternative and complementary therapies on the professional level, go to www.naturalstandard.com. Selected references are listed below.

Corletto F. [Female climacteric osteoporosis therapy with titrated horsetail (Equisetum arvense) extract plus calcium (osteosil calcium): randomized double blind study]. Miner Ortoped Traumatol 1999;50:201-206.

Fabre B, Geay B, Beaufils P. Thiaminase activity in *Equisetum arvense* and its extracts. Plant Med Phytother 1993;26:190-197.

Gibelli C. The hemostatic action of Equisetum. Arch Intern Pharmacodynam 1931;41:419-429.

Graefe EU, Veit M. Urinary metabolites of flavonoids and hydroxycinnamic acids in humans after application of a crude extract from Equisetum arvense. Phytomedicine 1999 Oct;6(4): 239-246.

Henderson JA, Evans EV, McIntosh RA. The antithiamine action of Equisetum. J Amer Vet Med Assoc 1952;120:375-378.

Joksic G, Stankovic M, Novak A. Antibacterial medicinal plants Equiseti herba and Ononidis radix modulate micronucleus formation in human lymphocytes *in vitro*. J Environ Pathol Toxicol Oncol 2003;22(1):41-48.

Katikova OIu, Kostin IaV, Tishkin VS. Hepatoprotective effect of plant preparations [Article in Russian]. Eksp Klin Farmakol. 2002 Jan-Feb;65(1):41-43.

Maeda H, Miyamoto K, Sano T. Occurrence of dermatitis in rats fed a cholesterol diet containing field horsetail (Equisetum arvense L.). J Nutr Sci Vitaminol (Tokyo). 1997 Oct;43(5):553-563.

Nitta A, Yoshida S, Tagaeto T. A comparative study of crude drugs in Southeast Asia. X. Crude drugs derived from Equisetum species. Chem Pharm Bull (Tokyo) 1977;25(5):1135-1139.

Perez Gutierrez RM, Laguna GY, Walkowski A. Diuretic activity of Mexican equisetum. J Ethnopharmacol 1985;14(2-3):269-272.

Revilla MC, Andrade-Cetto A, Islas S, Wiedenfeld H. Hypoglycemic effect of Equisetum myriochaetum aerial parts on type 2 diabetic patients. J Ethnopharmacol. 2002 Jun;81(1): 117-120.

Sudan BJ. Seborrhoeic dermatitis induced by nicotine of horsetails (*Equisetum arvense* L.). Contact Dermatitis 1985;13(3):201-202.

Tiktinskii OL, Bablumian IuA. Therapeutic action of Java tea and field horsetail in uric acid diathesis [Article in Russian]. Urol Nefrol (Mosk) 1983 Jan-Feb;(1):47-50.

Hoxsey Formula

BACKGROUND

- "Hoxsey formula" is a misleading name because it is not a single formula, but rather is a therapeutic regimen consisting of an oral tonic, topical (on the skin) preparations, and supportive therapy. The tonic is individualized for cancer patients based on general condition, location of cancer, and previous history of treatment. An ingredient that usually remains constant for every patient is potassium iodide. Other ingredients are then added and may include licorice, red clover, burdock, stillingia root, berberis root, pokeroot, cascara, Aromatic USP 14, prickly ash bark, and buckthorn bark. A red paste may be used, which tends to be caustic (irritating) and contains antimony trisulfide, zinc chloride, and bloodroot. A topical yellow powder may be used, and contains arsenic sulfide, talc, sulfur, and a "yellow precipitate." A clear solution may also be administered, and contains trichloroacetic acid.

USES BASED ON SCIENTIFIC EVIDENCE	Grade*
Cancer The original "Hoxsey formula" was developed in the mid-1800s, when a horse belonging to John Hoxsey was observed to recover from cancer after feeding in a field of wild plants. These plants were collected and used to create a remedy that was initially given to ill animals. Different historical accounts state various herbs included in the original formula. The formula was passed down in the Hoxsey family, and John Hoxsey's great-grandson Harry Hoxsey, an Illinois coal miner, marketed an herbal mixture for cancer and promoted himself as an herbal healer. The first Hoxsey clinic opened in the 1920s in Illinois, and Hoxsey therapy became popular for cancer in the U.S. during the 1940s and 1950s, with clinics operating in multiple states. The Hoxsey clinic in Dallas was one of the largest privately owned cancer hospitals in the world. However, after legal conflicts with the American Medical Association and U.S. Food and Drug Administration, the last U.S. clinic closed in the 1950s. The formula was passed to Mildred Nelson, a nurse in the clinic, who used the formula to open and operate a Hoxsey clinic in Tijuana, Mexico. The modern Hoxsey formula consists of a tonic taken by mouth, preparations placed on the skin, and other supportive therapies. The tonic is individualized for each patient according to cancer type and medical history. An ingredient often present is potassium iodide. Other ingredients are then added and may include licorice, red clover, burdock, stillingia root, berberis root, pokeroot, cascara, Aromatic USP	C

Continued

14, prickly ash bark, and buckthorn bark. A red paste may be used, which tends to be caustic (irritating), and contains antimony trisulfide, zinc chloride, and bloodroot. A topical yellow powder may be used, and contains arsenic sulfide, talc, sulfur, and a "yellow precipitate." A clear solution may also be administered, and contains trichloroacetic acid.
There are no well-designed human studies evaluating the safety or effectiveness of Hoxsey formula. A small number of individual human cases and case series have reported miraculous cancer cures with the treatment. However, many of the included patients did not have biopsy-proven cancer, were treated with other therapies at the same time as Hoxsey formula, still had cancer after treatment, or died. Because the formula is individualized for each patient, it is not clear which ingredient(s) may be beneficial. Without further well-designed research, a firm conclusion cannot be reached.

*Key to grades: *A:* Strong scientific evidence for this use; *B:* Good scientific evidence for this use; *C:* Unclear scientific evidence for this use; *D:* Fair scientific evidence against this use (it may not work); *F:* Strong scientific evidence against this use (it likely does not work). For a more detailed explanation of efficacy criteria, see "Natural Standard Evidence-Based Validated Grading Rationale" in the Introduction.

Uses Based on Tradition, Theory, or Limited Scientific Evidence

Breast cancer, cervical cancer, colon cancer, elimination of toxins, improving/normalizing cell metabolism, lung cancer, lymphoma, melanoma, mouth cancer, prostate cancer, sarcomas, tumor regression.

DOSING

Many herbal components of the Hoxsey formula have not been thoroughly tested, and their safety and effectiveness may not be proven. Formulas are tailored for individual patients and may be made differently, with variable ingredients even within the same formula. It is important to always read product labels and discuss doses with a qualified healthcare provider before therapy is started.

Adults (18 Years and Older)

- **Cancer:** No specific doses can be recommended, based on human use or scientific study.

Children (Younger Than 18 Years)

- There is no reliable scientific evidence to support the safe or effective use of the Hoxsey formula in children.

SAFETY

The U.S. Food and Drug Administration does not strictly regulate herbs and supplements. There is no guarantee of the strength, purity, or safety of products, and effects may vary. It is important to always read product labels. People who have a medical condition, or are taking other drugs, herbs, or supplements, should consult a qualified healthcare provider before starting a new therapy. A healthcare provider should be contacted immediately about any side effects.

Allergies

- People with known allergy/hypersensitivity to burdock root, potassium iodide, licorice, red clover, stillingia root, berberis root, pokeroot, cascara, prickly ash bark, or buckthorn bark (any of which may be contained in the oral Hoxsey tonic) should avoid the use of the Hoxsey formula.

Side Effects and Warnings

- Although no serious side effects have been reported, thorough safety studies of the Hoxsey formula have not been conducted. It is not known if concentrations of the various ingredients are great enough to cause side effects that may be associated with those ingredients when used alone in therapeutic amounts.

Pregnancy and Breastfeeding

- There is no reliable scientific study of the safety of the Hoxsey formula in women who are pregnant or breastfeeding. Therefore, use cannot be recommended.

INTERACTIONS

Most herbs and supplements have not been thoroughly tested for interactions with other herbs, supplements, drugs, or foods. It is important to always read product labels. People who have a medical condition, or are taking other drugs, herbs, or supplements, should consult a qualified healthcare provider before starting a new therapy.

Interactions with Drugs

- There is no published scientific evidence of drug interactions with the Hoxsey formula. It is not known if concentrations of the various ingredients are great enough to cause interactions that may be associated with those ingredients when used alone in therapeutic amounts. The formula may include antimony trisulfide, aromatic USP 14, arsenic sulfide, berberis root, bloodroot, buckthorn bark, burdock, licorice, pokeroot, cascara, potassium iodide, prickly ash bark, red clover, stillingia root, sulfur, talc, trichloroacetic acid, and/or zinc chloride.

Interactions with Herbs and Dietary Supplements

- There is no published scientific evidence of interactions of herbs or supplements with the Hoxsey formula. It is not known if concentrations of the various ingredients are great enough to cause interactions that may be associated with those ingredients when used alone in therapeutic amounts. The formula may include administration of antimony trisulphide, Aromatic USP 14, arsenic sulfide, berberis root, bloodroot, buckthorn bark, burdock, licorice, pokeroot, cascara, potassium iodide, prickly ash bark, red clover, stillingia root, sulfur, talc, trichloroacetic acid, and/or zinc chloride.

Interactions with Foods

- According to Mildred Nelson, who founded a Hoxsey clinic in Mexico, patients on Hoxsey therapy should not consume tomatoes, alcohol, artificial sweeteners, carbonated beverages, pork, bleached flour, salt, sugar, or vinegar to avoid negating the formula's effects. There is no available scientific evidence supporting such interactions.

Selected References

Natural Standard developed the preceding evidence-based information based on a systematic review of the published literature. For comprehensive information about alternative and complementary therapies on the professional level, go to www.naturalstandard.com. Selected references are listed here.

Austin S, Baumgartner E, DeKadt S. Long term follow-up of cancer patients using Contreras, Hoxsey and Gerson therapies. J Naturopathic Med 1995; 5(1):74-76.

Gebland H. The Hoxsey treatment. Unconventional Cancer Treatments. Washington, DC: U.S. Government Printing Office, 1990:75-81.

Hartwell JL. Plants used against cancer. A survey. Lloydia 1971;34(1):103-160.

Morton JF. Medicinal plants—old and new. Bull Med Libr Assoc 1968;56(2):161-167.

Kava

(*Piper methysticum* G. Forst)

RELATED TERMS

- Ava, ava pepper, ava pepper shrub, ava root, awa, cavain, gea, gi, intoxicating long pepper, intoxicating pepper, kao, kavakava, kava kava rhizome, kavapiper, kavarod, kava root, kavain, kave-kave, kawa, kawa kawa, kawa pepper, kawa pfeffer, kew, malohu, maluk, maori kava, meruk, milik, pepe kava, piperis methystici rhizoma, rauschpfeffer, rhizoma piperis methystici, sakua, tonga, yagona, yangona, yaqona.

BACKGROUND

- Kava beverages, made from dried roots of the shrub *Piper methysticum*, have been used ceremonially and socially in the South Pacific for hundreds of years, and in Europe since the 1700s. Currently, pharmaceutical preparations of the herb are widely used in Europe and the United States as anxiolytics but have recently been withdrawn from several European markets because of safety concerns.
- Several well-conducted human trials and a meta-analysis have demonstrated kava's efficacy in the treatment of anxiety, with effects observed after as few as one or two doses, and progressive improvement over 1 to 4 weeks. Preliminary evidence suggests possible equivalence to benzodiazepines.
- Many experts believe that kava is neither sedating nor tolerance-forming in recommended doses. Some trials report occasional mild sedation, although preliminary data from small studies suggest lack of neurologic-or psychologic impairment.
- There is growing concern regarding the potential hepatotoxicity of kava. More than 30 cases of liver damage have been reported in Europe, including hepatitis, cirrhosis, and fulminant liver failure. Kava has been removed from shelves in several countries because of safety concerns. The U.S. Food and Drug Administration has issued warnings to consumers and physicians. It is not clear what dose or duration of use is correlated with the risk of liver damage. The quality of these case reports has been variable; several are vague, describe use of products that do not actually list kava as an ingredient, or include patients who also ingest large quantities of alcohol. Nonetheless, caution is warranted.
- Chronic or heavy use of kava has been associated with cases of neurotoxicity, pulmonary hypertension, and dermatologic changes. Most trials in humans have been less than 2 months, with the longest study being 6 months in duration.

USES BASED ON SCIENTIFIC EVIDENCE	Grade*
Anxiety Studies in humans have found at least moderate benefit of kava in the treatment of anxiety, and preliminary evidence suggests that kava may be equivalent to benzodiazepine drugs such as diazepam (Valium). In one study, kava's effects were reported to be similar to those of the	A

Continued

prescription drug buspirone (BuSpar) when used for generalized anxiety disorder (GAD). However, there is concern regarding kava's potential toxicity, based on multiple reports of liver damage in Europe and a number of cases in the United States, including hepatitis, cirrhosis, and liver failure. The U.S. Food and Drug Administration has issued warnings to consumers and physicians. Many products containing kava have been pulled from the market.

*Key to grades: *A:* Strong scientific evidence for this use; *B:* Good scientific evidence for this use; *C:* Unclear scientific evidence for this use; *D:* Fair scientific evidence against this use (it may not work); *F:* Strong scientific evidence against this use (it likely does not work). For a more detailed explanation of efficacy criteria, see "Natural Standard Evidence-Based Validated Grading Rationale" in the Introduction.

Uses Based on Tradition, Theory, or Limited Scientific Evidence

Anesthesia, anorexia, antifungal, antipsychotic, aphrodisiac, arthritis, asthma, birth control, brain damage, cancer, colds, cystitis, depression, diuretic, dizziness, gonorrhea, hemorrhoids, infections, jet lag, joint pain and stiffness, kidney disorders, leprosy, menopause, menstrual disorders, migraine headache, pain, premenstrual syndrome (PMS), premenstrual dysphoric disorder (PMDD), seizures, spasm, stomach upset, syphilis, toothache, tuberculosis, urinary tract disorders, uterus inflammation, vaginal prolapse, vaginitis, weight reduction, wound healing.

DOSING

The following doses are based on scientific research, publications, traditional use, or expert opinion. Many herbs and supplements have not been thoroughly tested, and their safety and effectiveness may not be proven. Brands may be made differently, with variable ingredients even within the same brand. The doses shown may not apply to all products. It is important to always read product labels and discuss doses with a qualified healthcare provider before therapy is started.

Standardization

- Standardization involves measuring the amounts of certain chemicals in products to try to make different preparations similar to each other. It is not always known if the chemicals being measured are the "active" ingredients.
- Kava extract typically is standardized to 30% kava lactones. The actual lactone content of the root can vary between 3% and 20%. Many brands use the standardized preparation WS 1490. A review of standardized kava brands in the United States found 50 to 110 mg of kava lactones per tablet/capsule. Actual (measured) and labeled amounts of kava lactones were approximately equal in 13 products.

Adults (18 Years and Older)

- **Anxiety:** 300 mg of kava extract daily (standardized WS 1490 preparation) taken by mouth in three divided doses has been found beneficial in studies in humans. Typical doses range from 70 to 280 mg of kava lactones daily, as a single bedtime dose or in divided doses, using a lower dose first and increasing slowly if necessary. Doses as high as 800 mg daily of kava extract have been taken for short periods but have not been studied over the long term, and safety is not clear.

Children (Younger Than 18 Years)

- There is insufficient scientific evidence to recommend the use of kava in children.

SAFETY

The U.S. Food and Drug Administration does not strictly regulate herbs and supplements. There is no guarantee of the strength, purity, or safety of products, and effects may vary. It is important to always read product labels. People who have a medical condition, or are taking other drugs, herbs, or supplements, should consult a qualified healthcare provider before starting a new therapy. A healthcare provider should be contacted immediately about any side effects.

Allergies

- Allergic skin rashes have occasionally been reported.

Side Effects and Warnings

- Until recently, kava was generally believed to be safe when used over short periods of time (1 to 2 months) at recommended doses. Two brief studies of several thousand patients taking either 105 mg daily of a 75% kavalactone extract or 800 mg daily of a 30% kavalactone extract reported side effects in only a small number of subjects (1.5% to 2.3%). Side effects were primarily gastrointestinal (stomach) upset, allergic rash, and mild headache. However, more recently there have been numerous reports of severe liver problems in people using kava. More than 25 cases have been reported in Europe of liver toxicity, including liver failure, following use of kava. Two cases in Switzerland involved a specific brand (Leitan, Schwabe, Germany). In heavy kava users, abnormal blood levels of liver enzymes have occurred. It is not clear what dose or duration of use may raise the risk of liver damage, in part because most case reports have been vague or included patients who also drink large amounts of alcohol. The U.S. Food and Drug Administration has issued warnings to consumers and physicians, and has requested that physicians report cases of liver toxicity that may be related to kava use.
- Although many natural medicine experts believe that kava is safe at recommended doses, there is not enough scientific information to draw a clear conclusion. Kava should be used only under the supervision of a qualified healthcare provider, should never be taken above recommended doses, and should be avoided by people with liver problems or taking drugs that affect the liver.
- Other serious side effects have been observed with chronic or heavy use of kava, including skin disorders, blood abnormalities, abnormal muscle movements, apathy, kidney damage, seizures, psychotic syndromes, and increased blood pressure in the lungs (pulmonary hypertension). Skin disorders observed with chronic use of kava are commonly called "kava dermopathy" (or *kani* in Fiji). Dry, scaly skin or yellow skin discoloration may occur. The effects seem to be reversible upon stopping use. Blood disorders observed with chronic and heavy kava use include increased red blood cell size, reduced blood platelet size, reduced white blood cell numbers, and reduced blood protein levels. Blood in the urine has also been reported.
- Several cases of people with abnormal muscle movements have been reported after short-term use of kava (1 to 4 days), including tightening, twisting, or locking of

the muscles of the mouth, neck (torticollis) and eyes (oculogyric crisis). Worsening of symptoms of Parkinson's disease, as well as abnormal whole body movements (choreoathetosis), following high doses of kava have also been noted. Tremor, poor coordination, headache, drowsiness, and fatigue have uncommonly been reported, particularly with large doses. Muscle cell breakdown (rhabdomyolysis) was reported in a 29-year-old man after taking an herbal combination of ginkgo, guarana, and kava.

- Sedation (drowsiness) has occasionally been reported with kava use, although there is early evidence from several small studies in humans that kava may not significantly cause this effect. In two studies, no effect of kava on motor vehicle driving performance was found. However, there were two cases in the state of California of drivers being arrested for "driving under the influence" after drinking kava tea (neither case resulted in successful prosecution). Because this issue remains unclear, use of kava is not recommended in people who are driving or operating heavy machinery.
- Eye disturbances and irritation have rarely been associated with chronic or heavy kava use. There is one report of impaired eye focus, and increased pupil size following one-time use of kava. Rapid heart rate, electrocardiogram abnormalities, and shortness of breath have been reported in heavy kava users, perhaps related to abnormally high blood pressure in the lungs (pulmonary hypertension). Laboratory studies suggest that kava may increase the risk of bleeding through effects on blood platelets. However, evidence in humans is lacking in this area, and there are no reports of significant bleeding in the scientific literature.

Pregnancy and Breastfeeding

- Use of kava cannot be recommended in women who are pregnant. There may be a decrease in the muscle strength of the uterus with the use of kava, which may have harmful effects on pregnancy. Chemicals in kava may pass into breast milk, with unknown effects, and therefore this herb should be avoided in women who are breastfeeding.

INTERACTIONS

Most herbs and supplements have not been thoroughly tested for interactions with other herbs, supplements, drugs, or foods. The interactions listed here are based on reports in scientific publications, laboratory experiments, or traditional use. It is important to always read product labels. People who have a medical condition, or are taking other drugs, herbs, or supplements, should consult a qualified healthcare provider before starting a new therapy.

Interactions with Drugs

- Based on multiple reports of liver toxicity in humans, including hepatitis, cirrhosis, and liver failure, theoretically there is an increased risk of liver damage if kava is taken with drugs that may injure the liver, such as anabolic steroids, amiodarone, methotrexate, acetaminophen (Tylenol), and antifungal medications taken by mouth (e.g., ketoconazole).
- In theory, kava may increase the effects of alcohol and drugs that cause sedation (drowsiness). Examples of such drugs are barbiturates such as phenobarbital, and benzodiazepines such as lorazepam (Ativan) and diazepam (Valium). Lethargy and confusion were reported in a 54-year-old man taking kava with the benzodiazepine alprazolam (Xanax).

- In theory, kava may interfere with the effects of dopamine or drugs that are similar to dopamine, and may worsen the neurologic side effects of drugs that block dopamine such as haloperidol (Haldol) and metoclopramide (Reglan).
- Kava may have chemical properties similar to those of antidepressant drugs called monoamine oxidase inhibitors (MAOIs). Thus, theoretically kava may add to the effects of MAOI antidepressants such as isocarboxazid (Marplan), phenelzine (Nardil), and tranylcypromine (Parnate). Because of this possible effect, kava may prolong the effects of anesthesia, and some practitioners recommend stopping the use of kava 2 to 3 days before surgery.
- Laboratory studies suggest that kava may increase the risk of bleeding through its effects on blood platelets. However, evidence from studies in humans is lacking in this area, and there are no reports of significant bleeding in the scientific literature. People using anticoagulants (blood thinners) such as warfarin (Coumadin) and heparin, antiplatelet drugs such as clopidogrel (Plavix), or aspirin should be aware of possible interactions.

Interactions with Herbs and Dietary Supplements

- Based on multiple human reports of liver toxicity, including hepatitis, cirrhosis, and liver failure, theoretically there is an increased risk of liver damage if kava is taken with herbs or supplements that may injure the liver. Examples of such agents are ackee, bee pollen, birch oil, blessed thistle, borage, bush tea, butterbur, chaparral, coltsfoot, comfrey, dehydroepiandrosterone (DHEA), *Echinacea purpurea*, *Echium* spp., germander, *Heliotropium* spp., horse chestnut, jin-bu-huan (*Lycopodium serratum*), lobelia, L-tetrahydropalmatine (THP), mate, niacin (vitamin B_3), niacinamide, Paraguay tea, periwinkle, *Plantago lanceolata*, pride of Madeira, rue, sassafras, scullcap, *Senecio* spp./groundsel, tansy ragwort, turmeric/curcumin, tu-san-chi (*Gynura segetum*), uva ursi, and valerian.
- In theory, kava may increase the sedation (drowsiness) caused by some herbs and supplements. Examples of agents with possible sedative effects are calamus, calendula, California poppy, catnip, capsicum, celery, couch grass, dogwood, elecampane, German chamomile, goldenseal, gotu kola, hops, lemon balm, melatonin, sage, sassafras, scullcap, shepherd's purse, Siberian ginseng, stinging nettle, St. John's wort, valerian, wild carrot, wild lettuce, withania root, and yerba mansa.
- Kava may have chemical properties similar to those of antidepressant drugs called monoamine oxidase inhibitors (MAOIs). In theory, kava may add to the effects of herbs and supplements with possible MAOI activity, such as chromium, dehydroepiandrosterone (DHEA), DL-phenylalanine (DLPA), ephedra, evening primrose oil, fenugreek, *Ginkgo biloba*, hops, 5-hydroxytryptophan (5-HTP), *S*-adenosylmethionine (SAMe), St. John's wort, tyrosine, valerian, vitamin B_6, and yohimbe, as well as homeopathic remedies such as aurum metcallicum, kali bromatum, and sepia.
- Laboratory studies suggest that kava may increase the risk of bleeding through its effects on blood platelets. However, evidence from studies in humans is lacking in this area, and there are no published reports available of significant bleeding. People using other herbs or supplements that may increase the risk of bleeding should consult a qualified healthcare provider before starting kava. Multiple cases of bleeding have been reported with the use of *Ginkgo biloba*, fewer cases with garlic, and two cases with saw palmetto. Numerous other agents may theoretically increase the risk of bleeding, although this has not been proven in most cases.

Examples of such agents are alfalfa, American ginseng, angelica, anise, *Arnica montana*, asafetida, aspen bark, bilberry, birch, black cohosh, bladderwrack, bogbean, boldo, borage seed oil, bromelain, capsicum, cat's claw, celery, chamomile, chaparral, clove, coleus, cordyceps, danshen, devil's claw, dong quai, evening primrose, fenugreek, feverfew, flaxseed/flax powder (not a concern with flaxseed oil), ginger, grapefruit juice, grape seed, green tea, guggul, gymnestra, horse chestnut, horseradish, licorice root, lovage root, male fern, meadowsweet, nor-dihydroguaiaretic acid (NDGA), onion, *Panax ginseng*, papain, parsley, passion flower, poplar, prickly ash, propolis, quassia, red clover, reishi, rue, Siberian ginseng, sweet birch, sweet clover, turmeric, vitamin E, white willow, wild carrot, wild lettuce, willow, wintergreen, and yucca.
- There has been one self-report of nausea, sweating, muscle cramping, weakness and increased pulse and blood pressure after a single dose of a combination of St. John's wort, kava, and valerian.

Interactions with Foods

- Kava may have chemical properties similar to a type of antidepressant drug called monoamine oxidase inhibitors (MAOIs). Foods that contain tyramine or tryptophan may cause dangerously high blood pressure when taken with drugs, herbs, or supplements with MAOI properties. In the case of kava, this is theoretical, and no reliable reports of human cases have been reported. Examples of foods that may react with MAOIs are anchovies, avocados, bananas, bean curd, beer, caffeine (large amounts), caviar, champagne, cheeses (particularly aged, processed, and strong varieties), chocolate, dry sausage/salami/bologna, fava beans, figs, liver (particularly chicken), meat tenderizers, papaya, pickled herring, protein extracts/powder, raisins, shrimp paste, sour cream, soy sauce, wine (particularly chianti), yeast extracts, and yogurt.

Selected References

Natural Standard developed the preceding evidence-based information based on a systematic review of more than 400 scientific articles. For comprehensive information about alternative and complementary therapies on the professional level, go to www.naturalstandard.com. Selected references are listed here.

Abebe W. Herbal medication: potential for adverse interactions with analgesic drugs. J Clin Pharm Ther 2002;27(6):391-401.

Almeida JC, Grimsley EW. Coma from the health food store: interaction between kava and alprazolam. Ann Intern Med 1996;125(11):940-941.

Boerner RJ, Sommer H, Berger W, et al. Kava-Kava extract LI 150 is as effective as Opipramol and Buspirone in Generalised Anxiety Disorder—an 8-week randomized, double-blind multi-centre clinical trial in 129 out-patients. Phytomedicine 2003;10(Suppl 4):38-49.

Brauer RB, Stangl M, Stewart JR, et al. Acute liver failure after administration of herbal tranquilizer kava-kava (*Piper methysticum*). J Clin Psychiatry 2003;64(2):216-218.

Bujanda L, Palacios A, Silvarino R, et al. Kava-induced acute icteric hepatitis [article in Spanish]. Gastroenterol Hepatol 2002;25(6):434-435.

Cagnacci A, Arangino S, Renzi A, et al. Kava-Kava administration reduces anxiety in perimenopausal women. Maturitas 2003;44(2):103-109.

Cairney S, Clough AR, Maruff P, et al. Saccade and cognitive function in chronic kava users. Neuropsychopharmacology. 2003;28(2):389-396.

Campo JV, McNabb J, Perel JM, et al. Kava-induced fulminant hepatic failure. J Am Acad Child Adolesc Psychiatry 2002;41(6):631-632.

Clough AR, Wang Z, Bailie RS, et al. Case-control study of the association between kava use

and pneumonia in eastern Arnhem and Aboriginal communities (Northern Territory, Australia). Epidemiol Infect 2003;131(1):627-635.
Clough AR, Jacups SP, Wang Z, et al. Health effects of kava use in an eastern Arnhem Land Aboriginal community. Intern Med J 2003;33(8):336-340.
Connor KM, Davidson JR. A placebo-controlled study of Kava kava in generalized anxiety disorder. Int Clin Psychopharmacol 2002;17(4):185-188.
Cropley M, Cave Z, Ellis J, Middleton RW. Effect of kava and valerian on human physiological and psychological responses to mental stress assessed under laboratory conditions. Phytother Res 2002;16(1):23-27.
Currie BJ, Clough AR. Kava hepatotoxicity with Western herbal products: does it occur with traditional kava use? Med J Aust 2003;178(9):421-422. Comment in: Med J Aust 2003; 178(9):442-443 and Med J Aust 2003;178(9):451-453.
De Smet PA. Safety concerns about kava not unique. Lancet 2002;360(9342):1336. Comment in: Lancet 2002;359(9320):1865.
Dietlein G, Schroder-Bernhardi D. Doctors' prescription behaviour regarding dosage recommendations for preparations of kava extracts. Pharmacoepidemiol Drug Saf 2003;12(5): 417-421.
Ernst E. Safety concerns about kava. Lancet 2002;359(9320):1865. Comment in: Lancet 2002; 360(9342):1336.
Escher M, Desmeules J, Giostra E, et al. Hepatitis associated with kava, a herbal remedy for anxiety. BMJ 2001;322(7279):139.
Estes JD, Stolpman D, Olyaei A, et al. High prevalence of potentially hepatotoxic herbal supplement use in patients with fulminant hepatic failure. Arch Surg 2003;138(8):852-858.
Garrett KM, Basmadjian G, Khan IA, et al. Extracts of kava (*Piper methysticum*) induce acute anxiolytic-like behavioral changes in mice. Psychopharmacology (Berl) 2003 [Epub ahead of print].
Girman A, Lee R, Kligler B. An integrative medicine approach to premenstrual syndrome. Am J Obstet Gynecol 2003;188(5 Suppl):S56-S65.
Gow PJ, Connelly NJ, Hill RL, et al. Fatal fulminant hepatic failure induced by a natural therapy containing kava. Med J Aust 2003;178(9):442-443. Comment in: Med J Aust 2003; 178(9):421-422.
Jappe U, Franke I, Reinhold D, et al. Sebotropic drug reaction resulting from kava-kava extract therapy: a new entity? J Am Acad Dermatol 1998;38(1):104-106.
Humberston CL, Akhtar J, Krenzelok EP. Acute hepatitis induced by kava kava. J Toxicol Clin Toxicol. 2003;41(2):109-113.
Pittler MH, Ernst E. Efficacy of kava extract for treating anxiety: systematic review and meta-analysis. J Clin Psychopharmacol 2000;20(1):84-89.
Russmann S, Lauterburg BH, Helbling A. Kava hepatotoxicity. Ann Intern Med 2001; 135(1):68-69.
Scherer J. Kava-kava extract in anxiety disorders: an outpatient observational study. Adv Ther 1998;15(4):261-269.
Schmidt P, Boehncke WH. Delayed-type hypersensitivity reaction to kava-kava extract. Contact Dermatitis 2000;42(6):363-364.
Spillane PK, Fisher DA, Currie BJ. Neurological manifestations of kava intoxication. Med J Aust 1997;167(3):172-173.
Stafford N. Germany may ban kava kava herbal supplement. Reuter's News Service, Germany, Nov. 19, 2001.
Volz HP, Kieser M. Kava-kava extract WS 1490 versus placebo in anxiety disorders: a randomized placebo-controlled 25-week outpatient trial. Pharmacopsychiatry 1997; 30(1):1-5.

Lavender

(*Lavandula angustifolia* Miller)

RELATED TERMS

- Common lavender, English lavender, garden lavender, *Lavandula burnamii, Lavandula dentate, Lavandula dhofarensis, Lavandula latifolia*, *Lavandula officinalis* L., *Lavandula stoechas*, limonene, perillyl alcohol (POH), pink lavender, true lavender, white lavender.

BACKGROUND

- Lavender is native to the Mediterranean, the Arabian Peninsula, Russia, and Africa. It has been used cosmetically and medicinally throughout history. In modern times, lavender is cultivated around the world and the fragrant oils of its flowers are used in aromatherapy, baked goods, candles, cosmetics, detergents, jellies, massage oils, perfumes, powders, shampoo, soap, and tea. English lavender (*L. angustifolia*) is the most common species of lavender, although other species are used, including *Lavandula burnamii, L. dentate, L. dhofarensis, L. latifolia*, and *L. stoechas.*
- Many people find lavender aromatherapy to be relaxing, and in several small, methodologically flawed trials it was reported to have anxiolytic effects. Overall, the weight of the evidence suggests a small positive effect, although additional data from well-designed studies are required before the evidence can be considered strong.
- Lavender aromatherapy is also used as a hypnotic, although there is insufficient evidence in support of this use.
- Small phase-I trials in humans of the lavender constituent perillyl alcohol (POH) as cancer therapy have reported safety and tolerability (up to 1200 mg per square meter of body surface, four times daily), although efficacy has not been demonstrated.

USES BASED ON SCIENTIFIC EVIDENCE	Grade*
Anxiety (lavender aromatherapy) Lavender aromatherapy is traditionally used for relaxation. In several small studies, it was reported to help relieve anxiety. However, negative results were reported in other studies. Better-quality research is needed before a strong recommendation can be made.	B
Antibacterial (lavender used on the skin) Preliminary laboratory studies suggest that lavender oils may have antibiotic activity. However, this has not been well tested in studies in animals and humans.	C

Continued

Cancer (perillyl alcohol) Studies in animals suggest that perillyl alcohol (POH), derived from lavender, may be beneficial in the treatment of some types of cancer. This research has focused on cancers of the pancreas, breast, and intestine. Preliminary small studies in humans suggest safety and tolerability of POH, but effectiveness has not been established.	C
Dementia Small, randomized controlled trials investigating the effects of lavender aromatherapy on agitation and behavior in patients with Alzheimer's dementia reported conflicting results. Better-quality studies are necessary before a firm conclusion can be drawn.	C
Depression Preliminary research suggests that lavender may be helpful as an adjunct to prescription antidepressant medications. Additional research is necessary before a firm conclusion can be drawn.	C
Hypnotic/sleep aid (lavender aromatherapy) Lavender aromatherapy is often promoted as a sleep aid. Although early evidence suggests possible benefits, more research is needed before a firm conclusion can be drawn.	C
Perineal discomfort after childbirth (lavender added to bath) Lavender has been evaluated as an additive to bathwater to relieve pain in the perineal area (between the vagina and anus) in women after childbirth. Preliminary, poor-quality research reports no benefits. Better-quality research is needed before a firm conclusion can be drawn.	C

*Key to grades: *A:* Strong scientific evidence for this use; *B:* Good scientific evidence for this use; *C:* Unclear scientific evidence for this use; *D:* Fair scientific evidence against this use (it may not work); *F:* Strong scientific evidence against this use (it likely does not work). For a more detailed explanation of efficacy criteria, see "Natural Standard Evidence-Based Validated Grading Rationale" in the Introduction.

Uses Based on Tradition, Theory, or Limited Scientific Evidence

Acne, antifungal, anti-inflammatory, antioxidant, anxiety, aphrodisiac, appetite stimulant, asthma, bronchitis, carpal tunnel syndrome, circulation problems, colic, common cold, diabetes, diuretic, dizziness, douche, exercise recovery, fatigue, fever, flatulence (gas), hair loss, hangover, heartburn, HIV infection, indigestion, infertility, insect repellent, lice, low blood pressure, menopause, menstrual period problems, migraine headache, minor burns, motion sickness, muscle spasm, nausea, neuroprotection, pain, parasites/worms, psychosis, seizures/epilepsy, snake repellent, sores, sprains, tension headache, toothache, varicose veins, vomiting, wound healing.

L

DOSING

The following doses are based on scientific research, publications, traditional use, or expert opinion. Many herbs and supplements have not been thoroughly tested, and their safety and effectiveness may not be proven. Brands may be made differently, with variable ingredients even within the same brand. The doses shown may not apply to all products. It is important to always read product labels and discuss doses with a qualified healthcare provider before therapy is started.

Adults (18 Years and Older)

- **Tea:** 1 to 2 teaspoons (5 to 10 g) of lavender leaves steeped in 1 cup (250 ml) of boiling water for 15 minutes has been used.
- **Inhalation (aromatherapy):** 2 to 4 drops of lavender oil is placed in 2 to 3 cups of boiling water, and the vapors are inhaled. This can be repeated daily or as needed.
- **Bath additive:** To reduce perineal discomfort after childbirth, 6 drops of lavender oil are added to a bath. Another technique is to add ¼ to ½ cup of dried lavender flowers to hot bath water.
- **Massage therapy:** A technique that has been used is to add 1 to 4 drops of lavender oil per tablespoon of base massage oil.
- **Cancer therapy:** Doses of 800 to 1200 mg of perillyl alcohol (POH) per square meter of body surface have been taken by mouth, four times daily, in a 50:50 POH:soybean oil preparation.

Children (Younger Than 18 years)

- There is insufficient scientific evidence regarding the safety of lavender to recommend its use in children.

SAFETY

The U.S. Food and Drug Administration does not strictly regulate herbs and supplements. There is no guarantee of the strength, purity, or safety of products, and effects may vary. It is important to always read product labels. People who have a medical condition, or are taking other drugs, herbs, or supplements, should consult a qualified healthcare provider before starting a new therapy. A healthcare provider should be contacted immediately about any side effects.

Allergies

- People with allergies to lavender may experience skin irritation after contact and should avoid lavender in all forms.

Side Effects and Warnings

- Mild rash can develop after applying lavender oil. Reports describe increased sun sensitivity and changes in skin pigmentation after applying products containing lavender oil. Nausea, vomiting, loss of appetite, constipation, headache, chills, confusion, and drowsiness are sometimes reported after inhaling lavender or absorbing it through the skin, or after large doses of lavender (more than 5 g daily) or perillyl alcohol (POH) (derived from lavender) are taken by mouth. The essential oil of lavender may be poisonous if taken by mouth.
- Drowsiness may occur after lavender aromatherapy. More severe drowsiness or sedation may occur when lavender is used with other sedating agents. Caution is advised in people who are driving or operating heavy machinery.
- In theory, lavender taken by mouth may increase the risk of bleeding. Caution is advised in people with bleeding disorders or taking drugs that may increase bleeding. Dosing adjustments may be necessary.

- Some cancer patients have experienced low blood cell counts (neutropenia) after taking high doses of perillyl alcohol (POH) by mouth.

Pregnancy and Breastfeeding

- Studies regarding the safety of lavender are lacking, and therefore its use is not recommended in women who are pregnant or breastfeeding.

INTERACTIONS

Most herbs and supplements have not been thoroughly tested for interactions with other herbs, supplements, drugs, or foods. The interactions listed here are based on reports in scientific publications, laboratory experiments, or traditional use. It is important to always read product labels. People who have a medical condition, or are taking other drugs, herbs, or supplements, should consult a qualified healthcare provider before starting a new therapy.

Interactions with Drugs

- Studies suggest that lavender used as aromatherapy or by mouth may increase the amount of drowsiness caused by some drugs. Examples include alcohol, some antidepressants, barbiturates such as phenobarbital, benzodiazepines such as lorazepam (Ativan) and diazepam (Valium), and narcotics such as codeine. Drowsiness caused by some seizure medications may also be increased. Caution is advised in people who are driving or operating machinery.
- In theory, lavender may add to the effects of cholesterol-lowering drugs.
- Lavender may have additive effects when used with antidepressants such as imipramine.

L

Interactions with Herbs and Dietary Supplements

- Lavender used as aromatherapy or taken by mouth may increase the amount of drowsiness caused by some herbs or supplements. Examples of herbs that may cause sedation are calamus, calendula, California poppy, capsicum, catnip, celery, couchgrass, dogwood, elecampane, German chamomile, goldenseal, gotu kola, hops, kava, lemon balm, sage, sassafras, scullcap, shepherd's purse, Siberian ginseng, stinging nettle, St. John's wort, valerian, wild carrot, wild lettuce, withania root, and yerba mansa. Caution is advised in people who are driving or operating machinery.
- In theory, lavender may add to the cholesterol-lowering effects of some herbs or supplements, such as fish oil, garlic, guggul, and niacin.

Selected References

Natural Standard developed the preceding evidence-based information based on a systematic review of more than 150 scientific articles. For comprehensive information about alternative and complementary therapies on the professional level, go to www.naturalstandard.com. Selected references are listed here.

Akhondzadeh S, Kashani L, Fotouhi A, et al. Comparison of *Lavandula angustifolia* Mill. tincture and imipramine in the treatment of mild to moderate depression: a double-blind, randomized trial. Prog Neuropsychopharmacol Biol Psychiatry 2003;27(1):123-127.

Buyukokuroglu ME, Gepdiremen A, Hacimuftuoglu A, et al. The effects of aqueous extract of *Lavandula angustifolia* flowers in glutamate-induced neurotoxicity of cerebellar granular cell culture of rat pups. J Ethnopharmacol. 2003;84(1):91-94.

Clark L, Shivik J. Aerosolized essential oils and individual natural product compounds as brown treesnake repellents. Pest Manag Sci 2002;58(8):775-783.

Dale A, Cornwell S. The role of lavender oil in relieving perineal discomfort following childbirth: a blind randomized clinical trial. J Adv Nurs 1994;19(1):89-96.

Diego MA, Jones NA, Field T, et al. Aromatherapy positively affects mood, EEG patterns of alertness and math computations. Int J Neurosci 1998;96(3-4):217-224.

Dunn C, Sleep J, Collett D. Sensing an improvement: an experimental study to evaluate the use of aromatherapy, massage and periods of rest in an intensive care unit. J Adv Nurs 1995; 21(1):34-40.

Graham PH, Browne L, Cox H, et al. Inhalation aromatherapy during radiotherapy: results of a placebo-controlled double-blind randomized trial. J Clin Oncol 2003;21(12):2372-2376.

Gray SG, Clair AA. Influence of aromatherapy on medication administration to residential-care residents with dementia and behavioral challenges. Am J Alzheimers Dis Other Demen 2002;17(3):169-174.

Hardy M, Kirk-Smith MD, Stretch DD. Replacement of drug treatment for insomnia by ambient odour. Lancet 1995;346(8976):701.

Holmes C, Hopkins V, Hensford C, et al. Lavender oil as a treatment for agitated behaviour in severe dementia: a placebo controlled study. Int J Geriatr Psychiatry 2002;17(4):305-308.

Ripple GH, Gould MN, Arzoomanian RZ, et al. Phase I clinical and pharmacokinetic study of perillyl alcohol administered four times a day. Clin Cancer Res 2000;6(2):390-396.

Romine IJ, Bush AM, Geist CR. Lavender aromatherapy in recovery from exercise. Percept Mot Skills 1999;88(3 Pt 1):756-758.

Saeki Y. The effect of foot-bath with or without the essential oil of lavender on the autonomic nervous system: a randomized trial. Complement Ther Med 2000;8(1):2-7.

Licorice

(*Glycyrrhiza glabra* L.)

RELATED TERMS

- Bois doux, fabaceae, gan cao, glucoliquiritin, glycyrrhetenic acid, glycyrrhiza, *Glycyrrhiza uralensis,* glycyrrhizin, kanzo, lakrids, lakritzenwurzel, leguminose, licorice root, liquiritiae radix, *Liquiritia officinalis,* liquirizia, liquorice, prenyllicoflavone, radix glycyrrhizae, réglisse, sussholzwurzel, sweet root, sweet wood.

BACKGROUND

- Licorice is harvested from the root and dried rhizomes of the low-growing shrub *Glycyrrhiza glabra*. Currently, most licorice is produced in Greece, Turkey, and Asia.
- Licorice was used in ancient Greece, China, and Egypt, primarily for gastritis and ailments of the upper respiratory tract. Ancient Egyptians prepared a licorice drink for ritual use to honor spirits of the pharaohs.
- During World War II, the Dutch physician F. E. Revers observed improvement in patients with peptic ulcer disease who were taking a licorice preparation. He also noted facial and peripheral edema, sparking scientific investigation into licorice's properties and adverse effects. In the 1950s, there were reports that patients with Addison's disease had a "craving" for licorice candy, viewed by some as early evidence of steroid-modulating properties of licorice.
- In addition to its medicinal uses, licorice has been used as a flavoring agent, valued for sweetness (glycyrrhizin, a component of licorice, is 50 times sweeter than table sugar). The generic name *glycyrrhiza* stems from ancient Greek, meaning "sweet root." It was originally used as flavoring for licorice candies, although most licorice candy is now flavored with anise oil. Licorice is still used in subtherapeutic doses as a sweetening agent in herbal medicines, lozenges, and tobacco products (doses low enough that significant adverse effects are unlikely).
- Licorice has a long history of medicinal use in Europe and Asia. At high doses, potentially severe side effects have been reported, including high blood pressure, hypokalemia (low blood potassium levels) and fluid retention. Most adverse effects have been attributed to the chemical component glycyrrhiza (or glycyrrhizic acid). Licorice can be processed to remove the glycyrrhiza, resulting in deglycyrrhizinated licorice (DGL), which does not appear to have the metabolic disadvantages of unprocessed licorice.
- In Europe, licorice has most often been used to treat cough, bronchitis, gastritis, and peptic ulcer disease. In Chinese medicine, it is felt to benefit *qi*, reduce "fire poison" (sore throat, skin eruptions), and diminish "heat." Specific conditions treated by Chinese herbalists include abdominal pain, abscesses and sores, gastric and duodenal ulcers, pharyngitis, malaria, and tuberculosis,. In Ayurveda (traditional medicine practice in India), licorice is believed to be effective in the treatment of constipation, inflamed joints, peptic ulcer disease, and diseases of the eye.

USES BASED ON SCIENTIFIC EVIDENCE	Grade
Aphthous ulcers/canker sores Some research studies suggested that the licorice extracts deglycyrrhizinated licorice (DGL) and carbenoxolone may be beneficial in the treatment of canker sores. However, the studies were small, with design flaws. The safety of DGL makes it an attractive therapy, but it is not clear at this time whether there is truly any benefit.	C
Bleeding stomach ulcers caused by aspirin Although there has been some study of DGL in this area, it is not clear what effects DGL has on gastrointestinal bleeding.	C
Familial Mediterranean fever (FMF) A small clinical pilot study and laboratory study of a multi-ingredient preparation containing licorice, called Immunoguard, suggests possible effects in the management of FMF. Well-designed studies of licorice alone are necessary before a recommendation can be made.	C
Herpes simplex virus infection Laboratory studies have found that DGL may hinder the spread and infection of herpes simplex virus. Studies in humans have been small, but they suggest that topical application of carbenoxolone cream may improve healing and prevent recurrence.	C
High potassium levels resulting from hypoaldosteronism In theory, because of the known effects of licorice, there may be some benefits of licorice in the treatment of high potassium levels caused by hypoaldosteronism (abnormally low aldosterone levels). There is early evidence in humans in support of this use. However, research is preliminary and a qualified healthcare provider should supervise treatment.	C
Peptic ulcer disease The licorice extracts DGL and carbenoxolone have been studied for treatment of peptic ulcers. DGL (but not carbenoxolone) may offer some benefits. However, these studies have been small, with design flaws, and results of different studies have disagreed. Therefore, it is unclear whether there is any benefit from licorice for this condition.	C
Viral hepatitis The licorice extracts DGL and carbenoxolone have been proposed as possible therapies for viral hepatitis. Studies in animals have investigated the mechanism of licorice in hepatitis, and studies in humans have shown some benefits with a patented intravenous licorice preparation that is not available in the United States. Studies using oral licorice have been small, with design flaws. Therefore, it is not clear whether there is any benefit from oral licorice for hepatitis treatment.	C
Genital herpes Available studies have not found any benefit from carbenoxolone cream when applied topically (to the skin) to treat genital herpes infections.	D

Uses Based on Tradition, Theory, or Limited Scientific Evidence

Adrenal insufficiency (Addison's disease), antimicrobial, antioxidant, antispasmodic, aplastic anemia, asthma, bacterial infections, bad breath, body fat reducer, bronchitis, cancer, chronic fatigue syndrome, colitis, colorectal cancer, constipation, coronavirus, cough, dental hygiene, depression, detoxification, diabetes, diuretic, diverticulitis, dropped head syndrome, eczema, Epstein-Barr virus infection, fever, gastroesophageal reflux disease, gentamicin-induced kidney damage, graft healing, high cholesterol, HIV infection, hormone regulation, inflammation, inflammatory skin disorders, laryngitis, liver protection, lung cancer, menopausal symptoms, metabolic abnormalities, methicillin-resistant *Staphylococcus aureus*, muscle cramps, obesity, osteoarthritis, plaque, polycystic ovarian syndrome, rheumatoid arthritis, severe acute respiratory syndrome (SARS), skin disorders, sore throat, stomach upset, urinary tract inflammation.

L

DOSING

The following doses are based on scientific research, publications, traditional use, or expert opinion. Many herbs and supplements have not been thoroughly tested, and their safety and effectiveness may not be proven. Brands may be made differently, with variable ingredients even within the same brand. The doses shown may not apply to all products. It is important to always read product labels and discuss doses with a qualified healthcare provider before therapy is started.

Standardization

- Standardization involves measuring the amounts of certain chemicals in products to try to make different products similar to each other. It is not always known if the chemicals being measured are the "active" ingredients.
- The expert panel German Commission E recommends that licorice be used for only 4 to 6 weeks unless it is administered under direct medical supervision. However, this is based on the use of relatively large daily doses (5 to 15 g daily). Many experts believe that extended treatments may be safe if lower doses are used. In a 4-week study in healthy individuals, recommended doses were well tolerated, with few adverse effects. There are no standard or well-studied doses of licorice, and many different doses are used traditionally.

Adults (18 Years and Older)

- **Licorice powdered root (4% to 9% glycyrrhizin):** Doses of 1 to 4 g taken by mouth daily, divided into three or four doses, have been used.
- **Licorice fluid extract (10% to 20% glycyrrhizin):** Doses of 2 to 4 ml daily have been taken by mouth.
- **DGL extract tablets:** Doses of 380 to 1140 mg three times daily taken by mouth 20 minutes before meals have been used.
- **Carbenoxolone gel or cream:** A 2% cream or gel has been applied five times a day for 7 to 14 days for herpes simplex virus skin lesions.

Children (Younger Than 18 Years)

- Licorice is not recommended for use in children because of potential side effects.

SAFETY

The U.S. Food and Drug Administration does not strictly regulate herbs and supplements. There is no guarantee of the strength, purity, or safety of products, and effects may vary. It is important to always read product labels. People who have a medical condition, or are taking other drugs, herbs, or supplements, should consult a qualified healthcare provider before starting a new therapy. A healthcare provider should be contacted immediately about any side effects.

Allergies

- People should avoid the use of licorice if they have a known allergy to licorice, any component of licorice, or any member of the Fabaceae (Leguminosae) plant family (pea family). In one case report, a rash occurred after application of a cosmetic product containing licorice to the skin.

Side Effects and Warnings

- Licorice contains a chemical called glycyrrhizic acid, which is responsible for many of its reported side effects. Deglycyrrhizinated licorice (DGL) has had the glycyrrhizic acid removed and therefore is considered safer for use.
- Many of the adverse effects of licorice result from actions on hormone levels in the body. By altering the activities of certain hormones, licorice may cause electrolyte disturbances. Possible effects include sodium and fluid retention, low potassium levels, and metabolic alkalosis.
- Licorice has been reported to cause dangerously high blood pressure with symptoms such as headache, nausea, vomiting, and hypertensive encephalopathy with stroke-like effects (for example, one-sided weakness).
- Electrolyte abnormalities may also lead to irregular heartbeats, heart attack, kidney damage, muscle weakness, and muscle breakdown. Licorice should be used cautiously by people with congestive heart failure, coronary heart disease, kidney or liver disease, fluid retention (edema), high blood pressure, underlying electrolyte disturbances, or hormonal abnormalities, and by people taking diuretics.
- Hormonal imbalances have been reported with the use of licorice, such as abnormally low testosterone levels in men and high prolactin and estrogen levels in women. These adverse effects may reduce fertility or cause menstrual abnormalities.
- Reduced body fat mass has been observed with the use of licorice.
- High doses of licorice may cause temporary vision problems or loss.

Pregnancy and Breastfeeding

- Licorice cannot be recommended for use in women who are pregnant or breastfeeding because of possible alterations of hormone levels and the possibility of premature labor.
- Hormonal imbalances reported with the use of licorice include abnormally low testosterone levels in men and high prolactin levels/estrogen levels in women.

INTERACTIONS

Most herbs and supplements have not been thoroughly tested for interactions with other herbs, supplements, drugs, or foods. The interactions listed here are based on reports in scientific publications, laboratory experiments, or traditional use. It is important to always read product labels. People who have a medical condition, or are taking other drugs, herbs, or supplements, should consult a qualified healthcare provider before starting a new therapy.

Interactions with Drugs

- In general, prescription drugs should be taken 1 hour before taking licorice or 2 hours after taking licorice because licorice may increase the absorption of many drugs. Increased absorption may increase the activities and side effects of some drugs (for example, nitrofurantoin). Phosphate salts have been shown to increase licorice absorption.
- Because the toxicity of digoxin (Lanoxin) is increased when potassium levels are low, people who take digoxin and are interested in using licorice should discuss this with their healthcare provider. Increased monitoring may be necessary. Other drugs that may increase the tendency for irregular heart rhythms are also best avoided when using licorice.
- Licorice may reduce the effects of blood-pressure or diuretic (urine-producing) drugs, including hydrochlorothiazide and spironolactone. Use of licorice with the diuretics hydrochlorothiazide or furosemide (Lasix) may cause potassium levels to fall very low and lead to dangerous complications. Other drugs that can also cause potassium levels to fall and are best avoided when using licorice include insulin, sodium polystyrene (Kayexalate), and laxatives. Chewing tobacco may increase the toxicity of licorice gums by causing electrolyte disturbances.
- Licorice may increase the adverse effects associated with corticosteroids such as prednisolone, and monoamine oxidase inhibitors such as isocarboxazid (Marplan), phenelzine (Nardil), and tranylcypromine (Parnate).
- Licorice may reduce the effects of birth control pills, hormone replacement therapies, and testosterone therapy.
- In theory, licorice may increase the risk of bleeding when used with anticoagulants (blood thinners) or antiplatelet drugs. Examples of such drugs are warfarin (Coumadin), heparin, clopidogrel (Plavix), and aspirin.

Interactions with Herbs and Dietary Supplements

- Herbs with potential laxative properties may add to the potassium-lowering effects of licorice. Examples include alder buckthorn, aloe dried leaf sap, black root, blue flag rhizome, butternut bark, cascara bark, castor oil, chasteberry, colocynth fruit pulp, dandelion, dong quai, European buckthorn, eyebright, gamboges bark, horsetail, jalap root, manna bark, plantain leaf, podophyllum root, psyllium, rhubarb, senna, wild cucumber fruit, and yellow dock root.
- Herbs with potential diuretic properties may increase adverse effects associated with licorice. Examples are artichoke, celery, corn silk, couchgrass, dandelion, elder flower, horsetail, juniper berry, kava, shepherd's purse, uva ursi, and yarrow.
- Herbs and supplements that lower blood pressure may add to the blood pressure–lowering effects of licorice. Examples of such agents are aconite/monkshood, arnica, baneberry, betel nut, bilberry, black cohosh, bryony, calendula, California poppy, coleus, curcumin, eucalyptol, eucalyptus oil, flaxseed/flaxseed oil, garlic, ginger, ginkgo, goldenseal, green hellebore, hawthorn, Indian tobacco, jaborandi, mistletoe, night-blooming cereus, oleander, pasque flower, periwinkle, pleurisy root, *Polypodium vulgare*, shepherd's purse, Texas milkweed, turmeric, and wild cherry.
- Herbs with monoamine oxidase inhibitor (MAOI) activity may worsen side effects when used at the same time as licorice. Examples of such herbs are California poppy, chromium, dehydroepiandrosterone (DHEA), DL-phenylalanine (DLPA),

ephedra, evening primrose oil, fenugreek, *Ginkgo biloba*, hops, 5-hydroxytryptophan (5-HTP), mace, *S*-adenosylmethionine (SAMe), sepia, St. John's wort, tyrosine, valerian, vitamin B_6, and yohimbe bark extract.

- In theory, herbs and supplements that increase the risk of bleeding may further increase the risk of bleeding when taken with licorice. Multiple cases of bleeding have been reported with the use of *Ginkgo biloba*, and fewer cases with garlic and saw palmetto. Numerous other agents may theoretically increase the risk of bleeding, although this has not been proven in most cases. Examples of such agents are alfalfa, American ginseng, angelica, anise, *Arnica montana*, asafetida, aspen bark, bilberry, birch, black cohosh, bladderwrack, bogbean, boldo, borage seed oil, bromelain, capsicum, cat's claw, celery, chamomile, chaparral, clove, coleus, cordyceps, danshen, devil's claw, dong quai, eicosapentaenoic acid (EPA), evening primrose oil, fenugreek, feverfew, fish oil, flaxseed/flax powder (not a concern with flaxseed oil), ginger, grapefruit juice, grape seed, green tea, guggul, gymnestra, horse chestnut, horseradish, lovage root, male fern, meadowsweet, nordihydroguaiaretic acid (NDGA), omega-3 fatty acids, onion, *Panax ginseng*, papain, parsley, passionflower, poplar, prickly ash, propolis, quassia, red clover, reishi, rue, Siberian ginseng, sweet birch, sweet clover, turmeric, vitamin E, white willow, wild carrot, wild lettuce, willow, wintergreen, and yucca.

Interactions with Laboratory Values

- Licorice may decrease cortisol, ACTH, aldosterone, and potassium levels in the blood. Increases in renin and sodium levels also have been observed.

Selected References

Natural Standard developed the preceding evidence-based information based on a systematic review of more than 350 articles. For comprehensive information about alternative and complementary therapies on the professional level, go to www.naturalstandard.com. Selected references are listed here.

Amaryan G, Astvatsatryan V, Gabrielyan E, et al. Double-blind, placebo-controlled, randomized, pilot clinical trial of ImmunoGuard—a standardized fixed combination of *Andrographis paniculata* Nees, with *Eleutherococcus senticosus* Maxim, *Schizandra chinensis* Bail. and *Glycyrrhiza glabra* L. extracts in patients with Familial Mediterranean Fever. Phytomed 2003;10(4):271-285.

Arase Y, Ikeda K, Murashima N, et al. The long term efficacy of glycyrrhizin in chronic hepatitis C patients. Cancer 1997;79(8):1494-1500.

Carbonell-Barrachina AA, Aracil P, Garcia E, Burlo F, et al. Source of arsenic in licorice confectionery products. J Agric Food Chem 2003;51(6):1749-1752.

Cinatl J, Morgenstern B, Bauer G, et al. Glycyrrhizin, an active component of liquorice roots, and replication of SARS-associated coronavirus. Lancet 2003;361(9374):2045-2046.

Elinav E, Chajek-Shaul T. Licorice consumption causing severe hypokalemic paralysis. Mayo Clin Proc 2003;78(6):767-768.

Eriksson JW, Carlberg B, Hillorn V. Life-threatening ventricular tachycardia due to liquorice-induced hypokalaemia. J Intern Med 1999;245(3):307-310.

Fujioka T, Kondou T, Fukuhara A, et al. Efficacy of a glycyrrhizin suppository for the treatment of chronic hepatitis C: a pilot study. Hepatol Res 2003;26(1):10-14.

Harada T, Ohtaki E, Misu K, et al. Congestive heart failure caused by digitalis toxicity in an elderly man taking a licorice-containing Chinese herbal laxative. Cardiology 2002;98(4):218.

Hinoshita F, Ogura Y, Suzuki Y, et al. Effect of orally administered shao-yao-gan-cao-tang (Shakuyaku-kanzo-to) on muscle cramps in maintenance hemodialysis patients: a preliminary study. Am J Chin Med. 2003;31(3):445-453.

Hughes J, Sellick S, King R, et al. Re: "preterm birth and licorice consumption during pregnancy". Am J Epidemiol. 2003;158(2):190-191; author reply, 191.
Kamei J, Nakamura R, Ichiki H, et al. Antitussive principles of Glycyrrhizae radix, a main component of the Kampo preparations Bakumondo-to (Mai-men-dong-tang). Eur J Pharmacol. 2003;469(1-3):159-163.
Kang DG, Sohn EJ, Mun YJ, et al. Glycyrrhizin ameliorates renal function defects in the early-phase of ischemia-induced acute renal failure. Phytother Res 2003;17(8):947-951.
Kang DG, Sohn EJ, Lee HS. Effects of glycyrrhizin on renal functions in association with the regulation of water channels. Am J Chin Med 2003;31(3):403-413.
Lin JC. Mechanism of action of glycyrrhizic acid in inhibition of Epstein-Barr virus replication *in vitro*. Antiviral Res 2003;59(1):41-47.
Liu J, Manheimer E, Tsutani K, et al. Medicinal herbs for hepatitis C virus infection: a Cochrane hepatobiliary systematic review of randomized trials. Am J Gastroenterol 2003;98(3): 538-544.
Nokhodchi A, Nazemiyeh H, Ghafourian T, et al. The effect of glycyrrhizin on the release rate and skin penetration of diclofenac sodium from topical formulations. Farmaco 2002; 57(11):883-888.
Ofir R, Tamir S, Khatib S, Vaya J. Inhibition of serotonin re-uptake by licorice constituents. J Mol Neurosci 2003;20(2):135-140.
Oganesyan KR. Antioxidant effect of licorice root on blood catalase activity in vibration stress. Bull Exp Biol Med 2002;134(2):135-136.
Russo S, Mastropasqua M, Mosetti MA, et al. Low doses of liquorice can induce hypertension encephalopathy. Am J Nephrol 2000;20(2):145-148.
Sasaki H, Takei M, Kobayashi M, et al. Effect of glycyrrhizin, an active component of licorice roots, on HIV replication in cultures of peripheral blood mononuclear cells from HIV-seropositive patients. Pathobiol 2002-2003;70(4):229-236.
Serra A, Uehlinger DE, Ferrari P, et al. Glycyrrhetinic Acid decreases plasma potassium concentrations in patients with anuria. J Am Soc Nephrol 2002;13(1):191-196.
Sigurjonsdottir HA, Manhem K, Axelson M, et al. Subjects with essential hypertension are more sensitive to the inhibition of 11 beta-HSD by liquorice. J Hum Hypertens 2003;17(2): 125-131.
Sohn EJ, Kang DG, Lee HS. Protective effects of glycyrrhizin on gentamicin-induced acute renal failure in rats. Pharmacol Toxicol 2003;93(3):116-122.
Strandberg TE, Andersson S, Jarvenpaa AL. Risk factors for preterm delivery. Lancet 2003; 361(9355):436; author reply, 436-437.
van Rossum TG, Vulto AG, Hop WC, et al. Glycyrrhizin-induced reduction of ALT in European patients with chronic hepatitis C. Am J Gastroenterol 2001;96(8):2432-2437.

L

Lycopene

(Tomato [*Lycopersicon esculentum*])

RELATED TERMS

- ψ, ψ-carotene, all-trans lycopene, lycopersicon, solanorubin, tomato.

BACKGROUND

- Lycopene is a carotenoid and is present in human serum, liver, adrenal glands, lungs, prostate, colon, and skin at higher levels than other carotenoids. Lycopene has been found to possess antioxidant and antiproliferative properties in animal and *in vitro* studies, although activity in humans remains controversial.
- Numerous epidemiologic investigations have correlated high intake of lycopene-containing foods or high lycopene serum levels with reduced incidence of cancer, cardiovascular disease, and macular degeneration. However, estimates of lycopene consumption have been based on reported tomato intake, not on the use of lycopene supplements. Because tomatoes are sources of other nutrients, including vitamin C, folate, and potassium, it is not clear whether lycopene itself is beneficial.
- There is no established definition of "lycopene deficiency," and no direct evidence that repletion of low lycopene levels has any benefit.

USES BASED ON SCIENTIFIC EVIDENCE	Grade*
Age-related macular degeneration prevention Based on antioxidant properties observed in laboratory studies, lycopene has been suggested as a preventive therapy for age-related macular degeneration. Preliminary studies in humans overall have not found a clear benefit. More research is needed before a recommendation can be made.	C
Antioxidant Laboratory research suggests that lycopene, like other carotenoids, may have antioxidant properties. However, it is not clear if lycopene has these effects in humans. Results of different studies do not agree, and better-quality research is needed before a firm conclusion can be drawn.	C
Atherosclerosis ("clogged" arteries) and high cholesterol It has been suggested that lycopene may be helpful in people with atherosclerosis or high cholesterol, possibly because of lycopene's antioxidant properties. Several studies have been published in this area, most using tomato juice as a treatment. Results are inconsistent, and this issue remains unclear.	C

Continued

Breast cancer prevention Research in animals and observations of large human populations have examined the relationship between developing breast cancer and tomato intake or lycopene levels in the body. The evidence in this area is not clear, and further studies are needed before a firm conclusion can be drawn.	C
Cancer prevention (general) Studies have examined large populations to identify which lifestyle factors affect health. Many of these "epidemiologic" or "population" studies suggest a link between diets high in fruits and vegetables and a decreased risk of developing cancer. However, it is not entirely clear which foods are most beneficial, or if the reduced risk of developing cancer is due to other (non-dietary) aspects of a "healthy lifestyle." High levels of lycopene are found in tomatoes and in tomato-based products. Tomatoes are sources of other nutrients such as vitamin C, folate, and potassium. Several laboratory studies and studies in humans that examined tomato-based products and blood lycopene levels suggest that lycopene may be associated with a lower risk of developing cancer. However, because of a lack of well-designed human research using lycopene supplements, this issue remains unclear.	C
Cervical cancer prevention Observations of large human populations suggest possible benefits of tomato product intake in preventing cervical cancer. However, other studies report no benefits. Research that specifically studies lycopene supplements is lacking.	C
Exercise-induced asthma Laboratory research suggests that lycopene, like other carotenoids, may have antioxidant properties. It has been suggested that antioxidants may be helpful in the prevention of exercise-induced asthma. There is limited, poor-quality research in this area, and further evidence is needed before a recommendation can be made.	C
Gastrointestinal tract and colorectal cancer prevention Multiple studies have examined whether intake of tomatoes or tomato-based products helps prevent gastrointestinal tract cancers, including oral, pharyngeal, esophageal, gastric, colon, and rectal cancers. Results have been inconsistent, with some studies reporting significant benefits and others finding no effects. Research that specifically studies lycopene supplements is limited, and more research is needed in this area before a conclusion can be drawn.	C
Lung cancer prevention Several studies observing large populations report a lower risk of developing lung cancer in people who regularly eat tomatoes. However, other studies report no benefits of tomato consumption. Research that specifically studies lycopene supplements is lacking.	C

L

Continued

Prostate cancer prevention Studies of large populations report mixed results as to whether eating tomatoes or tomato-based products reduces the risk of developing prostate cancer. Research that specifically studies lycopene supplements is lacking.	C
Sun protection Lycopene in combination with other carotenoids such as beta-carotene, vitamins C and E, selenium, and proanthocyanidins, may help in reducing sunburn. Selected protective effects from ultraviolet (UV) rays have been observed in small, short-term studies. More research is needed before a firm conclusion can be drawn.	C
Immunostimulation It has been proposed that lycopene and other carotenoids such as beta-carotene may stimulate the immune system. However, several studies of lycopene supplements and tomato juice intake in humans report no effects on the immune system.	D

*Key to grades: *A:* Strong scientific evidence for this use; *B:* Good scientific evidence for this use; *C:* Unclear scientific evidence for this use; *D:* Fair scientific evidence against this use (it may not work); *F:* Strong scientific evidence against this use (it likely does not work). For a more detailed explanation of efficacy criteria, see "Natural Standard Evidence-Based Validated Grading Rationale" in the Introduction.

Uses Based on Tradition, Theory, or Limited Scientific Evidence

AIDS, bladder cancer, breast cancer, cataracts, cognitive function, diabetes mellitus, esophageal cancer, heart disease, inflammatory conditions, laryngeal cancer, mesothelioma, melanoma, ovarian cancer, pancreatic cancer, pancreatitis, Parkinson's disease, periodontal disease, pharyngeal cancer, rheumatoid arthritis, skin cancer, stomach cancer, stroke prevention, urinary tract cancer.

DOSING

The following doses are based on scientific research, publications, traditional use, or expert opinion. Many herbs and supplements have not been thoroughly tested, and safety and effectiveness may not be proven. Brands may be made differently, with variable ingredients even within the same brand. The doses shown may not apply to all products. It is important to always read product labels and discuss doses with a qualified healthcare provider before therapy is started.

Adults (18 Years and Older)

- **Cancer prevention:** Most research examining the prevention of cancer has studied tomato and tomato-based products (tomato sauce or juice), not lycopene supplements specifically. Effectiveness has not been proven.

- **Immune system enhancement:** 13.3 mg of lycopene daily, supplied as Lyco-O-Pen (LycoRed Natural Products Industries Ltd., Israel), has been studied.
- **Asthma (exercise-induced):** 30 mg of lycopene daily, supplied as Lyc-O-Mato (LycoRed Natural Products Industries Ltd., Israel), has been studied.
- **Atherosclerosis prevention:** 1.243 g of 6% lycopene oleoresin capsules daily (LycoRed Natural Products Industries Ltd., Israel) has been studied.
- **Sun protection:** 8 mg of lycopene in combination with other antioxidants has been studied.

Children (Younger Than 18 Years)

- There is insufficient scientific evidence to recommend the use of lycopene supplements in children.

SAFETY

The U.S. Food and Drug Administration does not strictly regulate herbs and supplements. There is no guarantee of strength, purity, or safety of products, and effects may vary. It is important to always read product labels. People who have a medical condition, or are taking other drugs, herbs, or supplements, should consult a qualified healthcare provider before starting a new therapy. A healthcare provider should be contacted immediately about any side effects.

Allergies

- People with allergy/hypersensitivity to lycopene or tomatoes should avoid the use of lycopene.

Side Effects and Warnings

- The safety of lycopene supplements has not been thoroughly studied. There are no reports in the available scientific literature of serious toxicity or adverse effects from eating tomatoes or tomato-based products or taking lycopene supplements. Tomatoes and tomato-based products may be acidic and can irritate stomach ulcers.

Pregnancy and Breastfeeding

- There is insufficient scientific evidence to recommend the use of lycopene supplements by women who are pregnant or breastfeeding. In one study, lycopene components were found in samples of human breast milk, at approximately 10% of blood concentrations. Amounts of lycopene found in foods are usually assumed to be safe.

INTERACTIONS

Most herbs and supplements have not been thoroughly tested for interactions with other herbs, supplements, drugs, or foods. The interactions listed here are based on reports in scientific publications, laboratory experiments, or traditional use. It is important to always read product labels. People who have a medical condition, or are taking other drugs, herbs, or supplements, should consult a qualified healthcare provider before starting a new therapy.

Interactions with Drugs

- Some drugs that lower cholesterol levels in the blood may also reduce levels of carotenoids such as lycopene. Examples of cholesterol-lowering drugs include "statin" drugs such as lovastatin (Mevacor) and atorvastatin (Lipitor), cholestyramine

(Questran, Prevalite, LoCHOLEST), and colestipol (Cholestid). There is no evidence that replacing lycopene levels with supplements has any benefit in people using these drugs. Some studies suggest that lycopene may add to the cholesterol-lowering effects of statin drugs.
- It has been proposed that nicotine (cigarette smoking) and alcohol may lower lycopene levels in the body, although this has not been proven.

Interactions with Herbs and Dietary Supplements

- Studies report mixed effects of taking lycopene with beta-carotene. Some studies report higher levels of lycopene, while others note no change or decreased levels. Canthaxanthin, a carotenoid, has been shown to reduce lycopene uptake from dietary sources, and may result in decreased lycopene levels in the blood.
- Laboratory studies suggest possible interactions between lycopene and other vitamins or supplements, although the significance of these interactions in the human body is not known. Examples include increased antioxidant effects when lycopene is combined with lutein and decreased growth of cancer-like cells when lycopene is used with vitamin D or vitamin E.

Interactions with Foods

- Based on studies in humans, the fat substitute product Olestra may decrease levels of lycopene in the blood. Olestra is an ingredient of many commercially available reduced-fat foods.
- In theory, lycopene may be assimilated better when taken with fatty foods. However, studies comparing the effects of a fatty diet and of a reduced-fat diet on lycopene blood levels did not find any significant differences.

Selected References

Natural Standard developed the preceding evidence-based information based on a systematic review of more than 600 scientific articles. For comprehensive information about alternative and complementary therapies on the professional level, go to www.naturalstandard.com. Selected references are listed here.

Agarwal S, Rao AV. Tomato lycopene and low density lipoprotein oxidation: a human dietary intervention study. Lipids 1998;33(10):981-984.

Barber N. The tomato: an important part of the urologist's diet? BJU Int 2003;91(4): 307-309.

Bowen P, Chen L, Stacewicz-Sapuntzakis M, et al. Tomato sauce supplementation and prostate cancer: lycopene accumulation and modulation of biomarkers of carcinogenesis. Exp Biol Med (Maywood) 2002;227(10):886-893.

Broekmans WM, Klopping-Ketelaars IA, Weststrate JA, et al. Decreased carotenoid concentrations due to dietary sucrose polyesters do not affect possible markers of disease risk in humans. J Nutr 2003;133(3):720-726.

Bureau I, Laporte F, Favier M, et al. No antioxidant effect of combined HRT on LDL oxidizability and oxidative stress biomarkers in treated post-menopausal women. J Am Coll Nutr 2002;21(4):333-338.

Cerhan JR, Saag KG, Merlino LA, et al. Antioxidant micronutrients and risk of rheumatoid arthritis in a cohort of older women. Am J Epidemiol 2003;157(4):345-354.

Chen G, Djuric Z. Detection of 2,6-cyclolycopene-1,5-diol in breast nipple aspirate fluids and plasma: a potential marker of oxidative stress. Cancer Epidemiol Biomarkers Prev 2002; 11(12):1592-1596.

Clarke R, Armitage J. Antioxidant vitamins and risk of cardiovascular disease. Review of large-scale randomized trials. Cardiovasc Drugs Ther 2002;16(5):411-415.

Corridan BM, O'Donoghue M, Hughes DA, et al. Low-dose supplementation with lycopene or beta-carotene does not enhance cell-mediated immunity in healthy free-living elderly humans. Eur J Clin Nutr 2001;55(8):627-635.

Dietrich M, Block G, Norkus EP, et al. Smoking and exposure to environmental tobacco smoke decrease some plasma antioxidants and increase gamma-tocopherol in vivo after adjustment for dietary antioxidant intakes. Am J Clin Nutr 2003;77(1):160-166.

Djuric Z, Uhley VE, Naegeli L, et al. Plasma carotenoids, tocopherols, and antioxidant capacity in a 12-week intervention study to reduce fat and/or energy intakes. Nutrition 2003;19(3): 244-249.

Dorgan JF, Sowell A, Swanson CA, et al. Relationships of serum carotenoids, retinol, alpha-tocopherol, and selenium with breast cancer risk: results from a prospective study in Columbia, Missouri (United States). Cancer Causes Control 1998;9(1):89-97.

Edwards AJ, Vinyard BT, Wiley ER, et al. Consumption of watermelon juice increases plasma concentrations of lycopene and beta-carotene in humans. J Nutr 2003;133(4):1043-1050.

Flood V, Smith W, Wang JJ, et al. Dietary antioxidant intake and incidence of early age-related maculopathy: the Blue Mountains Eye Study. Ophthalmology 2002;109(12):2272-2278.

Franceschi S, Bidoli E, La Vecchia C, et al. Tomatoes and risk of digestive-tract cancers. Int J Cancer 1994;59(2):181-184.

Gianetti J, Pedrinelli R, Petrucci R, et al. Inverse association between carotid intima-media thickness and the antioxidant lycopene in atherosclerosis. Am Heart J 2002;143(3):467-474.

Giovannucci E, Clinton SK. Tomatoes, lycopene, and prostate cancer. Proc Soc Exp Biol Med 1998;218(2):129-139.

Giovannucci E. Tomatoes, tomato-based products, lycopene, and cancer: review of the epidemiologic literature. J Natl Cancer Inst 1999;91(4):317-331.

Giovannucci E, Rimm EB, Liu Y, et al. A prospective study of tomato products, lycopene, and prostate cancer risk. J Natl Cancer Inst 2002;94(5):391-398.

Greul AK, Grundmann JU, Heinrich F, et al. Photoprotection of UV-irradiated human skin: an antioxidative combination of vitamins E and C, carotenoids, selenium and proanthocyanidins. Skin Pharmacol Appl Skin Physiol 2002;15(5):307-315.

Gross M, Yu X, Hannan P, et al. Lipid standardization of serum fat-soluble antioxidant concentrations: the YALTA study. Am J Clin Nutr 2003;77(2):458-466.

Hadley CW, Clinton SK, Schwartz SJ. The consumption of processed tomato products enhances plasma lycopene concentrations in association with a reduced lipoprotein sensitivity to oxidative damage. J Nutr 2003;133(3):727-732.

Hak AE, Stampfer MJ, Campos H, et al. Plasma carotenoids and tocopherols and risk of myocardial infarction in a low-risk population of US male physicians. Circulation 2003; 108(7):802-807. Epub 2003 Aug 04. Comment in: Circulation 2003;108(7):e9012-e9013.

Heinrich U, Gartner C, Wiebusch M, et al. Supplementation with beta-carotene or a similar amount of mixed carotenoids protects humans from UV-induced erythema. J Nutr 2003;133(1):98-101.

Holick CN, Michaud DS, Stolzenberg-Solomon R, et al. Dietary carotenoids, serum beta-carotene, and retinol and risk of lung cancer in the alpha-tocopherol, beta-carotene cohort study. Am J Epidemiol 2002;156(6):536-547.

Huang HY, Alberg AJ, Norkus EP, et al. Prospective study of antioxidant micronutrients in the blood and the risk of developing prostate cancer. Am J Epidemiol 2003;157(4):335-344. Erratum in: Am J Epidemiol 2003;157(12):1126.

Hughes DA, Wright AJ, Finglas PM, et al. Comparison of effects of beta-carotene and lycopene supplementation on the expression of functionally associated molecules on human monocytes. Biochem Soc Trans 1997;25(2):206S.

Neuman I, Nahum H, Ben Amotz A. Reduction of exercise-induced asthma oxidative stress by lycopene, a natural antioxidant. Allergy 2000;55(12):1184-1189.

Porrini M, Riso P. Lymphocyte lycopene concentration and DNA protection from oxidative damage is increased in women after a short period of tomato consumption. J Nutr 2000; 130(2):189-192.

Schmidt R, Hayn M, Reinhart B, et al. Plasma antioxidants and cognitive performance in middle-aged and older adults: results of the Austrian Stroke Prevention Study. J Am Geriatr Soc 1998;46(11):1407-1410.

Simon MS, Djuric Z, Dunn B, et al. An evaluation of plasma antioxidant levels and the risk of breast cancer: A Pilot Case Control Study. Breast J 2000;6(6):388-395.

Smith-Warner SA, Elmer PJ, Tharp TM, et al. Increasing vegetable and fruit intake: randomized intervention and monitoring in an at-risk population. Cancer Epidemiol Biomarkers Prev 2000;9(3):307-317.

Steinberg FM, Chait A. Antioxidant vitamin supplementation and lipid peroxidation in smokers. Am J Clin Nutr 1998;68(2):319-327.

Sutherland WH, Walker RJ, De Jong SA, et al. Supplementation with tomato juice increases plasma lycopene but does not alter susceptibility to oxidation of low-density lipoproteins from renal transplant recipients. Clin Nephrol 1999;52(1):30-36.

Vogel S, Contois JH, Tucker KL, et al. Plasma retinol and plasma and lipoprotein tocopherol and carotenoid concentrations in healthy elderly participants of the Framingham Heart Study. Am J Clin Nutr 1997;66(4):950-958.

Watzl B, Bub A, Blockhaus M, et al. Prolonged tomato juice consumption has no effect on cell-mediated immunity of well-nourished elderly men and women. J Nutr 2000;130(7):1719-1723.

Wright AJ, Hughes DA, Bailey AL, et al. Beta-carotene and lycopene, but not lutein, supplementation changes the plasma fatty acid profile of healthy male non-smokers. J Lab Clin Med 1999;134(6):592-598.

Maitake Mushroom

(*Grifola frondosa*)

RELATED TERMS

- Beta-glucan, cloud mushroom, dancing mushroom, grifolan, Grifon Pro Maitake D-Fraction Extract, king of mushroom, Maitake Gold 404, MD-fraction, MDF, my-take.

BACKGROUND

- "Maitake" is the Japanese name for the edible fungus *Grifola frondosa*, which is characterized by a large fruiting body and overlapping caps. Maitake has been used traditionally both as a food and for medicinal purposes. Polysaccharide constituents of maitake have been associated in animal studies with multiple bioactive properties. Extracts of maitake mushroom, particularly the beta-glucan polysaccharide constituent, have been associated with immune modulation in preclinical studies and are hypothesized to exert antitumor effects as a result of these immune properties. Human data are limited, and at this time there is insufficient evidence to recommend for or against the use of oral maitake for any indication.

M

USES BASED ON SCIENTIFIC EVIDENCE	Grade*
Cancer "Maitake" is the Japanese name for the edible fungus *Grifola frondosa*, which is notable for its large fruiting body and overlapping caps. Maitake has been used traditionally both as a food and for medicinal purposes. Early studies in the laboratory as well as in humans suggest that beta-glucan extracts from maitake may increase the body's ability to fight cancer. However, these studies have not been well designed, and better research is needed before the use of maitake for cancer can be recommended.	C
Diabetes In animal studies, maitake extracts are reported to lower blood sugar levels. However, little is known about the effect of maitake on blood sugar in humans.	C
Immune enhancement Animal and laboratory studies suggest that beta-glucan extracts from maitake may alter the immune system. However, no reliable studies in humans are available.	C

*Key to grades: *A:* Strong scientific evidence for this use; *B:* Good scientific evidence for this use; *C:* Unclear scientific evidence for this use; *D:* Fair scientific evidence against this use (it may not work); *F:* Strong scientific evidence against this use (it likely does not work). For a more detailed explanation of efficacy criteria, see "Natural Standard Evidence-Based Validated Grading Rationale" in the Introduction.

Uses Based on Tradition, Theory, or Limited Scientific Evidence
Arthritis, bacterial infection, high blood pressure, high cholesterol, HIV infection, liver inflammation (hepatitis), weight loss.

DOSING

The following doses are based on scientific research, publications, traditional use, or expert opinion. Many herbs and supplements have not been thoroughly tested, and their safety and effectiveness may not be proven. Brands may be made differently, with variable ingredients even within the same brand. The doses shown may not apply to all products. It is important to always read product labels and discuss doses with a qualified healthcare provider before therapy is started.

Standardization

- Standardization involves measuring the amount of certain chemicals in products to try to make different preparations similar to each other. It is not always known if the chemicals being measured are the "active" ingredients.
- Standardized maitake products are not widely available. Amounts of the ingredient beta-glucan may vary between preparations. Various chemicals from maitake can be prepared by standardized processes, but it is not known if these products have the same effects.

Adults (18 Years and Older)

- **Capsules, tablets, or liquid extract:** Doses of beta-glucan from maitake range from 0.5 to 1 mg/kg daily, taken in divided doses. Few studies in humans are available, and it is not known what doses may be safe or effective.
- **Raw mushroom:** It is not known what doses are safe or effective.

Children (Younger Than 18 Years)

- Little information is available about the safety of beta-glucan in children. Therefore, its use cannot be recommended.

SAFETY

The U.S. Food and Drug Administration does not strictly regulate herbs and supplements. There is no guarantee of strength, purity or safety of products, and effects may vary. It is important to always read product labels. People who a medical condition, or are taking other drugs, herbs, or supplements, should consult a qualified healthcare provider before starting a new therapy. A healthcare provider should be consulted immediately about any side effects.

Allergies

- No reliable scientific information is available about allergies to maitake or beta-glucan.

Side Effects and Warnings

- Maitake has not been studied thoroughly in humans, and its effects are not well known. Because maitake has been used historically as a food, it is thought that low doses may be safe. Studies in animals suggest that it may lower blood pressure. However, no information about these effects is reported for humans. Individuals who take blood pressure medications should use caution. Animal studies report that maitake may lower blood sugar levels. Caution is advised in patients with diabetes or hypoglycemia, and in those taking drugs, herbs, or supplements that affect blood sugar. Blood glucose levels may need to be monitored by a healthcare provider, and medication adjustments may be necessary.

Pregnancy and Breastfeeding

- Little is known about the safety of maitake in pregnancy and breastfeeding, and therefore its use as a supplement cannot be recommended.

INTERACTIONS

Most herbs and supplements have not been thoroughly tested for interactions with other herbs, supplements, drugs, or foods. The interactions listed here are based on reports in scientific publications, laboratory experiments, or traditional use. It is important to always read product labels. People who have a medical condition, or are taking other drugs, herbs, or supplements, should consult a qualified healthcare provider before starting a new therapy.

Interactions with Drugs

- Based on animal studies, maitake may lower blood sugar levels. Caution is advised when using medications that may also lower blood sugar. Patients taking drugs for diabetes by mouth or insulin should be monitored closely by a qualified healthcare provider. Medication adjustments may be necessary. Animal studies also suggest that maitake may lower blood pressure. Persons taking medications for blood pressure should use caution and should first discuss the use of maitake with a qualified healthcare provider.

Interactions with Herbs and Dietary Supplements

- Based on animal studies, maitake may lower blood sugar levels. Caution is advised when using herbs or supplements that may also lower blood sugar. Blood glucose levels may require monitoring, and doses may need adjustment. Possible examples of herbs and supplements that may affect blood sugar levels include *Aloe vera*, American ginseng, bilberry, bitter melon, burdock, fenugreek, fish oil, gymnema, horse chestnut seed extract (HCSE), marshmallow, milk thistle, *Panax ginseng*, rosemary, Siberian ginseng, stinging nettle, and white horehound.
- Animal studies suggest that maitake may lower blood pressure. Use caution when combining maitake with other herbs that can lower blood pressure. Some examples are aconite/monkshood, arnica, baneberry, betel nut, bilberry, black cohosh, bryony, calendula, California poppy, coleus, curcumin, eucalyptol, eucalyptus oil, garlic, ginger, ginkgo, goldenseal, green hellebore, hawthorn, Indian tobacco, jaborandi, mistletoe, night-blooming cereus, oleander, pasque flower, periwinkle, pleurisy root, shepherd's purse, Texas milkweed, turmeric, and wild cherry.

Selected References

Natural Standard developed the preceding evidence-based information based on a systematic review of more than 50 scientific articles. For comprehensive information about alternative and complementary therapies on the professional level, go to www.naturalstandard.com. Selected references are listed here.

Fullerton SA, Samadi AA, Tortorelis DG, et al. Induction of apoptosis in human prostatic cancer cells with beta-glucan (Maitake mushroom polysaccharide). Mol Urol 2000;4(1):7-13.

Kodama N, Komuta K, Nanba H. Can maitake MD-fraction aid cancer patients? Altern Med Rev 2002;7(3):236-239.

Konno S, Tortorelis DG, Fullerton SA, et al. A possible hypoglycaemic effect of maitake mushroom on Type 2 diabetic patients. Diabet Med 2001;18(12):1010.

Kubo K, Aoki H, Nanba H. Anti-diabetic activity present in the fruit body of *Grifola frondosa* (Maitake). I. Biol Pharm Bull 1994;17(8):1106-1110.

Kubo K, Nanba H. Anti-hyperliposis effect of maitake fruit body (*Grifola frondosa*). I. Biol Pharm Bull 1997;20(7):781-785.

Kubo K, Nanba H. The effect of maitake mushrooms on liver and serum lipids. Altern Ther Health Med 1996;2(5):62-66.

Li X, Rong J, Wu M, et al. [Anti-tumor effect of polysaccharide from *Grifola frondosa* and its influence on immunological function] Zhong Yao Cai 2003;26(1):31-32.

Matsui K, Kodama N, Nanba H. Effects of maitake (*Grifola frondosa*) D-fraction on the carcinoma angiogenesis. Cancer Lett 2001;172(2):193-198.

Marshmallow

(*Althaea officinalis* L.)

RELATED TERMS

- Althaea leaf, althaea root, *Althaea officinalis* L. var *robusta*, althaeae folium, althaeae radi, althaea radix, Althea, althea leaf, althea root, Altheia, Apothekerstockmalve (German), bismalva (Italian), buonvischio (Italian), cheeses, Eibischwurzel (German), guimauve (French), gul hatem (Turkish), herba malvae, hitmi (Turkish), kitmi (Turkish), mallards, Malvaceae (family), malvacioni (Italian), malvavisco (Spanish), malve, mortification root, racine de guimauve, sweet weed, witte malve, wymote.
- *Note:* Not to be confused with mallow leaf and mallow flower. Not to be confused with confectionery marshmallows; although confectionery marshmallows were once made from the *Althaea officinalis* plant, they now contain mostly sugar.

BACKGROUND

- Both the leaf and the root of marshmallow (*Althaea officinalis*) are used in commercial preparations. Herbal formulations are made from either the dried root or leaf (unpeeled or peeled). The actual mucilaginous content of the commercial product may vary according to the time of collection.
- No clinical trials assessing marshmallow monotherapy (used alone) have been conducted for any specific health condition. Medicinal uses of marshmallow are supported principally by traditional use and laboratory research. Limited human evidence is available studying the effects of marshmallow-containing combination products in dermatologic conditions.
- Although this effect is clinically unproven, marshmallow may interfere with the absorption of medications taken by mouth. Therefore, ingestion of marshmallow several hours before or after ingestion of other medicinal agents may be warranted.
- Marshmallow is generally regarded as safe, and literature review reveals no documented adverse reactions in case reports. However, the potential for marshmallow to cause allergic reactions or low blood sugar has been noted anecdotally.

USES BASED ON SCIENTIFIC EVIDENCE	Grade*
Inflammatory skin conditions (eczema, psoriasis) Marshmallow extracts have traditionally been used on the skin to treat inflammation. Several laboratory experiments, mostly from the 1960s, reported marshmallow to have anti-inflammatory activity. There was one human research study done in 1968. Safety, dosing, and effectiveness compared with those of other anti-inflammatory agents have not been examined.	C

*Key to grades: *A:* Strong scientific evidence for this use; *B:* Good scientific evidence for this use; *C:* Unclear scientific evidence for this use; *D:* Fair scientific evidence against this use (it may not work); *F:* Strong scientific evidence against this use (it likely does not work). For a more detailed explanation of efficacy criteria, see "Natural Standard Evidence-Based Validated Grading Rationale" in the Introduction.

Uses Based on Tradition, Theory, or Limited Scientific Evidence

Abscesses (topical), antidote to poisons, aphrodisiac, arthritis, bee stings, bronchitis, boils (topical), bruises (topical), burns (topical), cancer, chilblains, colitis, congestion, constipation, cough, Crohn's disease, cystitis, demulcent, dermatitis (topical), diarrhea, diuretic, diverticulitis, cough, duodenal ulcer, emollient, enteritis, expectorant, gastroenteritis, immunostimulant, impotence, indigestion, inflammation, insect bites, intestinal inflammation (small intestine), irritable bowel syndrome, kidney stones, laxative, minor wounds, mouthwash, mucilage, muscular pain, pap smear (abnormal), peptic ulcer disease, polyuria, skin ulcers (topical), soothing agent, sore throat, sprains, toothache, ulcerative colitis, urethritis, urinary tract irritation, urinary tract infection, varicose ulcers (topical), vomiting, whooping cough, wound healing.

DOSING

The following doses are based on scientific research, publications, traditional use, or expert opinion. Many herbs and supplements have not been thoroughly tested, and their safety and effectiveness may not be proven. Brands may be made differently, with variable ingredients even within the same brand. The doses shown may not apply to all products. It is important to always read product labels and discuss doses with a qualified healthcare provider before therapy is started.

Standardization

- Standardization involves measuring the amount of certain chemicals in products to try to make different preparations similar to each other. It is not always known if the chemicals being measured are the "active" ingredients.
- Pharmacopoeia-grade marshmallow must be properly identified by the naked eye and by microscope. The British Pharmacopoeia requires marshmallow leaf to be harvested before the flowering period, and to pass specific scientific tests for identification.

Adults (18 Years and Older)

- **Skin inflammatory conditions (eczema, psoriasis):** Historically, 5 to 10 g of marshmallow in ointment or cream base or 5% powdered marshmallow leaf has been applied to the skin three times daily. Daily oral doses of 5 g of marshmallow leaf or 6 g of marshmallow root have been suggested.
- **Oral and pharyngeal irritation:** A dose of 2 g of marshmallow in 1 cup of cold water, soaked for 2 hours and then gargled, has been used but is not supported by scientific evidence.

Children (Younger Than 18 Years)

- There are not enough scientific data to recommend marshmallow for use in children.

SAFETY

The U.S. Food and Drug Administration does not strictly regulate herbs and supplements. There is no guarantee of strength, purity, or safety of products, and effects may vary. It is important to always read product labels. People who have a medical condition, or are taking other drugs, herbs, or supplements, should consult a qualified healthcare provider before starting a new therapy. A healthcare provider should be consulted immediately about any side effects.

Allergies

- Although there are no known reports or studies about marshmallow allergy, allergic reactions to marshmallow may occur.

Side Effects and Warnings

- Historically, marshmallow is generally regarded as being safe in healthy individuals. However, because studies have not evaluated the safety of marshmallow, proper doses and duration in humans are not known. Allergic reactions may occur.
- Based on animal study, marshmallow may lower blood glucose levels. Caution is advised in patients with diabetes or hypoglycemia, and in those taking drugs, herbs, or supplements that affect blood sugar. Serum glucose levels should be monitored closely, and medication adjustments may be necessary.

Pregnancy and Breastfeeding

- There is not enough scientific evidence to support the safe use of marshmallow during pregnancy or breastfeeding.

INTERACTIONS

Most herbs and supplements have not been thoroughly tested for interactions with other herbs, supplements, drugs, or foods. The interactions listed here are based on reports in scientific publications, laboratory experiments, or traditional use. It is important to always read product labels. People who have a medical condition, or are taking other drugs, herbs, or supplements, should consult a qualified healthcare provider before starting a new therapy.

Interactions with Drugs

- Based on animal study, marshmallow may lower blood sugar levels. Caution is advised when using medications that may also lower blood sugar. A qualified healthcare provider should closely monitor patients taking drugs for diabetes by mouth or insulin. Medication adjustments may be necessary.
- Marshmallow may interfere with the absorption of other drugs and therefore should be taken 1 hour before or 2 hours after ingestion of other drugs.

Interactions with Herbs and Dietary Supplements

- Based on animal study, marshmallow may lower blood sugar levels. Caution is advised when using herbs or supplements that may also lower blood sugar. Blood glucose levels may require monitoring, and doses may need adjustment. Possible examples include *Aloe vera*, American ginseng, bilberry, bitter melon, burdock, fenugreek, fish oil, gymnema, horse chestnut seed extract (HCSE), milk thistle, *Panax ginseng*, rosemary, Siberian ginseng, stinging nettle, and white horehound. Agents that may raise blood sugar levels include arginine, cocoa, and ephedra (when combined with caffeine).
- Marshmallow may interfere with the absorption of other agents and therefore should be taken 1 hour before or 2 hours after ingestion of other herbs and supplements.

Selected References

Natural Standard developed the preceding evidence-based information based on a systematic review of more than 40 scientific articles. For comprehensive information about alternative and complementary therapies on the professional level, go to www.naturalstandard.com. Selected references are listed here.

Bone K. Marshmallow soothes cough. Br J Phytother 1993;3(2):93.

Kobayashi A, Hachiya A, Ohuchi A, et al. Inhibitory mechanism of an extract of *Althaea officinalis* L. on endothelin-1–induced melanocyte activation. Biol Pharm Bull 2002;25(2): 229-234.

Robertson CS, Smart H, Amar SS, et al. Oesophageal transit of marshmallow after the Angelchik procedure. Br J Surg 1989;76(3):245-247.

Tomoda M, Shimizu N, Oshima Y, et al. Hypoglycemic activity of twenty plant mucilages and three modified products. Planta Med 1987;53(1):8-12.

Melatonin

RELATED TERMS

- Acetamide, BMS-214778, luzindole, mel, MEL, melatonine, 5-methoxy-*N*-acetyltryptamine, MLT, *N*-acetyl-5-methoxytryptamine, *N*-2-(5-methoxyindol-3-ethyl)-acetamide.

BACKGROUND

- Melatonin is a neurohormone produced in the brain by the pineal gland, from the amino acid tryptophan. The synthesis and release of melatonin are stimulated by darkness and suppressed by light, suggesting the involvement of melatonin in circadian rhythm and regulation of diverse body functions. Levels of melatonin in the blood are highest before bedtime.
- Synthetic melatonin supplements have been used for a variety of medical conditions, most notably for disorders related to sleep.
- Melatonin possesses antioxidant activity, and many of its proposed therapeutic or preventive uses are based on this property.
- New drugs that block the effects of melatonin are in development, such as BMS-214778 or luzindole, and may have uses in various disorders.

USES BASED ON SCIENTIFIC EVIDENCE	Grade*
Jet lag Several randomized, placebo controlled human trials suggest that melatonin taken by mouth, started on the day of travel (close to the target bedtime at the destination) and continued for several days, reduces the number of days required to establish a normal sleep pattern, diminishes the time it takes to fall asleep ("sleep latency"), improves alertness, and reduces daytime fatigue. Effects may be greatest with eastward travel and with crossing of more than four time zones (results may be less impressive with westward travel or crossing of fewer time zones). Combination with prescription sleep aids such as zolpidem (Ambien) may add to these effects, although side effects such as morning sleepiness may occur. Although these results are compelling, a majority of studies have had methodologic problems with their designs and reporting, and some trials have not found benefits. Overall, the scientific evidence does suggest benefits of melatonin in up to half of people who take it for jet lag. Further well-designed trials are necessary to confirm these findings, to determine optimal dosing, and to evaluate use in combination with prescription sleep aids.	A

Continued

Preliminary research reports that starting melatonin on the day of travel, rather than before travel, may yield superior results. Higher doses (such as 5 mg nightly) may be slightly more effective than lower doses (for example, 0.1 to 0.5 mg nightly) for improvement of sleep quality and latency, although this area remains controversial, with some studies suggesting no differences. Slow-release melatonin may not be as effective as standard (quick-release) formulations. If the dose is taken too early in the day, it may actually result in excessive daytime sleepiness and greater difficulty adapting to the destination time zone.	
Delayed sleep phase syndrome Delayed sleep phase syndrome (DSPS) is a condition that results in delayed sleep onset, despite normal sleep architecture and sleep duration. Several small controlled studies and case series in healthy volunteers and in patients with DSPS have used 5 to 6 mg of melatonin, with reported improvements in sleep latency. Although these results are promising, additional research with large, well-designed controlled studies is needed before a stronger recommendation can be made.	**B**
Insomnia in the elderly Several human studies report that melatonin taken by mouth 30 to 120 minutes before bedtime decreases the amount of time it takes to fall asleep (sleep latency) in elderly individuals with insomnia. It is not clear if melatonin increases the length of time people are able to stay asleep. Low doses (0.1 to 0.3 mg taken nightly) appear to be as effective as higher doses (3 to 5 mg nightly). However, most studies have not been of high quality in design, and some research has found limited or no benefits. A majority of trials have been brief in duration (several days long), and long-term effects are not known. Although the evidence overall does suggest short-term benefits, additional study is needed before a strong recommendation can be made. It is not known how melatonin compares with standard therapies for insomnia—for example, use of benzodiazepines such as diazepam (Valium) and lorazepam (Ativan), or other sleep aids such as zolpidem (Ambien).	**B**
Sleep disturbances in children with neuropsychiatric disorders There are multiple controlled trials and several case reports of melatonin use in children with various neuropsychiatric disorders, including mental retardation, autism, psychiatric disorders, visual impairment, and epilepsy. Studies have demonstrated reduced time to fall asleep (sleep latency) and increased sleep duration. Oral doses of melatonin have ranged between 2.5 and 10 mg administered at the desired bedtime. Well-designed controlled trials in select patient populations are needed before a stronger or more specific recommendation can be made.	**B**

Continued

Sleep enhancement in healthy people Multiple human studies have measured the effects of melatonin supplements on sleep in healthy individuals. A wide range of doses has been used, from 0.1 to 1.0 mg ("low-dose" melatonin) up to doses between 5 and 10 mg, often taken by mouth 30 to 60 minutes before sleep time. Most trials have been small and brief in duration (often single-dose studies) and have not been rigorously designed or reported (inadequate blinding and randomization). However, the weight of scientific evidence does suggest that melatonin decreases the time it takes to fall asleep (sleep latency), increases the feeling of "sleepiness," and may increase the duration of sleep. Better-quality research is needed in this area. It is not known how melatonin compares with standard therapies for insomnia—for example, use of benzodiazepines such as diazepam (Valium) and lorazepam (Ativan), or other sleep aids such as zolpidem (Ambien).	B
Alzheimer's disease (sleep disorders) There is limited study of melatonin for management of sleep disorders associated with Alzheimer's disease (including nighttime agitation and poor sleep quality in patients with dementia). It has been reported that natural melatonin levels are altered in people with Alzheimer's disease, although it remains unclear if supplementation with melatonin is beneficial. Further research is needed in this area before a firm conclusion can be reached.	C
Antioxidant (free radical scavenging) There are well over 100 laboratory and animal studies of the antioxidant (free radical–scavenging) properties of melatonin. As a result, melatonin has been proposed as a supplement to prevent or treat many conditions that are associated with oxidative damage. However, there are no well-designed trials in humans that have demonstrated benefits of melatonin as an antioxidant for any health problem.	C
Attention deficit hyperactivity disorder There is limited research of the use of melatonin in children with attention deficit hyperactivity disorder (ADHD). A clear conclusion cannot be reached at this time.	C
Benzodiazepine tapering A small amount of research has examined the use of melatonin to assist with tapering or cessation of benzodiazepines such as diazepam (Valium) or lorazepam (Ativan). Although preliminary results are promising, because of weaknesses in the design and reporting of this research, further study is necessary before a firm conclusion can be reached.	C
Bipolar disorder (sleep disturbances) There is limited study of melatonin given to patients with sleep disturbances (such as insomnia or irregular sleep patterns) associated with bipolar disorder. No clear benefits have been reported. Further research is needed in this area before a clear conclusion can be reached.	C

M

Continued

Cancer treatment There are several early-phase and controlled human trials of melatonin in patients with various advanced-stage malignancies, including brain, breast, colorectal, gastric, liver, lung, pancreatic, and testicular cancers, as well as lymphoma, melanoma, renal cell carcinoma, and soft-tissue sarcoma. Many of these studies have been conducted by the same research group. In this research, melatonin has been combined with other types of treatment, including radiation therapy, chemotherapy (such as with cisplatin, etoposide, or irinotecan), hormonal treatments (such as with tamoxifen), or immune therapy such as with interferon, interleukin-2, or tumor necrosis factor. Most of these trials have been published by the same research group and have involved giving melatonin orally, intravenously, or injected into muscle. Results have been mixed, with some patients stabilizing and others demonstrating tumor progression. There are some promising reported results, including small significant improvements in the survival of patients with non–small cell lung cancer given oral melatonin with chemotherapy (using cisplatin and etoposide). However, the design and results of this research are not sufficient to provide definitive evidence in favor of safe and effective use of melatonin in cancer patients. High-quality follow-up trials are necessary to confirm these preliminary results. It has been proposed that melatonin may benefit cancer patients through antioxidant, immune-enhancing, hormonal, anti-inflammatory, antiangiogenic, apoptotic, or direct cytotoxic (cancer cell–killing) effects, and there are many ongoing laboratory and animal studies in these areas. Some experts believe that antioxidants can improve the effectiveness of chemotherapy drugs and reduce side effects, whereas others suggest that antioxidants may actually interfere with the effectiveness of chemotherapies. Currently, no clear conclusion can be drawn in this area. There is not enough definitive scientific evidence to discern if melatonin is beneficial against any type of cancer, whether it increases (or decreases) the effectiveness of other cancer therapies, or if it safely reduces chemotherapy side effects.	C
Chemotherapy side effects Several human trials have examined the effects of melatonin on side effects associated with use of various cancer chemotherapy agents (such as carboplatin, cisplatin, daunorubicin, doxorubicin, epirubicin, etoposide, 5-fluorouracil, gemcitabine, and mitoxantrone). Most of these studies are published by the same research group and involve giving melatonin through a vein or injected into muscle. Studies have included patients with advanced lung, breast, gastrointestinal, prostate, and head and neck cancers, as well as lymphoma. Promising early results include reductions in nerve injury (neuropathy), mouth sores (stomatitis), wasting (cachexia), and platelet count drops	C

Continued

(thrombocytopenia) associated with various chemotherapy agents. Animal studies note reduced severity of heart damage from anthracycline drugs or lung damage from bleomycin. Some researchers attribute these reported benefits to antioxidant properties of melatonin. Overall, it remains controversial whether antioxidants increase effectiveness and reduce side effects of chemotherapy agents, or whether antioxidants actually reduce effectiveness of chemotherapy agents. Increased platelet counts after melatonin use have been observed in patients with decreased platelets due to cancer therapies (in several studies reported by the same author), and stimulation of platelet production (thrombopoiesis) has been suggested but not clearly demonstrated. Although these early reported benefits are promising, high-quality controlled trials are necessary before a clear conclusion can be reached in this area. It remains unclear if melatonin safely reduces side effects of various chemotherapy agents without altering effectiveness.	
Circadian rhythm entraining (in blind persons) In blind individuals, light and dark stimuli are not received by the eye to trigger melatonin release and the onset of sleep. In these patients, natural melatonin levels peak at a different hour every night, to the point where individuals may sleep during the day and be awake at night. This is commonly referred to as "free running" circadian rhythm. There are numerous published small case series and case reports in the literature, yet limited controlled trials to date in this population. Present studies and individual cases suggest that melatonin, administered in the evening, may correct circadian rhythm. Large, well-designed controlled trials are needed before a stronger recommendation can be made.	**C**
Depression (sleep disturbances) Depression can be associated with neuroendocrine and sleep abnormalities, such as reduced time before dream sleep (REM latency). Melatonin has been suggested for the improvement of sleep patterns in patients with depression, although research is limited in this area. Further studies are needed before a clear conclusion can be reached.	**C**
Glaucoma It has been theorized that as a result of effects on photoreceptor renewal in the eye, high doses of melatonin may increase intraocular pressure and the risk of glaucoma, age-related maculopathy and myopia, or retinal damage. However, there is preliminary evidence that melatonin may actually decrease intraocular pressure in the eye, and it has been suggested as a possible agent for therapy of glaucoma. Additional study is necessary in this area. Patients with glaucoma who are taking melatonin should be monitored by a healthcare professional.	**C**
Headache prevention Several small studies have examined the possible role of melatonin in preventing various forms of headache, including migraine, cluster, and	**C**

Continued

tension-type headaches (in people who suffer from regular headaches). Limited initial research suggests possible benefits in all three types of headache, although well-designed controlled studies are needed before a firm conclusion can be drawn.	
High blood pressure (hypertension) Several controlled studies in patients with high blood pressure report small reductions in diastolic and systolic blood pressure with use of melatonin taken by mouth (orally) or inhaled through the nose (intranasally). Most trials have been small and not well designed or reported. Better-designed research is necessary before a firm conclusion can be reached.	**C**
HIV infection/AIDS There is a lack of well-designed scientific evidence to recommend for or against the use of melatonin as a treatment for AIDS. Melatonin should not be used in place of more proven therapies, and patients with HIV infection/AIDS are advised to be treated under the supervision of a medical doctor.	**C**
Insomnia (of unknown origin in the nonelderly) There are several small controlled human trials and pilot research of melatonin taken by mouth in people with insomnia. Results have been inconsistent, with some studies reporting benefits on sleep latency and subjective sleep quality and other research finding no benefits. Most studies have been small and not rigorously designed or reported. Better research is needed before a firm conclusion can be drawn. Notably, several studies in elderly individuals with insomnia provide preliminary evidence of benefits on sleep latency (discussed earlier).	**C**
Parkinson's disease Because study to date has been very limited, a recommendation cannot be made for or against the use of melatonin in parkinsonism or Parkinson's disease. Better-designed research is needed before a firm conclusion can be reached in this area.	**C**
Periodic limb movement disorder There is very limited study to date for the use of melatonin as a treatment in periodic limb movement disorder. Better-designed research is needed before a recommendation can be made in this area.	**C**
Preoperative sedation/anxiolysis A small number of controlled studies have compared melatonin with placebo and standard drugs (benzodiazepines) for sedation and anxiety reduction (anxiolysis) before general anesthesia for surgery. Results are promising, with similar results reported for melatonin and for benzodiazepines such as midazolam (Versed), and superiority to placebo. There are also promising reports using melatonin for sedation/anxiolysis before magnetic resonance imaging (MRI). However, because of	**C**

Continued

weaknesses in the design and reporting of the available research, better studies are needed before a clear conclusion can be drawn.

Melatonin has also been suggested as a treatment for delirium following surgery, although there is little evidence in this area.

REM sleep behavior disorder Limited case reports describe benefits in patients with REM sleep behavior disorder who receive melatonin. However, better research is needed before a clear conclusion can be drawn.	C
Rett's syndrome Rett's syndrome is a presumably genetic disorder that affects female children, characterized by decelerated head growth and global developmental regression. There is limited study of the possible role of melatonin in improving sleep disturbance associated with Rett's syndrome. Further research is needed before a recommendation can be made in this area.	C
Schizophrenia (sleep disorders) There is limited study of melatonin for decreasing sleep latency (time to fall asleep) in patients with schizophrenia. Further research is needed in this area before a clear conclusion can be reached.	C
Seasonal affective disorder There are several small, brief studies of melatonin in patients with seasonal affective disorder (SAD). This research is not well designed or reported, and further study is necessary before a clear conclusion can be reached.	C
Seizure disorder (children) The role of melatonin in seizure disorder is controversial. There are several reported cases of children with intractable seizures or neurologic damage who improved with regular nighttime melatonin administration. Limited animal research also suggests possible antiseizure effects. However, there has also been a report that melatonin may actually lower seizure threshold and increase the risk of seizures. Better evidence is needed in this area before a clear conclusion can be drawn regarding the safety or effectiveness of melatonin in seizure disorder.	C
Sleep disturbances due to pineal region brain damage Several published cases report improvements in sleep patterns in young people with damage to the pineal gland area of the brain due to tumors or surgery. Because of the rarity of such disorders, controlled trials may not be possible. Use of melatonin in such patients should be under the direction of a qualified healthcare provider.	C
Smoking cessation A small amount of research has examined the use of melatonin to reduce symptoms associated with smoking cessation, such as anxiousness,	C

M

Continued

restlessness, irritability, and cigarette craving. Although preliminary results are promising, because of weaknesses in the design and reporting of this research, further study is necessary before a firm conclusion can be reached.	
Stroke It has been proposed that melatonin may reduce the amount of neurologic damage patients experience after stroke, because of its antioxidant properties. In addition, melatonin levels may be altered in people immediately after stroke, and it has thus been suggested that melatonin supplementation may be beneficial, although this effect has not been shown in humans. At this time, the effects of melatonin supplements immediately after stroke are not clear.	C
Tardive dyskinesia Tardive dyskinesia (TD) is a serious potential side effect of antipsychotic medications, characterized by involuntary muscle movements. Limited small studies of melatonin use in patients with TD report mixed findings. Additional research is necessary before a clear conclusion can be drawn.	C
Thrombocytopenia (low platelets) Increased platelet counts after melatonin use have been observed in patients with decreased platelets due to cancer therapies (in several studies reported by the same author). Stimulation of platelet production (thrombopoiesis) has been suggested but not clearly demonstrated. Additional research is necessary in this area before a clear conclusion can be drawn. Cases of idiopathic thrombocytopenic purpura (ITP) treated with melatonin have been reported.	C
Ultraviolet light skin damage protection Several small, randomized trials have examined the use of melatonin in protecting human skin against ultraviolet (UV) light damage. It has been proposed that antioxidant properties of melatonin may be protective. Although this preliminary research reports reductions in erythema (skin redness) with the use of melatonin, further study is necessary before a clear conclusion can be drawn about clinical effectiveness in humans.	C
Work shift sleep disorder There are several studies of melatonin use in people who work irregular shifts, such as emergency room personnel. Results are mixed, with some studies finding no significant benefits and others reporting benefits in sleep quality compared with that described for placebo. Because most published trials are small, with incomplete reporting of design or results, additional research is necessary before a clear conclusion can be drawn.	C

*Key to grades: *A:* Strong scientific evidence for this use; *B:* Good scientific evidence for this use; *C:* Unclear scientific evidence for this use; *D:* Fair scientific evidence against this use (it may not work); *F:* Strong scientific evidence against this use (it likely does not work). For a more detailed explanation of efficacy criteria, see "Natural Standard Evidence-Based Validated Grading Rationale" in the Introduction.

Uses Based on Tradition, Theory, or Limited Scientific Evidence

Acetaminophen toxicity, acute respiratory distress syndrome (ARDS), aging, aluminum toxicity, Alzheimer's disease, amikacin-induced kidney damage, asthma, beta-blocker sleep disturbance, cachexia, cancer prevention, cardiac syndrome, cognitive enhancement, colitis, contraception, coronary artery disease, critical illness/intensive care unit sleep disturbance, cyclosporine-induced kidney toxicity, depression, edema, erectile dysfunction, fibromyalgia, itching, intestinal motility disorders, gastroesophageal reflux disease (GERD), gentamicin-induced kidney damage, glaucoma, heart attack prevention, hyperpigmentation, immunostimulant, interstitial cystitis, lead toxicity, melatonin deficiency, memory enhancement, multiple sclerosis, neurodegenerative disorders, noise-induced hearing loss, pancreatitis, polycystic ovarian syndrome (PCOS), postmenopausal osteoporosis, postoperative adjunct, postoperative delirium, prevention of post–lung transplantation ischemia-reperfusion injury, rheumatoid arthritis, sarcoidosis, schistosomiasis, sedation, sexual activity enhancement, sudden infant death syndrome (SIDS) prevention, tachycardia, tinnitus, toxic kidney damage, toxic liver damage, tuberculosis, tuberous sclerosis, ulcerative colitis, withdrawal from narcotics, wound healing.

DOSING

The following doses are based on scientific research, publications, traditional use, or expert opinion. Many herbs and supplements have not been thoroughly tested, and their safety and effectiveness may not be proven. Brands may be made differently, with variable ingredients even within the same brand. The doses shown may not apply to all products. It is important to always read product labels and discuss doses with a qualified healthcare provider before therapy is started.

Standardization

- Standardization involves measuring the amount of certain chemicals in products to try to make different preparations similar to each other. It is not always known if the chemicals being measured are the "active" ingredients.
- There is no widely accepted standardization for melatonin. Experts have noted that most brands contain impurities that cannot be characterized, as well as dissimilar amounts of actual hormone.
- In 2002, ConsumerLab.com evaluated 18 melatonin-containing supplements (15 quick-release and 3 time-release products), of which 12 were melatonin-only products. It was reported that 16 of the 18 products contained between 100% and 135% of the claimed amount of melatonin, one rapid-release product contained only 83% of the claimed amount of melatonin, and another rapid-release product contained a small amount of lead (slightly more than 0.5 micrograms per daily recommended dose of the supplement). Among the 12 melatonin-only products that "passed" these standards are Nature's Bounty Melatonin 1-mg and 3-mg tablets, Puritan's Pride Inspired by Nature Melatonin 3-mg tablets, Twinlab Melatonin Caps, Highest Quality, Quick Acting 3-mg tablets.

Adults (18 Years and Older)

- **Alzheimer's disease (sleep disturbances):** Studies have evaluated 0.5 mg of melatonin taken nightly by mouth 1 hour before sleep.

- **Bipolar disorder (sleep disturbances):** Studies have evaluated 10 mg of melatonin taken nightly by mouth.
- **Cancer:** Various doses of melatonin have been studied in patients with cancer, usually given in addition to other standard treatments such as chemotherapy, radiation therapy, or immune therapy. Oral doses have ranged between 10 and 50 mg taken nightly, with the most common dose being 20 mg nightly. Intramuscular injections of 20 mg of melatonin have also been studied. In studies of patients with melanoma, melatonin preparations have been applied to the skin. Patients are advised to discuss cancer treatment plans with an oncologist before considering use of melatonin either alone or with other therapies. Safety and effectiveness are not proven, and melatonin should not be used instead of more proven therapies.
- **Circadian rhythm entraining (in blind persons):** Doses of 5 to 10 mg of melatonin taken by mouth, administered in the evening, have been studied in blind patients to set the circadian rhythm to a 24-hour schedule.
- **Critical illness/ICU sleep disturbance:** Studies have evaluated 3 mg of melatonin taken nightly by mouth.
- **Delayed sleep phase syndrome:** A dose of 5 mg of melatonin given by mouth 5 hours before bedtime has been studied.
- **Depression (sleep disturbances):** Studies have evaluated 5 mg of melatonin taken nightly by mouth.
- **Headache prevention:** Studies have evaluated regular use of 5 to 10 mg of melatonin taken nightly by mouth.
- **Hypertension:** Studies have evaluated 1 to 3 mg of melatonin taken daily by mouth for short periods of time. Intranasal melatonin (1% solution in ethanol) at a dose of 2 mg daily for 1 week has also been studied.
- **Insomnia in the elderly:** Studies have evaluated melatonin taken by mouth 30 to 120 minutes before bedtime for insomnia in the elderly. Low doses (0.1 to 0.3 mg taken nightly) appear to be as effective as higher doses (3 to 5 mg nightly).
- **Insomnia of unknown origin (in the nonelderly):** Doses ranging from 1 to 5 mg taken by mouth shortly before bedtime have been studied.
- **Jet lag:** Melatonin is usually started on the day of travel (close to the target bedtime at the destination), then taken every 24 hours for several days. Various doses have been used and studied, including low doses between 0.1 and 0.5 mg, a more common dose of 5 mg, and a higher dose of 8 mg. Overall, 0.5 mg appears to be slightly less effective than 5 milligrams for improvement of sleep quality and latency, although this area remains controversial and other research suggests no differences. Slow-release melatonin may not be as effective as standard (quick-release) formulations. If the dose is taken too early in the day, it may actually result in excessive daytime sleepiness and greater difficulty adapting to the destination time zone.
- **Schizophrenia (sleep disturbances):** Studies have evaluated 2 mg of controlled-release melatonin taken by mouth for 3 weeks.
- **Seasonal affective disorder:** Studies have evaluated 0.25 to 5 mg of melatonin daily by mouth.
- **Sleep enhancement in healthy people:** Various doses of melatonin taken by mouth 30 to 60 minutes before bedtime have been studied and reported to have beneficial effects, including 0.1, 0.3, 1, 3, 5, and 6 mg. Studies report that 0.1 to 0.3 mg may produce melatonin levels in the body within the normal physiologic range of nighttime melatonin and may be sufficient. Research suggests that quick-release melatonin may be more effective than sustained-release formulations.

- **Other:** There are other uses with limited study and unclear effectiveness or safety. Use of melatonin for these conditions should be discussed with a primary healthcare provider and should not be substituted for more proven therapies.

Children (Younger Than 18 Years)

- **General:** There is limited study of melatonin supplements in children, and safety is not established. Use of melatonin should be discussed with the child's physician before supplementation is started.
- **Circadian rhythm entraining in blind children:** Studies have evaluated 2.5 to 10 mg of melatonin taken nightly at the desired bedtime.
- **Seizure disorder in children:** Studies have evaluated 5 to 10 mg of melatonin taken nightly. Research is limited in this area, and there are other reports that melatonin may actually increase risk of seizure or lower seizure threshold. Therefore, caution is advised, and use of melatonin should be discussed with the child's physician.
- **Sleep disturbances in children with neuropsychiatric disorders (mental retardation, autism, psychiatric disorders):** Studies have evaluated 0.5 to 10 mg of melatonin taken nightly for reduced sleep latency and increased sleep duration. Fast-release melatonin may be most useful for sleep induction and the slow-release formulation for sleep maintenance.

SAFETY

The U.S. Food and Drug Administration does not strictly regulate herbs and supplements. There is no guarantee of strength, purity, or safety of products, and effects may vary. It is important to always read product labels. People who have a medical condition, or are taking other drugs, herbs, or supplements, should consult a qualified healthcare provider before starting a new therapy. A healthcare provider should be consulted immediately about any side effects.

Allergies

- There are rare reports of allergic skin reactions after taking melatonin by mouth. Melatonin has been linked to a case of autoimmune hepatitis.

Side Effects and Warnings

- **General:** Based on available studies and clinical use, melatonin is generally regarded as safe in recommended doses for short-term use. Available trials report that overall adverse effects are not significantly more common with melatonin than with placebo. However, case reports raise concerns about risks of blood clotting abnormalities (particularly in patients taking warfarin), increased risk of seizure, and disorientation with overdose.
- **Neurologic (general):** Commonly reported adverse effects include fatigue, dizziness, headache, irritability, and sleepiness, although these effects may occur as a result of jet lag and not from melatonin itself. Fatigue may particularly occur with morning use or high doses (greater than 50 mg), and irregular sleep-wake cycles may occur. Disorientation, confusion, sleepwalking, vivid dreams, and nightmares have also been noted, with effects often resolving after cessation of melatonin. Because of the risk of daytime sleepiness, caution should be taken by persons driving or operating heavy machinery. Headache has been reported. Ataxia (difficulties with walking and balance) may occur following overdose.
- **Neurologic (seizure risk):** It has been suggested that melatonin may lower seizure threshold and increase the risk of seizure, particularly in children with severe

neurologic disorders, as reported in four out of six children in one study, and in an adult in whom symptoms recurred when melatonin was given a second time. However, other studies actually report reduced incidence of seizure with regular melatonin use. This remains an area of controversy. Patients with seizure disorder taking melatonin should be monitored closely by a healthcare professional.

- **Psychiatric:** Mood changes have been reported, including giddiness and dysphoria (sadness). Psychotic symptoms have been reported in at least two cases, including hallucinations and paranoia, possibly as a result of overdose. Patients with underlying major depression or psychotic disorders taking melatonin should be monitored closely by a healthcare professional.
- **Hematologic (blood clotting abnormalities):** There are at least six reported cases of alterations in prothrombin time (PT), a measurement of blood-clotting ability, in patients taking both melatonin and the blood-thinning medication warfarin (Coumadin). The reports noted decreases in PT, which would tend to decrease the effects of warfarin and increase the risk of blood clots. However, blood clots have not been noted in these patients. Rather, minor bleeding was noted in two of these cases (nosebleed and internal eye bleed), which may have been due to the blood-thinning effects of warfarin alone without a relation to use of melatonin, or possibly to an interaction between melatonin and warfarin. It is not known if melatonin has effects on blood clotting in people who are not taking warfarin. As indicated by these reports, melatonin should be avoided in patients using warfarin, and possibly in patients taking other blood-thinning medications or in those with clotting disorders.
- **Cardiovascular:** Melatonin may cause drops in blood pressure, as observed in animals and in preliminary human research. Whether these reductions in blood pressure are clinically relevant is not clear. Caution is advised in patients taking medications that may also lower blood pressure. As indicated by preliminary evidence, increases in cholesterol levels may occur. Preliminary research suggests that regular use of melatonin may increase atherosclerotic plaque buildup in humans and animals. Caution is therefore advised in patients with high cholesterol levels or atherosclerosis, or those at risk for cardiovascular disease. There are several poorly described reports of abnormal heart rhythms, fast heart rate, or chest pain, although in most cases patients were taking other drugs that could account for these findings.
- **Endocrine (blood sugar elevations):** Elevated blood sugar levels (hyperglycemia) have been reported in patients with type 1 diabetes mellitus (insulin-dependent diabetes), and low doses of melatonin have reduced glucose tolerance and insulin sensitivity. Caution is advised in patients with diabetes or hypoglycemia, and in those taking drugs, herbs, or supplements that affect blood sugar. Serum glucose levels may need to be monitored by a healthcare provider, and medication adjustments may be necessary.
- **Endocrine (hormonal effects):** Hormonal effects are reported, including decreases or increases in levels of luteinizing hormone, progesterone, estradiol, thyroid hormones (thyroxine [T_4] and triiodothyronine [T_3]), growth hormone, prolactin, cortisol, oxytocin, and vasopressin, although there are other reports of no significant hormonal effects. Variations may be related to underlying patient characteristics. Gynecomastia (increased breast size) has been reported in men, as well as decreased sperm count (both abnormalities resolved with cessation of melatonin). Decreased sperm motility has been reported in rats and humans.

- **Gastrointestinal:** Mild gastrointestinal distress commonly occurs, including nausea, vomiting, or cramping. Melatonin has been linked to a case of autoimmune hepatitis and with triggering of Crohn's disease symptoms.
- **Ocular (glaucoma):** It has been theorized that as a result of effects on photoreceptor renewal in the eye, high doses of melatonin may increase intraocular pressure and the risk of glaucoma, age-related maculopathy and myopia, or retinal damage. However, there is preliminary evidence that melatonin may actually decrease intraocular pressure in the eye, and it has been suggested as a possible agent for therapy of glaucoma. Patients with glaucoma who are taking melatonin should be monitored by a healthcare professional.

Pregnancy and Breastfeeding

- Melatonin supplementation should be avoided in women who are pregnant or attempting to become pregnant, because of possible hormonal effects, including alterations in pituitary or ovarian function and potential inhibition of ovulation or uterine contractions. High levels of melatonin during pregnancy may increase the risk of developmental disorders. In animal studies, melatonin is detected in breast milk and therefore should be avoided during breastfeeding. In men, decreased sperm motility and decreased sperm count are reported with use of melatonin.

INTERACTIONS

Most herbs and supplements have not been thoroughly tested for interactions with other herbs, supplements, drugs, or foods. The interactions listed here are based on reports in scientific publications, laboratory experiments, or traditional use. It is important to always read product labels. People who have a medical condition, or are taking other drugs, herbs, or supplements, should consult a qualified healthcare provider before starting a new therapy.

Interactions with Drugs

- **Fluvoxamine and other P450 1A2–altering drugs:** Melatonin is broken down (metabolized) in the body by the liver enzyme cytochrome P450 1A2 (with a small contribution from P450 2C19). As a result, drugs that alter the activity of these enzymes may increase or decrease the effects of melatonin supplements. For example, the drug fluvoxamine, when given with melatonin, reduces the activity of P450 1A2, thereby increasing blood levels of melatonin and theoretically increasing the activity or side effects of melatonin. Other drugs that may increase melatonin levels (by inhibiting P450 1A2) include amiodarone, anastrozole, cimetidine, ciprofloxacin, citalopram, clarithromycin, diethyldithiocarbamate, diltiazem, enoxacin, erythromycin, ethinyl estradiol, fluoroquinolones, fluoxetine (in high doses), furafylline, interferon, isoniazid, ketoconazole, levofloxacin, methoxsalen, mexiletine, mibefradil, norfloxacin, paroxetine (in high doses), ritonavir, sertraline (effect is mild), tacrine, ticlopidine, tricyclic antidepressants (tertiary), and zileuton. There is a case of psychotic symptoms in a patient taking both melatonin and the antidepressant drug fluoxetine, which may be due to this interaction. Drugs that may reduce melatonin levels (by inducing P450 1A2) include carbamazepine, insulin, 3-methylcholanthrene, modafinil, nafcillin, nicotine, omeprazole, phenobarbital, phenytoin, primidone, rifampin, and ritonavir.
- **Zolpidem and other sedative drugs:** Increased daytime drowsiness is reported when melatonin is used at the same time as the prescription sleep aid zolpidem (Ambien), although it is not clear that effects are greater than with the use of

zolpidem alone. In theory, because of possible risk of daytime sleepiness, melatonin may increase the amount of drowsiness caused by some other drugs—for example, benzodiazepines such as lorazepam (Ativan) and diazepam (Valium), barbiturates such as phenobarbital, narcotics such as codeine, some antidepressants, and alcohol. Caution is advised in persons driving or operating machinery.

- **Warfarin and other blood-thinners:** Based on preliminary evidence, melatonin should be avoided in patients taking the blood-thinning medication warfarin (Coumadin), and possibly in patients using other blood thinners (anticoagulants) such as aspirin and heparin. There are at least six reported cases of alterations in PT (a measurement of blood clotting ability) in patients taking both melatonin and warfarin. The reports noted decreases in PT, which would tend to decrease the effects of warfarin and increase the risk of blood clots. However, blood clots have not been noted in these patients. Rather, minor bleeding was noted in two of these cases (nosebleed and internal eye bleed), which may have been due to the blood-thinning effects of warfarin alone, without a relation to use of melatonin, or possibly to an interaction between melatonin and warfarin.
- **Natural melatonin levels:** Multiple drugs are reported to lower natural levels of melatonin in the body. It is not clear that there are any health hazards of lowered melatonin levels, or if replacing melatonin with supplements is beneficial. Examples of drugs that may reduce production or secretion of melatonin are nonsteroidal anti-inflammatory drugs (NSAIDs) such as ibuprofen (Motrin, Advil) and naproxen (Naprosyn, Aleve); beta-blocker blood pressure medications such as atenolol (Tenormin) and metoprolol (Lopressor, Toprol); and medications that reduce levels of vitamin B_6 in the body (such as oral contraceptives, hormone replacement therapy, loop diuretics, hydralazine, and theophylline). Other agents that may alter synthesis or release of melatonin include diazepam, vitamin B_{12}, verapamil, temazepam, and somatostatin.
- **Antiseizure drugs:** As indicated by preliminary evidence, melatonin should be avoided in patients taking antiseizure medications. It has been suggested that melatonin may lower seizure threshold and increase the risk of seizure, particularly in children with severe neurologic disorders, as reported in four out of six children in one study, and in an adult in whom symptoms recurred when melatonin was given a second time. However, other studies actually report reduced incidence of seizure with regular melatonin use. This remains an area of controversy. Patients with seizure disorder taking melatonin should be monitored closely by a healthcare professional.
- **Blood pressure medications (antihypertensives):** Melatonin may cause drops in blood pressure, as observed in animals and in preliminary human research. It is not known if melatonin causes further drops in blood pressure when it is taken with antihypertensive drugs. In animals, melatonin reduces the effects of the alpha-blocker drugs clonidine and methoxamine. By contrast, in humans, blood pressure increases have been observed when melatonin 5 mg is taken at the same time as the calcium channel blocker nifedipine.
- **Diabetes medications:** Elevated blood sugar levels (hyperglycemia) have been reported in patients with type 1 diabetes mellitus (insulin-dependent diabetes), and low doses of melatonin have reduced glucose tolerance and insulin sensitivity. Caution is advised in patients taking drugs for diabetes by mouth or insulin. Serum glucose levels may need to be monitored by a healthcare provider, and medication adjustments may be necessary.

- **Caffeine:** It is not clear if caffeine alters the effects of melatonin supplements in humans. Caffeine is reported to raise natural melatonin levels in the body, possibly as a result of effects on the liver enzyme cytochrome P450 1A2. However, caffeine may also alter circadian rhythms in the body, with effects on melatonin secretion.
- **Succinylcholine:** As indicated by laboratory study, melatonin may increase the neuromuscular blocking effect of the muscle relaxant succinylcholine, but not that of vecuronium.
- **Methamphetamine:** As indicated by animal research, melatonin may increase the adverse effects of methamphetamine on the nervous system.
- **Haloperidol (Haldol) (positive interaction):** Preliminary reports suggest that melatonin may aid in reversing symptoms of tardive dyskinesia associated with haloperidol use.
- **Hormone replacement therapy (HRT):** HRT is reported to cause a decrease in daily melatonin secretion without disturbing circadian rhythm. Clinical implications are not clear.
- **Isoniazid (positive interaction):** As indicated by preliminary evidence, melatonin may increase the effects of isoniazid against *Mycobacterium tuberculosis.*

Interactions with Herbs and Dietary Supplements

- **Sedative herbs:** Melatonin may increase daytime sleepiness or sedation when taken with herbs or supplements that may cause sedation. Examples of such agents include ashwagandha root, calamus, calendula, California poppy, capsicum, celery, cough elecampane, German chamomile, goldenseal, hops, 5-hydroxytryptamine (5-HTP), kava, lemon balm, sage, sassafras, shepherd's purse, Siberian ginseng, skullcap, stinging nettle, valerian, wild carrot, wild lettuce, and yerba manse.
- **Herbs that affect blood sugar:** Elevated blood sugar levels (hyperglycemia) have been reported in patients with type 1 diabetes mellitus (insulin-dependent diabetes), and low doses of melatonin have reduced glucose tolerance and insulin sensitivity. Caution is advised when using herbs or supplements that may also raise blood sugar levels, such as arginine, cocoa, dehydroepiandrosterone (DHEA), and ephedra (when combined with caffeine).
- **Blood-thinning herbs/supplements:** Based on preliminary evidence of an interaction with the blood-thinning drug warfarin, and on isolated reports of minor bleeding, melatonin may increase the risk of bleeding when it is taken with herbs and supplements that are believed to increase the risk of bleeding. Multiple cases of bleeding have been reported with the use of *Ginkgo biloba*, and fewer cases with garlic and saw palmetto. Numerous other agents may theoretically increase the risk of bleeding, although this effect has not been proven in most cases. Some examples are alfalfa, American ginseng, angelica, anise, *Arnica montana*, asafetida, aspen bark, bilberry, birch, black cohosh, bladderwrack, bogbean, boldo, borage seed oil, bromelain, capsicum, cat's claw, celery, chamomile, chaparral, clove, coleus, cordyceps, danshen, devil's claw, dong quai, eicosapentaenoic acid (EPA) (found in fish oils), evening primrose oil, fenugreek, feverfew, fish oil, flaxseed/flax powder (not a concern with flaxseed oil), ginger, grapefruit juice, grapeseed, green tea, guggul, gymnestra, horse chestnut, horseradish, licorice root, lovage root, male fern, meadowsweet, nordihydroguaiaretic acid (NDGA), omega-3 fatty acids, onion, *Panax ginseng*, papain, parsley, passionflower, poplar, prickly ash, propolis, quassia, red clover, reishi, rue, Siberian ginseng, sweet birch, sweet clover, turmeric, vitamin E, white willow, wild carrot, wild lettuce, willow, wintergreen, and yucca.

- **Chasteberry (*Vitex agnus-castus*):** Chasteberry may increase natural secretion of melatonin in the body, as indicated by preliminary research.
- **Folate:** Severe folate deficiency may reduce the body's natural levels of melatonin, as indicated by preliminary study.
- **DHEA:** In mice, DHEA and melatonin have been noted to stimulate immune function, with slight additive effects when used together. Effects of this combination in humans are not clear.
- ***Echinacea purpurea*:** In mice, a combination of echinacea and melatonin has been noted to slow the maturation of some types of immune cells, which may reduce immune function. Effects of this combination in humans are not clear.
- **Caffeine:** It is not clear if caffeine alters the effects of melatonin supplements in humans. Caffeine is reported to raise natural melatonin levels in the body, possibly as a result of effects on the liver enzyme cytochrome P450 1A2. However, caffeine may also alter circadian rhythms in the body, with effects on melatonin secretion.

Interactions with Magnetic Fields

- It has been theorized that chronic exposure to magnetic fields or recurrent cellular telephone use may alter melatonin levels and circadian rhythms. However, several studies suggest that this is not the case.

Selected References

Natural Standard developed the preceding evidence-based information based on a systematic review of more than 1100 scientific articles. For comprehensive information about alternative and complementary therapies on the professional level, go to www.naturalstandard.com. Selected references are listed here.

Arendt J, Aldhous M. Further evaluation of the treatment of jet-lag by melatonin: a double-blind crossover study. Annu Rev Chronopharmacol 1988;5:53-55.

Arendt J, Aldhous M, Marks V. Alleviation of jet lag by melatonin: preliminary results of controlled double blind trial. Br Med J (Clin Res Ed) 1986;292(6529):1170.

Atkinson G, Buckley P, Edwards B, et al. Are there hangover-effects on physical performance when melatonin is ingested by athletes before nocturnal sleep? Int J Sports Med 2001;22(3): 232-234.

Attenburrow ME, Dowling BA, Sharpley AL, et al. Case-control study of evening melatonin concentration in primary insomnia. BMJ 1996;312(7041):1263-1264.

Avery D, Lenz M, Landis C. Guidelines for prescribing melatonin. Ann Med 1998;30(1): 122-130.

Baskett JJ, Broad JB, Wood PC, et al. Does melatonin improve sleep in older people? A randomised crossover trial. Age Ageing 2003;32(2):164-170.

Cajochen C, Krauchi K, von Arx MA, et al. Daytime melatonin administration enhances sleepiness and theta/alpha activity in the waking EEG. Neurosci Lett 1996;207(3):209-213.

Camfield P, Gordon K, Dooley J, et al. Melatonin appears ineffective in children with intellectual deficits and fragmented sleep: six "N of 1" trials. J Child Neurol 1996;11(4):341-343.

Claustrat B, Brun J, David M, et al. Melatonin and jet lag: confirmatory result using a simplified protocol. Biol Psychiatry 1992;32(8):705-711.

Dagan Y, Yovel I, Hallis D, et al. Evaluating the role of melatonin in the long-term treatment of delayed sleep phase syndrome (DSPS). Chronobiol Int 1998;15(2):181-190.

Dahlitz M, Alvarez B, Vignau J, et al. Delayed sleep phase syndrome response to melatonin. Lancet 1991;337(8750):1121-1124.

Dawson D, Rogers NL, van den Heuvel CJ, et al. Effect of sustained nocturnal transbuccal melatonin administration on sleep and temperature in elderly insomniacs. J Biol Rhythms 1998;13(6):532-538.

Dodge NN, Wilson GA. Melatonin for treatment of sleep disorders in children with developmental disabilities. J Child Neurol 2001;16(8):581-584.

Dollins AB, Zhdanova IV, Wurtman RJ, et al. Effect of inducing nocturnal serum melatonin concentrations in daytime on sleep, mood, body temperature, and performance. Proc Natl Acad Sci U S A 1994;91(5):1824-1828.

Garfinkel D, Laudon M, Zisapel N. Improvement of sleep quality by controlled-release melatonin in benzodiazepine-treated elderly insomniacs. Arch Gerontol Geriatr 1997;24:223-231.

Garfinkel D, Laudon M, Nof D, et al. Improvement of sleep quality in elderly people by controlled-release melatonin. Lancet 1995;346(8974):541-544.

Ghielmini M, Pagani O, de Jong J, et al. Double-blind randomized study on the myeloprotective effect of melatonin in combination with carboplatin and etoposide in advanced lung cancer. Br J Cancer 1999;80(7):1058-1061.

Gilbert SS, van den Heuvel CJ, Dawson D. Daytime melatonin and temazepam in young adult humans: equivalent effects on sleep latency and body temperatures. J Physiol 1999;514 (Pt 3):905-914.

Gordon K, Camfield P, Dooley J, et al. Dramatically successful treatment of severe sleep disturbance in developmentally handicapped children with melatonin [abstract]. Ann Neurol 1993;34:504.

Haimov I, Lavie P. Potential of melatonin replacement therapy in older patients with sleep disorders. Drugs Aging 1995;7(2):75-78.

Haimov I, Lavie P, Laudon M, et al. Melatonin replacement therapy of elderly insomniacs. Sleep 1995;18(7):598-603.

Hayashi E. Effect of melatonin on sleep-wake rhythm: the sleep diary of an autistic male. Psychiatry Clin Neurosci 2000;54(3):383-384.

Herxheimer A, Petrie KJ. Melatonin for the prevention and treatment of jet lag. Cochrane Database Syst Rev 2002;(2):CD001520.

Hughes RJ, Badia P. Sleep-promoting and hypothermic effects of daytime melatonin administration in humans. Sleep 1997;20(2):124-131.

Hughes RJ, Sack RL, Lewy AJ. The role of melatonin and circadian phase in age-related sleep-maintenance insomnia: assessment in a clinical trial of melatonin replacement. Sleep 1998;21(1):52-68.

Hung JC, Appleton RE, Nunn AJ, et al. The use of melatonin in the treatment of sleep disturbances in children with neurological or behavioural disorders. J Ped Pharm Practice 1998;3(5):250-256.

James SP, Mendelson WB, Sack DA, et al. The effect of melatonin on normal sleep. Neuropsychopharmacology 1987;1(1):41-44.

Jan JE, Espezel H, Appleton RE. The treatment of sleep disorders with melatonin. Dev Med Child Neurol 1994;36(2):97-107.

Jan JE, Freeman RD, Fast DK. Melatonin treatment of sleep-wake cycle disorders in children and adolescents. Dev Med Child Neurol 1999;41(7):491-500.

Jan JE, Hamilton D, Seward N, et al. Clinical trials of controlled-release melatonin in children with sleep- wake cycle disorders. J Pineal Res 2000;29(1):34-39.

Jan JE, O'Donnell ME. Use of melatonin in the treatment of paediatric sleep disorders. J Pineal Res 1996;21(4):193-199.

Jan MM. Melatonin for the treatment of handicapped children with severe sleep disorders. Pediatr Neurol 2000;23(3):229-232.

Jean-Louis G, von Gizycki H, Zizi F. Melatonin effects on sleep, mood, and cognition in elderly with mild cognitive impairment. J Pineal Res 1998;25(3):177-183.

Kayumov L, Brown G, Jindal R, et al. A randomized, double-blind, placebo-controlled crossover study of the effect of exogenous melatonin on delayed sleep phase syndrome. Psychosom Med 2001;63(1):40-48.

Lissoni P, Ardizzoia A, Barni S, et al. A randomized study of tamoxifen alone versus tamoxifen plus melatonin in estrogen receptor-negative heavily pretreated metastatic breast cancer patients. Oncology Reports 1995;2:871-873.

Lissoni P, Barni S, Ardizzoia A, et al. Immunotherapy with low-dose interleukin-2 in association with melatonin as salvage therapy for metastatic soft tissue sarcomas. Oncology Reports 1997;4:157-159.

Lissoni P, Barni S, Mandala M, et al. Decreased toxicity and increased efficacy of cancer chemotherapy using the pineal hormone melatonin in metastatic solid tumour patients with poor clinical status. Eur J Cancer 1999;35(12):1688-1692.

Lissoni P, Barni S, Meregalli S, et al. Modulation of cancer endocrine therapy by melatonin: a phase II study of tamoxifen plus melatonin in metastatic breast cancer patients progressing under tamoxifen alone. Br J Cancer 1995;71(4):854-856.

Lissoni P, Fumagalli L, Paolorossi F, et al. Anticancer neuroimmunomodulation by pineal hormones other than melatonin: preliminary phase II study of the pineal indole 5-methoxytryptophol in association with low-dose IL-2 and melatonin. J Biol Regul Homeost Agents 1997;11(3):119-122.

Lissoni P, Meregalli S, Nosetto L, et al. Increased survival time in brain glioblastomas by a radioneuroendocrine strategy with radiotherapy plus melatonin compared to radiotherapy alone. Oncology 1996;53(1):43-46.

Lissoni P, Paolorossi F, Tancini G, et al. A phase II study of tamoxifen plus melatonin in metastatic solid tumour patients. Br J Cancer 1996;74(9):1466-1468.

Lissoni P, Tancini G, Paolorossi F, et al. Chemoneuroendocrine therapy of metastatic breast cancer with persistent thrombocytopenia with weekly low-dose epirubicin plus melatonin: a phase II study. J Pineal Res 1999;26(3):169-173.

Masters KJ. Melatonin for sleep problems. J Am Acad Child Adolesc Psychiatry 1996;35(6):704.

Nagtegaal JE, Kerkhof GA, Smits MG, et al. Delayed sleep phase syndrome: A placebo-controlled cross-over study on the effects of melatonin administered five hours before the individual dim light melatonin onset. J Sleep Res 1998;7(2):135-143.

Nave R, Peled R, Lavie P. Melatonin improves evening napping. Eur J Pharmacol 1995;275(2): 213-216.

Neri B, Fiorelli C, Moroni F, et al. Modulation of human lymphoblastoid interferon activity by melatonin in metastatic renal cell carcinoma. A phase II study. Cancer 1994;73(12): 3015-3019.

Nickelsen T, Lang A, Bergau L. The effect of 6-, 9- and 11-hour time shifts on circadian rhythms: adaptation of sleep parameters and hormonal patterns following the intake of melatonin or placebo. *In* Arendt J, Pevet P (eds): Advances in Pineal Research. London, John Libbey, 1991, pp 303-306.

O'Callaghan FJ, Clarke AA, Hancock E, et al. Use of melatonin to treat sleep disorders in tuberous sclerosis. Dev Med Child Neurol 1999;41(2):123-126.

Paavonen EJ, Nieminen-Von Wendt T, Vanhala R, et al. Effectiveness of melatonin in the treatment of sleep disturbances in children with Asperger disorder. J Child Adolesc Psychopharmacol 2003;13(1):83-95.

Petrie K, Conaglen JV, Thompson L, et al. Effect of melatonin on jet lag after long haul flights. BMJ 1989;298(6675):705-707.

Petrie K, Dawson AG, Thompson L, et al. A double-blind trial of melatonin as a treatment for jet lag in international cabin crew. Biol Psychiatry 1993;33(7):526-530.

Pillar G, Shahar E, Peled N, et al. Melatonin improves sleep-wake patterns in psychomotor retarded children. Pediatr Neurol 2000;23(3):225-228.

Ross C, Morris B, Whitehouse W. Melatonin treatment of sleep-wake cycle disorders in children and adolescents. Dev Med Child Neurol 1999;41(12):850.

Satomura T, Sakamoto T, Shirakawa S, et al. Hypnotic action of melatonin during daytime administration and its comparison with triazolam. Psychiatry Clin Neurosci 2001;55(3): 303-304.

Schmitt-Mechelke TH, Steinlin M, Bolthauser E. [Melatonin for the treatment of insomnia in neuropediatric patients] [abstract]. Schweiz Med Wochenschr 1997;127(Suppl 87):9.

Siegrist C, Benedetti C, Orlando A, et al. Lack of changes in serum prolactin, FSH, TSH, and estradiol after melatonin treatment in doses that improve sleep and reduce benzodiazepine consumption in sleep-disturbed, middle-aged, and elderly patients. J Pineal Res 2001;30(1): 34-42.

Smits MG, Nagtegaal EE, van der HJ, et al. Melatonin for chronic sleep onset insomnia in children: a randomized placebo-controlled trial. J Child Neurol 2001;16(2):86-92.

Spitzer RL, Terman M, Malt U, et al. Failure of melatonin to affect jet lag in a randomized double blind trial. Abstracts of the Annual Meeting of the Society for Light Treatment and Biological Rhythms 1997;9:1.

Spitzer RL, Terman M, Williams JB, et al. Jet lag: clinical features, validation of a new syndrome-specific scale, and lack of response to melatonin in a randomized, double-blind trial. Am J Psychiatry 1999;156(9):1392-1396.

Suhner A, Schlagenhauf P, Hoefer I, et al. Efficacy and tolerability of melatonin and zolpidem for the alleviation of jet-lag [abstract 603]. Paper presented at the 6th Conference of the International Society of Travel Medicine, Montreal, Canada, 1999.

Suhner A, Schlagenhauf P, Johnson R, et al. Comparative study to determine the optimal melatonin dosage form for the alleviation of jet lag. Chronobiol Int 1998;15(6):655-666.

Tanaka H, Araki A, Ito J, et al. Improvement of hypertonus after treatment for sleep disturbances in three patients with severe brain damage. Brain Dev 1997;19(4):240-244.

Tzischinsky O, Lavie P. Melatonin possesses time-dependent hypnotic effects. Sleep 1994;17(7):638-645.

Vollrath L, Semm P, Gammel G. Sleep induction by intranasal application of melatonin. Adv Biosci 1981;29:327-329.

Waldhauser F, Saletu B, Trinchard-Lugan I. Sleep laboratory investigations on hypnotic properties of melatonin. Psychopharmacology (Berl) 1990;100(2):222-226.

Wurtman RJ, Zhdanova I. Improvement of sleep quality by melatonin. Lancet 1995; 346(8988):1491.

Wyatt JK, Dijk D, Ritz-De Cecco A, et al. Circadian phase-dependent hypnotic effect of exogenous melatonin [abstract]. Sleep 1999;22 Suppl:S4-S5.

Yang CM, Spielman AJ, D'Ambrosio P, et al. A single dose of melatonin prevents the phase delay associated with a delayed weekend sleep pattern. Sleep 2001;24(3):272-281.

Zhdanova IV, Wurtman RJ, Lynch HJ, et al. Sleep-inducing effects of low doses of melatonin ingested in the evening. Clin Pharmacol Ther 1995;57(5):552-558.

Zhdanova IV, Wurtman RJ, Morabito C, et al. Effects of low oral doses of melatonin, given 2-4 hours before habitual bedtime, on sleep in normal young humans. Sleep 1996;19(5): 423-431.

Zhdanova IV, Wurtman RJ, Regan MM, et al. Melatonin treatment for age-related insomnia. J Clin Endocrinol Metab 2001;86(10):4727-4730.

Zhdanova IV, Wurtman RJ, Wagstaff J. Effects of a low dose of melatonin on sleep in children with Angelman syndrome. J Pediatr Endocrinol Metab 1999;12(1):57-67.

Milk Thistle

(*Silybum marianum*)

RELATED TERMS

- Bull thistle, cardo blanco, Cardui mariae fructus, Cardui mariae herba, *Cardum marianum* L., *Carduus marianus* L., chardon-Marie, emetic root, Frauendistel, fructus silybi mariae, fruit de chardon Marie, heal thistle, holy thistle, isosilibinin, kanger, kocakavkas, kuub, lady's thistle, Marian thistle, mariana mariana, Mariendistel, Marienkrörner, Mary thistle, mild thistle, milk ipecac, pig leaves, royal thistle, shui fei ji, silidyanin, Silybi mariae fructus, silybin, silybinin, silychristin, silymarin, snake milk, sow thistle, St. Mary's thistle, variegated thistle, Venus thistle, wild artichoke.

BACKGROUND

- Milk thistle has been used medicinally for over 2000 years, most commonly for the treatment of liver and gallbladder disorders. A flavonoid complex called silymarin can be extracted from the seeds of milk thistle and is believed to be the biologically active component. The terms "milk thistle" and "silymarin" are often used interchangeably.
- Milk thistle products are popular in Europe and the United States for various types of liver disease. Although numerous human trials have been published, most studies have not been well designed or reported.

USES BASED ON SCIENTIFIC EVIDENCE	Grade*
Cirrhosis Numerous studies from Europe suggest benefits of oral milk thistle for cirrhosis. In experiments up to 5 years in duration, milk thistle has improved liver function and decreased the number of deaths that occur in cirrhotic patients. Although these results are promising, most studies have been poorly designed. Better research is necessary before a strong recommendation can be made.	B
Acute viral hepatitis Research on milk thistle for acute viral hepatitis has not provided clear results, and milk thistle cannot be recommended for this potentially life-threatening condition.	C
***Amanita phalloides* mushroom poisoning** Milk thistle has been used traditionally to treat *Amanita phalloides* mushroom poisoning, and several animal studies and isolated human cases have suggested possible benefits. However, there are not enough reliable studies in humans to support this use of milk thistle.	

Continued

Cancer prevention There are early reports from laboratory experiments that the chemicals silymarin and silybinin in milk thistle limit the growth of human breast, cervical, and prostate cancer cells. There is also one report of a patient with liver cancer who improved following treatment with milk thistle. However, this research is too early to permit firm conclusions to be drawn, and effects have not been shown in high-quality human trials.	C
Chronic hepatitis (liver inflammation) Several studies of oral milk thistle for hepatitis caused by viruses or alcohol report improvements in liver tests. However, most studies have been small and poorly designed. More research is needed before a recommendation can be made.	C
Diabetes (in patients with cirrhosis) A small number of studies suggest possible improvements of blood sugar control in cirrhotic patients with diabetes. However, there is not enough scientific evidence to recommend milk thistle for this use.	C
High cholesterol Although animal and laboratory research suggests cholesterol-lowering effects of milk thistle, human studies have provided unclear results. Further studies are necessary before a recommendation can be made.	C
Liver damage from drugs or toxins Several studies suggest possible benefits of milk thistle to treat or prevent liver damage caused by drugs or toxic chemicals. Results of this research are not clear, and most studies have been poorly designed. Therefore, there is not enough scientific evidence to recommend milk thistle for this use.	C

*Key to grades: *A:* Strong scientific evidence for this use; *B:* Good scientific evidence for this use; *C:* Unclear scientific evidence for this use; *D:* Fair scientific evidence against this use (it may not work); *F:* Strong scientific evidence against this use (it likely does not work). For a more detailed explanation of efficacy criteria, see "Natural Standard Evidence-Based Validated Grading Rationale" in the Introduction.

M

Uses Based on Tradition, Theory, or Limited Scientific Evidence

Amiodarone toxicity reactions, asthma, bleeding, bronchitis, cough, diabetic nerve pain, dyspepsia, gallstones, hemorrhoids, liver cancer, liver "cleansing," malaria, menstrual problems, plague, prostate cancer, psoriasis, radiation sickness, skin cancer, snakebite, spleen disorders, sunscreen, varicose veins.

DOSING

The following doses are based on scientific research, publications, traditional use, or expert opinion. Many herbs and supplements have not been thoroughly tested, and their safety and effectiveness may not be proven. Brands may be made differently, with variable ingredients even within the same brand. The doses shown may not apply to all products. It is important to always read product labels and discuss doses with a qualified healthcare provider before therapy is started.

Standardization

- Standardization involves measuring the amount of certain chemicals in products to try to make different preparations similar to each other. It is not always known if the chemicals being measured are the "active" ingredients.
- Milk thistle is often standardized to contain 70% to 80% silymarin. Silymarin is a mixture of three flavonolignans: silybin, silydianin, and silychristin. Despite standardization, different preparations and brands may have different effects in the body. Silipide (IdB 1016) is a special milk thistle product that is designed to be absorbed better into the body. Doses of Silipide are measured by "silybin equivalents."
- One study analyzing stability of milk thistle tincture found a shelf life of approximately 3 months.

Adults (18 Years and Older)

- **Cirrhosis:** Silymarin (Legalon) 280 to 420 mg per day divided into two or three doses. Up to 450 mg daily divided into three doses has been studied.
- **Hepatitis (chronic):** Silipide (IdB 1016) 160 to 480 mg per day in silybin equivalents, or silymarin (Legalon) 420 mg daily divided into three doses.
- **Hepatitis (acute, viral):** Silymarin 420 mg daily divided into three doses.
- **Drug/toxin-induced hepatotoxicity:** Silymarin (Legalon) 280 to 420 mg daily divided into three doses. Up to 800 mg daily has been studied.
- **High cholesterol:** Silymarin 420 mg per day has been studied.
- **Type 1 diabetes mellitus (insulin-dependent diabetes) associated with cirrhosis:** Silymarin (Legalon) 230 to 600 mg per day has been studied. Effectiveness and safety have not been proven.

Children (Younger Than 18 Years)

- There are not enough scientific data to recommend milk thistle for use in children.

SAFETY

The U.S. Food and Drug Administration does not strictly regulate herbs and supplements. There is no guarantee of strength, purity, or safety of products, and effects may vary. It is important to always read product labels. People who have a medical condition, or are taking other drugs, herbs, or supplements, should consult a qualified healthcare provider before starting a new therapy. A healthcare provider should be consulted immediately about any side effects.

Allergies

- People with allergies to plants in the aster family (Compositae, Asteraceae) or to daisies, artichokes, common thistle, or kiwi, or to any of milk thistle's constituents (silybinin, silychristin, silydianin, silymonin, siliandrin) may have allergic reactions to milk thistle. Anaphylactic shock (a severe allergic reaction) from milk thistle tea or tablets has been reported in several patients.

Side Effects and Warnings

- Milk thistle appears to be well tolerated in recommended doses for up to 6 years. Some patients in studies have experienced stomach upset, headache, and itching.

There are rare reports of appetite loss, gas, heartburn, diarrhea, joint pain, and impotence with milk thistle use. One person experienced sweating, nausea, stomach pain, diarrhea, vomiting, weakness, and collapse after taking milk thistle. This reaction may have been due to an allergic reaction; the patient improved after 24 hours. High liver enzyme levels in one person taking milk thistle returned to normal after the person stopped taking the herb.

- In theory, milk thistle may lower blood sugar levels. Caution is advised in patients with diabetes or hypoglycemia, and in those taking drugs, herbs, or supplements that affect blood sugars. Serum glucose levels may need to be monitored by a healthcare provider, and medication adjustments may be necessary.

Pregnancy and Breastfeeding

- Milk thistle has been used historically to improve breast milk flow, and two brief studies of milk thistle in pregnant women reported no side effects. However, there is not enough scientific evidence to support the safe use of milk thistle during pregnancy or breastfeeding at this time.

INTERACTIONS

Most herbs and supplements have not been thoroughly tested for interactions with other herbs, supplements, drugs, or foods. The interactions listed here are based on reports in scientific publications, laboratory experiments, or traditional use. It is important to always read product labels. People who have a medical condition, or are taking other drugs, herbs, or supplements, should consult a qualified healthcare provider before starting a new therapy.

Interactions with Drugs

- Animal studies suggest that milk thistle may interfere with how the body uses the liver's cytochrome P450 system to process components of some drugs. As a result, blood levels of these components may be elevated, causing increased effects or potentially serious adverse reactions. Many types of drugs may be affected. A qualified healthcare provider should be consulted to obtain a list of these drugs and their possible interactions. In theory, milk thistle may lower blood sugar levels. Caution is advised when using medications that may also lower blood sugar. Patients taking drugs for diabetes by mouth or insulin should be monitored closely by a qualified healthcare provider. Medication adjustments may be necessary.
- A possible interaction with phenytoin (Dilantin) has been reported with milk thistle. However, the facts are unclear.
- Milk thistle ingredients have been reported to prevent amiodarone toxicity in animal studies.

Interactions with Herbs and Dietary Supplements

- Animal studies suggest that milk thistle may interfere with how the body uses the liver's cytochrome P450 enzyme system to process components of certain herbs or supplements. As a result, blood levels of these components may be too high. Milk thistle may also alter the effects of other herbs or supplements on the P450 system, such as bloodroot, cat's claw, chamomile, chaparral, chasteberry, damiana, *Echinacea angustifolia*, goldenseal, grapefruit, licorice, oregano, red clover, St. John's wort, wild cherry, and yucca.
- Milk thistle may lower blood sugar levels. Caution is advised when using herbs or supplements that may also lower blood sugar. Blood glucose levels may require

monitoring, and doses may need adjustment. Some examples are *Aloe vera*, American ginseng, bilberry, bitter melon, burdock, fenugreek, fish oil, gymnema, horse chestnut/horse chestnut seed extract (HCSE), marshmallow, *Panax ginseng*, rosemary, Siberian ginseng, stinging nettle, and vitamin E.
- Silymarin and vitamin E have been reported to prevent amiodarone toxicity in animal studies.

Selected References

Natural Standard developed the preceding evidence-based information based on a systematic review of more than 250 scientific articles. For comprehensive information about alternative and complementary therapies on the professional level, go to www.naturalstandard.com. Selected references are listed here.

Agoston M, Orsi F, Feher E, et al. Silymarin and vitamin E reduce amiodarone-induced lysosomal phospholipidosis in rats. Toxicology 2003;190(3):231-241.

Allain H, Schuck S, Lebreton S, et al. Aminotransferase levels and silymarin in de novo tacrine-treated patients with Alzheimer's disease. Dement Geriatr Cogn Disord 1999;10(3): 181-185.

Bettini R, Gorini M. [Use of ursodeoxycholic acid combined with silymarin in the treatment of chronic ethyl-toxic hepatopathy]. Clin Ter 2002;153(5):305-307.

Bilia AR, Bergonzi MC, Gallori S, et al. Stability of the constituents of calendula, milk-thistle and passionflower tinctures by LC-DAD and LC-MS. J Pharm Biomed Anal 2002 Oct 15;30(3):613-624.

Breschi MC, Martinotti E, Apostoliti F, Nieri P. Protective effect of silymarin in antigen challenge- and histamine-induced bronchoconstriction in in vivo guinea-pigs. Eur J Pharmacol 2002 Feb 15;437(1-2):91-95.

Buzzelli G, Moscarella S, Giusti A, et al. A pilot study on the liver protective effect of silybinphosphatidylcholine complex (IdB1016) in chronic active hepatitis. Int J Clin Pharmacol Ther Toxicol 1993;31(9):456-460.

De Martiis M, Fontana M, Assogna G, et al. [Milk thistle (*Silybum marianum*) derivatives in the therapy of chronic hepatopathies]. Clin Ter 1980;94(3):283-315.

DiCenzo R, Shelton M, Jordan K, et al. Coadministration of milk thistle and indinavir in healthy subjects. Pharmacotherapy 2003 Jul;23(7):866-870.

Ferenci P, Dragosics B, Dittrich H, et al. Randomized controlled trial of silymarin treatment in patients with cirrhosis of the liver. J Hepatol 1989;9(1):105-113.

Flora K, Hahn M, Rosen H, et al. Milk thistle (*Silybum marianum*) for the therapy of liver disease. Am J Gastroenterol 1998; 93(2):139-143.

Lawrence V, Jacobs B, Dennehy C, et al. Report on milk thistle: effects on liver disease and cirrhosis and clinical adverse effects. Evidence Report/Technology Assessment No. 21 (Contract 290-97-0012 to the San Antonio Evidence-based Practice Center, based at the University of Texas Health Science Center at San Antonio, and The Veterans Evidence-based Research, Dissemination, and Implementation Center, a Veterans Affairs Services Research and Development Center of Excellence). AHRQ Publication No. 01-E025. Rockville, Md, Agency for Healthcare Research and Quality, October 2000.

Lirussi F, Nassuato G, Orlando R, et al. Treatment of active cirrhosis with ursodeoxycholic acid and a free radical scavenger: a two year prospective study. Med Sci Ress 1995;23:31-33.

Lucena MI, Andrade RJ, de la Cruz JP, et al. Effects of silymarin MZ-80 on oxidative stress in patients with alcoholic cirrhosis. Results of a randomized, double-blind, placebo-controlled clinical study. Int J Clin Pharmacol Ther 2002;40(1):2-8.

Madisch A, Melderis H, Mayr G, et al. [A plant extract and its modified preparation in functional dyspepsia. Results of a double-blind placebo controlled comparative study]. Z Gastroenterol 2001;39(7):511-517.

Marcelli R, Bizzoni P, Conte D, et al. Randomized controlled study of the efficacy and tolerability of a short course of IdB 1016 in the treatment of chronic persistent hepatitis. Eur Bull Drug Res 1992;1(3):131-135.

Palasciano G, Portincasa P, Palmieri V, et al. The effect of silymarin on plasma levels of malon-dialdehyde in patients receiving long-term treatment with psychotropic drugs. Curr Ther Res 1994;55(5):537-545.

Pares A, Planas R, Torres M, et al. Effects of silymarin in alcoholic patients with cirrhosis of the liver: results of a controlled, double-blind, randomized and multicenter trial. J Hepatol 1998; 28(4):615-621.

Piscitelli SC, Formentini E, Burstein AH, et al. Effect of milk thistle on the pharmacokinetics of indinavir in healthy volunteers. Pharmacotherapy 2002;22(5):551-556.

Salmi HA, Sarna S. Effect of silymarin on chemical, functional, and morphological alterations of the liver. A double-blind controlled study. Scand J Gastroenterol 1982;17(4):517-521.

Szilard S, Szentgyorgyi D, Demeter I. Protective effect of Legalon in workers exposed to organic solvents. Acta Med Hung 1988;45(2):249-256.

Velussi M, Cernigoi AM, De Monte A, et al. Long-term (12 months) treatment with an anti-oxidant drug (silymarin) is effective on hyperinsulinemia, exogenous insulin need and malondialdehyde levels in cirrhotic diabetic patients. J Hepatol 1997;26(4):871-879.

Velussi M, Cernigoi AM, Viezzoli L, et al. Silymarin reduces hyperinsulinemia, malondialdehyde levels, and daily insulin need in cirrhotic diabetic patients. Curr Ther Res 1993;53(5): 533-545.

Niacin

(Vitamin B_3, Nicotinic Acid, Niacinamide, and Inositol Hexanicotinate)

RELATED TERMS

- 3-Pyridine carboxamide, anti-blacktongue factor, antipellagra factor, B-complex vitamin, benicot, Efacin, ENDUR-ACIN, Enduramide, Hexopal, inositol hexaniacinate, NIAC, Niacor, Niaspan, Nicalex, nicamid, Nicamin, Nico-400, Nicobid, Nicolar, Nicotinex, nicosedine, Nico-Span, nicotinamide, nicotinic acid amide, nicotinic amide, nicotylamidum, Papulex, pellagra preventing factor, Slo-Niacin, Tega-Span, Tri-B3, Wampocap.

BACKGROUND

- Vitamin B_3 is made up of niacin (nicotinic acid) and its amide, niacinamide, and can be found in many foods, including yeast, meat, fish, milk, eggs, green vegetables, and cereal grains. Dietary tryptophan is also converted to niacin in the body. Vitamin B_3 is often found in combination with other B vitamins, including thiamine, riboflavin, pantothenic acid, pyridoxine, cyanocobalamin, and folic acid.

USES BASED ON SCIENTIFIC EVIDENCE	Grade*
High cholesterol (niacin) Niacin is a well-accepted treatment for high cholesterol. Multiple studies show that niacin (not niacinamide) has significant benefits on levels of high-density cholesterol (HDL or "good cholesterol"), with better results than prescription drugs such as "statins" like atorvastatin (Lipitor). There are also benefits on levels of low-density cholesterol (LDL or "bad cholesterol"), although these effects are less dramatic. Adding niacin to a second drug such as a statin may increase the effects on low-density lipoproteins. The use of niacin for the treatment of dyslipidemia associated with type 2 diabetes has been controversial because of the possibility of worsening glycemic control. However, a recent randomized controlled multicenter trial reports that of 148 patients, only 4 discontinued niacin because of inadequate glucose control. Doses of 1000-1500 mg per day (in a controlled-release formulation) were reported as a potential treatment option for type 2 diabetics with dyslipidemia by these researchers. Patients should check with a physician and pharmacist before starting niacin.	A
Pellagra (niacin) Niacin (vitamin B_3) and niacinamide are FDA approved for the treatment of niacin deficiency. Pellagra is a nutritional disease that develops due to insufficient dietary amounts of vitamin B_3 or the chemical it	A

Continued

is made from, tryptophan. Symptoms of pellagra include skin disease, diarrhea, dementia and depression.

Atherosclerosis (niacin) Niacin decreases blood levels of cholesterol and lipoprotein(a), which may reduce atherosclerosis ("hardening" of the arteries). However, niacin also can increase homocysteine levels, which may have the opposite effect. Overall, the scientific evidence supports the use of niacin in combination with other drugs (but not alone) to decrease cholesterol and slow the process of atherosclerosis. More research is needed in this area before a firm conclusion can be drawn.	B
Prevention of a second heart attack (niacin) Niacin decreases levels of cholesterol, lipoprotein(a), and fibrinogen, which can reduce the risk of heart disease. However, niacin also increases homocysteine levels, which can increase this risk. Numerous studies have looked at the effects of niacin, alone and in combination with other drugs, on the prevention of heart disease and fatal heart attacks. Overall, this research suggests benefits of niacin, especially when combined with other cholesterol-lowering drugs.	B
Osteoarthritis (niacinamide) Preliminary human studies suggest that niacinamide may be useful in the treatment of osteoarthritis. Further research is needed before a recommendation can be made.	C
Type 1 diabetes mellitus prevention (niacinamide) Animal research reports that niacinamide (not niacin) has a protective effect on insulin-producing cells of the pancreas and may delay the development of type 1 diabetes mellitus. Preliminary human research suggests that niacinamide lowers blood sugar, increases C-peptide levels, and allows people to reduce their insulin dosages. However, these studies have been poorly designed with mixed results. More research is necessary before firm conclusions can be drawn.	C

N

*Key to grades: *A:* Strong scientific evidence for this use; *B:* Good scientific evidence for this use; *C:* Unclear scientific evidence for this use; *D:* Fair scientific evidence against this use (it may not work); *F:* Strong scientific evidence against this use (it likely does not work). For a more detailed explanation of efficacy criteria, see "Natural Standard Evidence-Based Validated Grading Rationale" in the Introduction.

Uses Based on Tradition, Theory, or Limited Scientific Evidence

Acne, alcohol dependence, anti-aging, anxiety, arthritis, Bell's palsy, blood circulation improvement, blood vessel spasms, bone marrow damage from chemotherapy, cancer prevention, cataract prevention, central nervous system disorders, cholera diarrhea, chronic diarrhea, confusion, depression, diagnostic test for

Continued

Uses Based on Tradition, Theory, or Limited Scientific Evidence *(cont'd)*

schizophrenia, digestion improvement, drug-induced hallucinations, ear ringing, edema, glucose intolerance, hearing loss, heart attack prevention, HIV infection prevention, high blood pressure, hypothyroidism (reduced thyroid function), insomnia, intermittent claudication (painful legs from clogged arteries), "ischemia-reperfusion injury" prevention, kava-related skin disorders, leprosy, liver disease, low blood sugar, memory loss, Meniere's syndrome, migraine headache, motion sickness, multiple sclerosis, orgasm improvement, painful menstruation, peripheral vascular disease, photosensitivity, pregnancy problems, premenstrual headache prevention, premenstrual syndrome, prostate cancer, psoriasis, psychosis, Raynaud's phenomenon, schizophrenia, scleroderma, sedative, seizure, skin disorders, smoking cessation, stomach ulcer, tardive dyskinesia, taste disturbances, tuberculosis, tumor detection, vertigo.

DOSING

The following doses are based on scientific research, publications, traditional use, or expert opinion. Many herbs and supplements have not been thoroughly tested, and safety and effectiveness may not be proven. Brands may be made differently, with variable ingredients even within the same brand. The doses shown may not apply to all products. It is important to always read product labels and discuss doses with a qualified healthcare provider before therapy is started.

Adults (18 Years and Older)

- *Note:* Taking niacin with food may reduce stomach upset and the risk of stomach ulcer. Doses are usually started low and gradually increased to minimize the common side effect of skin flushing. Taking aspirin or nonsteroidal anti-inflammatory drugs (NSAIDs) at the same time during the first 1 to 2 weeks may reduce this flushing. Use of an antihistamine 15 minutes prior to a niacin dose may also be helpful. The flushing response may decrease on its own after 1 to 2 weeks of therapy. Extended-release niacin products may cause less flushing than immediate-release (crystalline) formulations but may have a higher risk of stomach upset or liver irritation. In general, not all niacin products are equivalent. Patients switching from one product to another may have an increase or decrease in side effects.
- **Dietary intake:** The dietary reference intake established by the Food and Nutrition Board for niacin (in the form of niacin equivalents, 1 mg of niacin = 60 mg tryptophan) ranges from 16 to 18 mg daily for adults, with a maximum intake of 35 mg daily.
- **High cholesterol:** Clinical trials have most commonly studied immediate release (crystalline) niacin at doses of 500 to 3000 mg taken by mouth daily. Dosing may be started at 100 mg three times daily and increased gradually to an average of 1000 mg three times daily, as tolerated. Significant increases in high-density lipoprotein (HDL) levels by up to 30% may occur at doses ranging from 1 to 1.5 g daily. Mild reductions in low-density lipoprotein (LDL) levels may occur at these doses, with stronger effects (up to 20%) occurring at higher doses (3 to 4.5 g daily), or when used with a "statin" drug or bile acid sequestrant. The maximum recommended daily dose is 3 g, although some studies have used 4.5 to 6 g daily. Extended- or sustained-release niacin may be started at a dose of 500 mg daily (or nightly), and increased to 1 to 2 g per day.

- **Pellagra (niacin deficiency):** Dosing in the range of 50 mg to 1 g daily has been studied.
- **Atherosclerosis:** Niacin in doses of 1 to 4 g daily has been studied.
- **Cardiovascular disease:** Niacin at a dose of 3 g daily has been studied.
- **Diabetes mellitus (type 1), preservation of β-islet cell function:** Niacinamide has been studied in the preservation of pancreas cell (β-islet) function in patients with newly diagnosed diabetes mellitus (type 1) in divided doses, up to 3 g daily.

Children (Younger Than 18 Years)

- There is not enough scientific evidence to recommend the safe use of niacin or niacinamide in children. Niacinamide has been studied in children at daily doses of 150 to 300 mg per year of the child's age, or 25 mg per kilogram daily, for the prevention of type 1 diabetes mellitus in "high-risk" individuals. No serious side effects have been reported, although safety and effectiveness are not clear. Patients should speak with a qualified healthcare provider if they are considering this therapy.
- Note that there are concerns about the lack of evidence regarding treatment of childhood lipid disorders, including long-term psychological and metabolic effects. For many disorders, dietary alteration is considered acceptable as first-line treatment, without the use of lipid-lowering drugs until adulthood is reached.

SAFETY

The U.S. Food and Drug Administration does not strictly regulate herbs and supplements. There is no guarantee of strength, purity, or safety of products, and effects may vary. It is important to always read product labels. People who have a medical condition, or are taking other drugs, herbs, or supplements, you should consult a qualified healthcare provider before starting a new therapy. A healthcare provider should be contacted immediately about any side effects.

Allergies

- Rarely, anaphylactic shock (severe allergic reaction) has been described after intravenous or oral niacin therapy.

Side Effects and Warnings

- Most people taking niacin experience skin flushing and a warm sensation, especially of the face, neck, and ears, when they begin treatment or increase dose. This reaction is usually mild but has been intolerable enough to cause up to half of participants in studies to stop therapy. Dry skin and itching is also commonly experienced. Taking aspirin or non-steroidal anti-inflammatory drugs such as ibuprofen (Advil, Motrin), naproxen (Naprosyn), or indomethacin (Indocin) can reduce the flushing. Use of an antihistamine 15 minutes prior to a niacin dose may also be helpful. Slow-release niacin products may have less skin flushing than regular-release niacin preparations or may simply delay the appearance of flushing. The flushing response often decreases on its own after 1 to 2 weeks of therapy. Mild stomach upset, nausea, vomiting, and diarrhea also may occur when beginning niacin therapy, and usually resolve with continued use.
- More serious side effects include liver toxicity, worsening of stomach ulcers, and altered blood chemistry levels (increased blood sugar and uric acid concentrations). Numerous case reports describe liver toxicity, including increased liver enzyme levels in the blood, skin yellowing (jaundice), fluid in the abdomen (ascites), and

liver failure. Monitoring of liver blood tests while using niacin is recommended. While slow-release niacin products may have less skin flushing than regular-release niacin preparations, they may worsen stomach and liver side effects.

- Niacin can cause significant alterations in blood sugar levels and insulin. This has been a potential concern in patients with diabetes, although a recent randomized controlled trial reports that of 148 patients, only 4 discontinued niacin because of inadequate glucose control (doses of 1000 to 1500 mg per day in a controlled-release formulation were used). Nonetheless, caution is advised in patients with diabetes or hypoglycemia, and in those taking insulin, drugs, herbs, or supplements that affect blood sugar levels. Serum glucose levels may need to be monitored by a healthcare provider, and medication adjustments may be necessary. Although niacinamide is generally not associated with other side effects, it may affect insulin and blood sugar levels.
- In theory, gout may occur during niacin treatment, because of increased blood uric acid levels. Lactic acidosis has been reported after taking sustained-release niacin. Niacin-induced muscle cell damage (myopathy) and increased blood levels of creatine kinase (a marker of muscle damage) have been reported in studies.
- Abnormal heart rhythms and heart palpitations have occurred in niacin studies. Based on human research, taking niacin alone or with colestipol may increase blood homocysteine levels. High levels of homocysteine have been associated with an increased risk of heart disease.
- Blood clotting problems have been reported during treatment with sustained-release niacin. Caution is advised in patients with bleeding disorders or taking drugs that may increase the risk of bleeding. Dosing adjustments may be necessary. Low white blood cell number (leukopenia) and slightly increased blood eosinophils have also been reported.
- Rarely reported side effects include headache, tooth or gum pain, dizziness, breathing difficulty, increased anxiety, panic attacks, and decreased thyroid function (hypothyroidism). There are published accounts of temporary side effects of the eye, including macular swelling and blurred vision as well as toxic amblyopia ("lazy eye"). These side effects resolved when niacin was stopped.

Pregnancy and Breastfeeding

- Use of niacin supplementation during pregnancy or breastfeeding is not recommended because of lack of sufficient research on safety and effectiveness.

INTERACTIONS

Most herbs and supplements have not been thoroughly tested for interactions with other herbs, supplements, drugs, or foods. The interactions listed here are based on reports in scientific publications, laboratory experiments, or traditional use. It is important to always read product labels. People who have a medical condition, or are taking other drugs, herbs, or supplements, should consult a qualified healthcare provider before starting a new therapy.

Interactions with Drugs

- In theory, there may be an increased risk of liver damage if niacin is taken with alcohol or drugs that are toxic to the liver. Niacin-induced flushing may be increased by simultaneous use of alcohol and nicotine.
- Based on human study, use of niacin with cholesterol-lowering drugs, such as "statins" (HMG-CoA reductase inhibitors), including lovastatin (Mevacor) and

atorvastatin (Lipitor), bile acid sequestrants like cholestyramine, probucol, and anti-lipid agents like gemfibrozil, may result in further reductions in cholesterol than caused by either agent alone. Use of niacin with HMG-CoA reductase inhibitors or gemfibrozil may increase the risk of serious side effects such as liver or muscle damage. The bile acid sequestrants cholestyramine and colestipol may reduce niacin absorption into the body.

- Based on human study, niacin may increase blood sugar levels and may require dosing adjustments of insulin or prescription diabetes drugs. In research on children, use of niacinamide and insulin together has been shown to lead to a reduction in insulin dosage in patients with type 1 (insulin-dependent) diabetes mellitus. Caution is advised when using medications that may affect blood sugar. Patients taking drugs for diabetes by mouth or insulin should be monitored closely by a qualified healthcare provider. Medication adjustments may be necessary.
- Antibiotics can lead to decreased amounts of B vitamins in the body. Conversely, based on animal study, pyrazinamide may increase niacin levels. Use of niacin with neomycin may add to the cholesterol-lowering effects of niacin. Based on laboratory study, niacinamide may interact with the antifungal drug griseofulvin (increases its solubility), with possible effects on its activity.
- In theory, niacin therapy may increase the risk of bleeding. There are published case reports of patients who developed reversible abnormal blood clotting (coagulopathy) conditions while taking sustained-release niacin. In addition, low blood platelet number (thrombocytopenia) has been observed in studies of niacin therapy. Some examples of drugs that may increase the risk of bleeding if taken with niacin include aspirin, anticoagulants ("blood thinners") such as warfarin (Coumadin) and heparin, antiplatelet drugs such as clopidogrel (Plavix), and nonsteroidal anti-inflammatory drugs such as ibuprofen (Motrin, Advil) and naproxen (Naprosyn, Aleve).
- Based on animal research, use of niacinamide with seizure medications like diazepam (Valium), carbamazepine (Tegretol), and sodium valproate (Depakote) may increase their anti-seizure action. In laboratory study, niacinamide has interacted with diazepam (increases its solubility), with uncertain overall effects. If taken with blood pressure–lowering drugs, niacinamide may cause a greater lowering of blood pressure.
- Based on human study, niacin may alter thyroid hormones and require dosing adjustment of thyroid medications. Based on laboratory research, niacinamide may interact with testosterone, estrogen, or progesterone. Use of birth control pills may increase the amount of niacin produced in the body, thus lowering the doses of niacin needed for treatment.

Interactions with Herbs and Dietary Supplements

- In theory, use of niacin or niacinamide with herbs or supplements that have potential to cause liver injury may cause greater risk of liver toxicity. Examples include ackee, bee pollen, birch oil, blessed thistle, borage, bush tea, butterbur, chaparral, coltsfoot, comfrey, DHEA, *Echinacea purpurea*, *Echium* spp., germander, *Heliotropium* spp., horse chestnut, jin-bu-huan (*Lycopodium serratum*), kava, lobelia, L-tetrahydropalmatine (THP), mate, Paraguay tea, periwinkle, *Plantago lanceolata*, pride of Madeira, rue, sassafras, scullcap, *Senecio* spp./groundsel, tansy ragwort, turmeric/curcumin, tu-san-chi (*Gynura segetum*), uva ursi, valerian, and white chameleon.

- Use of aspirin has been shown to reduce the tingling, itching, flushing, and warmth associated with oral niacin administration, an effect which may also result from use of possible salicylate-containing herbs like black cohosh, meadowsweet, poplar, sweet birch, willow bark, and wintergreen. However, levels of salicylates in herbs may vary or be too low to have this desired effect.
- Niacin may add to the effects of herbs that may lower blood cholesterol levels, including fish oil, garlic, and guggul. Based on human study, taking such combinations as chromium polynicotinate (niacin-bound chromium) with grape seed proanthocyanidin, or niacin with β-sitosterol and dihydro-β-sitosterol, may result in greater improvements in cholesterol than taking either agent alone.
- Antioxidants may reduce niacin's beneficial effects on cholesterol levels and heart disease, possibly by interfering with niacin's effects on high-density cholesterol (HDL). Recent research suggests that the addition of antioxidants to a combination of niacin plus simvastatin (Zocor) reduced the benefit of niacin on heart blood vessel plaques, suggesting possible interference by antioxidants. In other research, use of niacin with vitamin A and vitamin E had greater effects on cholesterol levels than niacin alone. Vitamin E in combination with colestipol and niacin has also been associated with greater benefits on heart blood vessel plaques. This remains an area of controversy.
- Based on human study, niacin may increase blood sugar levels, and may require dosing adjustments of hypoglycemic agents. In a study of children, use of niacinamide and insulin together has been shown to lead to a reduction in insulin dosage in patients with type 1 diabetes mellitus. Caution is advised when using herbs or supplements that may affect blood sugar. Blood glucose levels may require monitoring, and doses may need adjustment. Possible examples of herbs that may lower blood sugar include: *Aloe vera*, American ginseng, bilberry, bitter melon, burdock, fenugreek, fish oil, gymnema, horse chestnut seed extract (HCSE), marshmallow, milk thistle, *Panax ginseng*, rosemary, Siberian ginseng, stinging nettle, and white horehound. Agents that may raise blood sugar levels include arginine, cocoa, and ephedra (when combined with caffeine).
- In theory, niacin therapy may increase the risk of bleeding when taken with herbs and supplements that are believed to increase the risk of bleeding. There are published case reports of patients who developed reversible abnormal blood clotting (coagulopathy) conditions while taking sustained-release niacin. In addition, low blood platelet number (thrombocytopenia) has been observed in studies of niacin therapy. Multiple cases of bleeding have been reported with the use of *Ginkgo biloba*, and fewer cases with garlic or saw palmetto. Numerous other agents may theoretically increase the risk of bleeding, although this has not been proven in most cases. Some examples are alfalfa, American ginseng, angelica, anise, *Arnica montana*, asafetida, aspen bark, bilberry, birch, black cohosh, bladderwrack, bogbean, boldo, borage seed oil, bromelain, capsicum, cat's claw, celery, chamomile, chaparral, clove, coleus, cordyceps, danshen, devil's claw, dong quai, evening primrose, fenugreek, feverfew, flaxseed/flax powder (not a concern with flaxseed oil), ginger, grapefruit juice, grape seed, green tea, guggul, gymnestra, horse chestnut, horseradish, licorice root, lovage root, male fern, meadowsweet, nordihydroguaiaretic acid (NDGA), onion, papain, *Panax ginseng*, parsley, passion flower, poplar, prickly ash, propolis, quassia, red clover, reishi, rue, Siberian ginseng, sweet birch, sweet clover, turmeric, vitamin E, white willow, wild carrot, wild lettuce, willow, wintergreen, and yucca.

- Based on laboratory study, niacinamide may interact with herbs or supplements with estrogen-like properties and theoretically may increase the amount of niacin produced in the body (thus lowering the doses of niacin needed for treatment). Examples of herbs with possible estrogen properties include alfalfa, black cohosh, bloodroot, burdock, hops, kudzu, licorice, pomegranate, red clover, soy, thyme, white horehound, and yucca.
- Based on human study, niacin may interact with thyroid-active herbs or supplements such as bladderwrack and alter thyroid hormone blood tests. Preliminary human research reports that zinc sulfate increases the amount of niacin breakdown products in the urine, suggesting a possible interaction between the two agents.

Interactions with Foods

- Hot beverages, when taken with niacin, may worsen niacin-induced skin flushing.

Selected References

Natural Standard developed the preceding evidence-based information based on a systematic review of more than 100 scientific articles. For comprehensive information about alternative and complementary therapies on the professional level, go to www.naturalstandard.com. Selected references are listed here.

Arcavi L, Shahar A. [Drug related taste disturbances: emphasis on the elderly.] Harefuah, 2003; 142(6):446-450, 485, 484.

Ayyobi AF, Brunzell JD. Lipoprotein distribution in the metabolic syndrome, type 2 diabetes mellitus, and familial combined hyperlipidemia. Am J Cardiol 2003;92(4A):27J-33J.

Ballantyne CM, Corsini A, Davidson MH, et al. Risk for myopathy with statin therapy in high-risk patients. Comment in: Arch Intern Med. 2003;163(13):1615-1616; author reply, 1616. Arch Intern Med 2003;163(5):553-564.

Bays HE, Dujovne CA, McGovern ME, et al. ADvicor Versus Other Cholesterol-Modulating Agents Trial Evaluation. Comparison of once-daily, niacin extended-release/lovastatin with standard doses of atorvastatin and simvastatin (the ADvicor Versus Other Cholesterol-Modulating Agents Trial Evaluation [ADVOCATE]). Am J Cardiol 2003;91(6):667-672.

Bhatnagar D. Should pediatric patients with hyperlipidemia receive drug therapy? Paediatr Drugs 2002;4(4):223-230.

Brown BG, Zhao XQ, Chait A, et al. Simvastatin and niacin, antioxidant vitamins, or the combination for the prevention of coronary disease. N Engl J Med 2001;345(22): 1583-1592.

Bucher HC, Griffith LE, Guyatt GH. Systematic review on the risk and benefit of different cholesterol-lowering interventions. Arterioscler Thromb Vasc Biol 1999;19(2):187-195.

Capuzzi DM, Morgan JM, Weiss RJ, et al. Beneficial effects of rosuvastatin alone and in combination with extended-release niacin in patients with a combined hyperlipidemia and low high-density lipoprotein cholesterol levels. Am J Cardiol 2003;91(11):1304-1310.

Cheung MC, Zhao XQ, Chait A, et al. Antioxidant supplements block the response of HDL to simvastatin-niacin therapy in patients with coronary artery disease and low HDL. Arterioscler Thromb Vasc Biol 2001;21(8):1320-1326.

Elam MB, Hunninghake DB, Davis KB, et al. Effect of niacin on lipid and lipoprotein levels and glycemic control in patients with diabetes and peripheral arterial disease: the ADMIT study: a randomized trial. Arterial Disease Multiple Intervention Trial. JAMA 2000;284(10): 1263-1270.

Freedman JE. Antioxidant versus lipid-altering therapy: some answers, more questions. N Engl J Med 2001;345(22):1636-1637.

Goldberg A, Alagona P Jr., Capuzzi DM, et al. Multiple-dose efficacy and safety of an extended-release form of niacin in the management of hyperlipidemia. Am J Cardiol 2000;85(9): 1100-1105.

Grundy SM, Vega GL, McGovern ME, et al. Diabetes Multicenter Research Group. Efficacy, safety, and tolerability of once-daily niacin for the treatment of dyslipidemia associated with

N

type 2 diabetes: results of the assessment of diabetes control and evaluation of the efficacy of niaspan trial. Arch Intern Med 2002;162(14):1568-1576.

Guyton JR, Capuzzi DM. Treatment of hyperlipidemia with combined niacin-statin regimens. Am J Cardiol 1998;82(12A):82U-84U.

Guyton JR, Goldberg AC, Kreisberg RA, et al. Effectiveness of once-nightly dosing of extended-release niacin alone and in combination for hypercholesterolemia. Am J Cardiol 1998;82(6):737-743.

Guyton JR, Blazing MA, Hagar J, et al. Extended-release niacin vs. gemfibrozil for the treatment of low levels of high-density lipoprotein cholesterol: Niaspan-Gemfibrozil Study Group. Arch Intern Med 2000;160(8):1177-1184.

Hannan F, Davoren P. Use of nicotinic acid in the management of recurrent hypoglycemic episodes in diabetes. Diabetes Care 2001;24(7):1301.

Kashyap ML, McGovern ME, Berra K, et al. Long-term safety and efficacy of a once-daily niacin/lovastatin formulation for patients with dyslipidemia. Am J Cardiol 2002;89(6): 672-678.

McKenney JM, McCormick LS, Schaefer EJ, et al. Effect of niacin and atorvastatin on lipoprotein subclasses in patients with atherogenic dyslipidemia. Am J Cardiol 2001;88(3): 270-274.

Pozzilli P, Browne PD, Kolb H. Meta-analysis of nicotinamide treatment in patients with recent-onset IDDM: The Nicotinamide Trialists. Diabetes Care 1996;19(12):1357-1363.

Schectman G, Hiatt J. Dose-response characteristics of cholesterol-lowering drug therapies: implications for treatment. Ann Intern Med 1996;125(12):990-1000.

Sprecher DL. Raising high-density lipoprotein cholesterol with niacin and fibrates: a comparative review. Am J Cardiol 2000;86(12A):46L-50L.

Wink J, Giacoppe G, King J. Effect of very-low-dose niacin on high-density lipoprotein in patients undergoing long-term statin therapy. Am Heart J 2002;143(3):514-518.

Wolfe ML, Vartanian SF, Ross JL, et al. Safety and effectiveness of Niaspan when added sequentially to a statin for treatment of dyslipidemia. Am J Cardiol 2001;87(4):476-9, A7.

Oleander

(Nerium oleander, Thevetia peruviana)

RELATED TERMS

- Adelfa, adynerin, ahouai (Antilles), ahousin, Anvirzel, Apocyanaceae, ashwahan, ashwamarak (Sanskrit), be-still nuts (Hawaii), boissaisi (Haiti), cardenolides, cardiac glycosides, cascaveleira (Brazil), *Cerebra thevetia* (India), cerebrine, cerebrose, common oleander, corrigen, dehydroadynerigen, digitoxigenin, exile, folinerin, horse poison, joro-joro (Dutch Guiana), karier, karavira, kohilphin, kokilpal (India), laurier blane (Haiti), laurier bol, laurier desjundins, laurier rose, lorier bol, lucky seed (Jamaica), neriantin, neridiginoside, neridlenone A, neriifolin, neriine, nerin, nerioside, neritaloside, *Nerium indicum, Nerium odorum,* nerizoside, NOAG-II, odoroside H, oleanderblatter, oleandri folium, oleandrigenin, oleandrin, oleandrinogen, oleandroside, olinerin, peruvoside, pila kaner (India), pink oleander, rosa francesa, rosagenin, rosebay, rose laurel, rosen lorbeer, ruvoside, soland, strospeside, *Thevetia nerifolia, Thevetia neriifolia,* thevetin A, thevetin B, thevetine, L-thevetose, thevetoxin, triterpenes, white oleander, yee tho (Thailand), yellow oleander.

O

BACKGROUND

- The term "oleander" refers to two plant species, *Nerium oleander* (common oleander) and *Thevetia peruviana* (yellow oleander), which grow in temperate climates throughout the world. Both species contain chemicals called "cardiac glycosides" that have effects similar to the heart drug digoxin. Both species can be toxic when taken by mouth, with many documented reports of deaths.

USES BASED ON SCIENTIFIC EVIDENCE	Grade*
Cancer Laboratory studies of oleander suggest possible anti-cancer effects, although reliable research in humans has not yet been performed. There are reports that long-term use of oleander may have positive effects in patients with leiomyosarcoma, Ewing's sarcoma, and prostate and breast cancer. More research is needed before a recommendation can be made.	C
Congestive heart failure The term "oleander" refers to two plants, *Nerium oleander* (common oleander) and *Thevetia peruviana* (yellow oleander). Both plants contain heart-active "cardiac glycoside" chemicals (similar to the prescription drug digoxin) and have been associated with serious side effects in humans, including death. The plants have been used to treat heart failure in China and Russia for decades, but scientific evidence supporting use	C

Continued

is limited to small, poorly designed studies. Human research began in the 1930s, but was largely abandoned because of serious gastrointestinal and heart toxicity.
It should be noted that the commonly used prescription drug digoxin may improve symptoms of congestive heart failure, but does not improve mortality (length of life).

*Key to grades: *A:* Strong scientific evidence for this use; *B:* Good scientific evidence for this use; *C:* Unclear scientific evidence for this use; *D:* Fair scientific evidence against this use (it may not work); *F:* Strong scientific evidence against this use (it likely does not work). For a more detailed explanation of efficacy criteria, see "Natural Standard Evidence-Based Validated Grading Rationale" in the Introduction.

Uses Based on Tradition, Theory, or Limited Scientific Evidence

Abnormal menstruation, alcoholism, anorexia, anti-fertility, anti-parasitic, asthma, bacterial infections, cachexia (weight loss/wasting from some diseases), cathartic, corns, diuretic (increase urine flow), epilepsy (seizure), eye diseases, heart disease, hemorrhoids, indigestion, inflammation, insecticide, leprosy, malaria, menstrual stimulant, neurologic disorders, pregnancy termination, psychiatric disorders, rat poison, ringworm, sinus problems, skin diseases, skin eruptions, snake bites, swelling, venereal disease, vomiting, warts, weight gain.

DOSING

The following doses are based on scientific research, publications, traditional use, or expert opinion. Many herbs and supplements have not been thoroughly tested, and safety and effectiveness may not be proven. Brands may be made differently, with variable ingredients even within the same brand. The doses shown may not apply to all products. It is important to always read product labels and discuss doses with a qualified healthcare provider before therapy is started.

Standardization

- Standardization involves measuring the amounts of certain chemicals in products to try to make different preparations similar to each other. It is not always known if the chemicals being measured are the "active" ingredients. There is no widely accepted standardization for oleander.

Adults (18 Years and Older)

- **Congestive heart failure:** Safety has not been established for any dose of oleander. Peruvoside, a heart-active substance in yellow oleander kernels (similar to the drug digoxin), has been studied taken as 1.8 to 3.2 mg by mouth, as an initial dose, followed by an average daily dose of 0.6 mg.

Children (Younger Than 18 Years)

- Oleander is not recommended for use in children because of the risk of toxicity or death, and lack of scientific data.

SAFETY

The U.S. Food and Drug Administration does not strictly regulate herbs and supplements. There is no guarantee of strength, purity, or safety of products, and effects may vary. It is important to always read product labels. People who have a medical condition, or are taking other drugs, herbs, or supplements, should consult a qualified healthcare provider before starting a new therapy. A healthcare provider should be contacted immediately about any side effects.

Allergies

- People with allergy/hypersensitivity to oleander or other cardiac glycosides such as digoxin or digitoxin may have reactions to oleander. Skin contact with sap from oleander leaves may cause rash/dermatitis.

Side Effects and Warnings

- Common oleander contains a strychnine-like toxin, and a heart-active cardiac glycoside substance (similar to the prescription drug digoxin) that may cause the heart to beat rapidly or abnormally or to stop beating. Common oleander has been used as rat poison, insecticide, and fish poison and is toxic to mammals, including humans. Animals (sheep) have died after eating as little as two or three leaves of *Nerium oleander* (common oleander). Children may die after eating a single leaf of common oleander. Eating the leaves, flowers, or bark of common oleander may cause nausea, vomiting, stomach cramps and pain, fatigue, drowsiness, unsteadiness, bloody diarrhea, abnormal heart rhythms, seizures, liver or kidney damage, or unconsciousness. Death may occur within 1 day. Reports of toxicity and deaths in children and adults have been reported for decades in Australia, India, Sri Lanka and the United States.
- Fruits of *Thevetin peruviana* (yellow oleander) are thought to be even more toxic than common oleander to mammals, including humans. Based on human studies of intentional overdose (suicide attempts), eating eight or more seeds of yellow oleander may be fatal.
- Additional side effects of oleander ingestion include irritation and redness of the lips, gums, and tongue, nausea, vomiting, depression, irritability, fast breathing, sweating, stomach pain, diarrhea, headache, confusion, visual disturbances, and constricted pupils. Abnormal blood tests, including tests of liver and kidney function (potassium, bilirubin, creatinine, and blood urea) have been reported in humans.

Pregnancy and Breastfeeding

- Oleander is toxic and should be avoided by pregnant or breastfeeding women.

INTERACTIONS

Most herbs and supplements have not been thoroughly tested for interactions with other herbs, supplements, drugs, or foods. The interactions listed here are based on reports in scientific publications, laboratory experiments, or traditional use. It is important to always read product labels. People who have a medical condition, or are taking other drugs, herbs, or supplements, should consult a qualified healthcare provider before starting a new therapy.

Interactions with Drugs

- Based on animal and human studies, common oleander and yellow oleander contain heart-active cardiac glycoside substances similar to the drug digoxin. There

may be an increased risk of unwanted side effects or damage to the heart if oleander is taken with other heart-active drugs such as digoxin (Lanoxin) or anti-arrhythmics.
- Because oleander is similar to the drug digoxin, it may share some of the same interactions, although this has not been thoroughly studied. Digoxin interacts with many drugs, including acarbose, acetazolamide, activated charcoal, amiodarone, atorvastatin, azithromycin, azosemide, bepridil, beta-adrenergic blockers, bumetanide, canrenoate, cascara sagrada, cholestyramine, clarithromycin, cyclophosphamide, cyclosporine, diltiazem, erythromycin, ethacrynic acid, furosemide, hydroxychloroquine, indomethacin, itraconazole, kaolin, lornoxicam, metoclopramide, mibefradil, nefazodone, nifedipine, nilvadipine, nisoldipine, nitrendipine, paromomycin, penicillamine, piretanide, propafenone, propantheline, quinidine, quinine, spironolactone, succinylcholine, thiazide diuretics, torsemide, valspodar, verapamil, and vincristine.
- Low potassium levels in the blood may increase the dangerous side effects of oleander. Therefore, oleander should be used cautiously with drugs that may lower potassium levels, such as laxatives or some diuretics (drugs that increase urine flow).

Interactions with Herbs and Dietary Supplements

- Common oleander and yellow oleander contain heart-active cardiac glycoside substances. Herbs or supplements that may cause increased heart effects/damage if taken with oleander include adonis, balloon cotton, black hellebore root/melampode, black Indian hemp, bushman's poison, cactus grandifloris, convallaria, eyebright, figwort, foxglove/digitalis, frangipani, hedge mustard, hemp root/Canadian hemp root, king's crown, lily of the valley, motherwort, pheasant's eye plant, plantain leaf, pleurisy root, psyllium husks, redheaded cotton-bush, rhubarb root, rubber vine, sea-mango, senna fruit, squill, strophanthus, uzara, wallflower, wintersweet, and yellow dock root. Notably, bufalin/chan suis is a Chinese herbal formula that has been reported as toxic or fatal when taken with cardiac glycosides.
- Toxic effects of oleander on the heart may be increased if it is used with calcium supplements or herbs that lower potassium levels, such as licorice. Potassium levels theoretically may be reduced by herbs and supplements with laxative properties, such as senna and psyllium, or herbs and supplements with diuretic properties (increasing urine flow) such as artichoke, celery, corn silk, couchgrass, dandelion, elder flower, horsetail, juniper berry, kava, shepherd's purse, uva ursi, and yarrow. Potential laxative herbs may include alder buckthorn, aloe dried leaf sap, black root, blue flag rhizome, butternut bark, cascara bark, castor oil, chasteberry, colocynth fruit pulp, dandelion, dong quai, European buckthorn, eyebright, gamboges bark, horsetail, jalap root, manna bark, plantain leaf, podophyllum root, psyllium, rhubarb, senna, wild cucumber fruit, and yellow dock root.

Selected References

Natural Standard developed the preceding evidence-based information based on a systematic review of more than 160 scientific articles. For comprehensive information about alternative and complementary therapies on the professional level, go to www.naturalstandard.com. Selected references are listed here.

Arao T, Fuke C, Takaesu H, Nakamoto M, et al. Simultaneous determination of cardenolides by sonic spray ionization liquidchromatography-ion trap mass spectrometry—a fatal case of oleander poisoning. J Anal Toxicol 2002;26(4):222-227.

Bose TK, Basu RK, Biswas B, et al. Cardiovascular effects of yellow oleander ingestion. J Indian Med Assoc 1999;97(10):407-410.

de Silva HA, Fonseka MM, Pathmeswaran A, et al. Multiple-dose activated charcoal for treatment of yellow oleander poisoning: a single-blind, randomised, placebo-controlled trial. Lancet 2003;361(9373):1935-1938.

Eddleston M, Ariaratnam CA, Sjostrom L, et al. Acute yellow oleander (*Thevetia peruviana*) poisoning: cardiac arrhythmias, electrolyte disturbances, and serum cardiac glycoside concentrations on presentation to hospital. Heart 2000;83(3):301-306.

Eddleston M. Patterns and problems of deliberate self-poisoning in the developing world. QJM 2000;93(11):715-731.

Eddleston M, Warrell DA. Management of acute yellow oleander poisoning. QJM 1999; 92(9):483-485.

Eddleston M, Persson H. Acute plant poisoning and antitoxin antibodies. J Toxicol Clin Toxicol 2003;41(3):309-315.

Fonseka MM, Seneviratne SL, de Silva CE, et al. Yellow oleander poisoning in Sri Lanka: outcome in a secondary care hospital. Hum Exp Toxicol 2002;21(6):293-295.

Le Couteur DG, Fisher AA. Chronic and criminal administration of *Nerium* oleander. J Toxicol Clin Toxicol 2002;40(4):523-524.

Lim DC, Hegewald K, Dandamudi N. A suicide attempt with an oleander cocktail. Chest 1999;116(4):405S-406S.

Monzani V, Rovellini A, Schinco G, et al. Acute oleander poisoning after a self-prepared tisane. J Toxicol Clin Toxicol 1997;35(6):667-668.

Ni D, Madden TL, Johansen M, et al. Murine pharmacokinetics and metabolism of oleandrin, a cytotoxic component of *Nerium* oleander. J Exp Ther Oncol 2002;2(5):278-285.

Nishioka S, Resende ES. Transitory complete atrioventricular block associated to ingestion of *Nerium oleander*. Rev Assoc Med Bras 1995;41(1):60-62.

Passion Flower

(*Passiflora incarnata* L.)

RELATED TERMS

- Apricot vine, banana passion fruit (*Passiflora mollissima*), Calmanervin (combination product), Compoz (combination product), corona de cristo, EUP, Euphytose (combination product), fleischfarbige, fleur de la passion, flor de passion, granadilla, grenadille, Jamaican honeysuckle (*Passiflora laurifolia*), madre selva, maypops, Naturest, passiflora, passionflower, passion vine, passionsblume, purple passion flower, Sedacalm, water lemon, wild passion flower.

BACKGROUND

- The dried aerial parts of *Passiflora incarnata* have historically been used as a sedative and hypnotic (for insomnia) and for "nervous" gastrointestinal complaints. However, there is no clear controlled clinical evidence supporting any therapeutic use in humans. Pre-clinical studies provide preliminary support for a benzodiazepine-like calming action.
- Evidence for significant adverse effects is equally inconclusive and is complicated by the variety of poorly classified, potentially active constituents in different *Passiflora* species.
- Passion fruit (*Passiflora edulis* Sims), a related species, is used as a food flavoring.

USES BASED ON SCIENTIFIC EVIDENCE	Grade*
Congestive heart failure An extract containing passion flower and hawthorn has been studied in people with congestive heart failure for the treatment of shortness of breath and difficulty exercising. People using this combination of herbs have experienced improvements in these symptoms. However, any positive effects may have resulted from hawthorn, which is more commonly used for congestive heart failure. High-quality human research on passion flower alone and compared to prescription drugs used for this condition is needed before a recommendation can be made.	C
Sedation (agitation, anxiety, insomnia) Passion flower has a long history of use for symptoms of restlessness, anxiety, or agitation. There is preliminary evidence in support of these uses from animal research and from poor-quality human studies. Better research is needed before a firm conclusion can be drawn.	C

*Key to grades: *A:* Strong scientific evidence for this use; *B:* Good scientific evidence for this use; *C:* Unclear scientific evidence for this use; *D:* Fair scientific evidence against this use (it may not work); *F:* Strong scientific evidence against this use (it likely does not work). For a more detailed explanation of efficacy criteria, see "Natural Standard Evidence-Based Validated Grading Rationale" in the Introduction.

Uses Based on Tradition, Theory, or Limited Scientific Evidence

Alcohol withdrawal, anti-bacterial, anti-seizure, anti-spasm, aphrodisiac, asthma, attention deficit hyperactivity disorder (ADHD), burns (skin), cancer, chronic pain, cough, drug addiction, Epstein-Barr virus infection, hemorrhoids, high blood pressure, insomnia, nerve pain, pain (general), menopausal symptoms (hot flashes), gastrointestinal discomfort ("nervous stomach"), tension, wrinkle prevention.

DOSING

The following doses are based on scientific research, publications, traditional use, or expert opinion. Many herbs and supplements have not been thoroughly tested, and safety and effectiveness may not be proven. Brands may be made differently, with variable ingredients even within the same brand. The doses shown may not apply to all products. It is important to always read product labels and discuss doses with a qualified healthcare provider before therapy is started.

Standardization

- Standardization involves measuring the amounts of certain chemicals in products to try to make different preparations similar to each other. It is not always known if the chemicals being measured are the "active" ingredients. Although there is no widely accepted standardization for passion flower, the flavonoid components have been used for standardization in some commercial products.

P

Adults (18 Years and Older)

- **General:** Safety and effectiveness have not been established for any dose. There are no standard or well-studied doses of passion flower. Different preparations and doses have been used traditionally.
- **Dried herb:** 0.5 to 2 g taken three to four times daily by mouth has been used.
- **Tincture (1:8):** 1 to 4 ml taken three to four times daily by mouth has been used.
- **Tea:** Tea made from 4 to 8 g of dried herb taken daily has been used.
- **Infusion:** 2.5 g has been used three to four times daily.

Children (Younger Than 18 Years)

- There are not enough scientific data to recommend passion flower for use in children at any dose.

SAFETY

The U.S. Food and Drug Administration does not strictly regulate herbs and supplements. There is no guarantee of strength, purity, or safety of products, and effects may vary. It is important to always read product labels. People who have a medical condition, or are taking other drugs, herbs, or supplements, should consult a qualified healthcare provider before starting a new therapy. Aa healthcare provider should be contacted immediately about any side effects.

Allergies

- Hypersensitivity reaction with urticaria (hives) and skin blood vessel inflammation (vasculitis), as well as occupational asthma with runny nose, have been reported with the use of passion flower products.

Side Effects and Warnings

- Passion flower is generally considered to be a safe herb, with few reported serious adverse events. In cases of side effects, the products being used have rarely been tested for contamination (which may have been the cause). There is a report of children in Costa Rica who died from eating passiflora fruit (*P. adenopoda*) due to cyanide poisoning, derived from a substance (cyanogenic B-glycoside) in the fruit. However, in other studies, these substances (cyanogenic alkaloids) have not been found in passiflora fruit.
- Rapid heart rate and rhythm, nausea, and vomiting have been reported. Side effects may also include drowsiness/sedation and mental slowing. Use caution if you are driving or operating heavy machinery.
- Passion flower may theoretically increase the risk of bleeding and alter blood tests that measure blood clotting (international normalized ratio [INR]).
- There is a case report of liver failure and death of a patient taking a preparation of passion flower with kava. Patients should use caution with any kava-containing products, as kava has been associated with liver damage. The cause of the liver damage is less likely related to the presence of passion flower.

Pregnancy and Breastfeeding

- There is not enough scientific evidence to recommend the safe use of passion flower in any dose during pregnancy or breastfeeding. During the 1930s, animal studies found uterine stimulant action in components of *Passiflora*.
- Many tinctures contain high levels of alcohol and should be avoided during pregnancy.

INTERACTIONS

Most herbs and supplements have not been thoroughly tested for interactions with other herbs, supplements, drugs, or foods. The interactions listed here are based on reports in scientific publications, laboratory experiments, or traditional use. It is important to always read product labels. People who have a medical condition, or are taking other drugs, herbs, or supplements, you should consult a qualified healthcare provider before starting a new therapy.

Interactions with Drugs

- Certain substances (harmala alkaloids) with monoamine oxidase inhibitory (MAOI) action have been found in small amounts in some species of *Passiflora*. Although levels of these substances may be too low to cause noticeable effects, in theory, use of passion flower with MAOI drugs may cause additive effects. MAOI drugs include isocarboxazid (Marplan), phenelzine (Nardil), and tranylcypromine (Parnate).
- Based on animal research, use of passion flower with alcohol or other sedative-hypnotic drugs may increase the amount of drowsiness caused by some drugs. Examples include benzodiazepines such as lorazepam (Ativan) and diazepam (Valium), barbiturates such as phenobarbital, narcotics such as codeine, some antidepressants, and alcohol. Caution is advised while driving or operating machinery.
- Passion flower may in theory increase the risk of bleeding when taken with drugs that increase the risk of bleeding. Some examples include aspirin, anticoagulants ("blood thinners") such as warfarin (Coumadin) and heparin, antiplatelet drugs such as clopidogrel (Plavix), and nonsteroidal anti-inflammatory drugs such

as ibuprofen (Motrin, Advil) and naproxen (Naprosyn, Aleve). Literature review reveals no reported cases of significant bleeding in humans taking passion flower.
- Many tinctures contain high levels of alcohol and may cause nausea or vomiting when taken with metronidazole (Flagyl) or disulfiram (Antabuse).

Interactions with Herbs and Dietary Supplements

- Certain substances (harmala alkaloids) with monoamine oxidase inhibitory (MAOI) action have been found in small amounts in some species of *Passiflora.* Although levels of these substances may be too low to cause noticeable effects, in theory, use of passion flower with herbs or supplements with MAOI activity may cause additive effects. Herbs and supplements with possible MAOI activity include 5-HTP (5-hydroxytryptophan), California poppy, chromium, dehydroepiandrosterone (DHEA), DL-phenylalanine (DLPA), ephedra, evening primrose oil, fenugreek, *Ginkgo biloba*, hops, mace, SAMe (*S*-adenosylmethionine (SAMe), sepia, St. John's wort, tyrosine, valerian, vitamin B_6, and yohimbe bark extract. In theory, use of passion flower with caffeine, guarana, or ephedra (ma huang) may cause an increased risk of elevated blood pressure.
- Based on animal research, use of passion flower with sedative-hypnotic herbs or supplements may increase the amount of drowsiness caused by some herbs or supplements. Examples include calamus, calendula, California poppy, capsicum, catnip, celery, couchgrass, dogwood, elecampane, German chamomile, goldenseal, gotu kola, hops, kava (may help sleep without drowsiness), lavender aromatherapy, lemon balm, sage, sassafras, scullcap, shepherd's purse, Siberian ginseng, St. John's wort, stinging nettle, valerian, wild carrot, wild lettuce, withania root, and yerba mansa. Caution is advised while driving or operating machinery.
- Passion flower may in theory increase the risk of bleeding when taken with herbs or supplements that increase the risk of bleeding. Multiple cases of bleeding have been reported with the use of *Ginkgo biloba*, and fewer cases with garlic and saw palmetto. Numerous other agents may theoretically increase the risk of bleeding, although this has not been proven in most cases. Some examples include alfalfa, American ginseng, angelica, anise, *Arnica montana*, asafetida, aspen bark, bilberry, birch, black cohosh, bladderwrack, bogbean, boldo, borage seed oil, bromelain, capsicum, cat's claw, celery, chamomile, chaparral, clove, coleus, cordyceps, danshen, devil's claw, dong quai, evening primrose, fenugreek, feverfew, flaxseed/flax powder (not a concern with flaxseed oil), ginger, grapefruit juice, grape seed, green tea, guggul, gymnestra, horse chestnut, horseradish, licorice root, lovage root, male fern, meadowsweet, nordihydroguaiaretic acid (NDGA), onion, papain, *Panax ginseng*, parsley, poplar, prickly ash, propolis, quassia, red clover, reishi, rue, Siberian ginseng, sweet birch, sweet clover, turmeric, vitamin E, white willow, wild carrot, wild lettuce, willow, wintergreen, and yucca. Literature review reveals no reported cases of clinically significant bleeding in humans taking passion flower.

P

Interactions with Foods

- Certain substances (harmala alkaloids) with monoamine oxidase inhibitory (MAOI) action have been found in small amounts in some species of *Passiflora.* Although levels of these substances may be too low to cause noticeable effects, in theory, use of passion flower with tyramine/tryptophan containing–foods may cause an increased risk of dangerously high blood pressure (hypertensive crisis). These include protein foods that have been aged/preserved. Specific examples of such foods are anchovies, avocados, bananas, bean curd, beer (alcohol-free/reduced alcohol), caffeine (large amounts), caviar, champagne, cheeses (particularly aged, processed, or strong varieties), chocolate, dry sausage/salami/bologna, fava beans, figs, herring (pickled), liver (particularly chicken), meat tenderizers, papaya, protein extracts/powder, raisins, shrimp paste, sour cream, soy sauce, wine (particularly chianti), yeast extracts, and yogurt.

Selected References

Natural Standard developed the preceding evidence-based information based on a systematic review of more than 70 scientific articles. For comprehensive information about alternative and complementary therapies on the professional level, go to www.naturalstandard.com. Selected references are listed here.

Bilia AR, Bergonzi MC, Gallori S, et al. Stability of the constituents of Calendula, milk-thistle and passionflower tinctures by LC-DAD and LC-MS. J Pharm Biomed Anal 2002;30(3): 613-624.

Bourin M, Bougerol T, Guitton B, et al. A combination of plant extracts in the treatment of outpatients with adjustment disorder with anxious mood: controlled study versus placebo. Fundam Clin Pharmacol 1997;11(2):127-132.

Capasso A, Pinto A. Experimental investigations of the synergistic-sedative effect of *Passiflora* and kava. Acta Therapeutica 1995;21:127-140.

Carlini EA. Plants and the central nervous system. Pharmacol Biochem Behav 2003;75(3): 501-512.

Dattilio L, Suddaby B. Ventricular tachycardia in a neonate. Pediatr Nurs 2002;28(6): 612-613.

de Melo NF, Guerra M. Variability of the 5S and 45S rDNA sites in Passiflora L. species with distinct base chromosome numbers. Ann Bot (Lond) 2003;92(2):309-316.

Dhawan K, Kumar S, Sharma A. Antiasthmatic activity of the methanol extract of leaves of *Passiflora incarnata*. Phytother Res 2003;17(7):821-822.

Dhawan K, Dhawan S, Chhabra S. Attenuation of benzodiazepine dependence in mice by a tri-substituted benzoflavone moiety of *Passiflora incarnata* Linneaus: a non–habit forming anxiolytic. J Pharm Pharm Sci 2003;6(2):215-222.

Dhawan K, Kumar S, Sharma A. Aphrodisiac activity of methanol extract of leaves of *Passiflora incarnata* Linn in mice. Phytother Res 2003;17(4):401-403.

Dhawan K, Sharma A. Antitussive activity of the methanol extract of *Passiflora incarnata* leaves. Fitoterapia 2002;73(5):397-399.

Dhawan K, Kumar S, Sharma A. Suppression of alcohol-cessation-oriented hyper-anxiety by the benzoflavone moiety of *Passiflora incarnata* Linneaus in mice. J Ethnopharmacol 2002; 81(2):239-244.

Dhawan K, Kumar S, Sharma A. Comparative anxiolytic activity profile of various preparations of *Passiflora incarnata* Linneaus: a comment on medicinal plants' standardization. J Altern Complement Med 2002;8(3):283-291.

Dhawan K, Kumar S, Sharma A. Reversal of cannabinoids (delta9-THC) by the benzoflavone moiety from methanol extract of *Passiflora incarnata* Linneaus in mice: a possible therapy for cannabinoid addiction. J Pharm Pharmacol 2002;54(6):875-881.

Giavina-Bianchi PF Jr., Castro FF, Machado ML, et al. Occupational respiratory allergic disease induced by *Passiflora alata* and *Rhamnus purshiana*. Ann Allergy Asthma Immunol 1997; 79(5):449-454.

Gow PJ, Connelly NJ, Hill RL, et al. Fatal fulminant hepatic failure induced by a natural therapy containing kava. Med J Aust 2003;178(9):442-443. Comment in: Med J Aust 2003;178(9): 421-422.

Kapadia GJ, Azuine MA, Tokuda H, et al. Inhibitory effect of herbal remedies on 12-o-tetradecanoylphorbol-13-acetate-promoted Epstein-Barr virus early antigen activation. Pharmacol Res 2002;45(3):213-220.

Krenn L. Passion Flower (Passiflora incarnata L.)—a reliable herbal sedative [article in German]. Wien Med Wochenschr 2002;152(15-16):404-406.

Marchart E, Krenn L, Kopp B. Quantification of the flavonoid glycosides in *Passiflora incarnata* by capillary electrophoresis. Planta Med 2003;69(5):452-456.

Puricelli L, Dell'Aica I, Sartor L, et al. Preliminary evaluation of inhibition of matrix-metalloprotease MMP-2 and MMP-9 by *Passiflora edulis* and *P. foetida* aqueous extracts. Fitoterapia 2003;74(3):302-304.

Seigler DS, Pauli GF, Nahrstedt A, et al. Cyanogenic allosides and glucosides from *Passiflora edulis* and Carica papaya. Phytochemistry 2002;60(8):873-882.

Smith GW, Chalmers TM, Nuki G. Vasculitis associated with herbal preparation containing *Passiflora* extract. Br J Rheumatol 1993;32(1):87-88.

Speroni E, Minghetti A. Neuropharmacological activity of extracts from *Passiflora incarnata*. Planta Med 1988;54(6):488-491.

Talcott ST, Percival SS, Pittet-Moore J, et al. Phytochemical composition and antioxidant stability of fortified yellow passion fruit (*Passiflora edulis*). J Agric Food Chem 2003;51(4): 935-941.

Von Eiff M, Brunner H, Haegeli A, et al. Hawthorn/passion flower extract and improvement in physical exercise capacity of patients with dyspnoea class II of the NYHA functional classifications. Acta Therapeutica 1994;20:47-66.

P

PC-SPES

RELATED TERMS

- *Chrysanthemum morifolium* (chrysanthemum, mum, chu-hua); *Ganoderma lucidum* (reishi mushroom, ling zhi); *Glycyrrhiza glabra* (licorice); *Isatis indigotica* Fort (da qing ye, dyer's wood); *Panax pseudo-ginseng* (san qi); *Rabdosia rubescens* (rubescens, dong ling cao); *Scutellaria baicalensis* (scullcap, huang-chin); *Serenoa repens* (saw palmetto).
- Not to be confused with SPES (a different product), or with copycat products marketed with similar names.

BACKGROUND

- PC-SPES is an herbal combination product that was produced and marketed until early 2002 by BotanicLab, Inc. for the treatment of prostate cancer. The initials *PC* stand for "prostate cancer," and *spes* is Latin for "hope."
- Based on a Chinese herbal formula, the ingredients of PC-SPES were officially listed as including *Serenoa repens* (saw palmetto) and seven other herbs: *Chrysanthemum morifolium* (chrysanthemum, mum, chu-hua); *Ganoderma lucidum* (reishi mushroom, ling zhi); *Glycyrrhiza glabra* (licorice); *Isatis indigotica* Fort (da qing ye, dyer's wood); *Panax pseudo-ginseng* (san qi); *Rabdosia rubescens* (rubescens, dong ling cao); and *Scutellaria baicalensis* (scullcap, huang-chin).
- In low-quality studies, PC-SPES was observed to reduce serum prostate-specific antigen (PSA) levels, reduce evidence of metastatic disease, diminish pain, and improve quality of life in patients with prostate cancer. This evidence was viewed as promising by major cancer centers in the United States.
- However, in early 2002, the FDA Safety Information and Adverse Event Reporting Program issued a warning to consumers to avoid using PC-SPES, based on findings that the product contained the anticoagulant ("blood thinner") warfarin. Bleeding disorders had previously been reported with PC-SPES. The manufacturer voluntarily recalled the product. Samples of PC-SPES were later found to contain variable amounts of the nonsteroidal anti-inflammatory drug indomethacin, the synthetic estrogen diethylstilbestrol (DES), and the estrogen ethinyl estradiol.
- A study published in the September 2002 issue of the *Journal of the National Cancer Institute* analyzed lots of PC-SPES manufactured between 1996 and 2001. This evaluation found variable ingredients in PC-SPES between lots, with higher levels of indomethacin and DES after 1999. These post-1999 samples were found to have much greater estrogenic properties compared to earlier samples, and to possess a higher level of activity against prostate cell lines in laboratory tests. After 2001, greater amounts of the natural constituents licochalcone A and baicalin, as well as warfarin, were found in samples. These results suggest that PC-SPES produced at different times may not be equivalent or comparable, and that the "anti-cancer" effects of PC-SPES may have been due to undeclared prescription drug ingredients.
- Several other BotanicLab products have also been found to contain undeclared prescription drugs. It is not clear if these adulterants were present in raw materials

obtained by BotanicLab from other sources or were added later in the manufacturing process.

- Since BotanicLab closed its doors, several products with similar names have been introduced on the market, but none has been evaluated scientifically to the same extent as PC-SPES. The National Center for Complementary and Alternative Medicine (NCCAM) has expressed willingness to support future research on formulations that are true to the claimed ingredients and proven not to be contaminated.

USES BASED ON SCIENTIFIC EVIDENCE	Grade*
Prostate cancer	**C**

Uncontrolled human studies of PC-SPES have reported improvements in patients with both androgen-dependent and androgen-independent prostate cancer. Overall, these studies found prostate-specific antigen (PSA) levels to fall by greater than 50% in most patients, improvements in bone scans and x-rays, reductions in pain scores, and improvements in quality of life. In a 2002 preliminary report (conference abstract) of a comparison between PC-SPES and diethylstilbestrol (DES) in patients with androgen-independent metastatic prostate cancer, patients treated with PC-SPES had a greater reduction in PSA levels. However, the later finding that undeclared amounts of DES are present in some PC-SPES samples clouds these results.

Various explanations for the effectiveness of PC-SPES were initially proposed. Estrogen-like effects were reported prior to 1998. These may be due to herbs with estrogen-like effects or to undeclared estrogenic drugs. The constituent baicalin, a flavone found in *Scutellaria baicalensis*, was found in laboratory experiments to inhibit the enzymes 12-lipoxygenase, 5-alpha-reductase, and aromatase. In addition, PC-SPES extracts were reported to cause cell death (apoptosis) or to slow the growth of cancer cell lines.

The recent finding that different lots of PC-SPES produced between 1996 and 2001 contained different ingredients from each other has raised questions about whether studies of PC-SPES can be compared with each other. The discovery of undeclared prescription drug ingredients, including the nonsteroidal anti-inflammatory drug indomethacin, the synthetic estrogen diethylstilbestrol (DES), the estrogen ethinyl estradiol, and the anticoagulant warfarin, make it unclear if these constituents may have caused the observed clinical effects.

Because of these complicated circumstances, and the fact that PC-SPES has never been compared to placebo or standard cancer treatments in a well-reported study, the question of effectiveness remains unclear.

Due to known and theoretical safety concerns, samples of PC-SPES that may be in the possession of patients should not be used.

*Key to grades: *A:* Strong scientific evidence for this use; *B:* Good scientific evidence for this use; *C:* Unclear scientific evidence for this use; *D:* Fair scientific evidence against this use (it may not work); *F:* Strong scientific evidence against this use (it likely does not work). For a more detailed explanation of efficacy criteria, see "Natural Standard Evidence-Based Validated Grading Rationale" in the Introduction.

Uses Based on Tradition, Theory, or Limited Scientific Evidence

Benign prostatic hypertrophy, breast cancer, breast enlargement, cancer prevention, leukemia, lymphoma, melanoma, "prostate health."

DOSING

The following doses are based on scientific research, publications, traditional use, or expert opinion. Many herbs and supplements have not been thoroughly tested, and safety and effectiveness may not be proven. Brands may be made differently, with variable ingredients even within the same brand. The doses shown may not apply to all products. It is important to always read product labels and discuss doses with a qualified healthcare provider before therapy is started.

Adult Dosing (18 Years and Older)

- Based on known safety concerns associated with PC-SPES, no dosing regimen is recommended. Samples of PC-SPES that may be in the possession of patients should not be used.

SAFETY

The U.S. Food and Drug Administration does not strictly regulate herbs and supplements. There is no guarantee of strength, purity, or safety of products, and effects may vary. It is important to always read product labels. People who have a medical condition, or are taking other drugs, herbs, or supplements, you should consult a qualified healthcare provider before starting a new therapy. A healthcare provider should be contacted immediately about any side effects.

Allergies

- In one human study, allergic reactions were reported in 2% of patients, and treatment was stopped in one case because of throat swelling and shortness of breath. It is not clear which ingredient in PC-SPES might have been responsible. Products containing herbs similar to PC-SPES should be avoided by people with allergies to any of the included herbs.

Side Effects and Warnings

- PC-SPES has been recalled and should not be used. Undeclared prescription drug ingredients have been found in samples of PC-SPES, including indomethacin, diethylstilbestrol (DES), ethinyl estradiol, and warfarin.
- PC-SPES may increase the risk of blood clots. Several cases of blood clots, including life-threatening clots to the lungs, have been reported with PC-SPES use. In contrast, cases of bleeding have also been reported. These are theorized to be due to undeclared amounts of the prescription drug warfarin in some samples of PC-SPES, or to the presence of the PC-SPES ingredient saw palmetto which is associated with one report of bleeding. This would add to the risk of bleeding in patients with bleeding disorders or taking drugs that may increase the risk of bleeding. The bleeding disorder disseminated intravascular coagulation (DIC), that can include clotting, bleeding, or both, has also been reported.
- PC-SPES has also been associated with erectile dysfunction, loss of libido, hot flashes, breast/nipple tenderness, breast enlargement, water retention (edema), and leg cramps.

- Adverse effects associated with undeclared prescription drug ingredients in PC-SPES are possible, such as gastrointestinal distress from indomethacin.

Pregnancy and Breastfeeding

- PC-SPES has not been evaluated during pregnancy or breastfeeding and should be avoided. Estrogenic effects may be harmful. The undeclared prescription drug diethylstilbestrol (DES), discovered in some samples of PC-SPES, may increase the risk of reproductive tract abnormalities in daughters born to women taking this drug.

INTERACTIONS

Most herbs and supplements have not been thoroughly tested for interactions with other herbs, supplements, drugs, or foods. The interactions listed here are based on reports in scientific publications, laboratory experiments, or traditional use. It is important to always read product labels. People who have a medical condition, or are taking other drugs, herbs, or supplements, should consult a qualified healthcare provider before starting a new therapy.

Interactions with Drugs

- Based on reported cases of bleeding and inclusion of undeclared amounts of the prescription blood-thinner warfarin in some samples, PC-SPES may increase the risk of bleeding when taken with drugs that increase the risk of bleeding. Some examples include aspirin, anticoagulants ("blood thinners") such as warfarin (Coumadin) and heparin, antiplatelet drugs such as clopidogrel (Plavix), and non-steroidal anti-inflammatory drugs such as ibuprofen (Motrin, Advil) and naproxen (Naprosyn, Aleve). In contrast, PC-SPES has also been associated with an increased risk of blood clots, which may be due to estrogen-like effects. This would work against the action of blood-thinning medications.
- Based on the proposed anti-androgenic mechanism of action of saw palmetto, a major ingredient of PC-SPES, additive effects may occur with anti-androgen drugs such as the 5α-reductase inhibitor finasteride (Proscar); the androgen receptor antagonists bicalutamide (Casodex), flutamide (Eulexin), and nilutamide (Nilandron); and the GnRH antagonists leuprolide (Lupron), goserelin (Zoladex), and histrelin (Supprelin). Similarly, this therapy may decrease the effectiveness of therapeutic androgens such as testosterone (Androderm, Testoderm), methyltestosterone (Android, Testred, Virilon), fluoxymesterone (Halotestin), nandrolone decanoate (Deca-Dubrolin), and stanozolol (Winstrol).
- PC-SPES may add to the estrogenic effects of other drugs, based on estrogen-like effects reported in studies and on the presence of undeclared amounts of prescription estrogen drugs in some samples of PC-SPES.

Interactions with Herbs and Dietary Supplements

- Based on reported cases of bleeding and inclusion of undeclared amounts of the prescription blood thinner warfarin in some samples, PC-SPES may increase the risk of bleeding when taken with herbs and supplements that are believed to increase the risk of bleeding. Multiple cases of bleeding have been reported with the use of *Ginkgo biloba*, and fewer cases with garlic and saw palmetto. Numerous other agents may theoretically increase the risk of bleeding, although this has not been proven in most cases. Some examples include alfalfa, American ginseng, angelica, anise, *Arnica montana*, asafetida, aspen bark, bilberry, birch, black cohosh, bladderwrack, bogbean, boldo, borage seed oil, bromelain, capsicum, cat's claw, celery, chamomile, chaparral, clove, coleus, cordyceps, danshen, devil's claw, dong quai, EPA (eicosapentaenoic acid, found in deep-sea fish oils), evening primrose oil, fenugreek, feverfew, fish oil, flaxseed/flax powder (not a concern with flaxseed oil), ginger, grapefruit juice, grape seed, green tea, guggul, gymnestra, horse chestnut, horseradish, licorice root, lovage root, male fern, meadowsweet, nordihydroguaiaretic acid (NDGA), onion, papain, *Panax ginseng*, parsley, passionflower, poplar, prickly ash, propolis, quassia, red clover, reishi, rue, Siberian ginseng, sweet birch, sweet clover, turmeric, vitamin E, white willow, wild carrot, wild lettuce, willow, wintergreen, yucca. In contrast, PC-SPES has also been associated with an increased risk of blood clots, which may be due to estrogen-like effects. This would work against the action of blood-thinning agents.

- PC-SPES may add to the estrogenic effects of other agents, based on estrogen-like effects reported in studies and on the presence of undeclared amounts of prescription estrogen drugs in some samples. Possible examples include alfalfa, black cohosh, bloodroot, burdock, hops, kudzu, licorice, pomegranate, red clover, soy, thyme, white horehoumd, and yucca.

Selected References

Natural Standard developed the preceding evidence-based information based on a systematic review of more than 75 articles. For comprehensive information about alternative and complementary therapies on the professional level, go to www.naturalstandard.com. Selected references are listed here.

Burton TM. Prostate cancer herbs gone for good. Wall Street Journal 2002 (May 21):D4.

Cheema P, El Mefty O, Jazieh AR. Intraoperative haemorrhage associated with the use of extract of Saw Palmetto herb: a case report and review of literature. J Intern Med 2001; 250(2):167-169.

Darzynkiewicz Z, Traganos F, Wu JM, et al. Chinese herbal mixture PC SPES in treatment of prostate cancer. Int J Oncol 2000;17:729-736.

Davis NB, Nahlik L, Vogelzang NJ. Does PC-SPES interact with warfarin? J Urol 2002;167:1793.

de la Taille A, Buttyan R, Hayek O, et al. Herbal therapy PC-SPES: in vitro effects and evaluation of its efficacy in 69 patients with prostate cancer. J Urol 2000; 164(4):1229-1234.

de la Taille A, Hayek OR, Buttyan R, et al. Effects of a phytotherapeutic agent, PC-SPES, on prostate cancer: a preliminary investigation on human cell lines and patients. BJU Int 1999; 84:845-850.

Di Silverio F, D'Eramo G, Lubrano C, et al. Evidence that *Serenoa repens* extract displays an antiestrogenic activity in prostatic tissue of benign prostatic hypertrophy patients. Eur Urol 1992;21(4):309-314.

DiPaola RS, Zhang H, Lambert GH, et al. Clinical and biologic activity of an estrogenic herbal combination (PC-SPES) in prostate cancer. N Engl J Med 1998;339(12):785-791.

Duncan GG. Re: Does PC-SPES interact with warfarin? J Urol 2003;169(1):294-295.

Elghamry MI, Hansel R. Activity and isolated phytoestrogen of shrub palmetto fruits (*Serenoa repens* Small), a new estrogenic plant. Experientia 1969;25(8):828-829.

Food and Drug Administration. MedWatch. 2002 Safety information summaries. PC SPES, SPES (BotanicLab). http://www.fda.gov/medwatch/SAFETY/2002/safety02.htm#spes.

Geliebter J, Mittelman A, Tiwari RK. PC-SPES and prostate cancer. J Nutr 2001;131:164S-166S.

Halicka HD, Ardelt B, Juan G, et al. Apoptosis and cell cycle effects induced by extracts of the Chinese herbal preparation PC SPES. Int J Oncol 1997;11:437-448.

Hsieh T, Chen SS, Wang X, et al. Regulation of androgen receptor (AR) and prostate specific antigen (PSA) expression in the androgen-responsive human prostate LNCaP cells by ethanolic extracts of the Chinese herbal preparation, PC-SPES. Biochem Mol Biol Int 1997; 42:535-544.

Hsieh TC, Ng C, Chang CC, et al. Induction of apoptosis and down-regulation of bcl-6 in mutu I cells treated with ethanolic extracts of the Chinese herbal supplement PC-SPES. Int J Oncol 1998;13:1199-1202.

Ikezoe T, Chen S, Saito T, et al. PC-SPES decreases proliferation and induces differentiation and apoptosis of human acute myeloid leukemia cells. Int J Oncol 2003;23(4):1203-1211.

Ikezoe T, Chen SS, Heber D, et al. Baicalin is a major component of PC-SPES which inhibits the proliferation of human cancer cells via apoptosis and cell cycle arrest. Prostate 2001; 49:285-292.

Ikezoe T, Chen SS, Yang Y, et al. PC-SPES: Molecular mechanism to induce apoptosis and down-regulate expression of PSA in LNCaP human prostate cancer cells. Int J Oncol 2003; 23(5):1461-1470.

Ikezoe T, Yang Y, Heber D, et al. PC-SPES: a potent inhibitor of nuclear factor-kappaB rescues mice from lipopolysaccharide-induced septic shock. Mol Pharmacol 2003;64(6):1521-1529.

Kao GD, Devine P. Use of complementary health practices by prostate carcinoma patients undergoing radiation therapy. Cancer 2000;88:615-619.

Kao YC, Zhou C, Sherman M, et al. Molecular basis of the inhibition of human aromatase (estrogen synthetase) by flavone and isoflavone phytoestrogens: a site-directed mutagenesis study. Environ Health Perspect 1998;106:85-92.

Kitahara S, Umeda H, Yano H. Effects of intravenous administration of high dose diethylstilbestrol diphosphate on serum hormonal levels in patients with hormone-refractory prostate cancer. Endocr J 1999;46:659-664.

Ko R, Wilson RD, Loscutoff S. PC-SPES. Urology 2003;61(6):1292.

Kubota T, Hisatake J, Hisatake Y, et al. PC-SPES: a unique inhibitor of proliferation of prostate cancer cells *in vitro* and *in vivo*. Prostate 2000;42:163-171.

Lippert MC, McClain R, Boyd JC, et al. Alternative medicine use in patients with localized prostate carcinoma treated with curative intent. Cancer 1999;86:2642-2648.

Lock M, Loblaw DA, Choo R, et al. Disseminated intravascular coagulation and PC-SPES: a case report and literature review. Can J Urol 2001;8:1326-1329.

Lu X, Guo J, Hsieh TC. PC-SPES inhibits cell proliferation by modulating p21, cyclins D, E and B and multiple cell cycle-related genes in prostate cancer cells. Cell Cycle 2003;2(1):59-63.

Malkowicz SB. The role of diethylstilbestrol in the treatment of prostate cancer. Urology 2001;58:108-113.

National Center for Complementary and Alternative Medicine (NCCAM). Recall of PC SPES and SPES Dietary Supplements. http://nccam.nih.gov/health/alerts/spes/.

Oh WK, George DJ, Hackmann K, et al. Activity of the herbal combination, PC-SPES, in the treatment of patients with androgen-independent prostate cancer. Urology 2001;57(1):122-126.

Oh WK, George DJ, Kantoff PW. Rapid rise of serum prostate specific antigen levels after discontinuation of the herbal therapy PC-SPES in patients with advanced prostate carcinoma: report of four cases. Cancer 2002;94(3):686-689.

Pfeifer BL, Pirani JF, Hamann SR, et al. PC-SPES, a dietary supplement for the treatment of hormone-refractory prostate cancer. BJU Int 2000;85:481485.

Pirani JF. The effects of phytotherapeutic agents on prostate cancer: an overview of recent clinical trials of PC SPES. Urology 2001;58:36-38.

Reynolds T. Contamination of PC-SPES remains a mystery. J Natl Cancer Inst 2002;94(17): 1266-1268.

Robertson CN, Roberson KM, Padilla GM, et al. Induction of apoptosis by diethylstilbestrol in hormone-insensitive prostate cancer cells. J Natl Cancer Inst 1996;88:908-917.

Rosenbaum E, Wygoda M, Gips M, et al. Diethylstilbestrol is an active agent in prostatic cancer patients after failure to complete androgen blockade (abstract 1372). Proc ASCO 2000:19.

Schwarz RE, Donohue CA, Sadava D, et al. Pancreatic cancer in vitro toxicity mediated by Chinese herbs SPES and PC-SPES: implications for monotherapy and combination treatment. Cancer Lett 2003;189(1):59-68.

Small EJ, Frohlich MW, Bok R, et al. Prospective trial of the herbal supplement PC-SPES in patients with progressive prostate cancer. J Clin Oncol 2000;18(21):3595-3603.

Small EJ, Kantoff P, Weinberg VK, et al. A prospective multicenter randomized trial of the herbal supplement, PC-SPES vs. diethylstilbestrol (DES) in patients with advanced, androgen independent prostate cancer (AiPCa). Proc ASCO 2002;21:178a.

Sovak M, Seligson AL, Konas M, et al. Herbal composition PC-SPES for management of prostate cancer: identification of active principles. J Natl Cancer Inst 2002;94:1275-1281.

Stepanov VN, Siniakova LA, Sarrazin B, et al. Efficacy and tolerability of the lipidosterolic extract of *Serenoa repens* (Permixon) in benign prostatic hyperplasia: a double-blind comparison of two dosage regimens. Adv Ther 1999;16(5):231-241.

Tiwari RK, Geliebter J, Garikapaty VP, et al. Anti-tumor effects of PC-SPES, an herbal formulation in prostate cancer. Int J Oncol 1999;14:713-719.

Wadsworth T, Poonyagariyagorn H, Sullivan E, et al. In vivo effect of PC-SPES on prostate growth and hepatic CYP3A expression in rats. J Pharmacol Exp Ther 2003;306(1):187-194.

Wang L. Study finds additional evidence for contamination of herbal supplement for prostate cancer. J Natl Cancer Inst 2002;94(17):1259.

Weinrobe MC, Montgomery B. Acquired bleeding diathesis in a patient taking PC-SPES. N Engl J Med 2001;345:1213-1214.

White J. PC-SPES—A lesson for future dietary supplement research. J Natl Cancer Inst 2002; 94(17):1261-1262.

Wu J, Chen D, Zhang R. Study on the bioavailability of baicalin-phospholipid complex by using HPLC. Biomed Chromatogr 1999;13:493-495.

Yip I, Cudiamat M, Chim D. PC-SPES for treatment of prostate cancer: herbal medicine. Curr Urol Rep 2003;4(3):253-257.

Pennyroyal

(American Pennyroyal [*Hedeoma pulegioides* L.], European Pennyroyal [*Mentha pulegium* L.])

RELATED TERMS

- Aloe herbal horse spray, American pennyroyal, brotherwort, chasse-puces, churchwort, *Cunila pulegioides*, dictamne de Virginie, European pennyroyal, fleabane, flea mint, fretillet, *Hedeoma phlebitides*, herbal horsespray, herbe aux puces, herbe de Saint-Laurent, Labiatae, la menthe pouliot, Lamiacea, lurk-in-the-ditch, *Melissa pulegioides*, mentha pouillot, Miracle Coat spray-on dog shampoo, mock pennyroyal, mosquito plant, Old World pennyroyal, pennyroyal essential oil, petit baume, piliolerial, poley, pouliot royal, pudding herb, pudding grass, pulegium, pulegium oil, *Pulegium regium*, *Pulegium vulgare*, pulioll-royall, run-by-the-ground, squaw balm, squawmint, stinking balm, tickweed.

BACKGROUND

- The essential oil of pennyroyal is considered toxic. Death has been reported after consumption of half an ounce (15 ml) of the oil. A characteristic noted in most cases of pennyroyal overdose is a strong minty smell on the patient's breath. The active metabolite menthofuran can be detected by gas chromatography in urine, blood, or other tissues. Overdose management includes oral decontamination by lavage, and/or administration of activated charcoal.
- The similarity of the pathogenesis of pennyroyal-induced hepatic necrosis to that produced by acetaminophen suggests a possible role for *N*-acetylcysteine (NAC) in the management of pennyroyal overdose. However, this application has not been confirmed by animal or human studies.
- Anecdotal evidence and one case report suggest that the essential oil of pennyroyal may function as an abortifacient and emmenagogue (menstrual flow stimulant). However, it may do so at lethal or near-lethal doses, making this action unpredictable and dangerous. Future research to determine the safety and efficacy of the less toxic aerial parts of the pennyroyal plant on the menstrual cycle are needed before a recommendation can be made.

P

USES BASED ON SCIENTIFIC EVIDENCE	Grade*
Abortifacient (uterus contraction stimulant/abortion inducer) Folkloric use and several human case reports describe use of the essential oil of pennyroyal to cause abortion. However, it may do so at deadly or toxic doses, making this an unpredictable and dangerous use.	**C**
Menstrual flow stimulant (emmenagogue) Folkloric use and several human case reports describe use of the essential oil of pennyroyal as an emmenagogue (menstrual flow stimulant).	**C**

Continued

However, it may do so at lethal or near-lethal doses, making this action unpredictable and dangerous.

*Key to grades: *A:* Strong scientific evidence for this use; *B:* Good scientific evidence for this use; *C:* Unclear scientific evidence for this use; *D:* Fair scientific evidence against this use (it may not work); *F:* Strong scientific evidence against this use (it likely does not work). For a more detailed explanation of efficacy criteria, see "Natural Standard Evidence-Based Validated Grading Rationale" in the Introduction.

Uses Based on Tradition, Theory, or Limited Scientific Evidence

Acne, antiseptic, anti-spasm, anxiety, asthma, bruises and burns, cancer, chest congestion, colds, colic, cough, cramps, diarrhea, digestion, diuretic (increasing urine flow), dizziness, dysentery, fever, flatulence (gas) flavoring agent, flea control, flu, fragrance (detergents, perfumes, soaps), gallbladder disorders, gout, hallucinations, headache, hysteria, immortality, indigestion, insect repellent, intestinal disorders, itchy eyes, joint problems, kidney disease, leprosy, liver disease, menstrual irregularities (stimulant, regulator), mouth sores, muscle pain, nosebleeds, pneumonia, potpourri, pregnancy, premenstrual syndrome, preparing the uterus for labor, purifier (water, blood), refrigerant, respiratory ailments, sedative, skin ailments (itching, burning, bruising), snake bites (venomous), stimulant, stomach pain, sunstroke, sweating, syncope, toothache, uterine fibroids, whooping cough.

DOSING

The following doses are based on scientific research, publications, traditional use, or expert opinion. Many herbs and supplements have not been thoroughly tested, and safety and effectiveness may not be proven. Brands may be made differently, with variable ingredients even within the same brand. The doses shown may not apply to all products. It is important to always read product labels and discuss doses with a qualified healthcare provider before therapy is started.

Standardization

- Standardization involves measuring the amounts of certain chemicals in products to try to make different preparations similar to each other. It is not always known if the chemicals being measured are the "active" ingredients.
- American pennyroyal may contain up to 2% volatile oil and European pennyroyal may contain up to 1% volatile oil. Both oils are reported to contain 85% to 92% pulegone, a constituent of pennyroyal.

Adults (18 Years and Older)

- *Note*: No safe dose of pennyroyal has been established. The following doses have been used, but may be toxic.
- **Extract (1:2):** Doses of 20 to 40 ml per week of pennyroyal have been used but may be toxic.
- **Oil:** Doses of 0.5 to 3 drops of pennyroyal oil have been used but may be toxic.
- **Tea/infusion:** Based on traditional usage, 1 or 2 cups of tea per day made from 1 to 2 teaspoons of dried leaves per cup of boiling water, steeped for 10 to 15 minutes, have been used but may be toxic. Pennyroyal tincture in tea water at

doses of 0.25 to 0.5 teaspoonfuls (1.25 to 2.5 ml), up to twice daily for treating cough, congestion, and upset stomach, has been used but may be toxic.

- **Topical:** Crushed plant material has been rubbed on the body as an insect repellent. Use of pennyroyal tincture mixed with skin cream and rubbed on the body has also been reported.
- **Veterinary:** Pennyroyal has been used as an herbal flea collar for animals by hanging a bag of pennyroyal from a regular collar or using a pennyroyal garland. Safety and effectiveness of these preparations have not been proven.

Children (Younger Than 18 Years)

- Pennyroyal is not recommended in children due to lack of scientific study and potential toxicity.

SAFETY

The U.S. Food and Drug Administration does not strictly regulate herbs and supplements. There is no guarantee of strength, purity or safety of products, and effects may vary. It is important to always read product labels. People who have a medical condition, or are taking other drugs, herbs, or supplements, should consult a qualified healthcare provider before starting a new therapy. A healthcare provider should be contacted immediately about any side effects.

Allergies

- Allergic reactions to pennyroyal or to its components, including pulegone, may occur, although there are no reliable published reports.

P

Side Effects and Warnings

- Pennyroyal herb and volatile oils have been associated with multiple reports of toxicity and adverse effects, including seizures, loss of consciousness, and death. In animals, pennyroyal (taken by mouth or placed on the skin) has been associated with liver, lung, and brain toxicity. Doses greater than 10 ml of pennyroyal may be associated with death. Cases of human overdose and death have been reported in infants, children, and adults.
- Pennyroyal oil toxicity may cause nausea, vomiting, abdominal pain, burning in the throat, difficulty swallowing, diarrhea, excessive sweating, chills, fever, headache, ringing in the ears, dizziness, extreme thirst, muscle spasms, restlessness, tremor, excessive talkativeness, hallucinations, agitation, drowsiness, fatigue, confusion, mania, seizures, organ failure (brain, liver, lung, kidney, heart), altered (low or high) heart rate, altered (low or high) blood pressure, slow breathing, coma, loss of consciousness, and death. Typically, the first symptoms of poisoning, from either pennyroyal oil or pennyroyal leaves, occur in the stomach and bowels, and are often apparent soon after ingestion. Symptoms in pennyroyal overdose may mimic that of acetaminophen (Tylenol) overdose, and the use of *N*-acetylcysteine (an antidote used for acetaminophen toxicity) treatment may prove beneficial.
- Other side effects may include contact dermatitis, rash (when placed on the skin), malaise, lethargy, agitation, abnormal sensations, or change (increase or decrease) in pupil size. There are reports that pennyroyal may cause abortion. Pennyroyal has been used historically as an emmenagogue (menstrual stimulant) and may cause menstrual bleeding. There are reports that large amounts of pennyroyal may be irritating to the urinary tract. Pennyroyal may cause hypoglycemia (low blood sugar), hemolytic anemia (low red blood cell count due to destruction of cells),

disseminated intravascular coagulation (widespread abnormal clotting and/or bleeding), and metabolic acidosis.

Pregnancy and Breastfeeding

- Pennyroyal is not recommended during pregnancy or breastfeeding because of the risk of uterine contractions, stimulation of menstruation, and abortion.
- Many tinctures contain high levels of alcohol, and should be avoided during pregnancy.

INTERACTIONS

Most herbs and supplements have not been thoroughly tested for interactions with other herbs, supplements, drugs, or foods. The interactions listed here are based on reports in scientific publications, laboratory experiments, or traditional use. It is important to always read product labels. People who have a medical condition, or are taking other drugs, herbs, or supplements, should consult a qualified healthcare provider before starting a new therapy.

Interactions with Drugs

- In theory, the toxicity of pennyroyal may be increased when combined with acetaminophen (Tylenol). Pennyroyal may lower a liver substance (glutathione), which may increase the risk of acetaminophen toxicity. Based on animal and human cases, pennyroyal may cause increased risk of liver damage caused by other drugs.
- Based on animal research, pennyroyal may interfere with the way the body processes certain drugs using the liver's cytochrome P450 enzyme system. As a result, the levels of these drugs may be increased in the blood and may cause increased effects or potentially serious adverse reactions. People who are using any medications should always read the package insert and consult their healthcare provider or pharmacist about possible interactions.
- Based on human cases, pennyroyal may lower blood sugar levels. Caution is advised when using medications that may also lower blood sugar levels. Patients taking drugs for diabetes by mouth or insulin should be monitored closely by a qualified healthcare provider. Medication adjustments may be necessary.
- Based on animal research, pennyroyal may have antihistamine effects, and may cause increased effects if combined with drugs that have antihistamine action, such as diphenhydramine (Benadryl), fexofenadine (Allegra), and loratadine (Claritin).
- Many tinctures contain high levels of alcohol and may cause nausea or vomiting when taken with metronidazole (Flagyl) or disulfiram (Antabuse).

Interactions with Herbs and Dietary Supplements

- Based on animal and human cases, pennyroyal may increase the risk of liver damage when combined with some herbs or supplements. Examples of other herbs that may damage the liver include ackee, bee pollen, birch oil, blessed thistle, borage, bush tea, butterbur, chaparral, coltsfoot, comfrey, DHEA, *Echinacea purpurea*, *Echium* spp., germander, *Heliotropium* spp., horse chestnut, jin-bu-huan (*Lycopodium serratum*), kava, lobelia, L-tetrahydropalmatine (THP), mate, niacin (vitamin B_3), niacinamide, Paraguay tea, periwinkle, *Plantago lanceolata*, pride of Madeira, rue, sassafras, scullcap, *Senecio* spp./groundsel, tansy ragwort, turmeric/curcumin, tu-san-chi (*Gynura segetum*), uva ursi, valerian, and white chameleon.
- Based on animal research, pennyroyal may interfere with the way the body processes certain herbs or supplements using the liver's cytochrome P450 enzyme system.

As a result, the levels of these herbs or supplements may be increased in the blood, and may cause increased effects or potentially serious adverse reactions. It may also alter the effects that other herbs or supplements possibly have on the P450 system, such as bloodroot, cat's claw, chamomile, chaparral, chasteberry, damiana, *Echinacea angustifolia*, goldenseal, grapefruit juice, licorice, oregano, red clover, St. John's wort, wild cherry, and yucca. People who are using any herbal medications or dietary supplements should always read the package insert and consult their healthcare provider or pharmacist about possible interactions.

- Based on human cases, pennyroyal may lower blood sugar levels. Caution is advised when using herbs or supplements that may also lower blood sugar levels. Possible examples include *Aloe vera*, American ginseng, bilberry, bitter melon, burdock, fenugreek, fish oil, gymnema, horse chestnut seed extract (HCSE), marshmallow, milk thistle, *Panax ginseng*, rosemary, Siberian ginseng, stinging nettle, and white horehound.
- Pennyroyal and black cohosh have been taken together to induce abortion, and this combination has been associated with toxicity and death. Pennyroyal and blue cohosh have traditionally been taken together to normalize the menstrual cycle in women. In theory, the combination of the two herbs may act together to increase menstrual flow. Notably, blue cohosh has been associated with multiple dangerous effects including stroke.
- Based on human study, pennyroyal may reduce the body's ability to absorb iron in meals by up to 75%.

Selected References

P

Natural Standard developed the preceding evidence-based information based on a systematic review of more than 90 scientific articles. For comprehensive information about alternative and complementary therapies on the professional level, go to www.naturalstandard.com. Selected references are listed here.

Anderson IB, Nelson SD, Blanc PD. Pennyroyal metabolites in human poisoning. Ann Intern Med 1997;126(3):250-251.

Anderson IB, Mullen WH, Meeker JE et al. Pennyroyal toxicity: measurement of toxic metabolite levels in two cases and review of the literature. Ann Intern Med 1996;124(8): 726-734.

Bakerink JA, Gospe SM, Jr., Dimand RJ et al. Multiple organ failure after ingestion of pennyroyal oil from herbal tea in two infants. Pediatrics 1996;98(5):944-947.

Black DR. Pregnancy unaffected by pennyroyal usage. J Am Osteopath Assoc 1985;85(5):282.

Buechel DW, Haverlah VC, Gardner ME. Pennyroyal oil ingestion: report of a case. J Am Osteopath Assoc 1983;82(10):793-794.

Burkhard PR, Burkhardt K, Haenggeli CA, et al. Plant-induced seizures: reappearance of an old problem. J Neurol 1999;246(8):667-670.

Carmichael PG. Pennyroyal metabolites in human poisoning. Ann Intern Med 1997;126(3): 250-251.

Chen LJ, Lebetkin EH, Burka LT. Metabolism of (R)-(+)-menthofuran in Fischer-344 rats: identification of sulfonic acid metabolites. Drug Metab Dispos 2003;31(10):1208-1213.

Chen LJ, Lebetkin EH, Burka LT. Comparative disposition of (R)-(+)-pulegone in B6C3F1 mice and F344 rats. Drug Metab Dispos 2003;31(7):892-899.

Chen LJ, Lebetkin EH, Burka LT. Metabolism of (R)-(+)-pulegone in F344 rats. Drug Metab Dispos 2001;29(12):1567-1577.

Ciganda C, Laborde A. Herbal infusions used for induced abortion. J Toxicol Clin Toxicol 2003;41(3):235-239.

Conway GA, Slocumb JC. Plants used as abortifacients and emmenagogues by Spanish New Mexicans. J Ethnopharmacol 1979;1(3):241-261.

Giorgi DF, Lobel D, Morasco R et al. N-acetylcysteine for pennyroyal oil toxicity. Vet Human Toxicol 1994;36(4):358.

Gordon WP, Huitric AC, Seth CL, et al. The metabolism of the abortifacient terpene, (R)-(+)-pulegone, to a proximate toxin, menthofuran. Drug Metab Dispos 1987;15(5):589-594.

Gordon WP, Forte AJ, McMurtry RJ, et al. Hepatotoxicity and pulmonary toxicity of pennyroyal oil and its constituent terpenes in the mouse. Toxicol Appl Pharmacol 1982; 65(3):413-424.

Khojasteh-Bakht SC, Chen W, Koenigs LL, et al. Metabolism of (R)-(+)-pulegone and (R)-(+)-menthofuran by human liver cytochrome P-450s: evidence for formation of a furan epoxide. Drug Metab Dispos 1999;27(5):574-580.

Mack RB. "Boldly they rode ... into the mouth of hell". Pennyroyal oil toxicity. N C Med J 1997;58(6):456-457.

Martins HM, Martins ML, Dias MI, et al. Evaluation of microbiological quality of medicinal plants used in natural infusions. Int J Food Microbiol 2001;68(1-2):149-153.

Mazur LJ, De Ybarrondo L, Miller J, et al. Use of alternative and complementary therapies for pediatric asthma. Tex Med 2001;97(6):64-68.

Mizutani T, Nomura H, Nakanishi K, et al. Effects of drug metabolism modifiers on pulegone-induced hepatotoxicity in mice. Res Commun Chem Pathol Pharmacol 1987;58(1):75-83.

Sudekum M, Poppenga RH, Raju N, et al. Pennyroyal oil toxicosis in a dog. J Am Vet Med Assoc 1992;200(6):817-818.

Sullivan JB Jr, Rumack BH, Thomas H Jr, et al. Pennyroyal oil poisoning and hepatotoxicity. JAMA 1979;242(26):2873-2874.

Peppermint

(*Mentha x piperita* L.)

RELATED TERMS

- Balm mint, black peppermint, brandy mint, curled mint, feullis de menthe, Japanese peppermint, katzenkraut (German), lamb mint, *Mentha arvensis* L. var *piperascens*, menta prima (Italian), Menthae piperitae aetheroleum (peppermint oil), *Mentha piperita* var *officinalis*, Menthae piperitae folium (peppermint leaf), menthe anglaise, menthe poivre, menthe poivree, *Mentha piperita* var *vulgaris*, Our Lady's mint, pebermynte (Danish), pfefferminz (German), porminzen, schmecker, spearmint (*Mentha spicata* L.), water mint (*Mentha aquatica*), white peppermint, WS 1340.
- **Essential oil constituents:** Cineol, isomenthone, liminene, menthofuran, menthol, menthone, menthyl acetate, terpenoids.
- **Leaf constituents:** Caffeic acid, chlorogenic acid, luteolin, hesperidin, rutin, "volatile" oil.
- **Selected brand names:** Ben-Gay, Colpermin, China Maze, Cholaktol, Citaethol, Enteroplant (contains peppermint and caraway oil), Kiminto, Mentacur, Mentholatum, Mintec, Rhuli Gel, Robitussin cough drops, SX Mentha, Vicks VapoRub.
- **Combination products:** Absorbine Jr., Iberogast, Listerine.
- *Note: Mentha* x *villosa* L. is a different species of mint with a similar appearance, used primarily as a flavoring agent.

P

BACKGROUND

- Peppermint is a perennial flowering plant that grows throughout Europe and North America. Peppermint is widely cultivated for its fragrant oil, which is obtained through steam distillation of the fresh above-ground parts of the plant. Peppermint oil has been used historically for numerous health conditions, including common cold symptoms, cramps, headache, indigestion, joint pain, and nausea. Peppermint leaf has been used for stomach/intestinal disorders and for gallbladder disease.
- Mint plants such as peppermint and spearmint have a long history of medicinal use, dating back to ancient Egypt, Greece, and Rome. The scientific name for peppermint (*Mentha* x *piperita*) is derived from the name *Mintha*, a Greek mythological nymph who transformed herself into the plant, and from the Latin *piper*, meaning "pepper." Peppermint is believed to be a cross (hybrid) between spearmint and water mint that arose naturally.
- Peppermint oil is available in bulk herb oil, enteric-coated capsules, soft gelatin capsules, and liquid form. In small doses such as in tea or chewing gum, peppermint is generally believed to be safe in healthy, non-pregnant, non-allergic adults. The United States is a principal producer of peppermint, and the largest markets for peppermint oil are manufacturers of chewing gum, toothpaste, mouthwash, and pharmaceuticals.

USES BASED ON SCIENTIFIC EVIDENCE	Grade*
Antispasmodic (gastric spasm) One study reports that peppermint oil solution administered intraluminally can be used as an antispasmodic agent with superior efficacy and fewer side effects than hyoscine-*N*-butylbromide administered by intramuscular injection during upper endoscopy.	C
Indigestion (non-ulcer dyspepsia) Several human trials examined the effects of peppermint oil or a combination of peppermint/caraway oil on dyspepsia. Overall, these studies have not been well designed or reported, and it remains unclear if peppermint oil is beneficial for this condition.	C
Irritable bowel syndrome (IBS) There are several human trials of peppermint oil for the relief of IBS symptoms such as abdominal pain, bloating, diarrhea, and gas. Results have been mixed, with some studies reporting benefits, and others finding lack of effect. Overall, these trials have been small and not well designed or reported. Better scientific studies are necessary before a firm conclusion can be drawn.	C
Nasal congestion Menthol, a constituent of peppermint oil, is sometimes included in inhaled preparations for nasal congestion, including "rubs" that are applied to the skin and inhaled. Early research suggests that nose breathing may be improved, although it is not clear if there are true benefits on breathing or nasal congestion. High-quality research is lacking in this area.	C
Nausea Due to limited human study, there is not enough evidence to recommend for or against the use of peppermint oil in the treatment of nausea. Further research is needed before a recommendation can be made.	C
Tension headache Application of diluted peppermint oil to the forehead and temples has been tested in people with headache. Studies have not been well conducted, and it is not clear if this is an effective treatment.	C
Urinary tract infection There is limited study of peppermint tea added to other therapies for urinary tract infections. It is not clear if this is an effective treatment, and it is not recommended to rely on peppermint tea alone to treat this condition.	C

*Key to grades: *A:* Strong scientific evidence for this use; *B:* Good scientific evidence for this use; *C:* Unclear scientific evidence for this use; *D:* Fair scientific evidence against this use (it may not work); *F:* Strong scientific evidence against this use (it likely does not work). For a more detailed explanation of efficacy criteria, see "Natural Standard Evidence-Based Validated Grading Rationale" in the Introduction.

Uses Based on Tradition, Theory, or Limited Scientific Evidence

Antacid, anorexia, antiviral, arthritis, asthma, bile duct disorders, bronchial spasm, cancer, chickenpox, cholelithiasis (gallstones), colonic spasm (during colonoscopy or barium enema), common cold, cough, cramps, dysmenorrhea (menstrual pain), enteritis, fever, fibromyositis, gallbladder disorders, gas (flatulence), gastritis, gastrointestinal disorders, gonorrhea, head lice (*Pediculus humanus capitis*), ileus (postoperative), inflammation of oral mucosa, influenza, intestinal colic, laryngeal spasm, local anesthetic, morning sickness, motility disorders, mouthwash, musculo-skeletal pain, myalgia (muscle pain), neuralgia (nerve pain), postherpetic neuralgia, pruritus (itching), rheumatic pain, sun block, tendonitis, toothache, tuberculosis, urticaria (hives).

DOSING

The following doses are based on scientific research, publications, traditional use, or expert opinion. Many herbs and supplements have not been thoroughly tested, and safety and effectiveness may not be proven. Brands may be made differently, with variable ingredients even within the same brand. The doses shown may not apply to all products. It is important to always read product labels and discuss doses with a qualified healthcare provider before therapy is started.

Adults (18 Years and Older)

P

- **Peppermint oil:** Peppermint oil should be used cautiously, as doses of the constituent menthol over 1 gram per kilogram of body weight may be deadly. For intestinal/digestion disorders, doses of 0.2 to 0.4 ml of peppermint oil in enteric-coated capsules, dilute preparations, or suspensions taken three times daily by mouth have been used or studied. Lozenges containing 2 to 10 mg of peppermint oil have been used. 10% peppermint oil (in methanol) has been applied to the skin (forehead and temples) multiple times per day for headache relief. Some sources recommend using peppermint oil preparations on the skin no more than 3 to 4 times per day, although reliable safety information is limited in this area. For inhalation, 3 to 4 drops of oil added to 150 ml of hot water and inhaled up to three times per day or 1% to 5% essential oil as a nasal ointment has been used to relieve congestion. Enteric-coated peppermint oil capsules may be better tolerated than other dosage forms.
- **Peppermint leaf:** There is limited study of the safety/effectiveness of peppermint leaf preparations, and doses are based on traditional use or anecdote. As an infusion, 3 to 6 g of peppermint leaf has been used daily. Doses of other liquid preparations depend on concentration, for example, 2 to 3 ml of tincture (1:5 in 45% ethanol) three times daily, or 1 ml of spirits (10% oil and 1% leaf extract, mixed with water) has been taken. Various doses of dried herb extract have been noted traditionally, ranging from 0.8 g daily up to 4 g taken three times daily, although safety is not clear.

Children (Younger Than 18 Years)

- There is not enough scientific information available to recommend the safe use of peppermint leaf or oil in children.

SAFETY

The U.S. Food and Drug Administration does not strictly regulate herbs and supplements. There is no guarantee of strength, purity, or safety of products, and effects may vary. It is important to always read product labels. People who have a medical condition, or are taking other drugs, herbs, or supplements, should consult a qualified healthcare provider before starting a new therapy. A healthcare provider should be contacted immediately about any side effects.

Allergies

- Allergic/hypersensitivity reactions may occur from using peppermint or menthol by mouth or on the skin, including throat closing (laryngeal spasm), breathing problems (bronchial constriction/asthma symptoms), and skin rash/hives/contact dermatitis. People with known allergy/hypersensitivity to peppermint leaf or oil should avoid peppermint products.

Side Effects and Warnings

- Peppermint is generally regarded as being safe in non-allergic adults when taken in small doses, for example as tea.
- Peppermint oil may be safe in small doses, although multiple adverse effects are possible. When used on the skin, peppermint oil has been associated with allergic/hypersensitivity reactions, skin rash/hives/contact dermatitis, mouth ulcers/sores, and eye irritation. Peppermint oil taken by mouth may cause headache, dizziness, heartburn, anal burning, slow heart rate, or muscle tremor. Mouth sores may occur with peppermint oil-containing mouthwashes. There is report of asthma symptoms related to a mint-flavored toothpaste. Very large doses of peppermint oil taken by mouth in animals have resulted in muscle weakness, brain damage, and seizure. Peppermint oil should be used cautiously by people with G6PD deficiency (based on reports of jaundice in babies exposed to menthol) or gallbladder disease (gallstones, bile duct obstruction). Enteric-coated tablets have been recommended in those with hiatal hernia or heartburn/gastroesophageal reflux disease (GERD), over other dosage forms. Use in infants or children is discouraged because of potential toxicity, including when inhaled, taken by mouth, or used on the skin around the facial area.
- Menthol, a constituent of peppermint oil that is included in mouthwashes, toothpastes, mentholated cigarettes, and decongestant "rubs" or lozenges, has been associated with multiple adverse effects. Although small amounts may be safe in non-allergic adults, doses over 1 gram per kilogram of body weight may be deadly in humans, and toxic doses can be absorbed through the skin (and may be increased with local application of heat, such as with a heating pad). Serious breathing difficulties or triggering of asthma symptoms may occur with menthol use near the nose or on the chest. Mouth sores have been associated with use of mint-flavored toothpaste, mouthwash, or mentholated cigarettes. Mentholated cigarettes have been linked with skin bruising (purpura), although the exact cause has not been proven. Use on the skin of menthol or methyl salicylate (also a peppermint oil constituent) has rarely been associated with rash, severe skin damage (necrosis), or kidney damage (interstitial nephritis). Inhalation of large doses of menthol may lead to dizziness, confusion, muscle weakness, nausea, or double vision. High doses of menthol have caused brain damage in animal studies.

Pregnancy and Breastfeeding

- Peppermint oil and menthol should be avoided during pregnancy and breastfeeding because of insufficient information and potential for toxicity.

INTERACTIONS

Most herbs and supplements have not been thoroughly tested for interactions with other herbs, supplements, drugs, or foods. The interactions listed here are based on reports in scientific publications, laboratory experiments, or traditional use. It is important to always read product labels. People who have a medical condition, or are taking other drugs, herbs, or supplements, should consult a qualified healthcare provider before starting a new therapy.

Interactions with Drugs

- There is a preliminary report that taking peppermint oil by mouth may increase blood levels of the drugs felodipine (Plendil) and simvastatin (Zocor). In rats, peppermint oil increases levels of cyclosporine in the blood, although effects in humans are not clear. Based on rat research, peppermint oil used on the skin with 5-fluorouracil (5-FU) may increase the rate of absorption of 5-FU.
- Based on laboratory studies, peppermint oil may interfere with the way the body processes certain drugs using the liver's cytochrome P450 enzyme system. As a result, the levels of these drugs may be increased in the blood and may cause increased effects or potentially serious adverse reactions. People who are using any medications should always read the package insert and consult their healthcare provider or pharmacist about possible interactions.

P

Interactions with Herbs and Supplements

- Based on laboratory studies, peppermint oil may interfere with the way the body processes certain herbs or supplements using the liver's cytochrome P450 enzyme system. As a result, the levels of other herbs or supplements may be too high in the blood. It may also alter the effects that other herbs or supplements possibly have on the P450 system, such as bloodroot, cat's claw, chamomile, chaparral, chasteberry, damiana, *Echinacea angustifolia*, goldenseal, grapefruit juice, licorice, oregano, red clover, St. John's wort, wild cherry, and yucca. People who are using any medications should always read the package insert and consult their healthcare provider or pharmacist about possible interactions.

Selected References

Natural Standard developed the preceding evidence-based information based on a systematic review of more than 140 articles. For comprehensive information about alternative and complementary therapies on the professional level, go to www.naturalstandard.com. Selected references are listed here.

Abdullah D, Ping QN, Liu GJ. Enhancing effect of essential oils on the penetration of 5-fluorouracil through rat skin. Yao Xue Xue Bao (Acta Pharmaceutica Sinica) 1996;31(3): 214-221.

Barnick CG, Cardozo LD. The treatment of abdominal distension and dyspepsia with enteric coated peppermint oil following routine gynaecological intraperitoneal surgery. J Obstet Gynecol 1990;10(5):423-424.

Bell GD, Richmond CR, Somerville KW. Peppermint oil capsules (Colpermin) for the irritable bowel syndrome: a pharmacokinetic study. Br J Clin Pharmacol 1983;16:228P-229P.

Camarasa G, Alomar A. Menthol dermatitis from cigarettes. Contact Derm 1978;4:169-170.

Carling L, Svedberg L, Hultsen S. Short term treatment of the irritable bowel syndrome: a placebo-controlled trial of peppermint oil against hyoscyamine. Opuscula Med 1989;34:55-57.

Chrisman BR. Menthol and dermatitis. Arch Dermatol 1976;114:286.

Davies SJ, Harding LM, Baranowski AP. A novel treatment of postherpetic neuralgia using peppermint oil. Clin J Pain 2002;18(3):200-202.

Dew MJ, Evans BK, Rhodes J. Peppermint oil for the irritable bowel syndrome: a multicentre trial. Br J Clin Pract 1984;38(11-12):394-398.

Dresser GK, Wacher V, Ramtoola Z, et al. Peppermint oil increases the oral bioavailability of felodipine and simvastatin. Amer Soc Clin Pharmacol Ther Ann Meeting, March 24-27, 2002;TPII-95.

Dresser GK, Wacher V, Wong S, et al. Evaluation of peppermint oil and ascorbyl palmitate as inhibitors of cytochrome P4503A4 activity *in vitro* and *in vivo*. Clin Pharmacol Ther 2002;72(3):247-255.

Ebbinghaus K D. A 'tea' containing various plant products as adjuvant to chemotherapy of urinary tract infections. Therapiewoche 1985;35:2041-2051.

Evans BK, Levine DF, Mayberry JF, et al. Multicentre trial of peppermint oil capsules in irritable bowel syndrome. Scand J Gastroenterol 1982;17:503.

Feng XZ. [Effect of peppermint oil hot compresses in preventing abdominal distension in postoperative gynecological patients.] Zhonghua Hu Li Za Zhi 1997;32(10):577-578.

Freise J, Kohler S. [Peppermint oil-caraway oil fixed combination in non-ulcer dyspepsia—comparison of the effects of enteric preparations.] Pharmazie 1999;54(3):210-215.

Gobel H, Fresenius J, Heinze A, et al. [Effectiveness of Oleum menthae piperitae and paracetamol in therapy of headache of the tension type.] Nervenarzt 1996;67(8):672-681.

Gobel H, Schmidt G, Soyka D. Effect of peppermint and eucalyptus oil preparations on neurophysiological and experimental algesimetric headache parameters. Cephalalgia 1994;14(3): 228-234.

Goerg KJ, Spilker T. Effect of peppermint oil and caraway oil on gastrointestinal motility in healthy volunteers: a pharmacodynamic study using simultaneous determination of gastric and gall-bladder emptying and orocaecal transit time. Aliment Pharmacol Ther 2003; 17(3):445-451.

Heng MC. Local necrosis and interstitial nephritis due to topical methyl salicylate and menthol. Cutis 1987;39(5):442-444.

Hiki N, Kurosaka H, Tatsutomi Y, et al. Peppermint oil reduces gastric spasm during upper endoscopy: a randomized, double-blind, double-dummy controlled trial. Gastrointest Endosc 2003;57(4):475-482.

Holtman G, Gschossmann J, Buenger L, et al. Effects of a fixed peppermint oil caraway oil combination (FPCO) on symptoms of functional dyspepsia accentuated by pain or discomfort. Digestive Disease Week 2002.

Kawane H. Menthol and aspirin-induced asthma. Respir Med 1996;90(4):247.

Kline RM, Kline JJ, Di Palma J, et al. Enteric-coated, pH-dependent peppermint oil capsules for the treatment of irritable bowel syndrome in children. J Pediatr 2001;138(1):125-128.

Lawson MJ, Knight RE, Tran K, et al. Failure of enteric-coated peppermint oil in the irritable bowel syndrome: a randomized, double-blind crossover study. J Gastroenterol Hepatol 1988; 3(3):235-238.

Lech Y, Olesen KM, Hey H, et al. [Treatment of irritable bowel syndrome with peppermint oil. A double-blind study with a placebo.] Ugeskr Laeger 1988;150(40):2388-2389.

Leicester RJ, Hunt RH. Peppermint oil to reduce colonic spasm during endoscopy. Lancet 1982;2(8305):989.

Liu JH, Chen GH, Yeh HZ, et al. Enteric-coated peppermint-oil capsules in the treatment of irritable bowel syndrome: a prospective, randomized trial. J Gastroenterol 1997;32(6):765-768.

Madisch A, Heydenreich CJ, Wieland V, et al. Treatment of functional dyspepsia with a fixed peppermint oil and caraway oil combination preparation as compared to cisapride. A multicenter, reference-controlled double-blind equivalence study. Arzneimittelforschung 1999;49(11):925-932.

Mascher H, Kikuta Ch, Schiel H. [Pharmacokinetics of carvone and menthol after administration of peppermint oil and caraway oil containing enteric formulation.] [Article in German.] Wien Med Wochenschr 2002;152(15-16):432-436.

May B, Kohler S, Schneider B. Efficacy and tolerability of a fixed combination of peppermint oil and caraway oil in patients suffering from functional dyspepsia. Aliment Pharmacol Ther 2000;14(12):1671-1677.

May B, Kuntz HD, Kieser M, et al. Efficacy of a fixed peppermint oil/caraway oil combination in non-ulcer dyspepsia. Arzneimittelforschung 1996;46(12):1149-1153.

McGowan EM. Menthol urticaria. Arch Dermatol 1966;94:62-63.

Micklefield GH, Greving I, May B. Effects of peppermint oil and caraway oil on gastroduodenal motility. Phytother Res 2000;14(1):20-23.

Moghadam BK, Gier R, Thurlow T. Extensive oral mucosal ulcerations caused by misuse of a commercial mouthwash. Cutis 1999;64(2):131-134.

Morice AH, Marshall AE, Higgins KS, et al. Effect of inhaled menthol on citric acid induced cough in normal subjects. Thorax 1994;49(10):1024-1026.

Morton CA, Garioch J, Todd P, et al. Contact sensitivity to menthol and peppermint in patients with intra-oral symptoms. Contact Dermatitis 1995;32(5):281-284.

Nash P, Gould SR, Bernardo DE. Peppermint oil does not relieve the pain of irritable bowel syndrome. Br J Clin Pract 1986;40(7):292-293.

Nicolay K. [Double blind trial of metoclopramide and Iberogast in functional gastroenteropathy.] Gastro-Entero-Hepatologie 1984;4:24-28.

Papa CM, Shelly WB. Menthol hypersensitivity. JAMA 1964;189:546-548.

Pittler MH, Ernst E. Peppermint oil for irritable bowel syndrome: a critical review and meta-analysis. Am J Gastroenterol 1998;93(7):1131-1135.

Rees WD, Evans BK, Rhodes J. Treating irritable bowel syndrome with peppermint oil. Br Med J 1979;2(6194):835-836.

Rhodes J, Evans BK, Rees WD. Peppermint oil in enteric coated capsules for the treatment of irritable bowel syndrome: a double blind controlled trial. Hepato-Gastroenterol 1980;27(Suppl):252.

Shkurupii VA, Kazarinova NV, Ogirenko AP, et al. [Efficiency of the use of peppermint (*Mentha piperita* L) essential oil inhalations in the combined multi-drug therapy for pulmonary tuberculosis.] [Article in Russian.] Probl Tuberk 2002;(4):36-9.

Sparks MJ, O'Sullivan P, Herrington AA, et al. Does peppermint oil relieve spasm during barium enema? Br J Radiol 1995;68(812):841-843.

Subiza J, Subiza JL, Valdivieso R, et al. Toothpaste flavor-induced asthma. J Allergy Clin Immunol 1992;90(6 Pt 1):1004-1006.

Tamaoki J, Chiyotani A, Sakai A, et al. Effect of menthol vapour on airway hyperresponsiveness in patients with mild asthma. Respir Med 1995;89(7):503-504.

Tate S. Peppermint oil: a treatment for postoperative nausea. J Adv Nurs 1997;26(3):543-549.

Veal L. The potential effectiveness of essential oils as a treatment for headlice, *Pediculus humanus capitis*. Complement Ther Nurs Midwifery 1996;2(4):97-101.

Weston CF. Anal burning and peppermint oil. Postgrad Med J 1987;63(742):717.

Wilkinson SM, Beck MH. Allergic contact dermatitis from menthol in peppermint. Contact Dermatitis 1994;30(1):42-43.

Wolf E. Peppermint oil and caraway oil for the irritable stomach. Pharmazeutische Zeitung 2001;146(27):29-30.

Wyllie JP, Alexander FW. Nasal instillation of 'Olbas Oil' in an infant. Arch Dis Child 1994; 70(4):357-358.

Polypodium Leucotomos

(*Polypodium leucotomos* extract and anapsos)

RELATED TERMS

- Calaguala, ferns, samambaia, Polypodiaceae, *Polypodium cambricum*, *Polypodium decumanum*, *Polypodium vulgare.*

BACKGROUND

- Extracts of fern species (family Polypodiaceae) have been used traditionally for numerous indications, most commonly in South America and Europe.
- The South American species *Polypodium leucotomos* L. is commonly known as "calaguala." Extracts of this species, called "anapsos," have been marketed and used as a treatment for multiple indications. Although *in vitro* and animal studies have reported anti-inflammatory, cytokine-suppressing, and leukotriene inhibitory properties, the small number of available human trials have not demonstrated efficacy for any specific indication.

USES BASED ON SCIENTIFIC EVIDENCE	Grade*
Psoriasis Extracts of *Polypodium leucotomos* (called "anapsos") have been taken by mouth in Europe and South America for psoriasis since the 1970s. Poor-quality human studies report that anapsos may improve skin appearance. However, there is currently little information supporting the use of *Polypodium leucotomos* for psoriasis. More research is needed in this area before a recommendation can be made.	C
Atopic dermatitis (eczema) Laboratory and animal studies report that *Polypodium leucotomos* extract (anapsos) may reduce inflammation. However, there is little information about the effectiveness of anapsos taken by mouth in people with atopic dermatitis.	C
Dementia (memory loss, disorientation) Limited scientific information is available about the effectiveness of polypodium in the treatment of dementia.	C

*Key to grades: *A:* Strong scientific evidence for this use; *B:* Good scientific evidence for this use; *C:* Unclear scientific evidence for this use; *D:* Fair scientific evidence against this use (it may not work); *F:* Strong scientific evidence against this use (it likely does not work). For a more detailed explanation of efficacy criteria, see "Natural Standard Evidence-Based Validated Grading Rationale" in the Introduction.

Uses Based on Tradition, Theory, or Limited Scientific Evidence

Asthma, autoimmune diseases, cancer, fever, high blood pressure, immune system stimulation, inflammation, joint diseases, rheumatism, sunburn protection, upper respiratory tract infection, vitiligo (loss of pigment in the skin), water retention, whooping cough.

DOSING

The following doses are based on scientific research, publications, traditional use, or expert opinion. Many herbs and supplements have not been thoroughly tested, and safety and effectiveness may not be proven. Brands may be made differently, with variable ingredients even within the same brand. The doses shown may not apply to all products. It is important to always read product labels and discuss doses with a qualified healthcare provider before therapy is started.

Standardization

- Standardization involves measuring the amounts of certain chemicals in products to try to make different preparations similar to each other. It is not always known if the chemicals being measured are the "active" ingredients. There is no widely accepted standardization for the preparation of *Polypodium leucotomos* extracts.

Adults (18 Years and Older)

- **Oral (taken by mouth):** For psoriasis, a dose of 120 mg of anapsos (*Polypodium leucotomos* extract), taken daily, has been used for short periods of time in limited research. For dementia, preliminary research reports using 360 mg daily for 4 weeks. Safety and effectiveness are not clear.
- **Topical (applied to the skin):** No clear dosing regimen has been reported or established.

Children (Younger Than 18 Years)

- Little information is available about the use of polypodium in children, and safety is not clear.

SAFETY

The U.S. Food and Drug Administration does not strictly regulate herbs and supplements. There is no guarantee of strength, purity, or safety of products, and effects may vary. It is important to always read product labels. People who have a medical condition, or are taking other drugs, herbs, or supplements, should consult a qualified healthcare provider before starting a new therapy. A healthcare provider should be contacted immediately about any side effects.

Allergies

- People with allergies to ferns (family Polypodiaceae) should avoid polypodium.

Side Effects and Warnings

- Isolated reports of itching or stomach upset are published. Studies of a different fern species, *Polypodium vulgare*, report sedation, changes in heart function in animals, low blood pressure, and rapid heart rate. Avoid driving and use of heavy

P

machinery when taking *Polypodium leucotomos* extract because of theoretical sedative effects. People with heart disease or those being treated for heart disorders or high blood pressure should use caution.

Pregnancy and Breastfeeding

- The use of polypodium during pregnancy or breastfeeding is not recommended, because there is little information about its safety.

INTERACTIONS

Most herbs and supplements have not been thoroughly tested for interactions with other herbs, supplements, drugs, or foods. The interactions listed here are based on reports in scientific publications, laboratory experiments, or traditional use. It is important to always read product labels. People who have a medical condition, or are taking other drugs, herbs, or supplements, should consult a qualified healthcare provider before starting a new therapy.

Interactions with Drugs

- Polypodium may increase the amount of drowsiness caused by some drugs. Examples include benzodiazepines such as lorazepam (Ativan) and diazepam (Valium), barbiturates such as phenobarbital, narcotics such as codeine, some antidepressants, and alcohol. Caution is advised while driving or operating machinery.
- Most testing has been done with a related fern species, *Polypodium vulgare.* Animal studies show that this related plant can affect the function of the heart and lower blood pressure. In theory, the use of *Polypodium leucotomos* extract with medications that affect heart function or lower blood pressure may cause the effects of these drugs to increase. Use caution if combining polypodium with heart medications such as beta-blockers, calcium channel blockers, and digoxin.

Interactions with Herbs and Dietary Supplements

- In theory, polypodium may increase the amount of drowsiness caused by some herbs or supplements. Examples of agents that may cause sedation include calamus, calendula, California poppy, capsicum, catnip, celery, couchgrass, dogwood, elecampane, German chamomile, goldenseal, gotu kola, hops, kava (may help sleep without drowsiness), lavender aromatherapy, lemon balm, sage, sassafras, scullcap, shepherd's purse, Siberian ginseng, stinging nettle, St. John's wort, valerian, wild carrot, wild lettuce, withania root, and yerba mansa. Caution is advised while driving or operating machinery.
- In studies of a related fern species, *Polypodium vulgare*, animals treated with the herb developed low blood pressure and changes in heart function. In theory, the use of *Polypodium leucotomos* extract with herbs or supplements that lower blood pressure may cause the blood pressure to fall too low. Herbs with potential blood pressure–lowering effects include aconite/monkshood, arnica, baneberry, betel nut, bilberry, black cohosh, bryony, calendula, California poppy, coleus, curcumin, eucalyptol, evening primrose oil, eucalyptus oil, flaxseed, garlic, ginger, ginkgo, goldenseal, green hellebore, hawthorn, Indian tobacco, jaborandi, mistletoe, night-blooming cereus, oleander, pasque flower, periwinkle, pleurisy root, shepherd's purse, Texas milkweed, turmeric, and wild cherry.
- For the same reason, be cautious if using *Polypodium leucotomos* extract with herbs or supplements that have possible cardiac glycoside ingredients, which can affect the function of the heart. Such agents include Adonis, balloon cotton, black hellebore

root/melampode, black Indian hemp, bushman's poison, *Cactus grandifloris*, convallaria, eyebright, figwort, foxglove/digitalis, frangipani, hedge mustard, hemp root/Canadian hemp root, king's crown, lily of the valley, motherwort, oleander leaf, pheasant's eye plant, plantain leaf, pleurisy root, psyllium husks, redheaded cotton-bush, rhubarb root, rubber vine, sea-mango, senna fruit, squill, strophanthus, uzara, wallflower, white horehound, wintersweet, yellow dock root, and yellow oleander. Notably, bufalin/chan suis is a Chinese herbal formula that has been reported as toxic or fatal when taken with cardiac glycosides.

Selected References

Natural Standard developed the preceding evidence-based information based on a systematic review of more than 40 scientific articles. For comprehensive information about alternative and complementary therapies on the professional level, go to www.naturalstandard.com. Selected references are listed here.

Alvarez XA, Pichel V, Perez P, et al. Double-blind, randomized, placebo-controlled pilot study with anapsos in senile dementia: effects on cognition, brain bioelectrical activity and cerebral hemodynamics. Methods Find Exp Clin Pharmacol 2000;22(7):585-594.

Capella Perez MC, Castells RA. [Double-blind study using "anapsos" 120 mg in the treatment of psoriasis.] Actas Dermosifiliogr 1981;72(9-10):487-494.

Del P, De S, Colomo G. Comparison of *Polypodium leucotomos* extract with placebo in 37 cases of psoriasis. Med Cutan Iber Lat Am 1982;10:203-208.

Del Pino GJ, De Sambricio GF, Colomo GC. [Comparative study between 120 mg of anapsos and a placebo in 37 psoriasis patients.] Med Cutan Ibero Lat Am 1982;10(3):203-208.

Gonzalez S, Pathak MA, Cuevas J, et al. Topical or oral administration with an extract of *Polypodium leucotomos* prevents acute sunburn and psoralen-induced phototoxic reactions as well as depletion of Langerhans cells in human skin. Photodermatol Photoimmunol Photomed 1997;13(1-2):50-60.

Jimenez D, Naranjo R, Doblare E, et al. Anapsos, an antipsoriatic drug, in atopic dermatitis. Allergol Immunopathol (Madr) 1987;15(4):185-189.

Mercadal PO, Maesci CF. [Preliminary communication on the treatment of psoriasis with anapsos.] Actas Dermosifiliogr 1981;72(1-2):65-68.

Mohammad A. Vitiligo repigmentation with Anapsos (*Polypodium leucotomos*). Int J Dermatol 1989;28(7):479.

Navarro-Blasco FJ, Sempere JM. Modification of the inflammatory activity of psoriatic arthritis in patients treated with extract of *Polipodium leucotomos* (Anapsos). Br J Rheumatol 1998;37(8):912.

Nogal-Ruiz JJ, Gomez-Barrio A, Escario JA, et al. Modulation by *Polypodium leucotomos* extract of cytokine patterns in experimental trichomoniasis model. Parasite 2003;10(1):73-78.

Padilla H, Lainez H, Pacheco J. A new agent (hydrophilic fraction of *Polypodium leucotomos*) for management of psoriasis. Int J Derm 1974;13:276-282.

Pineiro AB. [2 years personal experience in anapsos treatment of psoriasis in various clinical forms.] Med Cutan Ibero Lat Am 1983;11(1):65-72.

Vasange-Tuominen M, Perera-Ivarsson P, Shen J, et al. The fern *Polypodium decumanum*, used in the treatment of psoriasis, and its fatty acid constituents as inhibitors of leukotriene B4 formation. Prostaglandins Leukot Essent Fatty Acids 1994;50(5):279-284.

P

Propolis

(Bee propolis)

RELATED TERMS

- Bee glue, bee propolis, bee putty, bienenharz (German), hive dross, propolisina (Spanish), propolis balsam, propolis resin, propolis wax, Russian penicillin.

BACKGROUND

- Propolis is a natural resin created by bees, used in the construction of hives. Propolis is produced from the buds of conifer and poplar tress, in combination with beeswax and other bee secretions. Historically, propolis was used in Greece to treat abscesses, by the Assyrians to heal wounds and tumors, and by the Egyptians for mummification. Today, propolis is commonly found in chewing gum, cosmetics, creams, lozenges, and ointments.
- Propolis has shown promise in dentistry for dental caries, as a natural sealant and enamel hardener. Effectiveness of propolis against herpes simplex virus (HSV) types 1 and 2 and parasitic infections has been demonstrated in preliminary studies. However, properly controlled randomized human trials are lacking, and further evidence is warranted in order to establish the therapeutic efficacy of propolis for any indication.
- Numerous case reports have demonstrated propolis to be a potent allergen and sensitizing agent, and therefore it should be used cautiously in hypersensitive individuals. Toxicity with propolis is rare, although there are multiple case reports of contact dermatitis, erythema, eczema, vesiculitis, and pruritus.

USES BASED ON SCIENTIFIC EVIDENCE	Grade*
Acute cervicitis Laboratory studies suggest antibacterial activity of propolis. Preliminary poor-quality research has examined the use of propolis (applied as a cream or ointment) for cervicitis. Further study is necessary before a recommendation can be made.	C
Burns Preliminary research reports that propolis may have a beneficial effect on the healing of partial-thickness burn wounds.	C
Cornea complications from zoster Laboratory studies suggest antiviral and anti-inflammatory activity of propolis. There is limited poor-quality study of propolis for the treatment of corneal complications of varicella zoster, reporting faster healing and improvement of sight. Better human research is needed before a recommendation can be made.	C

Continued

Dental pain There is preliminary evidence that propolis may reduce dental pain, for example with the use of a propolis gel. Additional research is needed before a clear recommendation can be made.	C
Dental plaque and gingivitis (mouthwash) Propolis is a natural resin created by bees, used in the construction of hives. Propolis is produced from the buds of conifer and poplar tress, in combination with beeswax and other bee secretions. Propolis has been suggested for multiple oral problems, including reduction of pain, treatment of infection, and sealing/helping bone to re-form. Laboratory studies suggest activity of propolis against bacteria found in the mouth. Although preliminary human studies report reduction in oral bacterial counts and short-term reduction of plaque formation, these experiments have been poorly designed. Without additional research in this area, the evidence cannot be considered conclusive.	C
Dental wound healing Propolis has been reported to assist in repair after tooth extraction in animal studies. Reliable human research is needed before a recommendation can be made.	C
Genital herpes simplex virus (HSV) infection Laboratory studies report antiviral activity of propolis, including against herpes simplex virus types 1 and 2. Preliminary results from poorly designed human studies suggest propolis used on the skin may improve lesions from genital herpes virus infections. However, without better human study, including comparisons to prescription drugs, firm conclusions cannot be drawn.	C
Infections Animal and laboratory studies suggest activity of propolis in the treatment of various types of infections. Initial human research reports possible benefits against oral/dental bacteria, genital herpes, urine bacteria, intestinal giardia infections, and *H. pylori*. Additional research is needed before a recommendation can be made.	C
Legg-Calve-Perthes disease/avascular hip necrosis These diseases are characterized by the death of bone at the hip joint (femoral head). There is limited human study of injection of propolis into the joint following hip replacement surgery for these conditions. However, without additional human study of safety and effectiveness, no clear conclusions can be drawn.	C
Prevention of colds Laboratory studies suggest anti-infectious activity of propolis. Limited research in humans does not provide clear conclusions.	C

Continued

Rheumatic diseases	C
Based on anti-inflammatory action observed in laboratory research, propolis has been proposed as a possible treatment for rheumatic and other inflammatory diseases. However, there is currently not enough scientific human study to make a clear recommendation.	

*Key to grades: *A:* Strong scientific evidence for this use; *B:* Good scientific evidence for this use; *C:* Unclear scientific evidence for this use; *D:* Fair scientific evidence against this use (it may not work); *F:* Strong scientific evidence against this use (it likely does not work). For a more detailed explanation of efficacy criteria, see "Natural Standard Evidence-Based Validated Grading Rationale" in the Introduction.

Uses Based on Tradition, Theory, or Limited Scientific Evidence

Acne, anticoagulant, antioxidant, anti-spasm, blood clots, bowel diseases, cancer, Crohn's disease, dermatitis, dilation of veins (vasorelaxant), diverticulitis, eczema, eye infections/inflammation, fungal infections, hepatoprotection, HIV, immune stimulation, laryngitis, low blood pressure, nasopharyngeal carcinoma, osteoporosis, pruritus (itching), psoriasis, rheumatoid arthritis, skin rejuvenator, stomach ulcer, thyroid disease, tuberculosis, ulcerative colitis, viral infections, wound healing.

DOSING

The following doses are based on scientific research, publications, traditional use, or expert opinion. Many herbs and supplements have not been thoroughly tested, and safety and effectiveness may not be proven. Brands may be made differently, with variable ingredients even within the same brand. The doses shown may not apply to all products. It is important to always read product labels and discuss doses with a qualified healthcare provider before therapy is started.

Adults (18 Years and Older)

- **Dental plaque:** 10 ml of 0.2% to 10% propolis ethanol extract mouthwash has been used in studies, swished in the mouth for 60 to 90 seconds, then spit, used once or twice daily.
- **Acute cervicitis:** 5% ointment/cream of propolis applied in the form of vaginal dressings daily for 10 days has been studied.
- **Infections:** Two 250 mg of propolis capsules taken by mouth, three times daily for 2 days has been used for treating bacteria in the urine. 20% to 30% propolis extract taken by mouth for 5 days has been studied for giardiasis (milligram dosing not clearly described). Safety and effectiveness have not been established.
- **Genital herpes simplex virus infection:** 3% propolis ointment (made from 75% to 85% concentrated propolis extract) applied topically four times daily for 10 days has been studied. In cases of cervical or vaginal lesions, the same amount of ointment has been applied to the tip of a tampon and inserted vaginally four times daily for 10 days. Safety and effectiveness have not been established.

Children (Younger Than 18 Years)

- **Infections:** 10% ethanol extract of propolis taken by mouth over 5 days has been studied for giardiasis (milligram dosing not established). Note that ethanol (alcohol) preparations should be used cautiously in children. Safety and effectiveness have not been established.
- **Rhinopharyngitis:** 0.5 ml of propolis nasal spray (Nivcrisol), once weekly for 5 months has been used in preschool children (mean age 6 years) and school-age children (mean age 9 years), over a 5-month period. Safety and effectiveness have not been established.

SAFETY

The U.S. Food and Drug Administration does not strictly regulate herbs and supplements. There is no guarantee of strength, purity, or safety of products, and effects may vary. It is important to always read product labels. People who have a medical condition, or are taking other drugs, herbs, or supplements, should consult a qualified healthcare provider before starting a new therapy. A healthcare provider should be contacted immediately about any side effects.

Allergies

- Patients should avoid propolis who have had an allergic/hypersensitivity reaction to propolis, *Populus nigra* L. (black poplar), poplar bud, bee stings/bee products (including honey), or balsam of Peru. There are multiple reports of swelling, fluid collection, redness, burning, eczema, swelling, fever and other allergic reactions with repeated use of propolis on the skin.

Side Effects and Warnings

- The safety of propolis has not been thoroughly studied. Although there are several case reports of allergic reactions to propolis, it is generally believed to be well tolerated in most adults. Case reports of irritation in and around the mouth have occurred after use of propolis lozenges or extract taken by mouth.
- Toxicity data for propolis are limited. Preliminary animal studies have found propolis to be relatively non-toxic.

Pregnancy and Breastfeeding

- There is not enough scientific evidence to recommend use of propolis during pregnancy or breastfeeding. Many tinctures contain high levels of alcohol, and should be avoided during pregnancy.

INTERACTIONS

Most herbs and supplements have not been thoroughly tested for interactions with other herbs, supplements, drugs, or foods. The interactions listed here are based on reports in scientific publications, laboratory experiments, or traditional use. It is important to always read product labels. People who have a medical condition, or are taking other drugs, herbs, or supplements, should consult a qualified healthcare provider before starting a new therapy.

Interactions with Drugs

- Many tinctures contain high levels of alcohol, and may cause nausea or vomiting when taken with metronidazole (Flagyl) or disulfiram (Antabuse).

Interactions with Herbs and Dietary Supplements

- Balsam of Peru and propolis are both known to cause allergic sensitization in some people, and have multiple compounds in common, such as benzyl benzoate, benzyl cinnamate, benzyl alcohol, benzoic acid, cinnamic acid, caffeic acid, cinnamic alcohol, and vinallin. An increased risk of allergic sensitization may occur if both products are used together.

Selected References

Natural Standard developed the preceding evidence-based information based on a systematic review of more than 280 scientific articles. For comprehensive information about alternative and complementary therapies on the professional level, go to www.naturalstandard.com. Selected references are listed here.

Abd El Hady FK, Hegazi AG. Egyptian propolis: 2. Chemical composition, antiviral and antimicrobial activities of East Nile Delta propolis. Z Naturforsch [C] 2002;57(3-4):386-394.

Akao Y, Maruyama H, Matsumoto K, et al. Cell growth inhibitory effect of cinnamic acid derivatives from propolis on human tumor cell lines. Biol Pharm Bull 2003;26(7):1057-1059.

Almas K, Mahmoud A, Dahlan A. A comparative study of propolis and saline application on human dentin: a SEM study. Indian J Dent Res 2001;12(1):21-27.

Ansorge S, Reinhold D, Lendeckel U. Propolis and some of its constituents down-regulate DNA synthesis and inflammatory cytokine production but induce TGF-beta1 production of human immune cells. Z Naturforsch [C] 2003;58(7-8):580-589.

Banskota AH, Nagaoka T, Sumioka LY, et al. Antiproliferative activity of the Netherlands propolis and its active principles in cancer cell lines. J Ethnopharmacol 2002;80(1):67-73.

Barak V, Birkenfeld S, Halperin T, et al. The effect of herbal remedies on the production of human inflammatory and anti-inflammatory cytokines. Isr Med Assoc J 2002;4(11 Suppl): 919-922. Comment in: Isr Med Assoc J 2002;4(11 Suppl):944-946.

Bazo AP, Rodrigues MA, Sforcin JM, et al. Protective action of propolis on the rat colon carcinogenesis. Teratog Carcinog Mutagen 2002;22(3):183-194.

Borrelli F, Izzo AA, Di Carlo G, et al. Effect of a propolis extract and caffeic acid phenethyl ester on formation of aberrant crypt foci and tumors in the rat colon. Fitoterapia 2002;73 Suppl 1:S38-43.

Borrelli F, Maffia P, Pinto L, et al. Phytochemical compounds involved in the anti-inflammatory effect of propolis extract. Fitoterapia 2002;73 Suppl 1:S53-63.

Boyanova L, Derejian S, Koumanova R, et al. Inhibition of *Helicobacter pylori* growth in vitro by Bulgarian propolis: preliminary report. J Med Microbiol 2003;52(Pt 5):417-419.

Cardile V, Panico A, Gentile B, et al. Effect of propolis on human cartilage and chondrocytes. Life Sci 2003;73(8):1027-1035.

Ceschel GC, Maffei P, Sforzini A, et al. *In vitro* permeation through porcine buccal mucosa of caffeic acid phenetyl ester (CAPE) from a topical mucoadhesive gel containing propolis. Fitoterapia 2002;73 Suppl 1:S44-52.

Chen CN, Wu CL, Shy HS, et al. Cytotoxic prenylflavanones from Taiwanese propolis. J Nat Prod 2003;66(4):503-506.

Cicala C, Morello S, Iorio C, et al. Vascular effects of caffeic acid phenethyl ester (CAPE) on isolated rat thoracic aorta. Life Sci 2003;73(1):73-80.

Cos P, Rajan P, Vedernikova I, et al. *In vitro* antioxidant profile of phenolic acid derivatives. Free Radic Res 2002;36(6):711-716.

Crisan I, Zaharia CN, Popovici F, et al. Natural propolis extract NIVCRISOL in the treatment of acute and chronic rhinopharyngitis in children. Rom J Virol 1995;46(3-4):115-133.

Eley BM. Antibacterial agents in the control of supragingival plaque: a review. Br Dent J 1999;186(6):286-296.

El-Khatib AS, Agha AM, Mahran LG, et al. Prophylactic effect of aqueous propolis extract against acute experimental hepatotoxicity *in vivo*. Z Naturforsch [C] 2002;57(3-4):379-385.

Gregory SR, Piccolo N, Piccolo MT, et al. Comparison of propolis skin cream to silver sulfadiazine: a naturopathic alternative to antibiotics in treatment of minor burns. J Altern Complement Med 2002;8(1):77-83.

Han S, Sung KH, Yim D, et al. Activation of murine macrophage cell line RAW 264.7 by Korean propolis. Arch Pharm Res 2002;25(6):895-902.

Havsteen BH. The biochemistry and medical significance of the flavonoids. Pharmacol Ther 2002;96(2-3):67.

Hegazi AG, Abd El Hady FK. Egyptian propolis: 3. Antioxidant, antimicrobial activities and chemical composition of propolis from reclaimed lands. Z Naturforsch [C] 2002;57(3-4): 395-402.

Henschel R, Agathos M, Breit R. Occupational contact dermatitis from propolis. Contact Dermatitis 2002;47(1):52.

Mahmoud AS, Almas K, Dahlan AA. The effect of propolis on dentinal hypersensitivity and level of satisfaction among patients from a university hospital Riyadh, Saudi Arabia. Indian J Dent Res 1999;10(4):130-137.

Murray MC, Worthington HV, Blinkhorn AS. A study to investigate the effect of a propolis-containing mouthrinse on the inhibition of de novo plaque formation. J Clin Periodontol 1997;24(11):796-798.

Park YK, Koo MH, Abreu JA, et al. Antimicrobial activity of propolis on oral microorganisms. Curr Microbiol 1998;36(1):24-28.

Steinberg D, Kaine G, Gedalia I. Antibacterial effect of propolis and honey on oral bacteria. Am J Dent 1996;9(6):236-239.

Vynograd N, Vynograd I, Sosnowski Z. A comparative multi-centre study of the efficacy of propolis, acyclovir and placebo in the treatment of genital herpes (HSV). Phytomed 2000; 7(1):1-6.

Psyllium

(*Plantago ovata, Plantago ispaghula*)

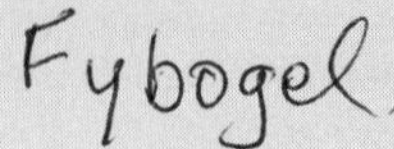

RELATED TERMS

- Bran Buds cereal, Effersyllium, Fiberall, flea seed, Fybogel, Heartwise cereal, Hydrocil, I-so-gel, ispaghula, ispaghula husk, ispaghula seed, Konsyl, Lunelax, Metamucil, Minolest, Natural Vegetable Laxative, Perdiem, *Plantago arenaria*, *Plantago psyllium*, Prodiem Plain, psyllion, psyllios, psyllium husk, psyllium seed, Regulan, Serutan, Vi-Siblin, Yerba Prima Psyllium hush powder.

BACKGROUND

- Psyllium, also referred to as *ispaghula*, is derived from the husks of the seeds of *Plantago ovata*. Psyllium contains a high level of soluble dietary fiber and is the chief ingredient in many commonly used bulk laxatives, including products such as Metamucil and Serutan.
- Psyllium has been studied as a "non-systemic" cholesterol-lowering agent, with generally modest effects seen on total cholesterol and high-density lipoprotein levels. Several psyllium-containing cereals such as Heartwise and Bran Buds have appeared in the United States marketplace during the last 15 years, and have been touted for their potential lipid-lowering and "heart health promoting" effects.
- Allergic reactions, including anaphylaxis, have been reported, particularly in health-care workers with previous experience preparing psyllium-containing bulk laxatives. Obstruction of the gastrointestinal tract by such laxatives has also been reported, particularly in patients with prior bowel surgeries or anatomic abnormalities, or when mixed with inadequate amounts of water.

USES BASED ON SCIENTIFIC EVIDENCE	Grade*
High cholesterol Psyllium is well studied as a lipid-lowering agent with generally modest reductions seen in blood levels of total cholesterol and low-density lipoprotein ("bad cholesterol"). Effects have been observed following 8 weeks of regular use. Psyllium does not appear to have significant effects on high-density lipoprotein ("good cholesterol") or triglyceride levels. Because only small reductions have been observed, people with high cholesterol should discuss the use of more potent agents with their healthcare provider. Effects have been observed in adults and children, although long-term safety in children is not established.	A
Constipation Psyllium has long been used as a chief ingredient in "bulk laxatives." Studies exploring the mechanisms of the laxative effects of psyllium are somewhat conflicting, but have generally revealed an increase in stool weight, an increase in bowel movements per day, and a decrease in total gut transit time.	B

Continued

Diarrhea Psyllium has been studied for the treatment of diarrhea, particularly in patients undergoing tube feeding. It has also been studied in addition to Orlistat therapy, in hopes of decreasing gastrointestinal effects (diarrhea and oily discharge) of this weight loss agent. An effective stool bulking effect has generally been found in scientific studies.	**B**
Fat excretion in stool Early research shows that dietary psyllium and chitosan supplementation may help to increase the excretion of fat in the stool.	**C**
Hyperglycemia (high blood sugar levels) Several studies have examined the administration of psyllium with meals or just prior to meals in order to measure effects on blood sugar levels. Measurements have been done immediately after meals and throughout the day. Effects of regular (chronic) psyllium use have also been investigated. In general, no immediate (acute) changes in blood sugar levels have been reported. Long-term effects have been inconsistent across studies, although modest reductions have been reported in some research. Better evidence is necessary before a firm conclusion can be drawn.	**C**
Inflammatory bowel disease There is limited and unclear evidence regarding the use of psyllium in patients with inflammatory bowel disease.	**C**
Irritable bowel syndrome Psyllium preparations have been studied for more than 20 years in the treatment of irritable bowel syndrome symptoms. Results of these trials have been conflicting. Better research is necessary before a firm conclusion can be reached.	**C**

*Key to grades: *A:* Strong scientific evidence for this use; *B:* Good scientific evidence for this use; *C:* Unclear scientific evidence for this use; *D:* Fair scientific evidence against this use (it may not work); *F:* Strong scientific evidence against this use (it likely does not work). For a more detailed explanation of efficacy criteria, see "Natural Standard Evidence-Based Validated Grading Rationale" in the Introduction.

Uses Based on Tradition, Theory, or Limited Scientific Evidence

Abscesses, anti-parasitic, atherosclerosis, bleeding hemorrhoids, boils, bronchitis, colon cancer prevention, Crohn's disease, cystitis, demulcent, diverticular disease, duodenal ulcer, dysentery, excessive menstrual bleeding, fecal (stool) incontinence, gallstones, hearing damage, high blood pressure, incontinence, leishmaniasis, obesity, poison ivy rash, primary biliary cirrhosis, psoriasis, radiation-induced colitis/diarrhea, sclerosing cholangitis, stomach ulcer, urethritis, wound healing (used on the skin).

DOSING

The following doses are based on scientific research, publications, traditional use, or expert opinion. Many herbs and supplements have not been thoroughly tested, and safety and effectiveness may not be proven. Brands may be made differently, with variable ingredients even within the same brand. The doses shown may not apply to all products. It is important to always read product labels and discuss doses with a qualified healthcare provider before therapy is started.

Standardization

- Standardization involves measuring the amounts of certain chemicals in products to try to make different preparations similar to each other. It is not always known if the chemicals being measured are the "active" ingredients.
- Psyllium products may contain husks of *Plantago ovata* seeds or the seeds themselves, with the husks being more commonly used. Amounts of psyllium in products are generally reported as total grams. Seed preparations contain approximately 47% soluble fiber by weight, while husk preparations generally contain 67 to 71% soluble fiber and 85% total fiber by weight.

Adults (18 Years and Older)

- **Dietary amounts:** Recommendations for dietary fiber intake for adults fall within the range of 20 to 35 g per day, or 10 to 13 g per 1,000 kilocalories ingested. However, popular U.S. foods are not high in dietary fiber, and common serving sizes of grains, fruits, and vegetables contain only 1 to 3 g of dietary fiber. The usual intake of dietary fiber in the U.S. remains lower than these recommended levels, averaging only 14 to 15 g daily.
- **General:** It is important to take laxatives such as psyllium with sufficient amounts of water or liquid in order to reduce the risk of bowel obstruction.
- **Cholesterol lowering:** A wide range of doses of psyllium has been studied, from 3.4 to 45 g per day, taken daily by mouth in two or three divided doses. Studies using psyllium-enriched cereals or other food products have administered preparations providing between 3 and 12 g of soluble fiber daily. Psyllium husk preparations have generally been used in cholesterol-lowering studies, although seed preparations have also been used.
- **Constipation:** Doses ranging from 7 to 30 g by mouth daily in single or divided doses have been used in studies.
- **Diarrhea:** Doses ranging from 7.5 to 30 g by mouth daily in single or divided doses have been used in studies.
- **Blood sugar lowering:** Doses ranging from 2.2 to 45 g by mouth daily in divided doses, often administered just prior to meals, have been used in studies. Blood sugar levels should be monitored by a qualified healthcare professional.
- **Inflammatory bowel disease:** 7 g by mouth daily in divided doses has been used in studies, although effects are not clearly established.
- **Irritable bowel syndrome:** Doses ranging from 6 to 30 g by mouth daily have been used in studies, although effects are not clearly established.

Children (Younger Than 18 Years)

- **High cholesterol:** 6 to 7 g by mouth daily of psyllium-enriched cereal has been studied, although more research is needed to establish benefits and long-term safety.
- **Diarrhea:** 3.4 g by mouth daily has been studied, although more research is needed to establish benefits and long-term safety.

- **Inflammatory bowel disease:** 16 g by mouth daily has been studied, although effects are not clearly established. More research is needed to establish potential benefits and long-term safety.

SAFETY

The U.S. Food and Drug Administration does not strictly regulate herbs and supplements. There is no guarantee of strength, purity, or safety of products, and effects may vary. It is important to always read product labels. People who have a medical condition, or are taking other drugs, herbs, or supplements, should consult a qualified healthcare provider before starting a new therapy. A healthcare provider should be contacted immediately about any side effects.

Allergies

- Serious allergic reactions, including anaphylaxis, difficulty breathing/wheezing, skin rash, and hives, have been reported after ingestion of psyllium products. Less severe hypersensitivity reactions have also been noted. Cross-sensitivity may occur in people with allergy to English plantain pollen (*Plantago lanceolata*), grass pollen, or melon. Plantain allergy may be associated with latex sensitivity, although it is not clear if this applies to psyllium as well. Workers in the healthcare and pharmaceutical industries can become sensitized and develop allergic respiratory (breathing) symptoms due to handling bulk laxatives containing psyllium powder. Occupational asthma associated with psyllium exposure has been observed. Reactions may also occur from breathing in the dust or from skin contact.

Side Effects and Warnings

- Psyllium-containing laxatives, cereals, and other products are generally believed to be safe. Important exceptions include those with repeated psyllium exposure (such as healthcare workers frequently handling bulk laxatives who are at risk for hypersensitivity reactions), and patients with significant pre-existing bowel abnormalities (such as gastrointestinal strictures or impaired motility) or prior bowel surgery.
- Obstruction of the gastrointestinal tract has been noted in numerous case reports of patients taking psyllium-containing laxatives, particularly in individuals with previous bowel surgery or problems, and/or when the laxatives are mixed with inadequate amounts of water.
- Gastrointestinal side effects are generally mild and have not prompted discontinuation of psyllium in most clinical trials. Flatulence (gas), bloating, diarrhea, and constipation have been reported, and all were less frequent when compared to wheat bran therapy in one study. Since many patients in studies of psyllium have pre-existing bowel concerns, it is difficult to discern which symptoms are caused by psyllium specifically. Esophageal obstruction has been reported in a patient with Parkinson's disease.
- Due to potential reductions in blood sugar levels caused by psyllium, blood glucose levels in diabetic patients should be closely monitored.

Pregnancy and Breastfeeding

- Psyllium-containing laxatives are considered class C-2 drugs in pregnancy, meaning that they appear to be safe in all three trimesters, although studies in pregnant humans and animals have not been done. Psyllium-containing products are considered class 1 (apparently safe) during breastfeeding.

INTERACTIONS

Most herbs and supplements have not been thoroughly tested for interactions with other herbs, supplements, drugs, or foods. The interactions listed here are based on reports in scientific publications, laboratory experiments, or traditional use. It is important to always read product labels. People who have a medical condition, or are taking other drugs, herbs, or supplements, should consult a qualified healthcare provider before starting a new therapy.

Interactions with Drugs

- Psyllium-containing products may delay gastric emptying time and reduce absorption of some drugs. For example, lithium, potassium-sparing diuretics such as spironolactone (Aldactone), carbamazepine, salicylates such as aspirin, tetracyclines, and nitrofurantoin may have decreased absorption when taken with psyllium. Digoxin (Lanoxin) levels may also be affected. It is advised that drugs be taken at separate administration times from psyllium to minimize potential interactions (for example, 1 hour before or a few hours after taking psyllium).
- Although no effect on warfarin (Coumadin) levels with co-administration of psyllium was reported in one study, administration of these agents should be separated until better research is available.
- Because of potential reductions in blood sugar levels caused by psyllium, requirements for insulin or other diabetes drugs in diabetic patients may be reduced. Blood glucose levels should be closely monitored, and dosing adjustments may be necessary.

Interactions with Herbs and Dietary Supplements

- Psyllium-containing products may delay gastric emptying time and reduce absorption of some herbs, supplements, vitamins, or minerals. For example, long-term use of psyllium can reduce absorption of iron, zinc, copper, magnesium and vitamin B_{12}. Absorption of calcium may also be affected. Other agents should be taken 1 hour before or a few hours after psyllium to avoid potential interactions.
- Psyllium and chitosan taken together may increase fat excretion in the stool.

Interactions with Foods

- Psyllium-containing products may delay gastric emptying time and reduce absorption of dietary carbohydrates. Long-term use of psyllium with meals may reduce nutrient absorption, requiring vitamin or mineral supplementation. However, in a review of eight human trials, the use of blond psyllium husk for up to 6 months did not alter vitamin or mineral status.

Selected References

Natural Standard developed the preceding evidence-based information based on a systematic review of more than 275 scientific articles. For comprehensive information about alternative and complementary therapies on the professional level, go to www.naturalstandard.com. Selected references are listed here.

Abraham ZD, Mehta T. Three-week psyllium-husk supplementation: effect on plasma cholesterol concentrations, fecal steroid excretion, and carbohydrate absorption in men. Am J Clin Nutr 1988;47(1):67-74.

Anderson JW, Allgood LD, Lawrence A, et al. Cholesterol-lowering effects of psyllium intake adjunctive to diet therapy in men and women with hypercholesterolemia: meta-analysis of 8 controlled trials. Am J Clin Nutr 2000;71(2):472-479.

Anderson JW, Allgood LD, Turner J, et al. Effects of psyllium on glucose and serum lipid responses in men with type 2 diabetes and hypercholesterolemia. Am J Clin Nutr 1999;70(4):466-473.

Anderson JW, Davidson MH, Blonde L, et al. Long-term cholesterol-lowering effects of psyllium as an adjunct to diet therapy in the treatment of hypercholesterolemia. Am J Clin Nutr 2000;71(6):1433-1438.

Anderson JW, Floore TL, Geil PB, et al. Hypocholesterolemic effects of different bulk-forming hydrophilic fibers as adjuncts to dietary therapy in mild to moderate hypercholesterolemia. Arch Intern Med 1991;151(8):1597-1602.

Arthurs Y, Fielding JF. Double blind trial of ispaghula/poloxamer in the irritable bowel syndrome. Ir Med J 1983;76(5):253.

Ashraf W, Park F, Lof J, et al. Effects of psyllium therapy on stool characteristics, colon transit and anorectal function in chronic idiopathic constipation. Aliment Pharmacol Ther 1995;9(6):639-647.

Ashraf W, Park F, Lof J, et al. Effects of psyllium therapy on stool characteristics, colon transit and anorectal function in chronic idiopathic constipation. Aliment Pharmacol Ther 1995;9(6):639-647.

Barroso Aranda J, Contreras F, Bagchi D, Preuss HG. Efficacy of a novel chitosan formulation on fecal fat excretion: a double-blind, crossover, placebo-controlled study. J Med 2002;33(1-4):209-225.

Belknap D, Davidson LJ, Smith CR. The effects of psyllium hydrophilic mucilloid on diarrhea in enterally fed patients. Heart Lung 1997;26(3):229-237.

Bhatnagar D. Should pediatric patients with hyperlipidemia receive drug therapy? Paediatr Drugs 2002;4(4):223-230.

Bianchi M, Capurso L. Effects of guar gum, ispaghula and microcrystalline cellulose on abdominal symptoms, gastric emptying, orocaecal transit time and gas production in healthy volunteers. Dig Liver Dis 2002;34(Suppl 2):S129-S133.

Burton R, Manninen V. Influence of a psyllium-based fibre preparation on faecal and serum parameters. Acta Med Scand Suppl 1982;668:91-94.

Campbell S. Dietary fibre supplementation with psyllium or gum arabic reduced incontinent stools and improved stool consistency in community living adults. Evid Based Nurs 2002;5(2):56.

Cavaliere H, Floriano I, Medeiros-Neto G. Gastrointestinal side effects of Orlistat may be prevented by concomitant prescription of natural fibers (psyllium mucilloid). Int J Obes Relat Metab Disord 2001;25(7):1095-1099.

Chan EK, Schroeder DJ. Psyllium in hypercholesterolemia. Ann Pharmacother 1995;29(6):625-628.

Chapman ND, Grillage MG, Mazumder R, et al. A comparison of mebeverine with high-fibre dietary advice and mebeverine plus ispaghula in the treatment of irritable bowel syndrome: an open, prospectively randomised, parallel group study. Br J Clin Pract 1990;44(11):461-466.

Cherbut C, Bruley d, V, Schnee M, et al. Involvement of small intestinal motility in blood glucose response to dietary fibre in man. Br J Nutr 1994;71(5):675-685.

Davidson MH, Dugan LD, Burns JH, et al. A psyllium-enriched cereal for the treatment of hypercholesterolemia in children: a controlled, double-blind, crossover study. Am J Clin Nutr 1996;63(1):96-102.

Davidson MH, Maki KC, Kong JC, et al. Long-term effects of consuming foods containing psyllium seed husk on serum lipids in subjects with hypercholesterolemia. Am J Clin Nutr 1998;67(3):367-376.

Dennison BA, Levine DM. Randomized, double-blind, placebo-controlled, two-period crossover clinical trial of psyllium fiber in children with hypercholesterolemia. J Pediatr 1993;123(1):24-29.

Dettmar PW, Sykes J. A multi-centre, general practice comparison of ispaghula husk with lactulose and other laxatives in the treatment of simple constipation. Curr Med Res Opin 1998;14(4):227-233.

Doerfler OC, Ruppert-Kohlmayr AJ, Reittner P, et al. Helical CT of the small bowel with an alternative oral contrast material in patients with Crohn's disease. Abdom Imaging 2003;28(3):313-318.

Eherer AJ, Santa Ana CA, Porter J, Fordtran JS. Effect of psyllium, calcium polycarbophil, and wheat bran on secretory diarrhea induced by phenolphthalein. Gastroenterology 1993; 104(4):1007-1012.

Everson GT, Daggy BP, McKinley C, Story JA. Effects of psyllium hydrophilic mucilloid on LDL-cholesterol and bile acid synthesis in hypercholesterolemic men. J Lipid Res 1992; 33(8):1183-1192.

Fernandez-Banares F, Hinojosa J, Sanchez-Lombrana JL, et al. Randomised clinical trial of Plantago ovata efficacy as compared to mesalazine in maintaining remission in ulcerative colitis. Gastroenterology 1997;112:A971.

Frape DL, Jones AM. Chronic and postprandial responses of plasma insulin, glucose and lipids in volunteers given dietary fibre supplements. Br J Nutr 1995;73(5):733-751.

Frati Munari AC, Benitez PW, Raul Ariza AC, et al. Lowering glycemic index of food by acarbose and Plantago psyllium mucilage. Arch Med Res 1998;29(2):137-141.

Frost GS, Brynes AE, Dhillo WS, Bloom SR, McBurney MI. The effects of fiber enrichment of pasta and fat content on gastric emptying, GLP-1, glucose, and insulin responses to a meal. Eur J Clin Nutr 2003;57(2):293-298.

Gaw A. A new reality: achieving cholesterol-lowering goals in clinical practice. Atheroscler Suppl 2002;2(4):5-8; discussion, 8-11.

Gelissen IC, Brodie B, Eastwood MA. Effect of *Plantago ovata* (psyllium) husk and seeds on sterol metabolism: studies in normal and ileostomy subjects. Am J Clin Nutr 1994; 59(2): 395-400.

Gupta RR, Agrawal CG, Singh GP, et al. Lipid-lowering efficacy of psyllium hydrophilic mucilloid in non-insulin dependent diabetes mellitus with hyperlipidaemia. Indian J Med Res 1994;100:237-241.

Hallert C, Kaldma M, Petersson BG. Ispaghula husk may relieve gastrointestinal symptoms in ulcerative colitis in remission. Scand J Gastroenterol 1991;26(7):747-750.

Heather DJ, Howell L, Montana M, et al. Effect of a bulk-forming cathartic on diarrhea in tube-fed patients. Heart Lung 1991;20(4):409-413.

Hermansen K, Dinesen B, Hoie LH, et al. Effects of soy and other natural products on LDL:HDL ratio and other lipid parameters: a literature review. Adv Ther 2003;20(1):50-78.

Hotz J, Plein K. [Effectiveness of plantago seed husks in comparison with wheat bran on stool frequency and manifestations of irritable colon syndrome with constipation.] Med Klin 1994;89(12):645-651.

Hunsaker DM, Hunsaker JC 3rd. Therapy-related cafe coronary deaths: two case reports of rare asphyxial deaths in patients under supervised care. Am J Forensic Med Pathol 2002; 23(2):149-154.

Jenkins DJ, Kendall CW, Vuksan V, et al. Soluble fiber intake at a dose approved by the US Food and Drug Administration for a claim of health benefits: serum lipid risk factors for cardiovascular disease assessed in a randomized controlled crossover trial. Am J Clin Nutr 2002;75(5):834-839.

Juarranz M, Calle-Puron ME, Gonzalez-Navarro A, et al. Physical exercise, use of *Plantago ovata* and aspirin, and reduced risk of colon cancer. Eur J Cancer Prev 2002;11(5):465-472.

Kanauchi O, Mitsuyama K, Araki Y, Andoh A. Modification of intestinal flora in the treatment of inflammatory bowel disease. Curr Pharm Des 2003;9(4):333-346.

Korula J. Dietary fiber supplementation with psyllium or gum arabic reduced fecal incontinence in community-living adults. ACP J Club 2002;136(1):23. Comment in: Nurs Res 2001; 50(4):203-213.

Kris-Etherton PM, Taylor DS, Smiciklas-Wright H, et al. High-soluble-fiber foods in conjunction with a telephone-based, personalized behavior change support service result in favorable changes in lipids and lifestyles after 7 weeks. J Am Diet Assoc 2002;102(4):503-10. Comment in: J Am Diet Assoc 2002; 102(12):1751.

Kumar A, Kumar N, Vij JC, et al. Optimum dosage of ispaghula husk in patients with irritable bowel syndrome: Correlation of symptom relief with whole gut transit time and stool weight. Gut 1987;28(2):150-155.

Longstreth GF, Fox DD, Youkeles L, et al. Psyllium therapy in the irritable bowel syndrome. A double-blind trial. Ann Intern Med 1981;95(1):53-56.

Maciejko JJ, Brazg R, Shah A, et al. Psyllium for the reduction of cholestyramine-associated gastrointestinal symptoms in the treatment of primary hypercholesterolemia. Arch Fam Med 1994;3(11):955-960.

MacMahon M, Carless J. Ispaghula husk in the treatment of hypercholesterolaemia: a double-blind controlled study. J Cardiovasc Risk 1998;5(3):167-172.

Marlett JA, Fischer MH. A poorly fermented gel from psyllium seed husk increases excreta moisture and bile acid excretion in rats. J Nutr 2002;132(9):2638-2643.

Marlett JA, Li BU, Patrow CJ, et al. Comparative laxation of psyllium with and without senna in an ambulatory constipated population. Am J Gastroenterol 1987;82(4):333-337.

McRorie JW, Daggy BP, More JG, et al. Psyllium is superior to docusate sodium for treatment of chronic constipation. Aliment Pharmacol Ther 1998;12(5):491-497.

Murphy J, Stacey D, Crook J, et al. Testing control of radiation-induced diarrhea with a psyllium bulking agent: a pilot study. Can Oncol Nurs J 2000;10(3):96-100.

Olson BH, Anderson SM, Becker MP, et al. Psyllium-enriched cereals lower blood total cholesterol and LDL cholesterol, but not HDL cholesterol, in hypercholesterolemic adults: results of a meta-analysis. J Nutr 1997;127(10):1973-1980.

Rai J, Singh J. Ispaghula husk. J Assoc Physicians India 2002;50:576-578.

Reid R, Fodor G, Lydon-Hassen K, et al. Dietary counselling for dyslipidemia in primary care: results of a randomized trial. Can J Diet Pract Res. 2002;63(4):169-75.

Rodriguez-Moran M, Guerrero-Romero F, Lazcano-Burciaga G. Lipid- and glucose-lowering efficacy of Plantago Psyllium in type II diabetes. J Diabetes Complications 1998;12(5): 273-278.

Romero AL, West KL, Zern T, Fernandez ML. The seeds from *Plantago ovata* lower plasma lipids by altering hepatic and bile acid metabolism in guinea pigs. J Nutr 2002;132(6): 1194-1198.

Roy S, Freake HC, Fernandez ML. Gender and hormonal status affect the regulation of hepatic cholesterol 7-alpha-hydroxylase activity and mRNA abundance by dietary soluble fiber in the guinea pig. Atherosclerosis 2002;163(1):29-37.

Sierra M, Garcia JJ, Fernandez N, et al. Therapeutic effects of psyllium in type 2 diabetic patients. Eur J Clin Nutr 2002;56(9):830-842.

Spence JD, Huff MW, Heidenheim P, et al. Combination therapy with colestipol and psyllium mucilloid in patients with hyperlipidemia. Ann Intern Med 1995;123(7):493-499.

van Rosendaal GM, Shaffer EA, Edwards AL et al. Issues raised by psyllium meta-analysis. Am J Clin Nutr 2001; 73(3):653-654.

Voderholzer WA, Schatke W, Muhldorfer BE, et al. Clinical response to dietary fiber treatment of chronic constipation. Am J Gastroenterol 1997;92(1):95-98.

Westerhof W, Das PK, Middelkoop E, et al. Mucopolysaccharides from psyllium involved in wound healing. Drugs Exp Clin Res. 2001;27(5-6):165-175.

Williams CL, Bollella M, Spark A, et al. Soluble fiber enhances the hypocholesterolemic effect of the step I diet in childhood. J Am Coll Nutr 1995;14(3):251-257.

Zaman V, Manzoor SM, Zaki M, et al. The presence of antiamoebic constituents in psyllium husk. Phytother Res 2002;16(1):78-79.

Pycnogenol
(*Pinus pinaster* ssp. atlantica)

RELATED TERMS

- Cocklebut, condensed tannins, French maritime pine bark extract, leucoanthocyanidins, *Pinus pinaster*, *Pinus maritime*, oligomeric proanthocyanidin complexes (OPCs), Pinaceae, proanthocyanidins, pygenol, stickwort.

BACKGROUND

- Pycnogenol is the patented trade name for a water extract of the bark of the French maritime pine (*Pinus pinaster* ssp. *atlantica*), which is grown in coastal southwest France. Pycnogenol contains oligomeric proanthocyanidins (OPCs) as well as several other bioflavonoids: catechin, epicatechin, phenolic fruit acids (such as ferulic acid and caffeic acid), and taxifolin.
- There has been some confusion in the U.S. market regarding OPC products containing Pycnogenol or grape seed extract (GSE), because one of the generic terms for chemical constituents ("pycnogenols") is the same as the patented trade name (Pycnogenol). Some GSE products were formerly erroneously labeled and marketed in the U.S. as containing "pycnogenols." Although GSE and Pycnogenol do contain similar chemical constituents (primarily in the OPC fraction), the chemical, pharmacologic, and clinical literature on the two products is distinct. The term Pycnogenol should therefore only be used to refer to this specific proprietary pine bark extract. Scientific literature regarding this product should not be referenced as a basis for the safety or effectiveness of GSE.

USES BASED ON SCIENTIFIC EVIDENCE	Grade*
Chronic venous insufficiency Chronic venous insufficiency (CVI) is a syndrome that includes leg swelling, varicose veins, pain, itching, skin changes, and skin ulcers. The term is more commonly used in Europe than in the United States. Pycnogenol used in people with chronic venous insufficiency is reported to reduce edema and pain. Pycnogenol may also be used in the management of other CVI symptoms.	**B**
ADHD (attention deficit hyperactivity disorder) Preliminary research comparing Pycnogenol vs. placebo in adults with ADHD reported improved concentration with both agents. After release of this study, Enfamol Nutraceuticals Inc. (maker of Efalex and Efalex Focus) and J&R Research (maker of Pycnogenol) settled a suit with the Federal Trade Commission (FTC) agreeing to no longer advertise these supplements as treatments for ADHD. The companies were not required to pay fines. FTC officials stated they are particularly concerned about dietary supplements with unproven claims being marketed for children.	**C**

Continued

Further research is necessary in this area before a firm conclusion can be reached.	
Antioxidant Due to conflicting study results, it is unclear if Pycnogenol has significant antioxidant effects in humans. Further research is necessary.	**C**
Asthma (chronic therapy) Pycnogenol is reported to reduce leukotriene levels in humans, suggesting possible benefits in the chronic management of asthma. Although these data are promising, well-designed controlled study is needed before a firm conclusion can be reached.	**C**
Erectile dysfunction Pycnogenol, in combination with L-arginine, may cause an improvement in sexual function in men with erectile dysfunction. It is not known what effect each of the individual compounds may have directly on this condition. Further research is needed.	**C**
Gingival bleeding/plaque Chewing gum containing 5 mg of Pycnogenol is reported to minimize gingival bleeding and plaque formation. Further research is needed to confirm these results.	**C**
High cholesterol One human trial reports Pycnogenol to significantly reduce low-density lipoprotein (LDL/"bad cholesterol") levels and increased high-density lipoprotein (HDL/"good cholesterol") levels. Other studies have reported decreases in total cholesterol and LDL levels with no change in HDL. Because of conflicting data and methodological problems with available research, further studies are necessary before clear conclusions can be drawn.	**C**
Male infertility Human studies report that Pycnogenol may improve sperm quality and function in sub-fertile men. Further research is needed to confirm these results.	**C**
Melasma (chloasma) Melasma (or chloasma) is a common disorder of hyperpigmentation of the skin predominately affecting sun-exposed areas in women. Formation of tan or brown patches/spots may occur. Pycnogenol has been reported to decrease the darkened area and the pigment intensity of melasma and improve symptoms of fatigue, constipation, body pains, and anxiety. Further well-designed research is needed before a clear recommendation can be made.	**C**
Platelet aggregation One human study reports reduced platelet aggregation in smokers. Further research is needed before a clear conclusion can be reached.	**C**

Continued

Retinopathy Several studies report benefits of Pycnogenol in the treatment and prevention of retinopathy, including slowing the progression of retinopathy in diabetics. Reported mechanisms include improvement of capillary resistance and reduction of leakage into the retina. Improvement of visual acuity has also been reported. Better-quality research is needed before a firm conclusion can be reached.	C
Sunburn Pycnogenol, taken orally, may reduce erythema (redness of the skin) caused by solar ultraviolet light. Further study is needed before a recommendation can be made.	C
Systemic lupus erythematosus (SLE) Preliminary human and non-human data suggest that Pycnogenol may be useful as a second-line therapy to reduce inflammatory features of SLE. Further research is needed before a recommendation can be made.	C

*Key to grades: *A:* Strong scientific evidence for this use; *B:* Good scientific evidence for this use; *C:* Unclear scientific evidence for this use; *D:* Fair scientific evidence against this use (it may not work); *F:* Strong scientific evidence against this use (it likely does not work). For a more detailed explanation of efficacy criteria, see "Natural Standard Evidence-Based Validated Grading Rationale" in the Introduction.

Uses Based on Tradition, Theory, or Limited Scientific Evidence

ACE-inhibitor activity, Alzheimer's disease, antihistamine, antiparasitic, atherosclerosis, autoimmune disorders, bone marrow production, cancer prevention, cancer treatment, cardiovascular disease, cerebral ischemia, chemotherapy side effects, exercise capacity, fat burning, G6PD deficiency, gout prevention (xanthine oxidase and dehydrogenase inhibitor), hemorrhoids, high blood pressure, hypoglycemic agent, immune enhancement, immune suppression, inflammation, inhibition of TNF-alpha, increased human growth hormone, lung cancer, premenstrual syndrome, macular degeneration, myocardial ischemia/reperfusion injury, night vision, pelvic pain, neurodegenerative diseases, prevention of fat formation, psoriasis, retinal protection, rheumatoid arthritis, sickle cell anemia, skin disorders, skin aging, vasorelaxant.

DOSING

The following doses are based on scientific research, publications, traditional use, or expert opinion. Many herbs and supplements have not been thoroughly tested, and safety and effectiveness may not be proven. Brands may be made differently, with variable ingredients even within the same brand. The doses shown may not apply to all products. It is important to always read product labels and discuss doses with a qualified healthcare provider before therapy is started.

Standardization

- Standardization involves measuring the amounts of certain chemicals in products to try to make different preparations similar to each other. It is not always known if the chemicals being measured are the "active" ingredients. Pycnogenol is a proprietary patented formula.

Adults (18 Years and Older)

- *Note*: Pycnogenol appears to be absorbed into the bloodstream in about 20 minutes. Once absorbed, therapeutic effects are purported to last for approximately 72 hours, followed by excretion in the urine. Because of its astringent taste and occasional minor stomach discomfort, it may be best to take Pycnogenol with or after meals.
- **Antioxidant/cholesterol reduction:** 150-360 mg/day for 4 to 6 weeks has been used.
- **Antiparasitic:** 30 mg/kg/day has been used.
- **Chronic venous insufficiency (CVI):** 100-360 mg/day in divided doses for 1 to 2 months has been used.
- **Asthma chronic therapy):** 1 mg/lb/day (maximum 200 mg/day) for up to 4 weeks has been used.
- **Erectile dysfunction:** A regimen combining Pycnogenol and L-arginine that has been used involves 1.7 g of L-arginine/day during month #1; 1.7 g of L-arginine/day and 40 mg of Pycnogenol 2 times/day during month #2; and 1.7 g of L-arginine/day and 40 mg of Pycnogenol 3 times/day during month #3.
- **Sunburn:** 1.10 mg/kg/day for 4 weeks, followed by 1.66 mg/kg/day for 4 weeks has been used.
- **Gum health (gingival bleeding/plaque):** 5 mg Pycnogenol in chewing gum for 14 days has been used.
- **Male infertility:** 200 mg/day of Pycnogenol for 90 days has been used.
- **Platelet aggregation reduction:** 100 to 200 mg/day has been used.
- **Melasma (chloasma):** 25-mg tablet with meals 3 times a day (75 mg/day) for 30 days has been used.
- **Retinopathy:** 50 mg taken three times a day for 2 months has been used.

Children (Younger Than 18 Years)

- Due to insufficient data, pycnogenol is not recommended for use by children.

SAFETY

The U.S. Food and Drug Administration does not strictly regulate herbs and supplements. There is no guarantee of strength, purity, or safety of products, and effects may vary. It is important to always read product labels. People who have a medical condition, or are taking other drugs, herbs, or supplements, should consult a qualified healthcare provider before starting a new therapy. A healthcare provider should be contacted immediately about any side effects.

Allergies

- Individuals should not take pycnogenol if allergic to it or any of its components.

Side Effects and Warnings

- Pycnogenol is generally reported as being well tolerated. Low acute and chronic toxicity with mild unwanted effects may occur in a small percentage of patients following oral administration. Because of Pycnogenol's astringent taste and occasional minor stomach discomfort, it may be best to take Pycnogenol with or after meals. To date, no serious adverse effects have been reported in the available scientific literature, although systematic study of safety is not available.

- In theory, Pycnogenol may alter blood sugar levels. Caution is advised in patients with diabetes or hypoglycemia, and in those taking drugs, herbs, or supplements that affect blood sugar. Serum glucose levels may need to be monitored by a healthcare provider, and medication adjustments may be necessary.
- In theory, Pycnogenol may increase the risk of bleeding. Caution is advised in patients with bleeding disorders or taking drugs that may increase the risk of bleeding. Dosing adjustments may be necessary.

Pregnancy and Breastfeeding

- Pycnogenol is not recommended during pregnancy or breastfeeding because of lack of scientific evidence.

INTERACTIONS

Most herbs and supplements have not been thoroughly tested for interactions with other herbs, supplements, drugs, or foods. The interactions listed here are based on reports in scientific publications, laboratory experiments, or traditional use. It is important to always read product labels. People who have a medical condition, or are taking other drugs, herbs, or supplements, should consult a qualified healthcare provider before starting a new therapy.

Interactions with Drugs

- Based on mechanism of action, there are potential interactions with other antihypertensive medications, specifically angiotensin-converting enzyme inhibitors (ACE-I) such as benazepril (Lotensin), captopril (Capoten), enalapril (Vasotec), fosinopril (Monopril), lisinopril (Prinivil), moexipril (Univasc), perindopril (Aceon), quinapril (Accupril), ramipril (Altace), trandolapril (Mavik), and angiotensin-converting enzyme receptor blockers such as losartan (Cozaar), irbesartan (Avapro), candesartan, cilexetil (Atacand), and valsartan (Diovan).
- Based on mechanism of action, Pycnogenol may lower blood sugar levels. Caution is advised when using medications that may also lower blood sugar levels. Patients taking drugs for diabetes by mouth (such as metformin, glyburide, glipizide) or insulin should be monitored closely by a qualified healthcare provider. Medication adjustments may be necessary.
- Based on mechanism of action, Pycnogenol may increase the risk of bleeding when taken with drugs that increase the risk of bleeding. Some examples include aspirin, anticoagulants ("blood thinners") such as warfarin (Coumadin) and heparin, antiplatelet drugs such as clopidogrel (Plavix), and nonsteroidal anti-inflammatory drugs such as ibuprofen (Motrin, Advil) and naproxen (Naprosyn, Aleve).
- Because of proposed immunomodulating activity, Pycnogenol may interfere with immunosuppressant or immunostimulant drugs.
- In theory, Pycnogenol and antioxidants may have additive effects.

Interactions with Herbs and Dietary Supplements

- Although data have yet to confirm this claim, it has been proposed that Pycnogenol may increase vitamin C levels.
- Based on mechanism of action, Pycnogenol may lower blood sugar levels. Caution is advised when using herbs or supplements that may also lower blood sugar levels. Blood glucose levels may require monitoring, and doses may need adjustment. Possible examples include *Aloe vera*, American ginseng, bilberry, bitter melon, burdock, dandelion, devil's claw, fenugreek, fish oil, gymnema, horse chestnut seed extract

(HCSE), maitake mushroom, marshmallow, melatonin, milk thistle, *Panax ginseng*, rosemary, shark cartilage, Siberian ginseng, stinging nettle, and white horehound.

- In theory, Pycnogenol may increase the risk of bleeding when taken with herbs and supplements that are believed to increase the risk of bleeding. Multiple cases of bleeding have been reported with the use of *Ginkgo biloba*, and fewer cases with garlic and saw palmetto. Numerous other agents may theoretically increase the risk of bleeding, although this has not been proven in most cases. Some examples include alfalfa, American ginseng, angelica, anise, *Arnica montana*, asafetida, aspen bark, bilberry, birch, black cohosh, bladderwrack, bogbean, boldo, borage seed oil, bromelain, capsicum, cat's claw, celery, chamomile, chaparral, clove, coleus, cordyceps, danshen, devil's claw, dong quai, EPA (eicosapentaenoic acid, found in fish oils), evening primrose oil, fenugreek, feverfew, fish oil, flaxseed/flax powder (not a concern with flaxseed oil), ginger, grapefruit juice, grape seed, green tea, guggul, gymnestra, horse chestnut, horseradish, licorice root, lovage root, male fern, meadowsweet, nordihydroguaiaretic acid (NDGA), omega-3 fatty acids, onion, papain, *Panax ginseng*, parsley, passion flower, poplar, prickly ash, propolis, quassia, red clover, reishi, rue, Siberian ginseng, sweet birch, sweet clover, turmeric, vitamin E, white willow, wild carrot, wild lettuce, willow, wintergreen, and yucca.
- In theory, Pycnogenol may interact with herbs and supplements that affect blood pressure. Potential hypotensive herbs include aconite/monkshood, arnica, baneberry, betel nut, bilberry, black cohosh, bryony, calendula, California poppy, coleus, curcumin, eucalyptol, eucalyptus oil, flaxseed/flaxseed oil, garlic, ginger, ginkgo, goldenseal, green hellebore, hawthorn, Indian tobacco, jaborandi, mistletoe, night-blooming cereus, oleander, pasque flower, periwinkle, pleurisy root, *Polypodium vulgare*, shepherd's purse, Texas milkweed, turmeric, wild cherry. Potential hypertensive herbs include American ginseng, arnica, bayberry, betel nut, blue cohosh, broom, cayenne, cola, coltsfoot, ephedra/ma huang, ginger, licorice, and yerba mate.
- Because of proposed immunomodulating activity, Pycnogenol may interfere with immunosuppressant or immunostimulant herbs and supplements.
- In theory, Pycnogenol and other antioxidants may have additive effects.

Selected References

Natural Standard developed the preceding evidence-based information based on a systematic review of more than 70 scientific articles. For comprehensive information about alternative and complementary therapies on the professional level, go to www.naturalstandard.com. Selected references are listed here.

Araghi-Niknam M, Hosseini S, Larson D, et al. Pine bark extract reduces platelet aggregation. Integr Med 2000;2(2):73-77.

Arcangeli P. Pycnogenol in chronic venous insufficiency. Fitoterapia 2000;71(3):236-244.

Bito T, Roy S, Sen CK, Packer L. Pine bark extract pycnogenol downregulates IFN-gamma-induced adhesion of T cells to human keratinocytes by inhibiting inducible ICAM-1 expression. Free Radic Biol Med 2000;28(2):219-227.

Bors W, Michel C, Stettmaier K. Electron paramagnetic resonance studies of radical species of proanthocyanidins and gallant esters. Arch Biochem Biophys 2000;374(2):347-355.

Buz'Zard AR, Peng Q, Lau BH. Kyolic and Pycnogenol increase human growth hormone secretion in genetically-engineered keratinocytes. Growth Horm IGF Res 2002;12(1):34-40.

Cheshier JE, Ardestani-Kaboudanian S, Liang B, et al. Immunomodulation by pycnogenol in retrovirus-infected or ethanol-fed mice. Life Sci 1996;58(5):PL 87-96.

Chida M, Suzuki K, Nakanishi-Ueda T, et al. *In vitro* testing of antioxidants and biochemical end-points in bovine retinal tissue. Ophthalmic Res 1999;31(6):407-415.

Cho KJ, Yun CH, Packer L, Chung AS. Inhibition mechanisms of bioflavonoids extracted from

P

the bark of *Pinus maritime* on the expression of proinflammatory cytokines. Ann N Y Acad Sci 2001;928:141-156.

Cho KJ, Yun CH, Yoon DY, et al. Effect of bioflavonoids extracted from the bark of *Pinus maritime* on proinflammatory cytokine interleukin-1 production in lipopolysaccharide-stimulated RAW 264.7. Toxicol Appl Pharmacol 2000;168(1):64-71.

Devaraj S, Vega-Lopez S, Kaul S, et al. Supplementation with a pine bark extract rich in polyphenols increases plasma antioxidant capacity and alters the plasma lipoprotein profile. Lipids 2002;37(10):931-934.

Feng WH, Wei HL, Liu GT. Effect of PYCNOGENOL on the toxicity of heart, bone marrow and immune organs as induced by antitumor drugs. Phytomedicine 2002;9(5):414-418.

Fitzpatrick DF, Bing B, Rohdewald P. Endothelium-dependent vascular effects of Pycnogenol. J Cardiovasc Pharmacol 1998;32(4):509-515.

Hasegawa N. Inhibition of lipogenesis by pycnogenol. Phytother Res 2000;14(6):472-473.

Hasegawa N. Stimulation of lipolysis by pycnogenol. Phytother Res 1999;13(7):619-620.

Horakova L, Licht A, Sandig G, et al. Standardized extracts of flavonoids increase the viability of PC12 cells treated with hydrogen peroxide: effects on oxidative injury. Arch Toxicol 2003;77(1):22-29.

Hosseini S, Pishnamazi S, Sadrzadeh SM, et al. Pycnogenol in the management of asthma. J Med Food 2001;4(4):201-209.

Huynh HT, Teel RW. Effects of intragastrically administered Pycnogenol on NNK metabolism in F344 rats. Anticancer Res 1999;19(3A):2095-2099.

Huynh HT, Teel RW. Effects of pycnogenol on the microsomal metabolism of the tobacco-specific nitrosamine NNK as a function of age. Cancer Lett 1998;132(1-2):135-139.

Huynh HT, Teel RW. Selective induction of apoptosis in human mammary cancer cells (MCF-7) by pycnogenol. Anticancer Res 2000;20(4):2417-2420.

Kim HC, Healey JM. Effects of pine bark extract administered to immunosuppressed adult mice infected with *Cryptosporidium parvum*. Am J Chin Med 2001;29(3-4):469-475.

Kim J, Chehade J, Pinnas JL, Mooradian AD. Effect of select antioxidants on malodialdehyde modification of proteins. Nutrition 2000;16(11-12):1079-1081.

Kimbrough C, Chun M, dela Roca G, Lau BH. Pycnogenol chewing gum minimizes gingival bleeding and plaque formation. Phytomedicine 2002;9(5):410-413.

Kobayashi MS, Han D, Packer L. Antioxidants and herbal extracts protect HT-4 neuronal cells against glutamate-induced cytotoxicity. Free Radic Res 2000;32(2):115-124.

Koch R. Comparative study of Venostasin and Pycnogenol in chronic venous insufficiency. Phytother Res 2002;16(Suppl 1):S1-S5.

Liu F, Lau BH, Peng Q, Shah V. Pycnogenol protects vascular endothelial cells from beta-amyloid-inducted injury. Biol Pharm Bull 2000;23(6):735-737.

Liu FJ, Zhang YX, Lau BH. Pycnogenol enhances immune and haemopoietic functions in senescence-accelerated mice. Cell Mol Life Sci 1998;54(10):1168-1172.

Macrides TA, Shihata A, Kalafatis N, Wright PF. A comparison of the hydroxyl radical scavenging properties of the shark bile steroid 5 beta-scymnol and plant pycnogenols. Biochem Mol Biol Int 1997;42(6):1249-1260.

Maritim A, Dene BA, Sanders RA, Watkins JB 3rd. Effects of pycnogenol treatment on oxidative stree in streptozotocin-induced diabetic rats. J Biochem Mol Toxicol 2003;17(3): 193-199.

Masquelier J. Flavonoids and pycnogenols. Int J Vitam Nutr Res 1979; 49:307-11.

Moini H, Guo Q, Packe L. Xanthine oxidase and xanthine dehydrogenase inhibition by the procyanidin-rich French maritime pine bark extract, pycnogenol: a protein binding effect. Adv Exp Med Biol 2002;505:141-149.

Moini H, Guo Q, Packer L. Enzyme inhibition and protein-binding action of procyanidin-rich French maritime pine bark extract, pycnogenol: effect on xanthine oxidase. J Agric Food Chem 2000;48(11):5630-5639.

Nelson A, Lau B, Ide N, Rong Y. Pycnogenol inhibits macrophage oxidative burst, lipoprotein oxidation, and hydroxyl radical induced DNA damage. Drug Devel Industr Pharm 1998; 24:139-144.

Ni Z, Mu Y, Gulati O. Treatment of melasma with Pycnogenol. Phytother Res 2002;16(6): 567-571.

Noda Y, Anzai K, Mori A, Kohno M, et al. Hydroxyl and superoxide anion radical scavenging activities of natural source antioxidants using the computerized JES-FR30 ESR spectrometer system. Biochem Mol Biol Int 1997;42(1):35-44.
Ohnishi ST, Ohnishi T, Ogunmola GB. Sickle cell anemia: a potential nutritional approach for a molecular disease. Nutrition 2000;16(5):330-338.
Packer L, Rimbach G, Virgili F. Antioxidant activity and biologic properties of a procyanidin-rich extract from pine (*Pinus maritime*) bark, pycnogenol. Free Radic Biol Med 1999; 27(5-6):704-724.
Park YC, Rimbach G, Saliou C, et al. Activity of monomeric, dimeric, and trimeric flavonoids on NO production, TNF-alpha secretion, and NF-kappaB-dependent gene expression in RAW 264.7 macrophages. FEBS Lett 2000;465(2-3):93-97.
Peng Q, Wei Z, Lau BH. Pycnogenol inhibits tumor necrosis factor-alpha-induced nuclear factor kappa B activation and adhesion molecule expression in human vascular endothelial cells. Cell Mol Life Sci 2000;57(5):834-841.
Peng QL, Buz'Zard AR, Lau BH. Pycnogenol protects neurons from amyloid-beta peptide-induced apoptosis. Brain Res Mol Brain Res 2002;104(1):55-65.
Petrassi C, Mastromarino A, Spartera C. Pycnogenol in chronic venous insufficiency. Phytomedicine 2000;7(5):383-388.
Putter M, Grotemeyer KH, Wurthwein G, et al. Inhibition of smoking-induced platelet aggregation by aspirin and pycnogenol. Thromb Res 1999;95(4):155-161.
Rihn B, Saliou C, Bottin MC, et al. From ancient remedies to modern therapeutics: pine bark uses in skin disorders revisited. Phytother Res 2001;15(1):76-78.
Rohdewald P. A review of the French maritime pine bark extract (Pycnogenol), a herbal medication with a diverse clinical pharmacology. Int J Clin Pharmacol Ther 2002;40(4):158-168.
Rong Y, Li L, Shah V, Lau BH. Pycnogenol protects vascular endothelial cells from t-butyl hydroperoxide induced oxidant injury. Biotechnol Ther 1994-95;5(3-4):117-126.
Roseff SJ. Improvement of sperm quality and function with French maritime pine tree bark extract. J Reprod Med 2002;47(10):821-824.
Saliou C, Rimbach G, Moini H, et al. Solar ultraviolet-induced erythema in human skin and nuclear factor-kappa-B-dependent gene expression in keratinocytes are modulated by a French maritime pine bark extract. Free Radic Biol Med 2001;30(2):154-160.
Schonlau F, Rohdewald P. Pycnogenol for diabetic retinopathy. A review. Int Ophthalmol 2001; 24(3):161-171.
Sharma SC, Sharma S, Gulati OP. Pycnogenol inhibits the release of histamine from mast cells. Phytother Res 2003;17(1):66-69.
Sharma SC, Sharma S, Gulati OP. Pycnogenol prevents haemolytic injury in G6PD deficient human erythrocytes. Phytother Res 2003;17(6):671-674.
Silliman K, Parry J, Kirk LL, Prior RL. Pycnogenol does not impact the antioxidant or vitamin C status of healthy young adults. J Am Diet Assoc 2003;103(1):67-72.
Spadea L, Balestrazzi E. Treatment of vascular retinopathies with Pycnogenol. Phytother Res 2001;15(3):219-223.
Stanislavov R, Nikolova V. Treatment of erectile dysfunction with pycnogenol and L-arginine. J Sex Marital Ther 2003;29(3):207-213.
Stefanescu M, Matach C, Onu A, et al. Pycnogenol efficacy in the treatment of systemic lupus erythematosus. Phytother Res 2001;15(8):698-704.
Suarez-Almazor ME, Kendall CJ, Dorgan M. Surfing the Net – information on the World Wide Web for persons with arthritis: patient empowerment or patient deceit? J Rheumatol 2001; 28(1):185-191.
Tenebaum S, Paull JC, Sparrow EP. An experimental comparison of Pycnogenol and methylphenidate in adults with Attention-Deficit/Hyperactivity Disorder (ADHD). J Atten Disord 2002;6(2):49-60.
van Jaarsveld H, Kuyl JM, Schulenburg DH, Wiid NM. Effect of flavonoids on the outcome of myocardial mitochondrial ischemia/reperfusion injury. Res Commun Mol Pathol Pharmacol 1996;91(1):65-75.
Veurink G, Liu D, Taddei K, et al. Reduction of inclusion body pathology in ApoE-deficient mice fed a combination of antioxidants. Free Radic Biol Med 2003;34(8):1070-1077.
Virgili F, Kim D, Packer L. Procyanidins extracted from pine bark protect alpha-tocopherol in

ECV 304 endothelial cells challenged by activated RAW 264.7 macrophages: role of nitric oxide and peroxynitrite. FEBS Lett 1998;431(3):315-318.

Virgili F, Kobuchi H, Packer L. Procyanidins extracted from *Pinus maritime* (Pycnogenol): scavengers of free radical species and modulators of nitrogen monoxide metabolism in activated murine RAW 264.7 macrophages. Free Radic Biol Med 1998;24(7-8):1120-1129.

Wang MY, Su C. Cancer preventive effect of *Morinda citrifolia* (Noni). Ann N Y Acad Sci 2001;952:161-168.

Watson, R. Reduction of cardiovascular disease risk factors by French Maritime Pine Bark Extract. Cardiovascular Reviews and Reports 1999; XX(VI): 326-329.

Wei Z, Peng Q, Lau B. Pycnogenol enhances endothelial cell antioxidant defenses. Redox Report 1997;3:219-24.

Pygeum

(*Prunus africanum, Pygeum africanum*)

RELATED TERMS

- African plum tree, African prune tree, African *Pygeum africanum* extract, alumty, iluo, kirah, Natal tree, *Pigeum africanum*, Pigenil, Pronitol, Provol, prunier d'afrique, *Pygeum africana*, Rosaceae, Tadenan, V1326, vla, wotangue.

BACKGROUND

- The *P. africanum* (African plum) tree is a tall evergreen of the family Rosaceae found in central and southern Africa. Its bark has been used medicinally for thousands of years. Traditional African healers have used the bark to treat bladder and micturition (urination) disorders, particularly symptoms associated with benign prostatic hypertrophy (BPH). Historically, the bark was powdered and used to make a tea which was taken by mouth for these conditions.
- The African plum tree has become endangered because of the demand for its bark to process *P. africanum* extract.
- The majority of trials conducted since the 1970s report improvements in BPH symptoms with the administration of *P. africanum* bark extract, including frequency of nocturia (nighttime urination), urine flow rate, and residual urine volume. This research has led some credibility to the common use of this agent in Europe for BPH. The herb is less commonly used in the United States, where prescription drugs or the herb saw palmetto is more commonly used.

P

USES BASED ON SCIENTIFIC EVIDENCE	Grade*
Benign prostatic hypertrophy/BPH symptoms Pygeum (*P. africanum* bark extract) has been observed to moderately improve urinary symptoms associated with enlargement of the prostate gland or prostate inflammation. Numerous controlled trials in humans, and studies that combine the results of other research (meta-analyses), report pygeum to significantly reduce the number of nighttime urinary episodes (nocturia), urinary hesitancy, urinary frequency, and dysuria (pain with urination) in men who experience mild-to-moderate symptoms. However, pygeum does not appear to reduce the size of the prostate gland or reverse the process of BPH. It is unclear how pygeum compares with the effectiveness or safety of other medical therapies, such as prescription drugs (such as alpha-adrenergic blockers or 5 alpha-reductase inhibitors), surgical approaches, and other herbs/supplements such as saw palmetto. Although many of the available studies are not well designed or reported, the weight of scientific evidence supports the benefits of pygeum. Better research would strengthen the scientific support for	**B**

Continued

this therapy, and there is ongoing study in this area. It is recommended that patients with BPH speak with their healthcare provider about the various available treatment options.

Most studies have used the European brand Tadenan. The mechanism of action of pygeum remains unclear. Early research reports reductions in urethral obstruction and improved bladder function. Laboratory studies report inhibition of enzymes including 5-lipoxygenase and 5 alpha-reductase, a mechanism similar to that of the prescription drug finasteride. Stimulation of secretory activity of the prostate and seminal vesicles is reported in rats and humans, and some estrogen-like properties are noted, as well as anti-inflammatory properties.

*Key to grades: *A:* Strong scientific evidence for this use; *B:* Good scientific evidence for this use; *C:* Unclear scientific evidence for this use; *D:* Fair scientific evidence against this use (it may not work); *F:* Strong scientific evidence against this use (it likely does not work). For a more detailed explanation of efficacy criteria, see "Natural Standard Evidence-Based Validated Grading Rationale" in the Introduction.

Uses Based on Tradition, Theory, or Limited Scientific Evidence

Aphrodisiac, bladder sphincter disorders, fever, impotence, inflammation, kidney disease, malaria, male baldness, partial bladder outlet obstruction, prostate cancer, prostatic adenoma, prostatitis, psychosis, sexual performance, stomach upset, urinary tract health.

DOSING

The following doses are based on scientific research, publications, traditional use, or expert opinion. Many herbs and supplements have not been thoroughly tested, and safety and effectiveness may not be proven. Brands may be made differently, with variable ingredients even within the same brand. The doses shown may not apply to all products. It is important to always read product labels and discuss doses with a qualified healthcare provider before therapy is started.

Standardization

- Standardization involves measuring the amounts of certain chemicals in products to try to make different preparations similar to each other. It is not always known if the chemicals being measured are the "active" ingredients.
- The active component(s) of *P. africanum* bark extract has not been identified.
- Tadenan (Laboratoires DEBAT, Garches, France), the most popular and commonly studied brand in Europe, is a lipophilic extract of *P. africanum* standardized to 13% total sterols. Other guidelines specify standardization to 14% triterpenes with 0.5% n-docosanol. One capsule of Tadenan contains 50 mg of standardized extract.
- Other studied brands include Pigenil (Inverni della Beffa, Milan, Italy), Harzol (Hoyer, Germany), and Prostatonin (Pharmaton SA, Lugano, Switzerland). Some brands may contain other herbs in addition to pygeum.
- Safety of use of pygeum beyond 12 months has not been reliably studied.

Adults (18 Years and Older)

- **Capsules:** For treating benign prostatic hypertrophy, 75- to 200-mg capsules of standardized pygeum extract taken daily by mouth, either as a single dose or divided into two equal doses, have been used and studied.

Children (Younger Than 18 Years)

- There are not enough scientific data to recommend pygeum for use in children, and pygeum is not recommended because of potential side effects.

SAFETY

The U.S. Food and Drug Administration does not strictly regulate herbs and supplements. There is no guarantee of strength, purity, or safety of products, and effects may vary. It is important to always read product labels. People who have a medical condition, or are taking other drugs, herbs, or supplements, should consult a qualified healthcare provider before starting a new therapy. A healthcare provider should be contacted immediately about any side effects.

Allergies

- People with known allergies to pygeum should avoid this herb.

Side Effects and Warnings

- Pygeum has been well tolerated in most studies, with adverse effects similar to placebo (sugar pill). Some people may experience stomach discomfort, including diarrhea, constipation, stomach pain, and nausea. Stomach upset is usually mild and does not typically cause people to stop using pygeum.
- Safety of use beyond 12 months has not been reliably studied.

Pregnancy and Breastfeeding

- Pygeum cannot be recommended during pregnancy or breastfeeding because of a lack of scientific information and possible hormonal effects.

INTERACTIONS

Most herbs and supplements have not been thoroughly tested for interactions with other herbs, supplements, drugs, or foods. The interactions listed here are based on reports in scientific publications, laboratory experiments, or traditional use. It is important to always read product labels. People who have a medical condition, or are taking other drugs, herbs, or supplements, should consult a qualified healthcare provider before starting a new therapy.

Interactions with Drugs

- Use of pygeum with other drugs commonly used to treat symptoms of prostate enlargement, called 5 alpha-reductase inhibitors, such as terazosin (Hytrin) and finasteride (Propecia, Proscar), may increase beneficial effects, although this is not well studied.
- In theory, pygeum may interact with estrogen or other hormones.

Interactions with Herbs and Dietary Supplements

- Pygeum may result in increased beneficial effects for the prostate if used with saw palmetto (*Serenoa repens*) or stinging nettle (*Urtica dioica*). Combination products are available containing both stinging nettle and pygeum.

- Pygeum may interact with herbs/supplements containing chemicals with estrogen-like effects (phytoestrogens). Possible examples include alfalfa, black cohosh, bloodroot, burdock, hops, kudzu, licorice, pomegranate, red clover, soy, thyme, white horehound, and yucca.

Selected References

Natural Standard developed the preceding evidence-based information based on a systematic review of more than 110 articles. For comprehensive information about alternative and complementary therapies on the professional level, go to www.naturalstandard.com. Selected references are listed here.

Andro M, Riffaud J. *Pygeum africanum* extract for the treatment of patients with benign prostatic hyperplasia: a review of 25 years of published experience. Curr Ther Res 1995; 56(8):796-817.

Barlet A, Albrecht J, Aubert A, et al. [Efficacy of *Pygeum africanum* extract in the medical therapy of urination disorders due to benign prostatic hyperplasia: evaluation of objective and subjective parameters. A placebo-controlled double-blind multicenter study]. Wien Klin Wochenschr 1990;102(22):667-673.

Bassi P, Artibani W, De L, V, et al. [Standardized extract of *Pygeum africanum* in the treatment of benign prostatic hypertrophy. Controlled clinical study versus placebo]. Minerva Urol Nefrol 1987;39(1):45-50.

Berges RR, Windeler J, Trampisch HJ, et al. Randomised, placebo-controlled, double-blind clinical trial of beta- sitosterol in patients with benign prostatic hyperplasia. Beta- sitosterol Study Group. Lancet 1995;345(8964):1529-1532.

Blitz M, Garbit JL, Masson JC, et al. [Controlled study on the effect of a medical treatment on subjects consulting for the first time for prostatic adenoma]. Lyon Mediterr Med 1985;21:11.

Bongi G. [Tadenan in the treatment of prostatic adenoma. Anatomo-clinical study]. Minerva Urol 1972;24(4):129-139.

Brackman F, Autet W. Once and twice daily dosage regimens of *Pygeum africanum* extract (PA): a double-blind study in patients with benign prostatic hyperplasia (BPH) [abstract]. J Urology 1999;161(4S):361.

Breza J, Dzurny O, Borowka A, et al. Efficacy and acceptability of tadenan (*Pygeum africanum* extract) in the treatment of benign prostatic hyperplasia (BPH): a multicentre trial in central Europe. Curr Med Res Opin 1998;14(3):127-139.

Chatelain C, Autet W, Brackman F. Comparison of once and twice daily dosage forms of *Pygeum africanum* extract in patients with benign prostatic hyperplasia: a randomized, double-blind study, with long-term open label extension. Urology 1999;54(3):473-478.

Choo M, Constantinou CE, Bellamy F. Beneficial effects of *Pygeum africanum* extract (PA) on dihydrotestosterone (DHT) induced modifications of micturition and prostate growth in rat [abstract]. J Urology 1999;161(4S):229.

Choo MS, Bellamy F, Constantinou CE. Functional evaluation of Tadenan on micturition and experimental prostate growth induced with exogenous dihydrotestosterone. Urology 2000; 55(2):292-298.

Clavert A, Cranz C, Riffaud JP, et al. [Effects of an extract of the bark of *Pygeum africanum* (V.1326) on prostatic secretions in the rat and in man]. Annales D'Urologie 1986;20(5): 341-343.

Donkervoort T, Sterling A, van Ness J, et al. A clinical and urodynamic study of tadenan in the treatment of benign prostatic hypertrophy. Eur Urol 1977;3(4):218-225.

Dufour B, Choquenet C, Revol M, et al. [Controlled study of the effects of *Pygeum africanum* extract on the functional symptoms of prostatic adenoma]. Ann Urol (Paris) 1984;18(3): 193-195.

Dutkiewicz S. Usefulness of Cernilton in the treatment of benign prostatic hyperplasia. Int Urol Nephrol 1996;28(1):49-53.

Frasseto G, Bertoglio S, Mancuso S, et al. [Study of the efficacy and tolerability of Tadenan 50 in patients with prostatic hypertrophy]. Progresso Medico 1986;42:49-53.

Gagliardi V, Apicella F, Pino P, et al. Terapia medica dell'ipertrofia prostatica. Sperimentazione clinica controllata. Arch Ital Urol Nefrol Andrologia 1983;55:51-59.

Giacobini S, von Heland M, de Natale G, et al. Valutazione clinica e morfo-funzionale del trattamento a doppio cieco con placebo, Tadenan 50 e Tadenan 50 associato a Farlutal nei pazienti con ipertrofia prostatica benigna. Antologia Medica Italiana 1986;6:1-10.

Ishani A, MacDonald R, Nelson D, et al. *Pygeum africanum* for the treatment of patients with benign prostatic hyperplasia: a systematic review and quantitative meta-analysis. Am J Med 2000;109(8):654-664.

Krzeski T, Kazon M, Borkowski A, et al. Combined extracts of Urtica dioica and *Pygeum africanum* in the treatment of benign prostatic hyperplasia: double-blind comparison of two doses. Clin Ther 1993;15(6):1011-1020.

Levin RM, Riffaud JP, Bellamy F, et al. Protective effect of Tadenan on bladder function secondary to partial outlet obstruction. J Urol 1996;155(4):1466-1470.

Levin RM, Das AK. A scientific basis for the therapeutic effects of *Pygeum africanum* and Serenoa repens. Urol Res 2000;28(3):201-209.

Mandressi A, Tarallo U, Maggioni A, et al. Terapia medica dell'adenoma prostatico: confronto della efficacia dell'estratto di Serenoa repens (Permixon) versus l'estratto di Pigeum africanum e placebo. Valutazione in doppio cieco. Urologia 1983;50(4):752-757.

Mathe G, Hallard M, Bourut CH, et al. A *Pygeum africanum* extract with so-called phyto-estrogenic action markedly reduces the volume of true and large prostatic hypertrophy. Biomed Pharmacother 1995;49(7-8):341-343.

Mathe G, Orbach-Arbouys S, Bizi E, et al. The so-called phyto-estrogenic action of *Pygeum africanum* extract. Biomed Pharmacother 1995;49(7-8):339-340.

Maver A. [Medical treatment of fibroadenomatous hypertrophy of the prostate with a new plant substance]. Minerva Med 1972;63(37):2126-2136.

Mehrsai AR, Pourmand G, Taheri M. Evaluation of the clinical and urodynamic effects of *Pygeum africanum* (Tadenan) in the treatment of benign prostatic hyperplasia (BPH) [abstract]. Br J Urol 1997;80(suppl 2):227.

Paubert-Braquet M, Cave A, Hocquemiller R, et al. Effect of *Pygeum africanum* extract on A23187-stimulated production of lipoxygenase metabolites from human polymorphonuclear cells. J Lipid Mediat Cell Signal 1994;9(3):285-290.

Ranno S, Minaldi G, Viscusi G, et al. [Efficacy and tolerability in the treatment of prostatic adenoma with Tadenan 50]. Progresso Medico 1986;42:165-169.

Rhodes L, Primka RL, Berman C, et al. Comparison of finasteride (Proscar), a 5 alpha reductase inhibitor, and various commercial plant extracts in in vitro and in vivo 5 alpha reductase inhibition. Prostate 1993;22(1):43-51.

Rigatti P, Zennaro F, Fraschini O, et al. L'impegio del Tadenan nell'adenoma prostatico. Ricerca clinica controllata. Atti della Accademia medica lombarda 1983;38:1-4.

Rizzo M. Terapia medica dell'adenoma della prostata: valutazione clinica comparativa tra estratto di *Pygeum africanum* ad alte dosi e placebo. Farmacia Terapia 1985;2:105-110.

Thieblot L, Grizard G, Boucher D. [Effect of V 1326 (active principle of *Pygeum africanum* bark extract) on hypophyseo-genito-adrenal axis in rats]. Therapie 1977;32(1):99-110.

Wilt T, Ishani A, Mac DR, et al. *Pygeum africanum* for benign prostatic hyperplasia (Cochrane Review). Cochrane Database Syst Rev 2002;(1):CD001044.

Yoshimura Y, Yamaguchi O, Bellamy F, et al. Effect of *Pygeum africanum* tadenan on micturition and prostate growth of the rat secondary to coadministered treatment and post-treatment with dihydrotestosterone. Urology 2003;61(2):474-478.

Yablonsky F, Nicolas V, Riffaud JP, et al. Antiproliferative effect of *Pygeum africanum* extract on rat prostatic fibroblasts. J Urol 1997;157(6):2381-2387.

P

Red Clover
(*Trifolium pratense*)

RELATED TERMS

- Ackerklee (German), beebread, cow clover, genistein, isoflavone, isoflavone clover extract (ICE), meadow clover, phytoestrogen, Promensil, purple clover, Rimostil, rotklee (German), trefoil, trefle des pres (French), trifolium pratense, Trinovin, wild clover.

BACKGROUND

- Red clover is a legume, which, like soy, contains phytoestrogens (plant-based chemicals that are similar to estrogen, and may act in the body like estrogen or may actually block the effects of estrogen). Red clover was traditionally used to treat asthma, pertussis, cancer, and gout. In modern times, isoflavone extracts of red clover are most often used to treat menopausal symptoms, as an alternative hormone replacement therapy, for high cholesterol, or to prevent osteoporosis. However, at this time, there are no high-quality human studies supporting the use of red clover for any medical condition.

USES BASED ON SCIENTIFIC EVIDENCE	Grade*
Cardiovascular—blood flow Red clover has been shown to improve the flow of blood through arteries and veins. However there is limited study in this area and more research is needed before a conclusion can be drawn.	C
Diabetes Red clover has been studied in patients with type 2 diabetes to determine potential benefits for diabetic complications such as high blood pressure and narrowing of the arteries and veins. A small randomized, controlled trial studied postmenopausal women with type 2 diabetes. Women were given red clover (approximately 50 mg/day) for 4 weeks and the effects were compared to placebo. Improvements were seen in blood pressure and in the function of the veins and arteries. Another small randomized, controlled clinical trial studied the effects of red clover (86 mg/day) on blood lipids and insulin in pre-menopausal women. The study followed 12 pre-menopausal women for 3 cycles and found that there was no change in the women's lipid profiles or their blood sugar or insulin levels. Further research is needed before a recommendation can be made. If you have diabetes you should contact your healthcare provider before taking red clover.	C

Continued

High cholesterol Red clover has not been clearly shown to have beneficial effects on blood cholesterol levels. One small randomized, controlled clinical trial studied the effects of red clover (86 mg/day) on blood lipids and insulin in pre-menopausal women. The study followed 12 pre-menopausal women for 3 cycles and found that there was no change in the women's lipid profile or their blood sugar or insulin levels. Due to conflicting study results, further research is needed in this area before a recommendation can be made.	C
Hormone replacement therapy (HRT) Laboratory research suggests that red clover isoflavones have estrogen-like activity. However, there is no clear evidence that isoflavones share the possible benefits of estrogens (such as beneficial effects on bone density). In addition, hormone replacement therapy itself is a controversial topic, with recent research reporting that the potential harm may outweigh any benefits.	C
Menopausal symptoms Laboratory research suggests that components of red clover called isoflavones have estrogen-like activity. Red clover isoflavones are proposed to reduce symptoms of menopause (such as hot flashes), and are popular for this use. However, most of the available human studies are poorly designed and short in duration (less than 12 weeks of treatment). In a well-conducted, multicenter randomized, controlled clinical trial the safety and efficacy of two brands of red clover were studied, as well as the effects of both brands compared to placebo on hot flashes. The two brands of red clover were Promensil (82 mg of red clover), and Rimostil (57 mg of red clover). The study included 252 postmenopausal women aged 45 to 60 years who were experiencing at least 35 hot flashes a week, and excluded vegetarians, those who consumed soy products more than once a week or those who took medications that would affect the absorption of the red clover. The study found that neither supplement had a significant effect on hot flashes or other symptoms of menopause. Another randomized, controlled clinical trial studied the effects of red clover (Promensil) vs. placebo on hot flashes. This was a smaller study and included only 30 postmenopausal women who were experiencing more than 5 hot flashes a week. This study found that red clover supplementation (Promensil, providing 80 mg of red clover) significantly decreased the amount of hot flashes that the women experienced. Because results of published studies conflict with each other, more research is needed before a clear conclusion can be drawn.	C
Osteoporosis It is not clear if red clover isoflavones have beneficial effects on bone density. Most studies of isoflavones in this area have looked at soy, which contains different amounts of isoflavones, as well as other non-isoflavone ingredients. More research is needed before a recommendation can be made.	C

R

Continued

Prostate cancer Red clover isoflavones may have estrogen-like properties in the body and have been proposed as a possible therapy for prostate cancer and related hot flashes. Some isoflavones have also been shown in laboratory studies to have anti-cancer properties. Because there is no well-designed human research in this area, a recommendation cannot be made.	C
Prostate enlargement (benign prostatic hypertrophy) There is only limited study of red clover for benign prostatic hypertrophy. More research is needed before a firm conclusion can be drawn.	C

*Key to grades: *A:* Strong scientific evidence for this use; *B:* Good scientific evidence for this use; *C:* Unclear scientific evidence for this use; *D:* Fair scientific evidence against this use (it may not work); *F:* Strong scientific evidence against this use (it likely does not work). For a more detailed explanation of efficacy criteria, see "Natural Standard Evidence-Based Validated Grading Rationale" in the Introduction.

Uses Based on Tradition, Theory, or Limited Scientific Evidence

Acne, AIDS, antibacterial, antioxidant, anti-spasm, appetite suppressant, arthritis, asthma, "blood purification," bronchitis, burns, cancer prevention, canker sores, chronic skin diseases, cough, diuretic (increasing urine flow), eczema, gout, hot flashes, indigestion, mastalgia (breast pain), premenstrual syndrome, psoriasis, sexually transmitted diseases, skin ulcers/sores, sore eyes, tuberculosis, whooping cough (pertussis).

DOSING

The following doses are based on scientific research, publications, traditional use, or expert opinion. Many herbs and supplements have not been thoroughly tested, and safety and effectiveness may not be proven. Brands may be made differently, with variable ingredients even within the same brand. The doses shown may not apply to all products. It is important to always read product labels and discuss doses with a qualified healthcare provider before therapy is started.

Standardization

- Standardization involves measuring the amounts of certain chemicals in products to try to make different preparations similar to each other. It is not always known if the chemicals being measured are the "active" ingredients.
- The brand of red clover extract used in most trials, and which is most commonly available, is Promensil. Each tablet, composed of 40 mg of total isoflavones, is standardized to contain the following components: 4 mg of genistein, 3.5 mg of daidzein, 24.5 mg of biochanin A, and 8.0 mg of formononetin.

Adults (18 Years and Older)

- **Menopausal symptoms:** 40 mg, 80 mg, or 160 mg of red clover isoflavones per day (Promensil) has been studied. Rimostil (57 mg of red clover) has also been used.
- **Hormone replacement:** 40 to 80 mg of red clover isoflavones per day (Promensil) has been studied.
- **High cholesterol:** 28 to 86 mg of red clover isoflavones per day (Rimostil) and 80 mg of red clover isoflavones per day (Promensil) have been studied.
- **Osteoporosis:** 40 mg of red clover isoflavones per day (Promensil) has been studied.
- **Benign prostatic hypertrophy:** 40 mg of red clover isoflavones per day (Trinovin) has been studied.
- **Diabetes:** 50 mg and 86 mg per day of red clover isoflavones per day have been studied for diabetic complications.

Children (Younger Than 18 Years)

- There is not enough scientific evidence to recommend use of red clover in children.

SAFETY

The U.S. Food and Drug Administration does not strictly regulate herbs and supplements. There is no guarantee of strength, purity, or safety of products, and effects may vary. It is important to always read product labels. People who have a medical condition, or are taking other drugs, herbs, or supplements, should consult a qualified healthcare provider before starting a new therapy. A healthcare provider should be contacted immediately about any side effects.

R

Allergies

- People with known allergies or reactions to products containing red clover or isoflavones should avoid taking red clover.

Side Effects and Warnings

- A small number of human studies using red clover extracts have all reported good tolerance, without serious side effects after up to 1 year of treatment. In theory, based on the estrogen-like action of red clover seen in laboratory studies, side effects may include weight gain and breast tenderness, although these have not been reported clearly in humans. In theory, menstrual changes and increased uterus cell growth (endometrial hyperplasia) may also occur, although preliminary short-term studies (less than 6 months) have found no increases in uterus wall (endometrial) thickness with red clover. Red clover may affect hormonal levels of gonadotropin-releasing hormone (GrH), follicle-stimulating hormone (FSH), and leutinizing hormone (LH), although early research has not found significant change in FSH or LH levels.
- In theory, red clover may increase the risk of bleeding. However, there are no reliable human reports of bleeding with red clover. Caution is advised in patients with bleeding disorders or taking drugs that may increase the risk of bleeding. Dosing adjustments may be necessary.
- Red clover has been studied for lowering blood sugar with inconclusive results. Caution is warranted until further research is available.

Pregnancy and Breastfeeding

- Red clover is not recommended during pregnancy and breastfeeding, because of its estrogen-like activity. Red clover has been reported as a possible cause of infertility and abortion in grazing livestock.

INTERACTIONS

Most herbs and supplements have not been thoroughly tested for interactions with other herbs, supplements, drugs, or foods. The interactions listed here are based on reports in scientific publications, laboratory experiments, or traditional use. It is important to always read product labels. People who have a medical condition, or are taking other drugs, herbs, or supplements, should consult a qualified healthcare provider before starting a new therapy.

Interactions with Drugs

- Based on laboratory studies, red clover may interfere with the way the liver processes some drugs using an enzyme called cytochrome P450 3A4. As a result, the levels of these drugs may be increased in the blood, and may cause increased effects or potentially serious adverse reactions. People who are using any medications should always read the package insert and consult their healthcare provider or pharmacist about possible interactions.
- In theory, red clover may increase the risk of bleeding when taken with drugs that increase the risk of bleeding. Some examples include aspirin, anticoagulants ("blood thinners") such as warfarin (Coumadin) or heparin, anti-platelet drugs such as clopidogrel (Plavix), and nonsteroidal anti-inflammatory drugs such as ibuprofen (Motrin, Advil) and naproxen (Naprosyn, Aleve). Because red clover contains estrogen-like chemicals, the effects of drugs with estrogen or estrogen-like properties may be altered, such as birth control pills or hormone replacement therapies like Premarin and Provera.
- Red clover has been studied for lowering blood sugar with inconclusive results. Caution is warranted if you are diabetic or taking other medications that may lower blood sugar until further research is available.

Interactions with Herbs and Dietary Supplements

- Based on laboratory studies, red clover may interfere with the way the liver processes some drugs using an enzyme called cytochrome P450 3A4. As a result, red clover may cause the levels of other herbs or supplements to be too high in the blood. It may also alter the effects that other herbs or supplements possibly have on the P450 system, such as bloodroot, cat's claw, chamomile, chaparral, chasteberry, damiana, *Echinacea angustifolia*, goldenseal, grapefruit juice, licorice, oregano, St. John's wort, wild cherry, and yucca. People who are using any herbal medications or dietary supplements should always read the package insert and consult their healthcare provider and pharmacist about possible interactions.
- In theory, red clover may increase the risk of bleeding when taken with herbs or supplements that increase the risk of bleeding. Multiple cases of bleeding have been reported with the use of *Ginkgo biloba*, fewer cases with garlic, and two cases with saw palmetto. Numerous other agents may theoretically increase the risk of bleeding, although this has not been proven in most cases. Some examples include alfalfa, American ginseng, angelica, anise, *Arnica montana*, asafetida, aspen bark, bilberry, birch, black cohosh, bladderwrack, bogbean, boldo, borage seed oil, bromelain, capsicum, cat's claw, celery, chamomile, chaparral, clove, coleus,

cordyceps, danshen, devil's claw, dong quai, evening primrose, fenugreek, feverfew, flaxseed/flax powder (not a concern with flaxseed oil), ginger, grapefruit juice, grape seed, green tea, guggul, gymnestra, horse chestnut, horseradish, licorice root, lovage root, male fern, meadowsweet, nordihydroguaiaretic acid (NDGA), onion, papain, *Panax ginseng*, parsley, passionflower, poplar, prickly ash, propolis, quassia, reishi, rue, Siberian ginseng, sweet birch, sweet clover, turmeric, vitamin E, white willow, wild carrot, wild lettuce, willow, wintergreen, and yucca.

- Because red clover contains estrogen-like chemicals, the effects of other agents believed to have estrogen-like properties may be altered. Possible examples include alfalfa, black cohosh, bloodroot, burdock, hops, kudzu, licorice, pomegranate, soy, thyme, white horehound, and yucca.
- Red clover has been studied for lowering blood sugar with inconclusive results. Caution is warranted if you are diabetic or taking other herbs or supplements that may lower blood sugar until further research is available.

Interactions with Foods

- Red clover has been on the U.S. Food and Drug Administration GRAS ("generally recognized as safe") list and is included in many beverages and teas. It is believed that the amounts found in these beverages may be too small to have significant effects in the body.

Selected References

Natural Standard developed the preceding evidence-based information based on a systematic review of more than 200 scientific articles. For comprehensive information about alternative and complementary therapies on the professional level, go to www.naturalstandard.com. Selected references are listed here.

R

Abernathy K, Brockie J, Suffling K, et al. An open study of the effects of a 40 mg isoflavone food supplement (derived from red clover), on menopausal symptoms [abstract]. Brit Menopause Soc (2001).

Atkinson C, Compston JE, Robins SP, et al. The effects of isoflavone phytoestrogens on bone: Preliminary results from a large randomized controlled trial. Endocr Soc Annu Meet Program 2000;82:196.

Baber RJ, Templeman C, Morton T, et al. Randomized placebo-controlled trial of an isoflavone supplement and menopausal symptoms in women. Climacteric 1999;2:85-92.

Barnes S. Phyto-oestrogens and osteoporosis: what is a safe dose? Br J Nutr. 2003 Jun;89(Suppl 1):S101-108.

Beck V, Unterrieder E, Krenn L, et al. Comparison of hormonal activity (estrogen, androgen and progestin) of standardized plant extracts for large scale use in hormone replacement therapy. J Steroid Biochem Mol Biol 2003;84(2-3):259-268.

Blakesmith SJ, Lyons-Wall PM, George C, et al. Effects of supplementation with purified red clover (*Trifolium pratense*) isoflavones on plasma lipids and insulin resistance in healthy premenopausal women. Br J Nutr 2003;89(4):467-474.

Boue SM, Wiese TE, Nehls S, et al. Evaluation of the estrogenic effects of legume extracts containing phytoestrogens. J Agric Food Chem 2003;51(8):2193-2199.

Clifton-Bligh PB, Baber RJ, Fulcher GR, et al. The effect of isoflavones extracted from red clover (Rimostil) on lipid and bone metabolism. Menopause 2001;8(4):259-265.

Garcia-Martinez MC, Hermenegildo C, Tarin JJ, Cano A. Phytoestrogens increase the capacity of serum to stimulate prostacyclin release in human endothelial cells. Acta Obstet Gynecol Scand 2003;82(8):705-710.

Gerber G, Lowe FC, Spigekman S. The use of a standardized extract of red clover isoflavones for the alleviation of BPH symptoms. The Endocrine Society's 82nd Annual Meeting 2000;82:2359.

Howes JB, Sullivan D, Lai N, et al. The effects of dietary supplementation with isoflavones from red clover on the lipoprotein profiles of post menopausal women with mild to moderate hypercholesterolaemia. Atherosclerosis 2000;152(1):143-147.
Howes JB, Tran D, Brillante D, Howes LG. Effects of dietary supplementation with isoflavones from red clover on ambulatory blood pressure and endothelial function in postmenopausal type 2 diabetes. Diabetes Obes Metab 2003;5(5):325-332.
Howes J, Waring M, Huang L, Howes LG. Long-term pharmacokinetics of an extract of isoflavones from red clover (*Trifolium pratense*). J Altern Complement Med 2002;8(2): 135-142.
Jarred RA, McPherson SJ, Jones ME, et al. Anti-androgenic action by red clover-derived dietary isoflavones reduces non-malignant prostate enlargement in aromatase knockout (ArKo) mice. Prostate 2003;56(1):54-64.
Jarred RA, Keikha M, Dowling C, et al. Induction of apoptosis in low to moderate-grade human prostate carcinoma by red clover-derived dietary isoflavones. Cancer Epidemiol Biomarkers Prev 2002;11(12):1689-1696.
Knight DC. The effect of Promensil, an isoflavone extract, on menopausal symptoms. Climacteric 1999;2:79-84.
Moyad MA. Complementary/alternative therapies for reducing hot flashes in prostate cancer patients: reevaluating the existing indirect data from studies of breast cancer and postmenopausal women. Urology 2002;59(4 Suppl 1):20-33.
Nachtigall LB, La Grega L, Lee WW, et al. The effects of isoflavones derived from red clover on vasomotor symptoms and endometrial thickness. 9th International Menopause Society World Congress on the Menopause 1999;331-336.
Nestel PJ, Pomeroy S, Kay S, et al. Isoflavones from red clover improve systemic arterial compliance but not plasma lipids in menopausal women. J Clin Endocrinol Metab 1999;84(3): 895-898.
Teede HJ, McGrath BP, DeSilva L, et al. Isoflavones reduce arterial stiffness: a placebo-controlled study in men and postmenopausal women. Arterioscler Thromb Vasc Biol 2003;23(6): 1066-1071. Epub 2003 Apr 24.
Tice JA, Ettinger B, Ensrud K, et al. Phytoestrogen supplements for the treatment of hot flashes: the Isoflavone Clover Extract (ICE) Study: a randomized controlled trial. JAMA 2003;290(2):207-214.
Umland EM, Cauffield JS, Kirk JK, et al. Phytoestrogens as therapeutic alternatives to traditional hormone replacement in postmenopausal women. Pharmacother 2000;20(8):981-990.
van de Weijer PH, Barentsen R. Isoflavones from red clover (Promensil) significantly reduce menopausal hot flush symptoms compared with placebo. Maturitas 2002;42(3):187-193.
Writing Group for the Women's Health Initiative Investigators. Risks and benefits of estrogen plus progestin in healthy postmenopausal women: principal results from the Women's Health Initiative randomized controlled trial. JAMA 2002;288(3):321-333.

Red Yeast

(*Monascus purpureus*)

RELATED TERMS

- Angkak, beni-koju, hong qu, hung-chu, monascus, red koji, red leaven, red rice, red rice yeast, red yeast, went, Xuezhikang, Zhitai.

BACKGROUND

- Red yeast rice (RYR) is the product of yeast (*Monascus purpureus*) grown on rice and serves as a dietary staple in some Asian countries. It contains several compounds collectively known as "monacolins," substances known to inhibit cholesterol synthesis. One of these, monacolin K, is a potent inhibitor of HMG-CoA reductase and is also known as mevinolin and lovastatin (Mevacor).
- Red yeast rice extract (RYRE) has been sold as a natural cholesterol-lowering agent in over-the-counter supplements such as Cholestin. However, there has been legal and industrial dispute as to whether RYR is a drug or a dietary supplement, involving the manufacturer of Cholestin (Pharmanex, Inc.), the U.S. Food and Drug Administration (FDA), and the pharmaceutical industry (particularly producers of HMG-CoA reductase inhibitor prescription drugs, or "statins").
- The use of RYR in China was first documented during the Tang Dynasty in 800 AD. A detailed description of its manufacture is found in the ancient Chinese pharmacopoeia, Ben Cao Gang Mu-Dan Shi Bu Yi, published during the Ming Dynasty (1368 to 1644). In this text, RYR is proposed to be a mild aid for gastric problems (indigestion, diarrhea), blood circulation, and spleen and stomach health. RYR in a dried, powdered form is called Zhitai. When extracted with alcohol it is called Xuezhikang.
- According to the Pharmanex Web site (accessed September 2004), new and improved Cholestin contains policosanol, a natural product from the wax of honey bees (*Apis mellifera*). It no longer contains any red yeast. Policosanols are potent inhibitors of cholesterol synthesis and have been well studied in clinical trials in Cuba and South America.

USES BASED ON SCIENTIFIC EVIDENCE	Grade*
High cholesterol Since the 1970s, human studies have reported that red yeast lowers blood levels of total cholesterol, low-density lipoprotein (LDL) ("bad cholesterol"), and triglyceride. In March 2001, a U.S. District Court ruled that the RYRE product Cholestin contains the same chemical as the prescription cholesterol-lowering drug lovastatin (Mevacor) and therefore cannot be sold without a prescription. Lovastatin, like other statin drugs, has been shown in multiple well-designed controlled trials to reduce total cholesterol and LDL levels. Cholestin has since been reformulated to contain different ingredients (such as policosanol).	**A**

Continued

Other products containing RYRE can still be purchased, mostly over the Internet. However, these products may not be standardized, and effects are not predictable. For lowering cholesterol, there is better evidence for using prescription drugs such as lovastatin.

*Key to grades: *A:* Strong scientific evidence for this use; *B:* Good scientific evidence for this use; *C:* Unclear scientific evidence for this use; *D:* Fair scientific evidence against this use (it may not work); *F:* Strong scientific evidence against this use (it likely does not work). For a more detailed explanation of efficacy criteria, see "Natural Standard Evidence-Based Validated Grading Rationale" in the Introduction.

Uses Based on Tradition, Theory, or Limited Scientific Evidence

Anthrax, blood circulation problems, bruised muscles, bruises, colic in children, diarrhea, dysentery (bloody diarrhea), hangover, high blood pressure, indigestion, postpartum problems, spleen problems, stomach problems, wounds.

DOSING

The following doses are based on scientific research, publications, traditional use, or expert opinion. Many herbs and supplements have not been thoroughly tested, and their safety and effectiveness may not be proven. Brands may be made differently, with variable ingredients even within the same brand. The doses shown may not apply to all products. It is important to always read product labels and discuss doses with a qualified healthcare provider before therapy is started.

Adults (18 Years and Older)

- *Capsules:* 1200 mg of concentrated red yeast powder two times per day by mouth with food has been used.

Children (Younger Than 18 Years)

- There is not enough scientific evidence to recommend red yeast for children.

SAFETY

The U.S. Food and Drug Administration does not strictly regulate herbs and supplements. There is no guarantee of strength, purity, or safety of products, and effects may vary. It is important to always read product labels. People who have a medical condition, or are taking other drugs, herbs, or supplements, should consult a qualified healthcare provider before starting a new therapy. A healthcare provider should be consulted immediately about any side effects.

Allergies

- There is one report of anaphylaxis (a severe allergic reaction) in a butcher who touched meat containing red yeast.

Side Effects and Warnings

- There is limited evidence about the side effects of red yeast. Mild headache and abdominal discomfort can occur. Side effects may be similar to those for the prescription drug lovastatin (Mevacor). Heartburn, gas, bloating, muscle pain, dizziness,

and kidney problems are possible. People with liver disease should not use red yeast products.
- In theory, red yeast may increase the risk of bleeding. Caution is advised in patients with bleeding disorders or taking drugs that may increase the risk of bleeding. Dosing adjustments may be necessary.

Pregnancy and Breastfeeding

- Prescription drugs with component chemicals similar to red yeast cannot be used during pregnancy. Therefore, it is strongly recommended that pregnant or breastfeeding women not take red yeast.

INTERACTIONS

Most herbs and supplements have not been thoroughly tested for interactions with other herbs, supplements, drugs, or foods. The interactions listed here are based on reports in scientific publications, laboratory experiments, or traditional use. It is important to always read product labels. People who have a medical condition, or are taking other drugs, herbs, or supplements, should consult a qualified healthcare provider before starting a new therapy.

Interactions with Drugs

- There are not many studies of the interactions of red yeast rice extract with drugs. However, because RYRE contains the same chemicals as the prescription drug lovastatin, the interactions may be the same. Alcohol and other drugs that may be toxic to the liver should be avoided with use of RYRE. Taking cyclosporine, ranitidine (Zantac), and certain antibiotics with red yeast rice extract may increase the risk of muscle breakdown or kidney damage.
- Certain drugs may interfere with how the body uses the liver's cytochrome P450 enzyme system to process red yeast. Inhibitors of cytochrome P450 may increase the chance of muscle and kidney damage if taken with red yeast. People using any medications should always read the package insert and consult their healthcare provider and pharmacist about possible interactions.
- In theory, red yeast may increase the risk of bleeding when taken with drugs that increase the risk of bleeding. Some examples are aspirin, anticoagulants (blood thinners) such as warfarin (Coumadin) and heparin, antiplatelet drugs such as clopidogrel (Plavix), and nonsteroidal anti-inflammatory drugs such as ibuprofen (Motrin, Advil) and naproxen (Naprosyn, Aleve).
- Red yeast may produce gamma-aminobutyric acid (GABA) and therefore can have additive effects when taken with drugs that affect GABA such as neurontin (Gabapentin).

Interactions with Herbs and Dietary Supplements

- Red yeast may interact with products that cause liver damage or are broken down in the liver. Grapefruit juice may increase the blood levels of red yeast. Milk thistle, St. John's wort, niacin, and vitamin A may interact with RYRE. Coenzyme Q levels may be lowered by RYRE.
- Certain herbs and supplements may interfere with how the body uses the liver's cytochrome P450 enzyme system to process red yeast. Inhibitors of cytochrome P450 may increase the chance of muscle and kidney damage if taken with red yeast. Examples are bloodroot, cat's claw, chamomile, chaparral, chasteberry, damiana, *Echinacea angustifolia*, goldenseal, grapefruit juice, licorice, oregano, red clover,

St. John's wort, wild cherry, and yucca. People who are using any other herbs or supplements should always read the package insert and consult their healthcare provider and pharmacist about possible interactions.
- In theory, red yeast may increase the risk of bleeding when taken with herbs and supplements that are believed to increase the risk of bleeding. Multiple cases of bleeding have been reported with the use of *Ginkgo biloba*, and fewer cases with garlic and saw palmetto. Numerous other agents may theoretically increase the risk of bleeding, although this has not been proven in most cases. Some examples include alfalfa, American ginseng, angelica, anise, *Arnica montana*, asafetida, aspen bark, bilberry, birch, black cohosh, bladderwrack, bogbean, boldo, borage seed oil, bromelain, capsicum, cat's claw, celery, chamomile, chaparral, clove, coleus, cordyceps, danshen, devil's claw, dong quai, EPA (eicosapentaenoic acid, found in fish oils), evening primrose oil, fenugreek, feverfew, fish oil, flaxseed/flax powder (not a concern with flaxseed oil), ginger, grapefruit juice, grapeseed, green tea, guggul, gymnestra, horse chestnut, horseradish, licorice root, lovage root, male fern, meadowsweet, nordihydroguaiaretic acid (NDGA), omega-3 fatty acids, onion, *Panax ginseng*, papain, parsley, passionflower, poplar, prickly ash, propolis, quassia, red clover, reishi, rue, Siberian ginseng, sweet birch, sweet clover, turmeric, vitamin E, white willow, wild carrot, wild lettuce, willow, wintergreen, and yucca.

Selected References

Natural Standard developed the preceding evidence-based information based on a systematic review of more than 160 articles. For comprehensive information about alternative and complementary therapies on the professional level, go to www.naturalstandard.com. Selected references are listed here.

Bonovich K, Colfer H, Petoskey MI, et al. A multi-center, self-controlled study of Cholestin in subjects with elevated cholesterol. J Invest Med 1999;47(2):54A.

Gavagan T. Cardiovascular disease. Prim Care 2002 Jun;29(2):323-338, vi.

Heber D, Yip I, Ashley JM, et al. Cholesterol-lowering effects of a proprietary Chinese red-yeast-rice dietary supplement. Am J Clin Nutr 1999;69(2):231-236.

Heber D. Dietary supplement or drug? The case for cholestin [letter]. Am J Clin Nutr 1999; 70(1):106-108.

Hsieh PS, Tai YH. Aqueous extract of *Monascus purpureus* M9011 prevents and reverses fructose-induced hypertension in rats. J Agric Food Chem 2003 Jul 2;51(14):3945-3950.

Liu L, Zhao SP, Cheng YC, Li YL. Xuezhikang decreases serum lipoprotein(a) and C-reactive protein concentrations in patients with coronary heart disease. Clin Chem 2003 Aug;49(8): 1347-1352.

Su YC, Wang JJ, Lin TT, Pan TM. Production of the secondary metabolites gamma-amino-butyric acid and monacolin K by *Monascus*. J Ind Microbiol Biotechnol 2003 Jan;30(1): 41-46. Epub 2003 Jan 03.

Thompson Coon JS, Ernst E. Herbs for serum cholesterol reduction: a systematic view. J Fam Pract 2003 Jun;52(6):468-478.

Wang J, Lu Z, Chi J, et al. Multicenter clinical trial of the serum lipid-lowering effects of a *Monascus purpureus* (red yeast) rice preparation from traditional Chinese medicine. Curr Ther Res 1997;58(12):964-978.

Wei W, Li C, Wang Y, et al. Hypolipidemic and anti-atherogenic effects of long-term Cholestin (*Monascus purpureus*-fermented rice, red yeast rice) in cholesterol fed rabbits. J Nutr Biochem 2003 Jun;14(6):314-318.

Wei J, Yang H, Zhang C, et al. A comparative study of xuezhikang and mevalotin in treatment of essential hyperlipidemia. Chin J New Drugs 1997;6:265-268.

Saw Palmetto

(*Serenoa repens* [Bartram] Small, *Sabal serrulata*)

RELATED TERMS

- American dwarf palm tree, Arecaceae (family), cabbage palm, dwarf palm, Elusan Prostate, IDS 89, LSESR, PA 109, Palmae (family), palmetto scrub, palmier de l'amerique du nord, palmier nain, Permixon, Prostagutt, Prostaserine, sabal, sabalfruchte, *Sabal fructus*, savpalme, saw palmetto berry, serenoa, *Serenoa serrulata* Hook F., SG 291, Strogen, WS 1473, zwegpalme.
- Also see information on pygeum (*Prunus africanum, Pygeum africanum*).

BACKGROUND

- Saw palmetto (*Serenoa repens, Sabal serrulata*) is used popularly in Europe for symptoms associated with benign prostatic hypertrophy (BPH) (enlargement of the prostate). Although use of saw palmetto is not considered standard of care in the United States, it is the most popular herbal treatment for this condition.
- Historical use of saw palmetto can be traced in the Americas to the Mayans, who used it as a tonic, and to the Seminoles, who took the berries as an expectorant and antiseptic.
- Saw palmetto was listed in the United States Pharmacopeia from 1906 to 1917, and in the National Formulary from 1926 to 1950. Saw palmetto extract is a licensed product in several European countries.
- Multiple mechanisms of action have been proposed, and saw palmetto appears to possess 5α-reductase inhibitory activity (thereby preventing the conversion of testosterone to dihydrotestosterone). Hormonal/estrogenic effects have also been reported, as well as direct inhibitory effects on androgen receptors and anti-inflammatory properties.

USES BASED ON SCIENTIFIC EVIDENCE	Grade*
Enlarged prostate (BPH) Numerous human trials report that saw palmetto reduces symptoms of BPH, such as nighttime urination and impaired urinary flow, and improves overall quality of life, although it may not greatly reduce the size of the prostate. It may be similar in effectiveness to the medication finasteride (Proscar), with fewer side effects. Although the quality of these studies has been variable, overall they suggest effectiveness. Saw palmetto has not been thoroughly compared with other types of drugs used for BPH, such as doxazosin (Cardura) or terazosin (Hytrin). Most available studies have assessed the standardized saw palmetto product Permixon. Although a 2003 study by Willetts et al. reports no difference between the effects of saw palmetto and placebo in 100 men over a 12-week period, overall the weight of available scientific evidence favors the effectiveness of saw palmetto.	A

Continued

Male pattern hair loss It has been suggested that saw palmetto may block some effects of testosterone and thereby reduce male pattern hair loss, similar to the medication finasteride (Propecia). More studies are necessary before saw palmetto can be recommended for this use.	C
Underactive bladder There is currently little information on the effectiveness of saw palmetto for the treatment of bladder disorders.	C
Prostatitis/chronic pelvic pain syndrome A prospective, randomized, open label, 1-year study was designed to assess the safety and efficacy of saw palmetto and finasteride in the treatment of men diagnosed with category III prostatitis/chronic pelvic pain (CP/CPPS). The men whose CP/CPPS was treated with saw palmetto had no appreciable long-term improvement. By contrast, patients whose CP/CPPS was treated with finasteride had significant and durable improvement in multiple parameters except for voiding.	D

*Key to grades: *A:* Strong scientific evidence for this use; *B:* Good scientific evidence for this use; *C:* Unclear scientific evidence for this use; *D:* Fair scientific evidence against this use (it may not work); *F:* Strong scientific evidence against this use (it likely does not work). For a more detailed explanation of efficacy criteria, see "Natural Standard Evidence-Based Validated Grading Rationale" in the Introduction.

Uses Based on Tradition, Theory, or Limited Scientific Evidence

Acne, aphrodisiac, asthma, bladder inflammation, breastfeeding, breast enlargement or reduction, bronchitis, cancer, cough, cystitis, diabetes, digestive aid, diarrhea, diuretic, dysentery, excess hair growth, expectorant, high blood pressure, hormone imbalances (estrogen or testosterone), immunostimulation, impotence, indigestion, inflammation, lactation stimulation, laryngitis, libido, menstrual pain, migraine headache, muscle or intestinal spasms, ovarian cysts, polycystic ovarian syndrome, postnasal drip, prostate cancer, reproductive organ problems, sedation, sexual vigor, sore throat, sperm production, testicular atrophy, upper respiratory tract infection, urethritis, urinary antiseptic, uterine or vaginal disorders.

DOSING

The following doses are based on scientific research, publications, traditional use, or expert opinion. Many herbs and supplements have not been thoroughly tested, and their safety and effectiveness may not be proven. Brands may be made differently, with variable ingredients even within the same brand. The doses shown may not apply to all products. It is important to always read product labels and discuss doses with a qualified healthcare provider before therapy is started.

Standardization

- Standardization involves measuring the amount of certain chemicals in products to try to make different preparations similar to each other. It is not always known if the chemicals being measured are the "active" ingredients.

- A standardized extract of saw palmetto containing 80% to 95% sterols and fatty acids (liposterolic content) is often recommended.
- One small study examining amounts of saw palmetto contained in preparations compared to amounts stated on labels reported a –97% to +140% difference compared with label claims. Half of the samples (three samples) contained less than 25% of the stated amounts. Although this study examined very few saw palmetto products, it is a noteworthy example of limited quality assurance.

Adults (18 Years and Older)

- **Oral (by mouth):** For enlarged prostate (benign prostatic hypertrophy), a dose of 320 mg daily, in one dose or two divided doses (80% to 90% liposterolic content), has been used in numerous studies. Reports suggest that 160 mg once daily may be as effective as twice daily. Traditional or other suggested doses that are less studied include 1 to 2 g of ground, dried, or whole berries daily; 2 to 4 ml of tincture (1:4) three times daily; 1 to 2 ml fluid extract of berry pulp (1:1) three times daily; or tea (2 teaspoons of dried berry with 24 ounces of water, simmered slowly until liquid is reduced by half) taken as 4 ounces three times daily. Teas prepared from saw palmetto berries are potentially not as effective because the active ingredients may not dissolve in water. Some experts believe that a preparation called lipidosterolic extract of *Serenoa repens* (LSESR) may cause fewer side effects.
- **Rectal (suppositories):** For enlarged prostate (BPH), limited research reports that rectal saw palmetto (640 mg once daily) extract is as effective as 160 mg taken by mouth four times daily.

Children (Younger Than 18 Years)

- Not enough information is available to recommend the use of saw palmetto in children.

S

Safety

The U.S. Food and Drug Administration does not strictly regulate herbs and supplements. There is no guarantee of strength, purity, or safety of products, and effects may vary. It is important to always read product labels. People who have a medical condition, or are taking other drugs, herbs, or supplements, should consult a qualified healthcare provider before starting a new therapy. A healthcare provider should be consulted immediately about any side effects.

Allergies

- Few allergic symptoms have been reported with saw palmetto. A study of people taking the combination product PC-SPES (no longer commercially available), which includes saw palmetto and seven other herbs, reports that three out of 70 people developed allergic reactions. In one case, the reaction included throat swelling and difficulty breathing.

Side Effects and Warnings

- Few severe side effects of saw palmetto are noted in the available scientific literature. The most common complaints involve the stomach and intestines and include stomach pain, nausea, vomiting, bad breath, constipation, and diarrhea. Stomach upset caused by saw palmetto may be reduced by taking it with food. Some reports suggest that there may be less abdominal discomfort with the preparation lipidosterolic extract of *Serenoa repens* (LSESR). A small number of reports describe

ulcers or liver damage and yellowing of the skin (jaundice), but the role of saw palmetto is not clear in these cases. Similarly, headache, dizziness, insomnia, depression, breathing difficulties, muscle pain, high blood pressure, chest pain, abnormal heart rhythm, and heart disease have been reported but are not clearly caused by saw palmetto. People with health conditions involving the stomach, liver, heart, or lungs should exercise caution regarding use of this herb.
- At least two case reports describe severe bleeding during saw palmetto use. Caution is advised in people scheduled to undergo some surgical procedures or dental work, who have bleeding disorders, or who are taking drugs that may increase the risk of bleeding. Dosing adjustments may be necessary. Several reports describe men with prostate cancer who developed blood clots in the legs and lung while taking saw palmetto. Since cancer may increase the risk of blood clots, it is not clear if saw palmetto was the cause.
- Some men using saw palmetto report difficulty with erections, testicular discomfort, breast tenderness or enlargement, and changes in sexual desire. Saw palmetto may have effects on the body's response to the sex hormones estrogen and testosterone, but no specific effect has been well demonstrated in humans. Men or women taking hormone medications (such as finasteride [Proscar/Propecia] or birth control pills) or who have hormone-sensitive conditions should exercise caution regarding use of this herb. Tinctures may contain high levels of alcohol and should be avoided in people who will be driving or operating heavy machinery.
- In theory, prostate-specific antigen (PSA) levels may be artificially lowered by saw palmetto, based on a proposed mechanism of action of saw palmetto (inhibition of 5 α-reductase). Therefore, there may be a delay in diagnosis of prostate cancer, or interference with following PSA levels during treatment or monitoring in men with known prostate cancer.
- The combination product PC-SPES, which contains saw palmetto and seven other herbs, has been found to contain prescription drugs including warfarin, a blood thinner. The U.S. Food and Drug Administration has issued a warning not to use PC-SPES for this reason, and it is no longer commercially available.

Pregnancy and Breastfeeding

- Because of possible hormonal activity, saw palmetto extract is not recommended for women who are pregnant or breast-feeding. Many tinctures contain high levels of alcohol, and should be avoided during pregnancy.

INTERACTIONS

Most herbs and supplements have not been thoroughly tested for interactions with other herbs, supplements, drugs, or foods. The interactions listed here are based on reports in scientific publications, laboratory experiments, or traditional use. It is important to always read product labels. People who have a medical condition, or are taking other drugs, herbs, or supplements, should consult a qualified healthcare provider before starting a new therapy.

Interactions with Drugs

- As indicated by at least two reports of serious bleeding, saw palmetto may increase the risk of bleeding when taken with drugs that increase the risk of bleeding. Some examples are aspirin, anticoagulants (blood thinners) such as warfarin (Coumadin) and heparin, antiplatelet drugs such as clopidogrel (Plavix), and nonsteroidal anti-inflammatory drugs such as ibuprofen (Motrin, Advil) and naproxen (Naprosyn,

Aleve). Some batches of the discontinued combination herbal preparation PC-SPES, which contains saw palmetto and seven other herbs, were found to contain several medications including the blood thinner warfarin.

- Saw palmetto should not be taken with drugs that affect the levels of male sex hormones (androgens), such as finasteride (Proscar, Propecia) or flutamide (Eulexin). In theory, saw palmetto may interfere with actions of birth control pills or hormone replacement therapy in women. Tinctures may contain high levels of alcohol and may cause nausea or vomiting when taken with metronidazole (Flagyl) or disulfiram (Antabuse).
- Study in normal volunteers reveals no effects of saw palmetto on cytochrome P450 3A4 or 2D6 activity.

Interactions with Herbs and Dietary Supplements

- As indicated by at least two reports of serious bleeding, saw palmetto may increase the risk of bleeding when taken with herbs and supplements that are believed to increase the risk of bleeding. Multiple cases of bleeding have been reported with the use of *Ginkgo biloba*, and fewer cases with garlic. Numerous other agents may theoretically increase the risk of bleeding, although this has not been proven in most cases. Some examples are alfalfa, American ginseng, angelica, anise, *Arnica montana*, asafetida, aspen bark, bilberry, birch, black cohosh, bladderwrack, bogbean, boldo, borage seed oil, bromelain, capsicum, cat's claw, celery, chamomile, chaparral, clove, coleus, cordyceps, danshen, devil's claw, dong quai, evening primrose, fenugreek, feverfew, flaxseed/flax powder (not a concern with flaxseed oil), ginger, grapefruit juice, grapeseed, green tea, guggul, gymnestra, horse chestnut, horseradish, licorice root, lovage root, male fern, meadowsweet, nordihydroguaiaretic acid (NDGA), onion, papain, *Panax ginseng*, parsley, passionflower, poplar, prickly ash, propolis, quassia, red clover, reishi, rue, Siberian ginseng, sweet birch, sweet clover, turmeric, vitamin E, white willow, wild carrot, wild lettuce, willow, wintergreen, and yucca.
- Because saw palmetto may have activity on the body's response to estrogen, the effects of other agents believed to have estrogen-like properties may be altered. Possible examples include alfalfa, black cohosh, bloodroot, burdock, hops, kudzu, licorice, pomegranate, red clover, soy, thyme, white horehound, and yucca.

Interactions with Foods

- Stomach upset caused by saw palmetto may be reduced by taking it with food. No published reports of specific interactions with foods are noted in the available scientific literature.

Selected References

Natural Standard developed the preceding evidence-based information based on a systematic review of more than 200 scientific articles. For comprehensive information about alternative and complementary therapies on the professional level, go to www.naturalstandard.com. Selected references are listed here.

Boyle P, Robertson C, Lowe F, et al. Meta-analysis of clinical trials of Permixon in the treatment of symptomatic benign prostatic hyperplasia. Urology 2000;55(4):533-539.

Braeckman J, Bruhwyler J, Vanderkerckhove K, et al. Efficacy and safety of the extract of *Serenoa repens* in the treatment of benign prostatic hyperplasia: therapeutic equivalence between twice and once daily dosage forms. Phytother Res 1997;11:558-563.

Braeckman J. A double-blind, placebo-controlled study of the plant extract *Serenoa repens* in the treatment of benign hyperplasia of the prostate. Eur J Clin Res 1997;9:247-259.

de la TA, Buttyan R, Hayek O, et al. Herbal therapy PC-SPES: in vitro effects and evaluation of its efficacy in 69 patients with prostate cancer. J Urol 2000;164(4):1229-1234.

Descotes J, Rambeaud J, Deschaseaux P, et al. Placebo-controlled evaluation of the efficacy and tolerability of Permixon in benign prostatic hyperplasia after exclusion of placebo responders. Clin Drug Invest 1995;9(5):291-297.

Feifer AH, Fleshner NE, Klotz L. Analytical accuracy and reliability of commonly used nutritional supplements in prostate disease. J Urol 2002;168(1):150-154; discussion 154.

Gerber GS, Kuznetsov D, Johnson BC, et al. Randomized, double-blind, placebo-controlled trial of saw palmetto in men with lower urinary tract symptoms. Urology 2001;58(6):960-964.

Gordon AE, Shaughnessy AF. Saw palmetto for prostate disorders. Am Fam Physician 2003; 67(6):1281-1283. Review.

Kaplan SA, Volpe MA, Te AE. A prospective, 1-year trial using saw palmetto versus finasteride in the treatment of category III prostatitis/chronic pelvic pain syndrome. J Urol 2004; 171(1):284-288.

Markowitz JS, Donovan JL, Devane CL, et al. Multiple doses of saw palmetto (*Serenoa repens*) did not alter cytochrome P450 2D6 and 3A4 activity in normal volunteers. Clin Pharmacol Ther 2003;74(6):536-542.

Oh WK, George DJ, Hackmann K, et al. Activity of the herbal combination, PC-SPES, in the treatment of patients with androgen-independent prostate cancer. Urology 2001;57(1): 122-126.

Pfeifer BL, Pirani JF, Hamann SR, et al. PC-SPES, a dietary supplement for the treatment of hormone-refractory prostate cancer. BJU Int 2000;85(4):481-485.

Shoskes DA. Phytotherapy and other alternative forms of care for the patient with prostatitis. Curr Urol Rep 2002;3(4):330-334.

Small EJ, Frohlich MW, Bok R, et al. Prospective trial of the herbal supplement PC-SPES in patients with progressive prostate cancer. J Clin Oncol 2000;18(21):3595-3603.

Talpur N, Echard B, Bagchi D, et al. Comparison of Saw palmetto (extract and whole berry) and Cernitin on prostate growth in rats. Mol Cell Biochem 2003;250(1-2):21-26.

Veltri RW, Marks LS, Miller MC, et al. Saw palmetto alters nuclear measurements reflecting DNA content in men with symptomatic BPH: evidence for a possible molecular mechanism. Urology 2002;60(4):617-622.

Willetts KE, Clements MS, Champion S, et al. *Serenoa repens* extract for benign prostate hyperplasia: a randomized controlled trial. BJU Int 2003;92(3):267-270.

Wilt TJ, Ishani A, Stark G, et al. Saw palmetto extracts for treatment of benign prostatic hyperplasia: a systematic review. JAMA 1998;280(18):1604-1609.

Shark Cartilage

RELATED TERMS

- AE-941, cartilage, haifischknorpel, Houtsmuller diet, Neovastat, shark, shark fin soup, *Sphyrna lewini* (hammerhead shark), squalamine, *Squalus acanthias* (spiny dogfish shark), U-955.
- *Note:* The product Catrix is made from cow cartilage, not from shark cartilage.

BACKGROUND

- Shark cartilage is one of the most popular supplements in the United States, with over 40 brand name products sold in 1995 alone. It is used primarily for cancer; this supplement became popular in the 1980s after several poor-quality studies reported "miracle" cancer cures.
- Laboratory research and animal studies of shark cartilage or the shark cartilage derivative product AE-941 (Neovastat) have demonstrated some anticancer (anti-angiogenic) and anti-inflammatory properties. However, there is currently not enough reliable human evidence to recommend for or against shark cartilage for any condition. There are several ongoing cancer studies. Many trials are supported by manufacturers of shark cartilage products, raising questions about impartiality.
- Commercial shark cartilage is primarily composed of chondroitin sulfate (a type of glycosaminoglycan), which is further broken down in the body into glucosamine and other end products. Although chondroitin and glucosamine have been extensively studied for osteoarthritis, there is no evidence supporting the use of unprocessed shark cartilage preparations for this condition. Shark cartilage also contains calcium (up to 600 to 780 mg of elemental calcium per daily dose). Manufacturers sometimes promote its use for calcium supplementation.
- Shark cartilage supplements at common doses can cost as much as $700 to $1000 per month.

S

USES BASED ON SCIENTIFIC EVIDENCE	Grade*
Arthritis Chondroitin sulfate, a component of shark cartilage, has been shown to benefit patients with osteoarthritis. However, the concentrations of chondroitin in shark cartilage products may be too small to be helpful. The ability of shark cartilage to block new blood vessel growth or reduce inflammation is proposed to be helpful in rheumatoid arthritis. However, there is limited research in these areas, and more studies are needed before a recommendation can be made.	C
Cancer For several decades, shark cartilage has been proposed as an agent for cancer treatment. Studies have shown shark cartilage or the shark	C

Continued

cartilage product AE-941 (Neovastat) to block the growth of new blood vessels, a process called "antiangiogenesis," which is believed to play a role in controlling growth of some tumors. There have also been several reports of successful treatment of end-stage cancer patients with shark cartilage, but these have not been well designed or included reliable comparisons with accepted treatments. Many studies have been supported by shark cartilage product manufacturers, which may influence the results. In the United States, shark cartilage products cannot claim to cure cancer, and the Food and Drug Administration (FDA) has sent warning letters to companies not to promote products in this way. Without further evidence from well-designed human trials, it remains unclear if shark cartilage is of any benefit in cancer and patients are advised to check with their doctor and pharmacist before taking shark cartilage.	
Macular degeneration It is proposed that shark cartilage or the shark cartilage product AE-941 (Neovastat) may be helpful in patients with macular degeneration. A small amount of research suggests possible benefits, but more study is needed before a recommendation can be made.	**C**
Pain As indicated by laboratory studies, shark cartilage may reduce inflammation. However, it is unclear if shark cartilage is a safe or helpful treatment for pain in humans.	**C**
Psoriasis Shark cartilage products have been tested by mouth or on the skin in people with psoriasis. However, no clear benefits have been shown. More research is needed before a conclusion can be drawn.	**C**

*Key to grades: *A:* Strong scientific evidence for this use; *B:* Good scientific evidence for this use; *C:* Unclear scientific evidence for this use; *D:* Fair scientific evidence against this use (it may not work); *F:* Strong scientific evidence against this use (it likely does not work). For a more detailed explanation of efficacy criteria, see "Natural Standard Evidence-Based Validated Grading Rationale" in the Introduction.

Uses Based on Tradition, Theory, or Limited Scientific Evidence

Allergic skin rashes, ankylosing spondylitis, atherosclerosis (hardening of the arteries), bacterial infections, diabetic retinopathy, diarrhea, immune system stimulant, intestinal disorders and inflammation, fungal infections, glaucoma, Kaposi's sarcoma, kidney stones, Reiter's syndrome, rheumatoid arthritis, sarcoidosis, scar healing, Sjögren's syndrome, skin rash, systemic lupus erythematosus (SLE), wound healing, wrinkle prevention.

DOSING

The following doses are based on scientific research, publications, traditional use, or expert opinion. Many herbs and supplements have not been thoroughly tested, and their safety and effectiveness may not be proven. Brands may be made differently, with variable ingredients even within the same brand. The doses shown may not apply to all products. It is important to always read product labels and discuss doses with a qualified healthcare provider before therapy is started.

Standardization

- Standardization involves measuring the amount of certain chemicals in products to try to make different preparations similar to each other. It is not always known if the chemicals being measured are the "active" ingredients.
- There is no well-accepted method of preparing or purifying shark cartilage products, although manufacturers may use specific procedures to control their own processes. Shark cartilage products are often made by sterilizing and grinding dried shark cartilage (hammerhead or spiny dogfish shark) into powder form. Some manufacturing processes can destroy the proteins that are believed to slow cancer growth. Analysis of one shark cartilage product found it to contain more than 99% water.

Adults (18 Years and Older)

- **Cancer:** Studied doses of ground cartilage extract include 80 to 100 g, or 1.0 to 1.3 g per kilogram of body weight, taken by mouth daily, divided into two to four doses. Doses of the shark cartilage derivative AE-941 (Neovastat), available in clinical trials, have ranged from 30 to 240 ml per day taken by mouth, or 20 ml per kilogram of body weight taken twice daily. Rectal doses of 15 g per day or 0.5 to 1.0 g per kilogram of body weight per day in two to three divided doses (prepared as an enema) have also been studied.
- **Arthritis:** Doses of 0.2 to 2.0 g per kilogram of body weight per day, taken by mouth in two to three divided doses, have been studied.
- **Psoriasis:** Doses of 0.4 to 0.5 g per kilogram of body weight per day, taken by mouth for 4 weeks, have been used. If skin lesions improve, doses have been reduced to 0.2 to 0.3 g per kilogram of body weight per day for 4 additional weeks. Creams applied to the skin with 5% to 30% shark cartilage are available and have been recommended by some practitioners for treatment of psoriasis alone or with shark cartilage by mouth, for 4 to 6 weeks. Studies have used 5% to 10% preparations applied daily.

S

Children (Younger Than 18 Years)

- Shark cartilage is not recommended in children because of lack of scientific study and a theoretical risk of blocking blood vessel growth. There is one report of a 9-year-old child with a brain tumor treated with shark cartilage who died 4 months later.

SAFETY

The U.S. Food and Drug Administration does not strictly regulate herbs and supplements. There is no guarantee of strength, purity, or safety of products, and effects may vary. It is important to always read product labels. People who have a medical condition, or are taking other drugs, herbs, or supplements, should consult a qualified healthcare provider before starting a new therapy. A healthcare provider should be consulted immediately about any side effects.

Allergies

- Allergic reactions to shark cartilage or to any of its ingredients are possible, although there is limited human information in this area.

Side Effects and Warnings

- A limited amount of published research suggests that shark cartilage is well tolerated in most people at recommended doses. An 18-month study in 330 people by the makers of the shark cartilage derivative Neovastat did not report any major toxic effects after exposure to the product for more than 4 years. The most common adverse effects reported are mild to moderate stomach upset and nausea. In several studies, 5% to 10% of patients stopped taking shark cartilage because of gastrointestinal distress (nausea, vomiting, constipation, dyspepsia), while 20% to 40% experienced milder symptoms of cramping or bloating. Gastrointestinal upset may be due to the high calcium concentration in some shark cartilage preparations. There is one report of liver damage in an elderly man using shark cartilage, which resolved 6 weeks after the supplement was stopped. One study reports taste alteration to be a frequent side effect, reported by up to 14% of patients.
- Uncommon side effects reported in studies or historically include confusion, decreased muscle strength, decreased sensation, weakness, dizziness, fatigue, increased or decreased blood sugar levels, and low blood pressure. Shark cartilage products may contain high levels of calcium, which may be harmful to patients with kidney disease, abnormal heart rhythms, or a tendency to form kidney stones, and those with cancers that raise calcium levels (breast cancer, prostate cancer, multiple myeloma, squamous cell lung cancer, and others). In theory, as a result of the blocking of new blood vessel growth, shark cartilage may be harmful in people with heart disease or narrowed blood vessels of the legs (peripheral vascular disease). In theory, wound healing and recovery from surgery or trauma may be reduced.
- Limited evidence suggests that shark cartilage may lower blood sugar levels. Caution is advised in patients with diabetes or hypoglycemia, and in those taking drugs, herbs, or supplements that affect blood sugar. Serum glucose levels may need to be monitored by a healthcare provider, and medication adjustments may be necessary.
- One case report implicates inhaled shark cartilage dust in an asthma exacerbation and resulting death of a 38-year-old male.

Pregnancy and Breastfeeding

- Shark cartilage is not recommended in pregnant or breastfeeding women. Shark cartilage may block the growth of new blood vessels, and drugs with similar properties, such as thalidomide, can cause birth defects. There is limited study of shark cartilage in these areas.

INTERACTIONS

Most herbs and supplements have not been thoroughly tested for interactions with other herbs, supplements, drugs, or foods. The interactions listed here are based on reports in scientific publications, laboratory experiments, or traditional use. It is important to always read product labels. People who have a medical condition, or are taking other drugs, herbs, or supplements, should consult a qualified healthcare provider before starting a new therapy.

Interactions with Drugs

- Shark cartilage products may contain high doses of calcium and may cause dangerously high blood calcium levels when taken with drugs known to increase blood calcium. For example, long-term use of thiazide diuretics such as chlorothiazide (Diuril) may lead to greatly increased blood calcium. In theory, shark cartilage may add to the effects of drugs and experimental agents that block new blood vessel growth. Examples are Ag3340, Bay12-9566, leflunomide (Arava), Marimastat, anti-VEGF (anti-vascular endothelial growth factor) antibody, carboxyaminotriazole, CGS 27023A, AGM-1470, SU5416, Vitaxin, EMD 121974, interleukin-12, CM 101, interferon alfa and beta, and thalidomide. Based on one animal study, the cancer drug cisplatin and shark cartilage may act together against tumors, although there is no reliable human supporting evidence.
- Limited evidence suggests that shark cartilage may lower blood sugar levels. Caution is advised with use of medications that may also lower blood sugar. Patients taking drugs for diabetes by mouth or insulin should be monitored closely by a qualified healthcare provider. Medication adjustments may be necessary.

Interactions with Herbs and Dietary Supplements

- Shark cartilage products may contain high doses of calcium and may cause dangerously high calcium levels in the blood when taken with calcium supplements or antacids such as Tums. Chondroitin sulfate, popular for treatment of osteoarthritis, is a component of shark cartilage. In theory, use of shark cartilage with chondroitin may lead to higher-than-expected blood levels of chondroitin, with unknown effects.
- Limited evidence suggests that shark cartilage may lower blood sugar levels. Caution is advised with use of herbs or supplements that may also lower blood sugar. Blood glucose levels may require monitoring, and doses may need adjustment. Possible examples include *Aloe vera*, American ginseng, bilberry, bitter melon, burdock, fenugreek, fish oil, gymnema, horse chestnut seed extract (HCSE), marshmallow, milk thistle, *Panax ginseng*, rosemary, Siberian ginseng, stinging nettle, and white horehound. Agents that may raise blood sugar levels include arginine, cocoa, and ephedra (when combined with caffeine).

Interactions with Foods

- Acidic fruit juices, such as apple, grape, or cranberry, may reduce the absorption of shark cartilage taken by mouth.

Selected References

Natural Standard developed the preceding evidence-based information based on a systematic review of more than 130 scientific articles. For comprehensive information about alternative and complementary therapies on the professional level, go to www.naturalstandard.com. Selected references are listed here.

Batist G, Patenaude F, Champagne P, et al. Neovastat (AE-941) in refractory renal cell carcinoma patients: report of a phase II trial with two dose levels. Ann Oncol 2002;13(8):1259-1263.

Beliveau R, Gingras D, Kruger EA, et al. The antiangiogenic agent Neovastat (AE-941) inhibits vascular endothelial growth factor–mediated biological effects. Clin Cancer Res 2002;8(4):1242-1250.

Berbari P, Thibodeau A, Germain L, et al. Antiangiogenic effects of the oral administration of liquid cartilage extract in humans. J Surg Res 1999;87(1):108-113.

Boivin D, Gendron S, Beaulieu E, et al. The antiangiogenic agent Neovastat (AE-941) induces endothelial cell apoptosis. Mol Cancer Ther 2002;1(10):795-802.

Bukowski RM. AE-941, a multifunctional antiangiogenic compound: trials in renal cell carcinoma. Expert Opin Invest Drugs 2003;12(8):1403-1411.

Dupont E, Falardeau P, Mousa SA, et al. Antiangiogenic and antimetastatic properties of Neovastat (AE-941), an orally active extract derived from cartilage tissue. Clin Exp Metastasis 2002;19(2):145-153.

Dupont E, Savard RE, Jourdain C, et al. Antiangiogenic properties of a novel shark cartilage extract: potential role in the treatment of psoriasis. J Cutan Med Surg 1998;2(3):146-152.

Escudier B, Patenaude F, Bukowski R, et al. Rationale for a phase III clinical trial with AE-941 (Neovastat®) in metastatic renal cell carcinoma patients refractory to immunotherapy. Ann Oncol 2000;11(suppl 4):143-144.

Gingras D, Boivin D, Deckers C, et al. Neovastat—a novel antiangiogenic drug for cancer therapy. Anticancer Drugs 2003;14(2):91-96.

Jagannath S, Champagne P, Hariton C, et al. Neovastat in multiple myeloma. Eur J Haematol 2003;70(4):267-268.

Jamali MA, Riviere P, Falardeau A, et al. Effect of AE-941 (Neovastat), an angiogenesis inhibitor, in the Lewis lung carcinoma metastatic model, efficacy, toxicity prevention and survival. Clin Invest Med 1998;(suppl):S16.

Kralovec JA, Guan Y, Metera K, et al. Immunomodulating principles from shark cartilage. Part 1. Isolation and biological assessment *in vitro*. Int Immunopharmacol 2003(5):657-669.

Lagman R, Walsh D. Dangerous nutrition? Calcium, vitamin D, and shark cartilage nutritional supplements and cancer-related hypercalcemia. Support Care Cancer 2003;11(4):232-235.

Leitner SP, Rothkopf MM, Haverstick DD, et al. Two phase II studies of oral dry shark cartilage powder (SCP) in patients with either metastatic breast or prostate cancer refractory to standard treatment. Amer Soc Clin Oncol 1998;17:A240.

Miller DR, Anderson GT, Stark JJ, et al. Phase I/II trial of the safety and efficacy of shark cartilage in the treatment of advanced cancer. J Clin Oncol 1998;16(11):3649-3655.

Ortega HG, Kreiss K, Schill DP, et al. Fatal asthma from powdering shark cartilage and review of fatal occupational asthma literature. Am J Ind Med 2002;42(1):50-54.

Riviere M, Alaoui-Jamali M, Falardeau P, et al. Neovastat: an inhibitor of angiogenesis with anti-cancer activity. Proc Am Assoc Cancer Res 1998;39:46.

Riviere M, Falardeau P, Latreille J, et al. Phase I/II lung cancer clinical trial results with AE-941 (Neovastat), an inhibitor of angiogenesis. J Clin Pharm 1998;38(9):860.

Riviere M, Latreille J, Falardeau P. AE-941 (Neovastat), an inhibitor of angiogenesis: phase I/II cancer clinical trial results. Cancer Invest 1999;17(suppl 1):16-17.20.

Sauder DN, Dekoven J, Champagne P, et al. Neovastat (AE-941), an inhibitor of angiogenesis: Randomized phase I/II clinical trial results in patients with plaque psoriasis. J Am Acad Dermatol 2002;47(4):535-41.

Sheu JR, Fu CC, Tsai ML, et al. Effect of U-995, a potent shark cartilage-derived angiogenesis inhibitor, on anti-angiogenesis and anti-tumor activities. Anticancer Res 1998;18(6A): 4435-4441.

Wilson JL. Topical shark cartilage subdues psoriasis. Altern Comp Ther 2000;6:291.

Slippery Elm

(Ulmus rubra, Ulmus fulva)

RELATED TERMS

- Indian elm, moose elm, red elm, rock elm, sweet elm, Ulmaceae, ulmi rubrae cortex, *Ulmus fulva* Michaux, winged elm.
- **Combination products:** Essiac, Robert's formula.
- *Note:* Inner bark of slippery elm should not be confused with the whole bark, which may be associated with significant risk of adverse effects. Bark of Californian slippery elm (*Fremontia californica*) is often used similarly medicinally, but it is not botanically related.

BACKGROUND

- Slippery elm inner bark has been used historically as a demulcent, emollient, nutritive, astringent, antitussive, and vulnerary (wound healer). It is included as one of four primary ingredients in the herbal cancer remedy Essiac and in a number of Essiac-like products such as Fluoressence. While anecdotal reports suggest that this combination formulation has anticancer activity, there are no reliable clinical trials to prove or discount this use.
- There are no scientific studies evaluating the common uses of this herb, but because of its high mucilage content, slippery elm bark may be a safe herbal remedy to treat irritations of the skin and mucous membranes.
- Although allergic reactions after contact have been reported, there is no known toxicity with typical dosing when products made only from the inner bark are used.
- In manufacturing, slippery elm is used in some baby foods and adult nutritionals, and in some oral lozenges for soothing throat pain. Avoid confusing whole bark with inner bark. Commercial lozenges containing slippery elm are preferred to the native herb when used for cough and sore throat, because they provide sustained release of mucilage to the throat.
- The slippery elm is native to eastern Canada, and the eastern and central United States, where it is found mostly in the Appalachian Mountains. Its name refers to the slippery consistency the inner bark attains when it is chewed or mixed with water. This property is responsible for the name used by the Iroquois Indians, do-hoosh-ah, which literally means "it slips." The tree can grow up to 18 to 20 meters in height and is found primarily in moist woodlands. It typically has spreading branches and an open crown with young branches that are orange to reddish brown in color. The bark is deeply fissured and the dark green leaves are 10 to 20 cm long with serrated edges. Supplies of slippery elm have dwindled as a result of devastation by Dutch elm disease. Slippery elm is easily mistaken for other elms.
- Native American healers have used the dried inner bark of slippery elm tree for centuries. Bark, collected in the spring, yields thick, viscous mucilage when mixed with water, which is used to treat conditions such as urinary tract inflammation, inflammation of the digestive tract, cold sores, boils, and irritated skin and mucous membranes. Poultices made from slippery elm bark were applied to bruises and black eyes and were recommended to help heal minor burns and abrasions. Ground bark was added to milk, which was taken as a nutrient by infants and chronically ill patients.

- Surgeons during the American Revolution used bark poultices as their primary treatment for gunshot wounds. As did Native American healers, physicians in the 19th century also recommended slippery elm broth for infants and chronically ill individuals, and slippery elm tea for patients with gastric ulcer and colitis.
- From 1820 to 1960, elm bark was listed in the United States Pharmacopoeia as a demulcent, emollient, and antitussive. In modern times, the powdered bark is included in herbal teas and throat lozenges used to soothe throat irritation. It is also an ingredient in herbal emollients and antitussives.

USES BASED ON SCIENTIFIC EVIDENCE	Grade*
Cancer Slippery elm is found as a common ingredient in a purported herbal anticancer product called Essiac and a number of Essiac-like products. These products contain other herbs such as rhubarb, sorrel, and burdock root. There is limited available human evidence regarding the efficacy or safety of Essiac or Essiac-like products. A laboratory at Memorial Sloan-Kettering Cancer Center tested Essiac on mice during the 1970s, although results were never formally published and remain controversial. Questions were raised about improper preparation of the formula. A human study was started in Canada in the late 1970s but was stopped early because of concerns about inconsistent preparation of the formula and inadequate study design. In the 1980s, the Canadian Department of National Health and Welfare collected information about 86 cancer patients who received Essiac. Results were inconclusive (17 patients had died at the time of the study, inadequate information was available for 8 patients, "no benefits" were found in 47 patients, 5 reported reduced need for pain medications, and 1 noted subjective improvement). Most individuals also received other cancer treatments such as chemotherapy, making the effects of Essiac impossible to isolate. Currently, there is not enough evidence to recommend for or against the use of this herbal mixture as a therapy for any type of cancer. Different brands may contain variable ingredients, and the comparative effectiveness of these formulas is not known. None of the individual herbs used in Essiac has been tested in rigorous human cancer trials (rhubarb has shown some antitumor properties in animal experiments, whereas slippery elm inner bark has not; sheep sorrel and burdock have been used traditionally in cancer remedies). Numerous patient testimonials and reports from manufacturers are available on the Internet, although these cannot be considered scientifically viable as evidence. Individuals with cancer are advised not to delay treatment with more proven therapies.	C

Continued

Diarrhea Traditionally, slippery elm has been used to treat diarrhea. While theoretically the tannins found in the herb may decrease water content of stool, and mucilage may act as a soothing agent on inflamed mucous membranes, there is no reliable scientific evidence to support this indication. Systematic research is necessary in this area before a clear conclusion can be drawn.	C
Gastrointestinal disorders Slippery elm is traditionally used to treat inflammatory conditions of the digestive tract such as gastritis, peptic ulcer disease, and enteritis. It may be taken alone or in combination with other herbs. While slippery elm is anecdotally reported to be effective, supporting evidence is largely based on traditional evidence and the fact that the mucilage contained in the herb appears to possess soothing properties. Scientific evidence is necessary in this area before a clear conclusion can be drawn.	C
Sore throat Slippery elm is commonly used to treat sore throats, most typically taken as a lozenge. While slippery elm is anecdotally reported to be effective, supporting evidence is largely based on traditional evidence and the fact that the mucilage contained in the herb appears to possess soothing properties. Scientific evidence is necessary in this area before a clear conclusion can be drawn.	C

*Key to grades: *A:* Strong scientific evidence for this use; *B:* Good scientific evidence for this use; *C:* Unclear scientific evidence for this use; *D:* Fair scientific evidence against this use (it may not work); *F:* Strong scientific evidence against this use (it likely does not work). For a more detailed explanation of efficacy criteria, see "Natural Standard Evidence-Based Validated Grading Rationale" in the Introduction.

Uses Based on Tradition, Theory, or Limited Scientific Evidence

Abscesses, abortifacient, abrasions, acidity, anal fissures, antihelminthic, antitussive, boils, bronchitis, burns, cancer, carbuncles, cleansing of impurities, colitis, cold sores, congestion, constipation, cough, Crohn's disease, cystitis, demulcent, diarrhea, diuretic, diverticulitis, duodenal ulcers, dysentery, emollient, enteritis, eruptions, esophageal reflex, expectorant, gastric catarrh, gastric ulcers, gastritis, gout, gynecologic disorders, heart burn, hemorrhoids, herpes, inflammation, irritable bowel syndrome, irritated mucous membranes, laxative, lung problems, milk tolerance, nutritive food, pleurisy, rheumatism, scalds, sore throat, stomach inflammation, suppuration, swollen glands, synovitis, syphilis, toothache, typhoid fever, ulcerative colitis, vaginitis, varicose ulcers, vulnerary, wounds.

DOSING

The following doses are based on scientific research, publications, traditional use, or expert opinion. Many herbs and supplements have not been thoroughly tested, and their safety and effectiveness may not be proven. Brands may be made differently, with variable ingredients even within the same brand. The doses shown may not apply to all products. It is important to always read product labels and discuss doses with a qualified healthcare provider before therapy is started.

Standardization

- There is no widely accepted standardization for slippery elm preparations. Amounts of slippery elm used in Essiac and Essiac-like products are proprietary and therefore not disclosed by the manufacturers.
- Mucilage U.S.P. is made by digesting 6 g of bruised slippery elm in 100 ml and heating in a closed vessel in a water bath for 1 hour, followed by straining.

Adults (18 Years and Older)

Oral (by mouth)

- **Powdered inner bark:** As a decoction (1:8), 4 to 16 ml (or 4 g in 500 ml of boiling water) three times daily has been used. For gastrointestinal upset, 7 g of slippery elm powder in 20 fluid ounces (1 pint) of boiling water has been used as a hot or cold infusion. For cough, 1 part powdered bark of slippery elm added to 8 parts water, or 1 teaspoon of slippery elm powder in 500 ml of water, one to three times daily has been used.
- **Tea:** Half a teaspoon of powdered bark in a cup of hot water taken twice or three times daily, or 0.5 to 1 g of the bark in 200 ml of water taken as 3 to 4 cups daily. For gastrointestinal upset, 1 teaspoon of slippery elm powder in 1 cup of boiling water taken multiple times during the day has been used.
- **Capsules/tablets:** 400- or 500-mg tablets or capsules taken three or four times daily, although strengths may vary because of lack of standardization. Lower doses of 200-mg capsules twice or three times per day have been used for bronchitis.

Topical (on the skin)

- Slippery elm has been used topically for wound care and inflammation. Typically, the coarse powdered inner bark is mixed with boiling water to make a paste. Various concentrations and application schedules have been used.

Children (Younger Than 18 Years)

- Traditionally it has been accepted that slippery elm can be used safely in children complaining of stomach upset and diarrhea. However, no safety studies have been conducted in this area, and therefore use in children should only be under the strict supervision of a licensed healthcare professional.

SAFETY

The U.S. Food and Drug Administration does not strictly regulate herbs and supplements. There is no guarantee of strength, purity, or safety of products, and effects may vary. It is important to always read product labels. People who have a medical condition, or are taking other drugs, herbs, or supplements, should consult a qualified healthcare provider before starting a new therapy. A healthcare provider should be consulted immediately about any side effects.

Allergies

- Known allergy/hypersensitivity such as hives (urticaria) have been reported with slippery elm; some persons may have contact sensitivity to elm tree pollen (or sensitivity on breathing it in), but the frequency of allergic reactions with medicinal use of elm bark products is extremely rare.

Side Effects and Warnings

- **Dermatologic:** Contact dermatitis and urticaria have been reported after exposure to slippery elm or an oleoresin contained in the slippery elm bark.
- **Genitourinary:** Based on historical accounts, whole bark of slippery elm (but not inner bark) may possess abortifacient properties.

Pregnancy and Breastfeeding

- Slippery elm should be avoided during pregnancy because of the risk of contamination with slippery elm whole bark, which may increase the risk of miscarriage.

INTERACTIONS

Most herbs and supplements have not been thoroughly tested for interactions with other herbs, supplements, drugs, or foods. The interactions listed here are based on reports in scientific publications, laboratory experiments, or traditional use. It is important to always read product labels. People who have a medical condition, or are taking other drugs, herbs, or supplements, should consult a qualified healthcare provider before starting a new therapy.

Interactions with Drugs/Herbs and Dietary Supplements

- Slippery elm could theoretically slow down or decrease absorption of other oral medications because it contains hydrocolloidal fibers, although no actual interactions have been reported. Slippery elm also contains tannins, which could theoretically decrease absorption of nitrogen-containing substances such as alkaloids, although no actual interactions have been reported.

Selected References

Natural Standard developed the preceding evidence-based information based on a systematic review of more than 50 articles. For comprehensive information about alternative and complementary therapies on the professional level, go to www.naturalstandard.com. Selected references are listed here.

Czarnecki D, Nixon R, Bekhor P, et al. Delayed prolonged contact urticaria from the elm tree. Contact Dermatitis 1993;28:196-197.

DeHaan RL. Home remedies for pets. J Am Holistic Veterinary Med Assoc 1994;12:26.

Ernst E, Cassileth BR. How useful are unconventional cancer treatments? Eur J Cancer 1999; 35(11):1608-1613.

Gallagher R. Use of herbal preparations for intractable cough. J Pain Symptom Manage 1997;14(1):1-2.

Kaegi E. Unconventional therapies for cancer: 1. Essiac. The Task Force on Alternative Therapies of the Canadian Breast Cancer Research Initiative. CMAJ 1998;158(7):897-902.

Karn H, Moore MJ. The use of the herbal remedy Essiac in an outpatient cancer population. Proc Annu Meet Am Soc Clin Oncol 1997;16:A245.

Kato A, Ando K, Tamura G, et al. Effects of some fatty acid esters on the viability and transplantability of Ehrlich ascites tumor cells. Cancer Res 1971;31(5):501-504.

Locock RA. Essiac. Can Pharm J 1997;130:18-20.

Luo W, Ang CY, Schmitt TC, et al. Determination of salicin and related compounds in botanical dietary supplements by liquid chromatography with fluorescence detection. J AOAC Int 1998;81(4):757-762.

Tamayo C, Richardson MA, Diamond S, et al. The chemistry and biological activity of herbs used in Flor-Essence herbal tonic and Essiac. Phytother Res 2000;14(1):1-14.

Soy

(*Glycine max* L. Merr.)

RELATED TERMS

- Coumestrol, daidzein, edamame, frijol de soya, genistein, greater bean, haba soya, hydrolyzed soy protein, isoflavone, isoflavonoid, legume, natto, phytoestrogen, plant estrogen, shoyu, soja, sojabohne, soybean, soy fiber, soy food, soy product, soy protein, soya, soya protein, ta-tou, texturized vegetable protein.
- **Selected brands used in human clinical trials:** Abalon (Nutri Pharma ASA, Oslo, Norway); SOYSELECT (Indena SpA, Milan, Italy); Takeda (Italia Farmaceutici, SpA, Catania, Italy); Osteofix (Chiesi, Parma, Italy); Piascledine 300 (Pharmascience Laboratories, Courbevoie, France); Isomil DF (Ross Products Division, Abbott Laboratories, Columbus, Ohio); Prosobee (Mead Johnson, Evansville, Indiana); Nursoy (Wyeth Laboratories); Nursoy Ready to Feed (Wyeth Laboratories); Isomil (Ross Laboratories, Columbus, Ohio); Hyprovit (Hayes Ltd., Ashdod, Israel); TakeCare (Protein Technology International, St. Louis, Missouri); Fibrim Brand Soy Fiber (Protein Technologies International); Purina 660 (Ralston Purina Company, St. Louis, Missouri); Supro 660 (Protein Technologies International); Supro 675 (Protein Technologies International); Supro 675 IF (Protein Technologies International); Supro Plus 675HG (Protein Technologies International); Temptein (Miles Laboratories, Elkhart, Indiana).

BACKGROUND

- Soy is a subtropical plant native to southeastern Asia. This member of the pea family (Fabaceae) grows from 1 to 5 feet tall and forms clusters of three to five pods, each containing two to four beans per pod. Soy has been a dietary staple in Asian countries for at least 5000 years, and during the Chou dynasty in China (1134 to 246 BC), fermentation techniques were discovered that allowed soy to be prepared in more easily digestible forms such as tempeh, miso, and tamari soy sauce. Tofu was invented in second century China.
- Soy was introduced to Europe in the 1700s, and to the United States in the 1800s. Large-scale soybean cultivation began in the United States during World War II. Currently, Midwestern U.S. growers produce approximately half of the world's supply of soybeans.
- Soy and components of soy called "isoflavones" have been studied scientifically for numerous health conditions. Isoflavones (such as genistein) are believed to have estrogen-like effects in the body and therefore are sometimes called "phytoestrogens." In laboratory studies, it is not clear if isoflavones stimulate or block the effects of estrogen, or both (acting as mixed receptor agonists/antagonists).

USES BASED ON SCIENTIFIC EVIDENCE	Grade*
Dietary source of protein Soy products such as tofu are high in protein and are an acceptable source of dietary protein.	A
High cholesterol Numerous human studies report that adding soy protein to the diet can moderately decrease blood levels of total cholesterol and low-density lipoprotein ("bad" cholesterol). Small reductions in triglycerides may also occur, while high-density lipoprotein ("good" cholesterol) does not seem to be significantly altered. The greatest effects seem to occur in people with elevated cholesterol levels, with benefits lasting as long as the diet is continued. Total replacement of dietary animal proteins with soy protein yields the greatest benefits. People on low-cholesterol diets experience further reductions in cholesterol levels by adding soy to the diet. Some scientists have proposed that specific components of soybean, such as the isoflavones genistein and daidzein, may be responsible for the cholesterol-lowering properties of soy. However, this has not been clearly demonstrated in research and remains controversial. It is not known if products containing isolated soy isoflavones have the same effects as those of regular dietary intake of soy protein. Dietary soy protein has not been proven to affect long-term cardiovascular outcomes such as heart attack or stroke.	A
Diarrhea (acute) in infants and young children Numerous studies report that infants and young children (ages 2 to 36 months) with diarrhea who are fed soy formula experience fewer bowel movements per day and fewer days of diarrhea. This research suggests soy to have benefits over other types of formula, including cow milk–based solutions. The addition of soy fiber to soy formula may increase the effectiveness. Although many of the trials in this area are not of high quality, and some report conflicting results (lack of benefits), overall the evidence supports this use of soy. Better-quality research is needed before a strong recommendation can be made. Parents are advised to consult a qualified healthcare provider if infants experience prolonged diarrhea, become dehydrated, demonstrate signs of infection such as fever, or have blood in the stool. A healthcare provider should be consulted for current breastfeeding recommendations, and to suggest long-term formulas with adequate nutritional value.	B
Menopausal hot flashes Soy products containing isoflavones have been studied for the reduction of menopausal symptoms such as hot flashes. The scientific evidence is mixed in this area, with several human trials suggesting reduced number of hot flashes and decrease in other menopausal symptoms, but with more recent research reporting no benefits. Overall, the scientific	B

S

Continued

evidence does suggest benefits, although better-quality studies are needed in this area in order to form a firm conclusion.

Many researchers have attributed these effects to the presence in soy of "phytoestrogens" (plant-based compounds with weak estrogen-like properties), such as isoflavones. An area of concern has been whether phytoestrogens carry the same risks as for prescription drug hormone replacement therapy (HRT), which includes estrogens. For example, HRT has been associated with increased risk for development of hormone-sensitive cancers (breast, ovarian, uterine) and of blood clots. This is an important area of concern for patients, as some women may consider soy as an alternative to HRT in order to avoid these risks. Early studies report that soy isoflavones do not cause the same thickening of the uterus lining (endometrium) as occurs with estrogen and therefore may not carry the same risks as those associated with HRT. In addition, some scientists theorize that isoflavones may actually reduce the risk of cancer by blocking estrogen effects in the body, based on laboratory studies showing isoflavones to partially block (noncompetitively inhibit) estrogen receptors. Additional research is needed in this area before a clear risk assessment can be conducted.

Breast cancer prevention C

Several large population studies have asked women about their eating habits and have reported higher soy intake (such as dietary tofu) to be associated with a decreased risk of developing breast cancer. However, this type of research (retrospective, case-control, epidemiologic) can only be considered preliminary, because people who choose to eat soy may also partake in other lifestyle decisions that may lower the risk of cancer. These other habits, rather than soy, could theoretically be the cause of the benefits seen in these studies (for example, lower fat intake, more frequent exercise, lack of smoking). Controlled human trials are necessary before a firm conclusion can be drawn.

Theoretical concerns have been raised that soy may actually *increase* the risk of breast cancer because of the presence in soy of phytoestrogens (plant-based compounds with weak estrogen-like properties), such as isoflavones. This possibility remains an area of controversy. Recently, some scientists have theorized that isoflavones may reduce the risk of cancer by blocking estrogen effects in the body, based on laboratory studies showing isoflavones to partially block (noncompetitively inhibit) estrogen receptors. In fact, early research suggests that soy isoflavones do not have the same effects on the body as those of estrogens, such as increasing the thickening of the uterus lining (endometrium). Genistein has been found in laboratory and animal studies to have other anticancer effects, such as blocking new blood vessel growth (antiangiogenesis), acting as a tyrosine kinase inhibitor (a mechanism of many new cancer treatments), or causing cancer cell death (apoptosis).

Until better research is available, it remains unclear if dietary soy or soy isoflavone supplements increase or decrease the risk of developing breast cancer.

Cancer treatment Genistein, an isoflavone found in soy, has been found in laboratory and animal studies to possess anticancer effects, such as blocking new blood vessel growth (antiangiogenesis), acting as a tyrosine kinase inhibitor (a mechanism of many new cancer treatments), or causing cancer cell death (apoptosis). By contrast, genistein has also been reported to *increase* the growth of pancreas tumor cells in laboratory research. None of these effects has been adequately assessed in humans. In the past, theoretical concerns have been raised that soy may increase the risk of hormone-sensitive cancers (for example, breast, ovarian, endometrial/uterine) because of the presence in soy of phytoestrogens (plant-based compounds with weak estrogen-like properties), such as isoflavones (genistein and others). This remains an area of controversy. Recently, some scientists have suggested that isoflavones may actually reduce the risk of hormone-sensitive cancers by blocking estrogen effects in the body, based on laboratory studies showing isoflavones to partially block (non-competitively inhibit) estrogen receptors. Preliminary human research suggests that soy isoflavones do not have the same effects on the body as those of estrogens, such as increasing the thickening of the uterus lining (endometrium). Until reliable human research is available, it remains unclear if dietary soy or soy isoflavone supplements are beneficial, harmful, or neutral in people with various types of cancer.	C
Cardiovascular disease Dietary soy protein has not been shown to affect long-term cardiovascular outcomes such as heart attack or stroke. Research does suggest cholesterol-lowering effects of dietary soy, which in theory may reduce cardiovascular risk. Soy has also been studied for blood pressure–lowering and blood sugar–reducing properties in people with type 2 diabetes, although the evidence is not definitive in these areas. Although the addition of soy to a regimen of exercise and diet may theoretically improve cardiovascular outcomes, this has not been scientifically proven. Some studies show an association between soy food consumption and lower risk of coronary heart disease in women, but further investigation is needed.	C
Cognitive function A recent study suggests that isoflavone supplementation in postmenopausal women may have favorable effects on cognitive function, particularly verbal memory. Further research is necessary before a firm conclusion can be drawn.	C
Colon cancer prevention There is not enough scientific evidence to determine if dietary intake of soy affects the risk of developing colon cancer.	C

Continued

Crohn's disease Due to limited human study, there is not enough evidence to recommend for or against the use of soy as a therapy in preventing Crohn's disease. Further research is needed before a recommendation can be made.	C
Cyclic breast pain It has been theorized that the presence in soy of phytoestrogens (plant-based compounds with weak estrogen-like properties) such as isoflavones may be beneficial to premenopausal women with cyclic breast pain. However, owing to limited human study, there is not enough evidence to recommend for or against the use of dietary soy protein as a therapy for this condition.	C
Diarrhea in adults Owing to limited human study, there is not enough evidence to recommend for or against the use of soy-polysaccharide/fiber in the treatment of diarrhea. Further research is needed before a recommendation can be made.	C
Endometrial cancer prevention Theoretical concerns have been raised that soy may actually *increase* the risk of endometrial cancer because of the presence in soy of phytoestrogens (plant-based compounds with weak estrogen-like properties), such as isoflavones. This remains an area of controversy. Recently, some scientists have theorized that isoflavones may reduce the risk of cancer by blocking estrogen effects in the body, based on laboratory studies showing isoflavones to partially block (noncompetitively inhibit) estrogen receptors. In fact, early research suggests that soy isoflavones do not have the same effects on the uterus as those of estrogens, such as increasing the thickening of the endometrium (lining of the uterus). Genistein has been found in laboratory and animal studies to have other anticancer effects, such as blocking new blood vessel growth (antiangiogenesis), acting as a tyrosine kinase inhibitor (a mechanism of many new cancer treatments), or causing cancer cell death (apoptosis).	C
Gallstones (cholelithiasis) Owing to limited human study, there is not enough evidence to recommend for or against the use of soy as a therapy in cholelithiasis. Further research is needed before a recommendation can be made.	C
High blood pressure Because of limited human study, the effects of dietary soy on blood pressure are not clear. Further research is necessary before any recommendation can be made.	C
Kidney disease (chronic renal failure, nephrotic syndrome, proteinuria) Because of limited human study, there is not enough evidence to recommend for or against the use of soy in the treatment of kidney	C

diseases such as nephrotic syndrome. People with kidney disease should consult their healthcare provider about recommended amounts of dietary protein and should bear in mind that soy is a high-protein food.	
Menstrual migraine One study of a phytoestrogen combination in the prophylactic treatment of menstrual migraines reduced the number of migraine attacks suffered. Further research is needed before a recommendation can be made.	C
Obesity, weight reduction Because of limited human study, there is not enough evidence to recommend for or against the use of soy for weight reduction. Further research is needed before a recommendation can be made.	C
Osteoporosis, postmenopausal bone loss It has been theorized that the presence in soy of phytoestrogens (plant-based compounds with weak estrogen-like properties) such as isoflavones may increase bone mineral density in postmenopausal women, reducing the risk of fractures. A small number of studies in this area report benefits, particularly in the lumbar spine (lower back). However, most studies have not been well designed or reported. Until better research is available, a firm conclusion cannot be drawn. Individuals at risk for osteoporosis should consult a qualified healthcare provider about the therapeutic options for increasing bone mineral density.	C
Prostate cancer prevention It has been theorized that the presence in soy of phytoestrogens (plant-based compounds with weak estrogen-like properties) such as isoflavones may be beneficial in the treatment of prostate cancer. In addition, the isoflavone genistein has been found in laboratory and animal studies to have anticancer effects, such as blocking new blood vessel growth (antiangiogenesis), acting as a tyrosine kinase inhibitor (a mechanism of many new cancer treatments), or causing cancer cell death (apoptosis). These mechanisms have not been clearly demonstrated to work in humans. Preliminary research has examined the effects of dietary soy intake on prostate cancer development in humans, but results have not been conclusive. Better study is needed before a recommendation can be made.	C
Stomach cancer Preliminary study suggests that intake of soy products may be associated with a reduced risk of death from stomach cancer. Further investigation is needed before a conclusion can be drawn.	C
Type 2 diabetes mellitus Several small studies have examined the effects of soy products on blood sugars in people with type 2 (adult-onset) diabetes mellitus. Results	C

Continued

are mixed, with some research reporting decreased blood glucose levels and other trials noting no effects. Overall, research in this area is not well designed or reported, and better information is needed before the effects of soy on blood sugar levels can be clearly described.

*Key to grades: *A:* Strong scientific evidence for this use; *B:* Good scientific evidence for this use; *C:* Unclear scientific evidence for this use; *D:* Fair scientific evidence against this use (it may not work); *F:* Strong scientific evidence against this use (it likely does not work). For a more detailed explanation of efficacy criteria, see "Natural Standard Evidence-Based Validated Grading Rationale" in the Introduction.

Uses Based on Tradition, Theory, or Limited Scientific Evidence

Anemia, anorexia, antifungal, antioxidant, antithrombotic, atherosclerosis, athletic endurance, attention deficit hyperactivity disorder (ADHD), autoimmune diseases, breast enlargement, cancer prevention (general), cystic fibrosis, diabetic neuropathy, fever, gastric cancer, gastrointestinal motility, headache, hepatitis (chronic), inflammation, insect repellent, lymphoma, memory enhancement, nosebleed (chronic), osteosarcoma, premature ovarian failure, rheumatoid arthritis, urinary tract cancer, vaginitis, vasoregulator.

DOSING

The following doses are based on scientific research, publications, traditional use, or expert opinion. Many herbs and supplements have not been thoroughly tested, and their safety and effectiveness may not be proven. Brands may be made differently, with variable ingredients even within the same brand. The doses shown may not apply to all products. It is important to always read product labels and discuss doses with a qualified healthcare provider before therapy is started.

Adults (18 Years and Older)

- **High cholesterol:** 30 to 50 g of soy protein taken daily by mouth has been studied in people with high cholesterol. Isoflavone content of the daily intake of soy has ranged from 60 to 80 mg per day. Cholesterol and low-density lipoprotein levels have been reduced in individuals ingesting 28 g daily of soy protein with a high isoflavone content, or with Abacor, a brand that contains 26 g of soy protein. There is limited study of soymilk (400 ml daily) in premenopausal women, with reported benefits on cholesterol levels.
- **Menopausal symptoms (hot flashes):** Isolated soy protein, such as Supro (60 g), soy flour (45 g), and a range of isoflavone products have been studied. Doses of 50 to 75 mg of isoflavones have been used in research.
- **Diarrhea:** In infants and young children (2 to 36 months of age), Hyprovit formula, Isomil formula, Nursoy formula or powder, and Prosobee formula taken by mouth have been studied. Because of potential safety concerns, a qualified healthcare provider should be consulted regarding the choice of infant formula. In adults, soy-derived diets and intake of soy polysaccharide/fiber have been studied, although benefits are not clear.

- **Cancer and cancer prevention:** Population and laboratory studies have examined levels of dietary soy intake. No specific doses can be recommended at this time.
- **Cardiovascular health:** Studies have examined regular intake of dietary soy, or 40 to 80 mg of isoflavones taken by mouth daily.
- **Osteoporosis/postmenopausal bone loss:** Isoflavones/isoflavone-rich soy (60 to 80 mg daily by mouth) and soy protein (for example, 40 g daily of Supro 675) have been studied.
- **Gallstones (cholelithiasis):** Dietary intake of soy has undergone limited study. Because of limited research in humans, no specific doses can be recommended at this time.
- **Crohn's disease:** Because of limited research in humans, no specific doses can be recommended at this time.
- **Cyclic breast pain:** A soy protein drink (17 g of soy protein per 200 ml) has undergone limited study.
- **Diabetes:** A fermented soybean-derived extract tea, various doses of soy protein (such as Abalon), and up to 7 g of soya fibers taken daily by mouth have undergone limited study in humans.
- **High blood pressure:** Soymilk (1000 ml daily for 3 months) for this indication has undergone limited study.
- **Kidney disease/chronic renal failure:** Soy-based diets have undergone limited study in people with kidney diseases such as the nephrotic syndrome. However, soy is a source of dietary protein, and low-protein diets may be more desirable in patients with kidney failure. People with kidney failure should consult a qualified healthcare provider before making any dietary changes.
- **Obesity:** A soy-derived diet has undergone limited study.

Children (Younger Than 18 Years)

- **Diarrhea:** In infants and young children (2 to 36 months of age), Hyprovit formula, Isomil formula, Nursoy formula or powder, and Prosobee formula taken by mouth have been studied. Because of potential safety concerns, a qualified healthcare provider should be consulted regarding the choice of infant formula.

S

SAFETY

Many complementary techniques are practiced by healthcare professionals with formal training, in accordance with the standards of national organizations. However, this is not universally the case, and adverse effects are possible. Because of limited research, in some cases only limited safety information is available.

Allergies

- Soy can act as a food allergen similar to milk, eggs, peanuts, fish, and wheat. The prevalence of soy allergy in children with positive skin tests has been reported as high as 6%. In limited research, soy has been well tolerated by most children with immunoglobulin E (IgE)-associated cow milk allergy (CMA), although allergic cross-reactivity has occasionally been reported. Rare allergic reactions have been reported in human research, and two subjects withdrew from a cholesterol study because of suspected allergy to soy. In a study involving young adults with asthma, soy beverages were associated with an increased risk of asthma. Asthma-like breathing problems have also been associated with inhaling soybean dust.

Side Effects and Warnings

- Soy has been a dietary staple in many countries for over 5000 years and is generally not regarded as having significant long-term toxicity. Limited side effects have been reported in infants, children, and adults.
- Soy protein taken by mouth has been associated with stomach and intestinal difficulties such as bloating, nausea, and constipation. More serious intestinal side effects have been uncommonly reported in infants fed soy protein formula, including vomiting, diarrhea, growth failure, and damage to or bleeding of the intestine walls. Soy protein fed to infants recovering from acute gastroenteritis may cause persistent intestinal damage and diarrhea. People who experience intestinal irritation (colitis) from cow milk may also react to soy formula.
- Based on human case reports and animal research, decreased thyroid hormone and increased thyroid-stimulating hormone (TSH) levels may occur during the use of soy formula in infants. This includes rare reports of goiter (enlargement in neck due to increased thyroid size). Hormone levels have become normal again after soy formula is stopped. Infants fed soy or cow milk formula may also have higher rates of atopic eczema than are seen in infants who are breastfed.
- Acute migraine headache has been reported with the use of a soy isoflavone product. Based on animal research, damage to the pancreas may theoretically occur from regularly eating raw soybeans or soy flour/protein powder made from raw, unroasted, or unfermented beans.
- The use of soy is often discouraged in patients with hormone-sensitive malignancies such as breast, ovarian, or uterine cancer, because of concerns about possible estrogen-like effects (which theoretically may stimulate tumor growth). Other hormone-sensitive conditions such as endometriosis may also theoretically be worsened. In laboratory studies, it is not clear if isoflavones stimulate or block the effects of estrogen, or both (acting as a receptor agonist/antagonist). Until additional research is available, patients with these conditions should exercise caution and consult a qualified healthcare practitioner before starting use of soy.
- It is not known if soy or soy isoflavones share the same side effects as those of estrogens, such as increased risk of blood clots. Preliminary studies suggest that soy isoflavones, unlike estrogens, do not cause the lining of the uterus (endometrium) to build up.

Pregnancy and Breastfeeding

- Soy as a part of the regular diet is traditionally considered to be safe during pregnancy and breastfeeding, although scientific research is limited in these areas. The effects of high doses of soy or soy isoflavones in humans are not clear, and therefore intake at these levels is not recommended.
- Recent study demonstrates that isoflavones, which may have estrogen-like properties, are transferred through breast milk from mothers to infants. High doses of isoflavones given to pregnant rats have resulted in tumors in female offspring, although this has not been tested in humans.
- In one human study, male infants born to women who ingested soymilk or soy products during pregnancy experienced more frequent hypospadias (a birth defect in which the urethral meatus, the opening from which urine passes, is abnormally positioned on the underside of the penis). However, other human and animal studies have examined males or females fed soy formula as infants and have not

found abnormalities in infant growth, head circumference, height, or weight, or in occurrence of puberty, menstruation, or reproductive ability.
- Research in children during the first year of life has found that the substitution of soy formula for cow milk may be associated with significantly lower bone mineral density. Parents considering the use of soy formula should consult a qualified healthcare practitioner to make sure the appropriate vitamins and minerals are provided in the formula.

INTERACTIONS

Most herbs and supplements have not been thoroughly tested for interactions with other herbs, supplements, drugs, or foods. The interactions listed here are based on reports in scientific publications, laboratory experiments, or traditional use. It is important to always read product labels. People who have a medical condition, or are taking other drugs, herbs, or supplements, should consult a qualified healthcare provider before starting a new therapy.

Interactions with Drugs

- **Estrogen:** Soy contains phytoestrogens (plant-based compounds with weak estrogen-like properties) such as isoflavones. In laboratory studies, it is not clear if isoflavones stimulate or block the effects of estrogen, or both (acting as a receptor agonist/antagonist). It is not known if taking soy or soy isoflavone supplements increases or decreases the effects of estrogen on the body, such as the risk of blood clots. It is unclear if taking soy alters the effectiveness of oral contraceptives containing estrogen.
- **Selective estrogen receptor modulators, aromatase inhibitors:** It is not known what the effects of soy phytoestrogens are on the antitumor effects of selective estrogen receptor modulators (SERMs) such as tamoxifen. The effects of aromatase inhibitors such as anastrozole (Arimidex), exemestane (Aromasin), and letrozole (Femara) may be reduced. Because of the potential estrogen-like properties of soy, people receiving these drugs should consult their oncologist before taking soy in amounts greater than normally found in the diet.
- **Warfarin (Coumadin):** Soy protein may interact with warfarin, although this potential interaction is not well characterized. Patients taking warfarin should consult their healthcare provider and pharmacist before taking soy supplementation.

S

Interactions with Herbs and Dietary Supplements

- **Iron:** The effects of soy protein or flour on iron absorption are not clear. Studies in the 1980s reported decreases in iron absorption, although more recent research has noted no effects or increased iron absorption in people taking soy. People using iron supplements as well as soy products should consult a qualified healthcare practitioner to follow blood iron levels.
- ***Panax ginseng*:** Some experts believe that there may be a potential interaction between soy extract and *Panax ginseng*, although this potential interaction is not well characterized.

Interactions with Laboratory Assays

- **Calcium, phosphate:** Animal research suggests that soy may possess estrogen-like effects that affect calcium and phosphate levels. Urinary calcium excretion may be reduced. Further study is needed before a firm conclusion can be drawn.

Interactions with Foods

- **Wheat:** Based on limited human study, reduced absorption of the soy isoflavone genistein (theorized to possess phytoestrogen properties) may occur when soy is taken in combination with wheat fiber.

Selected References

Natural Standard developed the preceding evidence-based information based on a systematic review of more than 600 published articles. For comprehensive information about alternative and complementary therapies on the professional level, go to www.naturalstandard.com. Selected references are listed here.

Adams KF, Newton KM, Chen C, et al. Soy isoflavones do not modulate circulating insulin-like growth factor concentrations in an older population in an intervention trial. J Nutr 2003; 133(5):1316-1319.

Albert A, Altabre C, Baro F, et al. Efficacy and safety of a phytoestrogen preparation derived from *Glycine max* (L.) Merr in climacteric symptomatology: a multicentric, open, prospective and non-randomized trial. Phytomedicine 2002;9(2):85-92.

Albertazzi P, Pansini F, Bonaccorsi G, et al. The effect of dietary soy supplementation on hot flushes. Obstet Gynecol 1998;91(1):6-11.

Alekel DL, Germain AS, Peterson CT, et al. Isoflavone-rich soy protein isolate attenuates bone loss in the lumbar spine of perimenopausal women. Am J Clin Nutr 2000;72(3):844-852.

Allen UD, McLeod K, Wang EE. Cow's milk versus soy-based formula in mild and moderate diarrhea: a randomized, controlled trial. Acta Paediatr 1994;83(2):183-187.

Allison DB, Gadbury, G, Schwartz LG, et al. A novel soy-based meal replacement formula for weight loss among obese individuals: a randomized controlled clinical trial. Eur J Clin Nutr 2003;57(4):514-522.

Andersson C, Servetnyk Z, Roomans GM. Activation of CFTR by genistein in human airway epithelial cell lines. Biochem Biophys Res Commun 2003;308(3):518-522.

Anderson GD, Rositio G, Mohustsy MA, et al. Drug interaction potential of soy extract and Panax ginseng. J Clin Pharmacol 2003;43(6):643-648.

Arjmandi BH, Khalil DA, Smith BJ, et al. Soy protein has a greater effect on bone in postmenopausal women not on hormone replacement therapy, as evidenced by reducing bone resorption and urinary calcium excretion. J Clin Endocrinol Metab 2003;88(3):1048-1054.

Atkinson C, Skor HE, Dawn Fitzgibbons E, et al. Urinary equol excretion in relation to 2-hydroxyestrone and 16-alpha-hydroxyestrone concentrations: an observational study of young to middle-aged women. J Steroid Biochem Mol Biol 2003;86(1):71-77.

Bakhit RM, Klein BP, Essex-Sorlie D, et al. Intake of 25 g of soybean protein with or without soybean fiber alters plasma lipids in men with elevated cholesterol concentrations. J Nutr 1994;124(2):213-222.

Baird DA, Umbach DM, Lansdell L, et al. Dietary intervention study to assess estrogenicity of dietary soy among postmenopausal women. J Clin Endorinol Metab 1995;80(5):1685-1690.

Baxa DM, Yoshimura FK. Genistein reduces NF-kappa B in T lymphoma cells via a caspase-mediated cleavage of I kappa B alpha. Biochem Pharmacol 2003;66(6):1009-1018.

Beck V, Unterrieder E, Krenn L, et al. Comparison of hormonal activity (estrogen, androgen, and progestin) of standardized plant extracts for large scale use in hormone replacement therapy. J Steroid Biochem Mol Biol 2003;84(2-3):259-268.

Blum A, Lang N, Peleg A, et al. Effects of oral soy protein on markers of inflammation in postmenopausal women with mild hypercholesteremia. Am Heart J 2003;145(2):e7.

Blum A, Lang N, Vigder F, et al. Effects of soy protein on endothelium-dependent vasodilation and lipid profile in postmenopausal women with mild hypercholesterolemia. Clin Invest Med 2003;26(1):20-26.

Blum A. Possible beneficial effects of soy protein on the vascular endothelium in postmenopausal women—future directions. Is Med Assoc J 2003;5(1):56-58.

Bos C, Metges CC, Gaudichon C, et al. Postprandial kinetics of dietary amino acids are the main determinant of their metabolism after soy or milk protein ingestion in humans. J Nutr 2003; 133(5):1308-1315.

Bowey E, Adlercreutz H, Rowland I. Metabolism of isoflavones and lignans by the gut microflora: a study in germ-free and human flora associated rats. Food Chem Toxicol 2003;41(5):631-636.

Burke BE, Olson RD, Cusack BJ. Randomized, controlled trial of phytoestrogen in the prophylactic treatment of menstrual migraine. Biomed Pharmacother 2002;56(6):283-288.

Burke GL, Legault C, Anthony M, et al. Soy protein and isoflavone effects on vasomotor symptoms in peri- and postmenopausal women: the Soy Estrogen Alternative Study. Menopause 2003;10(2):147-153.

Burks AW, Vanderhoof JA, Mehra S, et al. Randomized clinical trial of soy formula with and without added fiber in antibiotic-induced diarrhea. J Pediatr 2001;139(4):578-582.

Bus AE, Worsley A. Consumers' sensory and nutritional perceptions of three types of milk. Public Health Nutr 2003;6(2):201-208.

Cambria-Kiely JA. Effect of soy milk on warfarin efficacy. Ann Pharmacother 2002;36(12): 1893-1896.

Cassidy A. Potential risks and benefits of phytoestrogen-rich diets. Int J Vitam Nutr Res 2003;73(2):120-126.

Chavez M. Soybeans as an alternative to hormone replacement therapy. J Herbal Pharmacother 2002;1(1):91-99.

Chen HL, Huang YC. Fiber intake and food selection of the elderly in Taiwan. Nutrition 2003;19(4):332-336.

Chen WF, Huang MH, Tzang CH, et al. Inhibitory actions of genistein in human breast cancer (MCF-7) cells. Biochem Biophys Acta 2003;1638(2):187-196.

Chiechi LM, Secreto G, Vimercati A, et al. The effects of a soy rich diet on serum lipids: the Menfis randomized trial. Maturitas 2002;41(2):97-104.

Choi Em, Koo SJ. Effects of soybean ethanol extract on the cell survival and oxidative stress in osteoblastic cells. Phytother Res 2003;17(6):627-632.

Chorazy PA, Himelhoch S, Hopwood NJ, et al. Persistent hypothyroidism in an infant receiving a soy formula: case report and review of the literature. Pediatrics 1995;96(1 Pt 1):148-150.

Colquhoun D, Hicks BJ, Kelly GE. Lack of effect of isoflavones on human serum lipids and lipoproteins [abstract]. Atherosclerosis 1994;109:75.

Cressey PJ, Vannoort RW. Pesticide content of infant formulae and weaning foods available in New Zealand. Food Addit Contam 2003;20(1):57-64.

Crouse JR III, Morgan T, Terry JG, et al. A randomized trial comparing the effect of casein with that of soy protein containing varying amounts of isoflavones on plasma concentrations of lipids and lipoproteins. Arch Intern Med 1999;159(17):2070-2076.

Dalais FS, Ebeling PR, Kotsopoulos D, et al. The effects of soy protein containing isoflavones on lipids and indices of bone resorption in postmenopausal women. Clin Endocrinol 2003;58(6):704-709.

Dean TS, O'Reilly J, Bowey E, et al. The effects of soybean isoflavones on plasma HDL concentrations in healthy male and female subjects [abstract]. Proc Nutr Soc 1998;57:123A.

De Lemos ML. Effects of soy phytoestrogens genistein and daidzein on breast cancer growth. Ann Pharmacother 2001;35(9):1118-1121.

Demonty I, Lamrache B, Jones PJ. Role of isoflavones in the hypocholesterolemic effect of soy. Nutr Rev 2003;61(6 Pt 1):189-203.

Dewell A, Hollenbeck CB, Bruce B. The effects of soy-derived phytoestrogens on serum lipids and lipoproteins in moderately hypercholesterolemic postmenopausal women. J Clin Endocrinol Metab 2002;87(1):118-121.

Dreon DM, Slavin JL, Phinney SD. Oral contraceptive use and increased plasma concentration of C-reactive protein. Life Sci 2003;73(10):1245-1252.

Duncan AM, Underhill KEW, Xu X, et al. Modest hormonal effects of Soy isoflavones in postmenopausal women. J Clin Endocrinol Metab 1999;84(10):3479-3484.

Endres J, Barter S, Theodora P, et al. Soy-enhanced lunch acceptance by preschoolers. J Am Diet Assoc 2003;103(3):345-351.

Engel PA. New onset migraine associated with use of soy isoflavone supplements. Neurology 2002 Oct 22;59(8):1289-1290.

Fiocchi A, Restani P, Leo G, et al. Clinical tolerance to lactose in children with cow's milk allergy. Pediatrics 2003;112(2):359-362.

Fouillet H, Gaudichon C, Bos C, et al. Contribution of plasma proteins to splanchnic and total anabolic utilization of dietary nitrogen in humans. Am J Physiol Endocrinol Metab 2003; 285(1):E88-97.
Fowke JH, Chung FL, Jin F, et al. Urinary isothiocyanate levels, brassica, and human breast cancer. Cancer Res 2003;63(14):3980-3986.
Franke AA, Custer LJ, Tanaka Y. Isoflavones in human breast milk and other biological fluids. Am J Clin Nutr 1998;68(6 Suppl):1466S-1473S.
Frankenfeld CL, Patterson RE, Horner NK, et al. Validation of a soy food-frequency questionnaire and evaluation of correlates of plasma isoflavone concentrations in postmenopausal women. Am J Clin Nutr 2003;77(3):674-680.
Fujita H, Yamagami T, Ohshima K. Long-term ingestion of a fermented soybean-derived Touchi-extract with alpha-glucosidase inhibitory activity is safe and effective in humans with borderline and mild type-2 diabetes. J Nutr 2001;131(8):2105-2108.
Garcia-Martinez MC, Hermenegildo C, Tarin JJ, et al. Phytoestrogens increase the capacity of serum to stimulate prostacyclin release in human endothelial cells. Acta Obstet Gynecol Scand 2003;82(8):705-710.
Gentile MG, Manna G, D'Amico G. Soy consumption and renal function in patients with nephrotic syndrome: clinical effects and potential mechanism. Am J Clin Nutr 1998; 68(suppl):1516s.
Gentile MS, Vasu C, Green A, et al. Targeting colon cancer cells with genistein-17.1A immunoconjugate. Int J Oncol 2003;22(5):955-959.
Gianazza E, Eberini I, Arnoldi A, et al. A proteomic investigation of isolated soy proteins with variable effects in experimental and clinical studies. J Nutr 2003;133(1):9-14.
Goodman MT, Wilkens LR, Hankin JH, et al. Association of soy and fiber consumption with the risk of endometrial cancer. Am J Epidemiol 1997;146(4):294-306.
Greendale GA, FitzGerald G, Huang MH, et al. Dietary soy isoflavones and bone mineral density: results from the study of women's health across the nation. Am J Epidemiol 2002; 155(8):746-754.
Hargraves DF, Potten CF, Harding C, et al. Two-week dietary soy supplementation has an estrogenic effect on normal premenopausal breast. J Clin Endocrinol Metab 1999;84(11): 4017-4024.
Haselkorn T, Stewart SL, Horn-Ross PL. Why are thyroid cancer rates so high in Southeast Asian women living in the United States? The Bay Area Thyroid Cancer Study. Cancer Epidemiol Biomarkers Prev 2003;12(2):144-150.
Hedlund TE, Johannes WU, Miller GJ. Soy isoflavonoid equol modulates the growth of benign and malignant prostatic epithelial cells in vitro. Prostate 2003;54(1):68-78.
Hermansen K, Dinesen B, Hoie LH, et al. Effects of soy and other natural products on LDL:HDL ratio and other lipid parameters: a literature review. Adv Ther 2003;20(3):50-78.
Hermansen K, Sondergaard M, Hoie L, et al. Beneficial effects of a soy-based dietary supplement on lipid levels and cardiovascular risk markers in type 2 diabetic subjects. Diabetes Care 2001;24(2):228-233.
Hidvegi E, Arato A, Cserhati E, et al. Slight decrease in bone mineralization in cow milk-sensitive children. J Pediatr Gastroenterol Nutr 2003;36(1):44-49.
Ingram D, Sanders K, Kolybaba M, et al. Case-control study of phyto-oestrogens and breast cancer. Lancet 1997;350(9083):990-994.
Irvine C, Fitzpatrick M, Robertson I, et al. The potential adverse effects of soybean phytoestrogens in infant feeding. N Z Med J 1995;108(1000):208-209.
Ishikawa-Takata K, Ohta T. Relationship of lifestyle factors to bone mass in Japanese women. J Nutr Health Aging 2003;7(1):44-53.
Jacobsen BK, Knutsen SF, Fraser GE. Does high soy milk intake reduce prostate cancer incidence? The Adventist Health Study (United States). Cancer Causes Control 1998;9(6): 553-557.
Jenkins DJ, Kendall CW, Marchie A., et al. Effects of a dietary portfolio of cholesterol-lowering foods vs lovastatin on serum lipids and C-reactive protein. JAMA 2003;290(4):531-533.
Jenkins DJ, Kendall CW, Marchie A, et al. Type 2 diabetes and the vegetarian diet. Am J Clin Nutr 2003;78(3 Suppl):610S-616S.
Jenkins DJ, Kendall CW, D'Costa MA, et al. Soy consumption and phytoestrogens: effect on

serum prostate specific antigen when blood lipids and oxidized low-density lipoprotein are reduced in hyperlipidemic men. J Urol 2003;169(2):507-511.

Johns P, Dowlati L, Wargo W. Determination of isoflavones in ready-to-feed soy-based infant formula. J AOAC Int 2003;86(1):72-78.

Kazi A, Daniel KG, Smith DM, et al. Inhibition of the proteasome activity, a novel mechanism associated with tumor cell apoptosis-inducing ability of genistein. Biochem Pharmacol 2003; 66(6):965-976.

Knight DC, Howes JB, Eden JA, et al. Effects on menopausal symptoms and acceptability of isoflavone-containing soy powder dietary supplementation. Climacteric 2001;4(1):13-18.

Koo WW, Hammami M, Margeson DP, et al. Reduced bone mineralization in infants fed palm olein–containing formula; a randomized, double-blinded, prospective trial. Pediatrics 2003; 111(5 Pt 1):1017-1023.

Kritz-Silverstein D, Von Muhlen D, Barrett-Connor E, et al. Isoflavones and cognitive function in older women: the Soy and Postmenopausal Health In Aging (SOPHIA) Study. Menopause 2003;10(3)196-202.

Kurzer MS. Phytoestrogen supplement use by women. J Nutr 2003;133(6):1983S-1986S.

Lack G, Fox D, Northstone K, et al. Factors associated with the development of peanut allergy in childhood. N Engl J Med 2003;348(11):977-985.

LaCroix DE, Wolf WR. Determination of total fat in milk- and soy-based infant formula powder by supercritical fluid extraction. J AOAC Int 2003;86(1):86-95.

Lampe JW. Isoflavonoid and lignan phytoestrogens as dietary biomarkers. J Nutr 2003; 133(Suppl 3):956S-964S.

Laurin D, Jacques H, Moorjani S, et al. Effects of a soy-protein beverage on plasma lipoproteins in children with familial hypercholesterolemia. Am J Clin Nutr 1991;54(1):98-103.

Lombaert GA, Pellaers P, Roscoe V, et al. Mycotoxins in infant cereal foods from the Canadian retail market. Food Addit Contam 2003;20(5);494-504.

Macfarlane BJ, van der Riet WB, Bothwell TH, et al. Effect of traditional oriental soy products on iron absorption. Am J Clin Nutr 1990;51(5):873-880.

Mahady GB, Parrot J, Lee C, et al. Botanical dietary supplement use in peri- and post-menopausal women. Menopause 2003;10(1):65-72.

Maskirinec G, Robbins C, Riola B, et al. Three measures show high compliance in a soy intervention among premenopausal women. J Am Diet Assoc 2003;103(7):861-866.

Maskarinec G, Williams AE, Carlin L. Mammographic densities in a one-year isoflavone intervention. Eur J Cancer Prev 2003;12(2):165-169.

Maskarinec G, Williams AE, Inouye JS, et al. A randomized isoflavone intervention among premenopausal women. Cancer Epidemiol Biomarkers Prev 2002;11(2):195-201.

Maubach J, Bracke ME, Heyerick A, et al. Quantative of soy-derived phytoestrogens in human breast tissue and biological fluids by high-performance liquid chromatography. J Chromatogr B Analyt Technol Biomed Life Sci 2003;784(1):137-144.

McFadyen IJ, Chetty U, Setchell KDR, et al. A randomized double blind, cross over trial of soya protein for the treatment of cyclical breast pain. Breast 2000;9:271-276.

Merz-Demlow BE, Duncan AM, Wangen KE, et al. Soy isoflavones improve plasma lipids in normocholesterolemic, premenopausal women. Am J Clin Nutr 2000;71(6):1462-1469.

Messina M, Hughes C. Efficacy of soyfoods and soybean isoflavone supplements for alleviating menopausal symptoms is positively related to initial hot flush frequency. J Med Food 2003; 6(1):1-11.

Messina MJ. Emerging evidence on the role of soy in reducing prostate cancer risk. Nutr Rev 2003;61(4):117-131.

Migliaccio S, Anderon JJ. Isoflavones and skeletal health: are these molecules ready for clinical application? Osteoporos Int 2003;14(5):361-368.

Miltyk W, Craciunescu CN, Fischer L, et al. Lack of significant genotoxicity of purified soy isoflavones (genistein, daidzein, and glycitein) in 20 patients with prostate cancer. Am J Clin Nutr 2003;77(4):875-882.

Mimouni F, Campaigne B, Neylan M, et al. Bone mineralization in the first year of life in infants fed human milk, cow-milk formula, or soy-based formula. J Pediatr 1993;122(3): 348-354.

Moeller Le, Peterson CT, Hanson KB, et al. Isoflavone-rich soy protein prevents loss of hip lean

S

mass but does not prevent the shift in regional fat distribution in perimenopausal women. Menopause 2003;10(4):322-331.

Morens C, Bos C, Pueyo ME, et al. Increasing habitual protein intake accentuates differences in postprandial dietary nitrogen utilization between protein sources in humans. J Nutr 2003; 133(9):2733-2740.

Nagata C, Kabuto M, Kurisu Y, et al. Decreased serum estradiol concentration associated with high dietary intake of soy products in premenopausal Japanese women. Nutr Cancer 1997; 29(3):228-233.

Nagata C, Shimizu H, Takami R, et al. Association of blood pressure with intake of soy products and other food groups in Japanese men and women. Prev Med 2003;36(6):692-697.

Nagata C, Shimizu H, Takami R, et al. Soy product intake is inversely associated with serum homocysteine level in premenopausal Japanese women. J Nutr 2003;133(3):797-800.

Nagata C, Takatsuka N, Kawakami N, et al. A prospective cohort study of soy product intake and stomach cancer death. Br J Cancer 2002;87(1):31-36.

Nagata C, Takatsuka N, Kawakami N, et al. Soy product intake and hot flashes in Japanese women: results from a community-based prospective study. Am J Epidemiol 2001;153(8): 790-793.

Nagata C, Takatsuka N, Kurisu Y, et al. Decreased serum total cholesterol concentration is associated with high intake of soy products in Japanese men and women. J Nutr 1998;128(2): 209-213.

Nikitovic D, Tsatsakis AM, Karamanos NK, et al. The effects of genistein on the synthesis and distribution of glycosaminoglycans/proteoglycans by two osteosarcoma cell lines depends on tyrosine kinase and the estrogen receptor density. Anticancer Res 2003;23(1A):459-464.

North K, Golding J. A maternal vegetarian diet in pregnancy is associated with hypospadias. The ALSPAC Study Team. Avon Longitudinal Study of Pregnancy and Childhood. BJU Int 2000;85(1):107-113.

Nowak-Wegrzyn A, Sampson HA, Wood RA, et al. Food protein-induced enterocolitis syndrome caused by solid food proteins. Pediatrics 2003;111(4 Pt 1):829-835.

Oerter Klein K, Janfaza M, Wong JA, et al. Estrogen bioactivity in fo-ti and other herbs used for their estrogen-like effects as determined by a recombinant cell bioassay. J Clin Endocrinol Metab. 2003;88(9): 4075-4076.

Pathak SK, Sharma RA, Mellon JK. Chemoprevention of prostate cancer by diet-derived antioxidant agents and hormonal manipulation (Review). Int J Oncol 2003;22(1):5-13.

Penotti M, Fabio E, Modena AB, et al. Effect of soy-derived isoflavones on hot flushes, endometrial thickness, and the pulsatility index of the uterine and cerebral arteries. Fertil Steril 2003;79(5):1112-1117.

Pino AM, Vallardes LE, Palma MA, et al. Dietary isoflavones affect sex hormone-binding globulin levels in postmenopausal women. J Clin Endocrinol Metab 2000;85(8):2797-2800.

Potter SM, Bakshit RM, Essex-Sorlie DL, et al. Depression of plasma cholesterol in men by consumption of baked products containing soy protein. Am J Clin Nutr 1993;58(4): 501-506.

Potter SM, Baum JA, Teng H, et al. Soy protein and isoflavones: their effects on blood lipids and bone density in postmenopausal women. Am J Clin Nutr 1998;68(6 Suppl):1375S-1379S.

Puska P, Korpelainen V, Hoie LH, et al. Soy in hypercholesterolaemia: a double-blind, placebo-controlled trial. Eur J Clin Nutr 2002;56(4):352-357.

Quella SK, Loprinzi CL, Barton DL, et al. Evaluation of soy phytoestrogens for the treatment of hot flashes in breast cancer survivors: A North Central Cancer Treatment Group Trial. J Clin Oncol 2000;18(5):1068-1074.

Rajaram S. The effect of vegetarian diet, plant foods, and phytochemicals on hemostasis and thrombosis. Am J Clin Nutr 2003;78(3 Suppl):552S-558S.

Register TC, Jayo MJ, Anthony MS. Soy phytoestrogens do not prevent bone loss in post-menopausal monkeys. J Clin Endocrinol Metab 2003; 88(9):4362-4370.

Rivas M, Garay RP, Escanero JF, et al. Soy milk lowers blood pressure in men and women with mild to moderate essential hypertension. J Nutr 2002;132(7):1900-1902.

Rossi EA, Vendramini RC, Carlos IZ, et al. Effect of a new fermented soy milk product on serum lipid levels in normocholesterolemic adult men. Arch Latinoam Nutr 2003;53(1):47-51.

Santosham M, Goepp J, Burns B, et al. Role of a soy-based lactose-free formula in the outpatient management of diarrhea. Pediatrics 1991;87(5):619-622.

Scambia G, Mango D, Signorile PG, et al. Clinical effects of a standardized soy extract in postmenopausal women: a pilot study. Menopause 2000;7(2):105-111.

Scheiber MD, Liu JH, Subbiah MT, et al. Dietary inclusion of whole soy foods results in significant reductions in clinical risk factors for osteoporosis and cardiovascular disease in normal postmenopausal women. Menopause 2001;8(5):384-392.

Setchell KD, Brown NM, Desai PB, et al. Bioavailability, disposition, and dose-response effects of soy isoflavones when consumed by healthy women at physiologically typical dietary intakes. J Nutr 2003;133(4):1027-1035.

Setchell KD, Cassidy A. Dietary isoflavones: biological effects and relevance to human health. J Nutr 1999;129:758S-767S.

Setchell KD, Faughnan MS, Avades T, et al. Comparing the pharmacokinetics of daidzein and genistein with the use of ^{13}C-labeled tracers in premenopausal women. Am J Clin Nutr 2003;77(2):411-419.

Setchell KD, Lydeking-Olsen E. Dietary phytoestrogens and their effect on bone: evidence from *in vitro* and *in vivo*, human observational, and dietary intervention studies. Am J Clin 2003;78(3 Suppl):593S-609S.

Shimakawa Y, Matsubara S, Yuki N, et al. Evaluation of *Bifidobacterium breve* strain Yakult-fermented soymilk as a probiotic food. Int J Food Microbiol 2003;81(2):131-136.

Shu XO, Jin F, Dai Q, et al. Soyfood intake during adolescence and subsequent risk of breast cancer among Chinese women. Cancer Epidemiol Biomarkers Prev 2001;10(5):483-488.

Sirtori CR. Dubious benefits and potential risk of soy phyto-oestrogens. Lancet 2000; 355(9206):849.

Somekawa Y, Chiguchi M, Ishibashi T, et al. Soy intake related to menopausal symptoms, serum lipids, and bone mineral density in postmenopausal Japanese women. Obstet Gynecol 2001; 97(1):109-115.

Spilburg CA, Goldberg AC, McGill JB, et al. Fat-free foods supplemented with soy stanol-lecithin powder reduce cholesterol absorption and LDL cholesterol. J Am Diet Assoc 2003; 103(5):577-581.

St Germain A, Peterson CT, Robinson JG, et al. Isoflavone-rich or isoflavone-poor soy protein does not reduce menopausal symptoms during 24 weeks of treatment. Menopause 2001; 8(1):17-26.

Steichen JJ, Tsang RC. Bone mineralization and growth in term infants fed soy-based or cow milk-based formula. J Pediatr 1987;110(5):687-692.

Steinberg FM, Guthrie NL, Villablanca AC, et al. Soy protein with isoflavones has favorable effects on endothelial function that are independent of lipid and antioxidant effects in healthy postmenopausal women. Am J Clin Nutr 2003;78(1):123-130.

Strom BL, Schinnar R, Ziegler EE, et al. Exposure to soy-based formula in infancy and endocrinological and reproductive outcomes in young adulthood. JAMA 2001;286(7):807-814.

Strom SS, Yamamura Y, Duphorne CM, et al. Phytoestrogen intake and prostate cancer: a case-control study using a new database. Nutr Cancer 1999;33(1):20-25.

Taylor M. Alternatives to HRT: an evidence-based review. Int J Fertil Womens Med 2003; 48(2):64-68.

Teede HJ, Dalais FS, Kotsopoulos D, et al. Dietary soy has both beneficial and potentially adverse cardiovascular effects: a placebo-controlled study in men and postmenopausal women. J Clin Endocrinol Metab 2001;86(7):3053-3060.

Teixeira SR, Potter SM, Weigel R, et al. Effects of feeding 4 levels of soy protein for 3 and 6 wk on blood lipids and apolipoproteins in moderately hypercholesterolemic men. Am J Clin Nutr 2000;71(5):1077-1084.

Tice JA, Ettinger B, Ensrud K, et al. Phytoestrogen supplements for the treatment of hot flashes: the Isoflavone Clover Extract (ICE) Study: a randomized controlled trial. JAMA 2003;290(2):207-214.

Tonstad S, Smerud K, Hoie L. A comparison of the effects of 2 doses of soy protein or casein on serum lipids, serum lipoproteins, and plasma total homocysteine in hypercholesterolemic subjects. Am J Clin Nutr 2002;76(1):78-84.

Tsuchida K, Mizushima S, Toba M, et al. Dietary soybeans intake and bone mineral density among 995 middle-aged women in Yokohama. J Epidemiol 1999;9(1):14-19.

Turner NJ, Thomson BM, Shaw IC. Bioactive isoflavones in functional foods: the importance of gut microflora on bioavailability. Nutr Rev 2003;61(6 Pt 1):204-213.

Uesugi T, Fukui Y, Yamori Y. Beneficial effects of soybean isoflavone supplementation on bone metabolism and serum lipids in postmenopausal Japanese women: a four-week study. J Am Coll Nutr 2002;21(2):97-102.

Upmalis DH, Lobo R, Bradley L, et al. Vasomotor symptom relief by soy isoflavone extract tablets in postmenopausal women: a multicenter, double-blind, randomized, placebo-controlled study. Menopause 2000;7(4):236-242.

Van Patten CL, Olivotto IA, Chambers GK, et al. Effect of soy phytoestrogens on hot flashes in postmenopausal women with breast cancer: A randomized, controlled clinical trial. J Clin Oncol 2002;20(6):1449-1455.

Vanderhoof JA, Murray ND, Paule CL, et al. Use of soy fiber in acute diarrhea in infants and toddlers. Clin Pediatr (Phila) 1997;36(3):135-139.

Wangen KE, Duncan AM, Xu X, et al. Soy isoflavones improve plasma lipids in normocholesterolemic and mildly hypercholesterolemic postmenopausal women. Am J Clin Nutr 2001;73(2):225-231.

Watanabe S, Uesugi S, Zhuo X, et al. Phytoestrogens and cancer prevention. Gan To Kagaku Ryoho 2003;30(7):902-908.

White LR, Petrovitch H, Ross GW, et al. Brain aging and midlife tofu consumption. J Am Coll Nutr 2000;19(2):242-255.

Whitten PL, Lewis C, Russell E, et al. Potential adverse effects of phytoestrogens. J Nutr 1995;125(3 Suppl):771S-776S.

Wietzke JA, Welsh J. Phytoestrogen regulation of a vitamin D_3 receptor promoter and 1,25-dihydroxyvitamin D_3 actions in human breast cancer cells. J Steroid Biochem Mol Biol; 84(2-3):149-157.

Willett W. Lessons from dietary studies in Adventists and questions for the future. Am J Clin Nutr 2003;78(3 Suppl):539S-543S.

Wilson LC, Baek SJ, Call A, et al. Nonsteroidal anti-inflammatory drug-activated gene (NAG-1) is induced by genistein through the expression of p53 in colorectal cancer cells. Int J Cancer 2003;105(6):747-753.

Wong WW, Smith EO, Stuff JE, et al. Cholesterol-lowering effect of soy protein in normocholesterolemic and hypercholesterolemic men. Am J Clin Nutr 1998;68(6 Suppl): 1385S-1389S.

Woods RK, Walters EH, Raven JM. Food and nutrient intakes and asthma risk in young adults. Am J Clin Nutr 2003;78(3):414-423.

Wu AH, Yu MC, Tseng CC, et al. Green tea and risk of breast cancer in Asian Americans. Int J Cancer 2003;106(4):574-579.

Wu AH, Ziegler RG, Horn-Ross PL, et al. Tofu and risk of breast cancer in Asian-Americans. Cancer Epidemiol Biomarkers Prev 1996;5(11):901-906.

Yamamoto S, Sobue T, Kobayashi M, et al. Soy, isoflavones, and breast cancer risk in Japan. J Natl Cancer Inst 2003;95(12):906-913.

Yimyaem P, Chongsrisawat V, Vivatvakin B, et al. Gastrointestinal manifestations of cow's milk protein allergy during the first year of life. J Med Assoc Thai 2003;86(2):116-123.

Yu L, Blackburn GL, Zhou JR. Genistein and daidzein downregulate prostate androgen-regulated transcript-1 (PART-1) gene expression induced by dihydrotestosterone in human prostate LNCaP cancer cells. J Nutr 2003;133(2):389-392.

Zhang X, Shu XO, Gao YT, et al. Soy food consumption is associated with lower risk of coronary heart disease in Chinese women. J Nutr 2003;133(9):2874-2878.

Zhang Y, Hendrich S, Murphy PA. Glucuronides are the main isoflavone metabolites in women. J Nutr 2003;133(2):399-404.

Zhao XF, Hao LY, Yin SA, et al. Effect of long term supplementation of mineral-fortified dephytinized soy milk powder on biomarkers of bone turnover in boys aged 12 to 14 years. Zhonghua Yu Fang Yi Xue Za Zhi 2003;37(1):9-11.

Zhou JR, Yu L, Zhong Y, et al. Soy phytochemicals and tea bioactive components synergistically inhibit androgen-sensitive human prostate tumors in mice. J Nutr 2003;133(2):516-521.

Zubik L, Meydani M. Bioavailability of soybean isoflavones from aglycone and glucoside forms in American women. Am J Clin Nutr 2003;77(6):1459-1465.

Spirulina

(Aphanizomenon flos-aquae)

RELATED TERMS

- AFA, *Arthrospira platensis*, blue-green algae (BGA), cyanobacteria, dihe, klamath, *Microcystis aeruginosa*, *Microcystis wesenbergii*, Multinal, *Nostoc* spp., plant plankton, pond scum, *Spirulina fusiformis*, *Spirulina maxima*, *Spirulina platensis*, tecuitatl.
- *Note:* Non-*Spirulina* species, such as *Anabaena* species, *Aphanizomenon* species, and *Microcystis* species, are possibly unsafe because they are usually harvested naturally and may be subject to contamination.

BACKGROUND

- The term "spirulina" refers to any of a large number of cyanobacteria, or blue-green algae. Both Spirulina and non-Spirulina species fall into the classification of cyanobacteria and include *Aphanizomenon*, *Microcystis*, *Nostoc*, and *Spirulina* species. Most commercial products contain *Aphanizomenon flos-aquae*, *Spirulina maxima*, and/or *Spirulina platensis*. These algae are found in the warm, alkaline waters of the world, especially of Mexico and Central America. *Spirulina* algae are most often grown under controlled conditions and are subject to less contamination than the non-Spirulina algae that are harvested naturally.
- Spirulina is a rich source of nutrients, containing up to 70% protein, as well as B-complex vitamins, phycocyanin, chlorophyll, beta-carotene, vitamin E, and numerous minerals. In fact, spirulina contains more beta-carotene than carrots. Spirulina has been used since ancient times as a source of nutrients and has been said to possess a variety of medical uses, including as an antioxidant, antiviral, antineoplastic, weight loss aid, and lipid-lowering agent. Preliminary data from animal studies demonstrate effectiveness for some conditions as well as safety, although human evidence is lacking. On the basis of available research, no recommendation can be made either for or against the use of spirulina for any indication.

S

USES BASED ON SCIENTIFIC EVIDENCE	Grade*
Diabetes Preliminary study in people with type 2 diabetes mellitus reports that spirulina may reduce fasting blood sugar levels after 2 months of treatment. More research is needed before a firm conclusion can be drawn.	C
High cholesterol In animal studies, spirulina has been found to lower blood cholesterol and triglyceride levels. Preliminary poor-quality studies in humans suggest a similar effect. Better research is needed before a firm conclusion can be drawn.	C

Continued

Condition	Grade*
Oral leukoplakia (precancerous mouth lesions) Preliminary research has not clearly shown benefits of spirulina in the treatment of oral leukoplakia.	C
Weight loss Spirulina supplementation is a popular therapy for weight loss, and spirulina is sometimes marketed as a "vitamin-enriched" appetite suppressant. However, little scientific information is available on the effect of spirulina on weight loss in humans.	C
Malnutrition Spirulina has been studied as a food supplement in infant malnutrition. In a randomized controlled trial, 182 malnourished children younger than 2 years of age were given spirulina as a food supplement. The authors observed no added benefit of spirulina over traditional nutrition. Spirulina supplementation is often more costly and is currently not recommended for this condition.	D

*Key to grades: *A:* Strong scientific evidence for this use; *B:* Good scientific evidence for this use; *C:* Unclear scientific evidence for this use; *D:* Fair scientific evidence against this use (it may not work); *F:* Strong scientific evidence against this use (it likely does not work). For a more detailed explanation of efficacy criteria, see "Natural Standard Evidence-Based Validated Grading Rationale" in the Introduction.

Uses Based on Tradition, Theory, or Limited Scientific Evidence

Allergies, anaphylaxis (severe allergic reaction) prevention, anemia, antifungal, anti-inflammatory, antioxidant, antiviral, anxiety, atherosclerosis, attention deficit hyperactivity disorder (ADHD), bowel health, cancer prevention, cancer treatment, colitis, cytomegalovirus infection, depression, digestion, energy booster, fatigue, fatty liver, fibromyalgia, hair loss, heart disease, herpes simplex virus type 1 (HSV-1), high blood pressure, human immunodeficiency virus infection (HIV), immune system enhancement, influenza, iron deficiency, kidney disease, liver protection, measles, memory improvement, mood stimulant, mumps, obstetric and gynecologic disorders, premenstrual syndrome, radiation sickness, skin disorders, stomach acid excess, ulcers, vitamin and nutrient deficiency, warts, wound healing, yeast infection.

DOSING

The following doses are based on scientific research, publications, traditional use, or expert opinion. Many herbs and supplements have not been thoroughly tested, and their safety and effectiveness may not be proven. Brands may be made differently, with variable ingredients even within the same brand. The doses shown may not apply to all products. It is important to always read product labels and discuss doses with a qualified healthcare provider before therapy is started.

Standardization

- Standardization involves measuring the amount of certain chemicals in products to try to make different preparations similar to each other. It is not always known if the chemicals being measured are the "active" ingredients.
- There is no widely accepted standardization for spirulina products.

Adults (18 Years and Older)

- **High cholesterol:** 1.4 g of spirulina by mouth, three times daily with meals, for 8 weeks has been studied.
- **Diabetes mellitus (type 2):** 1 g of spirulina by mouth twice daily with meals has been studied.
- **Weight loss:** 200 mg of spirulina tablets by mouth three times daily, taken just before eating, has been studied.
- **Oral leukoplakia (precancerous mouth lesions):** 1 g of *Spirulina fusiformis* by mouth daily has been used for up to a year in one study.

Children (Younger Than 18 Years)

- Not enough scientific information is available to advise the safe use of spirulina in children.

SAFETY

The U.S. Food and Drug Administration does not strictly regulate herbs and supplements. There is no guarantee of strength, purity, or safety of products, and effects may vary. It is important to always read product labels. People who have a medical condition, or are taking other drugs, herbs, or supplements, should consult a qualified healthcare provider before starting a new therapy. A healthcare provider should be consulted immediately about any side effects.

Allergies

- Avoid use in individuals with known allergy to spirulina or blue-green algae species, or any of their constituents.

Side Effects and Warnings

- Few side effects have been reported with spirulina use in people. The most frequently reported adverse effects are headache, muscle pain, flushing of the face, sweating, and difficulty concentrating. These have been described in people taking 1 g of spirulina by mouth daily.
- Blue-green algae, especially types that are usually harvested in uncontrolled settings (*Anabaena* spp., *Aphanizomenon* spp., and *Microcystis* spp.), may be contaminated with heavy metals.
- The amino acid phenylalanine in blue-green algae may cause an adverse reaction in people with the genetic condition phenylketonuria (PKU); therefore, preparations containing these algae should be used cautiously by people with PKU.

Pregnancy and Breastfeeding

- There is not enough information to recommend the safe use of spirulina during pregnancy or breastfeeding. In mice, diets containing up to 30% spirulina are not reported to cause harmful effects to either the mother or the offspring. However, reliable human studies addressing safety during pregnancy or breastfeeding are not available.

INTERACTIONS

Most herbs and supplements have not been thoroughly tested for interactions with other herbs, supplements, drugs, or foods. The interactions listed here are based on reports in scientific publications, laboratory experiments, or traditional use. It is important to always read product labels. People who have a medical condition, or are taking other drugs, herbs, or supplements, should consult a qualified healthcare provider before starting a new therapy.

Interactions with Drugs

- Little information is available about the interactions of spirulina and other medications.

Interactions with Herbs and Dietary Supplements

- Small increases in calcium levels were reported in a weight loss study using 200-mg spirulina tablets for 4 weeks. However, the study also included a reduced-calorie diet that was not described. On the basis of this information, use of spirulina and calcium supplements together may further increase calcium levels.
- Blue-green algae may contain high levels of vitamin B_{12}.

Interactions with Foods

- Blue-green algae can contain high levels of the amino acid phenylalanine and may cause an adverse reaction in people with the genetic condition PKU. Individuals with PKU should use caution when taking spirulina and other foods with high levels of phenylalanine.

Selected References

Natural Standard developed the preceding evidence-based information based on a systematic review of more than 170 scientific articles. For comprehensive information about alternative and complementary therapies on the professional level, go to www.naturalstandard.com. Selected references are listed here.

Branger B, Cadudal JL, Delobel M, et al. [Spiruline as a food supplement in case of infant malnutrition in Burkina-Faso]. Arch Pediatr 2003;10(5):424-431.

Chamorro G, Salazar M, Araujo KG, et al. [Update on the pharmacology of *Spirulina* (*Arthrospira*), an unconventional food]. Arch Latinoam Nutr 2002;52(3):232-240.

Hernandez-Corona A, Nieves I, Meckes M, et al. Antiviral activity of *Spirulina maxima* against herpes simplex virus type 2. Antiviral Res 2002;56(3):279-85.

Hirahashi T, Matsumoto M, Hazeki K, et al. Activation of the human innate immune system by *Spirulina*: augmentation of interferon production and NK cytotoxicity by oral administration of hot water extract of *Spirulina platensis*. Int Immunopharmacol 2002;2(4):423-434.

Iwasa M, Yamamoto M, Tanaka Y, et al. Spirulina-associated hepatotoxicity. Am J Gastroenterol 2002;97(12):3212-3213.

Jensen GS, Ginsberg DI. Consumption of *Aphanizomenon flos aquae* has rapid effects on the circulation and function of immune cells in humans. J Am Nutraceut Assoc 2000;2(3):50-58.

Jensen GS, Ginsberg DI, Drapeau C. Blue-green algae as an immuno-enhancer and bio-modulator. J Am Nutraceut Assoc 2001;3(4):24-30.

Mani UV, Desai S, Iyer U. Studies on the long-term effect of spirulina supplementation on serum lipid profile and glycated proteins in NIDDM patients. J Nutraceut 2000;2(3):25-32.

Mathew B, Sankaranarayanan R, Nair PP, et al. Evaluation of chemoprevention of oral cancer with *Spirulina fusiformis*. Nutr Cancer 1995;24(2):197-202.

Mishima T, Murata J, Toyoshima M, et al. Inhibition of tumor invasion and metastasis by calcium spirulan (Ca-SP), a novel sulfated polysaccharide derived from a blue-green alga, *Spirulina platensis*. Clin Exp Metastasis 1998;16:541-550.

Romay C, Armesto J, Remirez D, et al. Antioxidant and anti-inflammatory properties of C-phycocyanin from blue- green algae. Inflamm Res 1998;47(1):36-41.
Samuels R, Mani UV, Iyer UM, et al. Hypocholesterolemic effect of spirulina in patients with hyperlipidemic nephrotic syndrome. J Med Food 2002;5(2):91-96.
Shih SR, Tsai KN, Li YS, et al. Inhibition of enterovirus 71-induced apoptosis by allophycocyanin isolated from a blue-green alga *Spirulina platensis.* J Med Virol 2003;70(1): 119-125.
Watanabe F, Takenaka S, Kittaka-Katsura H, et al. Characterization and bioavailability of vitamin B_{12}-compounds from edible algae. J Nutr Sci Vitaminol (Tokyo) 2002;48(5): 325-331.
Yang HN, Lee EH, Kim HM. *Spirulina platensis* inhibits anaphylactic reaction. Life Sci 1997; 61(13):1237-1244.

St. John's Wort

(*Hypericum perforatum* L.)

RELATED TERMS

- Amber touch-and-heal, balm-of-warrior's wound, balsana, bassant, blutkraut, bossant, corancillo, dendlu, devil's scourge, flor de Sao Joa, fuga daemonum, goatweed, hartheu, heofarigo on herba de millepertius, herba hyperici, herrgottsblut, hexenkraut, hierba de San Juan, hipericao, hiperico hipericon, isenblut, Johanniskraut, klammath weed, liebeskraut, LI 160, Lord God's wonder plant, millepertius pelicao, perforate, pinillo de oro, rosin rose, tenturotou, teufelsflucht, touch and heal, Walpurgiskraut, witcher's herb, WS 5572.

BACKGROUND

- Extracts of *Hypericum perforatum* L. (St. John's wort) have been recommended traditionally for a wide range of medical conditions. The most common modern-day use of St. John's wort is for the treatment of depression. Numerous studies report St. John's wort to be more effective than placebo and equally effective as tricyclic antidepressant drugs in the short-term treatment of mild to moderate major depression (1 to 3 months). It is not clear if St. John's wort is as effective as selective serotonin reuptake inhibitor (SSRI) antidepressants such as sertraline (Zoloft).
- Recently, controversy has been raised by two high-quality trials of St. John's wort for major depression that did not show any benefits. However, because of problems with the designs of these studies, they cannot be considered definitive. Overall, the scientific evidence supports the effectiveness of St. John's wort in mild to moderate major depression. The evidence in severe major depression remains unclear.
- St. John's wort can cause many serious interactions with prescription drugs, herbs, or supplements. Therefore, people using any medications should consult their healthcare provider and pharmacist prior to starting therapy.

USES BASED ON SCIENTIFIC EVIDENCE	Grade*
Depressive disorder (mild to moderate) St. John's wort has been extensively studied in Europe over the last two decades, with more recent research in the United States. Short-term studies (1 to 3 months) suggest that St. John's wort is more effective than placebo (sugar pill) and equally effective as tricyclic antidepressants (TCAs) in the treatment of mild to moderate major depression. Comparisons with the more commonly prescribed SSRI antidepressants, such as fluoxetine (Prozac) and sertraline (Zoloft), are more limited.	A
Anxiety disorder Several studies in patients with depression report that in addition to effects on depression, St. John's wort may also reduce anxiety symptoms. There is one study of St. John's wort (in a combination product with valerian) that specifically treated people with anxiety. It is important to realize that valerian alone is often used to treat anxiety, and	C

Continued

therefore any effects of the combination product may be due to valerian and not to St. John's wort. Therefore, there is currently not enough evidence to recommend St. John's wort for the primary treatment of anxiety disorders.	
Depressive disorder (severe) Studies of St. John's wort for severe depression have not provided clear evidence of effectiveness. A recent study reported that neither St. John's wort nor the SSRI drug sertraline (Zoloft) provided benefits over placebo for severe depression. Other recent well-designed research has suggested no benefit of St. John's wort for severe depression, although the evidence is still not completely clear in this area.	C
Obsessive-compulsive disorder There are a few reported cases of possible benefits of St. John's wort in patients with obsessive-compulsive disorder (OCD). However, because of a lack of large, controlled studies comparing St. John's wort with placebo or drugs, there is currently not enough scientific evidence to recommend St. John's wort for this condition.	C
Perimenopausal symptoms Several small studies suggest possible benefits of St. John's wort for psychological symptoms experienced around menopause. However, there is currently not enough scientific evidence to recommend St. John's wort for this indication.	C
Premenstrual syndrome One small study suggests that St. John's wort may be effective in reducing symptoms of premenstrual syndrome (PMS). Further studies are needed before a recommendation can be made.	C
Seasonal affective disorder Despite some promising early data, there is currently not enough evidence to recommend St. John's wort for depressive disorder with seasonal pattern, or seasonal affective disorder (SAD).	C
Human immunodeficiency virus infection Antiviral effects of St. John's wort have been observed in laboratory studies but were not found in one human study. Multiple reports of significant adverse effects and interactions with drugs used for HIV/AIDS, including protease inhibitors (PIs) and non-nucleoside reverse transcriptase inhibitors (NNRTIs), suggest that patients undergoing treatment for HIV/AIDS should avoid this herb. Therefore, there is evidence to recommend against using St. John's wort in patients with HIV/AIDS.	D

*Key to grades: *A:* Strong scientific evidence for this use; *B:* Good scientific evidence for this use; *C:* Unclear scientific evidence for this use; *D:* Fair scientific evidence against this use (it may not work); *F:* Strong scientific evidence against this use (it likely does not work). For a more detailed explanation of efficacy criteria, see "Natural Standard Evidence-Based Validated Grading Rationale" in the Introduction.

Uses Based on Tradition, Theory, or Limited Scientific Evidence

Abdominal discomfort or irritation, alcoholism, allergies, anti-inflammatory, antiviral, athletic performance enhancement, bacterial skin infections (topical), bed-wetting, bruises (topical), benzodiazepine withdrawal, burns (topical), cancer, chronic bowel irritation, chronic ear infections, dental pain, diarrhea, diuretic (increasing urine flow), Epstein-Barr virus infection, fatigue, glioma, heartburn, hemorrhoids, herpesvirus infection, influenza, insomnia, joint pain, liver protection from toxins, malaria treatment, menstrual pain, nerve pain, pain relief, rheumatism, snakebite, skin scrapes, sprains, ulcers, wound healing (topical).

DOSING

The following doses are based on scientific research, publications, traditional use, or expert opinion. Many herbs and supplements have not been thoroughly tested, and their safety and effectiveness may not be proven. Brands may be made differently, with variable ingredients even within the same brand. The doses shown may not apply to all products. It is important to always read product labels and discuss doses with a qualified healthcare provider before therapy is started.

Standardization

- Standardization involves measuring the amount of certain chemicals in products to try to make different preparations similar to each other. It is not always known if the chemicals being measured are the "active" ingredients.
- St. John's wort products are often standardized to contain 0.3% of one of the components called hypericin, although there has been a movement within the manufacturing industry to standardize to a different component called hyperforin (usually 2% to 5%). In one analysis of eight German St. John's wort products, large differences in hypericin and hyperforin content were found, and there was also variability within batches of the same brand.

Adults (18 Years and Older)

- **Depression:** *Starting dose:* 300 mg of St. John's wort, standardized to 0.3% hypericin extract, taken by mouth three times daily (may be standardized to 2% to 5% hyperforin as well) has been studied. *Maintenance dose:* 300 to 600 mg daily may be sufficient for maintenance therapy, although this has not been well studied. A liquid form may be used, taken three times daily and standardized to contain equivalent amounts of hypericin or hyperforin as noted previously. (*Note:* Clinical trials have used a range of doses, including 0.17 to 2.7 mg of hypericin, and 900 to 1450 mg of St. John's wort extract daily.)

Children (Younger Than 18 Years)

- There are not enough scientific data to recommend St. John's wort in children. One study of 101 children younger than 12 years of age with symptoms of depression used 300 to 1800 mg of St. John's wort extract daily for 4 to 6 weeks, with good tolerance.

SAFETY

The U.S. Food and Drug Administration does not strictly regulate herbs and supplements. There is no guarantee of strength, purity, or safety of products, and effects may vary. It is important to always read product labels. People who have a medical condition, or are taking other drugs, herbs, or supplements, should consult a qualified healthcare provider before starting a new therapy. A healthcare provider should be consulted immediately about any side effects.

Allergies

- Infrequent allergic skin reactions, including rash and itching, are reported in human studies. A drug-monitoring study of 3250 patients reported 17 cases of allergic reactions and 10 cases in which St. John's wort was stopped because of the allergy.

Side Effects and Warnings

- In published studies, St. John's wort has generally been well tolerated at recommended doses for up to 1 to 3 months. The most common adverse effects include gastrointestinal upset, skin reactions, fatigue/sedation, restlessness or anxiety, sexual dysfunction (including impotence), dizziness, headache, and dry mouth. Several recent studies suggest that side effects occur in 1% to 3% of patients taking St. John's wort, and that the number of adverse events may be similar to that with placebo (and less than with standard antidepressant drugs). Animal toxicity studies have found only nonspecific symptoms such as weight loss. One small study reported elevated thyroid-stimulating hormone (TSH) levels to be associated with ingestion of St. John's wort.

Pregnancy and Breastfeeding

- Insufficient data are available at this time to recommend use of St. John's wort during pregnancy or breastfeeding.

INTERACTIONS

Most herbs and supplements have not been thoroughly tested for interactions with other herbs, supplements, drugs, or foods. The interactions listed here are based on reports in scientific publications, laboratory experiments, or traditional use. It is important to always read product labels. People who have a medical condition, or are taking other drugs, herbs, or supplements, should consult a qualified healthcare provider before starting a new therapy.

Interactions with Drugs

- There is strong evidence from animal studies and multiple human cases that St. John's wort interferes with how the body uses the liver's cytochrome P450 enzyme system to process many drugs. As a result, blood levels of these drugs may be increased in the short term (causing increased effects or potentially serious adverse reactions), and/or decreased in the long term (which can reduce the intended effects). Examples of medications that may be affected by St. John's wort in this manner are birth control pills, carbamazepine, cyclosporine, irinotecan, midazolam, nifedipine, simvastatin, theophylline, tricyclic antidepressants, warfarin, and HIV drugs such as NNRTIs and PIs. The U.S. Food and Drug Administration suggests that patients with HIV/AIDS on PIs or NNRTIs should avoid taking St. John's wort.
- There are multiple case reports of significant reduction in cyclosporine drug levels and possible organ rejection following transplantation in people taking St. John's wort. Reports also exist of altered menstrual flow, bleeding, and unwanted pregnancies in women taking birth control pills and St. John's wort at the same time. Based on one human study, St. John's wort may interact with digoxin or digitoxin:

10 days of treatment with hypericum, a chemical in St. John's wort, resulted in a 25% decrease in digoxin blood concentration. In general, people who are using any medications should check the package insert and consult their healthcare provider or pharmacist about possible interactions with St. John's wort.

- Based on theory and human cases, taking St. John's wort with other antidepressants may lead to increased side effects, including serotonin syndrome and mania. Serotonin syndrome is a condition defined by muscle rigidity, fever, confusion, increased blood pressure and heart rate, and coma. Mania is defined by symptoms of elevated or irritable mood, rapid speech or thoughts, increased activity, and decreased need for sleep. These interactions may occur in people taking St. John's wort with SSRI antidepressants such as fluoxetine (Prozac) or sertraline (Zoloft), or with monoamine oxidase inhibitors (MAOIs) such as isocarboxazid (Marplan), phenelzine (Nardil), or tranylcypromine (Parnate). Using St. John's wort with MAOIs may also increase the risk of severely increased blood pressure.
- Based on animal and human cases, St. John's wort may lead to increased risk of sun sensitivity when taken with other drugs such as antibiotics or birth control pills. Based on theory and one human case, St. John's wort may interact with anesthetic drugs. A possible interaction with loperamide (Imodium) has been reported; confusion and agitation occurred in one patient taking St. John's wort, loperamide, and the herb valerian (*Valeriana officinalis*). Based on theory, St. John's wort may interact with triptan-type headache medications. Examples are naratriptan (Amerge), rizatriptan (Maxalt), sumatriptan (Imitrex), and zolmitriptan (Zomig). In theory, St. John's wort may also interact with certain chemotherapy drugs such as anthracyclines. St. John's wort may increase anti-inflammatory effects of COX-2 inhibitor drugs such as Vioxx, or NSAIDs such as ibuprofen (Motrin).

Interactions with Herbs and Dietary Supplements

- Based on animal studies and multiple human cases of drug interactions, St. John's wort may interfere with how the body uses the liver's cytochrome P450 enzyme system to process components of certain herbs and supplements. As a result, blood levels of these components may be increased in the short term, causing increased effects or potentially serious adverse reactions, or decreased in the long term, which can reduce the intended effects. Examples of herbs or supplements that may be affected by St. John's wort in this manner are bloodroot, cat's claw, chamomile, chaparral, chasteberry, damiana, *Echinacea angustifolia*, goldenseal, grapefruit, licorice, oregano, red clover, wild cherry, and yucca.
- Based on theory and human cases, taking St. John's wort with herbs or supplements with antidepressant activity may lead to increased side effects, including serotonin syndrome, mania, and severe increase in blood pressure. There is a particular risk of occurrence of these interactions with agents that possess possible MAOI-type properties, including 5-hydroxytryptophan (5-HTP), California poppy, chromium, dehydroepiandrosterone (DHEA), ephedra, evening primrose oil, fenugreek, *Ginkgo biloba*, hops, mace, DL-phenylalanine (DLPA), *S*-adenosylmethionine (SAMe), sepia, tyrosine, valerian, vitamin B_6, and yohimbe bark extract.
- Based on animal research and human cases, St. John's wort may lead to increased risk of sun sensitivity when taken with capsaicin or other photosensitizing products. Based on one human study of the cardiac glycoside drug digoxin, St. John's wort may interact with herbs that also possess cardiac glycoside properties: 10 days of

treatment with hypericum, a chemical extracted from St. John's wort, resulted in a 25% decrease in digoxin blood concentration. Herbs with possible cardiac glycoside properties include adonis, balloon cotton, black hellebore root/melampode, black Indian hemp, bushman's poison, *Cactus grandifloris*, convallaria, eyebright, figwort, foxglove/digitalis, frangipani, hedge mustard, hemp root/Canadian hemp root, king's crown, lily-of-the-valley, motherwort, oleander leaf, pheasant's eye plant, plantain leaf, pleurisy root; psyllium husks, redheaded cottonbush, rhubarb root, rubber vine, sea mango, senna fruit, squill, strophanthus, uzara, wallflower, wintersweet, yellow dock root, yellow oleander.

- A possible interaction with the herb valerian (*Valeriana officinalis*) has been reported: confusion and agitation occurred in one patient taking St. John's wort, loperamide (Imodium), and valerian. However, St. John's wort and valerian are often used together, with few reported adverse events. In theory, because of the presence of tannins, St. John's wort may inhibit the absorption of iron.

Interactions with Foods

- In theory, use of St. John's wort may require avoiding certain foods and beverages that interact with MAOIs. This is because St. John's wort has been theorized to possess MAOI activity. Although it has recently been suggested that St. John's wort may not have significant MAOI properties in the body, there were early reports of this type of activity, and it has not been fully disproven. Tyramine/tryptophan-containing foods may cause dangerously high blood pressure when taken at the same time as agents that have properties similar to those of MAOIs, and caution is indicated regarding consumption of such foods by those taking St. John's wort. These include protein foods that have been aged/preserved. Examples are anchovies, avocados, bananas, bean curd, beer (alcohol-free/reduced), caffeine (large amounts), caviar, champagne, cheeses (particularly aged, processed, or strong varieties), chocolate, dry sausage/salami/bologna, fava beans, figs, herring (pickled), liver (particularly chicken liver), meat tenderizers, papaya, protein extracts/powder, raisins, shrimp paste, sour cream, soy sauce, wine (particularly chianti), yeast extracts, and yogurt.

S

Selected References

Natural Standard developed the preceding evidence-based information based on a systematic review of more than 450 scientific articles. For comprehensive information about alternative and complementary therapies on the professional level, go to www.naturalstandard.com. Selected references are listed here.

Albert D, Zundorf I, Dingermann T, et al. Hyperforin is a dual inhibitor of cyclooxygenase-1 and 5-lipoxygenase. Biochem Pharmacol 2002;64(12):1767-1775.

Andelic S. [Bigeminy—the result of interaction between digoxin and St. John's wort]. Vojnosanit Pregl 2003;60(3):361-364.

Bauer S, Stormer E, Johne A, et al. Alterations in cyclosporin A pharmacokinetics and metabolism during treatment with St John's wort in renal transplant patients. Br J Clin Pharmacol 2003;55(2):203-211.

Behnke K, Jensen GS, Graubaum HJ, et al. *Hypericum perforatum* versus fluoxetine in the treatment of mild to moderate depression. Adv Ther 2002;19(1):43-52.

Dean AJ, Moses GM, Vernon JM. Suspected withdrawal syndrome after cessation of St. John's wort. Ann Pharmacother 2003;37(1):151.

Hammerness P, Basch E, Ulbricht C, et al. St. John's wort: a systematic review of adverse effects and drug interactions for the consultation psychiatrist. Psychosomatics 2003;44:271-282.

Kalb R, Trautmann-Sponsel RD, Kieser M. Efficacy and tolerability of hypericum extract WS 5572 versus placebo in mildly to moderately depressed patients: a randomized double-blind multicenter clinical trial. Pharmacopsych 2001;34(3):96-103.

Kim HL, Streltzer J, Goebert D. St. John's wort for depression: a meta-analysis of well-defined clinical trials. J Nerv Ment Dis 1999;187(9):532-539.

Linde K, Mulrow CD. St John's wort for depression. Cochrane Database Syst Rev 2000;(2): CD000448.

Linde K, Ramirez G, Mulrow CD, et al. St John's wort for depression: an overview and meta-analysis of randomised clinical trials. BMJ 1996;313(7052):253-258.

Miller LG. Drug interactions known or potentially associated with St. John's wort. J Herbal Pharmacother 2001;1(3):51-64.

Parker V, Wong AH, Boon HS, et al. Adverse reactions to St John's wort. Can J Psychiatry 2001;46(1):77-79.

Philipp M, Kohnen R, Hiller KO. Hypericum extract versus imipramine or placebo in patients with moderate depression: randomised multicentre study of treatment for eight weeks. BMJ 1999;319(7224):1534-1538.

Shelton RC, Keller MB, Gelenberg A, et al. Effectiveness of St John's wort in major depression: a randomized controlled trial. JAMA 2001;285(15):1978-1986.

Wheatley D. Safety of St John's wort (*Hypericum perforatum*). Lancet 2000;355(9203):576.

Sweet Almond

(*Prunus amygdalus dulcis*)

RELATED TERMS

- Almendra, almendra dulce, almond oil, amande, amande douce, amandel, amendoa, amêndoa doce, amigdalo, *Amygdalus communis, Amygdala dulcis*, badam, badami, badamo, badamshirin, bedamu, bian tao, bilati badam, cno ghreugach, expressed almond oil, fixed almond oil, harilik mandlipuu, Jordan almond, lawz, lozi, mandel, mandla, mandorla, mandorla dulce, mandula, mangel, mantelli, migdal, migdala, migdalo, mindal, Prunoidae (subfamily), *Prunus communis dulcis, Prunus dulcis var. dulcis*, Rosaceae (family), sladkiy mindal, sötmandel, süßmandel, sweet almond oil, tatli badem, tian wei bian tao, tian xing ren, vaadaam, vadumai, zoete amandel.
- *Note:* Sweet almond should not be confused with bitter almond, which contains amygdalin and can be broken down into the poisonous substance hydrocyanic acid (cyanide).

BACKGROUND

- The almond is closely related to the peach, apricot, and cherry (all classified as drupes). Unlike the fruit of the others, however, the outer layer of the almond is not edible. The edible portion of the almond is the seed.
- Sweet almonds are a popular nutritious food. Researchers are especially interested in their content of monounsaturated fats, as these appear to have a beneficial effect on blood lipids.
- Almond oil is widely used in lotions and cosmetics.

USES BASED ON SCIENTIFIC EVIDENCE	Grade*
High cholesterol (whole almonds) Early studies in humans and animals report that whole almonds may lower total cholesterol and low-density lipoprotein (LDL) ("bad" cholesterol) and raise high-density lipoprotein (HDL) ("good" cholesterol). It is not clear what dose may be safe or effective.	B
Radiation therapy skin reactions (used on the skin) In preliminary study, an ointment made of sweet almond has not shown a benefit when applied to the skin of patients receiving radiation therapy.	D

*Key to grades: *A:* Strong scientific evidence for this use; *B:* Good scientific evidence for this use; *C:* Unclear scientific evidence for this use; *D:* Fair scientific evidence against this use (it may not work); F: Strong scientific evidence against this use (it likely does not work). For a more detailed explanation of efficacy criteria, see "Natural Standard Evidence-Based Validated Grading Rationale" in the Introduction.

Uses Based on Tradition, Theory, or Limited Scientific Evidence

Antibacterial, aphrodisiac, bladder cancer, breast cancer, chapped lips, colon cancer, dilution of injected medications, emollient, heart disease, increasing sperm count, mild laxative, moisturizer, mouth and throat cancers, plant-derived estrogen, uterine cancer.

DOSING

The following doses are based on scientific research, publications, traditional use, or expert opinion. Many herbs and supplements have not been thoroughly tested, and their safety and effectiveness may not be proven. Brands may be made differently, with variable ingredients even within the same brand. The doses shown may not apply to all products. It is important to always read product labels and discuss doses with a qualified healthcare provider before therapy is started.

Standardization

- Standardization involves measuring the amount of certain chemicals in products to try to make different preparations similar to each other. It is not always known if the chemicals being measured are the "active" ingredients.
- Standardized sweet almond products are not widely available. Almond samples have been found to be contaminated with a dangerous molecule, aflatoxin. Aflatoxin is produced by Aspergillus fungus and is also present in small amounts in peanut products. The U.S. Department of Agriculture (USDA) is responsible for monitoring aflatoxin concentrations.

Adults (18 Years and Older)

- **High cholesterol:** Studies have used 84 to 100 g of whole almonds daily by mouth with no reported side effects.
- **Laxative:** 30 ml of sweet almond oil daily by mouth has been used.
- *Note:* A small randomized controlled trial showed the same cholesterol profile benefits in patients taking almond oil versus whole almonds, although dosing was based on a percentage of habitual fat intake and not on a specific weight of whole almonds or measure of almond oil. Sweet almonds and sweet almond oil should not be confused with bitter almonds or bitter almond oil, which can be dangerous in humans.

Children (Younger Than 18 Years)

- Little information is available for the use of sweet almonds in children, aside from the amounts normally eaten in the diet.

SAFETY

The U.S. Food and Drug Administration does not strictly regulate herbs and supplements. There is no guarantee of strength, purity, or safety of products, and effects may vary. It is important to always read product labels. People who have a medical condition, or are taking other drugs, herbs, or supplements, should consult a qualified healthcare provider before starting a new therapy. A healthcare provider should be consulted immediately about any side effects.

Allergies

- Allergies to almonds are common and can lead to severe reactions, including oral allergic syndrome (OAS), swelling of the lips and face, and closure of the throat. People who are allergic to one type of nut may also be allergic to other nuts. Avoid use in anyone with known allergy to almonds, almond products, or other nuts.

Side Effects and Warnings

- In most reports, sweet almond is generally considered to be safe when taken by mouth. Based on animal studies, sweet almond may lower blood sugar levels. Caution is advised in patients with diabetes or hypoglycemia, and in those taking drugs, herbs, or supplements that affect blood sugar. Serum glucose levels may need to be monitored by a healthcare provider, and medication adjustments may be necessary.
- Mice fed sweet almonds have been reported to lose weight, but it is not clear if this reflects a change in their diet or a specific effect of almonds. Almonds are reported to lower LDL ("bad cholesterol") and total cholesterol levels. One animal study reports that sweet almond may have estrogen-like activity. A study in mice reports hair loss and inflammation in the leg joints. There is a report of a fat embolism (fat bubbles traveling through the bloodstream, which is potentially dangerous) due to injection of almond oil into the penis.
- Theoretically, increased intake of almonds (and therefore increased intake of unsaturated fat) can lead to weight gain. However, a small randomized controlled trial reports that consuming approximately 320 calories of almonds daily for 6 months does not lead to statistically or biologically significant average changes in body weight and does increase the amount of unsaturated fats in the diet.

Pregnancy and Breastfeeding

- There is little information about the use of sweet almond during pregnancy or breastfeeding. It appears that almonds in regular dietary intake are safe for most nonallergic individuals.

S

INTERACTIONS

Most herbs and supplements have not been thoroughly tested for interactions with other herbs, supplements, drugs, or foods. The interactions listed here are based on reports in scientific publications, laboratory experiments, or traditional use. It is important to always read product labels. People who have a medical condition, or are taking other drugs, herbs, or supplements, should consult a qualified healthcare provider before starting a new therapy.

Interactions with Drugs

- Based on animal studies, sweet almond may lower blood sugar levels. Caution is advised when using medications that may also lower blood sugar. Patients taking drugs for diabetes by mouth or insulin should be monitored closely by a qualified healthcare provider. Medication adjustments may be necessary.
- Theoretically, almonds and cholesterol-lowering agents may have additive effects when taken together.

Interactions with Herbs and Dietary Supplements

- Based on animal studies, sweet almond may lower blood sugar levels. Caution is advised with use of herbs or supplements that may also lower blood sugar. Blood glucose levels may require monitoring, and doses may need adjustment. Possible examples include *Aloe vera*, American ginseng, bilberry, bitter melon, burdock, fenugreek, fish oil, gymnema, horse chestnut seed extract (HCSE), maitake mushroom, marshmallow, milk thistle, *Panax ginseng*, rosemary, Siberian ginseng, stinging nettle, and white horehound.

- Theoretically, almonds may add to the effects of herbs or supplements that lower blood cholesterol levels, such as fish oil, garlic, guggul, or niacin.

Selected References

Natural Standard developed the preceding evidence-based information based on a systematic review of more than 60 scientific articles. For comprehensive information about alternative and complementary therapies on the professional level, go to www.naturalstandard.com. Selected references are listed here.

Abbey M, Noakes M, Belling GB, et al. Partial replacement of saturated fatty acids with almonds or walnuts lowers total plasma cholesterol and low-density-lipoprotein cholesterol. Am J Clin Nutr 1994;59(5):995-999.

Clemetson CA, de Carlo SJ, Burney GA, et al. Estrogens in food: the almond mystery. Int J Gynaecol Obstet 1978;15(6):515-521.

Evans S, Skea D, Dolovich J. Fatal reaction to peanut antigen in almond icing. CMAJ 1988;139(3):231-232.

Fraser GE, Bennett HW, Jaceldo KB, Sabate J. Effect on body weight of a free 76 Kilojoule (320 calorie) daily supplement of almonds for six months. J Am Coll Nutr 2002;21(3): 275-283.

Hu FB, Stampfer MJ, Manson JE, et al. Frequent nut consumption and risk of coronary heart disease in women: prospective cohort study. BMJ 1998;317(7169):1341-1345.

Hyson DA, Schneeman BO, Davis PA. Almonds and almond oil have similar effects on plasma lipids and LDL oxidation in healthy men and women. J Nutr 2002;132(4):703-707.

Maiche A. Effect of chamomile cream and almond ointment on acute radiation skin reaction. Acta Oncol 1991;30(3):395-396.

Schade JE, McGreevy K, King AD Jr, et al. Incidence of aflatoxin in California almonds. Appl Microbiol 1975;29(1):48-53.

Spiller GA, Jenkins DA, Bosello O, et al. Nuts and plasma lipids: an almond-based diet lowers LDL-C while preserving HDL-C. J Am Coll Nutr 1998;17(3):285-290.

Spiller GA, Jenkins DJ, Cragen LN, et al. Effect of a diet high in monounsaturated fat from almonds on plasma cholesterol and lipoproteins. J Am Coll Nutr 1992;11(2):126-130.

Teotia S, Singh M, Pant MC. Effect of Prunus amygdalus seeds on lipid profile. Indian J Physiol Pharmacol 1997;41(4):383-389.

Thomas P, Boussuges A, Gainnier M, et al. [Fat embolism after intrapenile injection of sweet almond oil]. Rev Mal Respir 1998;15(3):307-308.

Tea Tree Oil

(*Melaleuca alternifolia* [Maiden & Betche] Cheel)

RELATED TERMS

- Australian tea tree oil, Bogaskin (veterinary formulation), Breathaway, Burnaid (40 mg/g of tea tree oil and 1 mg/g of triclosan), cymene, malaleuca, Melaleuca Alternifolia Hydrogel (burn dressing), melaleucae, melaleuca oil, oil of melaleuca, oleum, *Oleum melaleucae,* T36-C7, tea tree oil, Tebodont, teebaum, terpinen, terpinen-4-ol, terpinenol-4, ti tree.
- *Note:* Tea tree oil should not be confused with cajeput oil, niauouli oil, kanuka oil, or manuka oil obtained from other *Melaleuca* species.

BACKGROUND

- Tea tree oil is obtained by steam distillation of the leaves of *Melaleuca alternifolia.* Tea tree oil is purported to have antiseptic properties and has been used traditionally to prevent and treat infections. While numerous *in vitro* studies have demonstrated antimicrobial properties of tea tree oil (likely attributable to the constituent terpinen-4-ol), only a small number of randomized, controlled human trials have been published. Human studies have focused on the use of topical tea tree oil for fungal infections (including onychomycosis and tinea pedis), acne, and vaginal infections. However, no definitive evidence exists for the use of tea tree oil in any of these conditions, and further study is warranted.
- Oral use of tea tree oil should be avoided, as reports of toxicity after oral ingestion have been published. When used topically, tea tree oil is reported to be mildly irritating and has been associated with the development of allergic contact dermatitis, which may limit its potential as a topical agent for some patients.

T

USES BASED ON SCIENTIFIC EVIDENCE	Grade*
Acne vulgaris Although tea tree oil is available in many products, little information is available from human studies to evaluate the benefit of tea tree oil used on the skin for the treatment of acne. Tea tree oil may reduce the number of inflamed and noninflamed lesions.	C
Allergic skin reactions One small study shows that topical tea tree oil may reduce histamine-induced skin inflammation. Further research is needed to confirm these results.	C
Athlete's foot (tinea pedis) Preliminary studies report tea tree oil to have activity against several fungal species. However, at this time there is not sufficient information to make recommendations for or against the use of tea tree oil on the skin for this condition.	C

Continued

Dandruff Preliminary research reports that the use of 5% tea tree oil shampoo on mild to moderate dandruff may be effective and well tolerated. Further research is needed to confirm these results.	C
Fungal nail infection (onychomycosis) Although tea tree oil is thought to have activity against several fungus species, there is not sufficient information to make recommendations for or against the use of tea tree oil on the skin for onychomycosis.	C
Genital herpes Tea tree oil has activity against some viruses in laboratory studies, and it has been suggested that a tea tree gel may be useful as a treatment on the skin for genital herpes. However, there is currently not sufficient information to make recommendations for or against this use of tea tree oil.	C
Methicillin-resistant *Staphylococcus aureus* chronic infection (colonization) Laboratory studies report that tea tree oil has activity against methicillin-resistant *Staphylococcus aureus* (MRSA). It has been proposed that using tea tree oil ointment in the nose plus a tea tree body wash may treat colonization by this bacterium. However, there is currently not enough information from studies in humans to make recommendations for or against this use of tea tree oil.	C
Thrush (*Candida albicans* overgrowth in the mouth) In laboratory studies, tea tree oil can kill fungus and yeast such as *Candida albicans*. However, at this time there is not enough information available from studies in humans to make recommendations for or against this use of tea tree oil. Tea tree oil can be toxic when taken by mouth and therefore should not be swallowed.	C
Vaginal infections (yeast and bacteria) In laboratory studies, tea tree oil can kill yeast and certain bacteria. However, at this time there is not enough information available from studies in humans to make recommendations for or against this use of tea tree oil for vaginal infections. Although tea tree oil may reduce itching caused by yeast or bacteria, it may cause itching from dry skin or allergy.	C
Plaque One human study of a solution with tea tree oil utilized as ordinary mouthwash found no positive effect on the quantity or quality of supragingival plaque.	D

*Key to grades: *A:* Strong scientific evidence for this use; *B:* Good scientific evidence for this use; *C:* Unclear scientific evidence for this use; *D:* Fair scientific evidence against this use (it may not work); *F:* Strong scientific evidence against this use (it likely does not work). For a more detailed explanation of efficacy criteria, see "Natural Standard Evidence-Based Validated Grading Rationale" in the Introduction.

Uses Based on Tradition, Theory, or Limited Scientific Evidence

Antibacterial, antihistamine, anti-inflammatory, antioxidant, antiseptic, body odor, boils, bronchial congestion, bruises, burns, carbuncles, colds, contraction cessation, corns, cough, dental plaque, eczema, furuncles, gingivitis, immune system deficiencies, impetigo, insect bites/stings, lice, lung inflammation, mouth sores, muscle and joint pain, nose and throat irritation, periodontal disease, psoriasis, ringworm, root canal treatment, scabies, sinus infections, skin ailments/infections, solvent, sore throat, tonsillitis, warts, wound healing.

DOSING

The following doses are based on scientific research, publications, traditional use, or expert opinion. Many herbs and supplements have not been thoroughly tested, and their safety and effectiveness may not be proven. Brands may be made differently, with variable ingredients even within the same brand. The doses shown may not apply to all products. It is important to always read product labels and discuss doses with a qualified healthcare provider before therapy is started.

Standardization

- Standardization involves measuring the amount of certain chemicals in products to try to make different preparations similar to each other. It is not always known if the chemicals being measured are the "active" ingredients.
- The International Organization for Standardization has specified limits for 14 of the almost 100 ingredients that make up tea tree oil. By this standard, tea tree oil must contain terpinolene 1.5% to 5%, 1,8-cineole ≤15%, α-terpinene 5% to 13%, γ-terpinene 10% to 28%, p-cymene 0.5% to 12%, terpinen-4-ol ≥30%, α-terpineol 1.5% to 8%, limonene 0.5% to 4%, sabinene trace 3.5%, aromadendrene trace 7%, δ-cadinene trace 8%, globulol trace 3%, viridiflorol trace 1.5%, and α-pinene 1-6%. Prior to the development of the international standard (ISO 4730), an Australian standard existed (AS2782-1985) that required tea tree oil preparations to contain >30% terpinene-4-ol and <15% 1,8-cineole.

T

Adults (18 Years and Older)

- *Note:* Recommended doses are based on those used in studies. These doses have not necessarily been proven effective or safe. While 100% tea tree oil is sometimes used, it is often diluted with inactive ingredients. Because of reports of severe side effects after tea tree oil ingestion, it is strongly recommended that tea tree oil not be taken by mouth. Although tea tree oil solution has been used as a mouthwash, it should not be swallowed.
- **Acne:** Tea tree oil 5% gel, applied to acne-prone areas of the skin daily.
- **Athlete's foot (tinea pedis):** 10% tea tree oil cream, applied twice daily to the feet after they have been thoroughly washed and dried or 25% to 50% tea tree oil solution applied twice daily to the affected area for 4 weeks.
- **Burns:** It is recommended that tea tree oil products not be used on burn wounds because of the cytotoxicity of tea tree oil on human skin cells.
- **Dandruff:** 5% tea tree oil shampoo daily for at least 4 weeks has been used.
- **Fungal nail infection (onychomycosis):** 100% tea tree oil, applied to the affected area twice daily for 6 months.

- **Genital herpes:** 6% tea tree oil gel has been used.
- **MRSA:** 4% tea tree oil nasal ointment and 5% tea tree oil body wash has been used.
- **Thrush:** Alcohol-based or alcohol-free solution four times daily for 2 to 4 weeks.

Children (Younger Than 18 Years)

- There is insufficient research to recommend the safe use of tea tree oil in children.

SAFETY

The U.S. Food and Drug Administration does not strictly regulate herbs and supplements. There is no guarantee of strength, purity, or safety of products, and their effects may vary. It is important to always read product labels. People who have a medical condition, or are taking other drugs, herbs, or supplements, should consult a qualified healthcare provider before starting a new therapy. A healthcare provider should be consulted immediately about any side effects.

Allergies

- There are multiple reports of allergy to tea tree oil when taken by mouth or used on the skin. Skin reactions range from mild contact dermatitis to severe blistering rashes. People with a history of allergy to tea tree oil (*Melaleuca alternifolia*), to any of its components, or to plants that are members of the myrtle (Myrtaceae) family should not use tea tree oil. People with a history of allergy to tincture of benzoin or colophony (rosin) should not use tea tree oil products because cross-reactions have been reported. There is a case report of a patient with linear IgA disease, a subepidermal blistering disorder that can be precipitated by contact with tea tree oil.
- Caution is advised with use of tea tree oil in persons allergic to eucalyptol, as many tea tree oil preparations contain eucalyptol.

Side Effects and Warnings

- Tea tree oil taken by mouth is associated with potentially severe reactions, even when used in small quantities. Several reports describe development of severe rash, reduced immune system function, abdominal pain, diarrhea, lethargy, drowsiness, slow or uneven walking, confusion, or coma in people taking tea tree oil by mouth. There have also been reports of nausea, unpleasant taste, burning sensation, and bad breath associated with tea tree oil use. Many tea tree preparations contain large volumes of alcohol.
- When used on the skin, tea tree oil may cause allergic rash, redness, blistering, and itching. Use of tea tree oil inside of the mouth or in the eyes can cause irritation. One report describes a person with long-standing eczema (atopic dermatitis) who developed a severe flare after applying 100% tea tree oil mixed with honey to the skin. Animal research suggests that tea tree oil used on the skin in large quantities can cause serious reactions such as difficulty walking, weakness, muscle tremor, slowing of brain function, and poor coordination. When applied in the ears of animals, 100% tea tree oil has caused reduced hearing, although a 2% solution has not led to lasting changes in hearing. Effects of tea tree oil on hearing when used in the ears of humans are not known.

Pregnancy and Breastfeeding

- Not enough scientific information is available to recommend tea tree oil during pregnancy or breastfeeding. Animal studies suggest caution in the use of tea tree oil during childbirth, because tea tree oil has been reported to decrease the force of spontaneous contractions, which theoretically could put the baby and the mother at risk. Women who are breastfeeding should not apply tea tree oil to the breast or nipple, since it may be absorbed by the infant.

INTERACTIONS

Most herbs and supplements have not been thoroughly tested for interactions with other herbs, supplements, drugs, or foods. The interactions listed here are based on reports in scientific publications, laboratory experiments, or traditional use. It is important to always read product labels. People who have a medical condition, or are taking other drugs, herbs, or supplements, should consult a qualified healthcare provider before starting a new therapy.

Interactions with Drugs

- Tea tree oil skin products may result in drying of the skin and may worsen the drying caused by skin treatments such as tretinoin (Retin-A), benzoyl peroxide, salicylic acid, or isotretinoin (Accutane, taken by mouth).

Selected References

Natural Standard developed the preceding evidence-based information based on a systematic review of more than 100 scientific articles. For comprehensive information about alternative and complementary therapies on the professional level, go to www.naturalstandard.com. Selected references are listed here.

Arweiler NB, Donos N, Netuschil L, et al. Clinical and antibacterial effect of tea tree oil—a pilot study. Clin Oral Invest 2000;4(2):70-73.

Bassett IB, Pannowitz DL, Barnetson RS. A comparative study of tea-tree oil versus benzoyl peroxide in the treatment of acne. Med J Aust 1990;153(8):455-458.

Bhushan M, Beck MH. Allergic contact dermatitis from tea tree oil in a wart paint. Contact Derm 1997;36(2):117-118.

Brand C, Townley SL, Finlay-Jones JJ, Hart PH. Tea tree oil reduces histamine-induced oedema in murine ears. Inflamm Res 2002;51(6):283-289.

Buck DS, Nidorf DM, Addino JG. Comparison of two topical preparations for the treatment of onychomycosis: *Melaleuca alternifolia* (tea tree) oil and clotrimazole. J Fam Pract 1994; 38(6):601-605.

Budhiraja SS, Cullum ME, Sioutis SS, et al. Biological activity of *Melaleuca alternifola* (tea tree) oil component, terpinen-4-ol, in human myelocytic cell line HL-60. J Manipulative Physiol Ther 1999;22(7):447-453.

Caelli M, Porteous J, Carson CF, et al. Tea tree oil as an alternative topical decolonization agent for methicillin-resistant *Staphylococcus aureus.* J Hosp Infect 2000;46(3):236-237.

Caelli M, Riley T. Tea tree oil—an alternative topical decolonisation agent for adult inpatients with methicillin-resistant *Staphylococcus aureus* (MRSA)—a pilot study. J Hosp Infect 1998; 40(Suppl A):9.

Carson CF, Ashton L, Dry L, et al. *Melaleuca alternifolia* (tea tree) oil gel (6%) for the treatment of recurrent herpes labialis. J Antimicrob Chemother 2001;48(3):450-451.

Carson CF, Riley TV. Safety, efficacy and provenance of tea tree (*Melaleuca alternifolia*) oil. Contact Derm 2001;45(2):65-67.

Carson CF, Riley TV. Non-antibiotic therapies for infectious diseases. Commun Dis Intell 2003;27:S143-146.

Christoph F, Kaulfers PM, Stahl-Biskup E. A comparative study of the in vitro antimicrobial activity of tea tree with special reference to the activity of beta-triketones. Planta Med 2002;66(6):556-560.

Cox SD, Mann CM, Markham JL, et al. The mode of antimicrobial action of the essential oil of *Melaleuca alternifolia* (tea tree oil). J Appl Microbiol 2000;88(1):170-175.

Cox SD, Gustafson JE, Mann CM, et al. Tea tree oil causes K^+ leakage and inhibits respiration in *Escherichia coli.* Lett Appl Microbiol 1998;26(5):355-358.

Faogali J, George N, Leditschke JF. Does tea tree oil have a place in the topical treatment of burns? Burns 1997;23(4):349-351.

Fitzi J, Furst-Jucker J, Wegener T, et al. Phytotherapy of chronic dermatitis and pruritus of dogs with a topical preparation containing tea tree oil (Bogaskin). Schweiz Arch Tierheilkd 2002;144(5):223-231.

Gorduysus MO, Tasman F, Tuncer S, et al. Solubilizing efficiency of different gutta-percha solvents: a comparative study. J Nihon Univ Sch Dent 1997;39(3):133-135.

Groppo FC, Ramacciato JC, Simoes RP, et al. Antimicrobial activity of garlic, tea tree oil, and chlorhexidine against oral microorganisms. Int Dent J 2002;52(6):433-437.

Hada T, Inoue Y, Shiraishi A, et al. Leakage of K^+ ions from *Staphylococcus aureus* in response to tea tree oil. J Microbiol Methods 2003;53(3):309-312.

Hammer KA, Carson CF, Riley TV. Antifungal activity of the components of *Melaleuca alternifolia* (tea tree) oil. J Appl Microbiol 2003;95(4):853-860.

Hammer KA, Carson CF, Riley TV. Influence of organic matter, cations and surfactants on the antimicrobial activity of *Melaleuca alternifolia* (tea tree) oil in vitro. J Appl Microbiol 1999; 86(3):446-452.

Harkenthal M, Hausen BM, Reichling J. 1,2,4-Trihydroxy menthane, a contact allergen from oxidized Australian tea tree oil. Pharmazie 2000;55(2):153-154.

Hausen BM, Reichling J, Harkenthal M. Degradation products of monoterpenes are the sensitizing agents in tea tree oil. Am J Contact Dermat 1999;10(2):68-77.

Jandera V, Hudson DA, de Wet PM, et al. Cooling the burn wound: evaluation of different modalities. Burns 2000;26(3):265-270.

Jandourek A, Vaishampayan JK, Vazquez JA. Efficacy of melaleuca oral solution for the treatment of fluconazole refractory oral candidiasis in AIDS patients. AIDS 1998;12(9): 1033-1037.

Koh KJ, Pearce AL, Marshman G, et al. Tea tree oil reduces histamine-induced skin inflammation.Br J Dermatol 2002;147(6):1212-1217.

Kulik E, Lenkeit K, Meyer J. Antimicrobial effects of tea tree oil (*Melaleuca alternifolia*) on oral microorganisms. Schweiz Monatsschr Zahnmed 2000;110(11):125-130

McCage CM, Ward SM, Paling CA, et al. Development of a paw paw herbal shampoo for the removal of head lice. Phytomedicine 2002;9(8):743-748.

Mondello F, De Bernardis F, Girolamo A, et al. In vitro and *in vivo* activity of tea tree oil against azole-susceptible and -resistant human pathogenic yeasts. J Antimicrob Chemother 2003; 51(5):1223-1229.

Morris MC, Donoghue A, Markowitz JA, Osterhoudt KC. Ingestion of tea tree oil (*Melaleuca* oil) by a 4-year-old boy. Pediatr Emerg Care 2003;19(3):169-171.

Mozelsio NB, Harris KE, McGrath KG, Grammer LC. Immediate systemic hypersensitivity reaction associated with topical application of Australian tea tree oil. Allergy Asthma Proc 2003;24(1):73-75.

Nenoff P, Haustein UF, Brandt W. Antifungal activity of the essential oil of *Melaleuca alternifolia* (tea tree oil) against pathogenic fungi *in vitro*. Skin Pharmacol 1996;9(6):388-394.

Oliva B, Piccirilli E, Ceddia T. Antimycotic activity of *Melaleuca alternifolia* essential oil and its major components. Lett Appl Microbiol 2003;37(2):185-187.

Perrett CM, Evans AV, Russell-Jones R. Tea tree oil dermatitis associated with linear IgA disease. Clin Exp Dermatol 2003;28(2):167-170.

Pirotta MV, Gunn JM, Chondros P. "Not thrush again!" Women's experience of post-antibiotic vulvovaginitis. Med J Aust 2003;179(1):43-46.

Prensner R. Does 5% tea tree oil shampoo reduce dandruff? J Fam Pract 2003;52(4):285-286.

Rubel DM, Freeman S, Southwell IA. Tea tree oil allergy: what is the offending agent? Report of three cases of tea tree oil allergy and review of the literature. Australas J Dermatol 1998; 39(4):244-247.

Russell MF, Southwell I. Preferred age for assessment of qualitative and quantitative characteristics of the essential oil of tea tree (*Melaleuca alternifolia*) seedlings prior to plantation establishment. J Agric Food Chem 2003;51(15):4254-4257.

Russell MF, Southwell IA. Monoterpenoid accumulation in 1,8-cineole, terpinolene and terpinen-4-ol chemotypes of *Melaleuca alternifolia* seedlings. Phytochemistry 2003;62(5): 683-689.

Satchell AC, Saurajen A, Bell C, Barnetson RS. Treatment of dandruff with 5% tea tree oil shampoo. J Am Acad Dermatol 2002;47(6):852-855.
Satchell AC, Saurajen A, Bell C, Barnetson RS. Treatment of interdigital tinea pedis with 25% and 50% tea tree oil solution: a randomized, placebo-controlled, blinded study. Australas J Dermatol 2002;43(3):175-178.
Saxer UP, Stauble Z, Szabo SH, Menghini G. Effect of mouthwashing with tea tree oil on plaque and inflammation. Schweiz Monatsschr Zahnmed 2003;113(9):985-996.
Scardamaglia L, Nixon R, Fewings J. Compound tincture of benzoin: a common contact allergen? Australas J Dermatol 2003;44(3):180-184.
Schempp CM, Schopf E, Simon JC. Plant-induced toxic and allergic dermatitis (phytodermatitis). Hautarzt 2002;53(2):93-97.
Selvaag E, Eriksen B, Thune P. Contact allergy due to tea tree oil and cross-sensitization to colophony. Contact Dermatitis 1994;31(2):124-125.
Shin S. Anti-*Aspergillus* activities of plant essential oils and their combination effects with ketoconazole or amphotericin B. Arch Pharm Res 2003;26(5):389-393.
Syed TA, Qureshi ZA, Ali SM, et al. Treatment of toenail onychomycosis with 2% butenafine and 5% *Melaleuca alternifolia* (tea tree) oil in cream. Trop Med Int Health 1999;4(4): 284-287.
Tong MM, Altman PM, Barnetson RS. Tea tree oil in the treatment of tinea pedis. Australas J Dermatol 1992;33(3):145-149.
van der Valk PG, de Groot AC, Bruynzeel DP. Allergic contact eczema due to 'tea tree' oil. Ned Tijdschr Geneeskd 1994;138(16):823-825.
Vazquez JA, Vaishampayan J, Arganoza MT, et al. Use of an over the counter product, Breathaway (*Melaleuca* oral solution), as an alternative agent for refractory oropharyngeal candidiasis in AIDS patients [abstract]. Int Conf AIDS 1996;11:109.
Vazquez JA, Zawawi AA. Efficacy of alcohol-based and alcohol-free melaleuca oral solution for the treatment of fluconazole-refractory oropharyngeal candidiasis in patients with AIDS. HIV Clin Trials 2002;3(5):379-385.
Wolner-Hanssen P, Sjoberg I. Warning against a fashionable cure for vulvovaginitis. Tea tree oil may substitute *Candida* itching with allergy itching. Lakartidningen 1998;95(30-31): 3309-3310.

Turmeric
(*Curcuma longa* L.)

RELATED TERMS

- Amomoum curcuma, anlatone (constituent), curcuma, *Curcuma aromatica*, *Curcuma aromatica* Salisb., *Curcuma domestica*, *Curcuma domestica* Valet., curcuma oil, curcumae longae rhizoma, curcumin (I, II, III), diferuloylmethane, e zhu, gelbwurzel, gurkemeje, haldi, haridra, Indian saffron, Indian yellow root, jiang huang, kunir, kunyit, kurkumawurzelstock, kyoo, olena, radix zedoaria longa, rhizome de curcuma, safran des Indes, shati, turmeric root, tumerone (constituent), ukon, yellowroot, zedoary, Zingiberaceae (family), zingiberene (constituent), zitterwurzel.

BACKGROUND

- The rhizome (root) of turmeric (*Curcuma longa* L.) has long been used in traditional Asian medicine to treat gastrointestinal upset, arthritic pain, and "low energy." Laboratory and animal research has demonstrated anti-inflammatory, antioxidant, and anticancer properties of turmeric and its constituent curcumin. Preliminary human evidence, albeit of poor quality, suggests possible efficacy in the management of dyspepsia (heartburn), hyperlipidemia (high cholesterol), and scabies (with topical use). However, because of methodologic weaknesses in the available studies, an evidence-based recommendation cannot be made regarding the use of turmeric or curcumin for any specific indication.

USES BASED ON SCIENTIFIC EVIDENCE	Grade*
Cancer Several early animal and laboratory studies report anticancer (colon, skin, breast) properties of curcumin. Many mechanisms have been considered, including antioxidant activity, antiangiogenesis (prevention of new blood vessel growth), and direct effects on cancer cells. Reliable human studies are lacking in this area. It remains unclear if turmeric or curcumin has a role in preventing or treating human cancers.	C
Dyspepsia (heartburn) Turmeric has been traditionally used to treat stomach problems (such as indigestion from a fatty meal). There is preliminary evidence that turmeric may offer some relief from these stomach problems. However, at high doses or with prolonged use, turmeric may actually irritate or upset the stomach. Reliable human research is necessary before a recommendation can be made.	C
Gallstone prevention/bile flow stimulant It has been said that there are fewer people with gallstones in India, which is sometimes credited to turmeric in the diet. Early animal studies	C

Continued

report that curcumin, a chemical in turmeric, may decrease the occurrence of gallstones. Limited human research suggests that curcumin may stimulate squeezing (contraction) of the gallbladder and stimulate bile flow. However, reliable human studies are lacking in this area. The use of turmeric may be inadvisable in patients with active gallstones.	
High cholesterol Animal studies suggest that turmeric may lower levels of low-density lipoprotein ("bad cholesterol") and total cholesterol in the blood. Preliminary human research suggests a possible similar effect in people. Better human studies are needed before a recommendation can be made.	C
Human immunodeficiency virus infection Several laboratory studies suggest that curcumin, a component of turmeric, may have activity against human immunodeficiency virus (HIV) infection. However, reliable human studies are lacking in this area.	C
Inflammation Laboratory and animal studies show anti-inflammatory activity of turmeric and its constituent curcumin. Reliable human research is lacking.	C
Osteoarthritis Turmeric has been used historically to treat rheumatic conditions. Laboratory and animal studies show anti-inflammatory activity of turmeric and its constituent curcumin, which may be beneficial in people with osteoarthritis. Reliable human research is lacking.	C
Peptic ulcer disease (stomach ulcer) Turmeric has been used historically to treat stomach and duodenal ulcers. However, at high doses or with prolonged use, turmeric may actually further irritate or upset the stomach. In animals, turmeric taken by mouth protects against ulcers caused by irritating drugs or chemicals, and increases protective mucus. Currently, there is not enough human evidence to make a firm recommendation, and well-designed studies comparing turmeric with standard medical therapies are needed. Notably, the bacterium *H. pylori* is a common cause of ulcers, and treatment to eradicate *H. pylori* should be considered by people with ulcers, in consultation with a qualified healthcare provider.	C
Rheumatoid arthritis Turmeric has been used historically to treat rheumatic conditions and based on animal research may reduce inflammation. Reliable human studies are necessary before a recommendation can be made in this area.	C
Scabies Historically, turmeric has been used on the skin to treat chronic skin ulcers and scabies. It has also been used in combination with the leaves of the herb *Azadirachta indica* ADR (neem). Preliminary research	C

Continued

reports that this combination may help in treatment of scabies. It remains unclear if turmeric alone has beneficial effects. More research is necessary before a firm recommendation can be made.	
Uveitis (eye inflammation) Laboratory and animal studies show anti-inflammatory activity of turmeric and its constituent curcumin. A poorly designed human study suggests a possible benefit of curcumin in the treatment of uveitis. Reliable human research is necessary before a firm conclusion can be drawn.	**C**

*Key to grades: *A:* Strong scientific evidence for this use; *B:* Good scientific evidence for this use; *C:* Unclear scientific evidence for this use; *D:* Fair scientific evidence against this use (it may not work); *F:* Strong scientific evidence against this use (it likely does not work). For a more detailed explanation of efficacy criteria, see "Natural Standard Evidence-Based Validated Grading Rationale" in the Introduction.

Uses Based on Tradition, Theory, or Limited Scientific Evidence

Alzheimer's disease, antifungal, antispasmodic, antivenom, appetite stimulant, asthma, bleeding, bloating, boils, bruises, cataracts, colic, contraception, cough, diabetes, diarrhea, dizziness, epilepsy, gallstones, gas, gonorrhea, heart damage from doxorubicin (Adriamycin, Doxil), hepatitis, high blood pressure, increased sperm count/motility, insect bites, insect repellent, jaundice, kidney disease, lactation stimulant, leprosy, liver damage from toxins/drugs, liver protection, menstrual pain, menstrual period problems/lack of menstrual period, pain, parasites, ringworm.

DOSING

The following doses are based on scientific research, publications, traditional use, or expert opinion. Many herbs and supplements have not been thoroughly tested, and their safety and effectiveness may not be proven. Brands may be made differently, with variable ingredients even within the same brand. The doses shown may not apply to all products. It is important to always read product labels and discuss doses with a qualified healthcare provider before therapy is started.

Standardization

- Standardization involves measuring the amount of certain chemicals in products to try to make different preparations similar to each other. It is not always known if the chemicals being measured are the "active" ingredients.
- Turmeric may be standardized to contain 95% curcuminoids per dose. The dried root of turmeric is reported to contain 3% to 5% curcumin.
- Turmeric may be combined with bromelain, because it is believed that this will enhance absorption of turmeric into the body. A lipid base of lecithin, fish oils, or essential fatty acids may also be used to enhance absorption. Additional benefit from these special formulations is not proven.

Adults (18 Years and Older)

- **Oral (by mouth):** Traditional doses range from 1.5 to 3 g of turmeric root daily, divided into several doses. Studies have used 750 mg to 1.5 g of turmeric daily in three to four divided doses, with doses up to 8 g daily used for the treatment of duodenal ulcer. As a tea, 1 to 1.5 g of dried root may be steeped in 150 ml of water for 15 minutes and taken twice daily. Average dietary intake of turmeric in the Indian population may range between 2 and 2.5 g, corresponding to 60 to 200 mg of curcumin daily.
- **Topical (for treatment of scabies):** One reported method is to cover affected areas once daily with a paste consisting of a 4:1 mixture of *Azadirachta indica* ADR (neem) and turmeric, for up to 15 days. Scabies should be treated under the supervision of a qualified healthcare provider.

Children (Younger Than 18 Years)

- **Topical (for treatment of scabies):** One reported method is to cover affected areas once daily with a paste consisting of a 4:1 mixture of *Azadirachta indica* ADR (neem) and turmeric, for up to 15 days. Scabies should be treated under the supervision of a qualified healthcare provider.

SAFETY

The U.S. Food and Drug Administration does not strictly regulate herbs and supplements. There is no guarantee of strength, purity, or safety of products, and effects may vary. It is important to always read product labels. People who have a medical condition, or are taking other drugs, herbs, or supplements, should consult a qualified healthcare provider before starting a new therapy. A healthcare provider should be consulted immediately about any side effects.

Allergies

- Allergic reactions to turmeric may occur, including contact dermatitis (an itchy rash) after skin or scalp exposure. People with allergies to plants in the *Curcuma* family are more likely to have an allergic reaction to turmeric. Caution is indicated with use in patients allergic to turmeric or any of its constituents (including curcumin), to yellow food colorings, or to plants in the Zingiberaceae (ginger) family.

Side Effects and Warnings

- Turmeric may cause an upset stomach, especially in high doses or if taken over a long period of time. Heartburn has been reported by patients receiving turmeric for treatment of stomach ulcers. Since turmeric is sometimes used for the treatment of heartburn or ulcers, caution may be necessary in some patients. Nausea and diarrhea have also been reported.
- Based on laboratory and animal studies, turmeric may increase the risk of bleeding. Caution is advised in patients with bleeding disorders or taking drugs that may increase the risk of bleeding. Dosing adjustments may be necessary.
- Limited animal studies show that a component of turmeric, curcumin, may increase liver enzymes measured by liver function tests. However, one human study reports that turmeric has no effect on these tests. Turmeric or curcumin may cause gallbladder squeezing (contraction) and may not be advised in patients with gallstones. In animal studies, hair loss (alopecia) and lowering of blood pressure have been reported. In theory, turmeric may weaken the immune system and should be used cautiously in patients with immune system deficiencies.

Pregnancy and Breastfeeding

- Historically, turmeric has been considered safe when used as a spice in foods during pregnancy and breastfeeding. However, turmeric has been found to cause uterine stimulation and to stimulate menstrual flow, and caution is therefore warranted during pregnancy. Animal studies have not found turmeric taken by mouth to cause abnormal fetal development.

INTERACTIONS

Most herbs and supplements have not been thoroughly tested for interactions with other herbs, supplements, drugs, or foods. The interactions listed here are based on reports in scientific publications, laboratory experiments, or traditional use. It is important to always read product labels. People who have a medical condition, or are taking other drugs, herbs, or supplements, should consult a qualified healthcare provider before starting a new therapy.

Interactions with Drugs

- Based on laboratory and animal studies, turmeric may inhibit platelets in the blood, thereby increasing the risk of bleeding caused by other drugs. Some examples are aspirin, anticoagulants (blood thinners) such as warfarin (Coumadin) and heparin, antiplatelet drugs such as clopidogrel (Plavix), and nonsteroidal anti-inflammatory drugs (NSAIDs) such as ibuprofen (Motrin, Advil) and naproxen (Naprosyn, Aleve).
- Based on animal studies, turmeric may interfere with how the body uses the liver's cytochrome P450 enzyme system to process components of certain drugs. As a result, blood levels of these components may be increased, which may cause increased effects or potentially serious adverse reactions. People who are using any medications should always read the package insert and consult their healthcare provider or pharmacist about possible interactions.
- Turmeric may lower blood levels of low-density lipoprotein (LDL) ("bad" cholesterol) and increase high-density lipoprotein (HDL) ("good" cholesterol). Thus, turmeric may increase the effects of cholesterol-lowering drugs such as lovastatin (Mevacor) and atorvastatin (Lipitor).
- In animals, turmeric protects against stomach ulcers caused by NSAIDs such as indomethacin (Indocin), and against heart damage caused by the chemotherapy drug doxorubicin (Adriamycin).

Interactions with Herbs and Dietary Supplements

- Based on animal studies, turmeric may increase the risk of bleeding when taken with herbs and supplements that are believed to increase the risk of bleeding. Multiple cases of bleeding have been reported with the use of *Ginkgo biloba*, some cases with garlic, and fewer cases with saw palmetto. Numerous other agents may theoretically increase the risk of bleeding, although this effect has not been proven in most cases. Some examples are alfalfa, American ginseng, angelica, anise, *Arnica montana*, asafetida, aspen bark, bilberry, birch, black cohosh, bladderwrack, bogbean, boldo, borage seed oil, bromelain, capsicum, cat's claw, celery, chamomile, chaparral, clove, coleus, cordyceps, danshen, devil's claw, dong quai, evening primrose, fenugreek, feverfew, flaxseed/flax powder (not a concern with flaxseed oil), ginger, grapefruit juice, grapeseed, green tea, guggul, gymnestra, horse chestnut, horseradish, licorice root, lovage root, male fern, meadowsweet, nordihydroguaiaretic acid (NDGA), onion, *Panax ginseng*, papain, parsley, passionflower, poplar, prickly ash, propolis, quassia, red clover, reishi, rue, Siberian ginseng, sweet birch, sweet clover, vitamin E, white willow, wild carrot, wild lettuce, willow, wintergreen, and yucca.

- Based on animal studies, turmeric may interfere with how the body uses the liver's cytochrome P450 enzyme system to process certain herbs or supplements. As a result, blood levels of chemical components of other herbs or supplements may be too high. It may also alter the effects of other herbs or supplements on the P450 system, such as bloodroot, cat's claw, chamomile, chaparral, chasteberry, damiana, *Echinacea angustifolia*, goldenseal, grapefruit juice, licorice, oregano, red clover, St. John's wort, wild cherry, and yucca.
- Turmeric may lower blood levels of LDL) ("bad" cholesterol) and increase HDL ("good" cholesterol). Thus, turmeric may increase the effects of cholesterol-lowering herbs or supplements such as fish oil, garlic, guggul, and niacin.

Selected References

Natural Standard developed the preceding evidence-based information based on a systematic review of more than 350 scientific articles. For comprehensive information about alternative and complementary therapies on the professional level, go to www.naturalstandard.com. Selected references are listed here.

Aggarwal BB, Kumar A, Bharti AC. Anticancer potential of curcumin: preclinical and clinical studies. Anticancer Res 2003;23(1A):363-398.

Braga ME, Leal PF, Carvalho JE, et al. Comparison of yield, composition, and antioxidant activity of turmeric (*Curcuma longa* L.) extracts obtained using various techniques. J Agric Food Chem 2003;51(22):6604-6611.

Chainani-Wu N. Safety and anti-inflammatory activity of curcumin: a component of tumeric (*Curcuma longa*). J Altern Complement Med 2003;9(1):161-168.

Deodhar SD, Sethi R, Srimal RC. Preliminary study on antirheumatic activity of curcumin (diferuloyl methane). Indian J Med Res 1980;71:632-634.

Di GH, Li HC, Shen ZZ, et al. [Analysis of anti-proliferation of curcumin on human breast cancer cells and its mechanism]. Zhonghua Yi Xue Za Zhi 2003;83(20):1764-1768.

Gao C, Ding Z, Liang B, et al. [Study on the effects of curcumin on angiogenesis]. Zhong Yao Cai 2003;26(7):499-502.

Kositchaiwat C, Kositchaiwat S, Havanondha J. *Curcuma longa* Linn. in the treatment of gastric ulcer comparison to liquid antacid: a controlled clinical trial. J Med Assoc Thai 1993;76(11): 601-605.

Kulkarni RR, Patki PS, Jog VP, et al. Treatment of osteoarthritis with a herbomineral formulation: a double-blind, placebo-controlled, cross-over study. J Ethnopharmacol 1991; 33(1-2):91-95.

Leu TH, Su SL, Chuang YC, et al. Direct inhibitory effect of curcumin on Src and focal adhesion kinase activity. Biochem Pharmacol 2003;66(12):2323-2331.

Ohashi Y, Tsuchiya Y, Koizumi K, et al. Prevention of intrahepatic metastasis by curcumin in an orthotopic implantation model. Oncology 2003;65(3):250-258.

Rasyid A, Lelo A. The effect of curcumin and placebo on human gallbladder function: an ultrasound study. Aliment Pharmacol Ther 1999;13(2):245-249.

Rithaporn T, Monga M, Rajasekaran M. Curcumin: a potential vaginal contraceptive. Contraception 2003;68(3):219-223.

Satoskar RR, Shah SJ, Shenoy SG. Evaluation of anti-inflammatory property of curcumin (diferuloyl methane) in patients with postoperative inflammation. Int J Clin Pharmacol Ther Toxicol 1986;24(12):651-654.

Taher MM, Lammering G, Hershey C, et al. Curcumin inhibits ultraviolet light induced human immunodeficiency virus gene expression. Mol Cell Biochem 2003;254(1-2):289-297.

Thamlikitkul V, Bunyapraphatsara N, Dechatiwongse T, et al. Randomized double blind study of *Curcuma domestica* Val. for dyspepsia. J Med Assoc Thai 1989;72(11):613-620.

Van Dau N, Ngoc Ham N, Huy Khac D, et al. The effects of a traditional drug, turmeric (*Curcuma longa*), and placebo on the healing of duodenal ulcer. Phytomedicine 1998; 5(1):29-34.

Valerian

(*Valeriana officinalis* L.)

RELATED TERMS

- All-heal, amantilla, balderbrackenwurzel, baldrian, baldrianwurzel, baldrion, Belgian valerian, capon's tail, common valerian, fragrant valerian, garden heliotrope, garden valerian, great wild valerian, heliotrope, herba benedicta, Indian valerian, Jacob's ladder, Japanese valerian, katzenwurzel, laege-baldrian, Mexican valerian, Nervex, Neurol, Orasedon, Pacific valerian, phu, phu germanicum, phu parvum, pinnis dentatis, racine de valériane, red valerian, Sanox-N, Sedonium, setewale, setwall, setwell, theriacaria, Ticalma, *Valeriana edulis, Valeriana faurieri*, *Valeriana foliis pinnatis, Valeriana jatamansi, Valeriana sitchensis, Valeriana wallichii*, Valerianaceae (family), Valerianaheel, valeriane, Valmane, vandal root.

BACKGROUND

- Valerian is a herb native to Europe and Asia and now grows in most parts of the world. The name is believed to come from the Latin word *valere*, meaning "to be healthy or strong." The root of the plant is believed to contain its active constituents. Use of valerian as a sedative and antianxiety treatment has been reported for more than 2000 years. For example, in the 2nd century AD, Galen recommended valerian as a treatment for insomnia. Related species have been used in traditional Chinese and Indian Ayurvedic medicine. Preparations for use on the skin have been used to treat sores and acne, and valerian by mouth has been used for other conditions such as digestive problems, flatulence (gas), congestive heart failure, urinary tract disorders, and angina.
- Valerian extracts became popular in the United States and Europe in the mid-1800s and continued to be used by both physicians and the lay public until it was widely replaced by prescription sedative drugs.
- Valerian remains popular in North America, Europe, and Japan and is widely used to treat insomnia and anxiety. Although the active ingredients in valerian are not known, preparations are often standardized to the content of valerenic acid.

USES BASED ON SCIENTIFIC EVIDENCE	Grade*
Insomnia Several studies in adults suggest that valerian improves the quality of sleep and reduces the time to fall asleep (sleep latency), for up to 4 to 6 weeks. Ongoing nightly use may be more effective than single-dose use, with increasing effects over 4 weeks. Better effects have been found in poor sleepers. However, most studies have not used scientific ways of measuring sleep improvements, such as sleep pattern data in a sleep laboratory. Studies of combination valerian–hops or valerian–St. John's wort products are promising, but further study is needed before a	**B**

Continued

strong recommendation can be made. It is not clear how valerian compares with prescription sleep aids. Initial research suggests that valerian may also be helpful in children with sleep disorders.	
Anxiety disorder Several studies of valerian have reported benefits in reducing nonspecific anxiety symptoms. Valerian has also been given in combination with other herbs, such as passionflower and St. John's wort, to treat anxiety. However, most studies have been small and poorly designed. More research is needed before a recommendation can be made.	C
Sedation Although valerian has not been studied specifically as a sedative, evidence from studies conducted for other purposes suggests that valerian may not have significant sedative effects when used at recommended doses. Therefore, even though valerian could be helpful as a sleep aid, it does not appear to cause sedation.	D

*Key to grades: *A:* Strong scientific evidence for this use; *B:* Good scientific evidence for this use; *C:* Unclear scientific evidence for this use; *D:* Fair scientific evidence against this use (it may not work); *F:* Strong scientific evidence against this use (it likely does not work). For a more detailed explanation of efficacy criteria, see "Natural Standard Evidence-Based Validated Grading Rationale" in the Introduction.

Uses Based on Tradition, Theory, or Limited Scientific Evidence

Acne, amenorrhea (lack of menstruation), angina, anorexia, anti-seizure, antiperspirant, antiviral, anxiety, arthritis, asthma, bloating, bronchospasm/asthma, congestive heart failure, constipation, cough, cramping (abdominal, pelvic, menstrual), depression, digestive problems, diuretic (increasing urine flow), dysmenorrhea (pain with menstrual cycle), emmenagogue (stimulating menstrual blood flow), fatigue, fever, flatulence (gas), hangovers, headache, heart disease, heartburn, high blood pressure, human immunodeficiency virus (HIV) infection, hypochondria, irritable bowel syndrome, liver disorders, measles, memory enhancement, menopause, migraine, mood enhancement, muscle pain/spasm/tension, nausea, nerve pain, pain relief, premenstrual syndrome (PMS), restless legs syndrome, restlessness, rheumatic pain, skin disorders, stomach ulcers, stress, urinary tract disorders, vaginal infections, vertigo, viral gastroenteritis, vision problems, withdrawal from tranquilizers.

DOSING

The following doses are based on scientific research, publications, traditional use, or expert opinion. Many herbs and supplements have not been thoroughly tested, and their safety and effectiveness may not be proven. Brands may be made differently, with variable ingredients even within the same brand. The doses shown may not apply to all products. It is important to always read product labels and discuss doses with a qualified healthcare provider before therapy is started.

Standardization

- Standardization involves measuring the amount of certain chemicals in products to try to make different preparations similar to each other. It is not always known if the chemicals being measured are the "active" ingredients.
- Some valerian products are standardized to contain 0.8% to 0.3% valerenic or valeric acid, although other chemical components may be responsible for valerian's activity in the body.

Adults (18 Years and Older)

- **Insomnia:** Studied doses range from 400 to 900 mg of an aqueous or aqueous-ethanolic extract (corresponding to 1.5 to 3 g of herb), taken 30 to 60 minutes before going to bed. The better-designed studies have used 600 mg daily, taken 1 hour before bedtime. Valerian has historically been used in the form of a tea (1.5 to 3 g of root steeped for 5 to 10 minutes in 150 ml of boiling water), although this formulation has not been studied.
- **Sedation/anxiety:** One study evaluated the effect of 100 mg of aqueous or aqueous-ethanolic extract before a stressful event. Valerian is also used traditionally as a relaxant in the form of a tea (1.5 to 3 g of root steeped for 5 to 10 minutes in 150 ml of boiling water), although this formulation has not been studied.

Children (Younger Than 18 Years)

- There is not enough scientific evidence to recommend use of valerian in children.

SAFETY

The U.S. Food and Drug Administration does not strictly regulate herbs and supplements. There is no guarantee of strength, purity, or safety of products, and effects may vary. It is important to always read product labels. People who have a medical condition, or are taking other drugs, herbs, or supplements, should consult a qualified healthcare provider before starting a new therapy. A healthcare provider should be consulted immediately about any side effects.

Allergies

- People with allergies to plants in the Valerianaceae family may be allergic to valerian.

Side Effects and Warnings

- Studies report that valerian is generally well tolerated for up to 4 to 6 weeks in recommended doses, and side effects may occur no more often than with placebo (sugar pill). Valerian has occasionally been reported to cause headache, excitability, stomach upset, uneasiness, dizziness, unsteadiness (ataxia), and low body temperature (hypothermia). Chronic use (longer than 2 to 4 months) may result in insomnia. Slight reductions in concentration or complicated thinking may occur for a few hours after valerian is taken. Caution is advised in persons who will be driving or operating heavy machinery. Some research suggests that valerian may not cause sedation.
- A drug "hangover" effect has been reported in people taking high doses of valerian extracts. "Valerian withdrawal" may occur in people who stop using valerian suddenly after chronic high-dose use, including confusion (delirium) and rapid heartbeat. These symptoms may subside with the use of benzodiazepines such as lorazepam (Ativan). Although unknown, valerian may have similar brain activity as benzodiazepines (which are commonly used to treat anxiety and insomnia), through effects on the brain chemical gamma-aminobutyric acid (GABA).

- Valerian has been on the U.S. Food and Drug Administration's GRAS (generally regarded as safe) list, and no deaths due to overdose have been reported. Symptoms with overdose or chronic use may include low blood pressure, slow or abnormal heart rhythm, chest tightness, lightheadedness, constipation, excitability, blurred vision, tremor, headache, hypersensitivity (allergic) reactions, insomnia, and stomach upset.
- Liver toxicity has been associated with some multiherb preparations that include valerian. However, the contribution of valerian itself is not clear, due to the potential liver toxicity of other included ingredients, or the possibility of contamination with unlisted herbs.

Pregnancy and Breastfeeding

- Because human safety data are limited, valerian use during pregnancy and breastfeeding is not recommended. There are theoretical concerns over the adverse effects of chemical components that are toxic in laboratory studies.

INTERACTIONS

Most herbs and supplements have not been thoroughly tested for interactions with other herbs, supplements, drugs, or foods. The interactions listed here are based on reports in scientific publications, laboratory experiments, or traditional use. It is important to always read product labels. People who have a medical condition, or are taking other drugs, herbs, or supplements, should consult a qualified healthcare provider before starting a new therapy.

Interactions with Drugs

- Based on animal and human studies, valerian may increase the amount of drowsiness caused by some drugs, although this is an area of controversy. Examples are benzodiazepines such as lorazepam (Ativan) and diazepam (Valium), barbiturates such as phenobarbital, narcotics such as codeine, some antidepressants, and alcohol. Caution is advised in people who will be driving or operating machinery. In one human study, a combination of valerian and 20 mg of the beta-blocker drug propranolol (Inderal) reduced concentration levels more than valerian alone. A brief episode of confusion was reported in one patient using valerian with loperamide (Imodium) and St. John's wort (*Hypericum perforatum* L.).
- An episode of agitation, anxiety, and self-injury was reported in a patient after taking valerian with fluoxetine (Prozac) for a mood disorder (the person was also drinking alcohol). In theory, valerian may interact with antiseizure medications, although there are no human data on such an interaction. Valerian tinctures may have a high alcohol content (15% to 90%) and theoretically may cause vomiting if taken with metronidazole (Flagyl) or disulfiram (Antabuse).

Interactions with Herbs and Dietary Supplements

- Based on theoretical concerns, valerian may increase the amount of drowsiness caused by some herbs or supplements. Examples are calamus, calendula, California poppy, capsicum, catnip, celery, couchgrass, dogwood, elecampane, German chamomile, goldenseal, gotu kola, hops, kava (may promote sleep without causing drowsiness), lavender aromatherapy, lemon balm, sage, sassafras, scullcap, shepherd's purse, Siberian ginseng, St. John's wort, stinging nettle, wild carrot, wild lettuce, withania root, and yerba mansa. Caution is advised in persons who will be driving or operating heavy machinery.

- A brief episode of confusion was reported in one patient during use of valerian with loperamide (Imodium) and St. John's wort (*Hypericum perforatum* L.). Nausea, sweating, muscle cramping, weakness, elevated pulse, and high blood pressure were reported after a single dose of a combination product containing St. John's wort, kava, and valerian.

Selected References

Natural Standard developed the preceding evidence-based information based on a systematic review of more than 345 scientific articles. For comprehensive information about alternative and complementary therapies on the professional level, go to www.naturalstandard.com. Selected references are listed here.

Abebe W. An overview of herbal supplement utilization with particular emphasis on possible interactions with dental drugs and oral manifestations. J Dent Hyg 2003;77(1):37-46.

Abebe W. Herbal medication: potential for adverse interactions with analgesic drugs. J Clin Pharm Ther 2002;27(6):391-401.

Andreatini R, Sartori VA, Seabra ML, et al. Effect of valepotriates (valerian extract) in generalized anxiety disorder: a randomized placebo-controlled pilot study. Phytother Res 2002; 16(7):650-654.

Chan TY. An assessment of the delayed effects associated with valerian overdose. Int J Clin Pharmacol Ther 1998;36(10):569.

Chen D, Klesmer J, Giovanniello A, et al. Mental status changes in an alcohol abuser taking valerian and gingko biloba. Am J Addict 2002;11(1):75-77.

Cropley M, Cave Z, Ellis J, Middleton RW. Effect of kava and valerian on human physiological and psychological responses to mental stress assessed under laboratory conditions. Phytother Res 2002;16(1):23-27.

De Feo V, Faro C. Pharmacological effects of extracts from *Valeriana adscendens* Trel. II. Effects on GABA uptake and amino acids. Phytother Res 2003;17(6):661-664.

Dergal JM, Gold JL, Laxer DA, et al. Potential interactions between herbal medicines and conventional drug therapies used by older adults attending a memory clinic. Drugs Aging 2002;19(11):879-886.

Dominguez RA, Bravo-Valverde RL, Kaplowitz BR, et al. Valerian as a hypnotic for Hispanic patients. Cultur Divers Ethnic Minor Psychol 2000;6(1):84-92.

Donath F, Quispe S, Diefenbach K, et al. Critical evaluation of the effect of valerian extract on sleep structure and sleep quality. Pharmacopsychiatry 2000;33(2):47-53.

Francis AJ, Dempster RJ. Effect of valerian, *Valeriana edulis*, on sleep difficulties in children with intellectual deficits: randomized trial. Phytomedicine 2002;9(4):273-279.

Garges HP, Varia I, Doraiswamy PM. Cardiac complications and delirium associated with valerian root withdrawal. JAMA 1998;280(18):1566-1567.

Giedke H, Breyer-Pfaff U. Critical evaluation of the effect of valerian extract on sleep structure and sleep quality. Pharmacopsychiatry 2000;33(6):239.

Glass JR, Sproule BA, Herrmann N, et al. Acute pharmacological effects of temazepam, diphenhydramine, and valerian in healthy elderly subjects. J Clin Psychopharmacol 2003; 23(3):260-268.

Hadley S, Petry JJ. Valerian. Am Fam Physician 2003;67(8):1755-1758.

Hariya T, Kobayashi Y, Aihara M, et al. [Effects of sedative odorant inhalation on patients with atopic dermatitis]. Arerugi 2002;51(11):1113-1122.

Houghton PJ. The scientific basis for the reputed activity of valerian. J Pharm Pharmacol 1999;51(5):505-512.

Kapadia GJ, Azuine MA, Tokuda H, et al. Inhibitory effect of herbal remedies on 12-*o*-tetradecanoylphorbol-13-acetate–promoted Epstein-Barr virus early antigen activation. Pharmacol Res 2002;45(3):213-220.

Kuhlmann J, Berger W, Podzuweit H, et al. The influence of valerian treatment on "reaction time, alertness and concentration" in volunteers. Pharmacopsychiatry 1999;32(6):235-241.

Morozova SV, Zaitseva OV. Correction of autonomic sensory disorders in middle ear diseases [Article in Russian]. Vestn Otorinolaringol 2002;(3):38-41.

Muller D, Pfeil T, von den Driesch V. Treating depression comorbid with anxiety—results of an open, practice-oriented study with St John's wort WS 5572 and valerian extract in high doses. Phytomedicine 2003;10(Suppl 4):25-30.

Murakami N, Ye Y, Kawanishi M, et al. New Rev-transport inhibitor with anti-HIV activity from Valerianae Radix. Bioorg Med Chem Lett 2002;12(20):2807-2810.

Poyares DR, Guilleminault C, Ohayon MM, Tufik S. Can valerian improve the sleep of insomniacs after benzodiazepine withdrawal? Prog Neuropsychopharmacol Biol Psychiatry 2002(3):539-545.

Spinella M. The importance of pharmacological synergy in psychoactive herbal medicines. Altern Med Rev 2002;7(2):130-7.

Stevinson C, Ernst E. Valerian for insomnia: systematic review of randomized clinical trials. Sleep Med 2000;1:91-99.

Sun J. Morning/Evening menopausal formula relieves menopausal symptoms: a pilot study. J Altern Complement Med 2003;9(3):403-409.

Wheatley D. Stress-induced insomnia treated with kava and valerian: singly and in combination. Hum Psychopharmacol Clin Exp 2001;16(4):353-356.

Ziegler G, Ploch M, Miettinen-Baumann A, et al. Efficacy and tolerability of valerian extract LI 156 compared with oxazepam in the treatment of non-organic insomnia—a randomized, double-blind, comparative clinical study. Eur J Med Res 2002;7(11):480-486.

White Horehound

(*Marrubium vulgare* L.)

RELATED TERMS

- Andorn, blanc rubi, bonhomme, bouenriblé, bull's blood, common hoarhound/ horehound, eye of the star, grand bon-homme (grand-bonhomme), haran haran, herbe aux crocs, herbe vierge, hoarhound, horehound, hound-bane, houndsbane, Labiatae (family), Lamiaceae (family), llwyd y cwn, maltrasté, mapiochin, mariblé marinclin, marrochemin, marroio, marroio blanco, marromba, marrube, marrube blanc, marrube commun, marrube des champs, marrube officinal, marrube vulgaire, marrubii herba, marrubio, marrubium, maruil, marvel, mastranzo, mont blanc, Ricola, seed of Horus, soldier's tea, weisser andorn.
- *Note:* White horehound should not be confused with black horehound (*Ballota nigra*) or water horehound (*Lycopus americanus*, also known as bugleweed).

BACKGROUND

- Since the time of ancient Egypt, white horehound (*Marrubium vulgare* L.) has been used as an expectorant (to facilitate removal of mucus from the lungs or throat). Ayurvedic, Native American, and Australian Aboriginal medicines have traditionally used white horehound to treat respiratory (lung) conditions. The U.S. Food and Drug Administration (FDA) banned horehound from cough drops in 1989 because of insufficient evidence supporting its efficacy. However, horehound is currently widely used in Europe and can be found in European-made herbal cough remedies sold in the United States (for example, Ricola).
- There is no well-defined clinical evidence to support any therapeutic use of white horehound. The expert panel German Commission E has approved white horehound as a choleretic, for lack of appetite and dyspepsia (heartburn). There is promising early evidence favoring the use of white horehound as a hypoglycemic agent for diabetes mellitus, and as a nonopioid pain reliever.
- There is limited evidence on safety or toxicity in humans. White horehound has been reported to cause hypotension (low blood pressure), hypoglycemia (low blood sugar), and arrhythmias (abnormal heart rhythms) in animal studies

USES BASED ON SCIENTIFIC EVIDENCE	Grade*
Cough Since the time of ancient Egypt, white horehound has been used as an expectorant. Ayurvedic, Native American, and Australian Aboriginal medicines have traditionally used white horehound to treat respiratory (lung) conditions. The FDA banned horehound from cough drops in 1989 because of insufficient evidence supporting its effectiveness. However, horehound is currently widely used in Europe and can be found in European-made herbal cough remedies sold in the United States (for example, Ricola).	C

Continued

Diabetes White horehound has been used for diabetes in some countries, including Mexico. Animal studies suggest that white horehound may lower blood sugar levels. However, there are no reliable studies available in humans.	C
Heartburn/poor appetite In Germany, white horehound is approved for the treatment of heartburn and lack of appetite, based on historical use. There is not enough information from scientific studies to evaluate the effectiveness of white horehound for these conditions.	C
Intestinal disorders/antispasmodic White horehound has been used traditionally to treat intestinal disorders. However, there are few well-designed studies in this area, and little information is available about the effectiveness of white horehound for this use.	C
Pain White horehound has traditionally been used for pain and spasms from menstruation or intestinal conditions. There are no reliable human studies on safety or effectiveness for this use.	C

*Key to grades: *A:* Strong scientific evidence for this use; *B:* Good scientific evidence for this use; *C:* Unclear scientific evidence for this use; *D:* Fair scientific evidence against this use (it may not work); *F:* Strong scientific evidence against this use (it likely does not work). For a more detailed explanation of efficacy criteria, see "Natural Standard Evidence-Based Validated Grading Rationale" in the Introduction.

Uses Based on Tradition, Theory, or Limited Scientific Evidence

Asthma, bile secretion, bloating, bronchitis, blood vessel relaxation, cancer, cathartic, colic, congestion, constipation, chronic obstructive pulmonary disease (COPD), debility, diarrhea, digestive aid, fever reduction, flatulence, food flavoring, gallbladder complaints, heart rate abnormalities, indigestion, intestinal parasites, jaundice (yellowing of the skin), laxative, liver disease, lung congestion, morning sickness, pneumonia, rabies, respiratory (lung) spasms, skin conditions, snake poisoning, sore throat, sweat stimulation, tuberculosis, upper respiratory tract infection, vomiting stimulant, warts, water retention, wheezing, whooping cough, wound healing.

DOSING

The following doses are based on scientific research, publications, traditional use, or expert opinion. Many herbs and supplements have not been thoroughly tested, and their safety and effectiveness may not be proven. Brands may be made differently, with variable ingredients even within the same brand. The doses shown may not apply to all products. It is important to always read product labels and discuss doses with a qualified healthcare provider before therapy is started.

Standardization

- Standardization involves measuring the amount of certain chemicals in products to try to make different preparations similar to each other. It is not always known if the chemicals being measured are the "active" ingredients.
- There is no widely accepted standardization for white horehound. The maximum average concentration in candy is reported as 0.073%. Crude white horehound has previously been an official compound for pharmacists and listed in the United States Pharmacopia (USP). Strength of extracts can be expressed in terms of flavor intensity or weight-to-weight ratio.
- *Caution:* Black horehound (*Ballota nigra*) may be found in compounds reported to contain only white horehound.

Adults (18 Years and Older)

- **Cough/throat ailments:** Doses that have been used include 10 to 40 drops of extract in water up to three times a day and lozenges dissolved in the mouth as needed. Ricola drops are recommended by the manufacturer at a maximum of 2 lozenges every 1 to 2 hours as needed.
- **Heartburn/appetite stimulant:** Doses recommended by the expert German panel Commission E include 4.5 g daily of cut herb and 2 to 6 tablespoons of fresh plant juice daily. Other traditional dosing suggestions are 1 to 2 g of dried herb and the same amount taken as an infusion three times daily.

Children (Younger Than 18 Years)

- There is not enough information to recommend the safe use of white horehound in children.

SAFETY

The U.S. Food and Drug Administration does not strictly regulate herbs and supplements. There is no guarantee of strength, purity, or safety of products, and effects may vary. It is important to always read product labels. People who have a medical condition, or are taking other drugs, herbs, or supplements, should consult a qualified healthcare provider before starting a new therapy. A healthcare provider should be consulted immediately about any side effects.

Allergies

- In theory, white horehound may cause an allergic reaction in persons with known allergy or hypersensitivity to members of the Lamiaceae family (mint family) or any white horehound components.

Side Effects and Warnings

- White horehound is generally considered to be safe when used as a flavoring agent in foods. However, there is limited scientific study of safety, and most available information is from animal (not human) research. Reported side effects include rash at areas of direct contact with white horehound plant juice, abnormal heart rhythms, low blood pressure, and decreased blood sugar (seen in animals with high blood sugar). White horehound may cause vomiting and diarrhea. Caution is warranted in people with heart disease or gastrointestinal disorders. Caution may also be advisable in persons with diabetes or hypoglycemia, and in those taking drugs, herbs, or supplements that affect blood sugar. Serum glucose levels may need to be monitored by a healthcare provider, and medication adjustments may be necessary.

- Theoretically, white horehound may interfere with the body's response to the hormone aldosterone, which affects the ability of the kidneys to control the body's levels of water and electrolytes. These theoretical effects may cause high blood pressure, high blood sodium, low potassium, leg swelling, and muscle weakness. Individuals who have high or unstable blood pressure, high sodium, or low potassium or who are taking medications that reduce the amount of water in the body (diuretics, or "water pills") should use caution. White horehound may contain estrogen-like chemicals that have either stimulatory or inhibitory effects on estrogen-sensitive parts of the body. It is unclear what effects may occur in hormone-sensitive conditions such as some cancers (breast, ovarian, uterine) and endometriosis, or in people using hormone replacement therapy/birth control pills.

Pregnancy and Breastfeeding

- White horehound is not recommended during pregnancy or breastfeeding. Animal studies suggest that white horehound may cause miscarriage.

INTERACTIONS

Most herbs and supplements have not been thoroughly tested for interactions with other herbs, supplements, drugs, or foods. The interactions listed here are based on reports in scientific publications, laboratory experiments, or traditional use. It is important to always read product labels. People who have a medical condition, or are taking other drugs, herbs, or supplements, should consult a qualified healthcare provider before starting a new therapy.

Interactions with Drugs

- Because white horehound is thought to act as an expectorant in the treatment of cough or congestion, its use with cold medications that have expectorant ingredients may cause added effects. Theoretically, white horehound may reduce the effects of some medications given for vomiting (serotonin receptor antagonist drugs such as granisetron and ondansetron), or migraine headache (ergot alkaloids such as bromocriptine, dihydroergotamine, and ergotamine), and of antidepressants that possess serotonin activity (selective serotonin reuptake inhibitors [SSRIs] such as Prozac, Paxil, and Zoloft). White horehound may affect the ability of the body to excrete penicillin. Because white horehound may cause diarrhea, an excessive response may result when this herb is combined with stool softeners or laxatives.
- Large amounts of white horehound may increase the risk of abnormal heart rhythms and should be avoided by people taking drugs that affect heart rhythm. Animal studies suggest that use of white horehound with medications that lower blood pressure may cause a larger-than-expected drop in blood pressure. White horehound contains glycoside compounds that act on the heart, and these theoretically could affect the activity of glycoside medications such as digoxin (Lanoxin). Theoretically, white horehound may increase the action of the hormone aldosterone on the kidneys, and it may interact with some diuretic medications.
- Based on animal studies, white horehound may lower blood sugar levels. Caution is advised with use of medications that may also lower blood sugar. Patients taking drugs for diabetes by mouth or insulin should be monitored closely by a qualified healthcare provider. Medication adjustments may be necessary. In theory, white horehound may also interact with medications used to treat thyroid disorders such as iodine, liothyronine (triiodothyronine [T_3]) (Cytomel); methimazole (Tapazole); propylthiouracil (PTU); thyroxine (T_4) (Levoxyl, Synthroid); Thyrolar (T_4 plus T_3).

- White horehound may contain estrogen-like chemicals that have either stimulatory or inhibitory effects on estrogen-sensitive parts of the body. It is unclear what effects may occur in women using hormonal agents such as birth control pills or receiving hormone replacement therapy.

Interactions with Herbs and Dietary Supplements

- In theory, white horehound may lower blood pressure and may cause increased urine production. Caution is advised with use of herbs or supplements that also lower blood pressure or increase urination. Agents that may lower blood pressure include aconite/monkshood, arnica, baneberry, betel nut, bilberry, black cohosh, bryony, calendula, California poppy, coleus, curcumin, eucalyptol, eucalyptus oil, evening primrose oil, flaxseed/flaxseed oil, garlic, ginger, ginkgo, goldenseal, green hellebore, hawthorn, Indian tobacco, jaborandi, mistletoe, night-blooming cereus, oleander, pasque flower, periwinkle, pleurisy root, shepherd's purse, Texas milkweed, turmeric, and wild cherry. Supplements that may increase urine production include artichoke, celery, corn silk, couchgrass, dandelion, elder flower, horsetail, juniper berry, kava, shepherd's purse, uva ursi, and yarrow.
- White horehound may contain glycoside chemicals that affect the heart and therefore should be used with caution by people taking other supplements that have glycoside ingredients. Such agents include adonis, balloon cotton, black hellebore root/melampode, black Indian hemp, bushman's poison, *Cactus grandifloris*, convallaria, eyebright, figwort, foxglove/digitalis, frangipani, hedge mustard, hemp root/Canadian hemp root, king's crown, lily-of-the-valley, motherwort, oleander leaf, pheasant's eye plant, plantain leaf, pleurisy root, psyllium husks, redheaded cotton-bush, rhubarb root, rubber vine, sea mango, senna fruit, squill, strophanthus, uzara, wallflower, wintersweet, yellow dock root, and yellow oleander. Notably, Chan Su is a Chinese herbal formula containing bufalin that has been reported to be toxic or fatal when taken with cardiac glycosides.
- Because white horehound may cause diarrhea, caution is advised with use of other laxative herbs, such as alder buckthorn, aloe dried leaf sap, black root, blue flag rhizome, butternut bark, dong quai, European buckthorn, eyebright, cascara bark, castor oil, chasteberry, colocynth fruit pulp, dandelion, gamboges bark, horsetail, jalap root, manna bark, plantain leaf, podophyllum root, psyllium, rhubarb, senna, wild cucumber fruit, and yellow dock root.
- Animal studies suggest that white horehound may lower blood sugar levels. Caution is advised with use of herbs or supplements that may also lower blood sugar. Blood glucose levels may require monitoring, and doses may need adjustment. Possible examples include *Aloe vera*, American ginseng, bilberry, bitter melon, burdock, fenugreek, fish oil, gymnema, horse chestnut seed extract (HCSE), marshmallow, milk thistle, *Panax ginseng*, rosemary, Siberian ginseng, and stinging nettle.
- Because white horehound may contain estrogen-like chemicals, the effects of other agents believed to have estrogen-like properties may be altered. Possible examples include alfalfa, black cohosh, bloodroot, burdock, flaxseed, hops, kudzu, licorice, pomegranate, red clover, soy, thyme, and yucca. Theoretically, white horehound may interact with agents that affect serotonin activity, such as antidepressant herbs or supplements with possible SSRI properties, such as ephedra, evening primrose oil, fenugreek, *Ginkgo biloba*, hops, St. John's wort, tyrosine, valerian, and yohimbe. In theory, white horehound may interact with agents that affect the thyroid, such as bladderwrack.

Selected References

Natural Standard developed the preceding evidence-based information based on a systematic review of more than 40 scientific articles. For comprehensive information about alternative and complementary therapies on the professional level, go to www.naturalstandard.com. Selected references are listed here.

Cahen R. [Pharmacologic spectrum of *Marrubium vulgare* L.]. C R Seances Soc Biol Fil 1970;164(7):1467-1472.

De Jesus RA, Cechinel-Filho V, Oliveira AE, et al. Analysis of the antinociceptive properties of marrubiin isolated from *Marrubium vulgare*. Phytomedicine 2000;7(2):111-115.

De Souza MM, De Jesus RA, Cechinel-Filho V, et al. Analgesic profile of hydroalcoholic extract obtained from *Marrubium vulgare*. Phytomed 1998;5(2):103-107.

El Bardai S, Morel N, Wibo M, et al. The vasorelaxant activity of marrubenol and marrubiin from *Marrubium vulgare*. Planta Med 2003;69(1):75-77.

El Bardai S, Wibo M, Hamaide MC, et al. Characterisation of marrubenol, a diterpene extracted from *Marrubium vulgare*, as an L-type calcium channel blocker. Br J Pharmacol 2003; 140(7):1211-1216.

Karriyvev MO, Bairiyev CB, Atayeva AS. [On the curative properties and phytochemistry of *Marribum vulgare*]. Izvestiia Akademii Nauk Turkmenskoi SSR, Seriia Biol Nauk 1976; 3:86-88.

Karryvev MO, Bairyev CB, Ataeva AS. Some therapeutic properties of common horehound. Chem Abstr 1977;86:2355.

Roman RR, Alarcon-Aguilar F, Lara-Lemus A, et al. Hypoglycemic effect of plants used in Mexico as antidiabetics. Arch Med Res 1992;23(1):59-64.

Saleh MM, Glombitza KW. Volatile oil of *Marrubium vulgare* and its anti-schistosomal activity. Planta Med 1989;55:105.

Schlemper V, Ribas A, Nicolau M, et al. Antispasmodic effects of hydroalcoholic extract of *Marrubium vulgare* on isolated tissues. Phytomed 1996;3(2):211-216.

Wild Yam

(*Dioscorea villosa* L.)

RELATED TERMS

- Atlantic yam, barbasco, China root, colic root, devil's bones, dioscorea, *Dioscorea barbasco, Dioscorea hypoglauca, Dioscorea macrostachya, Dioscorea opposita, Dioscorea villosa*, *Dioscoreae*, diosgenin, Mexican yam, natural dehydroepiandrosterone (DHEA), phytoestrogen, rheumatism root, shan yao, wild yam root, yam, yuma.
- *Note:* "Yams" sold in the supermarket are members of the sweet potato family and are not true yams.

USES BASED ON SCIENTIFIC EVIDENCE	Grade*
High cholesterol Animal studies have shown that wild yam can reduce absorption of cholesterol from the gut. Early studies in humans have shown changes in the levels of certain sub-types of cholesterol, including decreases in low-density lipoprotein (LDL), or "bad" cholesterol, and triglycerides and increases in high-density lipoprotein (HDL), or "good" cholesterol. However, no changes in the total amount of blood cholesterol have been found. More studies are needed in this area.	C
Menopausal symptoms Studies have not shown a benefit from wild yam, either given by mouth or used as a vaginal cream, in reducing menopausal symptoms.	C
Hormonal properties (to mimic estrogen, progesterone, or DHEA) Despite popular belief, no natural progestins, estrogens, or other reproductive hormones are found in wild yam. Its active ingredient, diosgenin, is not converted to hormones in the human body. Artificial progesterone has been added to some wild yam products. The belief that there are hormones in wild yam may be due to the historical fact that progesterone, androgens, and cortisone were chemically manufactured from Mexican wild yam in the 1960s.	D

*Key to grades: *A:* Strong scientific evidence for this use; *B:* Good scientific evidence for this use; *C:* Unclear scientific evidence for this use; *D:* Fair scientific evidence against this use (it may not work); *F:* Strong scientific evidence against this use (it likely does not work). For a more detailed explanation of efficacy criteria, see "Natural Standard Evidence-Based Validated Grading Rationale" in the Introduction.

Uses Based on Tradition, Theory, or Limited Scientific Evidence

Antifungal, anti-inflammatory, asthma, bile flow improvement, biliary colic, breast enlargement, childbirth, cramps, croup, decreased perspiration, diverticulitis, energy enhancement, excessive perspiration, expectorant, flatus prevention, intestinal spasm, irritable bowel syndrome, joint pain, libido, liver protection, low blood sugar, menopause, menstrual pain or irregularities, morning sickness, nerve pain, osteoporosis, pelvic cramps, pancreatic enzyme inhibitor, postmenopausal vaginal dryness, premenstrual syndrome, rash, spasms, urinary tract disorders, uterus contraction, vomiting.

DOSING

The following doses are based on scientific research, publications, traditional use, or expert opinion. Many herbs and supplements have not been thoroughly tested, and their safety and effectiveness may not be proven. Brands may be made differently, with variable ingredients even within the same brand. The doses shown may not apply to all products. It is important to always read product labels and discuss doses with a qualified healthcare provider before therapy is started.

Standardization

- Standardization involves measuring the amount of certain chemicals in products to try to make different preparations similar to each other. It is not always known if the chemicals being measured are the "active" ingredients.
- Typical standardization of wild yam products is 10% diosgenin per dose. Diosgenin is considered the primary active ingredient in wild yam and is similar in structure to cholesterol. There are reports that synthetic progesterone has been added to some wild yam products.

Adults (18 Years and Older)

Topical (on the skin)

- **Cream:** Vaginal creams containing wild yam are available, but there is no widely accepted dose. Effects from absorption into the bloodstream have not been shown. Some products may contain synthetic progesterone, a steroid hormone with potential activity in vaginal changes.

Oral (by mouth)

- *Note:* Safety and effectiveness of oral doses have not been proven.
- **Dried root:** 2 to 4 g or one to two teaspoons daily in two or three divided doses is sometimes recommended.
- **Capsules:** 250 mg of wild yam taken one to three times daily is often recommended, or 450 to 900 mg per day of dioscorea extract from wild yam.
- **Liquid** (1:1 in 45% alcohol): 2 to 4 ml daily in three divided doses has been used.
- **Tincture:** 4 to 12 drops or 2 to 4 ml taken three to five times daily has been used.

Children (Younger Than 18 Years)

- Not enough evidence is available to recommend use of wild yam in children. In unofficial reports, doses in children have been calculated in proportion to the weight of the child relative to a 70-kg (150-lb) adult, as follows: The child's weight in kilograms is divided by 70 (or weight in pounds by 150); this number multiplied by the recommended adult dose equals the child's dose. Safety and effectiveness have not been proven, and dosing should be supervised by a licensed healthcare provider.

SAFETY

The U.S. Food and Drug Administration does not strictly regulate herbs and supplements. There is no guarantee of strength, purity, or safety of products, and effects may vary. It is important to always read product labels. People who have a medical condition, or are taking other drugs, herbs, or supplements, should consult a qualified healthcare provider before starting a new therapy. A healthcare provider should be consulted immediately about any side effects.

Allergies

- Rubbing the skin with *Dioscorea batatas* (a yam species related to *Dioscorea villosa*) has been reported to cause allergic rash. Workers exposed to *D. batatas* in large amounts and for a prolonged time have developed asthma that is made worse by exposure to the yam. A person who is known to have an allergy to *D. batatas* may also be allergic to other *Dioscorea* types.

Side Effects and Warnings

- Rubbing the skin with *D. batatas*, a related yam species, has been reported to cause a rash at the site of contact. Wild yam cream caused no rash in 23 healthy women in one reported study. In another study, wild yam given by mouth was reported to cause stomach upset at high doses.
- Wild yam was believed in the past to have properties similar to those of the reproductive hormone progesterone, but this has not been supported by scientific studies. It has been suggested that some wild yam creams might be tainted with artificial progesterone. In view of theoretical hormonal properties and because of possible progesterone contamination, people with hormone-sensitive conditions should use wild yam products with caution. This caution applies to people who have had blood clots or strokes and to women who receive hormone replacement therapy or who take birth control pills. In addition, women with fibroids, endometriosis, or cancer of the breast, uterus, or ovary should be aware that these are hormone-sensitive conditions that may be affected by agents with hormonal properties.
- In animal studies, compounds from the related species *Dioscorea dumentorum* (bitter or African yam) lower blood sugar levels. It is not clear whether wild yam (*D. villosa*) lowers blood sugar in humans. Caution is advised in patients with diabetes or hypoglycemia and in those taking drugs, herbs, or supplements that affect blood sugar. Blood sugar levels may need to be monitored by a healthcare provider, and medication adjustments may be necessary.

Pregnancy and Breastfeeding

- Use of wild yam is not recommended during pregnancy or breastfeeding because of lack of safety information. Wild yam is believed to cause uterine contractions, and therefore use is discouraged during pregnancy. Wild yam was once thought to have effects similar to those of reproductive hormones, although this has not been proven in scientific studies. Artificial progesterone may be added to some products.

INTERACTIONS

Most herbs and supplements have not been thoroughly tested for interactions with other herbs, supplements, drugs, or foods. The interactions listed here are based on reports in scientific publications, laboratory experiments, or traditional use. It is important to always read product labels. People who have a medical condition, or are taking other drugs, herbs, or supplements, should consult a qualified healthcare provider before starting a new therapy.

Interactions with Drugs

- In animals, wild yam lowers blood levels of indomethacin, a nonsteroidal anti-inflammatory drug, and reduces irritation of the intestine caused by indomethacin. Human studies have not been reported in this area, and it is not clear if wild yam affects the blood levels of other anti-inflammatory drugs such as ibuprofen (Advil, Motrin).
- An early study suggests that wild yam may interfere with the body's ability to control levels of the reproductive hormone progesterone. Progesterone is a key ingredient in some hormone replacement and birth control pills. There are reports that some wild yam products may be tainted with artificial progesterone. Women taking birth control pills or receiving hormone replacement therapy should consult a licensed healthcare provider before starting wild yam supplementation.
- It is not clear whether blood sugar is lowered by *D. villosa* (wild yam). Dioscoretine, a compound found in *D. dumentorum* (bitter or African yam), has been shown to lower blood sugar levels in rabbits, but this effect has not been shown for *D. villosa*. Effects on blood sugar in humans have not been reported. Nonetheless, caution is advised with use of medications that may also lower blood sugar. People taking diabetes drugs by mouth or insulin should be monitored closely by a qualified healthcare provider. Medication adjustments may be necessary.
- Diosgenin, thought to be the active substance in wild yam, has been found in animals to reduce absorption of cholesterol from the intestine and to lower total cholesterol levels in the blood. Studies in humans show no change in the total amount of cholesterol in the blood, although the amounts of specific types of cholesterol in the blood may be changed: LDL ("bad" cholesterol) and triglycerides may be lowered, and high-density lipoprotein (HDL) ("good" cholesterol) may be increased. It is thought that wild yam may enhance the effects of other cholesterol-lowering medications, including fibric acid derivatives such as clofibrate (Questran), gemfibrozil (Lopid), and fenofibrate (Tricor). In animals, wild yam has been found to improve the effect of clofibrate in lowering cholesterol levels.
- Tinctures of wild yam may contain high amounts of alcohol, which may lead to vomiting if these preparations are taken with disulfiram (Antabuse) or metronidazole (Flagyl).

W

Interactions with Herbs and Dietary Supplements

- In an early study, a wild yam preparation was reported to block the body's natural production of progesterone. However, this finding was not supported by later research. There have been several reports that some wild yam products are tainted with synthetic progesterone. Because wild yam may contain progesterone-like chemicals, the effects of other agents believed to have hormone-like properties, in particular those with estrogen-like properties, may be altered. Possible examples include alfalfa, black cohosh, bloodroot, burdock, hops, kudzu, licorice, pomegranate, red clover, soy, thyme, white horehound, and yucca.

- It is not clear whether *D. villosa* (wild yam) lowers blood sugar levels. Although dioscoretine, produced by *D. dumentorum* (bitter or African yam), has been shown to lower blood sugar in rabbits, this reaction has not been seen with *D. villosa* and has not been reported in humans. Nonetheless, caution is advised with use of herbs or supplements that may also lower blood glucose. Blood glucose levels may require monitoring, and doses may need adjustment. Possible examples include *Aloe vera*, American ginseng, bilberry, bitter melon, burdock, fenugreek, fish oil, gymnema, horse chestnut seed extract (HCSE), marshmallow, milk thistle, *Panax ginseng*, rosemary, Siberian ginseng, stinging nettle, and white horehound.
- Diosgenin, thought to be the active substance in wild yam, has been found in animals to reduce absorption of cholesterol from the intestine and to lower total cholesterol levels in the blood. Studies in humans show no change in the total amount of cholesterol in the blood, although the amounts of specific types of cholesterol in the blood may be changed: LDL ("bad" cholesterol) and triglycerides may be lowered, and HDL ("good" cholesterol) appears to be increased. In theory, wild yam may enhance the effects of other cholesterol-lowering agents, such as fish oil, garlic, guggul, and niacin. Vitamin C has been reported to enhance the ability of diosgenin to lower cholesterol. Further study is needed in this area.

Selected References

Natural Standard developed the preceding evidence-based information based on a systematic review of more than 50 scientific articles. For comprehensive information about alternative and complementary therapies on the professional level, go to www.naturalstandard.com. Selected references are listed here.

Araghiniknam M, Chung S, Nelson-White T, et al. Antioxidant activity of *Dioscorea* and dehydroepiandrosterone (DHEA) in older humans. Life Sciences 1996;59:L147-L157.

Hudson t, Standish L, Breed C, et al. Clinical and endocrinological effects of a menopausal botanical formula. J Naturopath Med 1997;7:73-77.

Komesaroff PA, Black CV, Cable V, et al. Effects of wild yam extract on menopausal symptoms, lipids and sex hormones in healthy menopausal women. Climacteric 2001;4(2):144-150.

Kubo Y, Nonaka S, Yoshida H. Allergic contact dermatitis from *Dioscorea batatas* Decaisne. Contact Derm 1988;18(2):111-112.

Yohimbe Bark Extract

(*Pausinystalia yohimbe* [K. Schumann] Pierre ex Beille)

RELATED TERMS

- Aphrodien, *Corynanthe johimbi*, *Corynanthe yohimbi* Schumann, corynine, johimbi, *Pausinystalia yohimbe*, quebrachine, Rubiaceae (family), yohimbehe, yohimbehe cortex, yohimbeherinde, yohimbene, yohimbime, yohimbine.

BACKGROUND

- The terms *yohimbine*, *yohimbine hydrochloride*, and *yohimbe bark extract* are related but not interchangeable. Yohimbine is an active chemical (indole alkaloid) found in the bark of the *Pausinystalia yohimbe* tree. Yohimbine hydrochloride is a standardized form of yohimbine that is available as a prescription drug in the United States and has been shown in human studies to be effective in the treatment of male impotence. Yohimbine hydrochloride has also been used for the treatment of sexual side effects caused by some antidepressants (selective serotonin reuptake inhibitors [SSRIs]) and female hyposexual disorder, as a blood pressure–boosting agent in autonomic failure, for relief of xerostomia, and as a probe for noradrenergic activity.

USES BASED ON SCIENTIFIC EVIDENCE	Grade*
Dry mouth (xerostomia) Studies report that yohimbine can increase saliva in animals and in humans. Based on these few studies, yohimbine has been used for the treatment of dry mouth caused by medications such as antidepressants. However, yohimbe bark extract may not contain significant amounts of yohimbine and therefore may not have these effects. More research is needed before a recommendation can be made.	C
Erectile dysfunction (male impotence) Yohimbine hydrochloride is a prescription drug that has been shown in multiple human trials to effectively treat male impotence. Although yohimbine is present in yohimbe bark extract, levels are variable and often very low. Yohimbe bark extract has not been shown to share the effects of yohimbine hydrochloride. Therefore, although yohimbe bark has been used traditionally to reduce male erectile dysfunction, there is not enough scientific evidence to form a firm conclusion in this area.	C
Libido (women) Yohimbine has been proposed to increase female libido (sexual interest). There is only limited poor-quality research in this area, and more study is needed before a recommendation can be made.	C

Continued

Y

Nervous system dysfunction (autonomic failure) It is theorized that yohimbine may improve orthostatic hypotension (lowering of blood pressure with standing) and relieve other symptoms of autonomic nervous system dysfunction. However, yohimbe bark extract may not contain significant amounts of yohimbine and therefore may not have these proposed effects. More research is needed before a recommendation can be made.	C
Sexual side effects of selective serotonin reuptake inhibitor antidepressants Yohimbine hydrochloride, a standardized form of yohimbine that is available as a prescription drug in the United States, has been suggested to treat sexual dysfunction due to SSRI antidepressants. However, research in this area is limited, and more study is needed before a recommendation can be made. In addition, yohimbe bark extract may not contain significant amounts of yohimbine and therefore may not have these proposed effects.	C

*Key to grades: *A:* Strong scientific evidence for this use; *B:* Good scientific evidence for this use; *C:* Unclear scientific evidence for this use; *D:* Fair scientific evidence against this use (it may not work); *F:* Strong scientific evidence against this use (it likely does not work). For a more detailed explanation of efficacy criteria, see "Natural Standard Evidence-Based Validated Grading Rationale" in the Introduction.

Uses Based on Tradition, Theory, or Limited Scientific Evidence

Alzheimer's disease, anesthetic, angina, aphrodisiac, clonidine overdose, cognition, coronary artery disease, cough, depression, diabetic complications, diabetic neuropathy, exhaustion, fevers, hallucinogenic, high cholesterol, insomnia, leprosy, low blood pressure, narcolepsy, obesity, panic disorder, Parkinson's disease, postural hypotension, pupil dilator, schizophrenia, syncope.

DOSING

The following doses are based on scientific research, publications, traditional use, or expert opinion. Many herbs and supplements have not been thoroughly tested, and their safety and effectiveness may not be proven. Brands may be made differently, with variable ingredients even within the same brand. The doses shown may not apply to all products. It is important to always read product labels and discuss doses with a qualified healthcare provider before therapy is started.

Standardization

- Standardization involves measuring the amount of certain chemicals in products to try to make different preparations similar to each other.
- There is no widely accepted standardization to regulate the production of yohimbe bark extract products, although yohimbine is believed to be the main ingredient of importance. A 1995 scientific analysis of 26 commercial yohimbe products reported that most products contained virtually no yohimbine.

- A 2003 scientific analysis of 20 commercial aphrodisiac preparations found that the amount of yohimbine measured and expressed as the maximal dose per day suggested on product labels ranged from 1.32 to 23.16 mg.

Adults (18 Years and Older)

- **Tea:** A tea can be prepared by simmering 5 to 10 teaspoons of shaved yohimbe bark in 1 pint of water (with a further recommendation of adding 0.5 to 1.0 g of vitamin C to the tea to make it more soluble). This traditional dose has not been tested in reliable human studies.
- **Tablets:** The following doses are based on human trials of pharmaceutical standardized yohimbine hydrochloride (available by prescription in the United States). No reliable clinical studies are available for administration of yohimbe bark extract. For erectile dysfunction (male impotence), 15 to 42 mg of yohimbine hydrochloride daily in three divided doses (for example, 5.4 to 10 mg three times daily) has been studied. For libido enhancement in women, 5.4 mg three times daily of yohimbine hydrochloride has been studied. For sexual side effects caused by antidepressant drugs, 2.7 to 16.2 mg of yohimbine hydrochloride has been studied. For autonomic dysfunction/orthostatic hypotension, 5.4 to 12 mg of daily yohimbine has been studied. For dry mouth (xerostomia), 6 mg three times daily of yohimbine hydrochloride has been studied.

Children (Younger Than 18 Years)

- Yohimbe and yohimbine hydrochloride are not recommended for use in children.

SAFETY

The U.S. Food and Drug Administration does not strictly regulate herbs and supplements. There is no guarantee of strength, purity, or safety of products, and effects may vary. It is important to always read product labels. People who have a medical condition, or are taking other drugs, herbs, or supplements, should consult a qualified healthcare provider before starting a new therapy. A healthcare provider should be consulted immediately about any side effects.

Allergies

- In theory, allergy/hypersensitivity to yohimbe or any of its constituents or to yohimbine-containing products may occur.

Side Effects and Warnings

- Yohimbe bark extract is traditionally said to cause occasional skin flushing, piloerection (standing up of body hair), painful urination, genital pain, reduced appetite, agitation, dizziness, headache, irritability, nervousness, tremors, or insomnia.
- Multiple adverse effects have been associated with the use of the drug yohimbine hydrochloride, although in recommended doses, it is usually tolerated. If adverse effects occur, discontinuing the drug will likely stop the effects. In theory, these same side effects may also occur with the use of yohimbe bark extract, which contains variable (usually low) amounts of yohimbine.
- There are reports of rash, flushing, breathing difficulty, cough, runny nose, nausea, vomiting, increased salivation, diarrhea, increased frequency of urination, kidney failure, muscle aches, and a lupus-like syndrome with the use of yohimbine hydrochloride. Yohimbine has also been associated with tremulousness, insomnia, anxiety, irritability, and excitability. Yohimbine may precipitate panic attacks, anxiety, manic episodes, or psychosis in patients with a history of mental illness.

- In animal research, yohimbine has been associated with increased motor activity and seizures at higher doses. In humans, yohimbine may change the seizure threshold (the likelihood that a seizure will happen in some people) and may cause blood pressure/heart rate increases, fluid retention, chest discomfort, and heart rhythm abnormalities. Higher doses may lower blood pressure. Yohimbine can enter the brain through the bloodstream. Yohimbine may increase the risk of bleeding by altering platelet function and may reduce the number of white blood cells to dangerously low levels (agranulocytosis).
- Symptoms of toxicity from yohimbine can include paralysis, dangerously low blood pressure, heart rhythm abnormalities, heart failure, and death. These same risks theoretically may also exist with yohimbe bark extract, depending on the concentration of yohimbine present and the amount ingested. Beta-blocker drugs such as metoprolol (Lopressor, Toprol) may be protective against yohimbine toxicity.

Pregnancy and Breastfeeding

- Yohimbe bark extract should be avoided during pregnancy because it may relax the uterus and may be toxic to the fetus. Yohimbe bark extra should be avoided during breastfeeding, because of reports of deaths in children.

INTERACTIONS

Most herbs and supplements have not been thoroughly tested for interactions with other herbs, supplements, drugs, or foods. The interactions listed here are based on reports in scientific publications, laboratory experiments, or traditional use. It is important to always read product labels. People who have a medical condition, or are taking other drugs, herbs, or supplements, should consult a qualified healthcare provider before starting a new therapy.

Interactions with Drugs

- Multiple drug interactions may occur with the use of yohimbine hydrochloride. In theory, these effects may also apply to yohimbe bark extract, which contains variable (usually low) amounts of yohimbine.
- Based on human study, yohimbine has been reported to block the effects of alpha-adrenergic drugs. Yohimbine may increase the effects of drugs that are antiadrenergic, such as clonidine or guanabenz. Use of yohimbine with central nervous system stimulants may have additive effects. In theory, due to inhibition of monoamine oxidase activity, use of yohimbine with monoamine oxidase inhibitor (MAOI) drugs such as isocarboxazid (Marplan), phenelzine (Nardil), tranylcypromine (Parnate), or linezolid (Zyvox) may produce additive side effects, such as an increased risk of extremely high blood pressure.
- Based on human study, use of ethanol (alcohol) with yohimbine may produce an additive effect of increasing intoxication. Based on human study, yohimbine may increase pain relief from morphine and may increase or decrease withdrawal symptoms caused by the medication naloxone. According to historical use and animal study, yohimbine may increase the effects of diabetic medications, including insulin, although there is no reliable scientific evidence in this area. Caution is advised with use of medications that may lower blood sugar. Patients taking drugs for diabetes by mouth or insulin should be monitored closely by a qualified healthcare provider. Medication adjustments may be necessary.
- Based on human study, use of yohimbine with physostigmine in patients with Alzheimer's disease may be associated with anxiety, agitation, restlessness, and chest

pain. Caution has been advised with use of yohimbine with antihistamines, although there is no reliable scientific evidence in this area. The combination of yohimbine with antimuscarinic agents may result in increased risk of toxicity. In theory, yohimbine may add to the effects of drugs that lower blood pressure.

- In theory, yohimbine may interfere with how the body uses the liver's cytochrome P450 enzyme system to process certain drugs. As a result, blood levels of these drugs (and of yohimbine) may be altered, which may cause increased or decreased effects or potentially serious adverse reactions. People who are using any medications should always read the package insert and consult their healthcare provider or pharmacist about possible interactions.

Interactions with Herbs and Dietary Supplements

- Multiple interactions may occur between the drug yohimbine hydrochloride and herbs or supplements. In theory, these effects may also apply to yohimbe bark extract, which contains variable (usually low) amounts of yohimbine.
- In theory, other over-the-counter products containing stimulants, including phenylephrine and phenylpropanolamine (removed from the U.S. market), may have additive effects when used in combination with yohimbine. Yohimbine theoretically may interfere with blood pressure control and should be used cautiously with other herbs or supplements that affect blood pressure.
- As a result of inhibition of monoamine oxidase, use of yohimbine with herbs or supplements with possible similar properties may produce additive effects, such as an increased risk of dangerously high blood pressure (hypertensive crisis). Such herbs and supplements include 5-hydroxytryptophan (5-HTP), California poppy, chromium, dehydroepiandrosterone (DHEA), ephedra, evening primrose oil, fenugreek, *Ginkgo biloba*, hops, mace, DL-phenylalanine (DLPA), St. John's wort, *S*-adenosylmethionine (SAMe), sepia, tyrosine, valerian, and vitamin B_6. In theory, caffeine-containing agents such as coffee, tea, cola, guarana, and mate may also increase the risk of hypertensive crisis when taken with yohimbine.
- Yohimbine theoretically may add to the effects of herbs or supplements that may lower blood sugar. Blood glucose levels may require monitoring, and doses may need adjustment. Possible examples include *Aloe vera*, American ginseng, bilberry, bitter melon, burdock, fenugreek, fish oil, gymnema, horse chestnut seed extract (HCSE), marshmallow, milk thistle, *Panax ginseng*, rosemary, Siberian ginseng, stinging nettle, and white horehound.
- In theory, yohimbine may interfere with how the body uses the liver's cytochrome P450 enzyme system to process herbs or supplements. As a result, blood levels of components of such herbs or supplements (and of yohimbine) may be altered, which may cause increased or decreased effects or potentially serious adverse reactions. Yohimbine may also alter the effects of other herbs or supplements on the P450 system, such as bloodroot, cat's claw, chamomile, chaparral, chasteberry, damiana, *Echinacea angustifolia*, goldenseal, grapefruit juice, licorice, oregano, red clover, St. John's wort, wild cherry, and yucca. People who are using any herbs or supplements should always read the package insert and consult their healthcare provider and pharmacist about possible interactions.

Interactions with Foods

- Yohimbine may inhibit monoamine oxidase; therefore, taking yohimbine with certain foods may carry a risk of dangerous reactions (high blood pressure). In theory, this effect may also apply to yohimbe bark extract, which contains variable (usually low) amounts of yohimbine. Examples of such foods are anchovies, avocados, bananas, bean curd, beer (alcohol-free/reduced), caffeine (large amounts), caviar, champagne, cheeses (particularly aged, processed, or strong varieties), chocolate, dry sausage/salami/bologna, fava beans, figs, herring (pickled), liver (particularly chicken liver), meat tenderizers, papaya, protein extracts/powder, raisins, shrimp paste, sour cream, soy sauce, wine (particularly chianti), yeast extracts, and yogurt.

Selected References

Natural Standard developed the preceding evidence-based information based on a systematic review of more than 400 scientific articles. For comprehensive information about alternative and complementary therapies on the professional level, go to www.naturalstandard.com. Selected references are listed here.

Bagheri H, Schmitt L, Berlan M, et al. A comparative study of the effects of yohimbine and anetholtrithione on salivary secretion in depressed patients treated with psychotropic drugs. Eur J Clin Pharmacol 1997;52(5):339-342.

Bagheri H, Schmitt L, Berlan M, et al. Effect of 3 weeks treatment with yohimbine on salivary secretion in healthy volunteers and in depressed patients treated with tricyclic antidepressants. Br J Clin Pharmacol 1992;34(6):555-558.

Balon R. Fluoxetine-induced sexual dysfunction and yohimbine. J Clin Psychiatry 1993; 54(4):161-162.

Betz JM, White KD, der Marderosian AH. Gas chromatographic determination of yohimbine in commercial yohimbe products. J AOAC Int 1995;78(5):1189-1194.

Brodde OE, Anlauf M, Arroyo J, et al. Hypersensitivity of adrenergic receptors and blood-pressure response to oral yohimbine in orthostatic hypotension. N Engl J Med 1983; 308(17):1033-1034.

Carey MP, Johnson BT. Effectiveness of yohimbine in the treatment of erectile disorder: four meta-analytic integrations. Arch Sex Behav 1996;25(4):341-360.

Ernst E, Pittler MH. Yohimbine for erectile dysfunction: a systematic review and meta-analysis of randomized clinical trials. J Urol 1998;159(2):433-436.

Friesen K, Palatnick W, Tenenbein M. Benign course after massive ingestion of yohimbine. J Emerg Med 1993;11(3):287-288.

Hollander E, McCarley A. Yohimbine treatment of sexual side effects induced by serotonin reuptake blockers. J Clin Psychiatry 1992;53(6):207-209.

Jacobsen FM. Fluoxetine-induced sexual dysfunction and an open trial of yohimbine. J Clin Psychiatry 1992;53(4):119-122.

Knoll LD, Benson RC, Jr., Bilhartz DL, et al. A randomized crossover study using yohimbine and isoxsuprine versus pentoxifylline in the management of vasculogenic impotence. J Urol 1996;155(1):144-146.

Kunelius P, Hakkinen J, Lukkarinen O. Is high-dose yohimbine hydrochloride effective in the treatment of mixed-type impotence? A prospective, randomized, controlled double-blind crossover study. Urology 1997;49(3):441-444.

Landis E, Shore E. Yohimbine-induced bronchospasm. Chest 1989;96(6):1424.

Montague DK, Barada JH, Belker AM, et al. Clinical guidelines panel on erectile dysfunction: summary report on the treatment of organic erectile dysfunction. The American Urological Association. J Urol 1996;156(6):2007-2011.

Morales A. Yohimbine in erectile dysfunction: the facts. Int J Impot Res 2000;12(Suppl 1): S70-S74.

Oliveto A, Sevarino K, McCance-Katz E, et al. Clonidine and yohimbine in opioid-dependent humans responding under a naloxone novel-response discrimination procedure. Behav Pharmacol 2003;14(2):97-109.

Price LH, Charney DS, Heninger GR. Three cases of manic symptoms following yohimbine administration. Am J Psychiatry 1984;141(10):1267-1268.

Rosen MI, Kosten TR, Kreek MJ. The effects of naltrexone maintenance on the response to yohimbine in healthy volunteers. Biol Psychiatry 1999;45(12):1636-1645.

Sandler B, Aronson P. Yohimbine-induced cutaneous drug eruption, progressive renal failure, and lupus-like syndrome. Urology 1993;41(4):343-345.

Vogt HJ, Brandl P, Kockott G, et al. Double-blind, placebo-controlled safety and efficacy trial with yohimbine hydrochloride in the treatment of nonorganic erectile dysfunction. Int J Impot Res 1997;9(3):155-161.

Zanolari B, Ndjoko K, Ioset JR, et al. Qualitative and quantitative determination of yohimbine in authentic yohimbe bark and in commercial aphrodisiacs by HPLC-UV-API/MS methods. Phytochem Anal 2003;14(4):193-201.

APPENDIX A
INTERACTIONS

HERBS WITH POTENTIAL HYPOGLYCEMIC OR HYPERGLYCEMIC PROPERTIES*

Possible Hypoglycemic Herbs

Based on expert opinion, anecdote, case reports, and/or preliminary trial evidence.

- Aloe vera, American ginseng (*Panax quinquefolius*), bilberry (*Vaccinium myrtillus*), bitter melon (*Momordica charantia*), burdock (*Arctium lappa*), dandelion, devil's claw, fenugreek (*Trigonella foenum-graecum*), fish oil, goldenseal (berberine), gymnema (*Gymnema sylvestre*), horse chestnut (*Aesculus hippocastanum*)/horse chestnut seed extract (HCSE), maitake mushroom (*Grifola frondosa*), marshmallow (*Althea officinalis*), melatonin, milk thistle (*Silybum marianum*), *Panax ginseng*, rosemary (*Rosmarinus officinalis*), Pycnogenol, shark cartilage, Siberian ginseng (*Eleutherococcus senticosus*), stinging nettle (*Urtica dioica*), white horehound (*Marrubium vulgare* L.).

Possible Hyperglycemic Herbs

Based on expert opinion, anecdote, case reports, and/or preliminary trial evidence.

- Arginine (L-arginine), cocoa, DHEA (dehydroepiandrosterone), ephedra (when combined with caffeine), melatonin.

HERBS AND SUPPLEMENTS WITH POTENTIAL HEPATOTOXIC EFFECTS

Use cautiously with other possible hepatotoxic agents, consider monitoring transaminase levels.

- Ackee (*Blighia sapida*), bee pollen, birch oil (*Betula lenta*), blessed thistle (*Cnicus benedictus*)†, borage (*Borago officinalis*), bush tea (*Crotalaria spp*)‡, butterbur (*Petasites hybridus*), chaparral (*Larrea tridentate*), coltsfoot (*Tussilago farfara*), comfrey (*Symphytum* spp.), DHEA, *Echinacea purpurea*, *Echium* spp.‡, germander (*Teucrium chamaedrys*), *Heliotropium* spp., horse chestnut parenteral preparations (*Aesculus hippocastanum*), Jin-bu-huan (*Lycopodium serratum*), kava (*Piper methysticum*), lobelia (*Lobelia inflata*), L-tetrahydropalmatine (THP), mate (*Ileus partaguayensis*)‡, niacin (vitamin B_3), niacinamide, Paraguay tea (*Ilex paraguayensis*), periwinkle (*Catharanthus roseus*), *Plantago lanceolata*†, pride of Madeira (*Echium fastuosum*)‡, rue (*Ruta graveolus*), sassafras (*Sassafras albidum*), scullcap (Scutellaria lateriflora), *Senecio* spp./groundsel (*Senecio jacobea, Senecio spartoides, Senecio vulgaris*)‡, tansy ragwort (*Senecio jacobea*)‡, turmeric (*Curcuma longa*), Tu-san-chi (*Gynura segetum*)‡, uva ursi (*Arctostaphylos uva-ursi* Spreng), valerian (*Valeriana officinalis*), white chameleon (*Atractylis gummifera*).

---

* *Note:* This is not an all-inclusive, comprehensive list of agents that may lower serum glucose. A qualified healthcare practitioner should be consulted with specific questions or concerns regarding potential effects on blood sugar or interactions.

†Contains tannins and may be hepatotoxic in large quantities.

‡Contains pyrrolizidine alkaloids, which may account for hepatotoxicity.

HERBS AND SUPPLEMENTS WITH POSSIBLE HYPOTENSIVE OR HYPERTENSIVE PROPERTIES

Hypotensive Herbs

Based on expert opinion, anecdote, case reports, and/or preliminary trial evidence.

- Aconite/monkshood (*Aconitum columbianum*), alpha-linolenic acid, arnica (*Arnica montana*), baneberry (*Actaea* spp.), betel nut (*Areca catechu*), bilberry (*Vaccinium myrtillus*), black cohosh (*Cimicifuga racemosa*), bryony (*Bryonia alba*), calendula (*Calendula officinalis*), California poppy (*Eschscholtzia californica*), coleus (*Coleus forskohlii*), curcumin, Danshen (*Salvia miltiorrhiza*), eucalyptol, eucalyptus oil (*Eucalyptus globulus*), evening primrose oil (*Oenothera biennis*), fish oils, flaxseed/flaxseed oil (*Linum usitatissimum*), garlic (*Allium sativum*), ginger (*Zingiber officinale* Roscoe), *Ginkgo biloba*, goldenseal (*Hydrastis canadensis*), green hellebore (*Veratrum alba*), hawthorn (*Crataegus oxyacantha*), Indian tobacco (*Lobelia inflata*), jaborandi (*Pilocarpus jaborandi*), maitake mushroom (*Grifola frondosa*), melatonin (N-acetyl-5-methoxytryptamine), mistletoe (*Viscum album*), night blooming cereus (*Cactus grandiflorus*), oleander (*Nerium oleander, Thevetia peruviana*), omega-3 fatty acids, pasque flower (*Anemone pulsatilla*), periwinkle (*Vinca major*), pleurisy root (*Asclepias tuberosa*), *Polypodium vulgare*, shepherd's purse (*Capsella bursa-pastoris*), Texas milkweed (*Asclepias asperula*), turmeric (*Curcuma longa*), wild cherry (*Prunus serotina*).

Hypertensive Herbs

Based on anecdotal or historical reports, pre-clinical data, or human studies.

- American ginseng *(Panax quinquifolium)*, *Arnica (Arnica chamissonis, Arnica cordifolia, Arnica fulgens, Arnica latifolia, Arnica montana, Arnica sororia)*, bayberry *(Myrica cerifera)*, betel nut (*Areca catechu*), blue cohosh *(Caulophyllum thalictroides)*, broom *(Sarothamnus scoparius)*, cayenne *(Capsicum annum)*, cola (*Cola* spp.), coltsfoot (*Tussilago farfara*), ephedra *(Ephedra sinica)*, ginger *(Zingiber officinale* Roscoe), licorice *(Glycyrrhiza glabra)*, yerba mate *(Ilex paraguariensis)*.

HERBS WITH POTENTIAL PROGESTATIONAL OR ESTROGENIC ACTIVITY

Phytoprogestin Herbs

Contain constituents reported to exhibit progestin-like activity in basic science and/or animal studies.

- Chasteberry (*Vitex agnus-castus*), bloodroot (*Sanguinaria canadensis*), damiana (*Turnera* spp), oregano (*Oregano* spp.), yucca (*Yucca* spp.).

Phytoestrogen Herbs

Contain constituents reported to act as estrogen receptor agonists and/or to exhibit estrogenic properties in basic science studies, animal research, or human trials.

- Alfalfa *(Medicago sativa)*, black cohosh *(Cimicifuga racemosa)**, bloodroot *(Sanguinaria canadensis)*, burdock *(Arctium lappa)*, hops (*Humulus lupulus*)[†], Kudzu *(Pueraria lobata)*[‡], licorice *(Glycyrrhiza glabra)*[†], pomegranate *(Punica granatum)*[†], red clover *(Trifolium pratense)*[‡], soy *(Glycine max)*[‡], thyme *(Thymus vulgaris)*, white horehound *(Marrubium vulgare* L.), yucca (*Yucca* spp).

---

*Estrogen and isoflavone constituents.
†Estriol, estrone, estradiol, or estrogen constituents.
‡Isoflavone constituents.

HERBS WITH KNOWN OR POTENTIAL DIURETIC PROPERTIES

Based on expert opinion, anecdote, case reports, and/or preliminary trial evidence.

- Artichoke *(Cynara scolymus)*, celery *(Apium graveolens)*, corn silk *(Zea mays)*, couchgrass *(Agropyron repens)*, dandelion *(Taraxacum officinale)*, elder flower *(Sambucus nigra/Sambucus canadensis)*, horsetail *(Equisetum arvense)*, juniper berry *(Juniperus communis)*, kava *(Piper methysticum)*, shepherd's purse *(Capsella bursa-pastoris)*, uva ursi leaf *(Arctostaphylos uva-ursi)*, yarrow flower *(Achillea millefolium)*.

HERBS WITH POSSIBLE SEDATING PROPERTIES

Based on expert opinion, anecdote, case reports, and/or preliminary trial evidence):

- 5-HTP, ashwagandha root, calamus, calendula, California poppy, capsicum, catnip, celery, couch grass, danshen, dogwood, elecampane, german chamomile, goldenseal, gotu kola (*Centella asiatica*), hops, kava (believed to be hypnotic/anxiolytic without significant sedation), lavender aromatherapy, lemon balm, melatonin, sage, sassafras, scullcap, shepherd's purse, Siberian ginseng, St. John's wort, stinging nettle, valerian, wild carrot, wild lettuce, Withania root, yerba mansa.

HERBS WITH POTENTIAL CARDIAC GLYCOSIDE PROPERTIES*

Based on expert opinion, anecdote, pre-clinical data, and/or preliminary human evidence.

- Adonis (*Adonis vernalis*), *Adonis microcarpa*, balloon cotton (*Asclepias friticosa*), black hellebore root/melampode (*Helleborus niger*), black Indian hemp (*Apocynum cannabinum*), bushman's poison (*Carissa acokanthera*), cactus grandifloris (*Selenicerus grandiflorus*), convallaria (*Convallaria majalis*), eyebright (*Euphrasia* spp.), figwort (Scrophulariaceae), foxglove/digitalis (*Digitalis purpurea*), frangipani (*Plumeria rubra*), hedgemustard (*Sisymbrium officinale*), *Helleborus viridus*, hemp root/Canadian hemp root, king's crown (*Calotropis procera*), lily-of-the-valley, motherwort (*Leonurus cardiaca*), oleander leaf (*Nerium oleander* L.), pheasant's eye plant (*Adonis aestivalis*), plantain leaf (*Plantago lanceolata*), pleurisy root, psyllium husks (*Plantago psyllium*), redheaded cotton-bush (*Asclepias currassavica*), rhubarb root (*Rheum palmatum*), rubber vine (*Cryptostegia grandifolia*), sea-mango (*Cerebra manghas*), senna fruit (*Cassia senna*), squill (*Urginea maritima*), strophanthus (*Strophanthus hispidus*, *Strophanthus kombe*), uzara (*Xysmalobium undulatum*), wallflower (*Cheirantus cheiri*), white horehound (*Marrubium vulgare*), wintersweet (*Carissa spectabilis*), yellow dock root (*Rumex crispus*), yellow oleander (*Thevetia peruviana*).

CYTOCHROME P450: SELECTED SUBSTRATES, INHIBITORS, AND INDUCERS

CYP 450 1A2: Substrates (Affected Herbs and Supplements)

- Melatonin (N-acetyl-5-methoxytryptamine)

---

*This is not an all-inclusive, comprehensive list of herbs that may contain clinically relevant levels of cardiac glycosides. A qualified healthcare practitioner should be consulted for specific questions or concerns regarding potential cardiac effects or interactions of specific agents.

Note: Bufalin/Chan Su (*Secretio bufonis*) is a Chinese herbal purported aphrodisiac that has been reported to be toxic or fatal when taken with cardiac glycosides. Reliable human data are limited.

CYP 450 1A2: Inducing Herbs/Foods

- Cabbage, broccoli, brussels sprouts, cauliflower, charbroiled meats, cigarette smoking.

CYP 450 1A2: Inhibiting Herbs

- Dandelion, chaparral component nordihydroguairetic acid (NDGA) inhibits cytochrome P450–mediated monoxygenase activity in rat hepatic microsomes.

CYP 450 2A6: Inhibiting Herbs

- American pennyroyal (*Hedeoma pulegioides* L.), European pennyroyal (*Mentha pulegium* L.).

CYP 450 2C19: Substrates (Affected Herbs and Supplements)

- Red yeast rice (*Monascus purpureus*): levels of lovastatin present in *Monascus purpureus* may be affected.

CYP 450 2C19: Inhibiting Herbs

- Chaparral component nordihydroguairetic acid (NDGA) inhibits cytochrome P450–mediated monoxygenase activity in rat hepatic microsomes.

CYP 450 2C9: Inhibiting Herbs

- Milk thistle (*Silybum marianum*)/silymarin, St. John's wort (*Hypericum perforatum)*, which is believed to exert more prominent effects on 3A4, has also been found i*n vivo* and *in vitro* to inhibit 2C9 and 2D6. The chaparral component nordihydroguairetic acid (NDGA) inhibits cytochrome P450–mediated monoxygenase activity in rat hepatic microsomes. *In vitro* inhibition of CYP 450 2C9 has also been reported for black tea, cat's claw (*Uncaria tomentosa, Uncaria guianensis*), chamomile (*Matricaria chamomilla*), clove, ginger, gotu kola, kava (weak), oregano (weak), sage, Siberian ginseng, thyme, and turmeric (weak), although interactions have not been demonstrated in humans.

CYP 450 2D6: Inhibiting Herbs

- *SSRI herbs* (in theory; see SSRI section below). St. John's wort, which is believed to exert more prominent effects on 3A4, has also been found i*n vivo* and *in vitro* to inhibit 2C9 and 2D6. The chaparral component nordihydroguairetic acid (NDGA) inhibits cytochrome P450–mediated monoxygenase activity in rat hepatic microsomes. *In vitro* inhibition of CYP 450 2D6 has also been reported for black tea, cat's claw (*Uncaria tomentosa, Uncaria guianensis*), chamomile (*Matricaria chamomilla*), clove, ginger, gotu kola, kava (weak), oregano, sage, thyme, and turmeric (weak), although interactions have not been demonstrated in humans.

CYP 450 2E1: Inhibiting Herbs

- Dandelion, chaparral component nordihydroguairetic acid (NDGA) inhibits cytochrome P450–mediated monoxygenase activity in rat hepatic microsomes.

CYP 450 3A (4,5,7): Substrates (Affected Herbs)

- DHEA, eucalyptol: initial evidence suggests that 1,8-cineole (eucalyptol), a principal constituent of eucalyptus oil, and a constituent of multiple other plants including tea tree oil, has been found in laboratory studies to be a substrate of CYP 450 3A.

CYP 450 3A (4,5,7): Inducing Herbs

- St. John's wort (*Hypericum perforatum*) appears to inhibit CYP 3A4 acutely and then to induce the enzyme with repeated administration. Hops (*Humulus lupuli*) have been demonstrated *in vitro* and *in vivo* to induce P450 3A and 2B. In theory, phytoprogestins (see above section) may induce CYP 3A4, although scientific data are lacking in this area. Examples include chasteberry (*Vitex agnus-castus*), bloodroot (*Sanguinaria canadensis*), oregano (*Oregano* spp.), damiana (*Turnera* spp.), and yucca (*Yucca* spp).

CYP 450 3A (4,5,7): Inhibiting Herbs/Foods

- Cannabinoids, ginseng (*Panax* and Siberian), grapefruit juice, milk thistle (*Silybum marianum*)/silymarin (although milk thistle has been found not to affect indinavir levels), peppermint oil, St. John's wort (*Hypericum perforatum*) appears to inhibit CYP 3A4 acutely and then to induce the enzyme with repeated administration. The chaparral component nordihydroguaiaretic acid (NDGA) inhibits cytochrome P450–mediated monoxygenase activity in rat hepatic microsomes. *In vitro* inhibition of CYP 450 3A4 has also been reported for black tea, cat's claw (*Uncaria tomentosa, Uncaria guianensis*), chamomile (*Matricaria chamomilla*), clove, *Echinacea angustifolia* root, ginger, goldenseal (*Hydrastis canadensis*), gotu kola, kava (weak), licorice (*Glycyrrhiza glabra*), oregano, sage, thyme, turmeric, and wild cherry (*Trifolium pratense*), although interactions have not been demonstrated in humans. No effect on P450 3A4 has been found in a human study of saw palmetto.

SELECTIVE SEROTONIN REUPTAKE INHIBITORS (SSRI): DRUGS, HERBS, VITAMINS, SUPPLEMENTS

Herbs/Supplements with Possible SSRI Effects

Based on preliminary evidence from basic science, human case reports/trials, and/or expert opinion.

- Ephedra, evening primrose oil (*Oenothera biennis*), fenugreek, ginkgo biloba, hops, St. John's wort, tyrosine, valerian, yohimbe.

Vitamins/Minerals with Possible SSRI Effects

Based on preliminary evidence from basic science, human case reports/trials, and/or expert opinion.

- 5-HTP (5-hydroxytryptophan), adrenal extract, chromium, DHEA (dehydroepiandrosterone), DLPA (DL phenylalanine), SAMe (S-adenosylmethionine), vitamin B_6.

Homeopathic Remedies with Possible SSRI Effects

Based on preliminary evidence from basic science, human case reports/trials, and/or expert opinion.

- Aurum metcallicum, Kali bromatum, Sepia.

MONOAMINE OXIDASE INHIBITORS (MAOIs)*

MAOI Drugs†

- Isocarboxazid (Marplan), phenelzine (Nardil), tranylcypromine (Parnate).

Herbs with Possible MAOI Effects

Based on preliminary evidence from basic science, human case reports/trials, and/or expert opinion.

- California poppy (*Eschscholtzia californica*), ephedra, evening primrose oil (*Oenothera biennis*), fenugreek (*Trigonella foenum-graecum*), ginkgo biloba, hops (*Humulus lupulus*), mace (*Myristica fragrans*), St. John's wort (*Hypericum perforatum*), valerian (*Valeriana officinalis*), yohimbe bark extract.

Supplements/Vitamins with Possible MAOI Effects

Based on preliminary evidence from basic science, human case reports/trials, and/or expert opinion.

- 5-HTP (5-hydroxytryptophan), adrenal extract, chromium, DHEA (dehydroepiandrosterone), DLPA (DL phenylalanine), SAMe (S-adenosylmethionine), vitamin B_6.

Homeopathic Remedies with Possible MAOI Effects

Based on preliminary evidence from basic science, human case reports/trials, and/or expert opinion

- Aurum metcallicum, kali bromatum, sepia.

TYRAMINE/TRYPTOPHAN-CONTAINING FOODS

May induce hypertensive crisis when taken concomitantly with MAOIs.

- Anchovies, avocados, bananas, bean curd, beer (alcohol-free/reduced), caffeine (large amounts), caviar, champagne, cheeses—particularly aged, processed, or strong varieties (e.g., camembert, cheddar, stilton)—chocolate, dry sausage/salami/bologna, fava beans, figs, herring (pickled), liver (particularly chicken), meat tenderizers, papaya, protein extracts/powder, raisins, shrimp paste, sour cream, soy sauce, wine (particularly chianti), yeast extracts, yogurt.

---

* *Warning*: Tyramine/tryptophan-containing foods may induce hypertensive crisis when taken concomitantly with MAOIs and should be avoided by individuals taking MAOIs. These include protein foods that have been aged/preserved. Specific examples of foods include anchovies, avocados, bananas, bean curd, beer (alcohol-free/reduced), caffeine (large amounts), caviar, champagne, cheeses—particularly aged, processed, or strong varieties (e.g., camembert, cheddar, stilton)—chocolate, dry sausage/salami/bologna, fava beans, figs, herring (pickled), liver (particularly chicken), meat tenderizers, papaya, protein extracts/powder, raisins, shrimp paste, sour cream, soy sauce, wine (particularly chianti), yeast extracts, yogurt. (Note: This is not a comprehensive, all-inclusive list of foods of concern, and a nutritionist or other qualified healthcare professional should be consulted for questions regarding potential drug-food or herb/supplement-food interactions.)

†Note: In general, patients taking monoamine oxidase inhibitors (MAOIs) should avoid protein foods that have been aged/preserved. This is not a comprehensive, all-inclusive list of foods of concern, and a nutritionist or other qualified healthcare professional should be consulted for questions regarding potential drug-food or herb/supplement-food interactions.

HERBS WITH LAXATIVE/STIMULANT LAXATIVE PROPERTIES*

Based on expert opinion, anecdote, case reports, and/or preliminary trial evidence.

- Alder buckthorn, aloe dried leaf sap (*Aloe* spp.), black root, blue flag rhizome, butternut bark, dong quai, European buckthorn, eyebright herb (*Euphrasia* spp.), cascara bark (*Rhamnus persiana*), castor oil, chasteberry (*Vitex agnus-castus*), colocynth fruit pulp, dandelion, gamboges bark exudates, horsetail (*Equisetum arvense*), jalap root, manna bark exudates, plantain leaf (*Plantago lanceolata*), podophyllum root, psyllium husks (*Plantago psyllium*), rhubarb (*Rheum palmatum*) root, senna (*Cassia senna*) fruit, wild cucumber fruit, yellow dock (*Rumex crispus*) root.

---

* *Note*: This informational page is not an all-inclusive, comprehensive list of laxative herbs. Other herbs and supplements may possess laxative qualities. A qualified healthcare practitioner should be consulted with specific questions or concerns regarding potential laxative effects of agents or interactions.

Appendix B
NATURAL STANDARD CONDITIONS TABLES

These tables are organized by specific health conditions and their related terms. Traditionally, ailments treated with herbs and supplements often are related to other illnesses, and these relationships are useful to consider. Each table is organized by level of evidence, according to the Natural Standard Evidence-Based Validated Grading Scale (see below), with therapies for which there is the best evidence graded higher on the table. Grades reflect the level of available scientific evidence in support of the efficacy of a given therapy for a specific indication. Evidence of harm is considered separately; the grades shown apply only to evidence of benefit. Note that these tables only consider therapies that are discussed in this text, and that there are other herbs and supplements not discussed in this book that are also used for many of these conditions.

Natural Standard Evidence-Based Validated Grading Rationale

Level of Evidence Grade	Criteria
A (Strong scientific evidence)	Statistically significant evidence of benefit from >2 randomized, controlled trials (RCTs), *or* evidence from 1 RCT *and* 1 properly conducted meta-analysis, *or* evidence from multiple RCTs with a clear majority of the trials showing statistically significant evidence of benefit, *and* with supporting evidence in basic science, animal studies, or theory.
B (Good scientific evidence)	Statistically significant evidence of benefit from 1 or 2 RCTs *or* evidence of benefit from >1 properly conducted meta-analysis, *or* evidence of benefit from >1 cohort/case-controlled/non-randomized trial, *and* with supporting evidence in basic science, animal studies, or theory.
C (Unclear or conflicting scientific evidence)	Evidence of benefit from ≥1 small RCT without adequate size, power, statistical significance, or quality of design by objective criteria,* *or* conflicting evidence from multiple RCTs without a clear majority of the properly conducted trials showing evidence of benefit or ineffectiveness, *or* evidence of

Continued

Natural Standard Evidence-Based Validated Grading Rationale—*cont'd*

	benefit from >1 cohort/case-controlled/non-randomized trial, *and* without supporting evidence in basic science, animal studies, or theory, *or* evidence of efficacy only from basic science, animal studies, or theory.
D (Fair negative scientific evidence)	Statistically significant negative evidence (i.e., lack of evidence of benefit) from cohort/case-controlled/non-randomized trials, *and* evidence in basic science, animal studies, or theory suggesting a lack of benefit.
F (Strong negative scientific evidence)	Statistically significant negative evidence (i.e., lack of evidence of benefit) from ≥1 properly randomized adequately powered trial of high-quality design by objective criteria.*
Lack of Evidence (Traditional/theoretical)	Unable to evaluate efficacy due to lack of adequate or available human data.

*Objective criteria are derived from validated instruments for evaluating study quality, including the 5-point scale developed by Jadad et al., in which a score below 4 is considered to indicate lesser quality methodologically (Jadad AR, Moore RA, Carroll D, et al. Assessing the quality of reports of randomized clinical trials: is blinding necessary? *Controlled Clinical Trials* 1996;17[1]:1-12).

ACNE AND RELATED CONDITIONS

Levels of Scientific Evidence for Specific Therapies

GRADE: C (Unclear or Conflicting Scientific Evidence)

Therapy	Specific Therapeutic Use(s)
Guggul (Commifora mukul)	Acne
Tea tree oil (*Melaleuca alternifolia* [Maiden & Betche] Cheel)	Acne vulgaris

TRADITIONAL OR THEORETICAL USES THAT LACK SUFFICIENT EVIDENCE

Therapy	Specific Therapeutic Use(s)
American pennyroyal (*Hedeoma pulegioides* L.), European pennyroyal (*Mentha pulegium* L.)	Acne
Boswellia (Boswellia serrata Roxb.)	Acne

Boswellia (*Boswellia serrata* Roxb.)	Pimples
Burdock (*Arctium lappa*)	Acne
Calendula (*Calendula officinalis* L.), marigold	Acne
Chamomile (*Matricaria recutita, Chamaemelum nobile*)	Acne
Dandelion (*Taraxacum officinale*)	Acne
Danshen (*Salvia miltiorrhiza*)	Acne
Echinacea (*Echinacea angustifolia* DC., *E. pallida, E. purpurea*)	Acne
Flaxseed and flaxseed oil (*Linum usitatissimum*)	Pimples
Goldenseal (*Hydrastis canadensis* L.), berberine	Acne
Hawthorn (*Crataegus laevigata, C. oxyacantha, C. monogyna, C. pentagyna*)	Acne
Lactobacillus acidophilus	Acne
Lavender (*Lavandula angustifolia* Miller)	Acne
Niacin (vitamin B_3, nicotinic acid), niacinamide, and inositol hexanicotinate	Acne
Propolis	Acne
Red clover (*Trifolium pratense*)	Acne
Saw palmetto (*Serenoa repens* [Bartram] Small)	Acne
Sorrel (*Rumex acetosa* L., *R. acetosella* L.), sinupret	Acne
Thyme (*Thymus vulgaris* L.), thymol	Acne
Valerian (*Valeriana officinalis* L.)	Acne

ADDICTION AND RELATED CONDITIONS

Levels of Scientific Evidence for Specific Therapies

GRADE: C (Unclear or Conflicting Scientific Evidence)

Therapy	Specific Therapeutic Use(s)
Globe artichoke (*Cynara scolymus* L.)	Alcohol-induced hangover
Goldenseal (*Hydrastis canadensis* L.), berberine	Narcotic concealment (urinalysis)
Melatonin	Benzodiazepine tapering
Melatonin	Smoking cessation

Continued

TRADITIONAL OR THEORETICAL USES THAT LACK SUFFICIENT EVIDENCE	
Therapy	Specific therapeutic Use(s)
Betel nut (*Areca catechu* L.)	Alcoholism
Black tea (*Camellia sinensis*)	Toxin/alcohol elimination from the body
Burdock (*Arctium lappa*)	Detoxification
Chamomile (*Matricaria recutita, Chamaemelum nobile*)	Delirium tremens (DTs)
Clay	Smoking
Dandelion (*Taraxacum officinale*)	Alcohol withdrawal
Dandelion (*Taraxacum officinale*)	Smoking cessation
Essiac	Detoxification
Evening primrose oil (*Oenothera biennis* L.)	Alcoholism
Evening primrose oil (*Oenothera biennis* L.)	Hangover remedy
Ginger (*Zingiber officinale* Roscoe)	Alcohol withdrawal
Ginkgo (*Ginkgo biloba* L.)	Alcoholism
Green tea (*Camellia sinensis*)	Alcohol intoxication
Green tea (*Camellia sinensis*)	Detoxification from alcohol or toxins
Lavender (*Lavandula angustifolia* Miller)	Hangover
Licorice (*Glycyrrhiza glabra* L.) and Deglycyrrhizinated licorice (DGL)	Detoxification
Melatonin	Withdrawal from narcotics
Niacin (vitamin B_3, nicotinic acid), niacinamide, and inositol hexanicotinate	Alcohol dependence
Niacin (vitamin B_3, nicotinic acid), niacinamide, and inositol hexanicotinate	Smoking cessation
Oleander (*Nerium oleander, Thevetia peruviana*)	Alcoholism
St. John's wort (*Hypericum perforatum* L.)	Alcoholism
St. John's wort (*Hypericum perforatum* L.)	Benzodiazepine withdrawal
Valerian (*Valeriana officinalis* L.)	Hangovers

AIDS/HIV AND RELATED CONDITIONS

Levels of Scientific Evidence for Specific Therapies

GRADE: C (Unclear or Conflicting Scientific Evidence)

Therapy	Specific therapeutic Use(s)
Aloe (*Aloe vera*)	HIV
Antineoplastons	HIV
Bitter melon (*Momordica charantia* L.) and MAP30	HIV
Coenzyme Q10	HIV/AIDS
DHEA (dehydroepiandrosterone)	HIV/AIDS
Flaxseed and flaxseed oil (*Linum usitatissimum*)	HIV/AIDS
Melatonin	HIV/AIDS
Turmeric (*Curcuma longa* L.), curcumin	HIV

GRADE: D (Fair Negative Scientific Evidence)

Therapy	Specific Therapeutic Use(s)
St. John's wort (*Hypericum perforatum* L.)	HIV

TRADITIONAL OR THEORETICAL USES THAT LACK SUFFICIENT EVIDENCE

Therapy	Specific Therapeutic Use(s)
Arginine (L-arginine)	AIDS/HIV
Astragalus (*Astragalus membranaceus*)	AIDS/HIV
Bromelain	AIDS
Burdock (*Arctium lappa*)	HIV
Calendula (*Calendula officinalis* L.), marigold	HIV
Dandelion (*Taraxacum officinale*)	AIDS
Danshen (*Salvia miltiorrhiza*)	HIV
DHEA (dehydroepiandrosterone)	Lipodystrophy in HIV
Echinacea (*Echinacea angustifolia* DC., *E. pallida*, *E. purpurea*)	HIV/AIDS

Continued

Elder (*Sambucus nigra* L.)	HIV
Essiac	AIDS/HIV
Eucalyptus oil (*Eucalyptus globulus* Labillardiere, *E. fructicetorum* F. Von Mueller, *E. smithii* R.T. Baker)	AIDS
Garlic (*Allium sativum* L.)	AIDS
Garlic (*Allium sativum* L.)	HIV
Ginseng (American ginseng, Asian ginseng, Chinese ginseng, Korean red ginseng, *Panax ginseng*: *Panax* spp. including *P. ginseng* C.C. Meyer and *P. quincefolium* L., excluding *Eleutherococcus senticosus*)	HIV
Goldenseal (*Hydrastis canadensis* L.), berberine	AIDS
Green tea (*Camellia sinensis*)	HIV/AIDS
Lactobacillus acidophilus	AIDS
Lavender (*Lavandula angustifolia* Miller)	HIV
Licorice (*Glycyrrhiza glabra* L.) and deglycyrrhizinated licorice (DGL)	HIV
Lycopene	AIDS
Maitake mushroom (*Grifola frondosa*) and beta-glucan	HIV
Niacin (vitamin B_3, nicotinic acid), niacinamide, and inositol hexanicotinate	HIV prevention
Omega-3 fatty acids, fish oil, alpha-linolenic acid	AIDS
Propolis	HIV
Red clover (*Trifolium pratense*)	AIDS
Spirulina	HIV

ALLERGIES AND RELATED CONDITIONS

Levels of Scientific Evidence for Specific Therapies

GRADE: B (Good Scientific Evidence)

Therapy	Specific Therapeutic Use(s)
Bromelain	Sinusitis

GRADE: C (Unclear or Conflicting Scientific Evidence)	
Therapy	Specific Therapeutic Use(s)
Elder (*Sambucus nigra* L.)	Bacterial sinusitis
Ephedra (Ephedra sinica) ma huang	Allergic rhinitis
Eucalyptus oil (*Eucalyptus globulus* Labillardiere, *E. fructicetorum* F. Von Mueller, *E. smithii* R.T. Baker)	Decongestant/expectorant
Sorrel (Rumex acetosa L., R. acetosella L.), Sinupret	Sinusitis

TRADITIONAL OR THEORETICAL USES THAT LACK SUFFICIENT EVIDENCE	
Therapy	Specific Therapeutic Use(s)
Alfalfa (*Medicago sativa* L.)	Allergies
Alfalfa (*Medicago sativa* L.)	Hay fever
Astragalus (*Astragalus membranaceus*)	Allergies
Belladonna (*Atropa belladonna* L. or its variety *acuminata* Royle ex Lindl)	Hay fever
Bromelain	Allergic rhinitis (hay fever)
Bromelain	Food allergies
Burdock (*Arctium lappa*)	Hives
Chamomile (*Matricaria recutita, Chamaemelum nobile*)	Hay fever
Chamomile (*Matricaria recutita, Chamaemelum nobile*)	Hives
Chamomile (*Matricaria recutita, Chamaemelum nobile*)	Sinusitis
Chaparral (*Larrea tridentata* DC. Coville, *L. divaricata* Cav.), nordihydroguaiaretic acid (NDGA)	Allergies
Clove (*Eugenia aromatica*)	Antihistamine
Dandelion (*Taraxacum officinale*)	Allergies
Devil's claw (*Harpagophytum procumbens* DC.)	Allergies
DHEA (dehydroepiandrosterone)	Allergic disorders
DHEA (dehydroepiandrosterone)	Angioedema

Continued

Dong quai (*Angelica sinensis* [Oliv.] Diels), Chinese angelica	Allergy
Dong quai (*Angelica sinensis* [Oliv.] Diels), Chinese angelica	Chronic rhinitis
Dong quai (*Angelica sinensis* [Oliv.] Diels), Chinese angelica	Hay fever
Echinacea (*Echinacea angustifolia* DC., *E. pallida*, *E. purpurea*)	Catarrh
Elder (*Sambucus nigra* L.)	Hay fever
Ephedra (*Ephedra sinica*)/ma huang	Acute coryza (rhinitis)
Ephedra (*Ephedra sinica*)/ma huang	Decongestant
Ephedra (*Ephedra sinica*)/ma huang	Hay fever
Ephedra (*Ephedra* sinica)/ma huang	Urticaria
Eucalyptus oil (*Eucalyptus globulus* Labillardiere, *E. fructicetorum* F. Von Mueller, *E. smithii* R.T. Baker)	Runny nose
Eucalyptus oil (*Eucalyptus globulus* Labillardiere, *E. fructicetorum* F. Von Mueller, *E. smithii* R.T. Baker)	Sinusitis
Eyebright (*Euphrasia officinalis*)	Allergies
Eyebright (*Euphrasia officinalis*)	Hay fever
Eyebright (*Euphrasia officinalis*)	Rhinitis
Eyebright (*Euphrasia officinalis*)	Sinusitis
Flaxseed and flaxseed oil (*Linum usitatissimum*)	Allergic reactions
Garlic (*Allium sativum* L.)	Allergies
Ginkgo (*Ginkgo biloba* L.)	Allergies
Ginkgo (*Ginkgo biloba* L.)	Chronic rhinitis
Ginseng (American ginseng, Asian ginseng, Chinese ginseng, Korean red ginseng, *Panax ginseng*: *Panax* spp. including *P. ginseng* C.C. *Meyer and P. quincefolium* L., excluding *Eleutherococcus senticosus*)	Allergies
Globe artichoke (*Cynara scolymus* L.)	Allergies
Goldenseal (*Hydrastis canadensis* L.), berberine	Antihistamine
Goldenseal (*Hydrastis canadensis* L.), berberine	Sinusitis

Guggul (*Commifora mukul*)	Rhinitis
Lactobacillus acidophilus	Allergies
Lactobacillus acidophilus	Hives
Oleander (*Nerium oleander*, *Thevetia peruviana*)	Sinus problems
Omega-3 fatty acids, fish oil, alpha-linolenic acid	Allergies
Omega-3 fatty acids, fish oil, alpha-linolenic acid	Hay fever
Saw palmetto (*Serenoa repens* [Bartram] Small)	Catarrh
Shark cartilage	Allergic skin rashes
Sorrel (*Rumex acetosa* L., *R. acetosella* L.), Sinupret	Sinusitis
Spirulina	Anaphylaxis (severe allergic reaction) prevention
Thyme (*Thymus vulgaris* L.), thymol	Sinusitis

ALOPECIA AND RELATED CONDITIONS

Levels of Scientific Evidence for Specific Therapies

GRADE: C (Unclear or Conflicting Scientific Evidence)

Therapy	Specific Therapeutic Use(s)
Saw palmetto (*Serenoa repens* [Bartram] Small)	Androgenetic alopecia (topical)
Thyme (Thymus vulgaris L.), thymol	Alopecia areata

TRADITIONAL OR THEORETICAL USES THAT LACK SUFFICIENT EVIDENCE

Therapy	Specific Therapeutic Use(s)
Aloe (*Aloe vera*)	Alopecia (hair loss)
Bladderwrack (*Fucus vesiculosus*)	Hair loss
Burdock (*Arctium lappa*)	Dandruff
Burdock (*Arctium lappa*)	Hair loss
Chaparral (*Larrea tridentata* DC. Coville, *L. divaricata* Cav.), nordihydroguaiaretic acid (NDGA)	Hair tonic
Coenzyme Q10	Hair loss from chemotherapy
Dandelion (*Taraxacum officinale*)	Dandruff

Continued

Elder (*Sambucus nigra* L.)	Hair dye
Fenugreek (*Trigonella foenum-graecum* L.)	Baldness
Garlic (*Allium sativum* L.)	Hair growth
Ginger (*Zingiber officinale* Roscoe)	Baldness
Goldenseal (*Hydrastis canadensis* L.), berberine	Dandruff
Gotu kola (*Centella asiatica* L.), total triterpenic fraction of *Centella asiatica* (TTFCA)	Hair growth promoter
Horsetail (*Equisetum arvense* L.)	Hair loss
Lavender (*Lavandula angustifolia* Miller)	Hair loss
Pygeum (*Prunus africana, Pygeum africanum*)	Male baldness
Seaweed, kelp, bladderwrack (*Fucus vesiculosus*)	Hair loss
Spirulina	Hair loss

ALZHEIMER'S DISEASE AND RELATED CONDITIONS

Levels of Scientific Evidence for Specific Therapies

GRADE: B (Good Scientific Evidence)

Therapy	Specific Therapeutic Use(s)
Ginkgo (*Ginkgo biloba* L.)	Cerebral insufficiency
Ginseng (American ginseng, Asian ginseng, Chinese ginseng, Korean red ginseng, *Panax ginseng*: *Panax* spp. including *P. ginseng* C.C. Meyer and *P. quincefolium* L., excluding *Eleutherococcus senticosus*)	Mental performance

GRADE: C (Unclear or Conflicting Scientific Evidence)

Therapy	Specific Therapeutic Use(s)
Black tea (*Camellia sinensis*)	Memory enhancement
Black tea (*Camellia sinensis*)	Mental performance/alertness
Boron	Improving cognitive function
Ginkgo (*Ginkgo biloba* L.)	Age-associated memory impairment (AAMI)
Ginkgo (*Ginkgo biloba* L.)	Memory enhancement (in healthy people)

Green tea (*Camellia sinensis*)	Memory enhancement
Green tea (*Camellia sinensis*)	Mental performance/alertness
Polypodium leucotomos extract, Anapsos	Dementia

GRADE: D (Fair Negative Scientific Evidence)

Therapy	Specific Therapeutic Use(s)
DHEA (dehydroepiandrosterone)	Brain function and well-being in the elderly

TRADITIONAL OR THEORETICAL USES THAT LACK SUFFICIENT EVIDENCE

Therapy	Specific Therapeutic Use(s)
Arginine (L-arginine)	Dementia
Astragalus (*Astragalus membranaceus*)	Dementia
Astragalus (*Astragalus membranaceus*)	Memory
Blessed thistle (*Cnicus benedictus* L.)	Memory improvement
Danshen (*Salvia miltiorrhiza*)	Anoxic brain injury
DHEA (dehydroepiandrosterone)	Dementia
Eyebright (*Euphrasia officinalis*)	Memory loss
Garlic (*Allium sativum* L.)	Age-related memory problems
Ginseng (American ginseng, Asian ginseng, Chinese ginseng, Korean red ginseng, *Panax ginseng*: *Panax* spp. including *P. ginseng* C.C. Meyer and *P. quincefolium* L., excluding *Eleutherococcus senticosus*)	Dementia
Ginseng (American ginseng, Asian ginseng, Chinese ginseng, Korean red ginseng, *Panax ginseng*: *Panax* spp. including *P. ginseng* C.C. Meyer and *P. quincefolium L.*, excluding *Eleutherococcus senticosus*)	Improved memory and thinking after menopause
Ginseng (American ginseng, Asian ginseng, Chinese ginseng, Korean red ginseng, *Panax ginseng*: *Panax* spp. including *P. ginseng* C.C. Meyer and *P. quincefolium* L., excluding *Eleutherococcus senticosus*)	Senile dementia
Gotu kola (*Centella asiatica* L.), total triterpenic fraction of *Centella asiatica* (TTFCA)	Memory enhancement
Green tea (*Camellia sinensis*)	Cognitive performance enhancement
Kava (*Piper methysticum* G. Forst)	Brain damage

Continued

Lycopene	Cognitive function
Melatonin	Cognitive enhancement
Melatonin	Memory enhancement
Niacin (vitamin B_3, nicotinic acid), niacinamide, and inositol hexanicotinate	Memory loss
Omega-3 fatty acids, fish oil, alpha-linolenic acid	Memory enhancement
Soy (*Glycine max* L. Merr.)	Cognitive function
Soy (*Glycine max* L. Merr.)	Memory enhancement
Spirulina	Memory improvement
Valerian (*Valeriana officinalis* L.)	Memory
Yohimbe bark extract (*Pausinystalia yohimbe* Pierre ex Beille)	Cognition

ANEMIA AND RELATED CONDITIONS

Levels of Scientific Evidence for Specific Therapies

GRADE: C (Unclear or Conflicting Scientific Evidence)

Therapy	Specific Therapeutic Use(s)
Antineoplastons	Sickle cell anemia/thalassemia
Betel nut (*Areca catechu* L.)	Anemia

TRADITIONAL OR THEORETICAL USES THAT LACK SUFFICIENT EVIDENCE

Therapy	Specific Therapeutic Use(s)
Arginine (L-arginine)	Beta-hemoglobinopathies
Arginine (L-arginine)	Sickle cell anemia
Astragalus (*Astragalus membranaceus*)	Anemia
Calendula (*Calendula officinalis* L.), marigold	Anemia
Dandelion (*Taraxacum officinale*)	Anemia
Dong quai (*Angelica sinensis* [Oliv.] Diels), Chinese angelica	Anemia

Dong quai (*Angelica sinensis* [Oliv.] Diels), Chinese angelica	Hemolytic disease of the newborn
Feverfew (*Tanacetum parthenium* L. Schultz-Bip.)	Anemia
Ginseng (American ginseng, Asian ginseng, Chinese ginseng, Korean red ginseng, *Panax ginseng*: Pa*n*ax spp. including *P. ginseng* C.C. Meyer and *P. quincefolium* L., excluding Eleutherococcus senticosus)	Anemia
Globe artichoke (*Cynara scolymus* L.)	Anemia
Gotu kola (*Centella asiatica* L.), total triterpenic fraction of *Centella asiatica* (TTFCA)	Anemia
Sorrel (*Rumex acetosa* L., *R. acetosella* L.), Sinupret	Anemia
Soy (*Glycine max* L. Merr.)	Anemia
Spirulina	Anemia

ANTI-AGING AND RELATED CONDITIONS

Levels of Scientific Evidence for Specific Therapies

TRADITIONAL OR THEORETICAL USES THAT LACK SUFFICIENT EVIDENCE

Therapy	Specific Therapeutic Use(s)
Antineoplastons	Aging
Arginine (L-arginine)	Anti-aging
Astragalus (*Astragalus membranaceus*)	Aging
DHEA (dehydroepiandrosterone)	Aging
Dong quai (*Angelica sinensis* [Oliv.] Diels), Chinese angelica	Anti-aging
Ginkgo (*Ginkgo biloba* L.)	Aging
Ginseng (American ginseng, Asian ginseng, Chinese ginseng, Korean red ginseng, *Panax ginseng*: *Panax* spp. including *P. ginseng* C.C. Meyer and *P. quincefolium* L., excluding *Eleutherococcus senticosus*)	Aging
Melatonin	Aging
Niacin (Vitamin B_3, nicotinic acid), niacinamide, and inositol hexanicotinate	Anti-aging

Continued

ANTICOAGULATION AND RELATED CONDITIONS

Levels of Scientific Evidence for Specific Therapies

GRADE: C (Unclear or Conflicting Scientific Evidence)

Therapy	Specific Therapeutic Use(s)
Bladderwrack (*Fucus vesiculosus*)	Anticoagulant (blood thinner)
Garlic (*Allium sativum* L.)	Antiplatelet effects (blood thinning)
Seaweed, kelp, bladderwrack (*Fucus vesiculosus*)	Anticoagulant
Yohimbe bark extract (*Pausinystalia yohimbe* Pierre ex Beille)	Inhibition of platelet aggregation

TRADITIONAL OR THEORETICAL USES THAT LACK SUFFICIENT EVIDENCE

Therapy	Specific therapeutic Use(s)
Alfalfa (*Medicago sativa* L.)	Blood clotting disorders
Astragalus (*Astragalus membranaceus*)	Blood thinner
Barley (*Hordeum vulgare* L.), germinated barley foodstuff (GBF)	Blood circulation
Bromelain	Blood clot treatment
Bromelain	Platelet inhibition (blood thinner)
Calendula (*Calendula officinalis* L.), marigold	Blood vessel clots
Clove (*Eugenia aromatica*)	Blood thinner (antiplatelet agent)
Danshen (*Salvia miltiorrhiza*)	Blood clotting disorders
Danshen (*Salvia miltiorrhiza*)	Hypercoagulability
Dong quai (*Angelica sinensis* [Oliv.] Diels), Chinese angelica	Blood clots
Dong quai (*Angelica sinensis* [Oliv.] Diels), Chinese angelica	Blood flow disorders
Dong quai (*Angelica sinensis* [Oliv.] Diels), Chinese angelica	Blood stagnation
Dong quai (*Angelica sinensis* [Oliv.] Diels), Chinese angelica	Blood vessel disorders
Elder (*Sambucus nigra* L.)	Blood vessel disorders

Flaxseed and flaxseed oil (*Linum usitatissimum*)	Blood thinner
Ginger (*Zingiber officinale* Roscoe)	Blood thinner
Ginkgo (*Ginkgo biloba* L.)	Blood clots
Ginkgo (*Ginkgo biloba* L.)	Blood vessel disorders
Goldenseal (*Hydrastis canadensis* L.), berberine	Anticoagulant (blood thinner)
Goldenseal (*Hydrastis canadensis* L.), berberine	Blood circulation stimulant
Green tea (*Camellia sinensis*)	Inhibition of platelet aggregation
Horse chestnut (*Aesculus hippocastanum* L.)	Lung blood clots (pulmonary embolism)
Niacin (vitamin B_3, nicotinic acid), niacinamide, and inositol hexanicotinate	Blood circulation improvement
Omega-3 fatty acids, fish oil, alpha-linolenic acid	Anticoagulation
Propolis	Anticoagulant
Red yeast rice (*Monascus purpureus*)	Blood circulation problems

ANTIDEPRESSANT AND RELATED CONDITIONS

Levels of scientific evidence for specific therapies

GRADE: A (Strong Scientific Evidence)

Therapy	Specific Therapeutic Use(s)
St. John's wort (*Hypericum perforatum* L.)	Depressive disorder (mild to moderate)

GRADE: C (UNCLEAR OR CONFLICTING SCIENTIFIC EVIDENCE)

Therapy	Specific Therapeutic Use(s)
DHEA (dehydroepiandrosterone)	Depression
Evening primrose Oil (*Oenothera biennis* L.) syndrome	Postviral/chronic fatigue
Ginkgo (*Ginkgo biloba* L.) affective disorder (SAD)	Depression and seasonal
Melatonin disturbances)	Bipolar disorder (sleep
Melatonin	Depression (sleep disturbances)

Continued

Melatonin	Seasonal affective disorder (SAD)
Omega-3 fatty acids, fish oil, alpha-linolenic acid	Bipolar disorder
Omega-3 fatty acids, fish oil, alpha-linolenic acid	Depression
St. John's wort (*Hypericum perforatum* L.)	Depressive disorder (severe)
St. John's wort (*Hypericum perforatum* L.)	Seasonal affective disorder (SAD)

TRADITIONAL OR THEORETICAL USES THAT LACK SUFFICIENT EVIDENCE

Therapy	Specific Therapeutic Use(s)
Black cohosh (*Cimicifuga racemosa* L. Nutt.)	Depression
Dong quai (*Angelica sinensis* [Oliv.] Diels), Chinese angelica	Anti-aging
Ginkgo (*Ginkgo biloba* L.)	Aging
Ginseng (American ginseng, Asian ginseng, Chinese ginseng, Korean red ginseng, *Panax ginseng*: *Panax* spp. including *P. ginseng* C.C. Meyer and *P. quincefolium* L., excluding *Eleutherococcus senticosus*)	Aging
Melatonin	Aging
Niacin (vitamin B_3, nicotinic acid), niacinamide, and inositol hexanicotinate	Anti-aging
Ginseng (American ginseng, Asian ginseng, Chinese ginseng, Korean red ginseng, *Panax ginseng*: *Panax* spp. *including P. ginseng* C.C. Meyer and *P. quincefolium* L., excluding *Eleutherococcus senticosus*)	Antidepressant
Gotu kola (*Centella asiatica* L.), total triterpenic fraction of *Centella asiatica* (TTFCA)	Antidepressant
Gotu kola (*Centella asiatica* L), total triterpenic fraction of *Centella asiatica* (TTFCA)	Mood disorders
Hops (*Humulus lupulus* L.)	Antidepressant
Hops (*Humulus lupulus* L.)	Mood disturbances
Kava (*Piper methysticum* G. Forst)	Depression
Lavender (*Lavandula angustifolia* Miller)	Depression
Licorice (*Glycyrrhiza glabra* L.) and deglycyrrhizinated licorice (DGL)	Depression
Melatonin	Depression

Milk thistle (*Silybum marianum*), silymarin	Depression
Niacin (vitamin B_3, nicotinic acid), niacinamide, and inositol hexanicotinate	Depression
Spirulina	Depression
Spirulina	Mood stimulant
Thyme (*Thymus vulgaris* L.), thymol	Depression
Valerian (*Valeriana officinalis* L.)	Mood enhancement
Yohimbe bark extract (*Pausinystalia yohimbe* Pierre ex Beille)	Depression
Yohimbe bark extract (*Pausinystalia yohimbe* Pierre ex Beille)	Depression

ANTI-INFLAMMATORY AND RELATED CONDITIONS

Levels of Scientific Evidence for Specific Therapies

GRADE: B (Good Scientific Evidence)

Therapy	Specific Therapeutic Use(s)
Bromelain	Inflammation

GRADE: C (Unclear or Conflicting Scientific Evidence)

Therapy	Specific Therapeutic Use(s)
Arginine (L-arginine)	Dental pain (ibuprofen arginate)
Black cohosh (*Cimicifuga racemosa* L. Nutt.)	Arthritis pain (rheumatoid arthritis, osteoarthritis)
Dandelion (*Taraxacum officinale*)	Anti-inflammatory
Eyebright (*Euphrasia officinalis*)	Anti-inflammatory
Propolis	Dental pain
Shark cartilage	Analgesia
Turmeric (*Curcuma longa* L.), curcumin	Inflammation
White horehound (*Marrubium vulgare*)	Pain

Continued

TRADITIONAL OR THEORETICAL USES THAT LACK SUFFICIENT EVIDENCE	
Therapy	Specific Therapeutic Use(s)
Alfalfa (*Medicago sativa* L.)	Inflammation
Arginine (L-arginine)	Pain
Astragalus (*Astragalus membranaceus*)	Myalgia (muscle pain)
Belladonna (*Atropa belladonna* L. or its variety *acuminata* Royle ex Lindl)	Anesthetic
Belladonna (*Atropa belladonna* L. or its variety *acuminata* Royle ex Lindl)	Inflammation
Belladonna (*Atropa belladonna* L. or its variety *acuminata* Royle ex Lindl)	Muscle and joint pain
Bitter almond (*Prunus amygdalus* Batch var. *amara* DC. Focke), Laetrile	Anti-inflammatory
Bitter Almond (*Prunus amygdalus* Batch var. *amara* DC. Focke), Laetrile	Local anesthetic
Bitter Almond (*Prunus amygdalus* Batch var. *amara* DC. Focke), Laetrile	Pain suppressant
Black cohosh (*Cimicifuga racemosa* L. Nutt.)	Inflammation
Black cohosh (*Cimicifuga racemosa* L. Nutt.)	Muscle pain
Black tea (*Camellia sinensis*)	Pain
Blessed thistle (*Cnicus benedictus* L.)	Inflammation
Bromelain	Pain
Bromelain	Pain (general)
Burdock (*Arctium lappa*)	Inflammation
Calendula (*Calendula officinalis* L.), marigold	Pain
Chamomile (*Matricaria recutita, Chamaemelum nobile*)	Anti-inflammatory
Chaparral (*Larrea tridentata* DC. Coville, *L. divaricata* Cav.), nordihydroguaiaretic acid (NDGA)	Anti-inflammatory
Chaparral (*Larrea tridentata* DC. Coville, *L. divaricata* Cav.), nordihydroguaiaretic acid (NDGA)	Pain
Clove (*Eugenia aromatica*)	Pain
Dandelion (*Taraxacum officinale*)	Analgesia
Devil's claw (*Harpagophytum procumbens* DC.)	Anti-inflammatory

Devil's claw (*Harpagophytum procumbens* DC.)	Muscle pain
Devil's claw (*Harpagophytum procumbens* DC.)	Pain
Dong quai (*Angelica sinensis* [Oliv.] Diels), Chinese angelica	Pain
Dong quai (*Angelica sinensis* [Oliv.] Diels), Chinese angelica	Pain from bruises
Echinacea (*Echinacea angustifolia* DC., *E. pallida*, *E. purpurea*)	Pain
Elder (*Sambucus nigra* L.)	Anti-inflammatory
Ephedra (*Ephedra sinica*)/ma huang	Anti-inflammatory
Eucalyptus oil (*Eucalyptus globulus* Labillardiere, *E. fructicetorum* F. Von Mueller, *E. smithii* R.T. Baker)	Inflammation
Eucalyptus oil (*Eucalyptus globulus* Labillardiere, *E. fructicetorum* F. Von Mueller, E. smithii R.T. Baker)	Muscle/joint pain (applied to the skin)
Evening primrose oil (*Oenothera biennis* L.)	Pain
Fenugreek (*Trigonella foenum-graecum* L. Leguminosae)	Inflammation
Feverfew (*Tanacetum parthenium* L. Schultz-Bip.)	Anti-inflammatory
Garlic (*Allium sativum* L.)	Dental pain
Ginger (*Zingiber officinale* Roscoe)	Pain relief
Ginseng (American ginseng, Asian ginseng, Chinese ginseng, Korean red ginseng, *Panax ginseng*: *Panax* spp. including *P. ginseng* C.C. Meyer and *P. quincefolium* L., excluding *Eleutherococcus senticosus*)	Inflammation
Ginseng (American ginseng, Asian ginseng, Chinese ginseng, Korean red ginseng, *Panax ginseng*: *Panax* spp. including *P. ginseng* C.C. Meyer and *P. quincefolium* L., excluding *Eleutherococcus senticosus*)	Pain relief
Goldenseal (*Hydrastis canadensis* L.), berberine	Anesthetic
Goldenseal (*Hydrastis canadensis* L.), berberine	Anti-inflammatory
Goldenseal (*Hydrastis canadensis* L.), berberine	Muscle pain
Goldenseal (*Hydrastis canadensis* L.), berberine	Pain
Gotu kola (*Centella asiatica* L), total triterpenic fraction of *Centella asiatica* (TTFCA)	Inflammation
Gotu kola (*Centella asiatica* L), total triterpenic fraction of *Centella asiatica* (TTFCA)	Pain
Guggul (*Commifora mukul*)	Pain

Continued

Hops (*Humulus lupulus* L.)	Anti-inflammatory
Hops (*Humulus lupulus* L.)	Pain
Kava (*Piper methysticum* G. Forst)	Anesthesia
Kava (*Piper methysticum* G. Forst)	Pain
Lavender (*Lavandula angustifolia* Miller)	Anti-inflammatory
Lavender (*Lavandula angustifolia* Miller)	Pain
Licorice (*Glycyrrhiza glabra* L.), deglycyrrhizinated licorice (DGL)	Inflammation
Marshmallow (*Althaea officinalis* L.)	Inflammation
Marshmallow (*Althaea officinalis* L.)	Muscular pain
Oleander (*Nerium oleander, Thevetia peruviana*)	Inflammation
Passionflower (*Passiflora incarnata* L.)	Chronic pain
Passionflower (*Passiflora incarnata* L.)	Pain (general)
Peppermint (*Mentha x piperita* L.)	Local anesthetic
Peppermint (*Mentha x piperita* L.)	Musculoskeletal pain
Peppermint (*Mentha x piperita* L.)	Myalgia (muscle pain)
Polypodium leucotomos extract, Anapsos	Inflammation
Pygeum (*Prunus africana, Pygeum africanum*)	Inflammation
Saw palmetto (*Serenoa repens* [Bartram] Small)	Anti-inflammatory
Slippery elm (*Ulmus rubra* Muhl., *U. fulva* Michx.)	Inflammation
Spirulina	Anti-inflammatory
St. John's wort (*Hypericum perforatum* L.)	Anti-inflammatory
St. John's wort (*Hypericum perforatum* L.)	Dental pain
St. John's wort (*Hypericum perforatum* L.)	Pain relief
Tea tree oil (*Melaleuca alternifolia* [Maiden & Betche] Cheel)	Anti-inflammatory
Tea tree oil (*Melaleuca alternifolia* [Maiden & Betche] Cheel)	Muscle and joint pain
Turmeric (*Curcuma longa* L.), curcumin	Pain
Valerian (*Valeriana officinalis* L.)	Anodyne (pain relief)

Valerian (*Valeriana officinalis* L.)	Muscle pain
Valerian (*Valeriana officinalis* L.)	Pain
White horehound (*Marrubium vulgare*)	Pain
Wild yam (*Dioscorea villosa*)	Anti-inflammatory

ANTIOXIDANT AND RELATED CONDITIONS

Levels of Scientific Evidence for Specific Therapies

GRADE: C (Unclear or Conflicting Scientific Evidence)

Therapy	Specific Therapeutic Use(s)
Bladderwrack (*Fucus vesiculosus*)	Antioxidant
Cranberry (*Vaccinium macrocarpon*)	Antioxidant
Dandelion (*Taraxacum officinale*)	Antioxidant
Globe artichoke (*Cynara scolymus* L.)	Antioxidant
Lycopene	Antioxidant
Melatonin	Antioxidant (free radical scavenging)
Seaweed, kelp, bladderwrack (*Fucus vesiculosus*)	Antioxidant

TRADITIONAL OR THEORETICAL USES THAT LACK SUFFICIENT EVIDENCE

Therapy	Specific Therapeutic Use(s)
Astragalus (*Astragalus membranaceus*)	Antioxidant
Black tea (*Camellia sinensis*)	Antioxidant
Coenzyme Q10	Antioxidant
Dandelion (*Taraxacum officinale*)	Antioxidant
Danshen (*Salvia miltiorrhiza*)	Antioxidant
Devil's claw (*Harpagophytum procumbens* DC.)	Antioxidant
Elder (*Sambucus nigra* L.)	Antioxidant
Garlic (*Allium sativum* L.)	Antioxidant
Ginger (*Zingiber officinale* Roscoe)	Antioxidant

Continued

Ginkgo (*Ginkgo biloba* L.)	Antioxidant
Green tea (*Camellia sinensis*)	Antioxidant
Horsetail (*Equisetum arvense* L.)	Antioxidant
Lavender (*Lavandula angustifolia* Miller)	Antioxidant
Licorice (*Glycyrrhiza glabra* L.), deglycyrrhizinated licorice (DGL)	Antioxidant
Propolis	Antioxidant
Red clover (*Trifolium pratense*)	Antioxidant
Spirulina	Antioxidant

ANTIPSYCHOTIC AND RELATED CONDITIONS

Levels of Scientific Evidence for Specific Therapies

GRADE: C (Unclear or Conflicting Scientific Evidence)

Therapy	Specific Therapeutic Use(s)
Betel nut (*Areca catechu* L.)	Schizophrenia
DHEA (dehydroepiandrosterone)	Schizophrenia
Melatonin	Schizophrenia (sleep disorders)
Omega-3 fatty acids, fish oil, alpha-linolenic acid	Schizophrenia

GRADE: D (Fair Negative Scientific Evidence)

Therapy	Specific Therapeutic Use(s)
Evening primrose oil (*Oenothera biennis* L.)	Schizophrenia

TRADITIONAL OR THEORETICAL USES THAT LACK SUFFICIENT EVIDENCE

Therapy	Specific Therapeutic Use(s)
American pennyroyal (*Hedeoma pulegioides* L.), European pennyroyal (*Mentha pulegium* L.)	Hallucinations
Chaparral (*Larrea tridentata* DC. Coville, *L. divaricata* Cav.), nordihydroguaiaretic acid (NDGA)	Hallucinations (including those due to LSD ingestion)
Coenzyme Q10	Psychiatric disorders
Ginkgo (*Ginkgo biloba* L.)	Schizophrenia

Ginseng (American ginseng, Asian ginseng, Chinese ginseng, Korean red ginseng, *Panax ginseng*: *Panax* spp. including *P. ginseng* C.C. Meyer and *P. quincefolium* L., excluding *Eleutherococcus senticosus*)	Psycho-asthenia
Gotu kola (*Centella asiatica* L), total triterpenic fraction of *Centella asiatica* (TTFCA)	Mental disorders
Kava (*Piper methysticum* G. Forst)	Antipsychotic
Lavender (*Lavandula angustifolia* Miller)	Psychosis
Niacin (vitamin B_3, nicotinic acid), niacinamide, and inositol hexanicotinate schizophrenia	Diagnostic test for
Niacin (vitamin B_3, nicotinic acid), niacinamide, and inositol hexanicotinate	Drug-induced hallucinations
Niacin (vitamin B_3, nicotinic acid), niacinamide, and inositol hexanicotinate	Psychosis
Niacin (vitamin B_3, nicotinic acid), niacinamide, and inositol hexanicotinate	Schizophrenia
Oleander (*Nerium oleander, Thevetia peruviana*)	Psychiatric disorders
Pygeum (*Prunus africana, Pygeum africanum*)	Psychosis
Yohimbe bark extract (*Pausinystalia yohimbe* Pierre ex Beille)	Hallucinogenic
Yohimbe bark extract (*Pausinystalia yohimbe* Pierre ex Beille)	Schizophrenia
Yohimbe bark extract (*Pausinystalia yohimbe* Pierre ex Beille)	Hallucinogenic

ANXIETY/STRESS AND RELATED CONDITIONS

Levels of Scientific Evidence for Specific Therapies

GRADE: A (Strong Scientific Evidence)

Therapy	Specific Therapeutic Use(s)
Kava (*Piper methysticum* G. Forst)	Anxiety

GRADE: B (Good Scientific Evidence)

Therapy	Specific Therapeutic Use(s)
Lavender (*Lavandula angustifolia* Miller)	Anxiety (lavender aromatherapy)

Continued

GRADE: C (Unclear or Conflicting Scientific Evidence)	
Therapy	**Specific Therapeutic Use(s)**
Gotu kola (*Centella asiatica* L), total triterpenic fraction of *Centella asiatica* (TTFCA)	Anxiety
St. John's wort (*Hypericum perforatum* L.)	Anxiety disorder
Valerian (*Valeriana officinalis* L.)	Anxiety

TRADITIONAL OR THEORETICAL USES THAT LACK SUFFICIENT EVIDENCE	
Therapy	**Specific Therapeutic Use(s)**
American pennyroyal (*Hedeoma pulegioides* L.), European pennyroyal (*Mentha pulegium* L.)	Anxiolytic
Belladonna (*Atropa belladonna* L. or its variety *acuminata* Royle ex Lindl)	Anxiety
Black cohosh (*Cimicifuga racemosa* L. Nutt.)	Anxiety
Black tea (*Camellia sinensis*)	Anxiety
Calendula (*Calendula officinalis* L.), marigold	Anxiety
Chamomile (*Matricaria recutita, Chamaemelum nobile*)	Anxiety
Danshen (*Salvia miltiorrhiza*)	Anxiety
DHEA (dehydroepiandrosterone)	Anxiety
DHEA (dehydroepiandrosterone)	Stress
Dong quai (*Angelica sinensis* [Oliv.] Diels), Chinese angelica	Anxiety
Dong quai (*Angelica sinensis* [Oliv.] Diels), Chinese angelica	Stress
Elder (*Sambucus nigra L.*)	Stress reduction
Eucalyptus oil (*Eucalyptus globulus* Labillardiere, *E. fructicetorum* F. Von Mueller, *E. smithii* R.T. Baker)	Aromatherapy
Garlic (*Allium sativum* L.)	Stress (anxiety)
Ginkgo (*Ginkgo biloba* L.)	Anxiety
Ginseng (American ginseng, Asian ginseng, Chinese ginseng, Korean red ginseng, *Panax ginseng*: *Panax* spp. including *P. ginseng* C.C. Meyer and *P. quincefolium* L., excluding *Eleutherococcus senticosus*)	Aggression

Ginseng (American ginseng, Asian ginseng, Chinese ginseng, Korean red ginseng, *Panax ginseng*: *Panax* spp. including *P. ginseng* C.C. Meyer and *P. quincefolium* L., excluding *Eleutherococcus senticosus*)	Anxiety
Ginseng (American ginseng, Asian ginseng, Chinese ginseng, Korean red ginseng, *Panax ginseng*: *Panax* spp. including *P. ginseng* C.C. Meyer and *P. quincefolium* L., excluding *Eleutherococcus senticosus*)	Stress
Goldenseal (*Hydrastis canadensis* L.), berberine	Anxiety
Gotu kola (*Centella asiatica* L), total triterpenic fraction of *Centella asiatica* (TTFCA)	Anxiety
Hops (*Humulus lupulus* L.)	Anxiety
Hops (*Humulus lupulus* L.)	Anxiety during menopause
Lavender (*Lavandula angustifolia* Miller)	Anxiety
Niacin (vitamin B_3, nicotinic acid), *Niacinamide, and Inositol hexanicotinate*	Anxiety
Omega-3 fatty acids, fish oil, alpha-linolenic acid	Panic disorder
Passionflower (*Passiflora incarnata* L.)	Tension
Spirulina	Anxiety
Thyme (*Thymus vulgaris* L.), thymol	Anxiety
Valerian (*Valeriana officinalis* L.)	Stress

ARRHYTHMIA AND RELATED CONDITIONS

Levels of Scientific Evidence for Specific Therapies

GRADE: C (Unclear or Conflicting Scientific Evidence)

Therapy	Specific Therapeutic Use(s)
Omega-3 fatty acids, fish oil, alpha-linolenic acid	Cardiac arrhythmias (abnormal heart rhythms)

TRADITIONAL OR THEORETICAL USES THAT LACK SUFFICIENT EVIDENCE

Therapy	Specific Therapeutic Use(s)
Astragalus (*Astragalus membranaceus*)	Palpitations
Black cohosh (*Cimicifuga racemosa* L. Nutt.)	Heart disease/palpitations
Clay	Heart disorders

Continued

Therapy	Specific Therapeutic Use(s)
Coenzyme Q10	Heart irregular beats
Danshen (*Salvia miltiorrhiza*)	Heart palpitations
Devil's claw (*Harpagophytum procumbens* DC.)	Irregular heartbeat
Dong quai (*Angelica sinensis* [Oliv.] Diels), Chinese angelica	Abnormal heart rhythms
Dong quai (*Angelica sinensis* [Oliv.] Diels), Chinese angelica	Palpitations
Garlic (*Allium sativum* L.)	Heart rhythm disorders
Ginkgo (*Ginkgo biloba* L.)	Cardiac rhythm abnormalities
Ginseng (American ginseng, Asian ginseng, Chinese ginseng, Korean red ginseng, *Panax ginseng*: *Panax* spp. including *P. ginseng* C.C. Meyer and *P. quincefolium* L., excluding *Eleutherococcus senticosus*)	Palpitations
Goldenseal (*Hydrastis Canadensis* L.), berberine	Abnormal heart rhythms
Valerian (*Valeriana officinalis* L.)	Nervous palpitation
Valerian (*Valeriana officinalis* L.)	Nervous tachycardia
White horehound (*Marrubium vulgare*)	Heart rate abnormalities

ASTHMA AND RELATED CONDITIONS

Levels of Scientific Evidence for Specific Therapies

GRADE: B (Good Scientific Evidence)

Therapy	Specific Therapeutic Use(s)
Boswellia (*Boswellia serrata* Roxb.)	Asthma (chronic therapy)
Ephedra (*Ephedra sinica*)/ma huang	Asthmatic bronchoconstriction

GRADE: C (Unclear or Conflicting Scientific Evidence)

Therapy	Specific Therapeutic Use(s)
Belladonna (*Atropa belladonna* L. or its variety *acuminata* Royle ex Lindl)	Airway obstruction
Black tea (*Camellia sinensis*)	Asthma
Bromelain	Chronic obstructive pulmonary disease (COPD)
Danshen (*Salvia miltiorrhiza*)	Asthmatic bronchitis

Therapy	Specific Therapeutic Use(s)
Green tea (*Camellia sinensis*)	Asthma
Lactobacillus acidophilus	Asthma
Lycopene	Asthma caused by exercise
Omega-3 fatty acids, fish oil, alpha-linolenic acid	Asthma

GRADE: D (Fair Negative Scientific Evidence)

Therapy	Specific Therapeutic Use(s)
Evening primrose oil (*Oenothera biennis* L.)	Asthma

GRADE: F (Strong Negative Scientific Evidence)

Therapy	Specific Therapeutic Use(s)
Arginine (L-arginine)	Asthma

TRADITIONAL OR THEORETICAL USES THAT LACK SUFFICIENT EVIDENCE

Therapy	Specific Therapeutic Use(s)
Alfalfa (*Medicago sativa* L.)	Asthma
Aloe (*Aloe vera*)	Asthma
Astragalus (*Astragalus membranaceus*)	Asthma
Astragalus (*Astragalus membranaceus*)	Shortness of breath
Barley (*Hordeum vulgare* L.), germinated barley foodstuff (GBF)	Asthma
Belladonna (*Atropa belladonna* L. or its variety *acuminata* Royle ex Lindl)	Asthma
Betel nut (*Areca catechu* L.)	Asthma
Black cohosh (*Cimicifuga racemosa* L. Nutt.)	Asthma
Boswellia (*Boswellia serrata* Roxb.)	Chronic obstructive pulmonary disease (COPD)
Clove (*Eugenia aromatica*)	Asthma
Coenzyme Q10	Asthma
Coenzyme Q10	Breathing difficulties
Coenzyme Q10	Chronic obstructive pulmonary disease (COPD)
DHEA (dehydroepiandrosterone)	Asthma

Continued

Dong quai (*Angelica sinensis* [Oliv.] Diels), Chinese angelica	Asthma
Dong quai (*Angelica sinensis* [Oliv.] Diels), Chinese angelica	Chronic obstructive pulmonary disease (COPD)
Elder (*Sambucus nigra* L.)	Asthma
Elder (*Sambucus nigra* L.)	Respiratory distress
Ephedra (*Ephedra sinica*)/ma huang	Dyspnea
Essiac	Asthma
Eucalyptus oil (Eucalyptus globulus Labillardiere, *E. fructicetorum* F. Von Mueller, *E. smithii* R.T. Baker)	Asthma
Eucalyptus oil (*Eucalyptus globulus* Labillardiere, *E. fructicetorum* F. Von Mueller, *E. smithii* R.T. Baker)	Chronic obstructive pulmonary disease (COPD)
Eucalyptus oil (*Eucalyptus globulus* Labillardiere, *E. fructicetorum* F. Von Mueller, *E. smithii* R.T. Baker)	Emphysema
Eyebright (*Euphrasia officinalis*)	Asthma
Feverfew (*Tanacetum parthenium* L. Schultz-Bip.)	Asthma
Flaxseed and flaxseed oil (*Linum usitatissimum*)	Bronchial irritation
Garlic (*Allium sativum* L.)	Asthma
Ginger (*Zingiber officinale* Roscoe)	Asthma
Ginkgo (*Ginkgo biloba* L.)	Asthma
Ginseng (American ginseng, Asian ginseng, Chinese ginseng, Korean red ginseng, *Panax ginseng*: *Panax* spp. including *P. ginseng* C.C. Meyer and *P. quincefolium* L., excluding *Eleutherococcus senticosus*)	Asthma
Ginseng (American ginseng, Asian ginseng, Chinese ginseng, Korean red ginseng, *Panax ginseng*: *Panax* spp. including *P. ginseng* C.C. Meyer and *P. quincefolium* L., excluding *Eleutherococcus senticosus*)	Breathing difficulty
Ginseng (American ginseng, Asian ginseng, Chinese ginseng, Korean red ginseng, *Panax ginseng*: *Panax* spp. including *P. ginseng* C.C. Meyer and *P. quincefolium* L., excluding *Eleutherococcus senticosus*)	Bronchodilation
Goldenseal (*Hydrastis canadensis* L.), berberine	Asthma

Gotu kola (*Centella asiatica* L.), total triterpenic fraction of *Centella asiatica* (TTFCA)	Asthma
Guggul (*Commifora mukul*)	Asthma
Hawthorn (*Crataegus laevigata*, *C. oxyacantha*, *C. monogyna*, *C. pentagyna*)	Asthma
Hawthorn (*Crataegus laevigata*, *C. oxyacantha*, *C. monogyna*, *C. pentagyna*)	Dyspnea
Kava (*Piper methysticum* G. Forst)	Asthma
Lavender (*Lavandula angustifolia* Miller)	Asthma
Licorice (Gly*cyrrhiza glabra* L.), deglycyrrhizinated licorice (DGL)	Asthma
Melatonin	Asthma
Oleander (*Nerium oleander*, *Thevetia peruviana*)	Asthma
Omega-3 fatty acids, fish oil, alpha-linolenic acid	Chronic obstructive pulmonary disease
Passionflower (*Passiflora incarnata* L.)	Asthma
Peppermint (*Mentha x piperita* L.)	Asthma
Polypodium leucotomos extract, Anapsos	Asthma
Red clover (*Trifolium pratense*)	Asthma
Saw palmetto (*Serenoa repens* [Bartram] Small)	Asthma
Slippery elm (*Ulmus rubra* Muhl., *U. fulva* Michx.)	Respiratory disorders
Thyme (*Thymus vulgaris* L.), Thymol	Asthma
Thyme (*Thymus vulgaris* L.), Thymol	Dyspnea
Turmeric (*Curcuma longa* L.), curcumin	Asthma
Valerian (*Valeriana officinalis* L.)	Asthma
Valerian (*Valeriana officinalis* L.)	Bronchospasm
White horehound (*Marrubium vulgare*)	Asthma
White horehound (*Marrubium vulgare*)	Chronic obstructive pulmonary disease (COPD)
White horehound (*Marrubium vulgare*)	Wheezing
Wild yam (*Dioscorea villosa*)	Asthma

ATHEROSCLEROSIS AND RELATED CONDITIONS

Levels of Scientific Evidence for Specific Therapies

GRADE: A (Strong Scientific Evidence)

Therapy	Specific Therapeutic Use(s)
Niacin (vitamin B_3, nicotinic acid), niacinamide, and inositol hexanicotinate	High cholesterol (niacin)
Omega-3 fatty acids, fish oil, alpha-linolenic acid)	Hypertriglyceridemia (fish oil/eicosapentaenoic acid [EPA] plus docosahexaenoic acid [DHA])
Omega-3 fatty acids, fish oil, alpha-linolenic acid	Secondary cardiovascular disease prevention (fish oil/eicosapentaenoic acid [EPA] plus docosahexaenoic acid [DHA])
Psyllium (*Plantago ovata*, *P. ispaghula*)	High cholesterol
Red yeast rice (*Monascus purpureus*)	High cholesterol
Soy (*Glycine max* L. Merr.)	High cholesterol

GRADE: B (Good Scientific Evidence)

Therapy	Specific Therapeutic Use(s)
Barley (*Hordeum vulgare* L.), germinated barley foodstuff (GBF)	High cholesterol
Garlic (*Allium sativum* L.)	High cholesterol
Niacin (vitamin B_3, nicotinic acid), niacinamide, and inositol hexanicotinate	Atherosclerosis (niacin)
Niacin (vitamin B_3, nicotinic acid), niacinamide, and inositol hexanicotinate	Prevention of a second heart attack (niacin)
Omega-3 fatty acids, fish oil, alpha-linolenic acid	Primary cardiovascular disease prevention (fish intake)
Sweet Almond (*Prunus amygdalus dulcis*)	High cholesterol (whole almonds)

GRADE: C (Unclear or Conflicting Scientific Evidence)

Therapy	Specific Therapeutic Use(s)
Alfalfa (*Medicago sativa* L.)	Atherosclerosis (cholesterol plaques in heart arteries)

Alfalfa (*Medicago sativa* L.)	High cholesterol
Arginine (L-arginine)	Coronary artery disease/angina
Arginine (L-arginine)	Heart protection during coronary artery bypass grafting (CABG)
Astragalus (*Astragalus membranaceus*)	Coronary artery disease
Bilberry *(Vaccinium myrtillus*)	Atherosclerosis (hardening of the arteries) and peripheral vascular disease
Black tea (*Camellia sinensis*)	Heart attack prevention
Coenzyme Q10	Angina (chest pain from clogged heart arteries)
Coenzyme Q10	Heart attack (acute myocardial infarction)
Coenzyme Q10	Heart protection during surgery
Danshen (*Salvia miltiorrhiza*)	Cardiovascular disease/angina
DHEA (dehydroepiandrosterone)	Atherosclerosis (cholesterol plaques in the arteries)
Dong quai (*Angelica sinensis* [Oliv.] Diels), Chinese angelica	Angina pectoris/coronary artery disease
Fenugreek (*Trigonella foenum-graecum* L.)	Hyperlipidemia
Flaxseed and flaxseed oil (*Linum usitatissimum*)	Heart disease (flaxseed and flaxseed oil)
Flaxseed and flaxseed oil (*Linum usitatissimum*)	High cholesterol or triglycerides (flaxseed and flaxseed oil)
Garlic (*Allium sativum* L.)	Atherosclerosis (hardening of the arteries)
Garlic (*Allium sativum* L.)	Familial hypercholesterolemia
Garlic (*Allium sativum* L.)	Heart attack prevention in patients with known heart disease
Ginseng (American ginseng, Asian ginseng, Chinese ginseng, Korean red ginseng, *Panax ginseng*: *Panax* spp. including *P. ginseng* C.C. Meyer and *P. quincefolium* L., excluding *Eleutherococcus senticosus*)	Coronary artery (heart) disease

Continued

Therapy	Specific Therapeutic Use(s)
Globe artichoke (*Cynara scolymus* L.)	Lipid-lowering (cholesterol and triglycerides)
Green tea (*Camellia sinensis*)	Heart attack prevention
Green tea (*Camellia sinensis*)	High cholesterol
Guggul (*Commifora mukul*)	Hyperlipidemia
Gymnema (*Gymnema sylvestre* R. Br.)	High cholesterol
Hawthorn (*Crataegus laevigata, C. oxyacantha, C. monogyna, C. pentagyna*)	Coronary artery disease (angina)
Lactobacillus acidophilus	High cholesterol
Lycopene	Atherosclerosis (clogged arteries) and high cholesterol
Milk thistle (*Silybum marianum*), silymarin	Hyperlipidemia
Omega-3 fatty acids, fish oil, alpha-linolenic acid	Angina pectoris
Omega-3 fatty acids, fish oil, alpha-linolenic acid	Atherosclerosis
Omega-3 fatty acids, fish oil, alpha-linolenic acid	Prevention of graft failure after heart bypass surgery
Omega-3 fatty acids, fish oil, alpha-linolenic acid	Prevention of restenosis after percutaneous transluminal coronary angioplasty (PTCA)
Red clover (*Trifolium pratense*)	High cholesterol
Soy (*Glycine max* L. Merr.)	Cardiovascular disease
Spirulina	High cholesterol
Turmeric (*Curcuma longa* L), curcumin	High cholesterol
Wild yam *(Dioscorea villosa)*	High cholesterol

GRADE: D (Fair Negative Scientific Evidence)

Therapy	Specific Therapeutic Use(s)
Omega-3 fatty acids, fish oil, alpha-linolenic acid	Hypercholesterolemia

TRADITIONAL OR THEORETICAL USES THAT LACK SUFFICIENT EVIDENCE

Therapy	Specific Therapeutic Use(s)
Aloe (*Aloe vera*)	Heart disease prevention
Antineoplastons	Cholesterol/triglyceride abnormalities

Arginine (L-arginine)	Cardiac syndrome X
Arginine (L-arginine)	Heart attack
Arginine (L-arginine)	High cholesterol
Astragalus (*Astragalus membranaceus*)	Angina
Astragalus (*Astragalus membranaceus*)	Heart attack
Astragalus (*Astragalus membranaceus*)	High cholesterol
Bilberry (*Vaccinium myrtillus*)	Angina
Bilberry (*Vaccinium myrtillus*)	Heart disease
Bilberry (*Vaccinium myrtillus*)	High cholesterol
Black cohosh (*Cimicifuga racemosa* L. Nutt.)	Cardiac diseases
Bladderwrack (*Fucus vesiculosus*)	Atherosclerosis
Bladderwrack (*Fucus vesiculosus*)	Heart disease
Bladderwrack (*Fucus vesiculosus*)	High cholesterol
Boron	High cholesterol
Bromelain	Angina
Bromelain	Atherosclerosis (hardening of the arteries)
Bromelain	Heart disease
Calendula (*Calendula officinalis* L.), marigold	Atherosclerosis (clogged arteries)
Calendula (*Calendula officinalis* L.), marigold	Heart disease
Clay	Cardiovascular disorders
Coenzyme Q10	High cholesterol
Dandelion (*Taraxacum officinale*)	Cardiovascular disorders
Dandelion (*Taraxacum officinale*)	Clogged arteries
Dandelion (*Taraxacum officinale*)	High cholesterol
Danshen (*Salvia miltiorrhiza*)	Clogged arteries
Danshen (*Salvia miltiorrhiza*)	High cholesterol
Devil's claw (*Harpagophytum procumbens* DC.)	Atherosclerosis (clogged arteries)

Continued

Devil's claw (*Harpagophytum procumbens* DC.)	High cholesterol
DHEA (dehydroepiandrosterone)	Heart attack
DHEA (dehydroepiandrosterone)	High cholesterol
Dong quai (*Angelica sinensis* [Oliv.] Diels), Chinese angelica	Atherosclerosis
Dong quai (*Angelica sinensis* [Oliv.] Diels), Chinese angelica	High cholesterol
Evening primrose oil (*Oenothera biennis* L.)	Atherosclerosis
Evening primrose oil (*Oenothera biennis* L.)	Heart disease
Evening primrose oil (*Oenothera biennis* L.)	High cholesterol
Fenugreek (*Trigonella foenum-graecum* L.)	Atherosclerosis
Ginger (*Zingiber officinale* Roscoe)	Atherosclerosis
Ginger (*Zingiber officinale* Roscoe)	Heart disease
Ginkgo (*Ginkgo biloba* L.)	Angina
Ginkgo (*Ginkgo biloba* L.)	Atherosclerosis (clogged arteries)
Ginkgo (*Ginkgo biloba* L.)	Heart attack
Ginkgo (*Ginkgo biloba* L.)	Heart disease
Ginkgo (*Ginkgo biloba* L.)	High cholesterol
Ginseng (American ginseng, Asian ginseng, Chinese ginseng, Korean red ginseng, *Panax ginseng*: *Panax* spp. including *P. ginseng* C.C. Meyer and *P. quincefolium* L., excluding *Eleutherococcus senticosus*)	Atherosclerosis
Ginseng (American ginseng, Asian ginseng, Chinese ginseng, Korean red ginseng, *Panax ginseng*: *Panax* spp. including *P. ginseng* C.C. Meyer and *P. quincefolium* L., excluding *Eleutherococcus senticosus*)	Heart damage
Globe artichoke (*Cynara scolymus* L.)	Atherosclerosis
Goldenseal (*Hydrastis canadensis* L.), berberine	Atherosclerosis (hardening of the arteries)
Goldenseal (*Hydrastis canadensis* L.), berberine	High cholesterol
Green tea (*Camellia sinensis*)	Heart disease
Gymnema (*Gymnema Sylvestre* R. Br.)	Cardiovascular disease

Hawthorn (*Crataegus laevigata*, *C. oxyacantha*, *C. monogyna*, *C. pentagyna*)	Angina
Hawthorn (*Crataegus laevigata*, C. oxyacantha, *C. monogyna*, *C. pentagyna*)	Cardiac murmurs
Lactobacillus acidophilus	Heart disease
Licorice (*Glycyrrhiza glabra* L.), deglycyrrhizinated licorice (DGL)	High cholesterol
Lycopene	Heart disease
Maitake mushroom (*Grifola frondosa*), beta-glucan	High cholesterol
Melatonin	Cardiac syndrome X
Melatonin	Coronary artery disease
Niacin (vitamin B_3, nicotinic acid), niacinamide, and inositol hexanicotinate	Heart attack prevention
Oleander (*Nerium oleander*, *Thevetia peruviana*)	Heart disease
Omega-3 fatty acids, fish oil, alpha-linolenic acid	Acute myocardial infarction (heart attack)
Psyllium (*Plantago ovata*, *P. ispaghula*)	Atherosclerosis
Seaweed, kelp, bladderwrack (*Fucus vesiculosus*)	Atherosclerosis
Seaweed, kelp, bladderwrack (*Fucus vesiculosus*)	Fatty heart
Seaweed, kelp, bladderwrack (*Fucus vesiculosus*)	Hyperlipemia
Shark cartilage	Atherosclerosis
Soy (*Glycine max* L. Merr.)	Atherosclerosis
Spirulina	Atherosclerosis
Spirulina	Heart disease
Sweet almond (*Prunus amygdalus dulcis*)	Heart disease
Valerian (*Valeriana officinalis* L.)	Angina pectoris
Valerian (*Valeriana officinalis* L.)	Heart disease
Yohimbe bark extract (*Pausinystalia yohimbe* Pierre ex Beille)	Angina
Yohimbe bark extract (*Pausinystalia yohimbe* Pierre ex Beille)	Coronary artery disease
Yohimbe bark extract (*Pausinystalia yohimbe* Pierre ex Beille)	High cholesterol

Continued

Yohimbe bark extract (*Pausinystalia yohimbe* Pierre ex Beille)	Angina
Yohimbe bark extract (*Pausinystalia yohimbe* Pierre ex Beille)	Atherosclerosis
Yohimbe bark extract (*Pausinystalia yohimbe* Pierre ex Beille)	Chest pain
Yohimbe bark extract (*Pausinystalia yohimbe* Pierre ex Beille)	Coronary artery disease
Yohimbe bark extract (*Pausinystalia yohimbe* Pierre ex Beillee)	Hyperlipidemia

ATTENTION DEFICIT HYPERACTIVITY DISORDER (ADHD) AND RELATED CONDITIONS

Levels of Scientific Evidence for Specific Therapies

GRADE: C (Unclear or Conflicting Scientific Evidence)

Therapy	Specific Therapeutic Use(s)
Melatonin	ADHD

GRADE: D (Fair Negative Scientific Evidence)

Therapy	Specific Therapeutic Use(s)
Evening primrose oil (*Oenothera biennis* L.)	ADHD

TRADITIONAL OR THEORETICAL USES THAT LACK SUFFICIENT EVIDENCE

Therapy	Specific Therapeutic Use(s)
Black tea (*Camellia sinensis*)	Hyperactivity (children)
Ginkgo (*Ginkgo biloba* L.)	ADHD
Ginseng (American ginseng, Asian ginseng, Chinese ginseng, Korean red ginseng, *Panax ginseng*: *Panax* spp. including *P. ginseng* C.C. Meyer and *P. quincefolium* L., excluding *Eleutherococcus senticosus*)	ADHD
Omega-3 fatty acids, fish oil, alpha-linolenic acid	ADHD
Passionflower (*Passiflora incarnata* L.)	ADHD
Soy (*Glycine max* L. Merr.)	ADHD
Spirulina	ADHD

BACK PAIN AND RELATED CONDITIONS

Levels of Scientific Evidence for Specific Therapies

GRADE: C (Unclear or Conflicting Scientific Evidence)

Therapy	Specific Therapeutic Use(s)
Devil's claw (*Harpagophytum procumbens* DC.)	Low back pain

TRADITIONAL OR THEORETICAL USES THAT LACK SUFFICIENT EVIDENCE

Therapy	Specific Therapeutic Use(s)
Belladonna (*Atropa belladonna* L. or its variety *acuminata* Royle ex Lindl)	Sciatica (back and leg pain)
Black cohosh (*Cimicifuga racemosa* L. Nutt.)	Back pain
Bromelain	Back pain
Bromelain	Sciatica
Burdock (*Arctium lappa*)	Back pain
Burdock (*Arctium lappa*)	Sciatica
Chamomile (*Matricaria recutita*, *Chamaemelum nobile*)	Back pain
Chamomile (*Matricaria recutita*, *Chamaemelum nobile*)	Sciatica
Dong quai (*Angelica sinensis* [Oliv.] Diels), Chinese angelica	Back pain
Dong quai (*Angelica sinensis* [Oliv.] Diels), Chinese angelica	Sciatica
Eucalyptus oil (Eucalyptus globulus Labillardiere, *E. fructicetorum* F. Von Mueller, *E. smithii* R.T. Baker)	Back pain
Goldenseal (*Hydrastis canadensis* L.), berberine	Sciatica

BACTERIAL INFECTIONS AND RELATED CONDITIONS

Levels of Scientific Evidence for Specific Therapies

GRADE: C (Unclear or Conflicting Scientific Evidence)

Therapy	Specific Therapeutic Use(s)
Bladderwrack (*Fucus vesiculosus*)	Antibacterial/antifungal
Blessed thistle (*Cnicus benedictus* L.)	Bacterial infections

Continued

Garlic (*Allium sativum* L.)	Cryptococcal meningitis
Goldenseal (*Hydrastis canadensis* L.), berberine	Trachoma (*Chlamydia trachomatosis* eye infection)
Lavender (*Lavandula angustifolia* Miller)	Antibacterial (lavender used on the skin)
Propolis	Infections
Seaweed, kelp, bladderwrack (*Fucus vesiculosus*)	Antibacterial
Sorrel (*Rumex acetosa* L., *R. acetosella* L.), Sinupret	Antibacterial
Tea tree oil (*Melaleuca alternifolia* [Maiden & Betche] Cheel)	Methicillin-resistant *Staphylococcus aureus* (MRSA) chronic infection (colonization)

TRADITIONAL OR THEORETICAL USES THAT LACK SUFFICIENT EVIDENCE

Therapy	Specific Therapeutic Use(s)
Aloe (*Aloe vera*)	Bacterial skin infections
American pennyroyal (*Hedeoma pulegioides* L.), European pennyroyal (*Mentha pulegium* L.)	Antiseptic
Astragalus (*Astragalus membranaceus*)	Antimicrobial
Bilberry (*Vaccinium myrtillus*)	Skin infections
Bitter almond (*Prunus amygdalus* Batch var. *amara* DC. Focke),d Laetrile	Antibacterial
Blessed thistle (*Cnicus benedictus* L.)	Bubonic plague
Boron	Antiseptic
Boswellia (*Boswellia serrata* Roxb.)	Antiseptic
Bromelain	Antibiotic absorption problems in the gut
Bromelain	Infections
Burdock (*Arctium lappa*)	Bacterial infections
Calendula (*Calendula officinalis* L.), marigold	Bacterial infections
Calendula (*Calendula officinalis* L.), marigold	Cholera
Calendula (*Calendula officinalis* L.), marigold	Tuberculosis
Chamomile (*Matricaria recutita*, *Chamaemelum nobile*)	Antibacterial

Chamomile (*Matricaria recutita*, *Chamaemelum nobile*)	Skin infections
Chaparral (*Larrea tridentata* DC. Coville, *L. divaricata* Cav.), nordihydroguaiaretic acid (NDGA)	Antibacterial
Chaparral (*Larrea tridentata* DC. Coville, *L. divaricata* Cav.), nordihydroguaiaretic acid (NDGA)	Tuberculosis
Clove (*Eugenia aromatica*)	Antiseptic
Dandelion (*Taraxacum officinale*)	Antibacterial
Dong quai (*Angelica sinensis* [Oliv.] Diels), Chinese angelica	Antibacterial
Dong quai (*Angelica sinensis* [Oliv.] Diels), Chinese angelica	Antiseptic
Dong quai (*Angelica sinensis* [Oliv.] Diels), Chinese angelica	Infections
Echinacea (*Echinacea angustifolia* DC., *E. pallida, E. purpurea*)	Bacterial infections
Ephedra (Ephedra sinica)/ma huang	Gonorrhea
Eucalyptus oil (*Eucalyptus globulus* Labillardiere, *E. fructicetorum* F. Von Mueller, *E. smithii* R.T. Baker)	Antibacterial
Eucalyptus oil (*Eucalyptus globulus* Labillardiere, *E.* fructicetorum F. Von Mueller, E. smithii R.T. Baker)	Skin infections in children
Eucalyptus oil (*Eucalyptus globulus* Labillardiere, E. *fructicetorum* F. Von Mueller, *E. smithii* R.T. Baker)	Tuberculosis
Eyebright (*Euphrasia officinalis*)	Antibacterial
Fenugreek (*Trigonella foenum-graecum* L.)	Cellulitis
Fenugreek (*Trigonella foenum-graecum* L.)	Infections
Fenugreek (*Trigonella foenum-graecum* L.)	Tuberculosis
Flaxseed and flaxseed oil (*Linum usitatissimum*)	Gonorrhea
Flaxseed and flaxseed oil (*Linum usitatissimum*)	Skin infections
Garlic (*Allium sativum* L.)	Cholera
Garlic (*Allium sativum* L.)	Cryptococcal meningitis
Garlic (*Allium sativum* L.)	Tuberculosis
Ginger (*Zingiber officinale* Roscoe)	Antiseptic
Ginger (*Zingiber officinale* Roscoe)	Cholera

Continued

Ginkgo (*Ginkgo biloba* L.)	Antibacterial
Goldenseal (*Hydrastis canadensis* L.), berberine	Antibacterial
Goldenseal (*Hydrastis canadensis* L.), berberine	Infections
Goldenseal (*Hydrastis canadensis* L.), berberine	Tuberculosis
Gotu kola (*Centella asiatica* L.), total triterpenic fraction of *Centella asiatica* (TTFCA)	Anti-infective
Gotu kola (*Centella asiatica* L.), total triterpenic fraction of *Centella asiatica* (TTFCA)	Cholera
Gotu kola (*Centella asiatica* L.), total triterpenic fraction of *Centella asiatica* (TTFCA)	Tuberculosis
Hawthorn (*Crataegus laevigata*, *C. oxyacantha*, *C. monogyna*, *C. pentagyna*)	Antibacterial
Hops (*Humulus lupulus* L.)	Antibacterial
Horsetail (*Equisetum arvense* L.)	Antibacterial
Horsetail (*Equisetum arvense* L.)	Gonorrhea
Horsetail (*Equisetum arvense* L.)	Tuberculosis
Kava (*Piper methysticum* G. Forst)	Gonorrhea
Kava (*Piper methysticum* G. Forst)	Infections
Kava (*Piper methysticum* G. Forst)	Tuberculosis
Lavender (*Lavandula angustifolia* Miller)	Antiseptic
Licorice (*Glycyrrhiza glabra* L.), deglycyrrhizinated licorice (DGL)	Antimicrobial
Licorice (*Glycyrrhiza glabra* L.), deglycyrrhizinated licorice (DGL)	Bacterial infections
Licorice (*Glycyrrhiza glabra* L.), deglycyrrhizinated licorice (DGL) staphylococcus aureus	Methicillin-resistant
Licorice (*Glycyrrhiza glabra* L.), deglycyrrhizinated licorice (DGL)	SARS
Maitake mushroom (*Grifola frondosa*), beta-glucan	Bacterial infection
Niacin (vitamin B_3, nicotinic acid), niacinamide, and inositol hexanicotinate	Tuberculosis
Oleander (*Nerium oleander*, *Thevetia peruviana*)	Bacterial infections
Omega-3 fatty acids, fish oil, alpha-linolenic acid	Bacterial infections

Passionflower (*Passiflora incarnata* L.)	Antibacterial
Peppermint (*Mentha x piperita* L.)	Gonorrhea
Propolis	Tuberculosis
Red clover (*Trifolium pratense*)	Antibacterial
Red clover (*Trifolium pratense*)	Tuberculosis
Red yeast rice (*Monascus purpureus*)	Anthrax
Shark cartilage	Bacterial infections
Slippery elm (*Ulmus rubra* Muhl., *U. fulva* Michx.)	Tuberculosis
St. John's wort (*Hypericum perforatum* L.)	Bacterial skin infections (topical)
Sweet almond (*Prunus amygdalus dulcis*)	Antibacterial
Tea tree oil (*Melaleuca alternifolia* [Maiden & Betche] Cheel)	Antibacterial
Thyme (*Thymus vulgaris* L.), thymol	Cellulitis
Turmeric (*Curcuma longa* L.), curcumin	Gonorrhea
White horehound (*Marrubium vulgare*)	Tuberculosis

BALANCE AND RELATED CONDITIONS

Levels of Scientific Evidence for Specific Therapies

GRADE: C (Unclear or Conflicting Scientific Evidence)

Therapy	Specific Therapeutic Use(s)
Coenzyme Q10	Exercise performance
DHEA (dehydroepiandrosterone)	Muscle mass/body mass
Ginseng (American ginseng, Asian ginseng, Chinese ginseng, Korean red ginseng, *Panax ginseng*: *Panax* spp. including *P. ginseng* C.C. Meyer and *P. quincefolium* L., excluding *Eleutherococcus senticosus*)	Exercise performance

GRADE: D (Fair Negative Scientific Evidence)

Therapy	Specific Therapeutic Use(s)
Boron	Bodybuilding aid (increasing testosterone)

Continued

TRADITIONAL OR THEORETICAL USES THAT LACK SUFFICIENT EVIDENCE	
Therapy	Specific Therapeutic Use(s)
Arginine (L-arginine)	Enhanced athletic performance
Arginine (L-arginine)	Increased muscle mass
Barley (*Hordeum vulgare* L.), germinated barley foodstuff (GBF)	Stamina/strength enhancer
DHEA (dehydroepiandrosterone)	Performance enhancement
Ephedra (*Ephedra sinica*)/ma huang	Bodybuilding
Essiac	Energy enhancement
Ginseng (American ginseng, Asian ginseng, Chinese ginseng, Korean red ginseng, *Panax ginseng*: *Panax* spp. including *P. ginseng* C.C. Meyer and *P. quincefolium* L., excluding *Eleutherococcus senticosus*)	Physical work capacity
Ginseng (American ginseng, Asian ginseng, Chinese ginseng, Korean red ginseng, *Panax ginseng*: *Panax* spp. including *P. ginseng* C.C. Meyer and *P. quincefolium* L., excluding *Eleutherococcus senticosus*)	Rehabilitation
Gotu kola (*Centella asiatica* L.), total triterpenic fraction of *Centella asiatica* (TTFCA)	Physical exhaustion
Lavender (*Lavandula angustifolia* Miller)	Exercise recovery
Soy (*Glycine max* L. Merr.)	Athletic endurance
St. John's wort (*Hypericum perforatum* L.)	Athletic performance enhancement
Wild yam (*Dioscorea villosa*)	Energy improvement

BEDWETTING AND RELATED CONDITIONS

Levels of Scientific Evidence for Specific Therapies

GRADE: C (Unclear or Conflicting Scientific Evidence)	
Therapy	Specific Therapeutic Use(s)
Cranberry (*Vaccinium macrocarpon*)	Reduction of odor from incontinence/bladder catheterization
Saw palmetto (*Serenoa repens* [Bartram] Small)	Hypotonic neurogenic bladder

TRADITIONAL OR THEORETICAL USES THAT LACK SUFFICIENT EVIDENCE	
Therapy	Specific Therapeutic Use(s)
Belladonna (*Atropa belladonna* L. or its variety *acuminata* Royle ex Lindl)	Bedwetting
Calendula (*Calendula officinalis* L.), marigold	Urinary retention
Ephedra (*Ephedra sinica*)/ma huang	Enuresis
Gotu kola (*Centella asiatica* L.), total triterpenic fraction of *Centella asiatica* (TTFCA)	Urinary retention
Horsetail (*Equisetum arvense* L.)	Urinary incontinence
Kava (*Piper methysticum* G. Forst)	Urinary incontinence
St. John's wort (*Hypericum perforatum* L.)	Bedwetting
Thyme (*Thymus vulgaris* L.), thymol	Enuresis

BENIGN PROSTATIC HYPERTROPHY (BPH) AND RELATED CONDITIONS

Levels of Scientific Evidence for Specific Therapies

GRADE: A (Strong Scientific Evidence)	
Therapy	Specific Therapeutic Use(s)
Saw palmetto (*Serenoa repens* [Bartram] Small)	BPH

GRADE: B (Good Scientific Evidence)	
Therapy	Specific Therapeutic Use(s)
Pygeum (*Prunus africana*, *Pygeum africanum*)	BPH symptoms

GRADE: C (Unclear or Conflicting Scientific Evidence)	
Therapy	Specific Therapeutic Use(s)
Red clover (*Trifolium pratense*)	Prostate enlargement (BPH)

TRADITIONAL OR THEORETICAL USES THAT LACK SUFFICIENT EVIDENCE	
Therapy	Specific Therapeutic Use(s)
Alfalfa (*Medicago sativa* L.)	Prostate disorders
Astragalus (*Astragalus membranaceus*)	Prostatitis

Continued

Bladderwrack (*Fucus vesiculosus*)	BPH
Calendula (*Calendula officinalis* L.), marigold	BPH
Calendula (*Calendula officinalis* L.), marigold	Prostatitis
Dandelion (*Taraxacum officinale*)	BPH
Flaxseed and flaxseed oil (*Linum usitatissimum*)	Enlarged prostate
Goldenseal (*Hydrastis canadensis* L.), berberine	Prostatitis
Horse chestnut (*Aesculus hippocastanum* L.)	BPH
Horsetail (*Equisetum arvense* L.)	Prostate inflammation
PC-SPES	BPH
Pygeum (*Prunus africana, Pygeum africanum*)	Prostatic adenoma
Pygeum (*Prunus africana, Pygeum africanum*)	Prostatitis
Seaweed, kelp, bladderwrack (*Fucus vesiculosus*)	BPH

BLADDER DISORDERS AND RELATED CONDITIONS

Levels of Scientific Evidence for Specific Therapies

GRADE: C (Unclear or Conflicting Scientific Evidence)

Therapy	Specific Therapeutic Use(s)
Chamomile (*Matricaria recutita, Chamaemelum nobile*)	Hemorrhagic cystitis (bladder irritation with bleeding)
Saw palmetto (*Serenoa repens* [Bartram] Small)	Underactive bladder

TRADITIONAL OR THEORETICAL USES THAT LACK SUFFICIENT EVIDENCE

Therapy	Specific Therapeutic Use(s)
Alfalfa (*Medicago sativa* L.)	Bladder disorders
Bladderwrack (*Fucus vesiculosus*)	Bladder inflammatory disease
Boswellia (*Boswellia serrata* Roxb.)	Cystitis
Burdock (*Arctium lappa*)	Bladder disorders
Calendula (*Calendula officinalis* L.), marigold	Bladder irritation
Dandelion (*Taraxacum officinale*)	Bladder irritation
Flaxseed and flaxseed oil (*Linum usitatissimum*)	Bladder inflammation

Globe artichoke (*Cynara scolymus* L.)	Cystitis
Goldenseal (*Hydrastis canadensis* L.), berberine	Cystitis
Hawthorn (*Crataegus laevigata, C. oxyacantha, C. monogyna, C. pentagyna*)	Bladder disorders
Horsetail (*Equisetum arvense* L.)	Bladder disturbances
Horsetail (*Equisetum arvense* L.)	Cystic ulcers
Kava (*Piper methysticum* G. Forst)	Cystitis
Marshmallow (*Althaea officinalis* L.)	Cystitis
Marshmallow (*Althaea officinalis* L.)	Urethritis
Psyllium (*Plantago ovata, P. ispaghula*)	Cystitis
Psyllium (*Plantago ovata, P. ispaghula*)	Urethritis
Pygeum (*Prunus africana, Pygeum africanum*)	Bladder sphincter disorders
Pygeum (*Prunus africana, Pygeum africanum*)	Partial bladder outlet obstruction
Saw palmetto (*Serenoa repens* [Bartram] Small)	Cystitis
Seaweed, kelp, bladderwrack (*Fucus vesiculosus*)	Bladder inflammatory disease
Slippery elm (*Ulmus rubra* Muhl., *U. fulva* Michx.)	Cystitis
Thyme (*Thymus vulgaris* L.), thymol	Cystitis
Thyme (*Thymus vulgaris* L.), thymol	Urethritis

BLEEDING AND RELATED CONDITIONS

Levels of Scientific Evidence for Specific Therapies

TRADITIONAL OR THEORETICAL USES THAT LACK SUFFICIENT EVIDENCE

Therapy	Specific Therapeutic Use(s)
Astragalus (*Astragalus membranaceus*)	Hemorrhage (bleeding)
Blessed thistle (*Cnicus benedictus* L.)	Bleeding
Cranberry (*Vaccinium macrocarpon*)	Blood disorders
Dong quai (*Angelica sinensis* [Oliv.] Diels), Chinese angelica	Hematopoiesis (stimulation of blood cell production)
Ginger (*Zingiber officinale* Roscoe)	Bleeding

Continued

Ginseng (American ginseng, Asian ginseng, Chinese ginseng, Korean red ginseng, *Panax ginseng*: *Panax* spp. including *P. ginseng* C.C. Meyer and *P. quincefolium* L., excluding *Eleutherococcus senticosus*)	Bleeding disorders
Glucosamine	Bleeding esophageal varices (blood vessels in the esophagus)
Goldenseal (*Hydrastis canadensis* L.), berberine	Anti-heparin
Goldenseal (*Hydrastis canadensis* L.), berberine	Hemorrhage (bleeding)
Guggul (*Commifora mukul*)	Bleeding
Horsetail (*Equisetum arvense* L.)	Bleeding
Milk thistle (*Silybum marianum*), silymarin	Hemorrhage
Sorrel (*Rumex acetosa* L., *R. acetosella* L.), Sinupret	Hemorrhage
Turmeric (*Curcuma longa* L.), curcumin	Bleeding

BREAST ENLARGEMENT AND RELATED CONDITIONS

Levels of Scientific Evidence for Specific Therapies

TRADITIONAL OR THEORETICAL USES THAT LACK SUFFICIENT EVIDENCE

Therapy	Specific Therapeutic Use(s)
Dandelion (*Taraxacum officinale*)	Breast augmentation
Dong quai (*Angelica sinensis* [Oliv.] Diels), Chinese angelica	Breast enlargement
Ginseng (American ginseng, Asian ginseng, Chinese ginseng, Korean red ginseng, *Panax ginseng*: *Panax* spp. including *P. ginseng* C.C. Meyer and *P. quincefolium* L., excluding *Eleutherococcus senticosus*)	Breast enlargement
PC-SPES	Breast enlargement
Saw palmetto (*Serenoa repens* [Bartram] Small)	Breast augmentation
Soy (*Glycine max* L. Merr.)	Breast enlargement
Wild yam (*Dioscorea villosa*)	Breast enlargement

BRUISES AND RELATED CONDITIONS

Levels of Scientific Evidence for Specific Therapies

TRADITIONAL OR THEORETICAL USES THAT LACK SUFFICIENT EVIDENCE

Therapy	Specific Therapeutic Use(s)
American pennyroyal (*Hedeoma pulegioides* L.), European pennyroyal (*Mentha pulegium* L.)	Bruises and burns
Bromelain	Bruises
Calendula (*Calendula officinalis* L.), Marigold	Bruises
Chaparral (*Larrea tridentata* DC. Coville, *L. divaricata* Cav.), nordihydroguaiaretic acid (NDGA)	Bruises
Dandelion (*Taraxacum officinale*)	Bruises
Danshen (*Salvia miltiorrhiza*)	Bruising
Evening primrose oil (*Oenothera biennis* L.)	Bruises (topical)
Gotu kola (*Centella asiatica* L.), total triterpenic fraction of *Centella asiatica* (TTFCA)	Bruises
Horse chestnut (*Aesculus hippocastanum* L.)	Bruising
Marshmallow (*Althaea officinalis* L.)	Bruises (topical)
Red yeast rice (*Monascus purpureus*)	Bruised muscles
Red yeast rice (*Monascus purpureus*)	Bruises
St. John's wort (*Hypericum perforatum* L.)	Bruises (topical)
Turmeric (*Curcuma longa* L.), curcumin	Bruises

BURNS AND RELATED CONDITIONS

Levels of Scientific Evidence for Specific Therapies

GRADE: C (Unclear or Conflicting Scientific Evidence)

Therapy	Specific Therapeutic Use(s)
Aloe (*Aloe vera*)	Skin burns
Arginine (L-arginine)	Burns
Danshen (*Salvia miltiorrhiza*)	Burn healing

Continued

TRADITIONAL OR THEORETICAL USES THAT LACK SUFFICIENT EVIDENCE	
Therapy	Specific Therapeutic Use(s)
Bromelain	Burn and wound care
Burdock (*Arctium lappa*)	Burns
Calendula (*Calendula officinalis* L.), marigold	Burns
Chamomile (*Matricaria recutita*, *Chamaemelum nobile*)	Burns
DHEA (dehydroepiandrosterone)	Burns
Echinacea (*Echinacea angustifolia* DC., *E. pallida*, *E. purpurea*)	Burn wounds
Elder (*Sambucus nigra* L.)	Burns
Eucalyptus oil (*Eucalyptus globulus* Labillardiere, *E. fructicetorum* F. Von Mueller, *E. smithii* R.T. Baker)	Burns
Fenugreek (*Trigonella foenum-graecum* L.)	Burns
Flaxseed and flaxseed oil (*Linum usitatissimum*)	Burns (poultice)
Ginger (*Zingiber officinale* Roscoe)	Burns (applied to the skin)
Ginseng (American ginseng, Asian ginseng, Chinese ginseng, Korean red ginseng, *Panax ginseng*: *Panax* spp. including *P. ginseng* C.C. Meyer and *P. quincefolium* L., excluding *Eleutherococcus senticosus*)	Burns
Marshmallow (*Althaea officinalis* L.)	Burns (topical)
Passionflower (*Passiflora incarnata* L.)	Burns (skin)
Red clover (*Trifolium pratense*)	Burns
Slippery elm (*Ulmus rubra* Muhl., *U. fulva* Michx.)	Burns
St. John's wort (*Hypericum perforatum* L.)	Burns (topical)
Tea tree oil (*Melaleuca alternifolia* [Maiden & Betche] Cheel)	Burns
Thyme (*Thymus vulgaris* L.), thymol	Burns

CANCER/CANCER PREVENTION AND RELATED CONDITIONS

Levels of Scientific Evidence for Specific Therapies

GRADE: C (Unclear or Conflicting Scientific Evidence)

Therapy	Specific Therapeutic Use(s)
Aloe (*Aloe vera*)	Cancer prevention
Antineoplastons	Cancer
Arginine (L-arginine)	Gastrointestinal cancer surgery
Astragalus (*Astragalus membranaceus*)	Cancer
Bitter melon (*Momordica charantia* L.), MAP30	Cancer
Black tea (*Camellia sinensis*)	Cancer prevention
Bladderwrack (*Fucus vesiculosus*)	Cancer
Bromelain	Cancer
Chaparral (*Larrea tridentata* DC. Coville, *L. divaricata* Cav.), nordihydroguaiaretic acid (NDGA)	Cancer
Coenzyme Q10	Breast cancer
Cranberry (*Vaccinium macrocarpon*)	Cancer prevention
Dandelion (*Taraxacum officinale*)	Cancer
DHEA (dehydroepiandrosterone)	Cervical dysplasia
Echinacea (*Echinacea angustifolia* DC., *E. pallida*, *E. purpurea*)	Cancer
Essiac	Cancer
Evening primrose oil (*Oenothera biennis* L.)	Breast cancer
Flaxseed and flaxseed oil (*Linum usitatissimum*)	Breast cancer (flaxseed, not flaxseed oil)
Garlic (*Allium sativum* L.)	Cancer prevention
Ginseng (American ginseng, Asian ginseng, Chinese ginseng, Korean red ginseng, *Panax ginseng*: *Panax* spp. including *P. ginseng* C.C. Meyer and *P. quincefolium* L., excluding *Eleutherococcus senticosus*)	Cancer prevention
Green tea (*Camellia sinensis*)	Cancer prevention
Hoxsey formula	Cancer

Continued

Lavender (*Lavandula angustifolia* Miller)	Cancer (perillyl alcohol)
Lycopene	Breast cancer prevention
Lycopene	Cancer prevention (general)
Lycopene	Cervical cancer prevention
Lycopene	Lung cancer prevention
Lycopene	Prostate cancer prevention
Maitake mushroom (*Grifola frondosa*), beta-glucan	Cancer
Melatonin	Cancer treatment
Milk thistle (*Silybum marianum*), silymarin	Cancer prevention
Oleander (*Nerium oleander, Thevetia peruviana*)	Cancer
Omega-3 fatty acids, fish oil, alpha-linolenic acid	Cancer prevention
Omega-3 fatty acids, fish oil, alpha-linolenic acid	Colon cancer
PC-SPES	Prostate cancer
Red clover (*Trifolium pratense*)	Prostate cancer
Seaweed, kelp, bladderwrack (*Fucus vesicu*losus)	Cancer
Shark cartilage	Cancer (solid tumors)
Slippery elm (*Ulmus rubra* Muhl., *U. fulva* Michx.)	Cancer
Sorrel (*Rumex acetosa* L., *R. acetosella* L.), Sinupret	Cancer
Soy (*Glycine max* L. Merr.)	Breast cancer prevention
Soy (*Glycine* max L. Merr.)	Cancer treatment
Soy (*Glycine max* L. Merr.)	Colon cancer prevention
Soy (*Glycine max* L. Merr.)	Endometrial cancer prevention
Soy (*Glycine max* L. Merr.)	Prostate cancer prevention
Spirulina	Oral leukoplakia/cancer
Turmeric (*Curcuma longa* L.), curcumin	Cancer

GRADE: D (Fair Negative Scientific Evidence)

Therapy	Specific Therapeutic Use(s)
Bitter almond (*Prunus amygdalus* Batch var. *amara* DC. Focke), Laetrile	Cancer (Laetrile)

Flaxseed and flaxseed oil (*Linum usitatissimum*)	Prostate cancer (flaxseed, not flaxseed oil)

TRADITIONAL OR THEORETICAL USES THAT LACK SUFFICIENT EVIDENCE

Therapy	Specific Therapeutic Use(s)
Aloe (*Aloe vera*)	Untreatable tumors
American pennyroyal (*Hedeoma pulegioides* L.), European pennyroyal (*Mentha pulegium* L.)	Cancer
Antineoplastons	Acute lymphocytic leukemia
Antineoplastons	Adenocarcinoma
Antineoplastons	Astrocytoma
Antineoplastons	Basal cell epithelioma
Antineoplastons	Bladder cancer
Antineoplastons	Chronic lymphocytic leukemia
Antineoplastons	Colon cancer
Antineoplastons	Glioblastoma
Antineoplastons	Hepatocellular carcinoma
Antineoplastons	Malignant melanoma
Antineoplastons	Medulloblastoma
Antineoplastons	Metastatic synovial sarcoma
Antineoplastons	Promyelocytic leukemia
Antineoplastons	Prostate cancer
Antineoplastons	Rectal cancer
Antineoplastons	Skin cancer
Arginine (L-arginine)	Cancer
Astragalus (*Astragalus membranaceus*)	Leukemia
Astragalus (*Astragalus membranaceus*)	Lung cancer
Barley (*Hordeum vulgare* L.), germinated barley foodstuff (GBF)	Colon cancer
Bilberry (*Vaccinium myrtillus*)	Cancer
Black cohosh (*Cimicifuga racemosa* L. Nutt.)	Cervical dysplasia (abnormal pap smear)

Continued

Black tea (*Camellia sinensis*)	Melanoma
Blessed thistle (*Cnicus benedictus* L.)	Cervical dysplasia
Boron	Breast cancer
Boron	Cancer
Boron	Leukemia
Bromelain	Cancer prevention
Burdock (*Arctium lappa*)	Cancer
Calendula (*Calendula officinalis* L.), marigold	Skin cancer
Chamomile (*Matricaria recutita*, *Chamaemelum nobile*)	Cancer
Clay	Cancer
Coenzyme Q10	Cancer
Coenzyme Q10	Lung cancer
Cranberry (*Vaccinium macrocarpon*)	Cancer treatment
Dandelion (*Taraxacum officinale*)	Breast cancer
Dandelion (*Taraxacum officinale*)	Leukemia
Danshen (*Salvia miltiorrhiza*)	Cancer
Danshen (*Salvia miltiorrhiza*)	Leukemia
Danshen (*Salvia miltiorrhiza*)	Liver cancer
DHEA (dehydroepiandrosterone)	Bladder cancer
DHEA (dehydroepiandrosterone)	Breast cancer
DHEA (dehydroepiandrosterone)	Colon cancer
DHEA (dehydroepiandrosterone)	Pancreatic cancer
DHEA (dehydroepiandrosterone)	Prostate cancer
Dong quai (*Angelica sinensis* [Oliv.] Diels), Chinese angelica	Cancer
Dong quai (*Angelica sinensis* [Oliv.] Diels), Chinese angelica	Stomach cancer
Echinacea (*Echinacea angustifolia* DC., *E. pallida*, *E. purpurea*)	Cancer
Elder (*Sambucus nigra* L.)	Cancer

Essiac	Bladder cancer
Essiac	Breast cancer
Essiac	Colon cancer
Essiac	Endometrial cancer
Essiac	Head/neck cancers
Essiac	Leukemia
Essiac	Lip cancer
Essiac	Liver cancer (hepatocellular carcinoma)
Essiac	Lung cancer
Essiac	Lymphoma
Essiac	Multiple myeloma
Essiac	Ovarian cancer
Essiac	Pancreatic cancer
Essiac	Prostate cancer
Essiac	Stomach cancer
Essiac	Throat cancer
Essiac	Tongue cancer
Eucalyptus oil (*Eucalyptus globulus* Labillardiere, *E. fructicetorum* F. Von Mueller, *E. smithii* R.T. Baker)	Cancer prevention
Evening primrose oil (*Oenothera biennis* L.)	Cancer
Evening primrose oil (*Oenothera biennis* L.)	Melanoma
Eyebright (*Euphrasia officinalis*)	Cancer
Flaxseed and flaxseed oil (*Linum usitatissimum*)	Colon cancer
Flaxseed and flaxseed oil (*Linum usitatissimum*)	Melanoma
Ginger (*Zingiber officinale* Roscoe)	Cancer
Ginkgo (*Ginkgo biloba* L.)	Cancer
Ginseng (American ginseng, Asian ginseng, Chinese ginseng, Korean red ginseng, *Panax ginseng*: *Panax* spp. including *P.* ginseng C.C. Meyer and *P. quincefolium* L., excluding *Eleutherococcus senticosus*)	Aplastic anemia

Continued

Ginseng (American ginseng, Asian ginseng, Chinese ginseng, Korean red ginseng, *Panax ginseng*: *Panax* spp. including *P. ginseng* C.C. Meyer and *P. quincefolium* L., excluding *Eleutherococcus senticosus*)	Breast cancer
Ginseng (American ginseng, Asian ginseng, Chinese ginseng, Korean red ginseng, *Panax ginseng*: *Panax* spp. including *P. ginseng* C.C. Meyer and *P. quincefolium* L., excluding *Eleutherococcus senticosus*)	Cancer prevention
Ginseng (American ginseng, Asian ginseng, Chinese ginseng, Korean red ginseng, *Panax ginseng*: *Panax* spp. including *P. ginseng* C.C. Meyer and *P. quincefolium* L., excluding *Eleutherococcus senticosus*)	Malignant tumors
Ginseng (American ginseng, Asian ginseng, Chinese ginseng, Korean red ginseng, *Panax ginseng*: *Panax* spp. including *P. ginseng* C.C. Meyer and *P. quincefolium* L., excluding *Eleutherococcus senticosus*)	Prostate cancer
Ginseng (American ginseng, Asian ginseng, Chinese ginseng, Korean red ginseng, *Panax ginseng*: *Panax* spp. including *P. ginseng* C.C. Meyer and *P. quincefolium* L., excluding *Eleutherococcus senticosus*)	Stomach cancer
Goldenseal (*Hydrastis canadensis* L.), berberine	Cancer
Green tea (*Camellia sinensis*)	Fibrosarcoma
Green tea (*Camellia sinensis*)	Liver cancer
Green tea (*Camellia sinensis*)	Lung cancer
Green tea (*Camellia sinensis*)	Ovarian cancer
Guggul (*Commifora mukul*)	Tumors
Gymnema (*Gymnema Sylvestre* R. Br.)	Cancer
Hawthorn (*Crataegus laevigata*, *C. oxyacantha*, *C. monogyna*, *C. pentagyna*)	Cancer
Hops (*Humulus lupulus* L.)	Breast cancer
Hops (*Humulus lupulus* L.)	Cancer (general)
Horsetail (*Equisetum arvense* L.)	Cancer
Hoxsey formula	Breast cancer
Hoxsey formula	Cervical cancer

Hoxsey formula	Colon cancer
Hoxsey formula	Lung cancer
Hoxsey formula	Lymphoma
Hoxsey formula	Melanoma
Hoxsey formula	Mouth cancer
Hoxsey formula	Prostate cancer
Hoxsey formula	Sarcomas
Kava (*Piper methysticum* G. Forst)	Cancer
Lactobacillus acidophilus	Cancer
Lactobacillus acidophilus	Colon cancer prevention
Licorice (*Glycyrrhiza glabra* L.), deglycyrrhizinated licorice (DGL)	Aplastic anemia
Licorice (*Glycyrrhiza glabra* L.), deglycyrrhizinated licorice (DGL)	Cancer
Licorice (*Glycyrrhiza glabra* L.), deglycyrrhizinated licorice (DGL)	Colorectal cancer
Licorice (*Glycyrrhiza glabra* L.), deglycyrrhizinated licorice (DGL)	Lung cancer
Lycopene	Bladder cancer
Lycopene	Breast cancer
Lycopene	Esophageal cancer
Lycopene	Laryngeal cancer
Lycopene	Melanoma
Lycopene	Mesothelioma
Lycopene	Ovarian cancer
Lycopene	Pancreatic cancer
Lycopene	Pharyngeal cancer
Lycopene	Skin cancer
Lycopene	Stomach cancer
Marshmallow (*Althaea officinalis* L.)	Cancer
Milk thistle (*Silybum marianum*), silymarin	Breast cancer

Continued

Milk thistle (*Silybum marianum*), silymarin	Liver cancer
Niacin (vitamin B_3, nicotinic acid), niacinamide, and inositol hexanicotinate	Cancer prevention
Niacin (vitamin B_3, nicotinic acid), niacinamide, and inositol hexanicotinate	Prostate cancer
Niacin (vitamin B_3, nicotinic acid), niacinamide, and inositol hexanicotinate	Tumor detection
Omega-3 fatty acids, fish oil, alpha-linolenic acid	Leukemia
Omega-3 fatty acids, fish oil, alpha-linolenic acid	Prostate cancer prevention
Passionflower (*Passiflora incarnata* L.)	Cancer
PC-SPES	Breast cancer
PC-SPES	Cancer prevention
PC-SPES	Leukemia
PC-SPES	Lymphoma
PC-SPES	Melanoma
Peppermint (*Mentha x piperita* L.)	Cancer
Polypodium leucotomos extract, Anapsos	Cancer
Propolis	Cancer
Propolis	Nasopharyngeal carcinoma
Psyllium (*Plantago ovata*, *P. ispaghula*)	Colon cancer prevention
Pygeum (*Prunus africana*, *Pygeum africanum*)	Prostate cancer
Red clover (*Trifolium pratense*)	Cancer prevention
Saw palmetto (*Serenoa repens* [Bartram] Small)	Cancer
Sorrel (*Rumex acetosa* L., *R. acetosella* L.), Sinupret	Skin cancer
Soy (*Glycine max* L. Merr.)	Cancer prevention (general)
Soy (*Glycine max* L. Merr.)	Gastric cancer
Soy (*Glycine max* L. Merr.)	Urinary tract cancer
Spirulina	Cancer prevention
St. John's wort (*Hypericum perforatum* L.)	Cancer
Sweet almond (*Prunus amygdalus dulcis*)	Bladder cancer

Sweet almond (*Prunus amygdalus dulcis*)	Breast cancer
Sweet almond (*Prunus amygdalus dulcis*)	Colon cancer
Sweet almond (*Prunus amygdalus dulcis*)	Mouth and throat cancers
White horehound (*Marrubium vulgare*)	Cancer

CARPAL TUNNEL SYNDROME AND RELATED CONDITIONS

Levels of Scientific Evidence for Specific Therapies

TRADITIONAL OR THEORETICAL USES THAT LACK SUFFICIENT EVIDENCE

Therapy	Specific Therapeutic Use(s)
Bromelain	Carpal tunnel syndrome
Chamomile (*Matricaria recutita, Chamaemelum nobile*)	Carpal tunnel syndrome
Lavender (*Lavandula angustifolia* Miller)	Carpal tunnel syndrome

CATARACTS AND RELATED CONDITIONS

Levels of Scientific Evidence for Specific Therapies

GRADE: C (Unclear or Conflicting Scientific Evidence)

Therapy	Specific Therapeutic Use(s)
Bilberry (*Vaccinium myrtillus*)	Cataracts
Danshen (*Salvia miltiorrhiza*)	Glaucoma
Ginkgo (*Ginkgo biloba* L.)	Glaucoma
Melatonin	Glaucoma

TRADITIONAL OR THEORETICAL USES THAT LACK SUFFICIENT EVIDENCE

Therapy	Specific Therapeutic Use(s)
Arginine (L-arginine)	Glaucoma
Belladonna (*Atropa belladonna* L. or its variety *acuminata* Royle ex Lindl)	Glaucoma
Betel nut (*Areca catechu* L.)	Glaucoma
Bilberry (*Vaccinium myrtillus*)	Glaucoma

Continued

Danshen (*Salvia miltiorrhiza*)	Cataracts
Dong quai (*Angelica sinensis* [Oliv.] Diels), Chinese angelica	Glaucoma
Eyebright (*Euphrasia officinalis*)	Cataracts
Green tea (*Camellia sinensis*)	Cataracts
Lycopene	Cataracts
Melatonin	Glaucoma
Niacin (vitamin B_3, nicotinic acid), niacinamide, and inositol hexanicotinate	Cataract prevention
Omega-3 fatty acids, fish oil, alpha-linolenic acid	Glaucoma
Shark cartilage	Glaucoma
Turmeric (*Curcuma longa* L.), curcumin	Cataracts

CEREBRAL INSUFFICIENCY AND RELATED CONDITIONS

Levels of Scientific Evidence for Specific Therapies

GRADE: B (Good Scientific Evidence)

Therapy	Specific Therapeutic Use(s)
Ginkgo (*Ginkgo biloba* L.)	Cerebral insufficiency
Ginseng (American ginseng, Asian ginseng, Chinese ginseng, Korean red ginseng, *Panax ginseng*: *Panax* spp. including *P. ginseng* C.C. Meyer and *P. quincefolium* L., excluding *Eleutherococcus senticosus*)	Mental performance

GRADE: C (Unclear or Conflicting Scientific Evidence)

Therapy	Specific Therapeutic Use(s)
Black tea (*Camellia sinensis*)	Memory enhancement
Black tea (*Camellia sinensis*)	Mental performance/alertness
Boron	Improving cognitive function
Ginkgo (*Ginkgo biloba* L.)	Age-associated memory impairment (AAMI)
Ginkgo (*Ginkgo biloba* L.)	Memory enhancement (in healthy people)

Therapy	Specific Therapeutic Use(s)
Green tea (*Camellia sinensis*)	Memory enhancement
Green tea (*Camellia sinensis*)	Mental performance/alertness
Polypodium leucotomos extract, Anapsos	Dementia

GRADE: D (Fair Negative Scientific Evidence)

Therapy	Specific Therapeutic Use(s)
DHEA (dehydroepiandrosterone)	Brain function and well-being in the elderly

TRADITIONAL OR THEORETICAL USES THAT LACK SUFFICIENT EVIDENCE

Therapy	Specific Therapeutic Use(s)
Arginine (L-arginine)	Dementia
Astragalus (*Astragalus membranaceus*)	Dementia
Astragalus (*Astragalus membranaceus*)	Memory
Blessed thistle (*Cnicus benedictus* L.)	Memory improvement
Danshen (*Salvia miltiorrhiza*)	Anoxic brain injury
DHEA (dehydroepiandrosterone)	Dementia
Eyebright (*Euphrasia officinalis*)	Memory loss
Garlic (*Allium sativum* L.)	Age-related memory problems
Ginseng (American ginseng, Asian ginseng, Chinese ginseng, Korean red ginseng, *Panax ginseng*: *Panax* spp. including *P. ginseng* C.C. Meyer and *P. quincefolium* L., excluding *Eleutherococcus senticosus*)	Dementia
Ginseng (American ginseng, Asian ginseng, Chinese ginseng, Korean red ginseng, *Panax ginseng*: *Panax* spp. including *P. ginseng* C.C. Meyer and *P. quincefolium* L., excluding *Eleutherococcus senticosus*)	Improved memory and thinking after menopause
Ginseng (American ginseng, Asian ginseng, Chinese ginseng, Korean red ginseng, *Panax ginseng*: *Panax* spp. including **P.** *ginseng* C.C. Meyer and *P. quincefolium* L., excluding *Eleutherococcus senticosus*)	Senile dementia
Gotu kola (*Centella asiatica* L.), total triterpenic fraction of *Centella asiatica* (TTFCA)	Memory enhancement
Green tea (*Camellia sinensis*)	Cognitive performance enhancement

Continued

Therapy	Specific Therapeutic Use(s)
Kava (*Piper methysticum* G. Forst)	Brain damage
Lycopene	Cognitive function
Melatonin	Cognitive enhancement
Melatonin	Memory enhancement
Niacin (vitamin B_3, nicotinic acid), niacinamide, and inositol hexanicotinate	Memory loss
Omega-3 fatty acids, fish oil, alpha-linolenic acid	Memory enhancement
Soy (*Glycine max* L. Merr.)	Cognitive function
Soy (*Glycine max* L. Merr.)	Memory enhancement
Spirulina	Memory improvement
Valerian (*Valeriana officinalis* L.)	Memory
Yohimbe bark extract (*Pausinystalia yohimbe* Pierre ex Beille)	Cognition

CEREBROVASCULAR ACCIDENT (STROKE) AND RELATED CONDITIONS

Levels of Scientific Evidence for Specific Therapies

GRADE: C (Unclear or Conflicting Scientific Evidence)

Therapy	Specific Therapeutic Use(s)
Betel nut (*Areca catechu* L.)	Stroke recovery
Danshen (*Salvia miltiorrhiza*)	Ischemic stroke
Melatonin	Stroke
Omega-3 fatty acids, fish oil, alpha-linolenic acid	Stroke prevention

GRADE: D (Fair Negative Scientific Evidence)

Therapy	Specific Therapeutic Use(s)
Ginkgo (*Ginkgo biloba* L.)	Stroke

TRADITIONAL OR THEORETICAL USES THAT LACK SUFFICIENT EVIDENCE

Therapy	Specific therapeutic Use(s)
Arginine (L-arginine)	Ischemic stroke

Arginine (L-arginine)	Stroke
Astragalus (*Astragalus membranaceus*)	Stroke
Dong quai (*Angelica sinensis* [Oliv.] Diels), Chinese angelica	Stroke
Garlic (*Allium sativum* L.)	Stroke
Ginseng (American ginseng, Asian ginseng, Chinese ginseng, Korean red ginseng, *Panax ginseng*: *Panax* spp. including *P. ginseng* C.C. Meyer and *P. quincefolium* L., excluding *Eleutherococcus senticosus*)	Strokes
Green tea (*Camellia sinensis*)	Ischemia-reperfusion injury protection
Green tea (*Camellia sinensis*)	Stroke prevention
Kava (*Piper methysticum* G. Forst)	Cerebral ischemia
Lycopene	Stroke prevention
Niacin (vitamin B_3, nicotinic acid), niacinamide, and inositol hexanicotinate	Ischemia-reperfusion injury prevention

CHEMOTHERAPY SIDE EFFECTS AND RELATED CONDITIONS

Levels of Scientific Evidence for Specific Therapies

GRADE: B (Good Scientific Evidence)

Therapy	Specific Therapeutic Use(s)
Omega-3 fatty acids, fish oil, alpha-linolenic acid	Protection from cyclosporine toxicity in organ transplant patients

GRADE: C (Unclear or Conflicting Scientific Evidence)

Therapy	Specific therapeutic Use(s)
Astragalus (*Astragalus membranaceus*)	Chemotherapy side effects
Coenzyme Q10	Anthracycline chemotherapy heart toxicity
Ginkgo (*Ginkgo biloba* L.)	Chemotherapy side effects
Melatonin	Chemotherapy side effects

Continued

TRADITIONAL OR THEORETICAL USES THAT LACK SUFFICIENT EVIDENCE	
Therapy	Specific Therapeutic Use(s)
Danshen (*Salvia miltiorrhiza*)	Bleomycin induced lung fibrosis
Dong quai (*Angelica sinensis* [Oliv.] Diels), Chinese angelica	Bleomycin-induced lung damage
Essiac	Chemotherapy side effects
Ginseng (American ginseng, Asian ginseng, Chinese ginseng, Korean red ginseng, *Panax ginseng*: *Panax* spp. including *P. ginseng* C.C. Meyer and *P. quincefolium* L., excluding *Eleutherococcus senticosus*)	Chemotherapy support
Omega-3 fatty acids, fish oil, alpha-linolenic acid	Anthracycline-induced cardiac toxicity
Omega-3 fatty acids, fish oil, alpha-linolenic acid	Protection from isotretinoin drug toxicity

CHOLELITHIASIS AND RELATED CONDITIONS

Levels of Scientific Evidence for Specific Therapies

GRADE: C (Unclear or Conflicting Scientific Evidence)	
Therapy	Specific Therapeutic Use(s)
Globe artichoke (*Cynara scolymus* L.)	Choleretic (bile flow stimulant)
Soy (*Glycine max* L. Merr.)	Gallstones (cholelithiasis)
Turmeric (*Curcuma longa* L.), curcumin	Gallstone prevention/bile flow stimulant
White horehound (*Marrubium vulgare*)	Choleretic (dyspepsia, appetite stimulation)

TRADITIONAL OR THEORETICAL USES THAT LACK SUFFICIENT EVIDENCE	
Therapy	Specific Therapeutic Use(s)
American pennyroyal (*Hedeoma pulegioides* L.), European pennyroyal (*Mentha pulegium* L.)	Gallbladder disorders
Black cohosh (*Cimicifuga racemosa* L. Nutt.)	Gallbladder disorders
Blessed thistle (*Cnicus benedictus* L.)	Choleretic (bile flow stimulant)

Blessed thistle (*Cnicus benedictus* L.)	Gallbladder disease
Cranberry (*Vaccinium macrocarpon*)	Gallbladder stones
Dandelion (*Taraxacum officinale*)	Bile flow stimulation
Dandelion (*Taraxacum officinale*)	Gallbladder disease
Dandelion (*Taraxacum officinale*)	Gallstones
Devil's claw (*Harpagophytum procumbens* DC.)	Choleretic (bile secretion)
Dong quai (*Angelica sinensis* [Oliv.] Diels), Chinese angelica	Cholagogue
Garlic (*Allium sativum* L.)	Bile secretion problems
Garlic (*Allium sativum* L.)	Gallstones
Ginger (*Zingiber officinale* Roscoe)	Bile secretion problems
Globe artichoke (*Cynara scolymus* L.)	Cholegogue
Globe artichoke (*Cynara scolymus* L.)	Cholelithiasis
Goldenseal (*Hydrastis canadensis* L.), berberine	Bile flow stimulant
Goldenseal (*Hydrastis canadensis* L.), berberine	Gallstones
Horse chestnut (*Aesculus hippocastanum* L.)	Gallbladder infection (cholecystitis)
Horse chestnut (*Aesculus hippocastanum* L.)	Gallbladder pain (colic)
Horse chestnut (*Aesculus hippocastanum* L.)	Gall ladder stones (cholelithiasis)
Lavender (*Lavandula angustifolia* Miller)	Cholagogue
Lavender (*Lavandula angustifolia* Miller)	Choleretic
Milk thistle (*Silybum marianum*), silymarin	Cholelithiasis
Omega-3 fatty acids, fish oil, alpha-linolenic acid	Gallstones
Peppermint (*Mentha x piperita* L.)	Bile duct disorders
Peppermint (*Mentha x piperita* L.)	Cholelithiasis (gallstones)
Peppermint (*Mentha x piperita* L.)	Gallbladder disorders
Psyllium (*Plantago ovata, P. ispaghula*)	Gallstones
Turmeric (*Curcuma longa* L.), curcumin	Gallstones
White horehound (*Marrubium vulgare*)	Bile secretion

Continued

White horehound (*Marrubium vulgare*)	Gallbladder complaints
Wild yam (*Dioscorea villosa*)	Bile flow improvement
Wild yam (*Dioscorea villosa*)	Biliary colic

CHRONIC OBSTRUCTIVE PULMONARY DISEASE AND RELATED CONDITIONS

Levels of Scientific Evidence for Specific Therapies

GRADE: B (Good Scientific Evidence)

Therapy	Specific therapeutic Use(s)
Boswellia (*Boswellia serrata* Roxb.)	Asthma (chronic therapy)
Ephedra (*Ephedra sinica*)/ma huang	Asthmatic bronchoconstriction

GRADE: C (Unclear or Conflicting Scientific Evidence)

Therapy	Specific Therapeutic Use(s)
Belladonna (*Atropa belladonna* L. or its variety *acuminata* Royle ex Lindl)	Airway obstruction
Black tea (*Camellia sinensis*)	Asthma
Bromelain	Chronic obstructive pulmonary disease (COPD)
Danshen (*Salvia miltiorrhiza*)	Asthmatic bronchitis
Green tea (*Camellia sinensis*)	Asthma
Lactobacillus acidophilus	Asthma
Lycopene	Asthma caused by exercise
Omega-3 fatty acids, fish oil, alpha-linolenic acid	Asthma

GRADE: D (Fair Negative Scientific Evidence)

Therapy	Specific Therapeutic Use(s)
Evening primrose oil (*Oenothera biennis* L.)	Asthma

GRADE: F (Strong Negative Scientific Evidence)

Therapy	Specific Therapeutic Use(s)
Arginine (L-arginine)	Asthma

TRADITIONAL OR THEORETICAL USES THAT LACK SUFFICIENT EVIDENCE

Therapy	Specific Therapeutic Use(s)
Alfalfa (*Medicago sativa* L.)	Asthma
Aloe (*Aloe vera*)	Asthma
Astragalus (*Astragalus membranaceus*)	Asthma
Astragalus (*Astragalus membranaceus*)	Shortness of breath
Barley (*Hordeum vulgare* L.), germinated barley foodstuff (GBF)	Asthma
Belladonna (*Atropa belladonna* L. or its variety *acuminata* Royle ex Lindl)	Asthma
Betel nut (*Areca catechu* L.)	Asthma
Black cohosh (*Cimicifuga racemosa* L. Nutt.)	Asthma
Boswellia (*Boswellia serrata* Roxb.)	Chronic obstructive pulmonary disease (COPD)
Clove (*Eugenia aromatica*)	Asthma
Coenzyme Q10	Asthma
Coenzyme Q10	Breathing difficulties
Coenzyme Q10	Chronic obstructive pulmonary disease (COPD)
DHEA (dehydroepiandrosterone)	Asthma
Dong quai (*Angelica sinensis* [Oliv.] Diels), Chinese angelica	Asthma
Dong quai (*Angelica sinensis* [Oliv.] Diels), Chinese angelica	Chronic obstructive pulmonary disease (COPD)
Elder (*Sambucus nigra L.*)	Asthma
Elder (*Sambucus nigra* L.)	Respiratory distress
Ephedra *(Ephedra sinica)*/ma huang	Dyspnea
Essiac	Asthma
Eucalyptus oil (*Eucalyptus globulus* Labillardiere, *E. fructicetorum* F. Von Mueller, E. *smithii* R.T. Baker)	Asthma
Eucalyptus oil (*Eucalyptus globulus* Labillardiere, *E. fructicetorum* F. Von Mueller, *E. smithii* R.T. Baker)	Chronic obstructive pulmonary disease (COPD)

Continued

Eucalyptus oil (*Eucalyptus globulus* Labillardiere, *E. fructicetorum* F. Von Mueller, *E. smithii* R.T. Baker)	Emphysema
Eyebright (*Euphrasia officinalis*)	Asthma
Feverfew (*Tanacetum parthenium* L. Schultz-Bip.)	Asthma
Flaxseed and flaxseed oil (*Linum usitatissimum*)	Bronchial irritation
Garlic (*Allium sativum* L.)	Asthma
Ginger (*Zingiber officinale* Roscoe)	Asthma
Ginkgo (*Ginkgo biloba* L.)	Asthma
Ginseng (American ginseng, Asian ginseng, Chinese ginseng, Korean red ginseng, *Panax ginseng*: *Panax* spp. including *P. ginseng* C.C. Meyer and *P. quincefolium* L., excluding *Eleutherococcus senticosus*)	Asthma
Ginseng (American ginseng, Asian ginseng, Chinese ginseng, Korean red ginseng, *Panax ginseng*: *Panax* spp. including *P. ginseng* C.C. Meyer and *P. quincefolium* L., excluding *Eleutherococcus senticosus*)	Breathing difficulty
Ginseng (American ginseng, Asian ginseng, Chinese ginseng, Korean red ginseng, *Panax ginseng*: *Panax* spp. including *P. ginseng* C.C. Meyer and *P. quincefolium* L., excluding *Eleutherococcus senticosus*)	Bronchodilation
Goldenseal (*Hydrastis canadensis* L.), berberine	Asthma
Gotu kola (*Centella asiatica* L.), total triterpenic fraction of *Centella asiatica* (TTFCA)	Asthma
Guggul (*Commifora mukul*)	Asthma
Hawthorn (*Crataegus laevigata*, *C. oxyacantha*, *C. monogyna*, *C. pentagyna*)	Asthma
Hawthorn (*Crataegus laevigata*, *C. oxyacantha*, *C. monogyna*, *C. pentagyna*)	Dyspnea
Kava (*Piper methysticum* G. Forst)	Asthma
Lavender (*Lavandula angustifolia* Miller)	Asthma
Licorice (*Glycyrrhiza glabra* L.), deglycyrrhizinated licorice (DGL)	Asthma
Melatonin	Asthma
Oleander (*Nerium oleander*, *Thevetia peruviana*)	Asthma

Omega-3 fatty acids, fish oil, alpha-linolenic acid	Chronic obstructive pulmonary disease (COPD)
Passionflower (*Passiflora incarnata* L.)	Asthma
Peppermint (*Mentha x piperita* L.)	Asthma
Polypodium leucotomos extract, Anapsos	Asthma
Red clover (*Trifolium pratense*)	Asthma
Saw palmetto (*Serenoa repens* [Bartram] Small)	Asthma
Slippery elm (*Ulmus rubra* Muhl., *U. fulva* Michx.)	Respiratory disorders
Thyme (*Thymus vulgaris* L.), thymol	Asthma
Thyme (*Thymus vulgaris* L.), thymol	Dyspnea
Turmeric (*Curcuma longa* L.), curcumin	Asthma
Valerian (*Valeriana officinalis* L.)	Asthma
Valerian (*Valeriana officinalis* L.)	Bronchospasm
White horehound (*Marrubium vulgare*)	Asthma
White horehound (*Marrubium vulgare*)	Chronic obstructive pulmonary disease (COPD)
White horehound (*Marrubium vulgare*)	Wheezing
Wild (*Dioscorea villosa*)	Asthma

CHRONIC VENOUS INSUFFICIENCY AND RELATED CONDITIONS

Levels of Scientific Evidence for Specific Therapies

GRADE: A (Strong Scientific Evidence)

Therapy	Specific Therapeutic Use(s)
Horse chestnut (*Aesculus hippocastanum* L.)	Chronic venous insufficiency

GRADE: B (Good Scientific Evidence)

Therapy	Specific Therapeutic Use(s)
Gotu kola (*Centella asiatica* L.), total triterpenic fraction of *Centella asiatica* (TTFCA)	Chronic venous insufficiency/varicose veins

Continued

GRADE: C (Unclear or Conflicting Scientific Evidence)	
Therapy	Specific Therapeutic Use(s)
Bilberry (*Vaccinium myrtillus*)	Chronic venous insufficiency
Glucosamine	Chronic venous insufficiency

TRADITIONAL OR THEORETICAL USES THAT LACK SUFFICIENT EVIDENCE	
Therapy	Specific Therapeutic Use(s)
Astragalus (Astragalus membranaceus)	Edema
Barley (*Hordeum vulgare* L.), germinated barley foodstuff (GBF)	Improved blood circulation
Bilberry (*Vaccinium myrtillus*)	Poor circulation
Black cohosh (*Cimicifuga racemosa* L. Nutt.)	Edema
Black tea (*Camellia sinensis*)	Circulatory/blood flow disorders
Bladderwrack (*Fucus vesiculosus*)	Edema
Bromelain	Varicose veins
Burdock (*Arctium lappa*)	Fluid retention
Calendula (*Calendula officinalis* L.), marigold	Circulation problems
Calendula (Calendula officinalis L.), marigold	Edema
Calendula (*Calendula officinalis* L.), marigold	Varicose veins
Dandelion (*Taraxacum officinale*)	Circulation
Dandelion (*Taraxacum officinale*)	Dropsy
Danshen (*Salvia miltiorrhiza*)	Circulation
Devil's claw (*Harpagophytum procumbens* DC.)	Edema
Dong quai (*Angelica sinensis* [Oliv.] Diels), Chinese angelica	Fluid retention
Elder (*Sambucus nigra* L.)	Circulatory stimulant
Elder (*Sambucus nigra* L.)	Edema
Ephedra (*Ephedra sinica*)/ma huang	Edema
Fenugreek (*Trigonella foenum-graecum* L.)	Dropsy
Ginkgo (*Ginkgo biloba* L.)	Swelling

Globe artichoke (*Cynara scolymus* L.)	Peripheral edema
Goldenseal (*Hydrastis canadensis* L.), berberine	Circulatory stimulant
Gotu kola (*Centella asiatica* L.), total triterpenic fraction of *Centella asiatica* (TTFCA)	Vascular fragility
Green tea (*Camellia sinensis*)	Improving blood flow
Hawthorn (*Crataegus laevigata*, *C. oxyacantha*, *C. monogyna*, *C. pentagyna*)	Edema
Horsetail (*Equisetum arvense* L.)	Dropsy
Lavender (*Lavandula angustifolia* Miller)	Circulation problems
Lavender (*Lavandula angustifolia* Miller)	Varicose veins
Melatonin	Edema
Milk thistle (*Silybum marianum*), silymarin	Edema
Niacin (Vitamin B_3, nicotinic acid), niacinamide, and inositol hexanicotinate	Edema
Oleander (*Nerium oleander*, *Thevetia peruviana*)	Swelling
Polypodium leucotomos extract, Anapsos	Water retention
Seaweed, kelp, bladderwrack (*Fucus vesiculosus*)	Edema
Slippery elm (*Ulmus rubra* Muhl., *U. fulva* Michx.)	Varicose ulcers
Thyme (*Thymus vulgaris* L.), thymol	Edema
White horehound (*Marrubium vulgare*)	Water retention

CIRRHOSIS AND RELATED CONDITIONS

Levels of Scientific Evidence for Specific Therapies

GRADE: B (Good Scientific Evidence)

Therapy	Specific Therapeutic Use(s)
Milk thistle (*Silybum marianum*), silymarin	Cirrhosis
Milk thistle (*Silybum marianum*), silymarin	Hepatitis (chronic)

GRADE: C (Unclear or Conflicting Scientific Evidence)

Therapy	Specific Therapeutic Use(s)
Astragalus (*Astragalus membranaceus*)	Liver protection
Clay	Protection from aflatoxins

Continued

Dandelion (*Taraxacum officinale*)	Hepatitis B
Danshen (*Salvia miltiorrhiza*)	Liver disease (cirrhosis/chronic hepatitis B)
Eyebright (*Euphrasia officinalis*)	Hepatoprotection
Lactobacillus acidophilus	Hepatic encephalopathy (confused thinking due to liver disorders)
Licorice (*Glycyrrhiza glabra* L.), deglycyrrhizinated licorice (DGL)	Viral hepatitis
Milk thistle (*Silybum marianum*), silymarin	Acute viral hepatitis
Milk thistle (*Silybum marianum*), silymarin	*Amanita phalloides* mushroom toxicity
Milk thistle (*Silybum marianum*), silymarin	Drug/toxin-induced hepatotoxicity

TRADITIONAL OR THEORETICAL USES THAT LACK SUFFICIENT EVIDENCE

Therapy	Specific Therapeutic Use(s)
Alfalfa (*Medicago sativa* L.)	Jaundice
Aloe (*Aloe vera*)	Hepatitis
American pennyroyal (*Hedeoma pulegioides* L.), European pennyroyal (Mentha pulegium L.)	Liver disease
Arginine (L-arginine)	Ammonia toxicity
Arginine (L-arginine)	Hepatic encephalopathy
Arginine (L-arginine)	Liver disease
Astragalus (*Astragalus membranaceus*)	Chronic hepatitis
Astragalus (*Astragalus membranaceus*)	Liver disease
Bilberry (*Vaccinium myrtillus*)	Liver disease
Black cohosh (*Cimicifuga racemosa* L. Nutt.)	Liver disease
Blessed thistle (*Cnicus benedictus* L.)	Jaundice
Blessed thistle (*Cnicus benedictus* L.)	Liver disorders
Burdock (*Arctium lappa*)	Liver protection
Calendula (*Calendula officinalis* L.), marigold	Jaundice
Calendula (*calendula officinalis* l.), marigold	Liver dysfunction
Chamomile (*Matricaria recutita*, *Chamaemelum nobile*)	Liver disorders

Coenzyme Q10	Hepatitis B
Coenzyme Q10	Liver enlargement or disease
Cranberry (*Vaccinium macrocarpon*)	Liver disorders
Dandelion (*Taraxacum officinale*)	Jaundice
Dandelion (*Taraxacum officinale*)	Liver cleansing
Dandelion (*Taraxacum officinale*)	Liver disease
Devil's claw (*Harpagophytum procumbens* DC.)	Liver and gallbladder tonic
DHEA (dehydroepiandrosterone)	Liver protection
Dong quai (*Angelica sinensis* [Oliv.] Diels), Chinese angelica	Chronic hepatitis
Dong quai (*Angelica sinensis* [Oliv.] Diels), Chinese angelica	Cirrhosis
Dong quai (*Angelica sinensis* [Oliv.] Diels), Chinese angelica	Liver protection
Elder (*Sambucus nigra* L.)	Liver disease
Eucalyptus oil (*Eucalyptus globulus* Labillardiere, *E. fructicetorum* F. Von Mueller, *E. smithii* R.T. Baker)	Liver protection
Evening primrose oil (*Oenothera biennis* L.)	Hepatitis B
Eyebright (*Euphrasia officinalis*)	Jaundice
Eyebright (*Euphrasia officinalis*)	Liver disease
Garlic (*Allium sativum* L.)	Antitoxin
Garlic (*Allium sativum* L.)	Hepatopulmonary syndrome
Garlic (*Allium sativum* L.)	Liver health
Ginger (*Zingiber officinale* Roscoe)	Liver disease
Ginkgo (*Ginkgo biloba* L.)	Hepatitis B
Ginseng (American ginseng, Asian ginseng, Chinese ginseng, Korean red ginseng, *Panax ginseng*: *Panax* spp. including *P. ginseng* C.C. Meyer and *P. quincefolium* L., excluding *Eleutherococcus senticosus*)	Hepatitis/hepatitis B infection
Ginseng (American ginseng, Asian ginseng, Chinese ginseng, Korean red ginseng, *Panax ginseng*: Panax *spp.* including *P. ginseng* C.C. Meyer and *P. quincefolium* L., excluding *Eleutherococcus senticosus*)	Liver disease

Continued

Ginseng (American ginseng, Asian ginseng, Chinese ginseng, Korean red ginseng, *Panax ginseng*: *Panax* spp. including *P. ginseng* C.C. Meyer and *P. quincefolium* L., excluding *Eleutherococcus senticosus*)	Liver health
Globe artichoke (*Cynara scolymus* L.)	Jaundice
Goldenseal (*Hydrastis canadensis* L.), berberine	Alcoholic liver disease
Goldenseal (*Hydrastis canadensis* L.), berberine	Hepatitis
Goldenseal (*Hydrastis canadensis* L.), berberine	Jaundice
Goldenseal (Hydrastis canadensis L.), berberine	Liver disorders
Gotu kola (*Centella asiatica* L.), total triterpenic fraction of *Centella asiatica* (TTFCA)	Hepatitis
Gotu kola (*Centella asiatica* L.), total triterpenic fraction of *Centella asiatica* (TTFCA)	Jaundice
Gymnema (*Gymnema Sylvestre* R. Br.)	Liver disease
Gymnema (*Gymnema Sylvestre* R. Br.)	Liver protection
Horse chestnut (*Aesculus hippocastanum* L.)	Liver congestion
Horsetail (*Equisetum arvense* L.)	Liver protection
Licorice (*Glycyrrhiza glabra* L.), deglycyrrhizinated licorice (DGL)	Liver protection
Maitake mushroom (*Grifola frondosa*), beta-glucan	Liver inflammation (hepatitis)
Melatonin	Toxic liver damage
Milk thistle (*Silybum marianum*), silymarin	Jaundice
Milk thistle (*Silybum Marianum*), silymarin	Liver-cleansing agent
Niacin (vitamin B_3, nicotinic acid), niacinamide, and inositol hexanicotinate	Liver disease
Omega-3 fatty acids, fish oil, alpha-linolenic acid	Cirrhosis

CLAUDICATION AND RELATED CONDITIONS

Levels of Scientific Evidence for Specific Therapies

GRADE: A (Strong Scientific Evidence)

Therapy	Specific Therapeutic Use(s)
Ginkgo (*Ginkgo biloba* L.)	Claudication (painful legs from clogged arteries)

GRADE: C (Unclear or Conflicting Scientific Evidence)	
Therapy	Specific Therapeutic Use(s)
Arginine (L-arginine)	Peripheral vascular disease/ claudication
Garlic (*Allium sativum* L.)	Peripheral vascular disease (blocked arteries in the legs)

TRADITIONAL OR THEORETICAL USES THAT LACK SUFFICIENT EVIDENCE	
Therapy	Specific Therapeutic Use(s)
Garlic (*Allium sativum* L.)	Claudication (leg pain due to poor blood flow)
Niacin (vitamin B_3, nicotinic acid), niacinamide, and inositol hexanicotinate	Peripheral vascular disease
Omega-3 fatty acids, fish oil, alpha-linolenic acid	Peripheral vascular disease

CONGESTIVE HEART FAILURE (CHF) AND RELATED CONDITIONS

Levels of Scientific Evidence for Specific Therapies

GRADE: A (Strong Scientific Evidence)	
Therapy	Specific Therapeutic Use(s)
Hawthorn (*Crataegus laevigata*, *C. oxyacantha*, *C. monogyna*, *C. pentagyna*)	CHF

GRADE: C (Unclear or Conflicting Scientific Evidence)	
Therapy	Specific Therapeutic Use(s)
Arginine (L-arginine)	Heart failure (CHF)
Astragalus (*Astragalus membranaceus*)	Heart failure
Coenzyme Q10	Cardiomyopathy (dilated, hypertrophic)
Coenzyme Q10	Heart failure
DHEA (dehydroepiandrosterone)	Heart failure
Ginseng (American ginseng, Asian ginseng, Chinese ginseng, Korean red ginseng, *Panax ginseng*: *Panax* spp. including *P. ginseng* C.C. Meyer and *P. quincefolium* L., excluding *Eleutherococcus senticosus*)	CHF

Continued

Hawthorn (*Crataegus laevigata, C. oxyacantha, C. monogyna, C. pentagyna*)	Functional cardiovascular disorders
Oleander (Nerium oleander, *Thevetia peruviana*)	CHF
Passionflower (*Passiflora incarnata* L.)	CHF (exercise capacity)

GRADE: D (Fair Negative Scientific Evidence)

TRADITIONAL OR THEORETICAL USES THAT LACK SUFFICIENT EVIDENCE

Therapy	Specific Therapeutic Use(s)
Dandelion (*Taraxacum officinale*)	CHF
Danshen (*Salvia miltiorrhiza*)	Left ventricular hypertrophy
Dong quai (*Angelica sinensis* [Oliv.] Diels), Chinese angelica	CHF
Ginkgo (*Ginkgo biloba* L.)	CHF
Goldenseal (*Hydrastis canadensis* L.), berberine	Heart failure
Horse chestnut (*Aesculus hippocastanum* L.)	Fluid in the lungs (pulmonary edema)
Horsetail (*Equisetum arvense* L.)	Fluid in the lungs
Omega-3 fatty acids, fish oil, alpha-linolenic acid	CHF
Passionflower (*Passiflora incarnata* L.)	CHF (exercise ability)
Valerian (*Valeriana officinalis* L.)	CHF

CONSTIPATION AND RELATED CONDITIONS

Levels of Scientific Evidence for Specific Therapies

GRADE: A (Strong Scientific Evidence)

Therapy	Specific Therapeutic Use(s)
Aloe (*Aloe vera*)	Constipation (laxative)

GRADE: B (Good Scientific Evidence)

Therapy	Specific Therapeutic Use(s)
Flaxseed and flaxseed oil (*Linum usitatissimum*)	Laxative (flaxseed, not flaxseed oil)
Psyllium (*Plantago ovata, P. ispaghula*)	Constipation

GRADE: C (Unclear or Conflicting Scientific Evidence)	
Therapy	Specific therapeutic Use(s)
Barley (*Hordeum vulgare* L.), germinated barley foodstuff (GBF)	Constipation

TRADITIONAL OR THEORETICAL USES THAT LACK SUFFICIENT EVIDENCE	
Therapy	Specific Therapeutic Use(s)
Astragalus (*Astragalus membranaceus*)	Laxative
Bladderwrack (*Fucus vesiculosus*)	Laxative
Bladderwrack (*Fucus vesiculosus*)	Stool softener
Burdock (*Arctium lappa*)	Laxative
Calendula (*Calendula officinalis* L.), marigold	Constipation
Chamomile (*Matricaria recutita*, *Chamaemelum nobile*)	Constipation
Clay	Constipation
Devil's claw (*Harpagophytum procumbens* DC.)	Constipation
Dong quai (*Angelica sinensis* [Oliv.] Diels), Chinese angelica	Constipation
Dong quai (*Angelica sinensis* [Oliv.] Diels), Chinese angelica	Laxative
Elder (*Sambucus nigra* L.)	Laxative
Fenugreek (*Trigonella foenum-graecum* L.)	Constipation
Feverfew (*Tanacetum parthenium* L. Schultz-Bip.)	Constipation
Ginger (*Zingiber officinale* Roscoe)	Laxative
Globe artichoke (*Cynara scolymus* L.)	Constipation
Goldenseal (Hydrastis Canadensis L.), Berberine	Constipation
Gymnema (*Gymnema Sylvestre* R. Br.)	Constipation
Gymnema (*Gymnema Sylvestre* R. Br.)	Laxative
Lactobacillus acidophilus	Constipation
Licorice (*Glycyrrhiza glabra* L.), deglycyrrhizinated licorice (DGL)	Constipation
Marshmallow (*Althaea officinalis* L.)	Constipation

Continued

Therapy	Specific Therapeutic Use(s)
Marshmallow (*Althaea officinalis* L.)	Laxative
Oleander (*Nerium oleander*, *Thevetia peruviana*)	Cathartic
Seaweed, kelp, bladderwrack (*Fucus vesiculosus*)	Bulk laxative
Seaweed, kelp, bladderwrack (*Fucus vesiculosus*)	Laxative
Seaweed, kelp, bladderwrack (*Fucus vesiculosus*)	Stool softener
Slippery elm (*Ulmus rubra* Muhl., *U. fulva* Michx.)	Constipation
Sorrel (*Rumex acetosa* L., *R. acetosella* L.), Sinupret	Constipation
Sweet almond (*Prunus amygdalus dulcis*)	Mild laxative
Valerian (*Valeriana officinalis* L.)	Constipation
White horehound (*Marrubium vulgare*)	Cathartic
White horehound (*Marrubium vulgare*)	Constipation
White horehound (*Marrubium vulgare*)	Laxative

CONTRACEPTIVE AND RELATED CONDITIONS

Levels of Scientific Evidence for Specific Therapies

TRADITIONAL OR THEORETICAL USES THAT LACK SUFFICIENT EVIDENCE

Therapy	Specific Therapeutic Use(s)
Blessed thistle (*Cnicus benedictus* L.)	Contraception
Kava (*Piper methysticum* G. Forst)	Contraception
Melatonin	Contraception
Oleander (*Nerium oleander*, *Thevetia peruviana*)	Anti-fertility
Turmeric (*Curcuma longa* L.), curcumin	Contraception

CORONARY ARTERY DISEASE AND RELATED CONDITIONS

Levels of Scientific Evidence for Specific Therapies

GRADE: A (Strong Scientific Evidence)

Therapy	Specific Therapeutic Use(s)
Niacin (vitamin B_3, nicotinic acid), niacinamide, and inositol hexanicotinate	High cholesterol (niacin)

Therapy	Specific Therapeutic Use(s)
Omega-3 fatty acids, fish oil, alpha-linolenic acid	Hypertriglyceridemia (fish oil/eicosapentaenoic acid [EPA] plus docosahexaenoic acid [DHA])
Omega-3 fatty acids, fish oil, alpha-linolenic acid	Secondary cardiovascular disease prevention (fish oil/eicosapentaenoic acid [EPA] plus docosahexaenoic acid [DHA])
Psyllium (*Plantago ovata*, *P. ispaghula*)	High cholesterol
Red yeast rice (*Monascus purpureus*)	High cholesterol
Soy (*Glycine max* L. Merr.)	High cholesterol

GRADE: B (Good Scientific Evidence)

Therapy	Specific Therapeutic Use(s)
Barley (*Hordeum vulgare* L.), germinated barley foodstuff (GBF)	High cholesterol
Garlic (*Allium sativum* L.)	High cholesterol
Niacin (vitamin B_3, nicotinic acid), niacinamide, and inositol hexanicotinate	Atherosclerosis (niacin)
Niacin (vitamin B_3, nicotinic acid), niacinamide, and inositol hexanicotinate	Prevention of a second heart attack (niacin)
Omega-3 fatty acids, fish oil, alpha-linolenic acid	Primary cardiovascular disease prevention (fish intake)
Sweet almond (*Prunus amygdalus dulcis*)	High cholesterol (whole almonds)

GRADE: C (Unclear or Conflicting Scientific Evidence)

Therapy	Specific Therapeutic Use(s)
Alfalfa (*Medicago sativa* L.)	Atherosclerosis (cholesterol plaques in heart arteries)
Alfalfa (*Medicago sativa* L.)	High cholesterol
Arginine (L-arginine)	Coronary artery disease/angina
Arginine (L-arginine)	Heart protection during coronary artery bypass grafting (CABG)
Astragalus (*Astragalus membranaceus*)	Coronary artery disease

Continued

Bilberry (*Vaccinium myrtillus*)	Atherosclerosis (hardening of the arteries) and peripheral vascular disease
Black tea (*Camellia sinensis*)	Heart attack prevention
Coenzyme Q10	Angina (chest pain from clogged heart arteries)
Coenzyme Q10	Heart attack (acute myocardial infarction)
Coenzyme Q10	Heart protection during surgery
Danshen (*Salvia miltiorrhiza*)	Cardiovascular disease/angina
DHEA (dehydroepiandrosterone)	Atherosclerosis (cholesterol plaques in the arteries)
Dong quai (*Angelica sinensis* [Oliv.] Diels), Chinese angelica	Angina pectoris/coronary artery disease
Fenugreek (*Trigonella foenum-graecum* L.)	Hyperlipidemia
Flaxseed and flaxseed oil (*Linum usitatissimum*)	Heart disease (flaxseed and flaxseed oil)
Flaxseed and flaxseed oil (*Linum usitatissimum*)	High cholesterol or triglycerides (flaxseed and flaxseed oil)
Garlic (*Allium sativum* L.)	Atherosclerosis (hardening of the arteries)
Garlic (*Allium sativum* L.)	Familial hypercholesterolemia
Garlic (*Allium sativum* L.)	Heart attack prevention in patients with known heart disease
Ginseng (American ginseng, Asian ginseng, Chinese ginseng, Korean red ginseng, *Panax ginseng*: *Panax* spp. including *P. ginseng* C.C. Meyer and *P. quincefolium* L., excluding *Eleutherococcus senticosus*)	Coronary artery (heart) disease
Globe artichoke (*Cynara scolymus* L.)	Lipid-lowering (cholesterol and triglycerides)
Green tea (*Camellia sinensis*)	Heart attack prevention
Green tea (*Camellia sinensis*)	High cholesterol
Guggul (*Commifora mukul*)	Hyperlipidemia
Gymnema (*Gymnema Sylvestre* R. Br.)	High cholesterol

Hawthorn (*Crataegus laevigata*, *C. oxyacantha*, *C. monogyna*, *C. pentagyna*)	Coronary artery disease (angina)
Lactobacillus acidophilus	High cholesterol
Lycopene	Atherosclerosis (clogged arteries) and high cholesterol
Milk thistle (*Silybum marianum*), silymarin	Hyperlipidemia
Omega-3 fatty acids, fish oil, alpha-linolenic acid	Angina pectoris
Omega-3 fatty acids, fish oil, alpha-linolenic acid	Atherosclerosis
Omega-3 fatty acids, fish oil, alpha-linolenic acid	Prevention of graft failure after heart bypass surgery
Omega-3 fatty acids, fish oil, alpha-linolenic acid	Prevention of restenosis after percutaneous transluminal coronary angioplasty (PTCA)
Red clover (*Trifolium pratense*)	High cholesterol
Soy (*Glycine max* L. Merr.)	Cardiovascular disease
Spirulina	High cholesterol
Turmeric (*Curcuma longa* L.), curcumin	High cholesterol
Wild yam (*Dioscorea villosa*)	High cholesterol

GRADE: D (Fair Negative Scientific Evidence)

Therapy	Specific Therapeutic Use(s)
Omega-3 fatty acids, fish oil, alpha-linolenic acid	Hypercholesterolemia

TRADITIONAL OR THEORETICAL USES THAT LACK SUFFICIENT EVIDENCE

Therapy	Specific therapeutic Use(s)
Aloe (*Aloe vera*)	Heart disease prevention
Antineoplastons	Cholesterol/triglyceride abnormalities
Arginine (L-arginine)	Cardiac syndrome X
Arginine (L-arginine)	Heart attack
Arginine (L-arginine)	High cholesterol
Astragalus (*Astragalus membranaceus*)	Angina
Astragalus (*Astragalus membranaceus*)	Heart attack

Continued

Astragalus (*Astragalus membranaceus*)	High cholesterol
Bilberry (*Vaccinium myrtillus*)	Angina
Bilberry (*Vaccinium myrtillus*)	Heart disease
Bilberry (*Vaccinium myrtillus*)	High cholesterol
Black cohosh (*Cimicifuga racemosa* L. Nutt.)	Cardiac diseases
Bladderwrack (*Fucus vesiculosus*)	Atherosclerosis
Bladderwrack (*Fucus vesiculosus*)	Heart disease
Bladderwrack (*Fucus vesiculosus*)	High cholesterol
Boron	High cholesterol
Bromelain	Angina
Bromelain	Atherosclerosis (hardening of the arteries)
Bromelain	Heart disease
Calendula (*Calendula officinalis* L.), marigold	Atherosclerosis (clogged arteries)
Calendula (*Calendula officinalis* L.), marigold	Heart disease
Clay	Cardiovascular disorders
Coenzyme Q10	High cholesterol
Dandelion (*Taraxacum officinale*)	Cardiovascular disorders
Dandelion (*Taraxacum officinale*)	Clogged arteries
Dandelion (*Taraxacum officinale*)	High cholesterol
Danshen (*Salvia miltiorrhiza*)	Clogged arteries
Danshen (*Salvia miltiorrhiza*)	High cholesterol
Devil's claw (*Harpagophytum procumbens* DC.)	Atherosclerosis (clogged arteries)
Devil's claw (*Harpagophytum procumbens* DC.)	High cholesterol
DHEA (dehydroepiandrosterone)	Heart attack
DHEA (dehydroepiandrosterone)	High cholesterol
Dong quai (*Angelica sinensis* [Oliv.] Diels), Chinese angelica	Atherosclerosis
Dong quai (*Angelica sinensis* [Oliv.] Diels), Chinese angelica	High cholesterol

Evening primrose oil (*Oenothera biennis* L.)	Atherosclerosis
Evening primrose oil (*Oenothera biennis* L.)	Heart disease
Evening primrose oil (*Oenothera biennis* L.)	High cholesterol
Fenugreek (*Trigonella foenum-graecum* L.)	Atherosclerosis
Ginger (*Zingiber officinale* Roscoe)	Atherosclerosis
Ginger (*Zingiber officinale* Roscoe)	Heart disease
Ginkgo (*Ginkgo biloba* L.)	Angina
Ginkgo (*Ginkgo biloba* L.)	Atherosclerosis (clogged arteries)
Ginkgo (*Ginkgo biloba* L.)	Heart attack
Ginkgo (*Ginkgo biloba* L.)	Heart disease
Ginkgo (*Ginkgo biloba* L.)	High cholesterol
Ginseng (American ginseng, Asian ginseng, Chinese ginseng, Korean red ginseng, *Panax ginseng*: *Panax* spp. including *P. ginseng* C.C. Meyer and *P. quincefolium* L., excluding *Eleutherococcus senticosus*)	Atherosclerosis
Ginseng (American ginseng, Asian ginseng, Chinese ginseng, Korean red ginseng, *Panax ginseng*: *Panax* spp. including *P. ginseng* C.C. Meyer and *P. quincefolium* L., excluding *Eleutherococcus senticosus*)	Heart damage
Globe artichoke (*Cynara scolymus* L.)	Atherosclerosis
Goldenseal (*Hydrastis canadensis* L.), berberine	Atherosclerosis (hardening of the arteries)
Goldenseal (*Hydrastis canadensis* L.), berberine	High cholesterol
Green tea (*Camellia sinensis*)	Heart disease
Gymnema (*Gymnema Sylvestre* R. Br.)	Cardiovascular disease
Hawthorn (*Crataegus laevigata*, *C. oxyacantha*, *C. monogyna*, *C. pentagyna*)	Angina
Hawthorn (*Crataegus laevigata*, *C. oxyacantha*, *C. monogyna*, *C. pentagyna*)	Cardiac murmurs
Lactobacillus acidophilus	Heart disease
Licorice (*Glycyrrhiza glabra* L.), deglycyrrhizinated licorice (DGL)	High cholesterol

Continued

Lycopene	Heart disease
Maitake mushroom (*Grifola frondosa*), beta-glucan	High cholesterol
Melatonin	Cardiac syndrome X
Melatonin	Coronary artery disease
Niacin (vitamin B_3, nicotinic acid), niacinamide, and inositol hexanicotinate	Heart attack prevention
Oleander (*Nerium oleander*, *Thevetia peruviana*)	Heart disease
Omega-3 fatty acids, fish oil, alpha-linolenic acid	Acute myocardial infarction (heart attack)
Psyllium (*Plantago ovata*, *P. ispaghula*)	Atherosclerosis
Seaweed, kelp, bladderwrack (*Fucus vesiculosus*)	Atherosclerosis
Seaweed, kelp, bladderwrack (*Fucus vesiculosus*)	Fatty heart
Seaweed, kelp, bladderwrack (*Fucus vesiculosus*)	Hyperlipemia
Shark cartilage	Atherosclerosis
Soy (*Glycine max* L. Merr.)	Atherosclerosis
Spirulina	Atherosclerosis
Spirulina	Heart disease
Sweet almond (*Prunus amygdalus dulcis*)	Heart disease
Valerian (*Valeriana officinalis* L.)	Angina pectoris
Valerian (*Valeriana officinalis* L.)	Heart disease
Yohimbe bark extract (*Pausinystalia yohimbe* Pierre ex Beille)	Angina
Yohimbe bark extract (*Pausinystalia yohimbe* Pierre ex Beille)	Coronary artery disease
Yohimbe bark extract (*Pausinystalia yohimbe* Pierre ex Beille)	High cholesterol
Yohimbe bark extract (*Pausinystalia yohimbe* Pierre ex Beille)	Angina
Yohimbe bark extract (*Pausinystalia yohimbe* Pierre ex Beille)	Atherosclerosis
Yohimbe bark extract (*Pausinystalia yohimbe* Pierre ex Beille)	Chest pain

Yohimbe bark extract (*Pausinystalia yohimbe* Pierre ex Beille)	Coronary artery disease
Yohimbe bark extract (*Pausinystalia yohimbe* Pierre ex Beille)	Hyperlipidemia

COUGH AND RELATED CONDITIONS

Levels of Scientific Evidence for Specific Therapies

GRADE: C (Unclear or Conflicting Scientific Evidence)

Therapy	Specific Therapeutic Use(s)
Eucalyptus oil (*Eucalyptus globulus* Labillardiere, *E. fructicetorum* F. Von Mueller, *E. smithii* R.T. Baker)	Decongestant-expectorant/ upper respiratory tract infection (oral/inhalation)
White horehound (*Marrubium vulgare* e)	Cough

TRADITIONAL OR THEORETICAL USES THAT LACK SUFFICIENT EVIDENCE

Therapy	Specific Therapeutic Use(s)
Alfalfa (*Medicago sativa* L.)	Cough
American pennyroyal (*Hedeoma pulegioides* L.), European pennyroyal (*Mentha pulegium* L.)	Cough
Betel nut (*Areca catechu* L.)	Cough
Bilberry (*Vaccinium myrtillus*)	Cough
Bitter almond (*Prunus amygdalus* Batch var. *amara* DC. Focke), Laetrile	Cough suppressant
Black cohosh (*Cimicifuga racemosa* L. Nutt.)	Pertussis (whooping cough)
Blessed thistle (*Cnicus benedictus* L.)	Expectorant
Boswellia (*Boswellia serrata* Roxb.)	Expectorant
Bromelain	Cough
Burdock (*Arctium lappa*)	Cough
Calendula (*Calendula officinalis* L.), marigold	Cough
Chaparral (*Larrea tridentata* DC. Coville, *L. divaricata* Cav.), nordihydroguaiaretic acid (NDGA)	Cough
Clove (*Eugenia aromatica*)	Cough

Continued

Clove (*Eugenia aromatica*)	Expectorant
Dong quai (*Angelica Sinensis* [Oliv.] Diels), Chinese angelica	Cough
Dong quai (*Angelica sinensis* [Oliv.] Diels), Chinese angelica	Expectorant
Echinacea (*Echinacea angustifolia* DC., *E. pallida*, *E. purpurea*)	Whooping cough (pertussis)
Elder (*Sambucus nigra* L.)	Cough suppressant
Ephedra (*Ephedra sinica*)/ma huang	Cough
Eucalyptus oil (*Eucalyptus globulus* Labillardiere, *E. fructicetorum* F. Von Mueller, *E. smithii* R.T. Baker)	Cough
Eucalyptus oil (*Eucalyptus globulus* Labillardiere, *E. fructicetorum* F. Von Mueller, *E. smithii* R.T. Baker)	Croup
Eucalyptus oil (*Eucalyptus globulus* Labillardiere, *E. fructicetorum* F. Von Mueller, *E. smithii* R.T. Baker)	Whooping cough
Evening primrose oil (*Oenothera biennis* L.)	Whooping cough
Eyebright (*Euphrasia officinalis*)	Cough
Eyebright (*Euphrasia officinalis*)	Expectorant
Fenugreek (*Trigonella foenum-graecum* L.)	Cough (chronic)
Flaxseed and flaxseed oil (*Linum usitatissimum*)	Antitussive
Flaxseed and flaxseed oil (*Linum usitatissimum*)	Cough
Flaxseed and flaxseed oil (*Linum usitatissimum*)	Expectorant
Garlic (*Allium sativum* L.)	Cough
Ginger (*Zingiber officinale* Roscoe)	Cough suppressant
Ginkgo (*Ginkgo biloba* L.)	Cough
Goldenseal (*Hydrastis canadensis* L.), berberine	Croup
Gymnema (*Gymnema Sylvestre* R. Br.)	Cough
Horse chestnut (*Aesculus hippocastanum* L.)	Cough
Licorice (*Glycyrrhiza glabra* L.), deglycyrrhizinated licorice (DGL)	Cough
Marshmallow (Althaea officinalis L.)	Cough
Marshmallow (*Althaea officinalis* L.)	Expectorant

Marshmallow (*Althaea officinalis* L.)	Whooping cough
Milk thistle (*Silybum marianum*), silymarin	Cough
Peppermint (*Mentha x piperita* L.)	Cough
Polypodium leucotomos extract, Anapsos	Pertussis
Red clover (*Trifolium pratense*)	Cough
Saw palmetto (*Serenoa repens* [Bartram] Small)	Cough
Saw palmetto (*Serenoa repens* [Bartram] Small)	Expectorant
Slippery elm (*Ulmus rubra* Muhl., *U. fulva* Michx.)	Cough
Tea tree oil (*Melaleuca alternifolia* [Maiden & Betche] Cheel)	Cough
Thyme (*Thymus vulgaris* L.), thymol	Pertussis
Turmeric (*Curcuma longa* L.), curcumin	Cough
Valerian (*Valeriana officinalis* L.)	Cough
White horehound (*Marrubium vulgare*)	Whooping cough
Wild yam (*Dioscorea villosa*)	Croup
Wild yam (*Dioscorea villosa*)	Expectorant
Yohimbe bark extract (*Pausinystalia yohimbe* Pierre ex Beille)	Cough
Yohimbe bark extract (*Pausinystalia yohimbe* Pierre ex Beille)	Coughs

CROHN'S DISEASE AND RELATED CONDITIONS

Levels of Scientific Evidence for Specific Therapies

GRADE: C (Unclear or Conflicting Scientific Evidence)

Therapy	Specific Therapeutic Use(s)
Barley (*Hordeum vulgare* L.), germinated barley foodstuff (GBF)	Ulcerative colitis
Betel nut (*Areca catechu* L.)	Ulcerative colitis
Boswellia (*Boswellia serrata* Roxb.)	Ulcerative colitis
Dandelion (*Taraxacum officinale*)	Colitis

Continued

Glucosamine	Inflammatory bowel disease
Licorice (*Glycyrrhiza glabra* L.), deglycyrrhizinated licorice (DGL)	Familial Mediterranean Fever (FMF)
Omega-3 fatty acids, fish oil, alpha-linolenic acid	Ulcerative colitis
Psyllium (*Plantago ovata*, *P. ispaghula*)	Inflammatory bowel disease

TRADITIONAL OR THEORETICAL USES THAT LACK SUFFICIENT EVIDENCE

Therapy	Specific Therapeutic Use(s)
Aloe (*Aloe vera*)	Inflammatory bowel disease
Arginine (L-arginine)	Inflammatory bowel disease
Barley (*Hordeum vulgare* L.), germinated barley foodstuff (GBF)	Inflammatory bowel disorders
Belladonna (*Atropa belladonna* L. or its variety *acuminata* Royle ex Lindl)	Colitis
Belladonna (*Atropa belladonna* L. or its variety *acuminata* Royle ex Lindl)	Ulcerative colitis
Bromelain	Colitis
Bromelain	Ulcerative colitis
Calendula (*Calendula officinalis* L.), marigold	Ulcerative colitis
DHEA (dehydroepiandrosterone)	Ulcerative colitis
Elder (*Sambucus nigra* L.)	Ulcerative colitis
Eucalyptus oil (*Eucalyptus globulus* Labillardiere, *E. fructicetorum* F. Von Mueller, *E. smithii* R.T. Baker)	Inflammatory bowel disease
Evening primrose oil (*Oenothera biennis* L.)	Ulcerative colitis
Flaxseed and flaxseed oil (*Linum usitatissimum*)	Ulcerative colitis
Ginkgo (*Ginkgo biloba* L.)	Ulcerative colitis
Ginseng (American ginseng, Asian ginseng, Chinese ginseng, Korean red ginseng, *Panax ginseng*: *Panax* spp. including *P. ginseng* C.C. Meyer and *P. quincefolium* L., excluding *Eleutherococcus senticosus*)	Colitis
Glucosamine	Inflammatory bowel disease
Glucosamine	Ulcerative colitis
Goldenseal (*Hydrastis canadensis* L.), berberine	Colitis

Guggul (*Commifora mukul*)	Colitis
Lactobacillus acidophilus	Colitis
Lactobacillus acidophilus	Ulcerative colitis
Licorice (*Glycyrrhiza glabra* L.), deglycyrrhizinated licorice (DGL)	Colitis
Marshmallow (*Althaea officinalis* L.)	Colitis
Marshmallow (*Althaea officinalis* L.)	Inflammation of the small intestine
Marshmallow (*Althaea officinalis* L.)	Ulcerative colitis
Melatonin	Colitis
Propolis	Ulcerative colitis
Slippery elm (*Ulmus rubra* Muhl., *U. fulva* Michx.)	Colitis
Slippery elm (*Ulmus rubra* Muhl., *U. fulva* Michx.)	Ulcerative colitis
Spirulina	Colitis
Thyme (*Thymus vulgaris* L.), thymol	Inflammation of the colon

DEEP VENOUS THROMBOSIS AND RELATED CONDITIONS

Levels of Scientific Evidence for Specific Therapies

GRADE: C (Unclear or Conflicting Scientific Evidence)

Therapy	Specific Therapeutic Use(s)
Bladderwrack (*Fucus vesiculosus*)	Anticoagulant (blood thinner)
Garlic (*Allium sativum* L.)	Antiplatelet effects (blood thinning)
Seaweed, kelp, bladderwrack (*Fucus vesiculosus*)	Anticoagulant
Yohimbe bark extract (*Pausinystalia yohimbe* Pierre ex Beille)	Inhibition of platelet aggregation

TRADITIONAL OR THEORETICAL USES THAT LACK SUFFICIENT EVIDENCE

Therapy	Specific Therapeutic Use(s)
Alfalfa (*Medicago sativa* L.)	Blood clotting disorders
Astragalus (*Astragalus membranaceus*)	Blood thinner

Continued

Barley (*Hordeum vulgare* L.), germinated barley foodstuff (GBF)	Blood circulation
Bromelain	Blood clot treatment
Bromelain	Platelet inhibition (blood thinner)
Calendula (*Calendula officinalis* L.), marigold	Blood vessel clots
Clove (*Eugenia aromatica*)	Blood thinner (antiplatelet agent)
Danshen (*Salvia miltiorrhiza*)	Blood clotting disorders
Danshen (*Salvia miltiorrhiza*)	Hypercoagulability
Dong quai (*Angelica Sinensis* [Oliv.] Diels), Chinese angelica	Blood clots
Dong quai (*Angelica sinensis* [Oliv.] Diels), Chinese angelica	Blood flow disorders
Dong quai (*Angelica sinensis* [Oliv.] Diels), Chinese angelica	Blood stagnation
Dong quai (*Angelica sinensis* [Oliv.] Diels), Chinese angelica	Blood vessel disorders
Elder (*Sambucus nigra* L.)	Blood vessel disorders
Flaxseed and flaxseed oil (*Linum usitatissimum*)	Blood thinner
Ginger (*Zingiber officinale* Roscoe)	Blood thinner
Ginkgo (*Ginkgo biloba* L.)	Blood clots
Ginkgo (*Ginkgo biloba* L.)	Blood vessel disorders
Goldenseal (*Hydrastis canadensis* L.), berberine	Anticoagulant (blood thinning)
Goldenseal (*Hydrastis canadensis* L.), berberine	Blood circulation stimulant
Green tea (*Camellia sinensis*)	Inhibition of platelet aggregation
Horse chestnut (*Aesculus hippocastanum* L.)	Lung blood clots (pulmonary embolism)
Niacin (vitamin B_3, nicotinic acid), niacinamide, and inositol hexanicotinate	Blood circulation improvement
Omega-3 fatty acids, fish oil, alpha-linolenic acid	Anticoagulation
Propolis	Anticoagulant
Red yeast rice (*Monascus purpureus*)	Blood circulation problems

DEMENTIA AND RELATED CONDITIONS

Levels of Scientific Evidence for Specific Therapies

GRADE: B (Good Scientific Evidence)

Therapy	Specific therapeutic Use(s)
Ginkgo (*Ginkgo biloba* L.)	Cerebral insufficiency
Ginseng (American ginseng, Asian ginseng, Chinese ginseng, Korean red ginseng, *Panax ginseng*: *Panax* spp. including *P. ginseng* C.C. Meyer and *P. quincefolium* L., excluding *Eleutherococcus senticosus*)	Mental performance

GRADE: C (Unclear or Conflicting Scientific Evidence)

Therapy	Specific Therapeutic Use(s)
Black tea (*Camellia sinensis*)	Memory enhancement
Black tea (*Camellia sinensis*)	Mental performance/alertness
Boron	Improving cognitive function
Ginkgo (*Ginkgo biloba* L.)	Age-associated memory impairment (AAMI)
Ginkgo (*Ginkgo biloba* L.)	Memory enhancement (in healthy people)
Green tea (*Camellia sinensis*)	Memory enhancement
Green tea (*Camellia sinensis*)	Mental performance/alertness
Polypodium leucotomos extract, Anapsos	Dementia

GRADE: D (Fair Negative Scientific Evidence)

Therapy	Specific Therapeutic Use(s)
DHEA (dehydroepiandrosterone)	Brain function and well-being in the elderly

TRADITIONAL OR THEORETICAL USES THAT LACK SUFFICIENT EVIDENCE

Therapy	Specific Therapeutic Use(s)
Arginine (L-arginine)	Dementia
Astragalus (*Astragalus membranaceus*)	Dementia

Continued

Astragalus (*Astragalus membranaceus*)	Memory
Blessed thistle (*Cnicus benedictus* L.)	Memory improvement
Danshen (*Salvia miltiorrhiza*)	Anoxic brain injury
DHEA (dehydroepiandrosterone)	Dementia
Eyebright (*Euphrasia officinalis*)	Memory loss
Garlic (*Allium sativum* L.)	Age-related memory problems
Ginseng (American ginseng, Asian ginseng, Chinese ginseng, Korean red ginseng, *Panax ginseng*: *Panax* spp. including *P. ginseng* C.C. Meyer and *P. quincefolium* L., excluding *Eleutherococcus senticosus*)	Dementia
Ginseng (American ginseng, Asian ginseng, Chinese ginseng, Korean red ginseng, *Panax ginseng*: *Panax* spp. including *P. ginseng* C.C. Meyer and *P. quincefolium* L., excluding *Eleutherococcus senticosus*)	Improved memory and thinking after menopause
Ginseng (American ginseng, Asian ginseng, Chinese ginseng, Korean red ginseng, *Panax ginseng*: Panax spp. including *P. ginseng* C.C. Meyer and *P. quincefolium* L., excluding *Eleutherococcus senticosus*)	Senile dementia
Gotu kola (*Centella asiatica* L.), total triterpenic fraction of *Centella asiatica* (TTFCA)	Memory enhancement
Green tea (*Camellia sinensis*)	Cognitive performance enhancement
Kava (*Piper methysticum* G. Forst)	Brain damage
Lycopene	Cognitive function
Melatonin	Cognitive enhancement
Melatonin	Memory enhancement
Niacin (vitamin B_3, nicotinic acid), niacinamide, and inositol hexanicotinate	Memory loss
Omega-3 fatty acids, fish oil, alpha-linolenic acid	Memory enhancement
Soy (*Glycine max* L. Merr.)	Cognitive function
Soy (*Glycine max* L. Merr.)	Memory enhancement
Spirulina	Memory improvement
Valerian (*Valeriana officinalis* L.)	Memory

Yohimbe bark extract (*Pausinystalia yohimbe* Pierre ex Beille)	Cognition

DENTAL CONDITIONS AND RELATED CONDITIONS

Levels of Scientific Evidence for Specific Therapies

GRADE: C (Unclear or Conflicting Scientific Evidence)

Therapy	Specific Therapeutic Use(s)
Betel nut (*Areca catechu* L.)	Dental cavities
Black tea (*Camellia sinensis*)	Dental cavity prevention
Coenzyme Q10	Gum disease (periodontitis)
Cranberry (*Vaccinium macrocarpon*)	Dental plaque
Eucalyptus oil (*Eucalyptus globulus* Labillardiere, *E. fructicetorum* F. Von Mueller, *E. smithii* R.T. Baker)	Dental plaque/gingivitis (mouthwash)
Green tea (*Camellia sinensis*)	Dental cavity prevention
Propolis	Dental plaque and gingivitis (mouthwash)
Thyme (*Thymus vulgaris* L.), thymol	Dental plaque

TRADITIONAL OR THEORETICAL USES THAT LACK SUFFICIENT EVIDENCE

Therapy	Specific Therapeutic Use(s)
Arginine (L-arginine)	Peritonitis
Astragalus (*Astragalus membranaceus*)	Denture adhesive (astragalus sap)
Bilberry (*Vaccinium myrtillus*)	Bleeding gums
Chamomile (*Matricaria recutita*, *Chamaemelum nobile*)	Gingivitis
Clove (*Eugenia aromatica*)	Cavities
Coenzyme Q10	Gingivitis
Echinacea (*Echinacea angustifolia* DC., *E. pallida*, *E. purpurea*)	Gingivitis
Goldenseal (*Hydrastis canadensis* L.), berberine	Gingivitis
Gotu kola (*Centella asiatica* L.), total triterpenic fraction of *Centella asiatica* (TTFCA)	Periodontal disease

Continued

Green tea (*Camellia sinensis*)	Bleeding of gums or tooth sockets
Green tea (*Camellia sinensis*)	Gum swelling
Guggul (*Commifora mukul*)	Gingivitis
Licorice (*Glycyrrhiza glabra* L.), deglycyrrhizinated licorice (DGL)	Dental hygiene
Licorice (*Glycyrrhiza glabra* L.), deglycyrrhizinated licorice (DGL)	Plaque
Lycopene	Periodontal disease
Milk thistle (*Silybum marianum*), silymarin	Peritonitis
Omega-3 fatty acids, fish oil, alpha-linolenic acid	Gingivitis
Tea tree oil (*Melaleuca alternifolia* [Maiden & Betche] Cheel)	Dental plaque
Tea tree oil (*Melaleuca alternifolia* [Maiden & Betche] Cheel)	Gingivitis
Tea tree oil (*Melaleuca alternifolia* [Maiden & Betche] Cheel)	Periodontal disease
Thyme (*Thymus vulgaris* L.), thymol	Gingivitis

DEPRESSION AND RELATED CONDITIONS

Levels of Scientific Evidence for Specific Therapies

GRADE: A (Strong Scientific Evidence)

Therapy	Specific Therapeutic Use(s)
St. John's wort (*Hypericum perforatum* L.)	Depressive disorder (mild to moderate)

GRADE: C (Unclear or Conflicting Scientific Evidence)

Therapy	Specific Therapeutic Use(s)
DHEA (dehydroepiandrosterone)	Depression
Evening primrose oil (*Oenothera biennis* L.)	Postviral/chronic fatigue syndrome
Ginkgo (*Ginkgo biloba* L.)	Depression and seasonal affective disorder (SAD)
Melatonin	Bipolar disorder (sleep disturbances)

Melatonin	Depression (sleep disturbances)
Melatonin	Seasonal affective disorder (SAD)
Omega-3 fatty acids, fish oil, alpha-linolenic acid	Bipolar disorder
Omega-3 fatty acids, fish oil, alpha-linolenic acid	Depression
St. John's wort (*Hypericum perforatum* L.)	Depressive disorder (severe)
St. John's wort (*Hypericum perforatum* L.)	Seasonal affective disorder (SAD)

TRADITIONAL OR THEORETICAL USES THAT LACK SUFFICIENT EVIDENCE

Therapy	Specific Therapeutic Use(s)
Black cohosh (*Cimicifuga racemosa* L.]Nutt.)	Depression
Ephedra (*Ephedra sinica*)/ma huang	Depression
Flaxseed and flaxseed oil (*Linum usitatissimum*)	Bipolar disorder
Flaxseed and flaxseed oil (*Linum usitatissimum*)	Depression
Ginger (*Zingiber officinale* Roscoe)	Depression
Ginkgo (*Ginkgo biloba* L.)	Mood disturbances
Ginseng (American ginseng, Asian ginseng, Chinese ginseng, Korean red ginseng, *Panax ginseng*: *Panax* spp. including *P. ginseng* C.C. Meyer and *P. quincefolium* L., excluding *Eleutherococcus* senticosus)	Antidepressant
Gotu kola (*Centella asiatica* L.), total triterpenic fraction of *Centella asiatica* (TTFCA)	Antidepressant
Gotu kola (*Centella asiatica* L.), total triterpenic fraction of *Centella asiatica* (TTFCA)	Mood disorders
Hops (*Humulus lupulus* L.)	Antidepressant
Hops (*Humulus lupulus* L.)	Mood disturbances
Kava (*Piper methysticum* G. Forst)	Depression
Lavender (*Lavandula angustifolia* Miller)	Depression
Licorice (*Glycyrrhiza glabra* L.), deglycyrrhizinated licorice (DGL)	Depression
Melatonin	Depression
Milk thistle (*Silybum marianum*), silymarin	Depression

Continued

Niacin (vitamin B_3, nicotinic acid), niacinamide, and inositol hexanicotinate	Depression
Spirulina	Depression
Spirulina	Mood stimulant
Thyme (*Thymus vulgaris* L.), thymol	Depression
Valerian (*Valeriana officinalis* L.)	Mood enhancement
Yohimbe bark extract (*Pausinystalia yohimbe* Pierre ex Beille)	Depression
Yohimbe bark extract (*Pausinystalia yohimbe* Pierre ex Beille)	Depression

DIABETES MELLITUS AND RELATED CONDITIONS

Levels of Scientific Evidence for Specific Therapies

GRADE: B (Good Scientific Evidence)

Therapy	Specific Therapeutic Use(s)
Bitter melon (*Momordica charantia* L.), MAP30	Diabetes (hypoglycemic agent)
Ginseng (American ginseng, Asian ginseng, Chinese ginseng, Korean red ginseng, *Panax ginseng*: Panax spp. including *P. ginseng* C.C. Meyer and *P. quincefolium* L., excluding *Eleutherococcus senticosus*)	Type 2 diabetes (adult onset)
Gymnema (*Gymnema Sylvestre* R. Br.)	Diabetes

GRADE: C (Unclear or Conflicting Scientific Evidence)

Therapy	Specific Therapeutic Use(s)
Alfalfa (*Medicago sativa* L.)	Diabetes
Aloe (*Aloe vera*)	Diabetes (type 2)
Barley (*Hordeum vulgare* L.), germinated barley foodstuff (GBF)	High blood sugar/glucose intolerance
Bilberry (*Vaccinium myrtillus*)	Diabetes
Bladderwrack (*Fucus vesiculosus*)	Diabetes
Burdock (*Arctium lappa*)	Diabetes
Dandelion (*Taraxacum officinale*)	Diabetes

Evening primrose oil (*Oenothera biennis* L.)	Diabetes
Fenugreek (*Trigonella foenum-graecum* L.)	Type 1 diabetes
Fenugreek (*Trigonella foenum-graecum* L.)	Type 2 diabetes
Flaxseed and flaxseed oil (*Linum usitatissimum*)	Diabetes (flaxseed, not flaxseed oil)
Gotu kola (*Centella asiatica* L.), total triterpenic fraction of *Centella asiatica* (TTFCA)	Diabetic microangiopathy
Maitake mushroom (*Grifola frondosa*), beta-glucan	Diabetes
Milk thistle (*Silybum marianum*), silymarin	Diabetes (associated with cirrhosis)
Niacin (vitamin B_3, nicotinic acid), niacinamide, and inositol hexanicotinate	Type 1 Diabetes prevention (niacinamide)
Psyllium (*Plantago ovata*, *P. ispaghula*)	Hyperglycemia (high blood sugar levels)
Red clover (*Trifolium pratense*)	Diabetes
Seaweed, kelp, bladderwrack (*Fucus vesiculosus*)	Hyperglycemia (diabetes)
Soy (*Glycine max* L. Merr.)	Type 2 diabetes
Spirulina	Diabetes
White horehound (*Marrubium vulgare*)	Diabetes

GRADE: D (Fair Negative Scientific Evidence)

Therapy	Specific Therapeutic Use(s)
Coenzyme Q10	Diabetes
Garlic (*Allium sativum* L.)	Diabetes
Omega-3 fatty acids, fish oil, alpha-linolenic acid	Diabetes

TRADITIONAL OR THEORETICAL USES THAT LACK SUFFICIENT EVIDENCE

Therapy	Specific Therapeutic Use(s)
Arginine (L-arginine)	Diabetes
Astragalus (*Astragalus membranaceus*)	Diabetes
Chaparral (*Larrea tridentata* DC. Coville, *L. divaricata* Cav.), nordihydroguaiaretic acid (NDGA)	Diabetes
Devil's claw (*Harpagophytum procumbens* DC.)	Diabetes

Continued

DHEA (dehydroepiandrosterone)	Diabetes
Dong quai (*Angelica sinensis* [Oliv.] Diels), Chinese angelica	Diabetes
Elder (*Sambucus nigra* L.)	Diabetes
Essiac	Diabetes
Eucalyptus oil (*Eucalyptus globulus* Labillardiere, *E. fructicetorum* F. Von Mueller, *E. smithii* R.T. Baker)	Diabetes
Evening primrose oil (*Oenothera biennis* L.)	Diabetes
Ginkgo (*Ginkgo biloba* L.)	Diabetes
Goldenseal (*Hydrastis canadensis* L.), berberine	Diabetes
Green tea (*Camellia sinensis*)	Diabetes
Guggul (*Commifora mukul*)	Diabetes
Hawthorn (*Crataegus laevigata*, *C. oxyacantha*, *C. monogyna*, *C. pentagyna*)	Diabetes mellitus
Hops (*Humulus lupulus* L.)	Diabetes
Horsetail (*Equisetum arvense* L.)	Diabetes
Lavender (*Lavandula angustifolia* Miller)	Diabetes
Licorice (*Glycyrrhiza glabra* L.), deglycyrrhizinated licorice (DGL)	Diabetes
Lycopene	Diabetes mellitus
Niacin (vitamin B_3, nicotinic acid), niacinamide, and inositol hexanicotinate	Type 1 diabetes
Niacin (vitamin B_3, nicotinic acid), niacinamide, and inositol hexanicotinate	Type 2 diabetes
Niacin (vitamin B_3, nicotinic acid), niacinamide, and inositol hexanicotinate	Low blood sugar
Saw palmetto (*Serenoa repens* [Bartram] Small)	Diabetes
Turmeric (*Curcuma longa* L.), curcumin	Diabetes
Wild yam (*Dioscorea villosa*)	Low blood sugar

DIABETIC COMPLICATIONS AND RELATED CONDITIONS

Levels of Scientific Evidence for Specific Therapies

GRADE: C (Unclear or Conflicting Scientific Evidence)

Therapy	Specific Therapeutic Use(s)
Bilberry (*Vaccinium myrtillus*)	Retinopathy
Evening primrose oil (*Oenothera biennis* L.)	Diabetic neuropathy (nerve damage)
Gotu kola (*Centella asiatica* L.), total triterpenic fraction of *Centella asiatica* (TTFCA)	Diabetic microangiopathy

TRADITIONAL OR THEORETICAL USES THAT LACK SUFFICIENT EVIDENCE

Therapy	Specific Therapeutic Use(s)
Astragalus (*Astragalus membranaceus*)	Diabetic foot ulcers
Astragalus (*Astragalus membranaceus*)	Diabetic neuropathy
Danshen (*Salvia miltiorrhiza*)	Diabetic nerve pain
Ginkgo (*Ginkgo biloba* L.)	Diabetic eye disease
Ginkgo (*Ginkgo biloba* L.)	Diabetic nerve damage (neuropathy)
Ginseng (American ginseng, Asian ginseng, Chinese ginseng, Korean red ginseng, *Panax ginseng*: *Panax* spp. including P. ginseng C.C. Meyer and *P. quincefolium* L., excluding *Eleutherococcus senticosus*)	Diabetic nephropathy (kidney disease)
Milk thistle (*Silybum marianum*), silymarin	Diabetic nerve pain
Omega-3 fatty acids, fish oil, alpha-linolenic acid	Diabetic nephropathy
Omega-3 fatty acids, fish oil, alpha-linolenic acid	Diabetic neuropathy
Shark cartilage	Diabetic retinopathy
Soy (*Glycine max* L. Merr.)	Diabetic neuropathy
Yohimbe bark extract (*Pausinystalia yohimbe* Pierre ex Beille)	Diabetic complications
Yohimbe bark extract (*Pausinystalia yohimbe* Pierre ex Beille)	Diabetic neuropathy
Yohimbe bark extract (*Pausinystalia yohimbe* Pierre ex Beille)	Diabetic complications

Continued

Yohimbe bark extract (*Pausinystalia yohimbe* Pierre ex Beille)	Diabetic neuropathy

DIARRHEA AND RELATED CONDITIONS

Levels of Scientific Evidence for Specific Therapies

GRADE: B (Good Scientific Evidence)

Therapy	Specific Therapeutic Use(s)
Psyllium (*Plantago ovata*, *P. ispaghula*)	Diarrhea
Soy (*Glycine max* L. Merr.)	Diarrhea (acute) in infants and young children

GRADE: C (Unclear or Conflicting Scientific Evidence)

Therapy	Specific Therapeutic Use(s)
Bilberry (*Vaccinium myrtillus*)	Diarrhea
Chamomile (*Matricaria recutita*, *Chamaemelum nobile*)	Diarrhea in children
Clay	Fecal incontinence associated with psychiatric disorders (encopresis): clay modeling therapy in children
Goldenseal (*Hydrastis canadensis* L.), berberine	Infectious diarrhea
Lactobacillus acidophilus	Diarrhea prevention
Lactobacillus acidophilus	Diarrhea treatment (children)
Lactobacillus acidophilus	Lactose intolerance
Slippery elm (*Ulmus rubra* Muhl., *U. fulva* Michx.)	Diarrhea
Soy (*Glycine max* L. Merr.)	Diarrhea in adults

TRADITIONAL OR THEORETICAL USES THAT LACK SUFFICIENT EVIDENCE

Therapy	Specific Therapeutic Use(s)
American pennyroyal (*Hedeoma pulegioides* L.), European pennyroyal (*Mentha pulegium* L.)	Dysentery
Astragalus (*Astragalus membranaceus*)	Diarrhea
Barley (*Hordeum vulgare* L.), germinated barley foodstuff (GBF)	Diarrhea

Belladonna (*Atropa belladonna* L. or its variety *acuminata* Royle ex Lindl)	Diarrhea
Bilberry (*Vaccinium myrtillus*)	Dysentery
Black cohosh (*Cimicifuga racemosa* L. Nutt.)	Diarrhea
Black tea (*Camellia sinensis*)	Diarrhea
Blessed thistle (*Cnicus benedictus* L.)	Diarrhea
Bromelain	Diarrhea
Chaparral (*Larrea tridentata* DC. Coville, *L. divaricata* Cav.), nordihydroguaiaretic acid (NDGA)	Diarrhea
Clay	Diarrhea
Clay	Dysentery
Clove (*Eugenia aromatica*)	Diarrhea
Dandelion (*Taraxacum officinale*)	Diarrhea
Devil's claw (*Harpagophytum procumbens* DC.)	Diarrhea
Dong quai (*Angelica sinensis* [Oliv.] Diels), Chinese angelica	Dysentery
Eucalyptus oil (*Eucalyptus globulus* Labillardiere, *E. fructicetorum* F. Von Mueller, *E. smithii* R.T. Baker)	Diarrhea
Fenugreek (*Trigonella foenum-graecum* L.)	Diarrhea
Fenugreek (*Trigonella foenum-graecum* L.)	Dysentery
Feverfew (*Tanacetum parthenium* L. Schultz-Bip.)	Diarrhea
Flaxseed and flaxseed oil (*Linum usitatissimum*)	Diarrhea
Garlic (*Allium sativum* L.)	Dysentery
Ginger (*Zingiber officinale* Roscoe)	Diarrhea
Ginkgo (*Ginkgo biloba* L.)	Dysentery (bloody diarrhea)
Ginseng (American ginseng, Asian ginseng, Chinese ginseng, Korean red ginseng, *Panax ginseng*: *Panax* spp. including *P. ginseng* C.C. Meyer and *P. quincefolium* L., excluding *Eleutherococcus senticosus*)	Dysentery
Goldenseal (*Hydrastis canadensis* L.), berberine	Diarrhea
Gotu kola (*Centella asiatica* L.), total triterpenic fraction of *Centella asiatica* (TTFCA)	Diarrhea

Continued

Gotu kola (*Centella asiatica* L.), total triterpenic fraction of *Centella asiatica* (TTFCA)	Dysentery
Green tea (*Camellia sinensis*)	Diarrhea
Hawthorn (*Crataegus laevigata, C. oxyacantha, C. monogyna, C. pentagyna*)	Diarrhea
Hawthorn (*Crataegus laevigata, C. oxyacantha, C. monogyna, C. pentagyna*)	Dysentery
Hops (*Humulus lupulus* L.)	Diarrhea caused by infection
Horse chestnut (*Aesculus hippocastanum* L.)	Diarrhea
Marshmallow (*Althaea officinalis* L.)	Diarrhea
Niacin (vitamin B_3, nicotinic acid), niacinamide, and inositol hexanicotinate	Cholera diarrhea
Niacin (vitamin B_3, nicotinic acid), niacinamide, and inositol hexanicotinate	Chronic diarrhea
Psyllium (*Plantago ovata, P. ispaghula*)	Dysentery
Psyllium (*Plantago ovata, P. ispaghula*)	Fecal (stool) incontinence
Red yeast rice (*Monascus purpureus*)	Diarrhea
Red yeast rice (*Monascus purpureus*)	Dysentery (bloody diarrhea)
Saw palmetto (*Serenoa repens* [Bartram] Small)	Dysentery
Slippery elm (*Ulmus rubra* Muhl., *U. fulva* Michx.)	Dysentery
Sorrel (*Rumex acetosa* L., *R. acetosella* L.), Sinupret	Diarrhea
St. John's wort (*Hypericum perforatum* L.)	Diarrhea
Thyme (*Thymus vulgaris* L.), thymol	Diarrhea
Turmeric (*Curcuma longa* L.), curcumin	Diarrhea
White horehound (*Marrubium vulgare*)	Diarrhea

DIURESIS AND RELATED CONDITIONS

Levels of Scientific Evidence for Specific Therapies

GRADE: B (Good Scientific Evidence)

Therapy	Specific Therapeutic Use(s)
Horsetail (*Equisetum arvense* L.)	Diuresis (increased urine)

GRADE: C (Unclear or Conflicting Scientific Evidence)	
Therapy	Specific Therapeutic Use(s)
Dandelion (*Taraxacum officinale*)	Diuretic (increased urine flow)

TRADITIONAL OR THEORETICAL USES THAT LACK SUFFICIENT EVIDENCE	
Therapy	Specific Therapeutic Use(s)
Alfalfa (*Medicago sativa* L.)	Diuresis (increasing urination)
American pennyroyal (*Hedeoma pulegioides* L.), European pennyroyal (*Mentha pulegium* L.)	Diuretic
Astragalus (*Astragalus membranaceus*)	Diuretic (urination stimulant)
Belladonna (*Atropa belladonna* L. or its variety *acuminata* Royle ex Lindl)	Diuretic (use as a water pill)
Betel nut (*Areca catechu* L.)	Diuretic
Black tea (*Camellia sinensis*)	Diuretic (increasing urine flow)
Blessed thistle (*Cnicus benedictus* L.)	Diuretic (increasing urine)
Boswellia (*Boswellia serrata* Roxb.)	Diuretic
Burdock (*Arctium lappa*)	Diuretic (increasing urine flow)
Calendula (*Calendula officinalis* L.), marigold	Diuretic
Chamomile (*Matricaria recutita*, *Chamaemelum nobile*)	Diuretic
Chaparral (*Larrea tridentata* DC. Coville, *L. divaricata* Cav.), nordihydroguaiaretic acid (NDGA)	Diuretic (increasing urine flow)
Cranberry (*Vaccinium macrocarpon*)	Diuresis (increasing urine flow)
Devil's claw (*Harpagophytum procumbens* DC.)	Diuretic
Dong quai (*Angelica sinensis* [Oliv.] Diels), Chinese angelica	Diuretic (increasing urination)
Elder (*Sambucus nigra* L.)	Diuresis (urine production)
Ephedra (*Ephedra sinica*)/ma huang	Diuretic
Garlic (*Allium sativum* L.)	Diuretic (water pill)
Ginger (*Zingiber officinale* Roscoe)	Diuresis
Ginseng (American ginseng, Asian ginseng, Chinese ginseng, Korean red ginseng, *Panax ginseng*: *Panax* spp. including *P. ginseng* C.C. Meyer and *P. quincefolium* L., excluding *Eleutherococcus senticosus*)	Diuretic (water pill)

Continued

Goldenseal (*Hydrastis canadensis* L.), berberine	Diuretic (increasing urine flow)
Gotu kola (*Centella asiatica* L.), total triterpenic fraction of *Centella asiatica* (TTFCA)	Diuretic
Green tea (*Camellia sinensis*)	Diuretic (increasing urine flow)
Green tea (*Camellia sinensis*)	Improving urine flow
Gymnema (*Gymnema Sylvestre* R. Br.)	Diuresis
Hawthorn (*Crataegus laevigata*, *C. oxyacantha*, *C. monogyna*, *C. pentagyna*)	Diuresis
Kava (*Piper methysticum* G. Forst)	Diuretic
Lavender (*Lavandula angustifolia* Miller)	Diuretic
Licorice (*Glycyrrhiza glabra* L.), deglycyrrhizinated licorice (DGL)	Diuretic
Marshmallow (*Althaea officinalis* L.)	Diuretic
Oleander (*Nerium oleander*, *Thevetia peruviana*)	Diuretic (increase urine flow)
Polypodium leucotomos extract, Anapsos	Diuretic
Red clover (*Trifolium pratense*)	Diuretic (increase urine flow)
Saw palmetto (*Serenoa repens* [Bartram] Small)	Diuretic
Slippery elm (*Ulmus rubra* Muhl., *U. fulva* Michx.)	Diuretic
Sorrel (*Rumex acetosa* L., *R. acetosella* L.), Sinupret	Diuresis
St. John's wort (*Hypericum perforatum* L.)	Diuretic (increasing urine flow)
Thyme (*Thymus vulgaris* L.), thymol	Diuresis
Valerian (*Valeriana officinalis* L.)	Diuretic
White horehound (*Marrubium vulgare*)	Diuresis

DIZZINESS AND RELATED CONDITIONS

Levels of Scientific Evidence for Specific Therapies

GRADE: C (Unclear or Conflicting Scientific Evidence)

Therapy	Specific Therapeutic Use(s)
Ginkgo (*Ginkgo biloba* L.)	Vertigo

TRADITIONAL OR THEORETICAL USES THAT LACK SUFFICIENT EVIDENCE	
Therapy	Specific therapeutic Use(s)
American pennyroyal (*Hedeoma pulegioides* L.), European pennyroyal (*Mentha pulegium* L.)	Dizziness
Black cohosh (*Cimicifuga racemosa* L. Nutt.)	Dizziness
Calendula (*Calendula officinalis* L.), marigold	Dizziness
Echinacea (*Echinacea angustifolia* DC., *E. pallida*, *E. purpurea*)	Dizziness
Feverfew (*Tanacetum parthenium* L. Schultz-Bip.)	Dizziness
Ginkgo (*Ginkgo biloba* L.)	Dizziness
Ginseng (American ginseng, Asian ginseng, Chinese ginseng, Korean red ginseng, *Panax ginseng*: *Panax* spp. including *P. ginseng* C.C. Meyer and *P. quincefolium* L., excluding *Eleutherococcus senticosus*)	Dizziness
Horse chestnut (*Aesculus hippocastanum* L.)	Dizziness
Kava (*Piper methysticum* G. Forst)	Dizziness
Lavender (*Lavandula angustifolia* Miller)	Dizziness
Niacin (vitamin B_3, nicotinic acid), niacinamide, and inositol hexanicotinate	Vertigo
Turmeric (*Curcuma longa* L.), curcumin	Dizziness
Valerian (*Valeriana officinalis* L.)	Vertigo

DRUG ADDICTION AND RELATED CONDITIONS

Levels of Scientific Evidence for Specific Therapies

GRADE: C (Unclear or Conflicting Scientific Evidence)	
Therapy	Specific Therapeutic Use(s)
Globe artichoke (*Cynara scolymus* L.)	Alcohol-induced hangover
Goldenseal (*Hydrastis canadensis* L.), berberine	Narcotic concealment (urinalysis)
Melatonin	Benzodiazepine tapering
Melatonin	Smoking cessation

Continued

TRADITIONAL OR THEORETICAL USES THAT LACK SUFFICIENT EVIDENCE	
Therapy	Specific Therapeutic Use(s)
Betel nut (*Areca catechu* L.)	Alcoholism
Black tea (*Camellia sinensis*)	Toxin/alcohol elimination from the body
Burdock (*Arctium lappa*)	Detoxification
Chamomile (*Matricaria recutita*, *Chamaemelum nobile*)	Delirium tremens (DTs)
Clay	Smoking
Dandelion (*Taraxacum officinale*)	Alcohol withdrawal
Dandelion (*Taraxacum officinale*)	Smoking cessation
Essiac	Detoxification
Evening primrose oil (*Oenothera biennis* L.)	Alcoholism
Evening primrose oil (*Oenothera biennis* L.)	Hangover remedy
Ginger (*Zingiber officinale* Roscoe)	Alcohol withdrawal
Ginkgo (*Ginkgo biloba* L.)	Alcoholism
Green tea (*Camellia sinensis*)	Alcohol intoxication
Green tea (*Camellia sinensis*)	Detoxification from alcohol or toxins
Lavender (*Lavandula angustifolia* Miller)	Hangover
Licorice (*Glycyrrhiza glabra* L.), deglycyrrhizinated licorice (DGL)	Detoxification
Melatonin	Withdrawal from narcotics
Niacin (vitamin B_3, nicotinic acid), niacinamide, and inositol hexanicotinate	Alcohol dependence
Niacin (vitamin B_3, nicotinic acid), niacinamide, and inositol hexanicotinate	Smoking cessation
Oleander (*Nerium oleander*, *Thevetia peruviana*)	Alcoholism
St. John's wort (*Hypericum perforatum* L.)	Alcoholism
St. John's wort (*Hypericum perforatum* L.)	Benzodiazepine withdrawal
Valerian (*Valeriana officinalis* L.)	Hangover

DYSMENORRHEA AND RELATED CONDITIONS

Levels of Scientific Evidence for Specific Therapies

GRADE: B (Good Scientific Evidence)

Therapy	Specific Therapeutic Use(s)
Black cohosh (*Cimicifuga racemosa* L.]Nutt.)	Menopausal symptoms
Soy (*Glycine max* L. Merr.)	Menopausal hot flashes

GRADE: C (Unclear or Conflicting Scientific Evidence)

Therapy	Specific Therapeutic Use(s)
American pennyroyal (*Hedeoma pulegioides* L.), European pennyroyal (*Mentha pulegium* L.)	Emmenagogue (menstrual flow stimulant)
Belladonna (*Atropa belladonna* L. or its variety *acuminata* Royle ex Lindl)	Premenstrual syndrome (PMS)
Bilberry (*Vaccinium myrtillus*)	Painful menstruation (dysmenorrhea)
DHEA (dehydroepiandrosterone)	Menopausal disorders
DHEA (dehydroepiandrosterone)	Ovulation disorders
Dong quai (*Angelica sinensis* [Oliv.] Diels), Chinese angelica	Amenorrhea (lack of menstrual period)
Dong quai (*Angelica sinensis* [Oliv.] Diels), Chinese angelica	Dysmenorrhea (painful menstruation)
Flaxseed and flaxseed oil (*Linum usitatissimum*)	Menstrual breast pain (flaxseed, not flaxseed oil)
Ginkgo (*Ginkgo biloba* L.)	Premenstrual syndrome (PMS)
Ginseng (American ginseng, Asian ginseng, Chinese ginseng, Korean red ginseng, *Panax ginseng*: *Panax* spp. including *P. ginseng* C.C. Meyer and *P. quincefolium* L., excluding *Eleutherococcus senticosus*)	Menopausal symptoms
Green tea (*Camellia sinensis*)	Menopausal symptoms
Omega-3 fatty acids, fish oil, alpha-linolenic acid	Dysmenorrhea (painful menstruation)
Red clover (*Trifolium pratense*)	Hormone replacement therapy (HRT)
Red clover (*Trifolium pratense*)	Menopausal symptoms

Continued

St. John's wort (*Hypericum perforatum* L.)	Perimenopausal symptoms
St. John's wort (*Hypericum perforatum* L.)	Premenstrual syndrome (PMS)
Wild yam (*Dioscorea villosa*)	Menopausal symptoms

GRADE: D (Fair Negative Scientific Evidence)

Therapy	Specific Therapeutic Use(s)
Belladonna (*Atropa belladonna* L. or its variety *acuminata* Royle ex Lindl)	Menopausal symptoms
Boron	Menopausal symptoms
Evening primrose oil (*Oenothera biennis* L.)	Menopause (flushing/bone metabolism)
Evening primrose oil (*Oenothera biennis* L.)	Premenstrual syndrome (PMS)
Wild yam (*Dioscorea villosa*)	Hormonal properties (to mimic estrogen, progesterone, or DHEA)

TRADITIONAL OR THEORETICAL USES THAT LACK SUFFICIENT EVIDENCE

Therapy	Specific Therapeutic Use(s)
Alfalfa (*Medicago sativa* L.)	Estrogen replacement
Alfalfa (*Medicago sativa* L.)	Menopausal symptoms
American pennyroyal (*Hedeoma pulegioides* L.), European pennyroyal (*Mentha pulegium* L.)	Cramps
American pennyroyal (*Hedeoma pulegioides* L.), European pennyroyal (*Mentha pulegium* L.)	Premenstrual syndrome (PMS)
Astragalus (*Astragalus membranaceus*)	Menstrual disorders
Astragalus (*Astragalus membranaceus*)	Pelvic congestion syndrome
Belladonna (*Atropa belladonna* L. or its variety *acuminata* Royle ex Lindl)	Abnormal menstrual periods
Betel nut (*Areca catechu* L.)	Excessive menstrual flow
Black cohosh (*Cimicifuga racemosa* L. Nutt.)	Endometriosis
Black cohosh (*Cimicifuga racemosa* L. Nutt.)	Menstrual period problems
Black cohosh (*Cimicifuga racemosa* L. Nutt.)	Ovarian cysts
Black cohosh (*Cimicifuga racemosa* L. Nutt.)	Premenstrual syndrome (PMS)
Bladderwrack (*Fucus vesiculosus*)	Menstruation irregularities

Blessed thistle (*Cnicus benedictus* L.)	Menstrual disorders
Blessed thistle (*Cnicus benedictus* L.)	Menstrual flow stimulant
Blessed thistle (*Cnicus benedictus* L.)	Painful menstruation
Boswellia (*Boswellia serrata* Roxb.)	Amenorrhea
Boswellia (*Boswellia serrata* Roxb.)	Emmenagogue (induces menstruation)
Bromelain	Menstrual pain
Calendula (*Calendula officinalis* L.), marigold	Cramps
Calendula (*Calendula officinalis* L.), marigold	Menstrual period abnormalities
Chamomile (*Matricaria recutita*, *Chamaemelum nobile*)	Dysmenorrhea
Chamomile (*Matricaria recutita*, *Chamaemelum nobile*)	Menstrual disorders
Chaparral (*Larrea tridentata* DC. Coville, *L. divaricata* Cav.), nordihydroguaiaretic acid (NDGA)	Menstrual cramps
Clay	Menstruation difficulties
Dandelion (*Taraxacum officinale*)	Menopause
Dandelion (*Taraxacum officinale*)	Premenstrual syndrome (PMS)
Danshen (*Salvia miltiorrhiza*)	Menstrual problems
Devil's claw (*Harpagophytum procumbens* DC.)	Menopausal symptoms
Devil's claw (*Harpagophytum procumbens* DC.)	Menstrual cramps
DHEA (dehydroepiandrosterone)	Amenorrhea associated with anorexia
DHEA (dehydroepiandrosterone)	Andropause/andrenopause
DHEA (dehydroepiandrosterone)	Premenstrual syndrome (PMS)
Dong quai (*Angelica sinensis* [Oliv.] Diels), Chinese angelica	Cramps
Dong quai (*Angelica sinensis* [Oliv.] Diels), Chinese angelica	Hormonal abnormalities
Dong quai (*Angelica sinensis* [Oliv.] Diels), Chinese angelica	Menorrhagia (heavy menstrual bleeding)
Dong quai (*Angelica sinensis* [Oliv.] Diels), Chinese angelica	Menstrual cramping
Dong quai (*Angelica sinensis* [Oliv.] Diels), Chinese angelica	Ovulation abnormalities

Continued

Dong quai (*Angelica sinensis* [Oliv.] Diels), Chinese angelica	Pelvic congestion syndrome
Dong quai (*Angelica sinensis* [Oliv.] Diels), Chinese angelica	Premenstrual syndrome (PMS)
Fenugreek (*Trigonella foenum-graecum* L.)	Menopausal symptoms
Fenugreek (*Trigonella foenum-graecum* L.)	Postmenopausal vaginal dryness
Feverfew (*Tanacetum parthenium* L. Schultz-Bip.)	Menstrual cramps
Feverfew (*Tanacetum parthenium* L. Schultz-Bip.)	Promotion of menstruation
Flaxseed and flaxseed oil (*Linum usitatissimum*)	Menstrual disorders
Flaxseed and flaxseed oil (*Linum usitatissimum*)	Ovarian disorders
Garlic (*Allium sativum* L.)	Emmenagogue
Ginger (*Zingiber officinale* Roscoe)	Dysmenorrhea
Ginger (*Zingiber officinale* Roscoe)	Promotion of menstruation
Ginkgo (*Ginkgo biloba* L.)	Menstrual pain
Ginseng (American ginseng, Asian ginseng, Chinese ginseng, Korean red ginseng, *Panax ginseng*: *Panax* spp. including *P. ginseng* C.C. Meyer and *P. quincefolium* L., excluding *Eleutherococcus senticosus*)	Menopausal symptoms
Goldenseal (*Hydrastis canadensis* L.), berberine	Menstruation problems
Goldenseal (*Hydrastis canadensis* L.), berberine	Premenstrual syndrome (PMS)
Gotu kola (*Centella asiatica* L.), total triterpenic fraction of *Centella asiatica* (TTFCA)	Amenorrhea
Gotu kola (*Centella asiatica* L.), total triterpenic fraction of *Centella asiatica* (TTFCA)	Hot flashes
Gotu kola (*Centella asiatica* L.), total triterpenic fraction of *Centella asiatica* (TTFCA)	Menstrual disorders
Guggul (*Commifora mukul*)	Menstrual disorders
Hawthorn (*Crataegus laevigata*, *C. oxyacantha*, *C. monogyna*, *C. pentagyna*)	Amenorrhea
Hops (*Humulus lupulus* L.)	Estrogenic effects
Horse chestnut (*Aesculus hippocastanum* L.)	Menstrual pain
Horsetail (*Equisetum arvense* L.)	Menstrual pain
Kava (*Piper methysticum* G. Forst)	Menopause

Kava (*Piper methysticum* G. Forst)	Menstrual disorders
Lavender (*Lavandula angustifolia* Miller)	Menopause
Lavender (*Lavandula angustifolia* Miller)	Menstrual period problems
Licorice (*Glycyrrhiza glabra* L.), deglycyrrhizinated licorice (DGL)	Hormone regulation
Licorice (*Glycyrrhiza glabra* L.), deglycyrrhizinated licorice (DGL)	Menopausal symptoms
Melatonin	Melatonin deficiency
Milk thistle (*Silybum marianum*), silymarin	Menstrual disorders
Niacin (vitamin B_3, nicotinic acid), niacinamide, and inositol hexanicotinate	Painful menstruation
Niacin (vitamin B_3, nicotinic acid), niacinamide, and inositol hexanicotinate	Premenstrual headache prevention
Niacin (vitamin B_3, nicotinic acid), niacinamide, and inositol hexanicotinate	Premenstrual syndrome (PMS)
Oleander (*Nerium oleander*, *Thevetia peruviana*)	Abnormal menstruation
Oleander (*Nerium oleander*, *Thevetia peruviana*)	Menstrual stimulant
Omega-3 fatty acids, fish oil, alpha-linolenic acid	Menopausal symptoms
Omega-3 fatty acids, fish oil, alpha-linolenic acid	Menstrual cramps
Omega-3 fatty acids, fish oil, alpha-linolenic acid	Premenstrual syndrome (PMS)
Passionflower (*Passiflora incarnata* L.)	Menopausal symptoms (hot flashes)
Peppermint (*Mentha x piperita* L.)	Cramps
Peppermint (*Mentha x piperita* L.)	Dysmenorrhea (menstrual pain)
Psyllium (*Plantago ovata*, *P. ispaghula*)	Excessive menstrual bleeding
Red clover (*Trifolium pratense*)	Hot flashes
Red clover (*Trifolium pratense*)	Premenstrual syndrome (PMS)
Saw palmetto (*Serenoa repens* [Bartram] Small)	Antiandrogen
Saw palmetto (*Serenoa repens* [Bartram] Small)	Antiestrogen
Saw palmetto (*Serenoa repens* [Bartram] Small)	Dysmenorrhea
Saw palmetto (*Serenoa repens* [Bartram] Small)	Estrogenic agent
Saw palmetto (*Serenoa repens* [Bartram] Small)	Ovarian cysts

Continued

Saw palmetto (*Serenoa repens* [Bartram] Small)	Pelvic congestive syndrome
Seaweed, kelp, bladderwrack (*Fucus vesiculosus*)	Menstrual irregularities (menorrhagia)
Slippery elm (*Ulmus rubra* Muhl., *U. fulva* Michx.)	Gynecologic disorders
Spirulina	Premenstrual syndrome (PMS)
St. John's wort (*Hypericum perforatum* L.)	Menstrual pain
Sweet Almond (*Prunus amygdalus dulcis*)	Plant-derived estrogen
Thyme (*Thymus vulgaris* L.), thymol	Dysmenorrhea
Turmeric (*Curcuma longa* L.), curcumin	Menstrual pain
Turmeric (*Curcuma longa* L.), curcumin	Menstrual period problems/ lack of menstrual period
Valerian (*Valeriana officinalis* L.)	Amenorrhea
Valerian (*Valeriana officinalis* L.)	Dysmenorrhea
Valerian (*Valeriana officinalis* L.)	Emmenagogue
Valerian (*Valeriana officinalis* L.)	Menopause
Valerian (*Valeriana officinalis* L.)	Premenstrual syndrome (PMS)
White horehound (*Marrubium vulgare*)	Dysmenorrhea
White horehound (*Marrubium vulgare*)	Menstrual pain
Wild yam (*Dioscorea villosa*)	Cramps
Wild yam (*Dioscorea villosa*)	Menopause
Wild yam (*Dioscorea villosa*)	Menstrual pain or irregularities
Wild yam (*Dioscorea villosa*)	Pelvic cramps
Wild yam (*Dioscorea villosa*)	Postmenopausal vaginal dryness
Wild yam (*Dioscorea villosa*)	Premenstrual syndrome (PMS)

ENERGY BOOSTER AND RELATED CONDITIONS

Levels of Scientific Evidence for Specific Therapies

GRADE: C (UNCLEAR OR CONFLICTING SCIENTIFIC EVIDENCE)

Therapy	Specific Therapeutic Use(s)
Betel nut (*Areca catechu* L.)	Stimulant
DHEA (dehydroepiandrosterone)	Chronic fatigue syndrome

Evening primrose oil (*Oenothera biennis* L.)	Chronic fatigue syndrome/ postviral infection symptoms
Ginseng (American ginseng, Asian ginseng, Chinese ginseng, Korean red ginseng, *Panax ginseng*: *Panax* spp. including *P. ginseng* C.C. Meyer and *P. quincefolium* L., excluding *Eleutherococcus senticosus*)	Fatigue

TRADITIONAL OR THEORETICAL USES THAT LACK SUFFICIENT EVIDENCE

Therapy	Specific Therapeutic Use(s)
Aloe (*Aloe vera*)	Chronic fatigue syndrome
American pennyroyal (*Hedeoma pulegioides* L.), European pennyroyal (*Mentha pulegium* L.)	Stimulant
Astragalus (*Astragalus membranaceus*)	Chronic fatigue syndrome
Astragalus (*Astragalus membranaceus*)	Fatigue
Black cohosh (*Cimicifuga racemosa* L. Nutt.)	Malaise
Bladderwrack (*Fucus vesiculosus*)	Fatigue
Calendula (*Calendula officinalis* L.), marigold	Fatigue
Coenzyme Q10	Chronic fatigue syndrome
Dandelion (*Taraxacum officinale*)	Chronic fatigue syndrome
Dandelion (*Taraxacum officinale*)	Stimulant
Dong quai (*Angelica sinensis* [Oliv.] Diels), Chinese angelica	Fatigue
Ephedra (Ephedra sinica)/ma huang	Energy enhancer
Ephedra (Ephedra sinica)/ma huang	Stimulant
Essiac	Chronic fatigue syndrome
Eucalyptus oil (*Eucalyptus globulus* Labillardiere, *E. fructicetorum* F. Von Mueller, *E. smithii* R.T. Baker)	Alertness
Eucalyptus oil (*Eucalyptus globulus* Labillardiere, *E. fructicetorum* F. Von Mueller, *E. smithii* R.T. Baker)	Stimulant
Garlic (*Allium sativum* L.)	Fatigue
Ginger (*Zingiber officinale* Roscoe)	Stimulant
Ginkgo (*Ginkgo biloba* L.)	Fatigue

Continued

Ginseng (American ginseng, Asian ginseng, Chinese ginseng, Korean red ginseng, *Panax ginseng*: *Panax* spp. including *P. ginseng* C.C. Meyer and *P. quincefolium* L., excluding *Eleutherococcus senticosus*)	Fatigue
Goldenseal (*Hydrastis canadensis* L.), berberine	Chronic fatigue syndrome
Goldenseal (*Hydrastis canadensis* L.), berberine	Stimulant
Gotu kola (*Centella asiatica* L.), total triterpenic fraction of *Centella asiatica* (TTFCA)	Energy
Gotu kola (*Centella asiatica* L.), total triterpenic fraction of *Centella asiatica* (TTFCA)	Fatigue
Green tea (*Camellia sinensis*)	Stimulant
Lavender (*Lavandula angustifolia* Miller)	Fatigue
Licorice (*Glycyrrhiza glabra* L.), deglycyrrhizinated licorice (DGL)	Chronic fatigue syndrome
Omega-3 fatty acids, fish oil, alpha-linolenic acid	Chronic fatigue syndrome
Seaweed, kelp, bladderwrack (*Fucus vesiculosus*)	Fatigue
Spirulina	Energy booster
Spirulina	Fatigue
St. John's wort (*Hypericum perforatum* L.)	Fatigue
Valerian (*Valeriana officinalis* L.)	Fatigue

ERECTILE DYSFUNCTION AND RELATED CONDITIONS

Levels of Scientific Evidence for Specific Therapies

GRADE: C (Unclear or Conflicting Scientific Evidence)

Therapy	Specific Therapeutic Use(s)
Arginine (L-arginine)	Erectile dysfunction
Clove (*Eugenia aromatica*)	Premature ejaculation
DHEA (dehydroepiandrosterone)	Sexual function/libido/erectile dysfunction
Ephedra (*Ephedra sinica*)/ma huang	Sexual arousal
Ginkgo (*Ginkgo biloba* L.)	Decreased libido/erectile dysfunction (impotence)

Therapy	Specific Therapeutic Use(s)
Ginseng (American ginseng, Asian ginseng, Chinese ginseng, Korean red ginseng, *Panax ginseng*: *Panax* spp. including *P. ginseng* C.C. Meyer and *P. quincefolium* L., excluding *Eleutherococcus senticosus*)	Erectile dysfunction
Yohimbe bark extract (*Pausinystalia yohimbe* Pierre ex Beille)	Erectile dysfunction (male impotence)
Yohimbe bark extract (*Pausinystalia yohimbe* Pierre ex Beille)	Libido (women)
Yohimbe bark extract (*Pausinystalia yohimbe* Pierre ex Beille)	Sexual side effects of selective serotonin reuptake inhibitor (SSRI) antidepressants

TRADITIONAL OR THEORETICAL USES THAT LACK SUFFICIENT EVIDENCE

Therapy	Specific Therapeutic Use(s)
Betel nut (Areca catechu L.)	Aphrodisiac
Betel nut (*Areca catechu* L.)	Impotence
Black cohosh (*Cimicifuga racemosa* L. Nutt.)	Aphrodisiac
Burdock (*Arctium lappa*)	Aphrodisiac
Burdock (*Arctium lappa*)	Impotence
Fenugreek (*Trigonella foenum-graecum* L.)	Impotence
Garlic (*Allium sativum* L.)	Aphrodisiac
Ginger (*Zingiber officinale* Roscoe)	Aphrodisiac
Ginger (*Zingiber officinale* Roscoe)	Impotence
Ginseng (American ginseng, Asian ginseng, Chinese ginseng, Korean red ginseng, *Panax ginseng*: *Panax* spp. including *P. ginseng* C.C. Meyer and *P. quincefolium* L., excluding *Eleutherococcus senticosus*)	Aphrodisiac
Ginseng (American ginseng, Asian ginseng, Chinese ginseng, Korean red ginseng, *Panax ginseng*: *Panax* spp. including *P. ginseng* C.C. Meyer and *P. quincefolium* L., excluding *Eleutherococcus senticosus*)	Premature ejaculation
Ginseng (American ginseng, Asian ginseng, Chinese ginseng, Korean red ginseng, *Panax ginseng*: *Panax* spp. including *P. ginseng* C.C. Meyer and *P. quincefolium* L., excluding *Eleutherococcus senticosus*)	Sexual arousal

Continued

Ginseng (American ginseng, Asian ginseng, Chinese ginseng, Korean red ginseng, *Panax ginseng*: *Panax* spp. including *P. ginseng* C.C. Meyer and *P. quincefolium* L., excluding *Eleutherococcus senticosus*)	Sexual symptoms
Gotu kola (*Centella asiatica* L.), total triterpenic fraction of *Centella asiatica* (TTFCA)	Aphrodisiac
Gotu kola (*Centella asiatica* L.), total triterpenic fraction of *Centella asiatica* (TTFCA)	Libido
Gymnema (*Gymnema Sylvestre* R. Br.)	Aphrodisiac
Hops (*Humulus lupulus* L.)	Aphrodisiac
Kava (*Piper methysticum* G. Forst)	Aphrodisiac
Lavender (*Lavandula angustifolia* Miller)	Aphrodisiac
Marshmallow (*Althaea officinalis* L.)	Aphrodisiac
Marshmallow (*Althaea officinalis* L.)	Impotence
Melatonin	Erectile dysfunction
Melatonin	Sexual activity enhancement
Niacin (vitamin B_3, nicotinic acid), niacinamide, and inositol hexanicotinate	Orgasm improvement
Pygeum (*Prunus africana*, *Pygeum africanum*)	Aphrodisiac
Pygeum (*Prunus africana*, *Pygeum africanum*)	Impotence
Pygeum (*Prunus africana*, *Pygeum africanum*)	Sexual performance
Saw palmetto (*Serenoa repens* [Bartram] Small)	Aphrodisiac
Saw palmetto (*Serenoa repens* [Bartram] Small)	Impotence
Saw palmetto (*Serenoa repens* [Bartram] Small)	Sexual vigor
Sweet almond (*Prunus amygdalus dulcis*)	Aphrodisiac
Wild yam (*Dioscorea villosa*)	Libido
Yohimbe bark extract (*Pausinystalia yohimbe* Pierre ex Beille)	Aphrodisiac

EYE DISORDERS AND RELATED CONDITIONS

Levels of Scientific Evidence for Specific Therapies

GRADE: C (Unclear or Conflicting Scientific Evidence)	
Therapy	Specific Therapeutic Use(s)
Eyebright (*Euphrasia officinalis*)	Conjunctivitis
Propolis	Cornea complications from zoster infection
Turmeric (*Curcuma longa* L.), curcumin	Uveitis (eye inflammation)

TRADITIONAL OR THEORETICAL USES THAT LACK SUFFICIENT EVIDENCE	
Therapy	Specific Therapeutic Use(s)
Belladonna (*Atropa belladonna* L. or its variety *acuminata* Royle ex Lindl)	Conjunctivitis
Bilberry (*Vaccinium myrtillus*)	Eye disorders
Boron	Eye cleansing
Calendula (*Calendula officinalis* L.), marigold	Conjunctivitis
Calendula (*Calendula officinalis* L.), marigold	Eye inflammation
Chamomile (*Matricaria recutita*, *Chamaemelum nobile*)	Eye infections
Clay	Eye disorders
Eyebright (*Euphrasia officinalis*)	Ocular compress
Eyebright (*Euphrasia officinalis*)	Ocular fatigue
Eyebright (*Euphrasia officinalis*)	Ocular rinse
Eyebright (*Euphrasia officinalis*)	Ophthalmia
Flaxseed and flaxseed oil (*Linum usitatissimum*)	Foreign body removal from the eye
Goldenseal (Hydrastis canadensis L.), berberine	Conjunctivitis
Goldenseal (*Hydrastis canadensis* L.), berberine	Eyewash
Goldenseal (*Hydrastis canadensis* L.), berberine	Keratitis (inflammation of the cornea of the eye)
Gotu kola (*Centella asiatica* L.), total triterpenic fraction of *Centella asiatica* (TTFCA)	Eye diseases

Continued

Green tea (*Camellia sinensis*)	Tired eyes
Oleander (*Nerium oleander*, *Thevetia peruviana*)	Eye diseases
Propolis	Eye infections/inflammation
Valerian (*Valeriana officinalis* L.)	Vision problems
Yohimbe bark extract (*Pausinystalia yohimbe* Pierre ex Beille)	Pupil dilator
Yohimbe bark extract (*Pausinystalia yohimbe* Pierre ex Beille)	Pupil dilator

FATIGUE AND RELATED CONDITIONS

Levels of Scientific Evidence for Specific Therapies

GRADE: C (Unclear or Conflicting Scientific Evidence)

Therapy	Specific Therapeutic Use(s)
Betel nut (*Areca catechu* L.)	Stimulant
DHEA (dehydroepiandrosterone)	Chronic fatigue syndrome
Evening primrose oil (*Oenothera biennis* L.)	Chronic fatigue syndrome/ post-viral infection symptoms
Ginseng (American ginseng, Asian ginseng, Chinese ginseng, Korean red ginseng, *Panax ginseng*: *Panax* spp. including *P. ginseng* C.C. Meyer and *P. quincefolium* L., excluding *Eleutherococcus senticosus*)	Fatigue

TRADITIONAL OR THEORETICAL USES THAT LACK SUFFICIENT EVIDENCE

Therapy	Specific Therapeutic Use(s)
Aloe (*Aloe vera*)	Chronic fatigue syndrome
American pennyroyal (*Hedeoma pulegioides* L.), European pennyroyal (*Mentha pulegium* L.)	Stimulant
Astragalus (*Astragalus membranaceus*)	Chronic fatigue syndrome
Astragalus (*Astragalus membranaceus*)	Fatigue
Black cohosh (*Cimicifuga racemosa* L. Nutt.)	Malaise
Bladderwrack (*Fucus vesiculosus*)	Fatigue
Calendula (*Calendula officinalis* L.), marigold	Fatigue

Coenzyme Q10	Chronic fatigue syndrome
Dandelion (*Taraxacum officinale*)	Chronic fatigue syndrome
Dandelion (*Taraxacum officinale*)	Stimulant
Dong quai (*Angelica sinensis* [Oliv.] Diels), Chinese angelica	Fatigue
Ephedra (*Ephedra sinica*)/ma huang	Energy enhancer
Ephedra (*Ephedra sinica*)/ma huang	Stimulant
Essiac	Chronic fatigue syndrome
Eucalyptus oil (*Eucalyptus globulus* Labillardiere, *E. fructicetorum* F. Von Mueller, *E. smithii* R.T. Baker)	Alertness
Eucalyptus oil (*Eucalyptus globulus* Labillardiere, *E. fructicetorum* F. Von Mueller, *E. smithii* R.T. Baker)	Stimulant
Garlic (*Allium sativum* L.)	Fatigue
Ginger (*Zingiber officinale* Roscoe)	Stimulant
Ginkgo (*Ginkgo biloba* L.)	Fatigue
Ginseng (American ginseng, Asian ginseng, Chinese ginseng, Korean red ginseng, *Panax ginseng*: *Panax* spp. including *P. ginseng* C.C. Meyer and *P. quincefolium* L., excluding *Eleutherococcus senticosus*)	Fatigue
Goldenseal (*Hydrastis canadensis* L.), berberine	Chronic fatigue syndrome
Goldenseal (*Hydrastis canadensis* L.), berberine	Stimulant
Gotu kola (*Centella asiatica* L.), total triterpenic fraction of *Centella asiatica* (TTFCA)	Energy
Gotu kola (*Centella asiatica* L.), total triterpenic fraction of *Centella asiatica* (TTFCA)	Fatigue
Green tea (*Camellia sinensis*)	Stimulant
Lavender (*Lavandula angustifolia* Miller)	Fatigue
Licorice (*Glycyrrhiza glabra* L.), deglycyrrhizinated licorice (DGL)	Chronic fatigue syndrome
Omega-3 fatty acids, fish oil, alpha-linolenic acid	Chronic fatigue syndrome
Seaweed, kelp, bladderwrack (*Fucus vesiculosus*)	Fatigue
Spirulina	Energy booster
Spirulina	Fatigue

Continued

St. John's wort (*Hypericum perforatum* L.)	Fatigue
Valerian (*Valeriana officinalis* L.)	Fatigue

FEVER AND RELATED CONDITIONS

Levels of Scientific Evidence for Specific Therapies

GRADE: C (Unclear or Conflicting Scientific Evidence)

Therapy	Specific Therapeutic Use(s)
Clove (*Eugenia aromatica*)	Fever reduction

TRADITIONAL OR THEORETICAL USES THAT LACK SUFFICIENT EVIDENCE

Therapy	Specific Therapeutic Use(s)
American pennyroyal (*Hedeoma pulegioides* L.), European pennyroyal (*Mentha pulegium* L.)	Diaphoretic
American pennyroyal (*Hedeoma pulegioides* L.), European pennyroyal (*Mentha pulegium* L.)	Fever
Astragalus (*Astragalus membranaceus*)	Fever
Belladonna (*Atropa belladonna* L. or its variety *acuminata* Royle ex Lindl)	Fever
Bilberry (*Vaccinium myrtillus*)	Fevers
Black cohosh (*Cimicifuga racemosa* L. Nutt.)	Fever
Blessed thistle (*Cnicus benedictus* L.)	Antipyretic
Blessed thistle (*Cnicus benedictus* L.)	Diaphoretic
Blessed thistle (*Cnicus benedictus* L.)	Fever
Burdock (*Arctium lappa*)	Fever
Calendula (*Calendula officinalis* L.), marigold	Fever
Chamomile (*Matricaria recutita*, *Chamaemelum nobile*)	Diaphoretic
Chamomile (*Matricaria recutita*, *Chamaemelum nobile*)	Fever
Clay	Fevers
Dandelion (*Taraxacum officinale*)	Fever reduction
Devil's claw (*Harpagophytum procumbens* DC.)	Fever
Elder (*Sambucus nigra* L.)	Fever

Ephedra (*Ephedra sinica*)/ma huang	Antipyretic
Ephedra (*Ephedra sinica*)/ma huang	Diaphoretic
Ephedra (*Ephedra sinica*)/ma huang	Fevers
Eucalyptus oil (*Eucalyptus globulus* Labillardiere, *E. fructicetorum* F. Von Mueller, *E. smithii* R.T. Baker)	Fever
Feverfew (*Tanacetum parthenium* L. Schultz-Bip.)	Fever
Garlic (*Allium sativum* L.)	Fever
Ginseng (American ginseng, Asian ginseng, Chinese ginseng, Korean red ginseng, *Panax ginseng*: *Panax* spp. including *P. ginseng* C.C. Meyer and *P. quincefolium* L., excluding *Eleutherococcus senticosus*)	Fever
Goldenseal (*Hydrastis canadensis* L.), berberine	Fever
Gotu kola (*Centella asiatica* L.), total triterpenic fraction of *Centella asiatica* (TTFCA)	Fever
Horse chestnut (*Aesculus hippocastanum* L.)	Fever
Horsetail (*Equisetum arvense* L.)	Fever
Lavender (*Lavandula angustifolia* Miller)	Fever
Licorice (*Glycyrrhiza glabra* L.), deglycyrrhizinated licorice (DGL)	Fever
Peppermint (*Mentha x piperita* L.)	Fever
Polypodium leucotomos extract, Anapsos	Fever
Pygeum (*Prunus africana*, *Pygeum africanum*)	Fever
Slippery elm (*Ulmus rubra* Muhl., *U. fulva* Michx.)	Fever
Sorrel (*Rumex acetosa* L., *R. acetosella* L.), Sinupret	Fever
Soy (*Glycine max* L. Merr.)	Fever
Thyme (*Thymus vulgaris* L.), thymol	Fever
Valerian (*Valeriana officinalis* L.)	Fever
White horehound (*Marrubium vulgare*)	Fever reduction
Yohimbe bark extract (*Pausinystalia yohimbe* Pierre ex Beille)	Fevers
Yohimbe bark extract (*Pausinystalia yohimbe* Pierre ex Beille)	Fevers

FIBROMYALGIA AND RELATED CONDITIONS

Levels of Scientific Evidence for Specific Therapies

TRADITIONAL OR THEORETICAL USES THAT LACK SUFFICIENT EVIDENCE

Therapy	Specific Therapeutic Use(s)
Black cohosh (*Cimicifuga racemosa* L. Nutt.)	Myalgia
Devil's claw (*Harpagophytum procumbens* DC.)	Fibromyalgia
Fenugreek (*Trigonella foenum-graecum* L.)	Myalgia
Ginseng (American ginseng, Asian ginseng, Chinese ginseng, Korean red ginseng, *Panax ginseng*: *Panax* spp. including	
P. ginseng C.C. Meyer and *P. quincefolium* L., excluding *Eleutherococcus senticosus*)	Fibromyalgia
Horse chestnut (*Aesculus hippocastanum* L.)	Nocturnal leg cramps
Melatonin	Fibromyalgia
Omega-3 fatty acids, fish oil, alpha-linolenic acid	Fibromyalgia
Peppermint (*Mentha x piperita* L.)	Fibromyositis
Spirulina	Fibromyalgia
Tea tree oil (*Melaleuca alternifolia* [Maiden & Betche] Cheel)	Muscle and joint distress

FLATULENCE AND RELATED CONDITIONS

Levels of Scientific Evidence for Specific Therapies

TRADITIONAL OR THEORETICAL USES THAT LACK SUFFICIENT EVIDENCE

Therapy	Specific Therapeutic Use(s)
American pennyroyal (*Hedeoma pulegioides* L.), European pennyroyal (*Mentha pulegium* L.)	Carminative
American pennyroyal (*Hedeoma pulegioides* L.), European pennyroyal (*Mentha pulegium* L.)	Flatulence
Betel nut (*Areca catechu* L.)	Gas
Boswellia (*Boswellia serrata* Roxb.)	Belching
Boswellia (*Boswellia serrata* Roxb.)	Carminative

Chamomile (*Matricaria recutita*, *Chamaemelum nobile*)	Gas
Chaparral (*Larrea tridentata* DC. Coville, *L. divaricata* Cav.), nordihydroguaiaretic acid (NDGA)	Gas
Clove (*Eugenia aromatica*)	Gas
Dandelion (*Taraxacum officinale*)	Gas
Devil's claw (*Harpagophytum procumbens* DC.)	Flatulence (gas)
Dong quai (*Angelica sinensis* [Oliv.] Diels), Chinese angelica	Flatulence (gas)
Fenugreek (*Trigonella foenum-graecum* L.)	Flatulence
Ginger (*Zingiber officinale* Roscoe)	Flatulence (gas)
Goldenseal (*Hydrastis canadensis* L.), berberine	Flatulence (gas)
Green tea (*Camellia sinensis*)	Flatulence
Lavender (*Lavandula angustifolia* Miller)	Gas
Peppermint (*Mentha x piperita* L.)	Gas (flatulence)
Thyme (*Thymus vulgaris* L.), thymol	Flatulence
Thyme (*Thymus vulgaris* L.), thymol	Gas
Turmeric (*Curcuma longa* L.), curcumin	Gas
Valerian (*Valeriana officinalis* L.)	Carminative
Valerian (*Valeriana officinalis* L.)	Flatulence
White horehound (*Marrubium vulgare*)	Flatulence
Wild Yam (*Dioscorea villosa*)	Flatus prevention

FLAVORING AGENT AND RELATED CONDITIONS

Levels of Scientific Evidence for Specific Therapies

TRADITIONAL OR THEORETICAL USES THAT LACK SUFFICIENT EVIDENCE

Therapy	Specific Therapeutic Use(s)
American pennyroyal (*Hedeoma pulegioides* L.), European pennyroyal (*Mentha pulegium* L.)	Flavoring agent
Clove (*Eugenia aromatica*)	Flavoring for food and cigarettes

Continued

Dandelion (*Taraxacum officinale*)	Coffee substitute
Dandelion (*Taraxacum officinale*)	Food uses
Elder (*Sambucus nigra* L.)	Flavoring
Eucalyptus oil (*Eucalyptus globulus* Labillardiere, *E. fructicetorum* F. Von Mueller, *E. smithii* R.T. Baker)	Flavoring
Eyebright (*Euphrasia officinalis*)	Flavoring agent
White horehound (*Marrubium vulgare*)	Food flavoring

FUNGAL INFECTIONS AND RELATED CONDITIONS

Levels of Scientific Evidence for Specific Therapies

GRADE: C (Unclear or Conflicting Scientific Evidence)

Therapy	Specific Therapeutic Use(s)
Garlic (*Allium sativum* L.)	Antifungal (applied to the skin)
Goldenseal (*Hydrastis canadensis* L.), berberine	Chloroquine-resistant malaria
Seaweed, kelp, bladderwrack (*Fucus vesiculosus*)	Antifungal
Tea tree oil (*Melaleuca alternifolia* [Maiden & Betche] Cheel)	Fungal nail infection (onychomycosis)
Tea tree oil (*Melaleuca alternifolia* [Maiden & Betche] Cheel)	Thrush (*Candida albicans* infection of the mouth)

TRADITIONAL OR THEORETICAL USES THAT LACK SUFFICIENT EVIDENCE

Therapy	Specific Therapeutic Use(s)
Aloe (*Aloe vera*)	Parasitic worm infections
Aloe (*Aloe vera*)	Yeast infections of the skin
Astragalus (*Astragalus membranaceus*)	Antifungal
Betel nut (*Areca catechu* L.)	Anthelminthic
Black cohosh (*Cimicifuga racemosa* L. Nutt.)	Malaria
Bladderwrack (*Fucus vesiculosus*)	Parasites
Blessed thistle (*Cnicus benedictus* L.)	Malaria
Burdock (*Arctium lappa*)	Fungal infections
Burdock (*Arctium lappa*)	Ringworm

Calendula (*Calendula officinalis* L.), marigold	Fungal infections
Chamomile (*Matricaria recutita*, *Chamaemelum nobile*)	Antifungal
Chamomile (*Matricaria recutita*, *Chamaemelum nobile*)	Fungal infections
Chamomile (*Matricaria recutita*, *Chamaemelum nobile*)	Malaria
Chamomile (*Matricaria recutita*, *Chamaemelum nobile*)	Parasites/worms
Chaparral (*Larrea tridentata* DC. Coville, *L. divaricata* Cav.), nordihydroguaiaretic acid (NDGA)	Antiparasitic
Clove (*Eugenia aromatica*)	Antifungal
Dandelion (*Taraxacum officinale*)	Antifungal
Devil's claw (*Harpagophytum procumbens* DC.)	Malaria
DHEA (dehydroepiandrosterone)	Malaria
Dong quai (*Angelica sinensis* [Oliv.] Diels), Chinese angelica	Antifungal
Dong quai (*Angelica sinensis* [Oliv.] Diels), Chinese angelica	Malaria
Echinacea (*Echinacea angustifolia* DC., *E. pallida*, *E. purpurea*)	Malaria
Eucalyptus oil (*Eucalyptus globulus* Labillardiere, *E. fructicetorum* F. Von Mueller, *E. smithii* R.T. Baker)	Antifungal
Eucalyptus oil (*Eucalyptus globulus* Labillardiere, *E. fructicetorum* F. Von Mueller, *E. smithii* R.T. Baker)	Hookworm
Eucalyptus oil (*Eucalyptus globulus* Labillardiere, *E. fructicetorum* F. Von Mueller, *E. smithii* R.T. Baker)	Parasitic infection
Eucalyptus oil (*Eucalyptus globulus* Labillardiere, *E. fructicetorum* F. Von Mueller, *E. smithii* R.T. Baker)	Ringworm
Eyebright (*Euphrasia officinalis*)	Anthelmintic
Garlic (*Allium sativum* L.)	Amoeba infections
Garlic (*Allium sativum* L.)	Malaria
Garlic (*Allium sativum* L.)	Parasites and worms
Garlic (*Allium sativum* L.)	Thrush
Ginger (*Zingiber officinale* Roscoe)	Fungal infections
Ginger (*Zingiber officinale* Roscoe)	Malaria
Ginkgo (*Ginkgo biloba* L.)	Antifungal

Continued

Ginkgo (*Ginkgo biloba* L.)	Antiparasitic
Ginkgo (*Ginkgo biloba* L.)	Filariasis
Goldenseal (*Hydrastis canadensis* L.), berberine	Antifungal
Goldenseal (*Hydrastis canadensis* L.), berberine	Thrush
Gotu kola (*Centella asiatica* L.), total triterpenic fraction of *Centella asiatica* (TTFCA)	Fungal infections
Gotu kola (*Centella asiatica* L.), total triterpenic fraction of *Centella asiatica* (TTFCA)	Malaria
Green tea (*Camellia sinensis*)	Fungal infections
Gymnema (*Gymnema Sylvestre* R. Br.)	Malaria
Hops (*Humulus lupulus* L.)	Parasites
Horsetail (*Equisetum arvense* L.)	Malaria
Kava (*Piper methysticum* G. Forst)	Antifungal
Lactobacillus acidophilus	Thrush
Lavender (*Lavandula angustifolia* Miller)	Antifungal
Lavender (*Lavandula angustifolia* Miller)	Parasites/worms
Milk thistle (*Silybum marianum*), silymarin	Malaria
Oleander (*Nerium oleander*, *Thevetia peruviana*)	Antiparasitic
Oleander (*Nerium oleander*, *Thevetia peruviana*)	Malaria
Oleander (*Nerium oleander*, *Thevetia peruviana*)	Ringworm
Omega-3 fatty acids, fish oil, alpha-linolenic acid	Malaria
Propolis	Fungal infections
Psyllium (*Plantago ovata*, *P. ispaghula*)	Antiparasitic
Pygeum (*Prunus africana*, *Pygeum africanum*)	Malaria
Seaweed, kelp, bladderwrack (*Fucus vesiculosus*)	Antiparasitic
Shark cartilage	Fungal infections
Sorrel (*Rumex acetosa* L., *R. acetosella* L.), Sinupret	Ringworm
Soy (*Glycine max* L. Merr.)	Antifungal
Spirulina	Antifungal
St. John's wort (*Hypericum perforatum* L.)	Antimalarial

Tea tree oil (*Melaleuca alternifolia* [Maiden & Betche] Cheel)	Ringworm
Turmeric (*Curcuma longa* L.), curcumin	Antifungal
Turmeric (*Curcuma longa* L.), curcumin	Parasites
Turmeric (*Curcuma longa* L.), curcumin	Ringworm
White horehound (*Marrubium vulgare*)	Anthelmintic
Wild yam (*Dioscorea villosa*)	Antifungal

GALLBLADDER DISORDERS AND RELATED CONDITIONS

Levels of Scientific Evidence for Specific Therapies

GRADE: C (Unclear or Conflicting Scientific Evidence)

Therapy	Specific Therapeutic Use(s)
Globe artichoke (*Cynara scolymus* L.)	Choleretic (bile-secretion stimulant)
Soy (*Glycine max* L. Merr.)	Gallstones (cholelithiasis)
Turmeric (*Curcuma longa* L.), curcumin	Gallstone prevention/bile flow stimulant
White horehound (*Marrubium vulgare*)	Choleretic (dyspepsia, appetite stimulation)

TRADITIONAL OR THEORETICAL USES THAT LACK SUFFICIENT EVIDENCE

Therapy	Specific Therapeutic Use(s)
American pennyroyal (*Hedeoma pulegioides* L.), European pennyroyal (*Mentha pulegium* L.)	Gallbladder disorders
Black cohosh (*Cimicifuga racemosa* L. Nutt.)	Gallbladder disorders
Blessed thistle (*Cnicus benedictus* L.)	Choleretic (bile flow stimulant)
Blessed thistle (*Cnicus benedictus* L.)	Gallbladder disease
Cranberry (*Vaccinium macrocarpon*)	Gallbladder stones
Dandelion (*Taraxacum officinale*)	Bile flow stimulation
Dandelion (*Taraxacum officinale*)	Gallbladder disease
Dandelion (*Taraxacum officinale*)	Gallstones

Continued

Devil's claw (*Harpagophytum procumbens* DC.)	Choleretic (bile secretion)
Dong quai (*Angelica sinensis* [Oliv.] Diels), Chinese angelica	Cholagogue
Garlic (*Allium sativum* L.)	Bile secretion problems
Garlic (*Allium sativum* L.)	Gallstones
Ginger (*Zingiber officinale* Roscoe)	Bile secretion problems
Globe artichoke (*Cynara scolymus* L.)	Cholegogue
Globe artichoke (*Cynara scolymus* L.)	Cholelithiasis
Goldenseal (*Hydrastis canadensis* L.), berberine	Bile flow stimulant
Goldenseal (*Hydrastis canadensis* L.), berberine	Gallstones
Horse chestnut (*Aesculus hippocastanum* L.)	Gallbladder infection (cholecystitis)
Horse chestnut (*Aesculus hippocastanum* L.)	Gallbladder pain (colic)
Horse chestnut (*Aesculus hippocastanum* L.)	Gallbladder stones (cholelithiasis)
Lavender (*Lavandula angustifolia* Miller)	Cholagogue
Lavender (*Lavandula angustifolia* Miller)	Choleretic
Milk thistle (*Silybum marianum*), silymarin	Cholelithiasis
Omega-3 fatty acids, fish oil, alpha-linolenic acid	Gallstones
Peppermint (*Mentha x piperita* L.)	Bile duct disorders
Peppermint (*Mentha x piperita* L.)	Cholelithiasis (gallstones)
Peppermint (*Mentha x piperita* L.)	Gallbladder disorders
Psyllium (*Plantago ovata, P. ispaghula*)	Gallstones
Turmeric (*Curcuma longa* L.), curcumin	Gallstones
White horehound (*Marrubium vulgare*)	Bile secretion
White horehound (*Marrubium vulgare*)	Gallbladder complaints
Wild yam (*Dioscorea villosa*)	Bile flow improvement
Wild yam (*Dioscorea villosa*)	Biliary colic

GASTROINTESTINAL DISORDERS AND RELATED CONDITIONS

Levels of Scientific Evidence for Specific Therapies

GRADE: C (Unclear or Conflicting Scientific Evidence)

Therapy	Specific Therapeutic Use(s)
Belladonna (*Atropa belladonna* L. or its variety *acuminata* Royle ex Lindl)	Irritable bowel syndrome
Chamomile (*Matricaria recutita*, *Chamaemelum nobile*)	Gastrointestinal conditions
Clay	Functional gastrointestinal disorders
Globe artichoke (*Cynara scolymus* L.)	Irritable bowel syndrome
Lactobacillus acidophilus	Irritable bowel syndrome
Lactobacillus acidophilus	Necrotizing enterocolitis prevention in infants
Peppermint (*Mentha x piperita* L.)	Irritable bowel syndrome
Psyllium (*Plantago ovata*, *P. ispaghula*)	Irritable bowel syndrome
Slippery elm (*Ulmus rubra* Muhl., *U. fulva* Michx.)	Gastrointestinal disorders
White horehound (*Marrubium vulgare*)	Intestinal disorders/ antispasmodic

TRADITIONAL OR THEORETICAL USES THAT LACK SUFFICIENT EVIDENCE

Therapy	Specific Therapeutic Use(s)
Alfalfa (*Medicago sativa* L.)	Gastrointestinal tract disorders
Aloe (*Aloe vera*)	Bowel disorders
American pennyroyal (*Hedeoma pulegioides* L.), European pennyroyal (*Mentha pulegium* L.)	Bowel disorders
American pennyroyal (*Hedeoma pulegioides* L.), European pennyroyal (*Mentha pulegium* L.)	Colic
American pennyroyal (*Hedeoma pulegioides* L.), European pennyroyal (*Mentha pulegium* L.)	Intestinal disorders
American pennyroyal (*Hedeoma pulegioides* L.), European pennyroyal (*Mentha pulegium* L.)	Stomach pain
American pennyroyal (*Hedeoma pulegioides* L.), European pennyroyal (*Mentha pulegium* L.)	Stomach spasms

Continued

Arginine (L-arginine)	Infantile necrotizing enterocolitis
Arginine (L-arginine)	Lower esophageal sphincter relaxation
Arginine (L-arginine)	Stomach motility disorders
Astragalus (*Astragalus membranaceus*)	Gastrointestinal disorders
Barley (*Hordeum vulgare* L.), germinated barley foodstuff (GBF)	Bowel/intestinal disorders
Belladonna (*Atropa belladonna* L. or its variety *acuminata* Royle ex Lindl)	Diverticulitis
Bilberry (*Vaccinium myrtillus*)	Stomach upset
Bitter melon (*Momordica charantia* L.), MAP30	Gastrointestinal cramps
Black tea (*Camellia sinensis*)	Stomach disorders
Bladderwrack (*Fucus vesiculosus*)	Stomach upset
Bromelain	Leaky gut syndrome
Calendula (*Calendula officinalis* L.), marigold	Bowel irritation
Calendula (*Calendula officinalis* L.), marigold	Gastrointestinal tract disorders
Chamomile (*Matricaria recutita*, *Chamaemelum nobile*)	Abdominal bloating
Chamomile (*Matricaria recutita*, *Chamaemelum nobile*)	Infantile colic
Chamomile (*Matricaria recutita*, *Chamaemelum nobile*)	Irritable bowel syndrome
Chaparral (*Larrea tridentata* DC. Coville, *L. divaricata* Cav.), nordihydroguaiaretic acid (NDGA)	Bowel cramps
Chaparral (*Larrea tridentata* DC. Coville, *L. divaricata* Cav.), nordihydroguaiaretic acid (NDGA)	Gastrointestinal disorders
Clay	Stomach disorders
Clove (*Eugenia aromatica*)	Abdominal pain
Clove (*Eugenia aromatica*)	Colic
Cranberry (*Vaccinium macrocarpon*)	Stomach ailments
Dandelion (*Taraxacum officinale*)	Stomachache
Devil's claw (*Harpagophytum procumbens* DC.)	Gastrointestinal disorders
Dong quai (*Angelica sinensis* [Oliv.] Diels), Chinese angelica	Abdominal pain

Dong quai (*Angelica sinensis* [Oliv.] Diels), Chinese angelica	Irritable bowel syndrome
Echinacea (*Echinacea angustifolia* DC., *E. pallida*, *E. purpurea*)	Stomach upset
Elder (*Sambucus nigra* L.)	Colic
Elder (*Sambucus nigra* L.)	Gut disorders
Evening primrose oil (*Oenothera biennis* L.)	Irritable bowel syndrome
Eyebright (*Euphrasia officinalis*)	Gastric acid secretion stimulation
Fenugreek (*Trigonella foenum-graecum* L.)	Colic
Feverfew (*Tanacetum parthenium* L. Schultz-Bip.)	Abdominal pain
Flaxseed and flaxseed oil (*Linum usitatissimum*)	Abdominal pain
Flaxseed and flaxseed oil (*Linum usitatissimum*)	Diverticulitis
Flaxseed and flaxseed oil (*Linum usitatissimum*)	Irritable bowel syndrome
Flaxseed and flaxseed oil (*Linum usitatissimum*)	Laxative-induced colon damage
Flaxseed and flaxseed oil (*Linum usitatissimum*)	Stomach upset
Garlic (*Allium sativum* L.)	Stomachache
Ginger (*Zingiber officinale* Roscoe)	Colic
Ginger (*Zingiber officinale* Roscoe)	Stomachache
Ginseng (American ginseng, Asian ginseng, Chinese ginseng, Korean red ginseng, *Panax ginseng*: *Panax* spp. including *P. ginseng* C.C. Meyer and *P. quincefolium* L., excluding *Eleutherococcus senticosus*)	Stomach upset
Goldenseal (*Hydrastis canadensis* L.), berberine	Stomachache
Green tea (*Camellia sinensis*)	Stomach disorders
Gymnema (*Gymnema Sylvestre* R. Br.)	Stomach ailments
Hawthorn (*Crataegus laevigata*, *C. oxyacantha*, *C. monogyna*, *C. pentagyna*)	Abdominal colic
Hawthorn (*Crataegus laevigata*, *C. oxyacantha*, *C. monogyna*, *C. pentagyna*)	Abdominal distention
Hawthorn (*Crataegus laevigata*, *C. oxyacantha*, *C. monogyna*, *C. pentagyna*)	Abdominal pain

Continued

Hawthorn (*Crataegus laevigata*, *C. oxyacantha*, *C. monogyna*, *C. pentagyna*)	Stomachache
Hops (*Humulus lupulus* L.)	Irritable bowel syndrome
Horsetail (*Equisetum arvense* L.)	Stomach upset
Kava (*Piper methysticum* G. Forst)	Stomach upset
Lactobacillus acidophilus	Diverticulitis
Lavender (*Lavandula angustifolia* Miller)	Colic
Licorice (*Glycyrrhiza glabra* L.), deglycyrrhizinated licorice (DGL)	Diverticulitis
Licorice (*Glycyrrhiza glabra* L.), deglycyrrhizinated licorice (DGL)	Stomach upset
Marshmallow (*Althaea officinalis* L.)	Diverticulitis
Marshmallow (*Althaea officinalis* L.)	Irritable bowel syndrome
Melatonin	Intestinal motility disorders
Passionflower (*Passiflora incarnata* L.)	Gastrointestinal discomfort (nervous stomach)
Peppermint (*Mentha x piperita* L.)	Gastrointestinal disorders
Peppermint (*Mentha x piperita* L.)	Ileus (postoperative)
Peppermint (*Mentha x piperita* L.)	Intestinal colic
Propolis	Diverticulitis
Pygeum (*Prunus africana*, *Pygeum africanum*)	Stomach upset
Red yeast rice (*Monascus purpureus*)	Colic in children
Red yeast rice (*Monascus purpureus*)	Stomach problems
Shark cartilage	Intestinal disorders and inflammation
Slippery elm (*Ulmus rubra* Muhl., *U. fulva* Michx.)	Colic
Slippery elm (*Ulmus rubra* Muhl., *U. fulva* Michx.)	Diverticulitis
Slippery elm (*Ulmus rubra* Muhl., *U. fulva* Michx.)	Irritable bowel syndrome
Sorrel (*Rumex acetosa* L., *R. acetosella* L.), Sinupret	Stimulation of secretion
Sorrel (*Rumex acetosa* L., *R. acetosella* L.), Sinupret	Ulcerated bowel
Soy (*Glycine max* L. Merr.)	Gastrointestinal motility

Spirulina	Bowel health
Thyme (*Thymus vulgaris* L.), thymol	Colic
Thyme (*Thymus vulgaris* L.), thymol	Stomach cramps
Turmeric (*Curcuma longa* L.), curcumin	Bloating
Turmeric (*Curcuma longa* L.), curcumin	Colic
Valerian (*Valeriana officinalis* L.)	Bloating
Valerian (*Valeriana officinalis* L.)	Colic
Valerian (*Valeriana officinalis* L.)	Intestinal disorders
Valerian (*Valeriana officinalis* L.)	Irritable bowel syndrome
Valerian (*Valeriana officinalis* L.)	Viral gastroenteritis
White horehound (*Marrubium vulgare*)	Bloating
White horehound (*Marrubium vulgare*)	Colic
Wild yam (*Dioscorea villosa*)	Diverticulitis
Wild yam (*Dioscorea villosa*)	Irritable bowel syndrom

GENERALIZED ANXIETY DISORDER AND RELATED CONDITIONS

Levels of Scientific Evidence for Specific Therapies

GRADE: A (Strong Scientific Evidence)

Therapy	Specific Therapeutic Use(s)
Kava (*Piper methysticum* G. Forst)	Anxiety

GRADE: B (Good Scientific Evidence)

Therapy	Specific therapeutic Use(s)
Lavender (*Lavandula angustifolia* Miller)	Anxiety (lavender aromatherapy)

GRADE: C (Unclear or Conflicting Scientific Evidence)

Therapy	Specific Therapeutic Use(s)
Gotu kola (*Centella asiatica* L.), total triterpenic fraction of *Centella asiatica* (TTFCA)	Anxiety

Continued

St. John's wort (*Hypericum perforatum* L.)	Anxiety disorder
Valerian (*Valeriana officinalis* L.)	Anxiety

TRADITIONAL OR THEORETICAL USES THAT LACK SUFFICIENT EVIDENCE

Therapy	Specific Therapeutic Use(s)
American pennyroyal (*Hedeoma pulegioides* L.), European pennyroyal (*Mentha pulegium* L.)	Anxiolytic
Belladonna (*Atropa belladonna* L. or its variety *acuminata* Royle ex Lindl)	Anxiety
Black cohosh (*Cimicifuga racemosa* L. Nutt.)	Anxiety
Black tea (*Camellia sinensis*)	Anxiety
Calendula (*Calendula officinalis* L.), marigold	Anxiety
Chamomile (*Matricaria recutita*, *Chamaemelum nobile*)	Anxiety
Danshen (*Salvia miltiorrhiza*)	Anxiety
DHEA (dehydroepiandrosterone)	Anxiety
DHEA (dehydroepiandrosterone)	Stress
Dong quai (*Angelica sinensis* [Oliv.] Diels), Chinese angelica	Anxiety
Dong quai (*Angelica sinensis* [Oliv.] Diels), Chinese angelica	Stress
Elder (*Sambucus nigra* L.)	Stress reduction
Eucalyptus oil (*Eucalyptus globulus* Labillardiere, *E. fructicetorum* F. Von Mueller, *E. smithii* R.T. Baker)	Aromatherapy
Garlic (*Allium sativum* L.)	Stress (anxiety)
Ginkgo (*Ginkgo biloba* L.)	Anxiety
Ginseng (American ginseng, Asian ginseng, Chinese ginseng, Korean red ginseng, *Panax ginseng*: *Panax* spp. including *P. ginseng* C.C. Meyer and *P. quincefolium* L., excluding *Eleutherococcus senticosus*)	Aggression
Ginseng (American ginseng, Asian ginseng, Chinese ginseng, Korean red ginseng, *Panax ginseng*: *Panax* spp. including *P. ginseng* C.C. Meyer and *P. quincefolium* L., excluding *Eleutherococcus senticosus*)	Anxiety

Ginseng (American ginseng, Asian ginseng, Chinese ginseng, Korean red ginseng, *Panax ginseng*: *Panax* spp. including *P. ginseng* C.C. Meyer and *P. quincefolium* L., excluding *Eleutherococcus senticosus*)	Stress
Goldenseal (*Hydrastis canadensis* L.), berberine	Anxiety
Gotu kola (*Centella asiatica* L.), total triterpenic fraction of *Centella asiatica* (TTFCA)	Anxiety
Hops (*Humulus lupulus* L.)	Anxiety
Hops (*Humulus lupulus* L.)	Anxiety during menopause
Lavender (*Lavandula angustifolia* Miller)	Anxiety
Niacin (vitamin B_3, nicotinic acid), niacinamide, and inositol hexanicotinate	Anxiety
Omega-3 fatty acids, fish oil, alpha-linolenic acid	Panic disorder
Passionflower (*Passiflora incarnata* L.)	Tension
Spirulina	Anxiety
Thyme (*Thymus vulgaris* L.), thymol	Anxiety
Valerian (*Valeriana officinalis* L.)	Stress
Yohimbe bark extract (*Pausinystalia yohimbe* Pierre ex Beille)	Panic disorder

GENITAL HERPES SIMPLEX VIRUS (HSV) INFECTION AND RELATED CONDITIONS

Levels of Scientific Evidence for Specific Therapies

GRADE: B (Good Scientific Evidence)

Therapy	Specific Therapeutic Use(s)
Aloe (*Aloe vera*)	Genital HSV infection

GRADE: C (Unclear or Conflicting Scientific Evidence)

Therapy	Specific Therapeutic Use(s)
Licorice (*Glycyrrhiza glabra* L.), deglycyrrhizinated licorice (DGL)	HSV infection
Propolis	Genital HSV infection

Continued

Tea tree oil (*Melaleuca alternifolia* [Maiden & Betche] Cheel)	Genital HSV infection

GRADE: D (FAIR NEGATIVE SCIENTIFIC EVIDENCE)

Therapy	Specific Therapeutic Use(s)
Echinacea (*Echinacea angustifolia* DC., *E. pallida*, *E. purpurea*)	Genital HSV infection
Licorice (*Glycyrrhiza glabra* L.), deglycyrrhizinated licorice (DGL)	Genital HSV infection

TRADITIONAL OR THEORETICAL USES THAT LACK SUFFICIENT EVIDENCE

Therapy	Specific Therapeutic Use(s)
Astragalus (*Astragalus membranaceus*)	Genital HSV infection
Belladonna (*Atropa belladonna* L. or its variety *acuminata* Royle ex Lindl)	Chickenpox
Bromelain	Shingles pain/postherpetic neuralgia
Calendula (*Calendula officinalis* L.), marigold	HSV infection
Chaparral (*Larrea tridentata* DC. Coville, *L. divaricata* Cav.), nordihydroguaiaretic acid (NDGA)	Chickenpox
Clove (*Eugenia aromatica*)	HSV infection
Elder (*Sambucus nigra* L.)	HSV infection
Eucalyptus oil (*Eucalyptus globulus* Labillardiere, *E. fructicetorum* F. Von Mueller, *E. smithii* R.T. Baker)	HSV infection
Eucalyptus oil (*Eucalyptus globulus* Labillardiere, *E. fructicetorum* F. Von Mueller, *E. smithii* R.T. Baker)	Shingles
Ginseng (American ginseng, Asian ginseng, Chinese ginseng, Korean red ginseng, *Panax ginseng*: *Panax* spp. including *P. ginseng* C.C. Meyer and *P. quincefolium* L., excluding *Eleutherococcus senticosus*)	HSV infection
Goldenseal (*Hydrastis canadensis* L.), berberine	Chickenpox
Goldenseal (*Hydrastis canadensis* L.), berberine	HSV infection
Gotu kola (*Centella asiatica* L.), total triterpenic fraction of *Centella asiatica* (TTFCA)	HSV-2 infection
Gotu kola (*Centella asiatica* L.), total triterpenic fraction of *Centella asiatica* (TTFCA)	Shingles (postherpetic neuralgia)

Peppermint (*Mentha x piperita* L.)	Chickenpox
Peppermint (*Mentha x piperita* L.)	Postherpetic neuralgia
Slippery elm (*Ulmus rubra* Muhl., *U. fulva* Michx.)	HSV infection
Spirulina	HSV-1 infection
St. John's wort (*Hypericum perforatum* L.)	HSV infection
Tea tree oil (*Melaleuca alternifolia* [Maiden & Betche] Cheel)	HSV infection

GLAUCOMA AND RELATED CONDITIONS

Levels of Scientific Evidence for Specific Therapies

GRADE: C (Unclear or Conflicting Scientific Evidence)

Therapy	Specific Therapeutic Use(s)
Bilberry (*Vaccinium myrtillus*)	Cataracts
Danshen (*Salvia miltiorrhiza*)	Glaucoma
Ginkgo (*Ginkgo biloba* L.)	Glaucoma
Melatonin	Glaucoma

TRADITIONAL OR THEORETICAL USES THAT LACK SUFFICIENT EVIDENCE

Therapy	Specific therapeutic Use(s)
Arginine (L-arginine)	Glaucoma
Belladonna (*Atropa belladonna* L. or its variety *acuminata* Royle ex Lindl)	Glaucoma
Betel nut (*Areca catechu* L.)	Glaucoma
Bilberry (*Vaccinium myrtillus*)	Glaucoma
Danshen (*Salvia miltiorrhiza*)	Cataracts
Dong quai (*Angelica sinensis* [Oliv.] Diels), Chinese angelica	Glaucoma
Eyebright (*Euphrasia officinalis*)	Cataracts
Green tea (*Camellia sinensis*)	Cataracts
Lycopene	Cataracts

Continued

Melatonin	Glaucoma
Niacin (vitamin B_3, nicotinic acid), niacinamide, and inositol hexanicotinate	Cataract prevention
Omega-3 fatty acids, fish oil, alpha-linolenic acid	Glaucoma
Shark cartilage	Glaucoma
Turmeric (*Curcuma longa* L.), curcumin	Cataracts

GOITER AND RELATED CONDITIONS

Levels of Scientific Evidence for Specific Therapies

GRADE: C (Unclear or Conflicting Scientific Evidence)

Therapy	Specific therapeutic Use(s)
Bladderwrack (*Fucus vesiculosus*)	Goiter (thyroid disease)

TRADITIONAL OR THEORETICAL USES THAT LACK SUFFICIENT EVIDENCE

Therapy	Specific Therapeutic Use(s)
Essiac	Thyroid disorders
Horsetail (*Equisetum arvense* L.)	Thyroid disorders
Niacin (vitamin B_3, nicotinic acid), niacinamide, and inositol hexanicotinate	Hypothyroidism
Propolis	Thyroid disease
Seaweed, kelp, bladderwrack (*Fucus vesiculosus*)	Exophthalmos
Seaweed, kelp, bladderwrack (*Fucus vesiculosus*)	Goiter
Seaweed, kelp, bladderwrack (*Fucus vesiculosus*)	Myxedema

GOUT AND RELATED CONDITIONS

Levels of Scientific Evidence for Specific Therapies

TRADITIONAL OR THEORETICAL USES THAT LACK SUFFICIENT EVIDENCE

Therapy	Specific Therapeutic Use(s)
American pennyroyal (*Hedeoma pulegioides* L.), European pennyroyal (*Mentha pulegium* L.)	Gout

Belladonna (*Atropa belladonna* L. or its variety *acuminata* Royle ex Lindl)	Gout
Bilberry (*Vaccinium myrtillus*)	Gout
Bromelain	Gout
Burdock (*Arctium lappa*)	Gout
Calendula (*Calendula officinalis* L.), marigold	Gout
Clove (Eugenia aromatica)	Gout
Dandelion (*Taraxacum officinale*)	Gout
Devil's claw (*Harpagophytum procumbens* DC.)	Gout
Ephedra (*Ephedra sinica*)/ma huang	Gout
Fenugreek (*Trigonella foenum-graecum* L.)	Gout
Globe artichoke (*Cynara scolymus* L.)	Gout
Gymnema (*Gymnema Sylvestre* R. Br.)	Gout
Horsetail (*Equisetum arvense* L.)	Gout
Omega-3 fatty acids, fish oil, alpha-linolenic acid	Gout
Red clover (*Trifolium pratense*)	Gout
Slippery elm (*Ulmus rubra* Muhl., *U. fulva* Michx.)	Gout
Thyme (*Thymus vulgaris* L.), thymol	Gout

HAIR LOSS AND RELATED CONDITIONS

Levels of Scientific Evidence for Specific Therapies

GRADE: C (UNCLEAR OR CONFLICTING SCIENTIFIC EVIDENCE)

Therapy	Specific Therapeutic Use(s)
Saw palmetto (*Serenoa repens* [Bartram] Small)	Androgenetic alopecia (topical)
Thyme (*Thymus vulgaris* L.), thymol	Alopecia areata

TRADITIONAL OR THEORETICAL USES THAT LACK SUFFICIENT EVIDENCE

Therapy	Specific Therapeutic Use(s)
Aloe (*Aloe vera*)	Alopecia (hair loss)
Bladderwrack (*Fucus vesiculosus*)	Hair loss

Continued

Therapy	Specific Therapeutic Use(s)
Burdock (*Arctium lappa*)	Dandruff
Burdock (*Arctium lappa*)	Hair loss
Chaparral (*Larrea tridentata* DC. Coville, *L. divaricata* Cav.), nordihydroguaiaretic acid (NDGA)	Hair tonic
Coenzyme Q10	Hair loss
Dandelion (*Taraxacum officinale*)	Dandruff
Elder (*Sambucus nigra* L.)	Hair dye
Fenugreek (*Trigonella foenum-graecum* L.)	Baldness
Garlic (*Allium sativum* L.)	Hair growth
Ginger (*Zingiber officinale* Roscoe)	Baldness
Goldenseal (*Hydrastis canadensis* L.), berberine	Dandruff
Gotu kola (*Centella asiatica* L.), total triterpenic fraction of *Centella asiatica* (TTFCA)	Hair growth promoter
Horsetail (*Equisetum arvense* L.)	Hair loss
Lavender (*Lavandula angustifolia* Miller)	Hair loss
Pygeum (*Prunus africana, Pygeum africanum*)	Male baldness
Seaweed, kelp, bladderwrack (*Fucus vesiculosus*)	Hair loss
Spirulina	Hair loss

HALITOSIS AND RELATED CONDITIONS

Levels of Scientific Evidence for Specific Therapies

TRADITIONAL OR THEORETICAL USES THAT LACK SUFFICIENT EVIDENCE

Therapy	Specific Therapeutic Use(s)
Clove (*Eugenia aromatica*)	Bad breath
Licorice (*Glycyrrhiza glabra* L.), deglycyrrhizinated licorice (DGL)	Bad breath
Thyme (*Thymus vulgaris* L.), thymol	Halitosis

HEADACHE AND RELATED CONDITIONS

Levels of Scientific Evidence for Specific Therapies

GRADE: B (Good Scientific Evidence)

Therapy	Specific Therapeutic Use(s)
Feverfew (*Tanacetum parthenium* L. Schultz-Bip.)	Migraine headache prevention

GRADE: C (Unclear or Conflicting Scientific Evidence)

Therapy	Specific Therapeutic Use(s)
Arginine (L-arginine)	Migraine headache
Belladonna (*Atropa belladonna* L. or its variety *acuminata* Royle ex Lindl)	Headache
Eucalyptus oil (*Eucalyptus globulus* Labillardiere, *E. fructicetorum* F. Von Mueller, *E. smithii* R.T. Baker)	Headache (applied to the skin)
Melatonin	Headache prevention
Peppermint (*Mentha x piperita* L.)	Tension headache

TRADITIONAL OR THEORETICAL USES THAT LACK SUFFICIENT EVIDENCE

Therapy	Specific Therapeutic Use(s)
American pennyroyal (*Hedeoma pulegioides* L.), European pennyroyal (*Mentha pulegium* L.)	Headache
Black cohosh (*Cimicifuga racemosa* L. Nutt.)	Headache
Black tea (*Camellia sinensis*)	Headache
Burdock (*Arctium lappa*)	Headache
Calendula (*Calendula officinalis* L.), marigold	Headache
Dandelion (*Taraxacum officinale*)	Headache
Devil's claw (*Harpagophytum procumbens* DC.)	Headache
Devil's claw (*Harpagophytum procumbens* DC.)	Migraine headache
Dong quai (*Angelica sinensis* [Oliv.] Diels), Chinese angelica	Headache
Dong quai (*Angelica sinensis* [Oliv.] Diels), Chinese angelica	Migraine headache

Continued

Echinacea (*Echinacea angustifolia* DC., *E. pallida*, *E. purpurea*)	Migraine headache
Elder (*Sambucus nigra* L.)	Headache
Elder (*Sambucus nigra* L.)	Migraine headache
Eyebright (*Euphrasia officinalis*)	Headache
Garlic (*Allium sativum* L.)	Headache
Ginger (*Zingiber officinale* Roscoe)	Headache
Ginger (*Zingiber officinale* Roscoe)	Migraine headache
Ginkgo (*Ginkgo biloba* L.)	Headache
Ginkgo (*Ginkgo biloba* L.)	Migraine headache
Ginseng (American ginseng, Asian ginseng, Chinese ginseng, Korean red ginseng, *Panax ginseng*: *Panax* spp. including *P. ginseng* C.C. Meyer and *P. quincefolium* L., excluding *Eleutherococcus senticosus*)	Headache
Ginseng (American ginseng, Asian ginseng, Chinese ginseng, Korean red ginseng, *Panax ginseng*: *Panax* spp. including *P. ginseng* C.C. Meyer and *P. quincefolium* L., excluding *Eleutherococcus senticosus*)	Migraine headache
Glucosamine	Migraine headache
Goldenseal (*Hydrastis canadensis* L.), berberine	Headache
Green tea (*Camellia sinensis*)	Headache
Kava (*Piper methysticum* G. Forst)	Migraine headache
Lavender (*Lavandula angustifolia* Miller)	Migraine headache
Lavender (*Lavandula angustifolia* Miller)	Tension headache
Niacin (vitamin B_3, nicotinic acid), niacinamide, and inositol hexanicotinate	Migraine headache
Omega-3 fatty acids, fish oil, alpha-linolenic acid	Headache
Saw palmetto (*Serenoa repens* [Bartram] Small)	Migraine headache
Soy (*Glycine max* L. Merr.)	Headache
Thyme (*Thymus vulgaris* L.), thymol	Headache
Valerian (*Valeriana officinalis* L.)	Migraine headache
Valerian (*Valeriana officinalis* L.)	Tension headaches

HEART FAILURE AND RELATED CONDITIONS

Levels of Scientific Evidence for Specific Therapies

GRADE: A (Strong Scientific Evidence)

Therapy	Specific Therapeutic Use(s)
Hawthorn (*Crataegus laevigata*, *C. oxyacantha*, *C. monogyna*, *C. pentagyna*)	Congestive heart failure

GRADE: C (Unclear or Conflicting Scientific Evidence)

Therapy	Specific Therapeutic Use(s)
Arginine (L-arginine)	Heart failure (congestive)
Astragalus (*Astragalus membranaceus*)	Heart failure
Coenzyme Q10	Cardiomyopathy (dilated, hypertrophic)
Coenzyme Q10	Heart failure
Dehydroepiandrosterone (DHEA)	Heart failure
Ginseng (American ginseng, Asian ginseng, Chinese ginseng, Korean red ginseng, *Panax ginseng*: *Panax* spp. including *P. ginseng* C.C. Meyer and *P. quinquefolium* L., excluding *Eleutherococcus senticosus*)	Congestive heart failure
Hawthorn (*Crataegus laevigata*, *C. oxyacantha*, *C. monogyna*, *C. pentagyna*)	Functional cardiovascular disorders
Oleander (*Nerium oleander*, *Thevetia peruviana*)	Congestive heart failure
Passionflower (*Passiflora incarnata* L.)	Congestive heart failure (exercise capacity)

GRADE: D (Fair Negative Scientific Evidence)

TRADITIONAL OR THEORETICAL USES THAT LACK SUFFICIENT EVIDENCE

Therapy	Specific Therapeutic Use(s)
Dandelion (*Taraxacum officinale*)	Congestive heart failure
Danshen (*Salvia miltiorrhiza*)	Left ventricular hypertrophy
Dong quai (*Angelica sinensis* [Oliv.] Diels), Chinese angelica	Congestive heart failure
Ginkgo (*Ginkgo biloba* L.)	Congestive heart failure

Continued

Goldenseal (*Hydrastis canadensis* L.), berberine	Heart failure
Horse chestnut (*Aesculus hippocastanum* L.)	Fluid in the lungs (pulmonary edema)
Horsetail (*Equisetum arvense* L.)	Fluid in the lungs
Omega-3 fatty acids, fish oil, alpha-linolenic acid	Congestive heart failure
Passionflower (*Passiflora incarnata* L.)	Congestive heart failure (exercise ability)
Valerian (*Valeriana officinalis* L.)	Congestive heart failure

HEARTBURN AND RELATED CONDITIONS

Levels of Scientific Evidence for Specific Therapies

GRADE: C (Unclear or Conflicting Scientific Evidence)

Therapy	Specific Therapeutic Use(s)
Bilberry (*Vaccinium myrtillus*)	Stomach ulcers (peptic ulcer disease)
Blessed thistle (*Cnicus benedictus* L.)	Indigestion and flatulence (gas)
Cranberry (*Vaccinium macrocarpon*)	Stomach ulcers caused by *Helicobacter pylori* bacteria
Globe artichoke (*Cynara scolymus* L.)	Nonulcer dyspepsia
Licorice (*Glycyrrhiza glabra* L.), deglycyrrhizinated licorice (DGL)	Bleeding stomach ulcers caused by aspirin
Licorice (*Glycyrrhiza glabra* L.), deglycyrrhizinated licorice (DGL)	Peptic ulcer disease
Peppermint (*Mentha* x *piperita* L.)	Indigestion (nonulcer dyspepsia)
Turmeric (*Curcuma longa* L.), curcumin	Dyspepsia (heartburn)
Turmeric (*Curcuma longa* L.), curcumin	Peptic ulcer disease (stomach ulcer)
White horehound (*Marrubium vulgare* L.)	Heartburn/poor appetite

GRADE: D (Fair Negative Scientific Evidence)

Therapy	Specific Therapeutic Use(s)
Garlic (*Allium sativum* L.)	Stomach ulcers caused by *Helicobacter pylori* bacteria

TRADITIONAL OR THEORETICAL USES THAT LACK SUFFICIENT EVIDENCE

Therapy	Specific Therapeutic Use(s)
Alfalfa (*Medicago sativa* L.)	Indigestion
Alfalfa (*Medicago sativa* L.)	Stomach ulcers
American pennyroyal (*Hedeoma pulegioides* L.), European pennyroyal (*Mentha pulegium* L.)	Indigestion
Arginine (L-arginine)	Stomach ulcer
Astragalus (*Astragalus membranaceus*)	Stomach ulcer
Barley (*Hordeum vulgare* L.), germinated barley foodstuff (GBF)	Gastritis
Barley (*Hordeum vulgare* L.), germinated barley foodstuff (GBF)	Gastrointestinal inflammation
Belladonna (*Atropa belladonna* L. or its variety *A. acuminata* Royle ex Lindl)	Stomach ulcers
Bilberry (*Vaccinium myrtillus*)	Dyspepsia
Bilberry (*Vaccinium myrtillus*)	Infantile dyspepsia
Bladderwrack (*Fucus vesiculosus*)	Heartburn
Bladderwrack (*Fucus vesiculosus*)	Ulcer
Boswellia (*Boswellia serrata* Roxb.)	Dyspepsia
Boswellia (*Boswellia serrata* Roxb.)	Peptic ulcer disease
Bromelain	Indigestion
Bromelain	Stomach ulcer/stomach ulcer prevention
Calendula (*Calendula officinalis* L.), marigold	Indigestion
Calendula (*Calendula officinalis* L.), marigold	Stomach ulcers
Chamomile (*Matricaria recutita*, *Chamaemelum nobile*)	Heartburn
Chaparral (*Larrea tridentata* DC. Coville, *L. divaricata* Cav), nordihydroguaiaretic acid (NDGA)	Heartburn
Chaparral (*Larrea tridentata* DC. Coville, *L. divaricata* Cav), nordihydroguaiaretic acid (NDGA)	Indigestion
Chaparral (*Larrea tridentata* DC. Coville, *L. divaricata* Cav), nordihydroguaiaretic acid (NDGA)	Stomach ulcer

Continued

Coenzyme Q10	Stomach ulcer
Dandelion (*Taraxacum officinale*)	Heartburn
Danshen (*Salvia miltiorrhiza*)	Gastric ulcers
Danshen (*Salvia miltiorrhiza*)	Stomach ulcers
Devil's claw (*Harpagophytum procumbens* DC.)	Dyspepsia
Devil's claw (*Harpagophytum procumbens* DC.)	Heartburn
Devil's claw (*Harpagophytum procumbens* DC.)	Indigestion
Dong quai (*Angelica sinensis* [Oliv.] Diels), Chinese angelica	Heartburn
Echinacea (*Echinacea angustifolia* DC., *E. pallida*, *E. purpurea*)	Dyspepsia
Evening primrose oil (*Oenothera biennis* L.)	Disorders of the stomach and intestines
Fenugreek (*Trigonella foenum-graecum* L.)	Dyspepsia
Fenugreek (*Trigonella foenum-graecum* L.)	Gastritis
Fenugreek (*Trigonella foenum-graecum* L.)	Indigestion
Flaxseed and flaxseed oil (*Linum usitatissimum*)	Enteritis
Flaxseed and flaxseed oil (*Linum usitatissimum*)	Gastritis
Garlic (*Allium sativum* L.)	Stomach acid reduction
Ginger (*Zingiber officinale* Roscoe)	Antacid
Ginger (*Zingiber officinale* Roscoe)	Dyspepsia
Ginger (*Zingiber officinale* Roscoe)	Helicobacter pylori infection
Ginger (*Zingiber officinale* Roscoe)	Stomach ulcers
Goldenseal (*Hydrastis canadensis* L.), berberine	Gastroenteritis
Goldenseal (*Hydrastis canadensis* L.), berberine	Indigestion
Goldenseal (*Hydrastis canadensis* L.), berberine	Stomach ulcers
Gotu kola (*Centella asiatica* L.) and total triterpenic fraction of *Centella asiatica* (TTFCA)	Gastritis
Green tea (*Camellia sinensis*)	Gastritis
Green tea (*Camellia sinensis*)	Helicobacter pylori infection
Hawthorn (*Crataegus laevigata*, *C. oxyacantha*, *C. monogyna*, *C. pentagyna*)	Dyspepsia

Hops (*Humulus lupulus* L.)	Indigestion
Horse chestnut (*Aesculus hippocastanum* L.)	Ulcers
Horsetail (*Equisetum arvense* L.)	Dyspepsia
Kava (*Piper methysticum* G. Forst)	Dyspepsia
Lactobacillus acidophilus	Heartburn
Lactobacillus acidophilus	Indigestion
Lactobacillus acidophilus	Stomach ulcer
Lavender (*Lavandula angustifolia* Miller)	Heartburn
Lavender (*Lavandula angustifolia* Miller)	Indigestion
Licorice (*Glycyrrhiza glabra* L.), deglycyrrhizinated licorice (DGL)	Gastroesophageal reflux disease
Marshmallow (*Althaea officinalis* L.)	Duodenal ulcer
Marshmallow (*Althaea officinalis* L.)	Enteritis
Marshmallow (*Althaea officinalis* L.)	Gastroenteritis
Marshmallow (*Althaea officinalis* L.)	Indigestion
Marshmallow (*Althaea officinalis* L.)	Peptic ulcer disease
Melatonin	Gastroesophageal reflux disease (GERD)
Niacin (vitamin B_3, nicotinic acid), niacinamide, inositol hexanicotinate	Stomach ulcer
Oleander (*Nerium oleander*, *Thevetia peruviana*)	Indigestion
Peppermint (*Mentha* x *piperita* L.)	Antacid
Peppermint (*Mentha* x *piperita* L.)	Enteritis
Peppermint (*Mentha* x *piperita* L.)	Gastritis
Propolis	Stomach ulcer
Psyllium (*Plantago ovata*, *P. ispaghula*)	Duodenal ulcer
Psyllium (*Plantago ovata*, *P. ispaghula*)	Stomach ulcer
Red clover (*Trifolium pratense*)	Indigestion
Red yeast rice (*Monascus purpureus*)	Indigestion
Saw palmetto (*Serenoa repens* [Bartram] Small)	Indigestion

Continued

Seaweed, kelp, bladderwrack (*Fucus vesiculosus*)	Dyspepsia
Seaweed, kelp, bladderwrack (*Fucus vesiculosus*)	Heartburn
Seaweed, kelp, bladderwrack (*Fucus vesiculosus*)	Ulcer
Shark cartilage	Enteritis
Slippery elm (*Ulmus rubra* Muhl. or *U. fulva* Michx.)	Duodenal ulcer
Slippery elm (*Ulmus rubra* Muhl. or *U. fulva* Michx.)	Enteritis
Slippery elm (*Ulmus rubra* Muhl. or *U. fulva* Michx.)	Gastric ulcer
Slippery elm (*Ulmus rubra* Muhl. or *U. fulva* Michx.)	Gastritis
Slippery elm (*Ulmus rubra* Muhl. or *U. fulva* Michx.)	Gastroesophageal reflux disease
Slippery elm (*Ulmus rubra* Muhl. or *U. fulva* Michx.)	Heartburn
Slippery elm (*Ulmus rubra* Muhl. or *U. fulva* Michx.)	Peptic ulcer disease
Spirulina	Stomach acid excess
Spirulina	Ulcers
St. John's wort (*Hypericum perforatum* L.)	Heartburn
St. John's wort (*Hypericum perforatum* L.)	Ulcers
Thyme (*Thymus vulgaris* L.), thymol	Dyspepsia
Thyme (*Thymus vulgaris* L.), thymol	Gastritis
Thyme (*Thymus vulgaris* L.), thymol	Heartburn
Thyme (*Thymus vulgaris* L.), thymol	Indigestion
Valerian (*Valeriana officinalis* L.)	Heartburn
Valerian (*Valeriana officinalis* L.)	Peptic ulcer disease
White horehound (*Marrubium vulgare* L.)	Indigestion

HEAVY METAL/LEAD TOXICITY AND RELATED CONDITIONS

Levels of Scientific Evidence for Specific Therapies

GRADE: C (Unclear or Conflicting Scientific Evidence)

Therapy	Specific Therapeutic Use(s)
Clay	Mercuric chloride poisoning

TRADITIONAL OR THEORETICAL USES THAT LACK SUFFICIENT EVIDENCE	
Therapy	**Specific Therapeutic Use(s)**
Belladonna (*Atropa belladonna* L. or its variety *A. acuminata* Royle ex Lindl)	Poisoning (especially by insecticides)
Clay	Poisoning
Essiac	Blood cleanser
Essiac	Chelating agent (heavy metals)
Hoxsey formula	Elimination of toxins
Marshmallow (*Althaea officinalis* L.)	Antidote to poisons
Melatonin	Aluminum toxicity
Melatonin	Lead toxicity

HEPATITIS AND RELATED CONDITIONS

Levels of Scientific Evidence for Specific Therapies

GRADE: B (Good Scientific Evidence)	
Therapy	Specific Therapeutic Use(s)
Milk thistle (*Silybum marianum*), silymarin	Cirrhosis
Milk thistle (*Silybum marianum*), silymarin	Hepatitis (chronic)

GRADE: C (Unclear or Conflicting Scientific Evidence)	
Therapy	**Specific Therapeutic Use(s)**
Astragalus (*Astragalus membranaceus*)	Liver protection
Clay	Protection from aflatoxins
Dandelion (*Taraxacum officinale*)	Hepatitis B
Danshen (*Salvia miltiorrhiza*)	Liver disease (cirrhosis/chronic hepatitis B)
Eyebright (*Euphrasia officinalis*)	Hepatoprotection
Lactobacillus acidophilus	Hepatic encephalopathy (confused thinking due to liver disorders)

Continued

Licorice (*Glycyrrhiza glabra* L.), deglycyrrhizinated licorice (DGL)	Viral hepatitis
Milk thistle (*Silybum marianum*), silymarin	Acute viral hepatitis
Milk thistle (*Silybum marianum*), silymarin	Amanita phalloides mushroom toxicity
Milk thistle (*Silybum marianum*), silymarin	Drug/toxin-induced hepatotoxicity

TRADITIONAL OR THEORETICAL USES THAT LACK SUFFICIENT EVIDENCE

Therapy	Specific Therapeutic Use(s)
Alfalfa (*Medicago sativa* L.)	Jaundice
Aloe (*Aloe vera*)	Hepatitis
American pennyroyal (*Hedeoma pulegioides* L.), European pennyroyal (*Mentha pulegium* L.)	Liver disease
Arginine (L-arginine)	Ammonia toxicity
Arginine (L-arginine)	Hepatic encephalopathy
Arginine (L-arginine)	Liver disease
Astragalus (*Astragalus membranaceus*)	Chronic hepatitis
Astragalus (*Astragalus membranaceus*)	Liver disease
Bilberry (*Vaccinium myrtillus*)	Liver disease
Black cohosh (*Cimicifuga racemosa* L. Nutt.)	Liver disease
Blessed thistle (*Cnicus benedictus* L.)	Jaundice
Blessed thistle (*Cnicus benedictus* L.)	Liver disorders
Burdock (*Arctium lappa*)	Liver protection
Calendula (*Calendula officinalis* L.), marigold	Jaundice
Calendula (*Calendula officinalis* L.), marigold	Liver dysfunction
Chamomile (*Matricaria recutita*, *Chamaemelum nobile*)	Liver disorders
Coenzyme Q10	Hepatitis B
Coenzyme Q10	Liver enlargement or disease
Cranberry (*Vaccinium macrocarpon*)	Liver disorders
Dandelion (*Taraxacum officinale*)	Jaundice

Dandelion (*Taraxacum officinale*)	Liver cleansing
Dandelion (*Taraxacum officinale*)	Liver disease
Devil's claw (*Harpagophytum procumbens* DC.)	Liver and gallbladder tonic
Dehydroepiandrosterone (DHEA)	Liver protection
Dong quai (*Angelica sinensis* [Oliv.] Diels), Chinese angelica	Chronic hepatitis
Dong quai (*Angelica sinensis* [Oliv.] Diels), Chinese angelica	Cirrhosis
Dong quai (*Angelica sinensis* [Oliv.] Diels), Chinese angelica	Liver protection
Elder (*Sambucus nigra* L.)	Liver disease
Eucalyptus oil (*Eucalyptus globulus* Labillardiere, *E. fructicetorum* F. Von Mueller, *E. smithii* R.T. Baker)	Liver protection
Evening primrose oil (*Oenothera biennis* L.)	Hepatitis B
Eyebright (*Euphrasia officinalis*)	Jaundice
Eyebright (*Euphrasia officinalis*)	Liver disease
Garlic (*Allium sativum* L.)	Antitoxin
Garlic (*Allium sativum* L.)	Hepatopulmonary syndrome
Garlic (*Allium sativum* L.)	Liver health
Ginger (*Zingiber officinale* Roscoe)	Liver disease
Ginkgo (*Ginkgo biloba* L.)	Hepatitis B
Ginseng (American ginseng, Asian ginseng, Chinese ginseng, Korean red ginseng, *Panax ginseng*: *Panax* spp. including *P. ginseng* C.C. Meyer and *P. quinquefolium* L., excluding *Eleutherococcus senticosus*)	Hepatitis/hepatitis B infection
Ginseng (American ginseng, Asian ginseng, Chinese ginseng, Korean red ginseng, *Panax ginseng*: *Panax* spp. including *P. ginseng* C.C. Meyer and *P. quinquefolium* L., excluding *Eleutherococcus senticosus*)	Liver diseases
Ginseng (American ginseng, Asian ginseng, Chinese ginseng, Korean red ginseng, *Panax ginseng*: *Panax* spp. including *P. ginseng* C.C. Meyer and *P. quinquefolium* L., excluding *Eleutherococcus senticosus*)	Liver health
Globe artichoke (*Cynara scolymus* L.)	Jaundice

Continued

Goldenseal (*Hydrastis canadensis* L.), berberine	Alcoholic liver disease
Goldenseal (*Hydrastis canadensis* L.), berberine	Hepatitis
Goldenseal (*Hydrastis canadensis* L.), berberine	Jaundice
Goldenseal (*Hydrastis canadensis* L.), berberine	Liver disorders
Gotu kola (*Centella asiatica* L.), total triterpenic fraction of *Centella asiatica* (TTFCA)	Hepatitis
Gotu kola (*Centella asiatica* L.), total triterpenic fraction of *Centella asiatica* (TTFCA)	Jaundice
Gymnema (*Gymnema sylvestre* R. Br.)	Liver disease
Gymnema (*Gymnema sylvestre* R. Br.)	Liver protection
Horse chestnut (*Aesculus hippocastanum* L.)	Liver congestion
Horsetail (*Equisetum arvense* L.)	Liver protection
Licorice (*Glycyrrhiza glabra* L.), deglycyrrhizinated licorice (DGL)	Liver protection
Maitake mushroom (*Grifola frondosa*), beta-glucan	Liver inflammation (hepatitis)
Melatonin	Toxic liver damage
Milk thistle (*Silybum marianum*), silymarin	Jaundice
Milk thistle (*Silybum marianum*), silymarin	Liver cleansing agent
Niacin (vitamin B_3, nicotinic acid), niacinamide, inositol hexanicotinate	Liver disease
Omega-3 fatty acids, fish oil, alpha-linolenic acid	Cirrhosis

HERPES SIMPLEX VIRUS AND RELATED CONDITIONS

Levels of Scientific Evidence for Specific Therapies

GRADE: B (Good Scientific Evidence)

Therapy	Specific Therapeutic Use(s)
Aloe (*Aloe vera*)	Genital herpes

GRADE: C (Unclear or Conflicting Scientific Evidence)

Therapy	Specific Therapeutic Use(s)
Licorice (*Glycyrrhiza glabra* L.), deglycyrrhizinated licorice (DGL)	Herpes simplex virus

Propolis	Genital herpes simplex virus (HSV) infection
Tea tree oil (*Melaleuca alternifolia* [Maiden & Betche] Cheel)	Genital herpes

GRADE: D (Fair Negative Scientific Evidence)

Therapy	Specific Therapeutic Use(s)
Echinacea (*Echinacea angustifolia* DC., *E. pallida, E. purpurea*)	Genital herpes
Licorice (*Glycyrrhiza glabra* L.), deglycyrrhizinated licorice (DGL)	Genital herpes

TRADITIONAL OR THEORETICAL USES THAT LACK SUFFICIENT EVIDENCE

Therapy	Specific Therapeutic Use(s)
Astragalus (*Astragalus membranaceus*)	Genital herpes
Belladonna (*Atropa belladonna* L. or its variety *A. acuminata* Royle ex Lindl)	Chickenpox
Bromelain	Shingles pain/postherpetic neuralgia
Calendula (*Calendula officinalis* L.), marigold	Herpes simplex virus infections
Chaparral (*Larrea tridentata* DC. Coville, *L. divaricata* Cav.), nordihydroguaiaretic acid (NDGA)	Chickenpox
Clove (*Eugenia aromatica*)	Herpes simplex virus infection
Elder (*Sambucus nigra* L.)	Herpes
Eucalyptus oil (*Eucalyptus globulus* Labillardiere, *E. fructicetorum* F. Von Mueller, *E. smithii* R.T. Baker)	Herpes
Eucalyptus oil (*Eucalyptus globulus* Labillardiere, *E. fructicetorum* F. Von Mueller, *E. smithii* R.T. Baker)	Shingles
Ginseng (American ginseng, Asian ginseng, Chinese ginseng, Korean red ginseng, *Panax ginseng*: *Panax* spp. including *P. ginseng* C.C. Meyer and *P. quinquefolium* L., excluding *Eleutherococcus senticosus*)	Herpes
Goldenseal (*Hydrastis canadensis* L.), berberine	Chickenpox
Goldenseal (*Hydrastis canadensis* L.), berberine	Herpes
Gotu kola (*Centella asiatica* L.), total triterpenic fraction of *Centella asiatica* (TTFCA)	Herpes simplex virus type 2 (HSV-2) infection

Continued

Gotu kola (*Centella asiatica* L.), total triterpenic fraction of *Centella asiatica* (TTFCA)	Shingles (postherpetic neuralgia)
Peppermint (*Mentha* x *piperita* L.)	Chickenpox
Peppermint (*Mentha* x *piperita* L.)	Postherpetic neuralgia
Slippery elm (*Ulmus rubra* Muhl. or *U. fulva* Michx.)	Herpes
Spirulina	Herpes simplex virus type 1 (HSV-1) infection
St. John's wort (*Hypericum perforatum* L.)	Herpesvirus infection
Tea tree oil (*Melaleuca alternifolia* [Maiden & Betche] Cheel)	Herpes simplex virus infection

HIGH CHOLESTEROL AND RELATED CONDITIONS

Levels of Scientific Evidence for Specific Therapies

GRADE: A (Strong Scientific Evidence)

Therapy	Specific Therapeutic Use(s)
Niacin (vitamin B_3, nicotinic acid), niacinamide, inositol hexanicotinate	High cholesterol (niacin)
Omega-3 fatty acids, fish oil, alpha-linolenic acid	Hypertriglyceridemia (fish oil/eicosapentaenoic acid [EPA] plus docosahexaenoic acid [DHA])
Omega-3 fatty acids, fish oil, alpha-linolenic acid	Secondary cardiovascular disease prevention (fish oil/eicosapentaenoic acid [EPA] plus docosahexaenoic acid [DHA])
Psyllium (*Plantago ovata*, *P. ispaghula*)	High cholesterol
Red yeast rice (*Monascus purpureus*)	High cholesterol
Soy (*Glycine max* L. Merr.)	High cholesterol

GRADE: B (Good Scientific Evidence)

Therapy	Specific Therapeutic Use(s)
Barley (*Hordeum vulgare* L.), germinated barley foodstuff (GBF)	High cholesterol
Garlic (*Allium sativum* L.)	High cholesterol

Niacin (vitamin B_3, nicotinic acid), niacinamide, and inositol hexanicotinate	Atherosclerosis (niacin)
Niacin (vitamin B_3, nicotinic acid), niacinamide, and inositol hexanicotinate	Prevention of a second heart attack (niacin)
Omega-3 fatty acids, fish oil, alpha-linolenic acid	Primary cardiovascular disease prevention (fish intake)
Sweet almond (*Prunus amygdalus dulcis*)	High cholesterol (whole almonds)

GRADE: C (Unclear or Conflicting Scientific Evidence)

Therapy	Specific Therapeutic Use(s)
Alfalfa (*Medicago sativa* L.)	Atherosclerosis (cholesterol plaques in heart arteries)
Alfalfa (*Medicago sativa* L.)	High cholesterol
Arginine (L-arginine)	Coronary artery disease/ angina
Arginine (L-arginine)	Heart protection during coronary artery bypass grafting (CABG)
Astragalus (*Astragalus membranaceus*)	Coronary artery disease
Bilberry (*Vaccinium myrtillus*)	Atherosclerosis (hardening of the arteries) and peripheral vascular disease
Black tea (*Camellia sinensis*)	Heart attack prevention
Coenzyme Q10	Angina (chest pain from clogged heart arteries)
Coenzyme Q10	Heart attack (acute myocardial infarction)
Coenzyme Q10	Heart protection during surgery
Danshen (*Salvia miltiorrhiza*)	Cardiovascular disease/angina
Dehydroepiandrosterone (DHEA)	Atherosclerosis (cholesterol plaques in the arteries)
Dong quai (*Angelica sinensis* [Oliv.] Diels), Chinese angelica	Angina pectoris/coronary artery disease
Fenugreek (*Trigonella foenum-graecum* L.)	Hyperlipidemia

Continued

Flaxseed and flaxseed oil (*Linum usitatissimum*)	Heart disease (flaxseed and flaxseed oil)
Flaxseed and flaxseed oil (*Linum usitatissimum*)	High cholesterol or triglycerides (flaxseed and flaxseed oil)
Garlic (*Allium sativum* L.)	Atherosclerosis (hardening of the arteries)
Garlic (*Allium sativum* L.)	Familial hypercholesterolemia
Garlic (*Allium sativum* L.)	Heart attack prevention in patients with known heart disease
Ginseng (American ginseng, Asian ginseng, Chinese ginseng, Korean red ginseng, *Panax ginseng*: *Panax* spp. including *P. ginseng* C.C. Meyer and *P. quinquefolium* L., excluding *Eleutherococcus senticosus*)	Coronary artery (heart) disease
Globe artichoke (*Cynara scolymus* L.)	Lipid lowering (cholesterol and triglycerides)
Green tea (*Camellia sinensis*)	Heart attack prevention
Green tea (*Camellia sinensis*)	High cholesterol
Guggul (*Commifora mukul*)	Hyperlipidemia
Gymnema (*Gymnema sylvestre* R. Br.)	High cholesterol
Hawthorn (*Crataegus laevigata*, *C. oxyacantha*, *C. monogyna*, *C. pentagyna*)	Coronary artery disease (angina)
Lactobacillus acidophilus	High cholesterol
Lycopene	Atherosclerosis (clogged arteries) and high cholesterol
Milk thistle (*Silybum marianum*), silymarin	Hyperlipidemia
Omega-3 fatty acids, fish oil, alpha-linolenic acid	Angina pectoris
Omega-3 fatty acids, fish oil, alpha-linolenic acid	Atherosclerosis
Omega-3 fatty acids, fish oil, alpha-linolenic acid	Prevention of graft failure after heart bypass surgery
Omega-3 fatty acids, fish oil, alpha-linolenic acid	Prevention of restenosis after coronary angioplasty (percutaneous transluminal coronary angioplasty [PTCA])
Red clover (*Trifolium pratense*)	High cholesterol

Soy (*Glycine max* L. Merr.)	Cardiovascular disease
Spirulina	High cholesterol
Turmeric (*Curcuma longa* L.), curcumin	High cholesterol
Wild yam (*Dioscorea villosa*)	High cholesterol

GRADE: D (Fair Negative Scientific Evidence)

Therapy	Specific Therapeutic Use(s)
Omega-3 fatty acids, fish oil, alpha-linolenic acid	Hypercholesterolemia

TRADITIONAL OR THEORETICAL USES THAT LACK SUFFICIENT EVIDENCE

Therapy	Specific Therapeutic Use(s)
Aloe (*Aloe vera*)	Heart disease prevention
Antineoplastons	Cholesterol/triglyceride abnormalities
Arginine (L-arginine)	Cardiac syndrome X
Arginine (L-arginine)	Heart attack
Arginine (L-arginine)	High cholesterol
Astragalus (*Astragalus membranaceus*)	Angina
Astragalus (*Astragalus membranaceus*)	Heart attack
Astragalus (*Astragalus membranaceus*)	High cholesterol
Bilberry (*Vaccinium myrtillus*)	Angina
Bilberry (*Vaccinium myrtillus*)	Heart disease
Bilberry (*Vaccinium myrtillus*)	High cholesterol
Black cohosh (*Cimicifuga racemosa* L. Nutt.)	Cardiac diseases
Bladderwrack (*Fucus vesiculosus*)	Atherosclerosis
Bladderwrack (*Fucus vesiculosus*)	Heart disease
Bladderwrack (*Fucus vesiculosus*)	High cholesterol
Boron	High cholesterol
Bromelain	Angina
Bromelain	Atherosclerosis (hardening of the arteries)

Continued

Bromelain	Heart disease
Calendula (*Calendula officinalis* L.), marigold	Atherosclerosis (clogged arteries)
Calendula (*Calendula officinalis* L.), marigold	Heart disease
Clay	Cardiovascular disorders
Coenzyme Q10	High cholesterol
Dandelion (*Taraxacum officinale*)	Cardiovascular disorders
Dandelion (*Taraxacum officinale*)	Clogged arteries
Dandelion (*Taraxacum officinale*)	High cholesterol
Danshen (*Salvia miltiorrhiza*)	Clogged arteries
Danshen (*Salvia miltiorrhiza*)	High cholesterol
Devil's claw (*Harpagophytum procumbens* DC.)	Atherosclerosis (clogged arteries)
Devil's claw (*Harpagophytum procumbens* DC.)	High cholesterol
Dehydroepiandrosterone (DHEA)	Heart attack
Dehydroepiandrosterone (DHEA)	High cholesterol
Dong quai (*Angelica sinensis* [Oliv.] Diels), Chinese angelica	Atherosclerosis
Dong quai (*Angelica sinensis* [Oliv.] Diels), Chinese angelica	High cholesterol
Evening primrose oil (*Oenothera biennis* L.)	Atherosclerosis
Evening primrose oil (*Oenothera biennis* L.)	Heart disease
Evening primrose oil (*Oenothera biennis* L.)	High cholesterol
Fenugreek (*Trigonella foenum-graecum* L.)	Atherosclerosis
Ginger (*Zingiber officinale* Roscoe)	Atherosclerosis
Ginger (*Zingiber officinale* Roscoe)	Heart disease
Ginkgo (*Ginkgo biloba* L.)	Angina
Ginkgo (*Ginkgo biloba* L.)	Atherosclerosis (clogged arteries)
Ginkgo (*Ginkgo biloba* L.)	Heart attack
Ginkgo (*Ginkgo biloba* L.)	Heart disease

Ginkgo (*Ginkgo biloba* L.)	High cholesterol
Ginseng (American ginseng, Asian ginseng, Chinese ginseng, Korean red ginseng, *Panax ginseng*: *Panax* spp. including *P. ginseng* C.C. Meyer and P. *quinquefolium* L., excluding *Eleutherococcus senticosus*)	Atherosclerosis
Ginseng (American ginseng, Asian ginseng, Chinese ginseng, Korean red ginseng, *Panax ginseng*: *Panax* spp. including *P. ginseng* C.C. Meyer *and P. quinquefolium* L., excluding *Eleutherococcus senticosus*)	Heart damage
Globe artichoke (*Cynara scolymus* L.)	Atherosclerosis
Goldenseal (*Hydrastis canadensis* L.), berberine	Atherosclerosis (hardening of the arteries)
Goldenseal (*Hydrastis canadensis* L.), berberine	High cholesterol
Green tea (*Camellia sinensis*)	Heart disease
Gymnema (*Gymnema sylvestre* R. Br.)	Cardiovascular disease
Hawthorn (*Crataegus laevigata*, *C. oxyacantha*, *C. monogyna*, *C.* pentagyna)	Angina
Hawthorn (*Crataegus laevigata*, *C. oxyacantha*, *C. monogyna*, *C. pentagyna*)	Cardiac murmurs
Lactobacillus acidophilus	Heart disease
Licorice (*Glycyrrhiza glabra* L.), deglycyrrhizinated licorice (DGL)	High cholesterol
Lycopene	Heart disease
Maitake mushroom (*Grifola frondosa*), beta-glucan	High cholesterol
Melatonin	Cardiac syndrome X
Melatonin	Coronary artery disease
Niacin (vitamin B_3, nicotinic acid), niacinamide, inositol hexanicotinate	Heart attack prevention
Oleander (*Nerium oleander*, *Thevetia peruviana*)	Heart disease
Omega-3 fatty acids, fish oil, alpha-linolenic acid	Acute myocardial infarction (heart attack)
Psyllium (*Plantago ovata, P. ispaghula*)	Atherosclerosis
Seaweed, kelp, bladderwrack (*Fucus vesiculosus*)	Atherosclerosis
Seaweed, kelp, bladderwrack (*Fucus vesiculosus*)	Fatty heart

Continued

Seaweed, kelp, bladderwrack (*Fucus vesiculosus*)	Hyperlipemia
Shark cartilage	Atherosclerosis
Soy (*Glycine max* L. Merr.)	Atherosclerosis
Spirulina	Atherosclerosis
Spirulina	Heart disease
Sweet almond (*Prunus amygdalus dulcis*)	Heart disease
Valerian (*Valeriana officinalis* L.)	Angina pectoris
Valerian (*Valeriana officinalis* L.)	Heart disease
Yohimbe bark extract (*Pausinystalia yohimbe* Pierre ex Beille)	Angina
Yohimbe bark extract (*Pausinystalia yohimbe* Pierre ex Beille)	Coronary artery disease
Yohimbe bark extract (*Pausinystalia yohimbe* Pierre ex Beille)	High cholesterol
Yohimbe bark extract (*Pausinystalia yohimbe* Pierre ex Beille)	Atherosclerosis
Yohimbe bark extract (*Pausinystalia yohimbe* Pierre ex Beille)	Chest pain
Yohimbe bark extract (*Pausinystalia yohimbe* Pierre ex Beille)	Coronary artery disease
Yohimbe bark extract (*Pausinystalia yohimbe* Pierre ex Beille)	Hyperlipidemia

HUMAN IMMUNODEFICIENCY VIRUS (HIV) INFECTION/AIDS AND RELATED CONDITIONS

Levels of Scientific Evidence for Specific Therapies

GRADE: C (Unclear or Conflicting Scientific Evidence)

Therapy	Specific Therapeutic Use(s)
Aloe (*Aloe vera*)	HIV infection
Antineoplastons	HIV infection
Bitter melon (*Momordica charantia* L.), MAP30	HIV infection
Coenzyme Q10	HIV infection/AIDS

Dehydroepiandrosterone (DHEA)	HIV infection/AIDS
Flaxseed and flaxseed oil (*Linum usitatissimum*)	HIV infection/AIDS
Melatonin	HIV infection/AIDS
Turmeric (*Curcuma longa* L.), curcumin	HIV infection

GRADE: D (Fair Negative Scientific Evidence)

Therapy	Specific Therapeutic Use(s)
St. John's wort (*Hypericum perforatum* L.)	HIV infection

TRADITIONAL OR THEORETICAL USES THAT LACK SUFFICIENT EVIDENCE

Therapy	Specific Therapeutic Use(s)
Arginine (L-arginine)	AIDS/HIV infection
Astragalus (*Astragalus membranaceus*)	AIDS/HIV infection
Bromelain	AIDS
Burdock (*Arctium lappa*)	HIV infection
Calendula (*Calendula officinalis* L.), marigold	HIV infection
Dandelion (*Taraxacum officinale*)	AIDS
Danshen (*Salvia miltiorrhiza*)	HIV infection
Dehydroepiandrosterone (DHEA)	Lipodystrophy in HIV infection
Echinacea (*Echinacea angustifolia* DC., *E. pallida*, *E. purpurea*)	HIV infection/AIDS
Elder (*Sambucus nigra* L.)	HIV infection
Essiac	AIDS/HIV infection
Eucalyptus oil (*Eucalyptus globulus* Labillardiere, *E. fructicetorum* F. Von Mueller, *E. smithii* R.T. Baker)	AIDS
Garlic (*Allium sativum* L.)	AIDS
Garlic (*Allium sativum* L.)	HIV infection
Ginseng (American ginseng, Asian ginseng, Chinese ginseng, Korean red ginseng, *Panax ginseng*: *Panax* spp. including *P. ginseng* C.C. Meyer and *P. quinquefolium* L., excluding *Eleutherococcus senticosus*)	HIV infection
Goldenseal (*Hydrastis canadensis* L.), berberine	AIDS

Continued

Green tea (*Camellia sinensis*)	HIV infection/AIDS
Lactobacillus acidophilus	AIDS
Lavender (*Lavandula angustifolia* Miller)	HIV infection
Licorice (*Glycyrrhiza glabra* L.), deglycyrrhizinated licorice (DGL)	HIV infection
Lycopene	AIDS
Maitake mushroom (*Grifola frondosa*), beta-glucan	HIV infection
Niacin (vitamin B_3, nicotinic acid), niacinamide, inositol hexanicotinate	HIV infection prevention
Omega-3 fatty acids, fish oil, alpha-linolenic acid	AIDS
Propolis	HIV infection
Red clover (*Trifolium pratense*)	AIDS
Spirulina	HIV infection

HYPERTENSION AND RELATED CONDITIONS

Levels of Scientific Evidence for Specific Therapies

GRADE: A (Strong Scientific Evidence)

Therapy	Specific therapeutic Use(s)
Omega-3 fatty acids, fish oil, alpha-linolenic acid	High blood pressure

GRADE: B (Good Scientific Evidence)

Therapy	Specific Therapeutic Use(s)
Coenzyme Q10	High blood pressure (hypertension)

GRADE: C (Unclear or Conflicting Scientific Evidence)

Therapy	Specific Therapeutic Use(s)
Arginine (L-arginine)	High blood pressure
Evening primrose oil (*Oenothera biennis* L.)	Preeclampsia/high blood pressure of pregnancy
Flaxseed and flaxseed oil (*Linum usitatissimum*)	High blood pressure (flaxseed, not flaxseed oil)

Garlic (*Allium sativum* L.)	High blood pressure
Ginseng (American ginseng, Asian ginseng, Chinese ginseng, Korean red ginseng, *Panax ginseng*: *Panax* spp. including *P. ginseng* C.C. Meyer and *P. quinquefolium* L., excluding *Eleutherococcus senticosus*)	High blood pressure
Melatonin	High blood pressure (hypertension)
Omega-3 fatty acids, fish oil, alpha-linolenic acid	Preeclampsia
Soy (*Glycine max* L. Merr.)	High blood pressure

TRADITIONAL OR THEORETICAL USES THAT LACK SUFFICIENT EVIDENCE

Therapy	Specific Therapeutic Use(s)
Arginine (L-arginine)	Preeclampsia
Astragalus (*Astragalus membranaceus*)	High blood pressure
Bilberry (*Vaccinium myrtillus*)	High blood pressure
Black cohosh (*Cimicifuga racemosa* L. Nutt.)	High blood pressure
Dandelion (*Taraxacum officinale*)	High blood pressure
Danshen (*Salvia miltiorrhiza*)	Preeclampsia
Dong quai (*Angelica sinensis* [Oliv.] Diels), Chinese angelica	High blood pressure
Fenugreek (*Trigonella foenum-graecum* L.)	Hypertension
Ginger (*Zingiber officinale* Roscoe)	High blood pressure
Ginkgo (*Ginkgo biloba* L.)	High blood pressure
Ginseng (American ginseng, Asian ginseng, Chinese ginseng, Korean red ginseng, *Panax ginseng*: *Panax* spp. including *P. ginseng* C.C. Meyer and *P. quinquefolium* L., excluding *Eleutherococcus senticosus*)	High blood pressure
Goldenseal (*Hydrastis canadensis* L.), berberine	High blood pressure
Gotu kola (*Centella asiatica* L.), total triterpenic fraction of *Centella asiatica* (TTFCA)	Hypertension
Gotu kola (*Centella asiatica* L.), total triterpenic fraction of *Centella asiatica* (TTFCA)	Peripheral vasodilator
Gymnema (*Gymnema sylvestre* R. Br.)	High blood pressure

Continued

Maitake mushroom (*Grifola frondosa*), beta-glucan	High blood pressure
Niacin (vitamin B_3, nicotinic acid), niacinamide, inositol hexanicotinate	High blood pressure
Passionflower (*Passiflora incarnata* L.)	High blood pressure
Polypodium leucotomos extract, Anapsos	Hypertension
Psyllium (*Plantago ovata*, *P. ispaghula*)	High blood pressure
Red yeast rice (*Monascus purpureus*)	High blood pressure
Saw palmetto (*Serenoa repens* [Bartram] Small)	High blood pressure
Spirulina	High blood pressure
Turmeric (*Curcuma longa* L.), curcumin	High blood pressure
Valerian (*Valeriana officinalis* L.)	Hypertension

HYPOTENSION AND RELATED CONDITIONS

Levels of Scientific Evidence for Specific Therapies

GRADE: C (Unclear or Conflicting Scientific Evidence)

Therapy	Specific Therapeutic Use(s)
Dehydroepiandrosterone (DHEA)	Septicemia (serious bacterial infections in the blood)
Ephedra (*Ephedra sinica*)/ma huang	Hypotension

TRADITIONAL OR THEORETICAL USES THAT LACK SUFFICIENT EVIDENCE

Therapy	Specific Therapeutic Use(s)
Arginine (L-arginine)	Sepsis
Dong quai (*Angelica sinensis* [Oliv.] Diels), Chinese angelica	Sepsis
Echinacea (*Echinacea angustifolia* DC., *E. pallida*, *E. purpurea*)	Septicemia
Ginger (*Zingiber officinale* Roscoe)	Low blood pressure
Ginkgo (*Ginkgo biloba* L.)	Acidosis
Ginkgo (*Ginkgo biloba* L.)	Sepsis
Lavender (*Lavandula angustifolia* Miller)	Low blood pressure

Propolis	Low blood pressure
Yohimbe bark extract (*Pausinystalia yohimbe* Pierre ex Beille)	Low blood pressure

HYPOTHYROIDISM AND RELATED CONDITIONS

Levels of Scientific Evidence for Specific Therapies

GRADE: C (Unclear or Conflicting Scientific Evidence)

Therapy	Specific Therapeutic Use(s)
Bladderwrack (*Fucus vesiculosus*)	Goiter (thyroid disease)

TRADITIONAL OR THEORETICAL USES THAT LACK SUFFICIENT EVIDENCE

Therapy	Specific Therapeutic Use(s)
Essiac	Thyroid disorders
Horsetail (*Equisetum arvense* L.)	Thyroid disorders
Niacin (vitamin B_3, nicotinic acid), niacinamide, inositol hexanicotinate	Hypothyroidism
Propolis	Thyroid disease
Seaweed, kelp, bladderwrack (*Fucus vesiculosus*)	Exophthalmos
Seaweed, kelp, bladderwrack (*Fucus vesiculosus*)	Goiter
Seaweed, kelp, bladderwrack (*Fucus vesiculosus*)	Myxedema

IMMUNOMODULATION AND RELATED CONDITIONS

Levels of Scientific Evidence for Specific Therapies

GRADE: C (UNCLEAR OR CONFLICTING SCIENTIFIC EVIDENCE)

Therapy	Specific Therapeutic Use(s)
Astragalus (*Astragalus membranaceus*)	Immunostimulation
Astragalus (*Astragalus membranaceus*)	Low white blood cell count
Ginseng (American ginseng, Asian ginseng, Chinese ginseng, Korean red ginseng, *Panax ginseng*: *Panax* spp. including *P. ginseng* C.C. Meyer and *P. quinquefolium* L., excluding *Eleutherococcus senticosus*)	Immune system enhancement

Continued

Therapy	Specific Therapeutic Use(s)
Ginseng (American ginseng, Asian ginseng, Chinese ginseng, Korean red ginseng, *Panax ginseng*: *Panax* spp. including *P. ginseng* C.C. Meyer and *P. quinquefolium* L., excluding *Eleutherococcus senticosus*)	Low white blood cell counts
Goldenseal (*Hydrastis canadensis* L.), berberine	Immune system stimulation
Maitake mushroom (*Grifola frondosa*), beta-glucan	Immunoenhancement

GRADE: D (Fair Negative Scientific Evidence)

Therapy	Specific Therapeutic Use(s)
Dehydroepiandrosterone (DHEA)	Immune system stimulant
Lycopene	Immunostimulation

TRADITIONAL OR THEORETICAL USES THAT LACK SUFFICIENT EVIDENCE

Therapy	Specific Therapeutic Use(s)
Arginine (L-arginine)	Enhanced immune function
Arginine (L-arginine)	Immunomodulation
Black tea (*Camellia sinensis*)	Immune enhancement/ improving resistance to disease
Bromelain	Immune system regulation
Calendula (*Calendula officinalis* L.), marigold	Immune system stimulant
Chaparral (*Larrea tridentata* DC. Coville, *L. divaricata* Cav.), nordihydroguaiaretic acid (NDGA)	Immune system disorders
Coenzyme Q10	Immune system diseases
Dandelion (*Taraxacum officinale*)	Immunostimulation
Elder (*Sambucus nigra* L.)	Immunostimulant
Essiac	Immune system enhancement
Garlic (*Allium sativum* L.)	Immune system stimulation
Ginger (*Zingiber officinale* Roscoe)	Immunostimulation
Gotu kola (*Centella asiatica* L.), total triterpenic fraction of *Centella asiatica* (TTFCA)	Immunomodulator
Green tea (*Camellia sinensis*)	Improving resistance to disease
Lactobacillus acidophilus	Immune system enhancement

Marshmallow (*Althaea officinalis* L.)	Immunostimulant
Melatonin	Immunostimulant
Omega-3 fatty acids, fish oil, alpha-linolenic acid	Immunosuppression
Polypodium leucotomos extract, Anapsos	Immunostimulation
Propolis	Immunostimulation
Saw palmetto (*Serenoa repens* [Bartram] Small)	Immunostimulation
Spirulina	Immune system enhancement
Tea tree oil (*Melaleuca alternifolia* [Maiden & Betche] Cheel)	Immune system deficiencies

INCONTINENCE AND RELATED CONDITIONS

Levels of Scientific Evidence for Specific Therapies

GRADE: C (Unclear or Conflicting Scientific Evidence)

Therapy	Specific Therapeutic Use(s)
Cranberry (*Vaccinium macrocarpon*)	Reduction of odor from incontinence/bladder catheterization
Saw palmetto (*Serenoa repens* [Bartram] Small)	Hypotonic neurogenic bladder

TRADITIONAL OR THEORETICAL USES THAT LACK SUFFICIENT EVIDENCE

Therapy	Specific Therapeutic Use(s)
Belladonna (*Atropa belladonna* L. or its variety *A. acuminata* Royle ex Lindl)	Bedwetting
Calendula (*Calendula officinalis* L.), marigold	Urinary retention
Ephedra (*Ephedra sinica*)/ma huang	Enuresis
Gotu kola (*Centella asiatica* L.), total triterpenic fraction of *Centella asiatica* (TTFCA)	Urinary retention
Horsetail (*Equisetum arvense* L.)	Urinary incontinence
Kava (*Piper methysticum* G. Forst)	Urinary incontinence
St. John's wort (*Hypericum perforatum* L.)	Bedwetting
Thyme (*Thymus vulgaris* L.), thymol	Enuresis

INFERTILITY AND RELATED CONDITIONS

Levels of Scientific Evidence for Specific Therapies

GRADE: D (Fair Negative Scientific Evidence)

Therapy	Specific Therapeutic Use(s)
Arginine (L-arginine)	Infertility

TRADITIONAL OR THEORETICAL USES THAT LACK SUFFICIENT EVIDENCE

Therapy	Specific Therapeutic Use(s)
Bitter melon (*Momordica charantia* L.), MAP30	Infertility
Black cohosh (*Cimicifuga racemosa* L. Nutt.)	Infertility
Burdock (*Arctium lappa*)	Sterility
Coenzyme Q10	Infertility
Dong quai (*Angelica sinensis* [Oliv.] Diels), Chinese angelica	Infertility
Ginseng (American ginseng, Asian ginseng, Chinese ginseng, Korean red ginseng, *Panax ginseng*: *Panax* spp. including *P. ginseng* C.C. Meyer and *P. quinquefolium* L., excluding *Eleutherococcus senticosus*)	Male infertility
Lavender (*Lavandula angustifolia* Miller)	Infertility
Omega-3 fatty acids, fish oil, alpha-linolenic acid	Male infertility
Sweet almond (*Prunus amygdalus dulcis*)	Increasing sperm count

INFLAMMATION AND RELATED CONDITIONS

Levels of Scientific Evidence for Specific Therapies

GRADE: B (Good Scientific Evidence)

Therapy	Specific Therapeutic Use(s)
Bromelain	Inflammation

GRADE: C (Unclear or Conflicting Scientific Evidence)

Therapy	Specific Therapeutic Use(s)
Arginine (L-arginine)	Dental pain (ibuprofen arginate)

Black cohosh (*Cimicifuga racemosa* L. Nutt.)	Arthritis pain (rheumatoid arthritis, osteoarthritis)
Dandelion (*Taraxacum officinale*)	Anti-inflammatory
Eyebright (*Euphrasia officinalis*)	Anti-inflammatory
Propolis	Dental pain
Shark cartilage	Analgesia
Turmeric (*Curcuma longa* L.), curcumin	Inflammation
White horehound (*Marrubium vulgare* L.)	Pain

TRADITIONAL OR THEORETICAL USES THAT LACK SUFFICIENT EVIDENCE

Therapy	Specific Therapeutic Use(s)
Alfalfa (*Medicago sativa* L.)	Inflammation
Arginine (L-arginine)	Pain
Astragalus (*Astragalus membranaceus*)	Myalgia (muscle pain)
Belladonna (*Atropa belladonna* L. or its variety *A. acuminata* Royle ex Lindl)	Anesthetic
Belladonna (*Atropa belladonna* L. or its variety *A. acuminata* Royle ex Lindl)	Inflammation
Belladonna (*Atropa belladonna* L. or its variety *A. acuminata* Royle ex Lindl)	Muscle and joint pain
Bitter almond (*Prunus amygdalus* Batch var. *amara* DC. Focke), Laetrile	Anti-inflammatory
Bitter almond (*Prunus amygdalus* Batch var. *amara* DC. Focke), Laetrile	Local anesthetic
Bitter almond (*Prunus amygdalus* Batch var. *amara* DC. Focke), Laetrile	Pain suppressant
Black cohosh (*Cimicifuga racemosa* L. Nutt.)	Inflammation
Black cohosh (*Cimicifuga racemosa* L. Nutt.)	Muscle pain
Black tea (*Camellia sinensis*)	Pain
Blessed thistle (*Cnicus benedictus* L.)	Inflammation
Bromelain	Pain
Bromelain	Pain (general)
Burdock (*Arctium lappa*)	Inflammation

Continued

Calendula (*Calendula officinalis* L.), marigold	Pain
Chamomile (*Matricaria recutita*, *Chamaemelum nobile*)	Anti-inflammatory
Chaparral (*Larrea tridentata* DC. Coville, *L. divaricata* Cav.), nordihydroguaiaretic acid (NDGA)	Anti-inflammatory
Chaparral (*Larrea tridentata* DC. Coville, *L. divaricata* Cav.), nordihydroguaiaretic acid (NDGA)	Pain
Clove (*Eugenia aromatica*)	Pain
Dandelion (*Taraxacum officinale*)	Analgesia
Devil's claw (*Harpagophytum procumbens* DC.)	Anti-inflammatory
Devil's claw (*Harpagophytum procumbens* DC.)	Muscle pain
Devil's claw (*Harpagophytum procumbens* DC.)	Pain
Dong quai (*Angelica sinensis* [Oliv.] Diels), Chinese angelica	Pain
Dong quai (*Angelica sinensis* [Oliv.] Diels), Chinese angelica	Pain from bruises
Echinacea (*Echinacea angustifolia* DC., *E. pallida*, *E. purpurea*)	Pain
Elder (*Sambucus nigra* L.)	Anti-inflammatory
Ephedra (*Ephedra sinica*)/ma huang	Anti-inflammatory
Eucalyptus oil (*Eucalyptus globulus* Labillardiere, *E. fructicetorum* F. Von Mueller, *E. smithii* R.T. Baker)	Inflammation
Eucalyptus oil (*Eucalyptus globulus* Labillardiere, *E. fructicetorum* F. Von Mueller, E. *smithii* R.T. Baker)	Muscle/joint pain (applied to the skin)
Evening primrose oil (*Oenothera biennis* L.)	Pain
Fenugreek (*Trigonella foenum-graecum* L.)	Inflammation
Feverfew (*Tanacetum parthenium* L. Schultz-Bip.)	Anti-inflammatory
Garlic (*Allium sativum* L.)	Dental pain
Ginger (*Zingiber officinale* Roscoe)	Pain relief
Ginseng (American ginseng, Asian ginseng, Chinese ginseng, Korean red ginseng, *Panax ginseng*: *Panax* spp. including *P. ginseng* C.C. Meyer and *P. quinquefolium* L., excluding *Eleutherococcus senticosus*)	Inflammation

Ginseng (American ginseng, Asian ginseng, Chinese ginseng, Korean red ginseng, *Panax ginseng*: *Panax* spp. including *P. ginseng* C.C. Meyer and *P. quinquefolium* L., excluding *Eleutherococcus senticosus*)	Pain relief
Goldenseal (*Hydrastis canadensis* L.), berberine	Anesthetic
Goldenseal (*Hydrastis canadensis* L.), berberine	Anti-inflammatory
Goldenseal (*Hydrastis canadensis* L.), berberine	Muscle pain
Goldenseal (*Hydrastis canadensis* L.), berberine	Pain
Gotu kola (*Centella asiatica* L.), total triterpenic fraction of *Centella asiatica* (TTFCA)	Inflammation
Gotu kola (*Centella asiatica* L.), total triterpenic fraction of *Centella asiatica* (TTFCA)	Pain
Guggul (*Commifora mukul*)	Pain
Hops (*Humulus lupulus* L.)	Anti-inflammatory
Hops (*Humulus lupulus* L.)	Pain
Kava (*Piper methysticum* G. Forst)	Anesthesia
Kava (*Piper methysticum* G. Forst)	Pain
Lavender (*Lavandula angustifolia* Miller)	Anti-inflammatory
Lavender (*Lavandula angustifolia* Miller)	Pain
Licorice (*Glycyrrhiza glabra* L.), deglycyrrhizinated licorice (DGL)	Inflammation
Marshmallow (*Althaea officinalis* L.)	Inflammation
Marshmallow (*Althaea officinalis* L.)	Muscular pain
Oleander (*Nerium oleander*, *Thevetia peruviana*)	Inflammation
Passionflower (*Passiflora incarnata* L.)	Chronic pain
Passionflower (*Passiflora incarnata* L.)	Pain (general)
Peppermint (*Mentha* x *piperita* L.)	Local anesthetic
Peppermint (*Mentha* x *piperita* L.)	Musculoskeletal pain
Peppermint (*Mentha* x *piperita* L.)	Myalgia (muscle pain)
Polypodium leucotomos extract, Anapsos	Inflammation
Pygeum (*Prunus africana*, *Pygeum africanum*)	Inflammation

Continued

Saw palmetto (*Serenoa repens* [Bartram] Small)	Anti-inflammatory
Slippery elm (*Ulmus rubra* Muhl. or *U. fulva* Michx.)	Inflammation
Spirulina	Anti-inflammatory
St. John's wort (*Hypericum perforatum* L.)	Anti-inflammatory
St. John's wort (*Hypericum perforatum* L.)	Dental pain
St. John's wort (*Hypericum perforatum* L.)	Pain relief
Tea tree oil (*Melaleuca alternifolia* [Maiden & Betche] Cheel)	Anti-inflammatory
Tea tree oil (*Melaleuca alternifolia* [Maiden & Betche] Cheel)	Muscle and joint pain
Turmeric (*Curcuma longa* L.), curcumin	Pain
Valerian (*Valeriana officinalis* L.)	Anodyne (pain relief)
Valerian (*Valeriana officinalis* L.)	Muscle pain
Valerian (*Valeriana officinalis* L.)	Pain
White horehound (*Marrubium vulgare* L.)	Pain
Wild yam (*Dioscorea villosa*)	Anti-inflammatory
Yohimbe bark extract (*Pausinystalia yohimbe* Pierre ex Beille)	Anesthetic

INSECT BITES AND STINGS AND RELATED CONDITIONS

Levels of Scientific Evidence for Specific Therapies

GRADE: C (Unclear or Conflicting Scientific Evidence)

Therapy	Specific Therapeutic Use(s)
Garlic (*Allium sativum* L.)	Tick repellent

TRADITIONAL OR THEORETICAL USES THAT LACK SUFFICIENT EVIDENCE

Therapy	Specific Therapeutic Use(s)
Alfalfa (*Medicago sativa* L.)	Insect bites
American pennyroyal (*Hedeoma pulegioides* L.), European pennyroyal (*Mentha pulegium* L.)	Flea control
American pennyroyal (*Hedeoma pulegioides* L.), European pennyroyal (*Mentha pulegium* L.)	Insect repellent

Black cohosh (*Cimicifuga racemosa* L. Nutt.)	Insect repellent
Chamomile (*Matricaria recutita*, *Chamaemelum nobile*)	Insect bites
Echinacea (*Echinacea angustifolia* DC., *E. pallida*, *E. purpurea*)	Bee stings
Elder (*Sambucus nigra* L.)	Mosquito repellent
Eucalyptus oil (*Eucalyptus globulus* Labillardiere, *E. fructicetorum* F. Von Mueller, *E. smithii* R.T. Baker)	Insect repellent
Feverfew (*Tanacetum parthenium* L. Schultz-Bip.)	Insect bites
Feverfew (*Tanacetum parthenium* L. Schultz-Bip.)	Insect repellent
Ginger (*Zingiber officinale* Roscoe)	Insecticide
Lavender (*Lavandula angustifolia* Miller)	Insect repellent
Marshmallow (*Althaea officinalis* L.)	Bee stings
Marshmallow (*Althaea officinalis* L.)	Insect bites
Oleander (*Nerium oleander*, *Thevetia peruviana*)	Insecticide
Soy (*Glycine max* L. Merr.)	Insect repellent
Tea tree oil (*Melaleuca alternifolia* [Maiden & Betche] Cheel)	Insect bites/stings
Thyme (*Thymus vulgaris* L.), thymol	Insect bites
Turmeric (*Curcuma longa* L.), curcumin	Insect bites
Turmeric (*Curcuma longa* L.), curcumin	Insect repellent

IRRITABLE BOWEL SYNDROME AND RELATED CONDITIONS

Levels of Scientific Evidence for Specific Therapies

GRADE: C (Unclear or Conflicting Scientific Evidence)

Therapy	Specific Therapeutic Use(s)
Belladonna (*Atropa belladonna* L. or its variety *A. acuminata* Royle ex Lindl)	Irritable bowel syndrome
Chamomile (*Matricaria recutita*, *Chamaemelum nobile*)	Gastrointestinal conditions
Clay	Functional gastrointestinal disorders
Globe artichoke (*Cynara scolymus* L.)	Irritable bowel syndrome

Continued

Lactobacillus acidophilus	Irritable bowel syndrome
Lactobacillus acidophilus	Necrotizing enterocolitis prevention in infants
Peppermint (*Mentha* x *piperita* L.)	Irritable bowel syndrome
Psyllium (*Plantago ovata, P. ispaghula*)	Irritable bowel syndrome
Slippery elm (*Ulmus rubra* Muhl. or *U. fulva* Michx.)	Gastrointestinal disorders
White horehound (*Marrubium vulgare* L.)	Intestinal disorders/ antispasmodic

TRADITIONAL OR THEORETICAL USES THAT LACK SUFFICIENT EVIDENCE

Therapy	Specific Therapeutic Use(s)
Alfalfa (*Medicago sativa* L.)	Gastrointestinal tract disorders
Aloe (*Aloe vera*)	Bowel disorders
American pennyroyal (*Hedeoma pulegioides* L.), European pennyroyal (*Mentha pulegium* L.)	Bowel disorders
American pennyroyal (*Hedeoma pulegioides* L.), European pennyroyal (*Mentha pulegium* L.)	Colic
American pennyroyal (*Hedeoma pulegioides* L.), European pennyroyal (*Mentha pulegium* L.)	Intestinal disorders
American pennyroyal (*Hedeoma pulegioides* L.), European pennyroyal (*Mentha pulegium* L.)	Stomach pain
American pennyroyal (*Hedeoma pulegioides* L.), European pennyroyal (*Mentha pulegium* L.)	Stomach spasms
Arginine (L-arginine)	Infantile necrotizing enterocolitis
Arginine (L-arginine)	Lower esophageal sphincter relaxation
Arginine (L-arginine)	Stomach motility disorders
Astragalus (*Astragalus membranaceus*)	Gastrointestinal disorders
Barley (*Hordeum vulgare* L.), germinated barley foodstuff (GBF)	Bowel/intestinal disorders
Belladonna (*Atropa belladonna* L. or its variety *A. acuminata* Royle ex Lindl)	Diverticulitis
Bilberry (*Vaccinium myrtillus*)	Stomach upset
Bitter melon (*Momordica charantia* L.), MAP30	Gastrointestinal cramps

Black tea (*Camellia sinensis*)	Stomach disorders
Bladderwrack (*Fucus vesiculosus*)	Stomach upset
Bromelain	Leaky gut syndrome
Calendula (*Calendula officinalis* L.), marigold	Bowel irritation
Calendula (*Calendula officinalis* L.), marigold	Gastrointestinal tract disorders
Chamomile (*Matricaria recutita*, *Chamaemelum nobile*)	Abdominal bloating
Chamomile (*Matricaria recutita*, *Chamaemelum nobile*)	Infantile colic
Chamomile (*Matricaria recutita*, *Chamaemelum nobile*)	Irritable bowel syndrome
Chaparral (*Larrea tridentata* DC. Coville, *L. divaricata* Cav.), nordihydroguaiaretic acid (NDGA)	Bowel cramps
Chaparral (*Larrea tridentata* DC. Coville, *L. divaricata* Cav.), nordihydroguaiaretic acid (NDGA)	Gastrointestinal disorders
Clay	Stomach disorders
Clove (*Eugenia aromatica*)	Abdominal pain
Clove (*Eugenia aromatica*)	Colic
Cranberry (*Vaccinium macrocarpon*)	Stomach ailments
Dandelion (*Taraxacum officinale*)	Stomach ache
Devil's claw (*Harpagophytum procumbens* DC.)	Gastrointestinal disorders
Dong quai (*Angelica sinensis* [Oliv.] Diels), Chinese angelica	Abdominal pain
Dong quai (*Angelica sinensis* [Oliv.] Diels), Chinese angelica	Irritable bowel syndrome
Echinacea (*Echinacea angustifolia* DC., *E. pallida*, *E. purpurea*)	Stomach upset
Elder (*Sambucus nigra* L.)	Colic
Elder (*Sambucus nigra* L.)	Gut disorders
Evening primrose oil (*Oenothera biennis* L.)	Irritable bowel syndrome
Eyebright (*Euphrasia officinalis*)	Gastric acid secretion stimulation
Fenugreek (*Trigonella foenum-graecum* L.)	Colic
Feverfew (*Tanacetum parthenium* L. Schultz-Bip.)	Abdominal pain
Flaxseed and flaxseed oil (*Linum usitatissimum*)	Abdominal pain

Continued

Flaxseed and flaxseed oil (*Linum usitatissimum*)	Diverticulitis
Flaxseed and flaxseed oil (*Linum usitatissimum*)	Irritable bowel syndrome
Flaxseed and flaxseed oil (*Linum usitatissimum*)	Laxative-induced colon damage
Flaxseed and flaxseed oil (*Linum usitatissimum*)	Stomach upset
Garlic (*Allium sativum* L.)	Stomachache
Ginger (*Zingiber officinale* Roscoe)	Colic
Ginger (*Zingiber officinale* Roscoe)	Stomachache
Ginseng (American ginseng, Asian ginseng, Chinese ginseng, Korean red ginseng, *Panax ginseng*: *Panax* spp. including *P. ginseng* C.C. Meyer and *P. quinquefolium* L., excluding *Eleutherococcus senticosus*)	Stomach upset
Goldenseal (*Hydrastis canadensis* L.), berberine	Stomachache
Green tea (*Camellia sinensis*)	Stomach disorders
Gymnema (*Gymnema sylvestre* R. Br.)	Stomach ailments
Hawthorn (*Crataegus laevigata*, C. *oxyacantha*, *C. monogyna*, *C. pentagyna*)	Abdominal colic
Hawthorn (*Crataegus laevigata*, *C. oxyacantha*, *C. monogyna*, *C. pentagyna*)	Abdominal distention
Hawthorn (*Crataegus laevigata*, *C. oxyacantha*, *C. monogyna*, *C. pentagyna*)	Abdominal pain
Hawthorn (*Crataegus laevigata*, *C. oxyacantha*, *C. monogyna*, *C. pentagyna*)	Stomachache
Hops (*Humulus lupulus* L.)	Irritable bowel syndrome
Horsetail (*Equisetum arvense* L.)	Stomach upset
Kava (*Piper methysticum* G. Forst)	Stomach upset
Lactobacillus acidophilus	Diverticulitis
Lavender (*Lavandula angustifolia* Miller)	Colic
Licorice (*Glycyrrhiza glabra* L.), deglycyrrhizinated licorice (DGL)	Diverticulitis
Licorice (*Glycyrrhiza glabra* L.), deglycyrrhizinated licorice (DGL)	Stomach upset
Marshmallow (*Althaea officinalis* L.)	Diverticulitis

Marshmallow (*Althaea officinalis* L.)	Irritable bowel syndrome
Melatonin	Intestinal motility disorders
Passionflower (*Passiflora incarnata* L.)	Gastrointestinal discomfort (nervous stomach)
Peppermint (*Mentha* x *piperita* L.)	Gastrointestinal disorders
Peppermint (*Mentha* x *piperita* L.)	Ileus (postoperative)
Peppermint (*Mentha* x *piperita* L.)	Intestinal colic
Propolis	Diverticulitis
Pygeum (*Prunus africana, Pygeum africanum*)	Stomach upset
Red yeast rice (*Monascus purpureus*)	Colic in children
Red yeast rice (*Monascus purpureus*)	Stomach problems
Shark cartilage	Intestinal disorders and inflammation
Slippery elm (*Ulmus rubra* Muhl. or *U. fulva* Michx.)	Colic
Slippery elm (*Ulmus rubra* Muhl. or *U. fulva* Michx.)	Diverticulitis
Slippery elm (*Ulmus rubra* Muhl. or *U. fulva* Michx.)	Irritable bowel syndrome
Sorrel (*Rumex acetosa* L., *R. acetosella* L.), Sinupret	Stimulation of secretion
Sorrel (*Rumex acetosa* L., *R. acetosella* L.), Sinupret	Ulcerated bowel
Soy (*Glycine max* L. Merr.)	Gastrointestinal motility
Spirulina	Bowel health
Thyme (*Thymus vulgaris* L.), thymol	Colic
Thyme (*Thymus vulgaris* L.), thymol	Stomach cramps
Turmeric (*Curcuma longa* L.), curcumin	Bloating
Turmeric (*Curcuma longa* L.), curcumin	Colic
Valerian (*Valeriana officinalis* L.)	Bloating
Valerian (*Valeriana officinalis* L.)	Colic
Valerian (*Valeriana officinalis* L.)	Intestinal disorders
Valerian (*Valeriana officinalis* L.)	Irritable bowel syndrome
Valerian (*Valeriana officinalis* L.)	Viral gastroenteritis
White horehound (*Marrubium vulgare* L.)	Bloating

Continued

White horehound (*Marrubium vulgare* L.)	Colic
Wild yam (*Dioscorea villosa*)	Diverticulitis
Wild yam (*Dioscorea villosa*)	Irritable bowel syndrome

KIDNEY DISEASE AND RELATED CONDITIONS

Levels of Scientific Evidence for Specific Therapies

GRADE: C (Unclear or Conflicting Scientific Evidence)

Therapy	Specific Therapeutic Use(s)
Astragalus (*Astragalus membranaceus*)	Renal failure
Danshen (*Salvia miltiorrhiza*)	Increased rate of peritoneal dialysis
Dong quai (*Angelica sinensis* [Oliv.] Diels), Chinese angelica	Glomerulonephritis
Flaxseed and flaxseed oil (*Linum usitatissimum*)	Kidney disease/lupus nephritis (flaxseed, not flaxseed oil)
Omega-3 fatty acids, fish oil, alpha-linolenic acid	IgA nephropathy
Omega-3 fatty acids, fish oil, alpha-linolenic acid	Nephrotic syndrome
Soy (*Glycine max* L. Merr.)	Kidney disease (chronic renal failure, nephrotic syndrome, proteinuria)

GRADE: D (Fair Negative Scientific Evidence)

Therapy	Specific Therapeutic Use(s)
Arginine (L-arginine)	Cyclosporine toxicity
Arginine (L-arginine)	Kidney disease
Arginine (L-arginine)	Kidney protection during angiography

TRADITIONAL OR THEORETICAL USES THAT LACK SUFFICIENT EVIDENCE

Therapy	Specific Therapeutic Use(s)
Alfalfa (*Medicago sativa* L.)	Kidney disorders
Aloe (*Aloe vera*)	Kidney or bladder stones
American pennyroyal (*Hedeoma pulegioides* L.), European pennyroyal (*Mentha pulegium* L.)	Kidney disease

Astragalus (*Astragalus membranaceus*)	Nephritis
Bilberry (*Vaccinium myrtillus*)	Kidney disease
Bilberry (*Vaccinium myrtillus*)	Urine blood
Black cohosh (*Cimicifuga racemosa* L. Nutt.)	Kidney inflammation
Bladderwrack (*Fucus vesiculosus*)	Kidney disease
Boswellia (*Boswellia serrata* Roxb.)	Nephritis
Burdock (*Arctium lappa*)	Kidney diseases
Coenzyme Q10	Kidney failure
Dandelion (*Taraxacum officinale*)	Kidney disease
Danshen (*Salvia miltiorrhiza*)	Gentamicin toxicity
Danshen (*Salvia miltiorrhiza*)	Kidney failure
Dong quai (*Angelica sinensis* [Oliv.] Diels), Chinese angelica	Kidney disease
Elder (*Sambucus nigra* L.)	Kidney disease
Ephedra (*Ephedra sinica*)/ma huang	Nephritis
Essiac	Kidney diseases
Flaxseed and flaxseed oil (*Linum usitatissimum*)	Glomerulonephritis
Garlic (*Allium sativum* L.)	Bloody urine
Garlic (*Allium sativum* L.)	Kidney damage from antibiotics
Garlic (*Allium sativum* L.)	Kidney problems
Garlic (*Allium sativum* L.)	Nephrotic syndrome
Ginger (*Zingiber officinale* Roscoe)	Kidney disease
Ginseng (American ginseng, Asian ginseng, Chinese ginseng, Korean red ginseng, *Panax ginseng*: *Panax* spp. including *P. ginseng* C.C. Meyer and *P. quinquefolium* L., excluding *Eleutherococcus senticosus*)	Diabetic nephropathy (kidney disease)
Ginseng (American ginseng, Asian ginseng, Chinese ginseng, Korean red ginseng, *Panax ginseng*: *Panax* spp. including *P. ginseng* C.C. Meyer and *P. quinquefolium* L., excluding *Eleutherococcus senticosus*)	Kidney disease
Globe artichoke (*Cynara scolymus* L.)	Nephrosclerosis

Continued

Hawthorn (*Crataegus laevigata, C. oxyacantha, C. monogyna, C. pentagyna*)	Nephrosis
Hops (*Humulus lupulus* L.)	Kidney disorders
Horse chestnut (*Aesculus hippocastanum* L.)	Kidney diseases
Horsetail (*Equisetum arvense* L.)	Kidney disease
Kava (*Piper methysticum* G. Forst)	Kidney disorders
Licorice (*Glycyrrhiza glabra* L.), deglycyrrhizinated licorice (DGL)	Gentamicin induced kidney damage
Melatonin	Gentamicin-induced kidney damage
Melatonin	Toxic kidney damage
Milk thistle (*Silybum marianum*), silymarin	Nephrotoxicity protection
Omega-3 fatty acids, fish oil, alpha-linolenic acid	Diabetic nephropathy
Omega-3 fatty acids, fish oil, alpha-linolenic acid	Glomerulonephritis
Omega-3 fatty acids, fish oil, alpha-linolenic acid	Hepatorenal syndrome
Omega-3 fatty acids, fish oil, alpha-linolenic acid	Kidney disease prevention
Pygeum (*Prunus africana, Pygeum africanum*)	Kidney disease
Spirulina	Kidney disease
Turmeric (*Curcuma longa* L.), curcumin	Kidney disease

LABOR AND DELIVERY AND RELATED CONDITIONS

Levels of Scientific Evidence for Specific Therapies

GRADE: C (Unclear or Conflicting Scientific Evidence)

Therapy	Specific Therapeutic Use(s)
American pennyroyal (*Hedeoma pulegioides* L.), European pennyroyal (*Mentha pulegium* L.)	Abortifacient (uterine contraction stimulant)
Blessed thistle (*Cnicus benedictus* L.)	Abortifacient

TRADITIONAL OR THEORETICAL USES THAT LACK SUFFICIENT EVIDENCE

Therapy	Specific Therapeutic Use(s)
American pennyroyal (*Hedeoma pulegioides* L.), European pennyroyal (*Mentha pulegium* L.)	Pregnancy

Arginine (L-arginine)	Preterm labor contractions
Astragalus (*Astragalus membranaceus*)	Postpartum fever
Astragalus (*Astragalus membranaceus*)	Postpartum urinary retention
Black cohosh (*Cimicifuga racemosa* L. Nutt.)	Labor induction
Blessed thistle (*Cnicus benedictus* L.)	Abortifacient
Bromelain	Shortening of labor
Dandelion (*Taraxacum officinale*)	Pregnancy
Danshen (*Salvia miltiorrhiza*)	Ectopic pregnancy
Danshen (*Salvia miltiorrhiza*)	Intrauterine growth restriction/retardation
Dong quai (*Angelica sinensis* [Oliv.] Diels), Chinese angelica	Labor aid
Dong quai (*Angelica sinensis* [Oliv.] Diels), Chinese angelica	Postpartum weakness
Dong quai (*Angelica sinensis* [Oliv.] Diels), Chinese angelica	Pregnancy support
Fenugreek (*Trigonella foenum-graecum* L.)	Abortifacient
Fenugreek (*Trigonella foenum-graecum* L.)	Labor induction (uterine stimulant)
Feverfew (*Tanacetum parthenium* L. Schultz-Bip.)	Abortifacient
Feverfew (*Tanacetum parthenium* L. Schultz-Bip.)	Labor induction
Garlic (*Allium sativum* L.)	Abortion
Ginkgo (*Ginkgo biloba* L.)	Labor induction
Goldenseal (*Hydrastis canadensis* L.), berberine	Abortifacient
Goldenseal (*Hydrastis canadensis* L.), berberine	Postpartum hemorrhage
Niacin (vitamin B_3, nicotinic acid), niacinamide, inositol hexanicotinate	Pregnancy problems
Oleander (*Nerium oleander*, *Thevetia peruviana*)	Pregnancy termination
Omega-3 fatty acids, fish oil, alpha-linolenic acid	Pregnancy nutritional supplement
Omega-3 fatty acids, fish oil, alpha-linolenic acid	Premature birth prevention
Red yeast rice (*Monascus purpureus*)	Postpartum problems

Continued

Saw palmetto (*Serenoa repens* [Bartram] Small)	Postnasal drip
Slippery elm (*Ulmus rubra* Muhl. or *U. fulva* Michx.)	Abortifacient
Spirulina	Obstetric and gynecologic disorders

LACTATION STIMULATION AND RELATED CONDITIONS

Levels of Scientific Evidence for Specific Therapies

TRADITIONAL OR THEORETICAL USES THAT LACK SUFFICIENT EVIDENCE

Therapy	Specific Therapeutic Use(s)
Alfalfa (*Medicago sativa* L.)	Increasing breast milk
Blessed thistle (*Cnicus benedictus* L.)	Breast milk stimulant
Fenugreek (*Trigonella foenum-graecum* L.)	Galactagogue (lactation stimulant)
Milk thistle (*Silybum marianum*), silymarin	Lactation stimulation
Saw palmetto (*Serenoa repens* [Bartram] Small)	Lactation
Turmeric (*Curcuma longa* L.), curcumin	Lactation stimulation

LAXATIVE AND RELATED CONDITIONS

Levels of Scientific Evidence for Specific Therapies

GRADE: A (Strong Scientific Evidence)

Therapy	Specific Therapeutic Use(s)
Aloe (*Aloe vera*)	Constipation (laxative)

GRADE: B (Good Scientific Evidence)

Therapy	Specific Therapeutic Use(s)
Flaxseed and flaxseed oil (*Linum usitatissimum*)	Laxative (flaxseed, not flaxseed oil)
Psyllium (*Plantago ovata*, *P. ispaghula*)	Constipation

GRADE: C (Unclear or Conflicting Scientific Evidence)

Therapy	Specific Therapeutic Use(s)
Barley (*Hordeum vulgare* L.), germinated barley foodstuff (GBF)	Constipation

TRADITIONAL OR THEORETICAL USES THAT LACK SUFFICIENT EVIDENCE	
Therapy	Specific Therapeutic Use(s)
Astragalus (*Astragalus membranaceus*)	Laxative
Bladderwrack (*Fucus vesiculosus*)	Laxative
Bladderwrack (*Fucus vesiculosus*)	Stool softener
Burdock (*Arctium lappa*)	Laxative
Calendula (*Calendula officinalis* L.), marigold	Constipation
Chamomile (*Matricaria recutita*, *Chamaemelum nobile*)	Constipation
Clay	Constipation
Devil's claw (*Harpagophytum procumbens* DC.)	Constipation
Dong quai (*Angelica sinensis* [Oliv.] Diels), Chinese angelica	Constipation
Dong quai (*Angelica sinensis* [Oliv.] Diels), Chinese angelica	Laxative
Elder (*Sambucus nigra* L.)	Laxative
Fenugreek (*Trigonella foenum-graecum* L.)	Constipation
Feverfew (*Tanacetum parthenium* L. Schultz-Bip.)	Constipation
Ginger (*Zingiber officinale* Roscoe)	Laxative
Globe artichoke (*Cynara scolymus* L.)	Constipation
Goldenseal (*Hydrastis canadensis* L.), berberine	Constipation
Gymnema (*Gymnema sylvestre* R. Br.)	Constipation
Gymnema (*Gymnema sylvestre* R. Br.)	Laxative
Lactobacillus acidophilus	Constipation
Licorice (*Glycyrrhiza glabra* L.), deglycyrrhizinated licorice (DGL)	Constipation
Marshmallow (*Althaea officinalis* L.)	Constipation
Marshmallow (*Althaea officinalis* L.)	Laxative
Oleander (*Nerium oleander*, *Thevetia peruviana*)	Cathartic
Seaweed, kelp, bladderwrack (*Fucus vesiculosus*)	Bulk laxative
Seaweed, kelp, bladderwrack (*Fucus vesiculosus*)	Laxative

Continued

Seaweed, kelp, bladderwrack (*Fucus vesiculosus*)	Stool softener
Slippery elm (*Ulmus rubra* Muhl. or *U. fulva* Michx.)	Constipation
Sorrel (*Rumex acetosa* L., *R. acetosella* L.) and Sinupret	Constipation
Sweet almond (*Prunus amygdalus dulcis*)	Mild laxative
Valerian (*Valeriana officinalis* L.)	Constipation
White horehound (*Marrubium vulgare* L.)	Cathartic
White horehound (*Marrubium vulgare* L.)	Constipation
White horehound (*Marrubium vulgare* L.)	Laxative

LIVER DISEASE AND RELATED CONDITIONS

Levels of Scientific Evidence for Specific Therapies

GRADE: B (Good Scientific Evidence)

Therapy	Specific Therapeutic Use(s)
Milk thistle (*Silybum marianum*), silymarin	Cirrhosis
Milk thistle (*Silybum marianum*), silymarin	Hepatitis (chronic)

GRADE: C (Unclear or Conflicting Scientific Evidence)

Therapy	Specific Therapeutic Use(s)
Astragalus (*Astragalus membranaceus*)	Liver protection
Clay	Protection from aflatoxins
Dandelion (*Taraxacum officinale*)	Hepatitis B
Danshen (*Salvia miltiorrhiza*)	Liver disease (cirrhosis/chronic hepatitis B)
Eyebright (*Euphrasia officinalis*)	Hepatoprotection
Lactobacillus acidophilus	Hepatic encephalopathy (confused thinking due to liver disorders)
Licorice (*Glycyrrhiza glabra* L.), deglycyrrhizinated licorice (DGL)	Viral hepatitis
Milk thistle (*Silybum marianum*), silymarin	Acute viral hepatitis
Milk thistle (*Silybum marianum*), silymarin	*Amanita phalloides* mushroom toxicity

Milk thistle (*Silybum marianum*), silymarin	Drug/toxin-induced hepatotoxicity

TRADITIONAL OR THEORETICAL USES THAT LACK SUFFICIENT EVIDENCE

Therapy	Specific Therapeutic Use(s)
Alfalfa (*Medicago sativa* L.)	Jaundice
Aloe (*Aloe vera*)	Hepatitis
American pennyroyal (*Hedeoma pulegioides* L.), European pennyroyal (*Mentha pulegium* L.)	Liver disease
Arginine (L-arginine)	Ammonia toxicity
Arginine (L-arginine)	Hepatic encephalopathy
Arginine (L-arginine)	Liver disease
Astragalus (*Astragalus membranaceus*)	Chronic hepatitis
Astragalus (*Astragalus membranaceus*)	Liver disease
Bilberry (*Vaccinium myrtillus*)	Liver disease
Black cohosh (*Cimicifuga racemosa* L. Nutt.)	Liver disease
Blessed thistle (*Cnicus benedictus* L.)	Jaundice
Blessed thistle (*Cnicus benedictus* L.)	Liver disorders
Burdock (*Arctium lappa*)	Liver protection
Calendula (*Calendula officinalis* L.), marigold	Jaundice
Calendula (*Calendula officinalis* L.), marigold	Liver dysfunction
Chamomile (*Matricaria recutita*, *Chamaemelum nobile*)	Liver disorders
Coenzyme Q10	Hepatitis B
Coenzyme Q10	Liver enlargement or disease
Cranberry (*Vaccinium macrocarpon*)	Liver disorders
Dandelion (*Taraxacum officinale*)	Jaundice
Dandelion (*Taraxacum officinale*)	Liver cleansing
Dandelion (*Taraxacum officinale*)	Liver disease
Devil's claw (*Harpagophytum procumbens* DC.)	Liver and gallbladder tonic
Dehydroepiandrosterone (DHEA)	Liver protection

Continued

Dong quai (*Angelica sinensis* [Oliv.] Diels), Chinese angelica	Chronic hepatitis
Dong quai (*Angelica sinensis* [Oliv.] Diels), Chinese angelica	Cirrhosis
Dong quai (*Angelica sinensis* [Oliv.] Diels), Chinese angelica	Liver protection
Elder (*Sambucus nigra* L.)	Liver disease
Eucalyptus oil (*Eucalyptus globulus* Labillardiere, *E. fructicetorum* F. Von Mueller, *E. smithii* R.T. Baker)	Liver protection
Evening primrose oil (*Oenothera biennis* L.)	Hepatitis B
Eyebright (*Euphrasia officinalis*)	Jaundice
Eyebright (*Euphrasia officinalis*)	Liver disease
Garlic (*Allium sativum* L.)	Antitoxin
Garlic (*Allium sativum* L.)	Hepatopulmonary syndrome
Garlic (*Allium sativum* L.)	Liver health
Ginger (*Zingiber officinale* Roscoe)	Liver disease
Ginkgo (*Ginkgo biloba* L.)	Hepatitis B
Ginseng (American ginseng, Asian ginseng, Chinese ginseng, Korean red ginseng, *Panax ginseng*: *Panax* spp. including *P. ginseng* C.C. Meyer and *P. quinquefolium* L., excluding *Eleutherococcus senticosus*)	Hepatitis/hepatitis B virus infection
Ginseng (American ginseng, Asian ginseng, Chinese ginseng, Korean red ginseng, *Panax ginseng*: *Panax* spp. including *P. ginseng* C.C. Meyer and *P. quinquefolium* L., excluding *Eleutherococcus senticosus*)	Liver diseases
Ginseng (American ginseng, Asian ginseng, Chinese ginseng, Korean red ginseng, *Panax ginseng*: *Panax* spp. including *P. ginseng* C.C. Meyer and *P. quinquefolium* L., excluding *Eleutherococcus senticosus*)	Liver health
Globe artichoke (*Cynara scolymus* L.)	Jaundice
Goldenseal (*Hydrastis canadensis* L.), berberine	Alcoholic liver disease
Goldenseal (*Hydrastis canadensis* L.), berberine	Hepatitis
Goldenseal (*Hydrastis canadensis* L.), berberine	Jaundice
Goldenseal (*Hydrastis canadensis* L.), berberine	Liver disorders

Gotu kola (*Centella asiatica* L.), total triterpenic fraction of *Centella asiatica* (TTFCA)	Hepatitis
Gotu kola (*Centella asiatica* L.), total triterpenic fraction of *Centella asiatica* (TTFCA)	Jaundice
Gymnema (*Gymnema sylvestre* R. Br.)	Liver disease
Gymnema (*Gymnema sylvestre* R. Br.)	Liver protection
Horse chestnut (*Aesculus hippocastanum* L.)	Liver congestion
Horsetail (*Equisetum arvense* L.)	Liver protection
Licorice (*Glycyrrhiza glabra* L.), deglycyrrhizinated licorice (DGL)	Liver protection
Maitake mushroom (*Grifola frondosa*), beta-glucan	Liver inflammation (hepatitis)
Melatonin	Toxic liver damage
Milk thistle (*Silybum marianum*), silymarin	Jaundice
Milk thistle (*Silybum marianum*), silymarin	Liver cleansing agent
Niacin (vitamin B_3, nicotinic acid), niacinamide, inositol hexanicotinate	Liver disease
Omega-3 fatty acids, fish oil, alpha-linolenic acid	Cirrhosis

LOWER BACK PAIN AND RELATED CONDITIONS

Levels of Scientific Evidence for Specific Therapies

GRADE: C (Unclear or Conflicting Scientific Evidence)

Therapy	Specific Therapeutic Use(s)
Devil's claw (*Harpagophytum procumbens* DC.)	Low back pain

TRADITIONAL OR THEORETICAL USES THAT LACK SUFFICIENT EVIDENCE

Therapy	Specific Therapeutic Use(s)
Belladonna (*Atropa belladonna* L. or its variety *A. acuminata* Royle ex Lindl)	Sciatica (back and leg pain)
Black cohosh (*Cimicifuga racemosa* L. Nutt.)	Back pain
Bromelain	Back pain
Bromelain	Sciatica

Continued

Burdock (*Arctium lappa*)	Back pain
Burdock (*Arctium lappa*)	Sciatica
Chamomile (*Matricaria recutita*, *Chamaemelum nobile*)	Back pain
Chamomile (*Matricaria recutita*, *Chamaemelum nobile*)	Sciatica
Dong quai (*Angelica sinensis* [Oliv.] Diels), Chinese angelica	Back pain
Dong quai (*Angelica sinensis* [Oliv.] Diels), Chinese angelica	Sciatica
Eucalyptus oil (*Eucalyptus globulus* Labillardiere, *E. fructicetorum* F. Von Mueller, *E. smithii* R.T. Baker)	Back pain
Goldenseal (*Hydrastis canadensis* L.), berberine	Sciatica

LOWER EXTREMEITY EDEMA AND RELATED CONDITIONS

Levels of Scientific Evidence for Specific Therapies

GRADE: A (Strong Scientific Evidence)

Therapy	Specific Therapeutic Use(s)
Horse chestnut (*Aesculus hippocastanum* L.)	Chronic venous insufficiency

GRADE: B (Good Scientific Evidence)

Therapy	Specific Therapeutic Use(s)
Gotu kola (*Centella asiatica* L.), total triterpenic fraction of *Centella asiatica* (TTFCA)	Chronic venous insufficiency/ varicose veins

GRADE: C (Unclear or Conflicting Scientific Evidence)

Therapy	Specific Therapeutic Use(s)
Bilberry (*Vaccinium myrtillus*)	Chronic venous insufficiency
Glucosamine	Chronic venous insufficiency

TRADITIONAL OR THEORETICAL USES THAT LACK SUFFICIENT EVIDENCE

Therapy	Specific Therapeutic Use(s)
Astragalus (*Astragalus membranaceus*)	Edema
Barley (*Hordeum vulgare* L.), germinated barley foodstuff (GBF)	Improved blood circulation

Bilberry (*Vaccinium myrtillus*)	Poor circulation
Black cohosh (*Cimicifuga racemosa* L. Nutt.)	Edema
Black tea (*Camellia sinensis*)	Circulatory/blood flow disorders
Bladderwrack (*Fucus vesiculosus*)	Edema
Bromelain	Varicose veins
Burdock (*Arctium lappa*)	Fluid retention
Calendula (*Calendula officinalis* L.), marigold	Circulation problems
Calendula (*Calendula officinalis* L.), marigold	Edema
Calendula (*Calendula officinalis* L.), marigold	Varicose veins
Dandelion (*Taraxacum officinale*)	Circulation
Dandelion (*Taraxacum officinale*)	Dropsy
Danshen (*Salvia miltiorrhiza*)	Circulation
Devil's claw (*Harpagophytum procumbens* DC.)	Edema
Dong quai (*Angelica sinensis* [Oliv.] Diels), Chinese angelica	Fluid retention
Elder (*Sambucus nigra* L.)	Circulatory stimulant
Elder (*Sambucus nigra* L.)	Edema
Ephedra (*Ephedra sinica*)/ma huang	Edema
Fenugreek (*Trigonella foenum-graecum* L.)	Dropsy
Ginkgo (*Ginkgo biloba* L.)	Swelling
Globe artichoke (*Cynara scolymus* L.)	Peripheral edema
Goldenseal (*Hydrastis canadensis* L.), berberine	Circulatory stimulant
Gotu kola (*Centella asiatica* L.), total triterpenic fraction of *Centella asiatica* (TTFCA)	Vascular fragility
Green tea (*Camellia sinensis*)	Improving blood flow
Hawthorn (*Crataegus laevigata*, *C. oxyacantha*, *C. monogyna*, *C. pentagyna*)	Edema
Horsetail (*Equisetum arvense* L.)	Dropsy
Lavender (*Lavandula angustifolia* Miller)	Circulation problems

Continued

Therapy	Specific Therapeutic Use(s)
Lavender (*Lavandula angustifolia* Miller)	Varicose veins
Melatonin	Edema
Milk thistle (*Silybum marianum*), silymarin	Edema
Niacin (vitamin B_3, nicotinic acid), niacinamide, inositol hexanicotinate	Edema
Oleander (*Nerium oleander*, *Thevetia peruviana*)	Swelling
Polypodium leucotomos extract, Anapsos	Water retention
Seaweed, kelp, bladderwrack (*Fucus vesiculosus*)	Edema
Slippery elm (*Ulmus rubra* Muhl. or *U. fulva* Michx.)	Varicose ulcers
Thyme (*Thymus vulgaris* L.), thymol	Edema
White horehound (*Marrubium vulgare* L.)	Water retention

LUNG DISEASE AND RELATED CONDITIONS

Levels of Scientific Evidence for Specific Therapies

GRADE: C (Unclear or Conflicting Scientific Evidence)

Therapy	Specific Therapeutic Use(s)

TRADITIONAL OR THEORETICAL USES THAT LACK SUFFICIENT EVIDENCE

Therapy	Specific Therapeutic Use(s)
American pennyroyal (*Hedeoma pulegioides* L.), European pennyroyal (*Mentha pulegium* L.)	Pneumonia
Blessed thistle (*Cnicus benedictus* L.)	Pneumonitis
Bromelain	Pneumonia
Burdock (*Arctium lappa*)	Pneumonia
Coenzyme Q10	Lung disease
Danshen (*Salvia miltiorrhiza*)	Lung fibrosis
Dong quai (*Angelica sinensis* [Oliv.] Diels), Chinese angelica	Lung disease

Dong quai (*Angelica sinensis* [Oliv.] Diels), Chinese angelica	Pleurisy
Garlic (*Allium sativum* L.)	Pneumonia
Goldenseal (*Hydrastis canadensis* L.), berberine	Pneumonia
Hops (*Humulus lupulus* L.)	Lung disease (from inhalation of silica dust or asbestos)
Melatonin	Sarcoidosis
Shark cartilage	Sarcoidosis
Slippery elm (*Ulmus rubra* Muhl. or *U. fulva* Michx.)	Lung diseases
Slippery elm (*Ulmus rubra* Muhl. or *U. fulva* Michx.)	Pleurisy
Tea tree oil (*Melaleuca alternifolia* [Maiden & Betche] Cheel)	Lung inflammation
White horehound (*Marrubium vulgare* L.)	Lung congestion
White horehound (*Marrubium vulgare* L.)	Pneumonia

MACULAR DEGENERATION AND RELATED CONDITIONS

Levels of Scientific Evidence for Specific Therapies

GRADE: C (Unclear or Conflicting Scientific Evidence)

Therapy	Specific Therapeutic Use(s)
Ginkgo (*Ginkgo biloba* L.)	Macular degeneration
Lycopene	Age-related macular degeneration prevention
Shark cartilage	Macular degeneration

TRADITIONAL OR THEORETICAL USES THAT LACK SUFFICIENT EVIDENCE

Therapy	Specific Therapeutic Use(s)
Coenzyme Q10	Macular degeneration
Omega-3 fatty acids, fish oil, alpha-linolenic acid	Age-related macular degeneration

MEMORY ENHANCEMENT AND RELATED CONDITIONS

Levels of Scientific Evidence for Specific Therapies

GRADE: B (Good Scientific Evidence)

Therapy	Specific Therapeutic Use(s)
Ginkgo (*Ginkgo biloba* L.)	Cerebral insufficiency
Ginseng (American ginseng, Asian ginseng, Chinese ginseng, Korean red ginseng, *Panax ginseng*: *Panax* spp. including *P. ginseng* C.C. Meyer and *P. quinquefolium* L., excluding *Eleutherococcus senticosus*)	Mental performance

GRADE: C (Unclear or Conflicting Scientific Evidence)

Therapy	Specific Therapeutic Use(s)
Black tea (*Camellia sinensis*)	Memory enhancement
Black tea (*Camellia sinensis*)	Mental performance/alertness
Boron	Improving cognitive function
Ginkgo (*Ginkgo biloba* L.)	Age-associated memory impairment (AAMI)
Ginkgo (*Ginkgo biloba* L.)	Memory enhancement (in healthy people)
Green tea (*Camellia sinensis*)	Memory enhancement
Green tea (*Camellia sinensis*)	Mental performance/alertness
Polypodium leucotomos extract, Anapsos	Dementia

GRADE: D (Fair Negative Scientific Evidence)

Therapy	Specific Therapeutic Use(s)
Dehydroepiandrosterone (DHEA)	Brain function and well-being in the elderly

TRADITIONAL OR THEORETICAL USES THAT LACK SUFFICIENT EVIDENCE

Therapy	Specific Therapeutic Use(s)
Arginine (L-arginine)	Dementia
Astragalus (*Astragalus membranaceus*)	Dementia
Astragalus (*Astragalus membranaceus*)	Memory

Blessed thistle (*Cnicus benedictus* L.)	Memory improvement
Danshen (*Salvia miltiorrhiza*)	Anoxic brain injury
Dehydroepiandrosterone (DHEA)	Dementia
Eyebright (*Euphrasia officinalis*)	Memory loss
Garlic (*Allium sativum* L.)	Age-related memory problems
Ginseng (American ginseng, Asian ginseng, Chinese ginseng, Korean red ginseng, *Panax ginseng*: *Panax* spp. including *P. ginseng* C.C. Meyer and *P. quinquefolium* L., excluding *Eleutherococcus senticosus*)	Dementia
Ginseng (American ginseng, Asian ginseng, Chinese ginseng, Korean red ginseng, *Panax ginseng*: *Panax* spp. including *P. ginseng* C.C. Meyer and *P. quinquefolium* L., excluding *Eleutherococcus senticosus*)	Improved memory and thinking after menopause
Ginseng (American ginseng, Asian ginseng, Chinese ginseng, Korean red ginseng, *Panax ginseng*: *Panax* spp. including *P. ginseng* C.C. Meyer and *P. quinquefolium* L., excluding *Eleutherococcus senticosus*)	Senile dementia
Gotu kola (*Centella asiatica* L.), total triterpenic fraction of *Centella asiatica* (TTFCA)	Memory enhancement
Green tea (*Camellia sinensis*)	Cognitive performance enhancement
Kava (*Piper methysticum* G. Forst)	Brain damage
Lycopene	Cognitive function
Melatonin	Cognitive enhancement
Melatonin	Memory enhancement
Niacin (vitamin B_3, nicotinic acid), niacinamide, inositol hexanicotinate	Memory loss
Omega-3 fatty acids, fish oil, alpha-linolenic acid	Memory enhancement
Soy (*Glycine max* L. Merr.)	Cognitive function
Soy (*Glycine max* L. Merr.)	Memory enhancement
Spirulina	Memory improvement
Valerian (*Valeriana officinalis* L.)	Memory
Yohimbe bark extract (*Pausinystalia yohimbe* Pierre ex Beille)	Cognition

Continued

MENOPAUSAL SYMPTOMS AND RELATED CONDITIONS

Levels of Scientific Evidence for Specific Therapies

GRADE: B (Good Scientific Evidence)	
Therapy	Specific Therapeutic Use(s)
Black cohosh (*Cimicifuga racemosa* L. Nutt.)	Menopausal symptoms
Soy (*Glycine max* L. Merr.)	Menopausal hot flashes

GRADE: C (Unclear or Conflicting Scientific Evidence)	
Therapy	Specific Therapeutic Use(s)
American pennyroyal (*Hedeoma pulegioides* L.), European pennyroyal (*Mentha pulegium* L.)	Emmenagogue (menstrual flow stimulant)
Belladonna (*Atropa belladonna* L. or its variety *A. acuminata* Royle ex Lindl)	Premenstrual syndrome
Bilberry (*Vaccinium myrtillus*)	Painful menstruation (dysmenorrhea)
Dehydroepiandrosterone (DHEA)	Menopausal disorders
Dehydroepiandrosterone (DHEA)	Ovulation disorders
Dong quai (*Angelica sinensis* [Oliv.] Diels), Chinese angelica	Amenorrhea (lack of menstrual period)
Dong quai (*Angelica sinensis* [Oliv.] Diels), Chinese angelica	Dysmenorrhea (painful menstruation)
Flaxseed and flaxseed oil (*Linum usitatissimum*)	Menstrual breast pain (flaxseed, not flaxseed oil)
Ginkgo (*Ginkgo biloba* L.)	Premenstrual syndrome
Ginseng (American ginseng, Asian ginseng, Chinese ginseng, Korean red ginseng, *Panax ginseng*: *Panax* spp. including *P. ginseng* C.C. Meyer and *P. quinquefolium* L., excluding *Eleutherococcus senticosus*)	Menopausal symptoms
Green tea (*Camellia sinensis*)	Menopausal symptoms
Omega-3 fatty acids, fish oil, alpha-linolenic acid	Dysmenorrhea (painful menstruation)
Red clover (*Trifolium pratense*)	Hormone replacement therapy (HRT)
Red clover (*Trifolium pratense*)	Menopausal symptoms

St. John's wort (*Hypericum perforatum* L.)	Perimenopausal symptoms
St. John's wort (*Hypericum perforatum* L.)	Premenstrual syndrome
Wild yam (*Dioscorea villosa*)	Menopausal symptoms

GRADE: D (Fair Negative Scientific Evidence)

Therapy	Specific Therapeutic Use(s)
Belladonna (*Atropa belladonna* L. or its variety *A. acuminata* Royle ex Lindl)	Menopausal symptoms
Boron	Menopausal symptoms
Evening primrose oil (*Oenothera biennis* L.)	Menopause (flushing/bone metabolism)
Evening primrose oil (*Oenothera biennis* L.)	Premenstrual syndrome
Wild yam (*Dioscorea villosa*)	Hormonal properties (to mimic estrogen, progesterone, or dehydroepiandrosterone [DHEA])

TRADITIONAL OR THEORETICAL USES THAT LACK SUFFICIENT EVIDENCE

Therapy	Specific Therapeutic Use(s)
Alfalfa (*Medicago sativa* L.)	Estrogen replacement
Alfalfa (*Medicago sativa* L.)	Menopausal symptoms
American pennyroyal (*Hedeoma pulegioides* L.), European pennyroyal (*Mentha pulegium* L.)	Cramps
American pennyroyal (*Hedeoma pulegioides* L.), European pennyroyal (*Mentha pulegium* L.)	Premenstrual syndrome
Astragalus (*Astragalus membranaceus*)	Menstrual disorders
Astragalus (*Astragalus membranaceus*)	Pelvic congestion syndrome
Belladonna (*Atropa belladonna* L. or its variety *A. acuminata* Royle ex Lindl)	Abnormal menstrual periods
Betel nut (*Areca catechu* L.)	Excessive menstrual flow
Black cohosh (*Cimicifuga racemosa* L. Nutt.)	Endometriosis
Black cohosh (*Cimicifuga racemosa* L. Nutt.)	Menstrual period problems
Black cohosh (*Cimicifuga racemosa* L. Nutt.)	Ovarian cysts
Black cohosh (*Cimicifuga racemosa* L. Nutt.)	Premenstrual syndrome

Continued

Bladderwrack (*Fucus vesiculosus*)	Menstruation irregularities
Blessed thistle (*Cnicus benedictus* L.)	Menstrual disorders
Blessed thistle (*Cnicus benedictus* L.)	Menstrual flow stimulant
Blessed thistle (*Cnicus benedictus* L.)	Painful menstruation
Boswellia (*Boswellia serrata* Roxb.)	Amenorrhea
Boswellia (*Boswellia serrata* Roxb.)	Emmenagogue (inducer of menstruation)
Bromelain	Menstrual pain
Calendula (*Calendula officinalis* L.), marigold	Cramps
Calendula (*Calendula officinalis* L.), marigold	Menstrual period abnormalities
Chamomile (*Matricaria recutita, Chamaemelum nobile*)	Dysmenorrhea
Chamomile (*Matricaria recutita, Chamaemelum nobile*)	Menstrual disorders
Chaparral (*Larrea tridentata* DC. Coville, *L. divaricata* Cav.), nordihydroguaiaretic acid (NDGA)	Menstrual cramps
Clay	Menstruation difficulties
Dandelion (*Taraxacum officinale*)	Menopause
Dandelion (*Taraxacum officinale*)	Premenstrual syndrome
Danshen (*Salvia miltiorrhiza*)	Menstrual problems
Devil's claw (*Harpagophytum procumbens* DC.)	Menopausal symptoms
Devil's claw (*Harpagophytum procumbens* DC.)	Menstrual cramps
Dehydroepiandrosterone (DHEA)	Amenorrhea associated with anorexia
Dehydroepiandrosterone (DHEA)	Andropause/andrenopause
Dehydroepiandrosterone (DHEA)	Premenstrual syndrome
Dong quai (*Angelica sinensis* [Oliv.] Diels), Chinese angelica	Cramps
Dong quai (*Angelica sinensis* [Oliv.] Diels), Chinese angelica	Hormonal abnormalities
Dong quai (*Angelica sinensis* [Oliv.] Diels), Chinese angelica	Menorrhagia (heavy menstrual bleeding)
Dong quai (*Angelica sinensis* [Oliv.] Diels), Chinese angelica	Menstrual cramping

Dong quai (*Angelica sinensis* [Oliv.] Diels), Chinese angelica	Ovulation abnormalities
Dong quai (*Angelica sinensis* [Oliv.] Diels), Chinese angelica	Pelvic congestion syndrome
Dong quai (*Angelica sinensis* [Oliv.] Diels), Chinese angelica	Premenstrual syndrome
Fenugreek (*Trigonella foenum-graecum* L.)	Menopausal symptoms
Fenugreek (*Trigonella foenum-graecum* L.)	Postmenopausal vaginal dryness
Feverfew (*Tanacetum parthenium* L. Schultz-Bip.)	Menstrual cramps
Feverfew (*Tanacetum parthenium* L. Schultz-Bip.)	Promotion of menstruation
Flaxseed and flaxseed oil (*Linum usitatissimum*)	Menstrual disorders
Flaxseed and flaxseed oil (*Linum usitatissimum*)	Ovarian disorders
Garlic (*Allium sativum* L.)	Emmenagogue
Ginger (*Zingiber officinale* Roscoe)	Dysmenorrhea
Ginger (*Zingiber officinale* Roscoe)	Promotion of menstruation
Ginkgo (*Ginkgo biloba* L.)	Menstrual pain
Ginseng (American ginseng, Asian ginseng, Chinese ginseng, Korean red ginseng, *Panax ginseng*: *Panax* spp. including *P. ginseng* C.C. Meyer and *P. quinquefolium* L., excluding *Eleutherococcus senticosus*)	Menopausal symptoms
Goldenseal (*Hydrastis canadensis* L.), berberine	Menstruation problems
Goldenseal (*Hydrastis canadensis* L.), berberine	Premenstrual syndrome
Gotu kola (*Centella asiatica* L.), total triterpenic fraction of *Centella asiatica* (TTFCA)	Amenorrhea
Gotu kola (*Centella asiatica* L.), total triterpenic fraction of *Centella asiatica* (TTFCA)	Hot flashes
Gotu kola (*Centella asiatica* L.), total triterpenic fraction of *Centella asiatica* (TTFCA)	Menstrual disorders
Guggul (*Commifora mukul*)	Menstrual disorders
Hawthorn (*Crataegus laevigata*, *C. oxyacantha*, *C. monogyna*, *C. pentagyna*)	Amenorrhea
Hops (*Humulus lupulus* L.)	Estrogenic effects
Horse chestnut (*Aesculus hippocastanum* L.)	Menstrual pain

Continued

Horsetail (*Equisetum arvense* L.)	Menstrual pain
Kava (*Piper methysticum* G. Forst)	Menopause
Kava (*Piper methysticum* G. Forst)	Menstrual disorders
Lavender (*Lavandula angustifolia* Miller)	Menopause
Lavender (*Lavandula angustifolia* Miller)	Menstrual period problems
Licorice (*Glycyrrhiza glabra* L.), deglycyrrhizinated licorice (DGL)	Hormone regulation
Licorice (*Glycyrrhiza glabra* L.), deglycyrrhizinated licorice (DGL)	Menopausal symptoms
Melatonin	Melatonin deficiency
Milk thistle (*Silybum marianum*), silymarin	Menstrual disorders
Niacin (vitamin B_3, nicotinic acid), niacinamide, inositol hexanicotinate	Painful menstruation
Niacin (vitamin B_3, nicotinic acid), niacinamide, inositol hexanicotinate	Premenstrual headache prevention
Niacin (vitamin B_3, nicotinic acid), niacinamide, inositol hexanicotinate	Premenstrual syndrome
Oleander (*Nerium oleander*, *Thevetia peruviana*)	Abnormal menstruation
Oleander (*Nerium oleander*, *Thevetia peruviana*)	Menstrual stimulant
Omega-3 fatty acids, fish oil, alpha-linolenic acid	Menopausal symptoms
Omega-3 fatty acids, fish oil, alpha-linolenic acid	Menstrual cramps
Omega-3 fatty acids, fish oil, alpha-linolenic acid	Premenstrual syndrome
Passionflower (*Passiflora incarnata* L.)	Menopausal symptoms (hot flashes)
Peppermint (*Mentha* x *piperita* L.)	Cramps
Peppermint (*Mentha* x *piperita* L.)	Dysmenorrhea (menstrual pain)
Psyllium (*Plantago ovata*, *P. ispaghula*)	Excessive menstrual bleeding
Red clover (*Trifolium pratense*)	Hot flashes
Red clover (*Trifolium pratense*)	Premenstrual syndrome
Saw palmetto (*Serenoa repens* [Bartram] Small)	Antiandrogen
Saw palmetto (*Serenoa repens* [Bartram] Small)	Antiestrogen

Saw palmetto (*Serenoa repens* [Bartram] Small)	Dysmenorrhea
Saw palmetto (*Serenoa repens* [Bartram] Small)	Estrogenic agent
Saw palmetto (*Serenoa repens* [Bartram] Small)	Ovarian cysts
Saw palmetto (*Serenoa repens* [Bartram] Small)	Pelvic congestive syndrome
Seaweed, kelp, bladderwrack (*Fucus vesiculosus*)	Menstrual irregularities (menorrhagia)
Slippery elm (*Ulmus rubra* Muhl. or *U. fulva* Michx.)	Gynecologic disorders
Spirulina	Premenstrual syndrome
St. John's wort (*Hypericum perforatum* L.)	Menstrual pain
Sweet almond (*Prunus amygdalus dulcis*)	Plant-derived estrogen
Thyme (*Thymus vulgaris* L.), thymol	Dysmenorrhea
Turmeric (*Curcuma longa* L.), curcumin	Menstrual pain
Turmeric (*Curcuma longa* L.), curcumin	Menstrual period problems/ lack of menstrual period
Valerian (*Valeriana officinalis* L.)	Amenorrhea
Valerian (*Valeriana officinalis* L.)	Dysmenorrhea
Valerian (*Valeriana officinalis* L.)	Emmenagogue
Valerian (*Valeriana officinalis* L.)	Menopause
Valerian (*Valeriana officinalis* L.)	Premenstrual syndrome
White horehound (*Marrubium vulgare* L.)	Dysmenorrhea
White horehound (*Marrubium vulgare* L.)	Menstrual pain
Wild yam (*Dioscorea villosa*)	Cramps
Wild yam (*Dioscorea villosa*)	Menopause
Wild yam (*Dioscorea villosa*)	Menstrual pain or irregularities
Wild yam (*Dioscorea villosa*)	Pelvic cramps
Wild yam (*Dioscorea villosa*)	Postmenopausal vaginal dryness
Wild yam (*Dioscorea villosa*)	Premenstrual syndrome

METABOLIC DISORDERS AND RELATED CONDITIONS

Levels of Scientific Evidence for Specific Therapies

GRADE: A (Strong Scientific Evidence)

Therapy	Specific Therapeutic Use(s)
Arginine (L-arginine)	Inborn errors of urea synthesis

GRADE: C (Unclear or Conflicting Scientific Evidence)

Therapy	Specific Therapeutic Use(s)
Coenzyme Q10	Mitochondrial diseases, Kearns-Sayre syndrome

TRADITIONAL OR THEORETICAL USES THAT LACK SUFFICIENT EVIDENCE

Therapy	Specific Therapeutic Use(s)
Astragalus (*Astragalus membranaceus*)	Metabolic disorders
Calendula (*Calendula officinalis* L.), marigold	Metabolic disorders
Coenzyme Q10	Mitochondrial encephalopathy–lactic acidosis–stroke-like symptoms (MELAS) syndrome
Ephedra (*Ephedra sinica*)/ma huang	Metabolic enhancement

MOUTH SORES AND RELATED CONDITIONS

Levels of Scientific Evidence for Specific Therapies

GRADE: C (UNCLEAR OR CONFLICTING SCIENTIFIC EVIDENCE)

Therapy	Specific Therapeutic Use(s)
Aloe (*Aloe vera*)	Canker sores (aphthous stomatitis)
Chamomile (*Matricaria recutita*, *Chamaemelum nobile*)	Mucositis from cancer treatment (mouth ulcers/ irritation)
Licorice (*Glycyrrhiza glabra* L.), deglycyrrhizinated licorice (DGL)	Aphthous ulcers/canker sores
Spirulina	Oral leukoplakia (precancerous mouth lesions)

TRADITIONAL OR THEORETICAL USES THAT LACK SUFFICIENT EVIDENCE	
Therapy	Specific Therapeutic Use(s)
American pennyroyal (*Hedeoma pulegioides* L.), European pennyroyal (*Mentha pulegium* L.)	Mouth sores
Bilberry (*Vaccinium myrtillus*)	Oral ulcers
Burdock (*Arctium lappa*)	Canker sores
Clove (*Eugenia aromatica*)	Mouth and throat inflammation
Dandelion (*Taraxacum officinale*)	Aphthous ulcers
Fenugreek (*Trigonella foenum-graecum* L.)	Aphthous ulcers
Fenugreek (*Trigonella foenum-graecum* L.)	Chapped lips
Goldenseal (*Hydrastis canadensis* L.), berberine	Canker sores
Green tea (*Camellia sinensis*)	Oral leukoplakia
Lactobacillus acidophilus	Canker sores
Peppermint (*Mentha* x *piperita* L.)	Inflammation of oral mucosa
Red clover (*Trifolium pratense*)	Canker sores
Sorrel (*Rumex acetosa* L., *R. acetosella* L.), Sinupret	Oral ulcers
Sweet almond (*Prunus amygdalus dulcis*)	Chapped lips
Tea tree oil (*Melaleuca alternifolia* [Maiden & Betche] Cheel)	Mouth sores
Thyme (*Thymus vulgaris* L.), thymol	Stomatitis

MULTIPLE SCLEROSIS (MS) AND RELATED CONDITIONS

Levels of Scientific Evidence for Specific Therapies

GRADE: C (UNCLEAR OR CONFLICTING SCIENTIFIC EVIDENCE)	
Therapy	Specific Therapeutic Use(s)
Evening primrose oil (*Oenothera biennis* L.)	Multiple sclerosis
Ginkgo (*Ginkgo biloba* L.)	Multiple sclerosis
Yohimbe bark extract (*Pausinystalia yohimbe* Pierre ex Beille)	Autonomic failure

Continued

TRADITIONAL OR THEORETICAL USES THAT LACK SUFFICIENT EVIDENCE	
Therapy	Specific Therapeutic Use(s)
Astragalus (*Astragalus membranaceus*)	Myasthenia gravis
Boswellia (*Boswellia serrata* Roxb.)	Multiple sclerosis
Dehydroepiandrosterone (DHEA)	Multiple sclerosis
Ephedra (*Ephedra sinica*)/ma huang	Myasthenia gravis
Evening primrose oil (*Oenothera biennis* L.)	Multiple sclerosis
Melatonin	Multiple sclerosis
Niacin (vitamin B_3, nicotinic acid), niacinamide, inositol hexanicotinate	Multiple sclerosis
Omega-3 fatty acids, fish oil, alpha-linolenic acid	Multiple sclerosis

MUSCULAR DYSTROPHY AND RELATED CONDITIONS

Levels of Scientific Evidence for Specific Therapies

GRADE: C (Unclear or Conflicting Scientific Evidence)	
Therapy	Specific Therapeutic Use(s)
Coenzyme Q10	Muscular dystrophies

TRADITIONAL OR THEORETICAL USES THAT LACK SUFFICIENT EVIDENCE	
Therapy	Specific Therapeutic Use(s)
Calendula (*Calendula officinalis* L.), marigold	Muscle wasting
Coenzyme Q10	Muscular dystrophy
Omega-3 fatty acids, fish oil, alpha-linolenic acid	Myopathy

MUSCULOSKELETAL DISORDERS AND RELATED CONDITIONS

Levels of Scientific Evidence for Specific Therapies

TRADITIONAL OR THEORETICAL USES THAT LACK SUFFICIENT EVIDENCE	
Therapy	Specific Therapeutic Use(s)
Bitter almond (*Prunus amygdalus* Batch var. *amara* DC. Focke) and Laetrile	Muscle relaxant

Black cohosh (*Cimicifuga racemosa* L. Nutt.)	Muscle spasms
Boswellia (*Boswellia serrata* Roxb.)	Bursitis
Boswellia (*Boswellia serrata* Roxb.)	Tendonitis
Bromelain	Bursitis
Bromelain	Sports or other physical injuries
Bromelain	Tendonitis
Clove (*Eugenia aromatica*)	Muscle spasm
Devil's claw (*Harpagophytum procumbens* DC.)	Tendonitis
Dong quai (*Angelica sinensis* [Oliv.] Diels), Chinese angelica	Muscle relaxant
Eucalyptus oil (*Eucalyptus globulus* Labillardiere, *E. fructicetorum* F. Von Mueller, *E. smithii* R.T. Baker)	Muscle spasm
Eucalyptus oil (*Eucalyptus globulus* Labillardiere, *E. fructicetorum* F. Von Mueller, *E. smithii* R.T. Baker)	Strains/sprains (applied to the skin)
Garlic (*Allium sativum* L.)	Muscle spasms
Goldenseal (*Hydrastis canadensis* L.), berberine	Muscle spasm
Hops (*Humulus lupulus* L.)	Muscle and joint disorders
Hops (*Humulus lupulus* L.)	Muscle spasm
Lavender (*Lavandula angustifolia* Miller)	Muscle spasm
Lavender (*Lavandula angustifolia* Miller)	Sprains
Licorice (*Glycyrrhiza glabra* L.), deglycyrrhizinated licorice (DGL)	Muscle cramps
Marshmallow (*Althaea officinalis* L.)	Sprains
Niacin (vitamin B_3, nicotinic acid), niacinamide, inositol hexanicotinate	Bursitis
Omega-3 fatty acids, fish oil, alpha-linolenic acid	Tennis elbow
Peppermint (*Mentha* x *piperita* L.)	Tendonitis
Saw palmetto (*Serenoa repens* [Bartram] Small)	Muscle or intestinal spasms
Slippery elm (*Ulmus rubra* Muhl. or *U. fulva* Michx.)	Synovitis
St. John's wort (*Hypericum perforatum* L.)	Sprains

Continued

Thyme (*Thymus vulgaris* L.), thymol	Sprains
Valerian (*Valeriana officinalis* L.)	Muscle pain/spasm/tension

NAUSEA AND RELATED CONDITIONS

Levels of Scientific Evidence for Specific Therapies

GRADE: B (Good Scientific Evidence)

Therapy	Specific Therapeutic Use(s)
Ginger (*Zingiber officinale* Roscoe)	Nausea (due to chemotherapy)
Ginger (*Zingiber officinale* Roscoe)	Nausea and vomiting of pregnancy (hyperemesis gravidarum)

GRADE: C (Unclear or Conflicting Scientific Evidence)

Therapy	Specific Therapeutic Use(s)
Ginger (*Zingiber officinale* Roscoe)	Nausea and vomiting (after surgery)
Peppermint (*Mentha* x *piperita* L.)	Nausea

TRADITIONAL OR THEORETICAL USES THAT LACK SUFFICIENT EVIDENCE

Therapy	Specific Therapeutic Use(s)
Belladonna (*Atropa belladonna* L. or its variety *A. acuminata* Royle ex Lindl)	Motion sickness
Black tea (*Camellia sinensis*)	Vomiting
Calendula (*Calendula officinalis* L.), marigold	Nausea
Chamomile (*Matricaria recutita*, *Chamaemelum nobile*)	Motion sickness
Chamomile (*Matricaria recutita*, *Chamaemelum nobile*)	Nausea
Chamomile (*Matricaria recutita*, *Chamaemelum nobile*)	Sea sickness
Chaparral (*Larrea tridentata* DC. Coville, *L. divaricata* Cav.), nordihydroguaiaretic acid (NDGA)	Vomiting
Clay	Vomiting
Clay	Vomiting/nausea during pregnancy

Clove (*Eugenia aromatica*)	Nausea or vomiting
Cranberry (*Vaccinium macrocarpon*)	Vomiting
Elder (*Sambucus nigra* L.)	Vomiting
Globe artichoke (*Cynara scolymus* L.)	Emesis
Lavender (*Lavandula angustifolia* Miller)	Motion sickness
Lavender (*Lavandula angustifolia* Miller)	Nausea
Lavender (*Lavandula angustifolia* Miller)	Vomiting
Marshmallow (*Althaea officinalis* L.)	Vomiting
Niacin (vitamin B_3, nicotinic acid), niacinamide, inositol hexanicotinate	Motion sickness
Oleander (*Nerium oleander*, *Thevetia peruviana*)	Vomiting
Valerian (*Valeriana officinalis* L.)	Nausea
White horehound (*Marrubium vulgare* L.)	Emetic
Wild yam (*Dioscorea villosa*)	Emetic

NEPHROLITHIASIS (KIDNEY STONES) AND RELATED CONDITIONS

Levels of Scientific Evidence for Specific Therapies

GRADE: C (Unclear or Conflicting Scientific Evidence)

Therapy	Specific Therapeutic Use(s)
Cranberry (*Vaccinium macrocarpon*)	Kidney stones

TRADITIONAL OR THEORETICAL USES THAT LACK SUFFICIENT EVIDENCE

Therapy	Specific Therapeutic Use(s)
Aloe (*Aloe vera*)	Urolithiasis (bladder stones)
Belladonna (*Atropa belladonna* L. or its variety *A. acuminata* Royle ex Lindl)	Kidney stones
Black tea (*Camellia sinensis*)	Kidney stone prevention
Burdock (*Arctium lappa*)	Kidney stones
Cranberry (*Vaccinium macrocarpon*)	Nephrolithiasis prevention

Continued

Evening primrose oil (*Oenothera biennis* L.)	Kidney stones
Globe artichoke (*Cynara scolymus* L.)	Nephrolithiasis
Globe artichoke (*Cynara scolymus* L.)	Urolithiasis
Glucosamine	Kidney stones
Green tea (*Camellia sinensis*)	Kidney stone prevention
Horsetail (*Equisetum arvense* L.)	Kidney stones
Marshmallow (*Althaea officinalis* L.)	Kidney stones
Omega-3 fatty acids, fish oil, alpha-linolenic acid	Kidney stones
Omega-3 fatty acids, fish oil, alpha-linolenic acid	Urolithiasis (bladder stones)
Shark cartilage	Nephrolithiasis
Sorrel (*Rumex acetosa* L., *R. acetosella* L.), Sinupret	Kidney stones
Valerian (*Valeriana officinalis* L.)	Urolithiasis

NEUROLOGIC DISORDERS AND RELATED CONDITIONS

Levels of Scientific Evidence for Specific Therapies

GRADE: C (Unclear or Conflicting Scientific Evidence)

Therapy	Specific Therapeutic Use(s)
Arginine (L-arginine)	Adrenoleukodystrophy
Belladonna (*Atropa belladonna* L. or its variety *A. acuminata* Royle ex Lindl)	Nervous system disorders
Dehydroepiandrosterone (DHEA)	Myotonic dystrophy
Dong quai (*Angelica sinensis* [Oliv.] Diels), Chinese angelica	Nerve pain
Melatonin	Periodic limb movement disorder
Yohimbe bark extract (*Pausinystalia yohimbe* Pierre ex Beille)	Nervous system dysfunction (autonomic failure)

TRADITIONAL OR THEORETICAL USES THAT LACK SUFFICIENT EVIDENCE

Therapy	Specific Therapeutic Use(s)
Belladonna (*Atropa belladonna* L. or its variety *A. acuminata* Royle ex Lindl)	Hyperkinesis (excessive motor function)

Belladonna (*Atropa belladonna* L. or its variety *A. acuminata* Royle ex Lindl)	Neuralgia
Black cohosh (*Cimicifuga racemosa* L. Nutt.)	Chorea
Black cohosh (*Cimicifuga racemosa* L. Nutt.)	Neurovegetative complaints
Black tea (*Camellia sinensis*)	Trigeminal neuralgia
Calendula (*Calendula officinalis* L.), marigold	Nervous system disorders
Chamomile (*Matricaria recutita*, *Chamaemelum nobile*)	Neuralgia (nerve pain)
Chaparral (*Larrea tridentata* DC. Coville, *L. divaricata* Cav.), nordihydroguaiaretic acid (NDGA)	Central nervous system disorders
Coenzyme Q10	Amyotrophic lateral sclerosis (ALS)
Coenzyme Q10	Cerebellar ataxia
Devil's claw (*Harpagophytum procumbens* DC.)	Nerve pain
Dehydroepiandrosterone (DHEA)	Movement disorders
Dong quai (*Angelica sinensis* [Oliv.] Diels), Chinese angelica	Age-related nerve damage
Dong quai (*Angelica sinensis* [Oliv.] Diels), Chinese angelica	Central nervous system disorders
Elder (*Sambucus nigra* L.)	Nerve pain
Eucalyptus oil (*Eucalyptus globulus* Labillardiere, *E. fructicetorum* F. Von Mueller, *E. smithii* R.T. Baker)	Nerve pain
Ginseng (American ginseng, Asian ginseng, Chinese ginseng, Korean red ginseng, *Panax ginseng*: *Panax* spp. including *P. ginseng* C.C. Meyer and *P. quinquefolium* L., excluding *Eleutherococcus senticosus*)	Neuralgia (pain due to nerve damage or inflammation)
Green tea (*Camellia sinensis*)	Neuroprotection
Guggul (*Commifora mukul*)	Neuralgia
Horse chestnut (*Aesculus hippocastanum* L.)	Nerve pain
Horsetail (*Equisetum arvense* L.)	Neurodermatitis
Licorice (*Glycyrrhiza glabra* L.), deglycyrrhizinated licorice (DGL)	Dropped head syndrome
Melatonin	Neurodegenerative disorders
Melatonin	Tuberous sclerosis

Continued

Niacin (vitamin B_3, nicotinic acid), niacinamide, inositol hexanicotinate	Central nervous system disorders
Oleander (*Nerium oleander*, *Thevetia peruviana*)	Neurologic disorders
Passionflower (*Passiflora incarnata* L.)	Nerve pain
Peppermint (*Mentha* x *piperita* L.)	Neuralgia (nerve pain)
St. John's wort (*Hypericum perforatum* L.)	Nerve pain
Thyme (*Thymus vulgaris* L.), thymol	Neuralgia
Valerian (*Valeriana officinalis* L.)	Nervous excitability
Valerian (*Valeriana officinalis* L.)	Neuralgia
Wild yam (*Dioscorea villosa*)	Nerve pain

NEUROPATHY AND RELATED CONDITIONS

Levels of Scientific Evidence for Specific Therapies

GRADE: C (Unclear or Conflicting Scientific Evidence)

Therapy	Specific Therapeutic Use(s)
Evening primrose oil (*Oenothera biennis* L.)	Diabetic neuropathy (nerve damage)

TRADITIONAL OR THEORETICAL USES THAT LACK SUFFICIENT EVIDENCE

Therapy	Specific Therapeutic Use(s)
Astragalus (*Astragalus membranaceus*)	Diabetic neuropathy
Belladonna (*Atropa belladonna* L. or its variety *A. acuminata* Royle ex Lindl)	Pain from nerve disorders
Danshen (*Salvia miltiorrhiza*)	Diabetic nerve pain
Ginkgo (*Ginkgo biloba* L.)	Diabetic nerve damage (neuropathy)
Milk thistle (*Silybum marianum*), silymarin	Diabetic nerve pain
Omega-3 fatty acids, fish oil, alpha-linolenic acid	Diabetic neuropathy
Omega-3 fatty acids, fish oil, alpha-linolenic acid	Neuropathy
Soy (*Glycine max* L. Merr.)	Diabetic neuropathy

Yohimbe bark extract (*Pausinystalia yohimbe* Pierre ex Beille)	Diabetic neuropathy

NOSEBLEED AND RELATED CONDITIONS

Levels of Scientific Evidence for Specific Therapies

TRADITIONAL OR THEORETICAL USES THAT LACK SUFFICIENT EVIDENCE

Therapy	Specific Therapeutic Use(s)
American pennyroyal (*Hedeoma pulegioides* L.), European pennyroyal (*Mentha pulegium* L.)	Nosebleed
Calendula (*Calendula officinalis* L.), marigold	Nosebleed
Horsetail (*Equisetum arvense* L.)	Nosebleed
Soy (*Glycine max* L. Merr.)	Nosebleed (chronic)

NUTRITIONAL DEFICIENCIES AND RELATED CONDITIONS

Levels of Scientific Evidence for Specific Therapies

GRADE: A (Strong Scientific Evidence)

Therapy	Specific Therapeutic Use(s)
Niacin (vitamin B_3, nicotinic acid), niacinamide, inositol hexanicotinate	Pellagra (niacin)
Soy (*Glycine max* L. Merr.)	Dietary source of protein

GRADE: C (Unclear or Conflicting Scientific Evidence)

Therapy	Specific Therapeutic Use(s)
Bromelain	Nutrition supplementation
Cranberry (*Vaccinium macrocarpon*)	Vitamin B_{12} absorption in people using antacids
Omega-3 fatty acids, fish oil, alpha-linolenic acid	Infant eye/brain development

GRADE: D (Fair Negative Scientific Evidence)

Therapy	Specific Therapeutic Use(s)
Omega-3 fatty acids, fish oil, alpha-linolenic acid	Appetite/weight loss in cancer patients

Continued

TRADITIONAL OR THEORETICAL USES THAT LACK SUFFICIENT EVIDENCE	
Therapy	Specific Therapeutic Use(s)
Alfalfa (*Medicago sativa* L.)	Appetite stimulant
Alfalfa (*Medicago sativa* L.)	Nutritional support
Arginine (L-arginine)	Supplementation to a low-protein diet
Astragalus (*Astragalus membranaceus*)	Anorexia
Betel nut (*Areca catechu* L.)	Appetite stimulant
Black cohosh (*Cimicifuga racemosa* L. Nutt.)	Appetite stimulant
Bladderwrack (*Fucus vesiculosus*)	Malnutrition
Blessed thistle (*Cnicus benedictus* L.)	Anorexia
Blessed thistle (*Cnicus benedictus* L.)	Appetite stimulant
Boron	Boron deficiency
Boron	Vitamin D deficiency
Burdock (*Arctium lappa*)	Anorexia nervosa
Calendula (*Calendula officinalis* L.), marigold	Appetite stimulant
Chamomile (*Matricaria recutita*, *Chamaemelum nobile*)	Anorexia
Clay	Nutrition
Coenzyme Q10	Nutrition
Cranberry (*Vaccinium macrocarpon*)	Anorexia
Dandelion (*Taraxacum officinale*)	Appetite stimulant
Dandelion (*Taraxacum officinale*)	Nutrition
Devil's claw (*Harpagophytum procumbens* DC.)	Appetite stimulant
Devil's claw (*Harpagophytum procumbens* DC.)	Loss of appetite
Dehydroepiandrosterone (DHEA)	Malnutrition
Dong quai (*Angelica sinensis* [Oliv.] Diels), Chinese angelica	Anorexia nervosa
Dong quai (*Angelica sinensis* [Oliv.] Diels), Chinese angelica	Vitamin E deficiency
Essiac	Appetite stimulant

Essiac	Nutritional supplement
Eyebright (*Euphrasia officinalis*)	Appetite stimulant
Fenugreek (*Trigonella foenum-graecum* L.)	Appetite stimulant
Fenugreek (*Trigonella foenum-graecum* L.)	Beriberi
Fenugreek (*Trigonella foenum-graecum* L.)	Rickets
Fenugreek (*Trigonella foenum-graecum* L.)	Vitamin deficiencies
Ginger (*Zingiber officinale* Roscoe)	Diminished appetite (anorexia)
Ginseng (American ginseng, Asian ginseng, Chinese ginseng, Korean red ginseng, *Panax ginseng*: *Panax* spp. including *P. ginseng* C.C. Meyer and *P. quinquefolium* L., excluding *Eleutherococcus senticosus*)	Appetite stimulant
Goldenseal (*Hydrastis canadensis* L.), berberine	Appetite stimulant
Hawthorn (*Crataegus laevigata*, *C. oxyacantha*, *C. monogyna*, *C. pentagyna*)	Appetite stimulant
Hops (*Humulus lupulus* L.)	Appetite stimulant
Kava (*Piper methysticum* G. Forst)	Anorexia
Lavender (*Lavandula angustifolia* Miller)	Appetite stimulant
Melatonin	Cachexia
Oleander (*Nerium oleander*, *Thevetia peruviana*)	Anorexia
Peppermint (*Mentha* x *piperita* L.)	Anorexia
Seaweed, kelp, bladderwrack (*Fucus vesiculosus*)	Malnutrition
Slippery elm (*Ulmus rubra* Muhl. or *U. fulva* Michx.)	Nutrition
Sorrel (*Rumex acetosa* L., *R. acetosella* L.), Sinupret	Appetite stimulation
Soy (*Glycine max* L. Merr.)	Anorexia
Spirulina	Iron deficiency
Spirulina	Vitamin and nutrient deficiency
Thyme (*Thymus vulgaris* L.), thymol	Appetite stimulant
Turmeric (*Curcuma longa* L.), curcumin	Appetite stimulant
Valerian (*Valeriana officinalis* L.)	Anorexia
White horehound (*Marrubium vulgare* L.)	Anorexia

Continued

OBSESSIVE-COMPULSIVE DISORDER AND RELATED CONDITIONS

Levels of Scientific Evidence for Specific Therapies

GRADE: C (Unclear or Conflicting Scientific Evidence)

Therapy	Specific Therapeutic Use(s)
St. John's wort (*Hypericum perforatum* L.)	Obsessive-compulsive disorder (OCD)

OSTEOARTHRITIS AND RELATED CONDITIONS

Levels of Scientific Evidence for Specific Therapies

GRADE: A (Strong Scientific Evidence)

Therapy	Specific Therapeutic Use(s)
Glucosamine	Knee osteoarthritis (mild to moderate)

GRADE: B (Good Scientific Evidence)

Therapy	Specific Therapeutic Use(s)
Devil's claw (*Harpagophytum procumbens* DC.)	Osteoarthritis
Glucosamine	Osteoarthritis (general)

GRADE: C (Unclear or Conflicting Scientific Evidence)

Therapy	Specific Therapeutic Use(s)
Black cohosh (*Cimicifuga racemosa* L. Nutt.)	Joint pain
Boron	Osteoarthritis
Boswellia (*Boswellia serrata* Roxb.)	Osteoarthritis
Chondroitin	Osteoarthritis
Glucosamine	Temporomandibular joint (TMJ) disorders
Guggul (*Commifora mukul*)	Osteoarthritis

Niacin (vitamin B_3, nicotinic acid), niacinamide, inositol hexanicotinate	Osteoarthritis (niacinamide)
Turmeric (*Curcuma longa* L.), curcumin	Osteoarthritis

TRADITIONAL OR THEORETICAL USES THAT LACK SUFFICIENT EVIDENCE

Therapy	Specific Therapeutic Use(s)
American pennyroyal (*Hedeoma pulegioides* L.), European pennyroyal (*Mentha pulegium* L.)	Joint problems
Astragalus (*Astragalus membranaceus*)	Joint pain
Betel nut (*Areca catechu* L.)	Joint pain/swelling
Black tea (*Camellia sinensis*)	Joint pain
Bromelain	Joint disease
Dandelion (*Taraxacum officinale*)	Osteoarthritis
Devil's claw (*Harpagophytum procumbens* DC.)	Hip pain
Devil's claw (*Harpagophytum procumbens* DC.)	Knee pain
Dehydroepiandrosterone (DHEA)	Joint diseases
Dong quai (*Angelica sinensis* [Oliv.] Diels), Chinese angelica	Joint pain
Elder (*Sambucus nigra* L.)	Joint swelling
Ephedra (*Ephedra sinica*), ma huang	Joint pain
Feverfew (*Tanacetum parthenium* L. Schultz-Bip.)	Joint pain
Glucosamine	Joint pain
Green tea (*Camellia sinensis*)	Joint pain
Horse chestnut (*Aesculus hippocastanum* L.)	Osteoarthritis
Kava (*Piper methysticum* G. Forst)	Joint pain and stiffness
Licorice (*Glycyrrhiza glabra* L.), deglycyrrhizinated licorice (DGL)	Osteoarthritis
Omega-3 fatty acids, fish oil, alpha-linolenic acid	Osteoarthritis
St. John's wort (*Hypericum perforatum* L.)	Joint pain
Wild yam (*Dioscorea villosa*)	Joint pain

OSTEOPOROSIS AND RELATED CONDITIONS

Levels of Scientific Evidence for Specific Therapies

GRADE: C (Unclear or Conflicting Scientific Evidence)

Therapy	Specific Therapeutic Use(s)
Black tea (*Camellia sinensis*)	Osteoporosis prevention
Boron	Osteoporosis
Dehydroepiandrosterone (DHEA)	Bone density
Horsetail (*Equisetum arvense* L.)	Osteoporosis (weakening of the bones)
Red clover (*Trifolium pratense*)	Osteoporosis
Soy (*Glycine max* L. Merr.)	Osteoporosis/postmenopausal bone loss

TRADITIONAL OR THEORETICAL USES THAT LACK SUFFICIENT EVIDENCE

Therapy	Specific Therapeutic Use(s)
Arginine (L-arginine)	Osteoporosis
Black cohosh (*Cimicifuga racemosa* L. Nutt.)	Bone diseases
Dehydroepiandrosterone (DHEA)	Bone diseases
Dehydroepiandrosterone (DHEA)	Bone loss associated with anorexia
Dehydroepiandrosterone (DHEA)	Osteoporosis
Dong quai (*Angelica sinensis* [Oliv.] Diels), Chinese angelica	Osteoporosis
Goldenseal (*Hydrastis canadensis* L.), berberine	Osteoporosis
Green tea (*Camellia sinensis*)	Bone density improvement
Melatonin	Postmenopausal osteoporosis
Omega-3 fatty acids, fish oil, alpha-linolenic acid	Osteoporosis
Propolis	Osteoporosis
Wild yam (*Dioscorea villosa*)	Osteoporosis

OTITIS MEDIA AND RELATED CONDITIONS

Levels of Scientific Evidence for Specific Therapies

GRADE: C (Unclear or Conflicting Scientific Evidence)

Therapy	Specific Therapeutic Use(s)
Belladonna (*Atropa belladonna* L. or its *variety A. acuminata* Royle ex Lindl)	Ear infection
Calendula (*Calendula officinalis* L.), marigold	Ear infection

TRADITIONAL OR THEORETICAL USES THAT LACK SUFFICIENT EVIDENCE

Therapy	Specific Therapeutic Use(s)
Belladonna (*Atropa belladonna* L. or its variety *A. acuminata* Royle ex Lindl)	Earache
Betel nut (*Areca catechu* L.)	Ear infections
Chamomile (*Matricaria recutita*, *Chamaemelum nobile*)	Ear infections
Eucalyptus oil (*Eucalyptus globulus* Labillardiere, *E. fructicetorum* F. Von Mueller, *E. smithii* R.T. Baker)	Ear infections
Eyebright (*Euphrasia officinalis*)	Earache
Garlic (*Allium sativum* L.)	Earache
Goldenseal (*Hydrastis canadensis* L.), berberine	Otorrhea
Kava (*Piper methysticum* G. Forst)	Otitis

PAIN AND RELATED CONDITIONS

Levels of Scientific Evidence for Specific Therapies

GRADE: B (GOOD SCIENTIFIC EVIDENCE)

Therapy	Specific Therapeutic Use(s)
Bromelain	Inflammation

GRADE: C (UNCLEAR OR CONFLICTING SCIENTIFIC EVIDENCE)

Therapy	Specific Therapeutic Use(s)
Arginine (L-arginine)	Dental pain (ibuprofen arginate)

Continued

Black cohosh (*Cimicifuga racemosa* L. Nutt.)	Arthritis pain (rheumatoid arthritis, osteoarthritis)
Dandelion (*Taraxacum officinale*)	Anti-inflammatory
Eyebright (*Euphrasia officinalis*)	Anti-inflammatory
Propolis	Dental pain
Shark cartilage	Analgesia
Turmeric (*Curcuma longa* L.), curcumin	Inflammation
White horehound (*Marrubium vulgare* L.)	Pain

TRADITIONAL OR THEORETICAL USES THAT LACK SUFFICIENT EVIDENCE

Therapy	Specific Therapeutic Use(s)
Alfalfa (*Medicago sativa* L.)	Inflammation
Arginine (L-arginine)	Pain
Astragalus (*Astragalus membranaceus*)	Myalgia (muscle pain)
Belladonna (*Atropa belladonna* L. or its variety *A. acuminata* Royle ex Lindl)	Anesthetic
Belladonna (*Atropa belladonna* L. or its variety *A. acuminata* Royle ex Lindl)	Inflammation
Belladonna (*Atropa belladonna* L. or its variety *A. acuminata* Royle ex Lindl)	Muscle and joint pain
Bitter almond (*Prunus amygdalus* Batch var. *amara* DC. Focke), Laetrile	Anti-inflammatory
Bitter almond (*Prunus amygdalus* Batch var. *amara* DC. Focke), Laetrile	Local anesthetic
Bitter almond (*Prunus amygdalus* Batch var. *amara* DC. Focke), Laetrile	Pain suppressant
Black cohosh (*Cimicifuga racemosa* L. Nutt.)	Inflammation
Black cohosh (*Cimicifuga racemosa* L. Nutt.)	Muscle pain
Black tea (*Camellia sinensis*)	Pain
Blessed thistle (*Cnicus benedictus* L.)	Inflammation
Bromelain	Pain
Bromelain	Pain (general)
Burdock (*Arctium lappa*)	Inflammation

Calendula (*Calendula officinalis* L.), marigold	Pain
Chamomile (*Matricaria recutita, Chamaemelum nobile*)	Anti-inflammatory
Chaparral (*Larrea tridentata* DC. Coville, *L. divaricata* Cav.), nordihydroguaiaretic acid (NDGA)	Anti-inflammatory
Chaparral (*Larrea tridentata* DC. Coville, *L. divaricata* Cav.), nordihydroguaiaretic acid (NDGA)	Pain
Clove (*Eugenia aromatica*)	Pain
Dandelion (*Taraxacum officinale*)	Analgesia
Devil's claw (*Harpagophytum procumbens* DC.)	Anti-inflammatory
Devil's claw (*Harpagophytum procumbens* DC.)	Muscle pain
Devil's claw (*Harpagophytum procumbens* DC.)	Pain
Dong quai (*Angelica sinensis* [Oliv.] Diels), Chinese angelica	Pain
Dong quai (*Angelica sinensis* [Oliv.] Diels), Chinese angelica	Pain from bruises
Echinacea (*Echinacea angustifolia* DC., *E. pallida, E. purpurea*)	Pain
Elder (*Sambucus nigra* L.)	Anti-inflammatory
Ephedra (*Ephedra sinica*), ma huang	Anti-inflammatory
Eucalyptus oil (*Eucalyptus globulus* Labillardiere, *E. fructicetorum* F. Von Mueller, *E. smithii* R.T. Baker)	Inflammation
Eucalyptus oil (*Eucalyptus globulus* Labillardiere, *E. fructicetorum* F. Von Mueller, *E. smithii* R.T. Baker)	Muscle/joint pain (applied to the skin)
Evening primrose oil (*Oenothera biennis* L.)	Pain
Fenugreek (*Trigonella foenum-graecum* L.)	Inflammation
Feverfew (*Tanacetum parthenium* L. Schultz-Bip.)	Anti-inflammatory
Garlic (*Allium sativum* L.)	Dental pain
Ginger (*Zingiber officinale* Roscoe)	Pain relief
Ginseng (American ginseng, Asian ginseng, Chinese ginseng, Korean red ginseng, *Panax ginseng*: *Panax* spp. including *P. ginseng* C.C. Meyer and *P. quinquefolium* L., excluding *Eleutherococcus senticosus*)	Inflammation

Continued

Ginseng (American ginseng, Asian ginseng, Chinese ginseng, Korean red ginseng, *Panax ginseng*: *Panax* spp. including *P. ginseng* C.C. Meyer and *P. quinquefolium* L., excluding *Eleutherococcus senticosus*)	Pain relief
Goldenseal (*Hydrastis canadensis* L.), berberine	Anesthetic
Goldenseal (*Hydrastis canadensis* L.), berberine	Anti-inflammatory
Goldenseal (*Hydrastis canadensis* L.), berberine	Muscle pain
Goldenseal (*Hydrastis canadensis* L.), berberine	Pain
Gotu kola (*Centella asiatica* L.), total triterpenic fraction of *Centella asiatica* (TTFCA)	Inflammation
Gotu kola (*Centella asiatica* L.), total triterpenic fraction of *Centella asiatica* (TTFCA)	Pain
Guggul (*Commifora mukul*)	Pain
Hops (*Humulus lupulus* L.)	Anti-inflammatory
Hops (*Humulus lupulus* L.)	Pain
Kava (*Piper methysticum* G. Forst)	Anesthesia
Kava (*Piper methysticum* G. Forst)	Pain
Lavender (*Lavandula angustifolia* Miller)	Anti-inflammatory
Lavender (*Lavandula angustifolia* Miller)	Pain
Licorice (*Glycyrrhiza glabra* L.), deglycyrrhizinated licorice (DGL)	Inflammation
Marshmallow (*Althaea officinalis* L.)	Inflammation
Marshmallow (*Althaea officinalis* L.)	Muscular pain
Oleander (*Nerium oleander*, *Thevetia peruviana*)	Inflammation
Passionflower (*Passiflora incarnata* L.)	Chronic pain
Passionflower (*Passiflora incarnata* L.)	Pain (general)
Peppermint (*Mentha* x *piperita* L.)	Local anesthetic
Peppermint (*Mentha* x *piperita* L.)	Musculoskeletal pain
Peppermint (*Mentha* x *piperita* L.)	Myalgia (muscle pain)
Polypodium leucotomos extract, Anapsos	Inflammation
Pygeum (*Prunus africana*, *Pygeum africanum*)	Inflammation

Saw palmetto (*Serenoa repens* [Bartram] Small)	Anti-inflammatory
Slippery elm (*Ulmus rubra* Muhl. or *U. fulva* Michx.)	Inflammation
Spirulina	Anti-inflammatory
St. John's wort (*Hypericum perforatum* L.)	Anti-inflammatory
St. John's wort (*Hypericum perforatum* L.)	Dental pain
St. John's wort (*Hypericum perforatum* L.)	Pain relief
Tea tree oil (*Melaleuca alternifolia* [Maiden & Betche] Cheel)	Anti-inflammatory
Tea tree oil (*Melaleuca alternifolia* [Maiden & Betche] Cheel)	Muscle and joint pain
Turmeric (*Curcuma longa* L.), curcumin	Pain
Valerian (*Valeriana officinalis* L.)	Anodyne (pain relief)
Valerian (*Valeriana officinalis* L.)	Muscle pain
Valerian (*Valeriana officinalis* L.)	Pain
White horehound (*Marrubium vulgare* L.)	Pain
Wild yam (*Dioscorea villosa*)	Anti-inflammatory
Yohimbe bark extract (*Pausinystalia yohimbe* Pierre ex Beille)	Anesthetic

PEPTIC ULCER DISEASE AND RELATED CONDITIONS

Levels of Scientific Evidence for Specific Therapies

GRADE: C (Unclear or Conflicting Scientific Evidence)

Therapy	Specific Therapeutic Use(s)
Bilberry (*Vaccinium myrtillus*)	Stomach ulcers (peptic ulcer disease)
Blessed thistle (*Cnicus benedictus* L.)	Indigestion and flatulence (gas)
Cranberry (*Vaccinium macrocarpon*)	Stomach ulcers caused by Helicobacter pylori bacteria
Globe artichoke (*Cynara scolymus* L.)	Nonulcer dyspepsia
Licorice (*Glycyrrhiza glabra* L.), deglycyrrhizinated licorice (DGL)	Bleeding stomach ulcers caused by aspirin

Continued

Therapy	Specific Therapeutic Use(s)
Licorice (*Glycyrrhiza glabra* L.), deglycyrrhizinated licorice (DGL)	Peptic ulcer disease
Peppermint (*Mentha* x *piperita* L.)	Indigestion (nonulcer dyspepsia)
Turmeric (*Curcuma longa* L.), curcumin	Dyspepsia (heartburn)
Turmeric (*Curcuma longa* L.), curcumin	Peptic ulcer disease (stomach ulcer)
White horehound (*Marrubium vulgare* L.)	Heartburn/poor appetite

GRADE: D (Fair Negative Scientific Evidence)

Therapy	Specific Therapeutic Use(s)
Garlic (*Allium sativum* L.)	Stomach ulcers caused by *Helicobacter pylori* bacteria

TRADITIONAL OR THEORETICAL USES THAT LACK SUFFICIENT EVIDENCE

Therapy	Specific Therapeutic Use(s)
Alfalfa (*Medicago sativa* L.)	Indigestion
Alfalfa (*Medicago sativa* L.)	Stomach ulcers
American pennyroyal (*Hedeoma pulegioides* L.), European pennyroyal (*Mentha pulegium* L.)	Indigestion
Arginine (L-arginine)	Stomach ulcer
Astragalus (*Astragalus membranaceus*)	Stomach ulcer
Barley (*Hordeum vulgare* L.), germinated barley foodstuff (GBF)	Gastritis
Barley (*Hordeum vulgare* L.), germinated barley foodstuff (GBF)	Gastrointestinal inflammation
Belladonna (*Atropa belladonna* L. or its variety *A. acuminata* Royle ex Lindl)	Stomach ulcers
Bilberry (*Vaccinium myrtillus*)	Dyspepsia
Bilberry (*Vaccinium myrtillus*)	Infantile dyspepsia
Bladderwrack (*Fucus vesiculosus*)	Heartburn
Bladderwrack (*Fucus vesiculosus*)	Ulcer
Boswellia (*Boswellia serrata* Roxb.)	Dyspepsia
Boswellia (*Boswellia serrata* Roxb.)	Peptic ulcer disease

Bromelain	Indigestion
Bromelain	Stomach ulcer/stomach ulcer prevention
Calendula (*Calendula officinalis* L.), marigold	Indigestion
Calendula (*Calendula officinalis* L.), marigold	Stomach ulcers
Chamomile (*Matricaria recutita, Chamaemelum nobile*)	Heartburn
Chaparral (*Larrea tridentata* DC. Coville, *L. divaricata* Cav.), nordihydroguaiaretic acid (NDGA)	Heartburn
Chaparral (*Larrea tridentata* DC. Coville, *L. divaricata* Cav.), nordihydroguaiaretic acid (NDGA)	Indigestion
Chaparral (*Larrea tridentata* DC. Coville, *L. divaricata* Cav.), nordihydroguaiaretic acid (NDGA)	Stomach ulcer
Coenzyme Q10	Stomach ulcer
Dandelion (*Taraxacum officinale*)	Heartburn
Danshen (*Salvia miltiorrhiza*)	Gastric ulcers
Danshen (*Salvia miltiorrhiza*)	Stomach ulcers
Devil's claw (*Harpagophytum procumbens* DC.)	Dyspepsia
Devil's claw (*Harpagophytum procumbens* DC.)	Heartburn
Devil's claw (*Harpagophytum procumbens* DC.)	Indigestion
Dong quai (*Angelica sinensis* [Oliv.] Diels), Chinese angelica	Heartburn
Echinacea (*Echinacea angustifolia* DC., *E. pallida, E. purpurea*)	Dyspepsia
Evening primrose oil (*Oenothera biennis* L.)	Disorders of the stomach and intestines
Fenugreek (*Trigonella foenum-graecum* L.)	Dyspepsia
Fenugreek (*Trigonella foenum-graecum* L.)	Gastritis
Fenugreek (*Trigonella foenum-graecum* L.)	Indigestion
Flaxseed and flaxseed oil (*Linum usitatissimum*)	Enteritis
Flaxseed and flaxseed oil (*Linum usitatissimum*)	Gastritis

Continued

Garlic (*Allium sativum* L.)	Stomach acid reduction
Ginger (*Zingiber officinale* Roscoe)	Antacid
Ginger (*Zingiber officinale* Roscoe)	Dyspepsia
Ginger (*Zingiber officinale* Roscoe)	*Helicobacter pylori* infection
Ginger (*Zingiber officinale* Roscoe)	Stomach ulcers
Goldenseal (*Hydrastis canadensis* L.), berberine	Gastroenteritis
Goldenseal (*Hydrastis canadensis* L.), berberine	Indigestion
Goldenseal (*Hydrastis canadensis* L.), berberine	Stomach ulcers
Gotu kola (*Centella asiatica* L.), total triterpenic fraction of *Centella asiatica* (TTFCA)	Gastritis
Green tea (*Camellia sinensis*)	Gastritis
Green tea (*Camellia sinensis*)	*Helicobacter pylori* infection
Hawthorn (*Crataegus laevigata, C. oxyacantha, C. monogyna, C. pentagyna*)	Dyspepsia
Hops (*Humulus lupulus* L.)	Indigestion
Horse chestnut (*Aesculus hippocastanum* L.)	Ulcers
Horsetail (*Equisetum arvense* L.)	Dyspepsia
Kava (*Piper methysticum* G. Forst)	Dyspepsia
Lactobacillus acidophilus	Heartburn
Lactobacillus acidophilus	Indigestion
Lactobacillus acidophilus	Stomach ulcer
Lavender (*Lavandula angustifolia* Miller)	Heartburn
Lavender (*Lavandula angustifolia* Miller)	Indigestion
Licorice (*Glycyrrhiza glabra* L.), deglycyrrhizinated licorice (DGL)	Gastroesophageal reflux disease
Marshmallow (*Althaea officinalis* L.)	Duodenal ulcer
Marshmallow (*Althaea officinalis* L.)	Enteritis
Marshmallow (*Althaea officinalis* L.)	Gastroenteritis
Marshmallow (*Althaea officinalis* L.)	Indigestion
Marshmallow (*Althaea officinalis* L.)	Peptic ulcer disease

Melatonin	Gastroesophageal reflux disease
Niacin (vitamin B_3, nicotinic acid), niacinamide, inositol hexanicotinate	Stomach ulcer
Oleander (*Nerium oleander*, *Thevetia peruviana*)	Indigestion
Peppermint (*Mentha* x *piperita* L.)	Antacid
Peppermint (*Mentha* x *piperita* L.)	Enteritis
Peppermint (*Mentha* x *piperita* L.)	Gastritis
Propolis	Stomach ulcer
Psyllium (*Plantago ovata*, *P. ispaghula*)	Duodenal ulcer
Psyllium (*Plantago ovata*, *P. ispaghula*)	Stomach ulcer
Red clover (*Trifolium pratense*)	Indigestion
Red yeast rice (*Monascus purpureus*)	Indigestion
Saw palmetto (*Serenoa repens* [Bartram] Small)	Indigestion
Seaweed, kelp, bladderwrack (*Fucus vesiculosus*)	Dyspepsia
Seaweed, kelp, bladderwrack (*Fucus vesiculosus*)	Heartburn
Seaweed, kelp, bladderwrack (*Fucus vesiculosus*)	Ulcer
Shark cartilage	Enteritis
Slippery elm (*Ulmus rubra* Muhl. or *U. fulva* Michx.)	Duodenal ulcer
Slippery elm (*Ulmus rubra* Muhl. or *U. fulva* Michx.)	Enteritis
Slippery elm (*Ulmus rubra* Muhl. or *U. fulva* Michx.)	Gastric ulcer
Slippery elm (*Ulmus rubra* Muhl. or *U. fulva* Michx.)	Gastritis
Slippery elm (*Ulmus rubra* Muhl. or *U. fulva* Michx.)	Gastroesophageal reflux disease
Slippery elm (*Ulmus rubra* Muhl. or *U. fulva* Michx.)	Heartburn
Slippery elm (*Ulmus rubra* Muhl. or *U. fulva* Michx.)	Peptic ulcer disease
Spirulina	Stomach acid excess
Spirulina	Ulcers
St. John's wort (*Hypericum perforatum* L.)	Heartburn
St. John's wort (*Hypericum perforatum* L.)	Ulcers
Thyme (*Thymus vulgaris* L.), thymol	Dyspepsia

Continued

Thyme (*Thymus vulgaris* L.), thymol	Gastritis
Thyme (*Thymus vulgaris* L.), thymol	Heartburn
Thyme (*Thymus vulgaris* L.), thymol	Indigestion
Valerian (*Valeriana officinalis* L.)	Heartburn
Valerian (*Valeriana officinalis* L.)	Peptic ulcer disease
White horehound (*Marrubium vulgare* L.)	Indigestion

PERIPHERAL VASCULAR DISEASE AND RELATED CONDITIONS

Levels of Scientific Evidence for Specific Therapies

GRADE: A (Strong Scientific Evidence)

Therapy	Specific Therapeutic Use(s)
Ginkgo (*Ginkgo biloba* L.)	Claudication (painful legs from clogged arteries)

GRADE: C (Unclear or Conflicting Scientific Evidence)

Therapy	Specific Therapeutic Use(s)
Arginine (L-arginine)	Peripheral vascular disease/ claudication
Garlic (*Allium sativum* L.)	Peripheral vascular disease (blocked arteries in the legs)

TRADITIONAL OR THEORETICAL USES THAT LACK SUFFICIENT EVIDENCE

Therapy	Specific Therapeutic Use(s)
Garlic (*Allium sativum* L.)	Claudication (leg pain due to poor blood flow)
Niacin (vitamin B_3, nicotinic acid), niacinamide, inositol hexanicotinate	Peripheral vascular disease
Omega-3 fatty acids, fish oil, alpha-linolenic acid	Peripheral vascular disease

PLAQUE/PERIODONTAL DISEASE AND RELATED CONDITIONS

Levels of Scientific Evidence for Specific Therapies

GRADE: C (Unclear or Conflicting Scientific Evidence)

Therapy	Specific Therapeutic Use(s)
Betel nut (*Areca catechu* L.)	Dental cavities
Black tea (*Camellia sinensis*)	Dental cavity prevention
Coenzyme Q10	Gum disease (periodontitis)
Cranberry (*Vaccinium macrocarpon*)	Dental plaque
Eucalyptus oil (*Eucalyptus globulus* Labillardiere, *E. fructicetorum* F. Von Mueller, *E. smithii* R.T. Baker)	Dental plaque/gingivitis (mouthwash)
Green tea (*Camellia sinensis*)	Dental cavity prevention
Propolis	Dental plaque and gingivitis (mouthwash)
Thyme (*Thymus vulgaris* L.), thymol	Dental plaque

TRADITIONAL OR THEORETICAL USES THAT LACK SUFFICIENT EVIDENCE

Therapy	Specific Therapeutic Use(s)
Arginine (L-arginine)	Peritonitis
Astragalus (*Astragalus membranaceus*)	Denture adhesive (astragalus sap)
Bilberry (*Vaccinium myrtillus*)	Bleeding gums
Chamomile (*Matricaria recutita, Chamaemelum nobile*)	Gingivitis
Clove (*Eugenia aromatica*)	Cavities
Coenzyme Q10	Gingivitis
Echinacea (*Echinacea angustifolia* DC., *E. pallida, E. purpurea*)	Gingivitis
Goldenseal (*Hydrastis canadensis* L.), berberine	Gingivitis
Gotu kola (*Centella asiatica* L.), total triterpenic fraction of *Centella asiatica* (TTFCA)	Periodontal disease
Green tea (*Camellia sinensis*)	Bleeding of gums or tooth sockets

Continued

Green tea (*Camellia sinensis*)	Gum swelling
Guggul (*Commifora mukul*)	Gingivitis
Licorice (*Glycyrrhiza glabra* L.), deglycyrrhizinated licorice (DGL)	Dental hygiene
Licorice (*Glycyrrhiza glabra* L.), deglycyrrhizinated licorice (DGL)	Plaque
Lycopene	Periodontal disease
Milk thistle (*Silybum marianum*), silymarin	Peritonitis
Omega-3 fatty acids, fish oil, alpha-linolenic acid	Gingivitis
Tea tree oil (*Melaleuca alternifolia* [Maiden & Betche] Cheel)	Dental plaque
Tea tree oil (*Melaleuca alternifolia* [Maiden & Betche] Cheel)	Gingivitis
Tea tree oil (*Melaleuca alternifolia* [Maiden & Betche] Cheel)	Periodontal disease
Thyme (*Thymus vulgaris* L.), thymol	Gingivitis

PNEUMONIA AND RELATED CONDITIONS

Levels of Scientific Evidence for Specific Therapies

TRADITIONAL OR THEORETICAL USES THAT LACK SUFFICIENT EVIDENCE

Therapy	Specific Therapeutic Use(s)
American pennyroyal (*Hedeoma pulegioides* L.), European pennyroyal (*Mentha pulegium* L.)	Pneumonia
Blessed thistle (*Cnicus benedictus* L.)	Pneumonitis
Bromelain	Pneumonia
Burdock (*Arctium lappa*)	Pneumonia
Coenzyme Q10	Lung disease
Danshen (*Salvia miltiorrhiza*)	Lung fibrosis
Dong quai (*Angelica sinensis* [Oliv.] Diels), Chinese angelica	Lung disease
Dong quai (*Angelica sinensis* [Oliv.] Diels), Chinese angelica	Pleurisy

Garlic (*Allium sativum* L.)	Pneumonia
Goldenseal (*Hydrastis canadensis* L.), berberine	Pneumonia
Hops (*Humulus lupulus* L.)	Lung disease (from inhalation of silica dust or asbestos)
Melatonin	Sarcoidosis
Shark cartilage	Sarcoidosis
Slippery elm (*Ulmus rubra* Muhl. or *U. fulva* Michx.)	Lung diseases
Slippery elm (*Ulmus rubra* Muhl. or *U. fulva* Michx.)	Pleurisy
Tea tree oil (*Melaleuca alternifolia* [Maiden & Betche] Cheel)	Lung inflammation
White horehound (*Marrubium vulgare* L.)	Lung congestion
White horehound (*Marrubium vulgare* L.)	Pneumonia

POISONING AND RELATED CONDITIONS

Levels of Scientific Evidence for Specific Therapies

GRADE: C (Unclear or Conflicting Scientific Evidence)

Therapy	Specific Therapeutic Use(s)
Clay	Mercuric chloride poisoning

TRADITIONAL OR THEORETICAL USES THAT LACK SUFFICIENT EVIDENCE

Therapy	Specific Therapeutic Use(s)
Belladonna (*Atropa belladonna* L. or its variety *A. acuminata* Royle ex Lindl)	Poisoning (especially by insecticides)
Clay	Poisoning
Essiac	Blood cleanser
Essiac	Chelating agent (heavy metals)
Hoxsey formula	Elimination of toxins
Marshmallow (*Althaea officinalis* L.)	Antidote to poisons
Melatonin	Aluminum toxicity
Melatonin	Lead toxicity

POLYCYSTIC OVARY SYNDROME AND RELATED CONDITIONS

Levels of Scientific Evidence for Specific Therapies

TRADITIONAL OR THEORETICAL USES THAT LACK SUFFICIENT EVIDENCE

Therapy	Specific Therapeutic Use(s)
Black cohosh (*Cimicifuga racemosa* L. Nutt.)	Polycystic ovary syndrome
Dehydroepiandrosterone (DHEA)	Polycystic ovary syndrome
Licorice (*Glycyrrhiza glabra* L.), deglycyrrhizinated licorice (DGL)	Polycystic ovary syndrome
Saw palmetto (*Serenoa repens* [Bartram] Small)	Polycystic ovary syndrome

PREMENSTRUAL SYNDROME AND RELATED CONDITIONS

Levels of Scientific Evidence for Specific Therapies

GRADE: B (Good Scientific Evidence)

Therapy	Specific Therapeutic Use(s)
Black cohosh (*Cimicifuga racemosa* L. Nutt.)	Menopausal symptoms
Soy (*Glycine max* L. Merr.)	Menopausal hot flashes

GRADE: C (Unclear or Conflicting Scientific Evidence)

Therapy	Specific Therapeutic Use(s)
American pennyroyal (*Hedeoma pulegioides* L.), European pennyroyal (*Mentha pulegium* L.)	Emmenagogue (menstrual flow stimulant)
Belladonna (*Atropa belladonna* L. or its variety *A. acuminata* Royle ex Lindl)	Premenstrual syndrome
Bilberry (*Vaccinium myrtillus*)	Painful menstruation (dysmenorrhea)
Dehydroepiandrosterone (DHEA)	Menopausal disorders
Dehydroepiandrosterone (DHEA)	Ovulation disorders
Dong quai (*Angelica sinensis* [Oliv.] Diels), Chinese angelica	Amenorrhea (lack of menstrual periods)
Dong quai (*Angelica sinensis* [Oliv.] Diels), Chinese angelica	Dysmenorrhea (painful menstruation)
Flaxseed and flaxseed oil (*Linum usitatissimum*)	Menstrual breast pain (flaxseed, not flaxseed oil)

Ginkgo (*Ginkgo biloba* L.)	Premenstrual syndrome
Ginseng (American ginseng, Asian ginseng, Chinese ginseng, Korean red ginseng, *Panax ginseng*: *Panax* spp. including *P. ginseng* C.C. Meyer and *P. quinquefolium* L., excluding *Eleutherococcus senticosus*)	Menopausal symptoms
Green tea (*Camellia sinensis*)	Menopausal symptoms
Omega-3 fatty acids, fish oil, alpha-linolenic acid	Dysmenorrhea (painful menstruation)
Red clover (*Trifolium pratense*)	Hormone replacement therapy (HRT)
Red clover (*Trifolium pratense*)	Menopausal symptoms
St. John's wort (*Hypericum perforatum* L.)	Perimenopausal symptoms
St. John's wort (*Hypericum perforatum* L.)	Premenstrual syndrome
Wild yam (*Dioscorea villosa*)	Menopausal symptoms

GRADE: D (Fair Negative Scientific Evidence)

Therapy	Specific Therapeutic Use(s)
Belladonna (*Atropa belladonna* L. or its variety *A. acuminata* Royle ex Lindl)	Menopausal symptoms
Boron	Menopausal symptoms
Evening primrose oil (*Oenothera biennis* L.)	Menopause (flushing/bone metabolism)
Evening primrose oil (*Oenothera biennis* L.)	Premenstrual syndrome
Wild yam (*Dioscorea villosa*)	Hormonal properties (to mimic estrogen, progesterone, or dehydroepiandrosterone [DHEA])

TRADITIONAL OR THEORETICAL USES THAT LACK SUFFICIENT EVIDENCE

Therapy	Specific Therapeutic Use(s)
Alfalfa (*Medicago sativa* L.)	Estrogen replacement
Alfalfa (*Medicago sativa* L.)	Menopausal symptoms
American pennyroyal (*Hedeoma pulegioides* L.), European pennyroyal (*Mentha pulegium* L.)	Cramps

Continued

American pennyroyal (*Hedeoma pulegioides* L.), European pennyroyal (*Mentha pulegium* L.)	Premenstrual syndrome
Astragalus (*Astragalus membranaceus*)	Menstrual disorders
Astragalus (*Astragalus membranaceus*)	Pelvic congestion syndrome
Belladonna (*Atropa belladonna* L. or its variety *A. acuminata* Royle ex Lindl)	Abnormal menstrual periods
Betel nut (*Areca catechu* L.)	Excessive menstrual flow
Black cohosh (*Cimicifuga racemosa* L. Nutt.)	Endometriosis
Black cohosh (*Cimicifuga racemosa* L. Nutt.)	Menstrual period problems
Black cohosh (*Cimicifuga racemosa* L. Nutt.)	Ovarian cysts
Black cohosh (*Cimicifuga racemosa* L. Nutt.)	Premenstrual syndrome
Bladderwrack (*Fucus vesiculosus*)	Menstruation irregularities
Blessed thistle (*Cnicus benedictus* L.)	Menstrual disorders
Blessed thistle (*Cnicus benedictus* L.)	Menstrual flow stimulant
Blessed thistle (*Cnicus benedictus* L.)	Painful menstruation
Boswellia (*Boswellia serrata* Roxb.)	Amenorrhea
Boswellia (*Boswellia serrata* Roxb.)	Emmenagogue (inducer of menstruation)
Bromelain	Menstrual pain
Calendula (*Calendula officinalis* L.), marigold	Cramps
Calendula (*Calendula officinalis* L.), marigold	Menstrual period abnormalities
Chamomile (*Matricaria recutita*, *Chamaemelum nobile*)	Dysmenorrhea
Chamomile (*Matricaria recutita*, *Chamaemelum nobile*)	Menstrual disorders
Chaparral (*Larrea tridentata* DC. Coville, *L. divaricata* Cav.), nordihydroguaiaretic acid (NDGA)	Menstrual cramps
Clay	Menstruation difficulties
Dandelion (*Taraxacum officinale*)	Menopause
Dandelion (*Taraxacum officinale*)	Premenstrual syndrome
Danshen (*Salvia miltiorrhiza*)	Menstrual problems
Devil's claw (*Harpagophytum procumbens* DC.)	Menopausal symptoms
Devil's claw (*Harpagophytum procumbens* DC.)	Menstrual cramps

Dehydroepiandrosterone (DHEA)	Amenorrhea associated with anorexia
Dehydroepiandrosterone (DHEA)	Andropause/andrenopause
Dehydroepiandrosterone (DHEA)	Premenstrual syndrome
Dong quai (*Angelica sinensis* [Oliv.] Diels), Chinese angelica	Cramps
Dong quai (*Angelica sinensis* [Oliv.] Diels), Chinese angelica	Hormonal abnormalities
Dong quai (*Angelica sinensis* [Oliv.] Diels), Chinese angelica	Menorrhagia (heavy menstrual bleeding)
Dong quai (*Angelica sinensis* [Oliv.] Diels), Chinese angelica	Menstrual cramping
Dong quai (*Angelica sinensis* [Oliv.] Diels), Chinese angelica	Ovulation abnormalities
Dong quai (*Angelica sinensis* [Oliv.] Diels), Chinese angelica	Pelvic congestion syndrome
Dong quai (*Angelica sinensis* [Oliv.] Diels), Chinese angelica	Premenstrual syndrome
Fenugreek (*Trigonella foenum-graecum* L.)	Menopausal symptoms
Fenugreek (*Trigonella foenum-graecum* L.)	Postmenopausal vaginal dryness
Feverfew (*Tanacetum parthenium* L. Schultz-Bip.)	Menstrual cramps
Feverfew (*Tanacetum parthenium* L. Schultz-Bip.)	Promotion of menstruation
Flaxseed and flaxseed oil (*Linum usitatissimum*)	Menstrual disorders
Flaxseed and flaxseed oil (*Linum usitatissimum*)	Ovarian disorders
Garlic (*Allium sativum* L.)	Emmenagogue
Ginger (*Zingiber officinale* Roscoe)	Dysmenorrhea
Ginger (*Zingiber officinale* Roscoe)	Promotion of menstruation
Ginkgo (*Ginkgo biloba* L.)	Menstrual pain
Ginseng (American ginseng, Asian ginseng, Chinese ginseng, Korean red ginseng, *Panax ginseng*: *Panax* spp. including *P. ginseng* C.C. Meyer and *P. quinquefolium* L., excluding *Eleutherococcus senticosus*)	Menopausal symptoms
Goldenseal (*Hydrastis canadensis* L.), berberine	Menstruation problems

Continued

Goldenseal (*Hydrastis canadensis* L.), berberine	Premenstrual syndrome
Gotu kola (*Centella asiatica* L.), total triterpenic fraction of *Centella asiatica* (TTFCA)	Amenorrhea
Gotu kola (*Centella asiatica* L.), total triterpenic fraction of *Centella asiatica* (TTFCA)	Hot flashes
Gotu kola (*Centella asiatica* L.), total triterpenic fraction of *Centella asiatica* (TTFCA)	Menstrual disorders
Guggul (*Commifora mukul*)	Menstrual disorders
Hawthorn (*Crataegus laevigata*, *C. oxyacantha*, *C. monogyna*, *C. pentagyna*)	Amenorrhea
Hops (*Humulus lupulus* L.)	Estrogenic effects
Horse chestnut (*Aesculus hippocastanum* L.)	Menstrual pain
Horsetail (*Equisetum arvense* L.)	Menstrual pain
Kava (*Piper methysticum* G. Forst)	Menopause
Kava (*Piper methysticum* G. Forst)	Menstrual disorders
Lavender (*Lavandula angustifolia* Miller)	Menopause
Lavender (*Lavandula angustifolia* Miller)	Menstrual period problems
Licorice (*Glycyrrhiza glabra* L.), deglycyrrhizinated licorice (DGL)	Hormone regulation
Licorice (*Glycyrrhiza glabra* L.), deglycyrrhizinated licorice (DGL)	Menopausal symptoms
Melatonin	Melatonin deficiency
Milk thistle (*Silybum marianum*), ,silymarin	Menstrual disorders
Niacin (vitamin B_3, nicotinic acid), niacinamide, inositol hexanicotinate	Painful menstruation
Niacin (vitamin B_3, nicotinic acid), niacinamide, inositol hexanicotinate	Premenstrual headache prevention
Niacin (vitamin B_3, nicotinic acid), niacinamide, inositol hexanicotinate	Premenstrual syndrome
Oleander (*Nerium oleander*, *Thevetia peruviana*)	Abnormal menstruation
Oleander (*Nerium oleander*, *Thevetia peruviana*)	Menstrual stimulant
Omega-3 fatty acids, fish oil, alpha-linolenic acid	Menopausal symptoms
Omega-3 fatty acids, fish oil, alpha-linolenic acid	Menstrual cramps

Omega-3 fatty acids, fish oil, alpha-linolenic acid	Premenstrual syndrome
Passionflower (*Passiflora incarnata* L.)	Menopausal symptoms (hot flashes)
Peppermint (*Mentha* x *piperita* L.)	Cramps
Peppermint (*Mentha* x *piperita* L.)	Dysmenorrhea (menstrual pain)
Psyllium (*Plantago ovata, P. ispaghula*)	Excessive menstrual bleeding
Red clover (*Trifolium pratense*)	Hot flashes
Red clover (*Trifolium pratense*)	Premenstrual syndrome
Saw palmetto (*Serenoa repens* [Bartram] Small)	Antiandrogen
Saw palmetto (*Serenoa repens* [Bartram] Small)	Antiestrogen
Saw palmetto (*Serenoa repens* [Bartram] Small)	Dysmenorrhea
Saw palmetto (*Serenoa repens* [Bartram] Small)	Estrogenic agent
Saw palmetto (*Serenoa repens* [Bartram] Small)	Ovarian cysts
Saw palmetto (*Serenoa repens* [Bartram] Small)	Pelvic congestive syndrome
Seaweed, kelp, bladderwrack (*Fucus vesiculosus*)	Menstrual irregularities (menorrhagia)
Slippery elm (*Ulmus rubra* Muhl. or *U. fulva* Michx.)	Gynecologic disorders
Spirulina	Premenstrual syndrome
St. John's wort (*Hypericum perforatum* L.)	Menstrual pain
Sweet almond (*Prunus amygdalus dulcis*)	Plant-derived estrogen
Thyme (*Thymus vulgaris* L.), thymol	Dysmenorrhea
Turmeric (*Curcuma longa* L.), curcumin	Menstrual pain
Turmeric (*Curcuma longa* L.), curcumin	Menstrual period problems/ lack of menstrual periods
Valerian (*Valeriana officinalis* L.)	Amenorrhea
Valerian (*Valeriana officinalis* L.)	Dysmenorrhea
Valerian (*Valeriana officinalis* L.)	Emmenagogue
Valerian (*Valeriana officinalis* L.)	Menopause
Valerian (*Valeriana officinalis* L.)	Premenstrual syndrome
White horehound (*Marrubium vulgare* L.)	Dysmenorrhea

Continued

White horehound (*Marrubium vulgare* L.)	Menstrual pain
Wild yam (*Dioscorea villosa*)	Cramps
Wild yam (*Dioscorea villosa*)	Menopause
Wild yam (*Dioscorea villosa*)	Menstrual pain or irregularities
Wild yam (*Dioscorea villosa*)	Pelvic cramps
Wild yam (*Dioscorea villosa*)	Postmenopausal vaginal dryness
Wild yam (*Dioscorea villosa*)	Premenstrual syndrome

PROSTATE DISORDERS AND RELATED CONDITIONS

Levels of Scientific Evidence for Specific Therapies

GRADE: A (Strong Scientific Evidence)

Therapy	Specific Therapeutic Use(s)
Saw palmetto (*Serenoa repens* [Bartram] Small)	Benign prostatic hypertrophy (BPH)

GRADE: B (Good Scientific Evidence)

Therapy	Specific Therapeutic Use(s)
Pygeum (*Prunus africana*, *Pygeum africanum*)	BPH symptoms

GRADE: C (Unclear or Conflicting Scientific Evidence)

Therapy	Specific Therapeutic Use(s)
Red clover (*Trifolium pratense*)	Prostate enlargement (BPH)

TRADITIONAL OR THEORETICAL USES THAT LACK SUFFICIENT EVIDENCE

Therapy	Specific Therapeutic Use(s)
Alfalfa (*Medicago sativa* L.)	Prostate disorders
Astragalus (*Astragalus membranaceus*)	Prostatitis
Bladderwrack (*Fucus vesiculosus*)	BPH
Calendula (*Calendula officinalis* L.), marigold	BPH
Calendula (*Calendula officinalis* L.), marigold	Prostatitis

Dandelion (*Taraxacum officinale*)	BPH
Flaxseed and flaxseed oil (*Linum usitatissimum*)	Enlarged prostate
Goldenseal (*Hydrastis canadensis* L.), berberine	Prostatitis
Horse chestnut (*Aesculus hippocastanum* L.)	BPH
Horsetail (*Equisetum arvense* L.)	Prostate inflammation
PC-SPES	BPH
Pygeum (*Prunus africana*, *Pygeum africanum*)	Prostatic adenoma
Pygeum (*Prunus africana*, *Pygeum africanum*)	Prostatitis
Seaweed, kelp, bladderwrack (*Fucus vesiculosus*)	BPH

PSYCHOSIS AND RELATED CONDITIONS

Levels of Scientific Evidence for Specific Therapies

GRADE: C (Unclear or Conflicting Scientific Evidence)

Therapy	Specific Therapeutic Use(s)
Betel nut (*Areca catechu* L.)	Schizophrenia
Dehydroepiandrosterone (DHEA)	Schizophrenia
Melatonin	Schizophrenia (sleep disorders)
Omega-3 fatty acids, fish oil, alpha-linolenic acid	Schizophrenia

GRADE: D (Fair Negative Scientific Evidence)

Therapy	Specific Therapeutic Use(s)
Evening primrose oil (*Oenothera biennis* L.)	Schizophrenia

TRADITIONAL OR THEORETICAL USES THAT LACK SUFFICIENT EVIDENCE

Therapy	Specific Therapeutic Use(s)
American pennyroyal (*Hedeoma pulegioides* L.), European pennyroyal (*Mentha pulegium* L.)	Hallucinations
Chaparral (*Larrea tridentata* DC. Coville, *L. divaricata* Cav.), nordihydroguaiaretic acid (NDGA)	Hallucinations (including those due to LSD ingestion)
Coenzyme Q10	Psychiatric disorders
Ginkgo (*Ginkgo biloba* L.)	Schizophrenia

Continued

Ginseng (American ginseng, Asian ginseng, Chinese ginseng, Korean red ginseng, *Panax ginseng*: *Panax* spp. including *P. ginseng* C.C. Meyer and *P. quinquefolium* L., excluding *Eleutherococcus senticosus*)	Psychoasthenia
Gotu kola (*Centella asiatica* L.), total triterpenic fraction of *Centella asiatica* (TTFCA)	Mental disorders
Kava (*Piper methysticum* G. Forst)	Antipsychotic
Lavender (*Lavandula angustifolia* Miller)	Psychosis
Niacin (vitamin B_3, nicotinic acid), niacinamide, inositol hexanicotinate	Diagnostic test for schizophrenia
Niacin (vitamin B_3, nicotinic acid), niacinamide, inositol hexanicotinate	Drug-induced hallucinations
Niacin (vitamin B_3, nicotinic acid), niacinamide, inositol hexanicotinate	Psychosis
Niacin (vitamin B_3, nicotinic acid), niacinamide, inositol hexanicotinate	Schizophrenia
Oleander (*Nerium oleander*, *Thevetia peruviana*)	Psychiatric disorders
Pygeum (*Prunus africana*, *Pygeum africanum*)	Psychosis
Yohimbe bark extract (*Pausinystalia yohimbe* Pierre ex Beille)	Hallucinogenic
Yohimbe bark extract (*Pausinystalia yohimbe* Pierre ex Beille)	Schizophrenia

PULMONARY EDEMA AND RELATED CONDITIONS

Levels of Scientific Evidence for Specific Therapies

GRADE: A (Strong Scientific Evidence)

Therapy	Specific Therapeutic Use(s)
Hawthorn (*Crataegus laevigata*, *C. oxyacantha*, *C. monogyna*, *C. pentagyna*)	Congestive heart failure

GRADE: C (Unclear or Conflicting Scientific Evidence)

Therapy	Specific Therapeutic Use(s)
Arginine (L-arginine)	Heart failure (congestive)
Astragalus (*Astragalus membranaceus*)	Heart failure

Coenzyme Q10	Cardiomyopathy (dilated, hypertrophic)
Coenzyme Q10	Heart failure
Dehydroepiandrosterone (DHEA)	Heart failure
Ginseng (American ginseng, Asian ginseng, Chinese ginseng, Korean red ginseng, *Panax ginseng*: *Panax* spp. including *P. ginseng* C.C. Meyer and *P. quinquefolium* L., excluding *Eleutherococcus senticosus*)	Congestive heart failure
Hawthorn (*Crataegus laevigata*, *C. oxyacantha*, *C. monogyna*, *C. pentagyna*)	Functional cardiovascular disorders
Oleander (*Nerium oleander*, *Thevetia peruviana*)	Congestive heart failure
Passionflower (*Passiflora incarnata* L.)	Congestive heart failure (exercise capacity)

TRADITIONAL OR THEORETICAL USES THAT LACK SUFFICIENT EVIDENCE

Therapy	Specific Therapeutic Use(s)
Dandelion (*Taraxacum officinale*)	Congestive heart failure
Danshen (*Salvia miltiorrhiza*)	Left ventricular hypertrophy
Dong quai (*Angelica sinensis* [Oliv.] Diels), Chinese angelica	Congestive heart failure
Ginkgo (*Ginkgo biloba* L.)	Congestive heart failure
Goldenseal (*Hydrastis canadensis* L.), berberine	Heart failure
Horse chestnut (*Aesculus hippocastanum* L.)	Fluid in the lungs (pulmonary edema)
Horsetail (*Equisetum arvense* L.)	Fluid in the lungs
Omega-3 fatty acids, fish oil, alpha-linolenic acid	Congestive heart failure
Passionflower (*Passiflora incarnata* L.)	Congestive heart failure (exercise ability)
Valerian (*Valeriana officinalis* L.)	Congestive heart failure

PULMONARY HYPERTENSION AND RELATED CONDITIONS

Levels of Scientific Evidence for Specific Therapies

GRADE: C (Unclear or Conflicting Scientific Evidence)

Therapy	Specific Therapeutic Use(s)
Dong quai (*Angelica sinensis* [Oliv.] Diels), Chinese angelica	Pulmonary hypertension

TRADITIONAL OR THEORETICAL USES THAT LACK SUFFICIENT EVIDENCE

Therapy	Specific Therapeutic Use(s)
Arginine (L-arginine)	Pulmonary hypertension (high blood pressure in the lungs)
Danshen (*Salvia miltiorrhiza*)	Pulmonary hypertension
Feverfew (*Tanacetum parthenium* L. Schultz-Bip.)	Blood vessel dilation (relaxation)
White horehound (*Marrubium vulgare* L.)	Vasodilator

QUALITY OF LIFE AND RELATED CONDITIONS

Levels of Scientific Evidence for Specific Therapies

GRADE: C (Unclear or Conflicting Scientific Evidence)

Therapy	Specific Therapeutic Use(s)
Chamomile (*Matricaria recutita*, *Chamaemelum nobile*)	Quality of life in cancer patients

TRADITIONAL OR THEORETICAL USES THAT LACK SUFFICIENT EVIDENCE

Therapy	Specific Therapeutic Use(s)
Essiac	Supportive care in advanced-cancer patients
Ginseng (American ginseng, Asian ginseng, Chinese ginseng, Korean red ginseng, *Panax ginseng*: *Panax* spp. including *P. ginseng* C.C. Meyer and P. *quinquefolium* L., excluding *Eleutherococcus senticosus*)	Qi deficiency and blood stasis syndrome in heart disease (Eastern medicine)
Ginseng (American ginseng, Asian ginseng, Chinese ginseng, Korean red ginseng, *Panax ginseng*: *Panax* spp. including *P. ginseng* C.C. Meyer and *P. quinquefolium* L., excluding *Eleutherococcus senticosus*)	Quality of life

RADIATION THERAPY SIDE EFFECTS AND RELATED CONDITIONS

Levels of Scientific Evidence for Specific Therapies

GRADE: C (Unclear or Conflicting Scientific Evidence)

Therapy	Specific Therapeutic Use(s)
Aloe (*Aloe vera*)	Radiation dermatitis
Belladonna (*Atropa belladonna* L. or its variety *A. acuminata* Royle ex Lindl)	Radiation therapy rash (radiation burn)
Echinacea (*Echinacea angustifolia* DC., *E. pallida*, *E. purpurea*)	Low white blood cell counts after x-ray treatment
Melatonin	Ultraviolet light skin damage protection

GRADE: D (Fair Negative Scientific Evidence)

Therapy	Specific Therapeutic Use(s)
Aloe (*Aloe vera*)	Radiation dermatitis
Sweet almond (*Prunus amygdalus dulcis*)	Radiation therapy skin reactions (used on the skin)

TRADITIONAL OR THEORETICAL USES THAT LACK SUFFICIENT EVIDENCE

Therapy	Specific Therapeutic Use(s)
Alfalfa (*Medicago sativa* L.)	Skin damage from radiation
Aloe (*Aloe vera*)	Skin protection during radiation therapy
Bladderwrack (*Fucus vesiculosus*)	Radiation protection
Danshen (*Salvia miltiorrhiza*)	Radiation-induced lung damage
Ginseng (American ginseng, Asian ginseng, Chinese ginseng, Korean red ginseng, *Panax ginseng*: *Panax* spp. including *P. ginseng* C.C. Meyer and *P. quinquefolium* L., excluding *Eleutherococcus senticosus*)	Recovery from radiation
Milk thistle (*Silybum marianum*), silymarin	Radiation sickness
Psyllium (*Plantago ovata*, *P. ispaghula*)	Radiation-induced colitis/diarrhea
Seaweed, kelp, bladderwrack (*Fucus vesiculosus*)	Radiation protection
Spirulina	Radiation sickness

Continued

RETINOPATHY AND RELATED CONDITIONS

Levels of Scientific Evidence for Specific Therapies

GRADE: C (Unclear or Conflicting Scientific Evidence)	
Therapy	Specific Therapeutic Use(s)
Bilberry (*Vaccinium myrtillus*)	Retinopathy

TRADITIONAL OR THEORETICAL USES THAT LACK SUFFICIENT EVIDENCE	
Therapy	Specific Therapeutic Use(s)
Ginkgo (*Ginkgo biloba* L.)	Diabetic eye disease
Shark cartilage	Diabetic retinopathy

RHEUMATOID ARTHRITIS AND RELATED CONDITIONS

Levels of Scientific Evidence for Specific Therapies

GRADE: B (GOOD SCIENTIFIC EVIDENCE)	
Therapy	Specific Therapeutic Use(s)
Omega-3 fatty acids, fish oil, alpha-linolenic acid	Rheumatoid arthritis (fish oil)

GRADE: C (Unclear or Conflicting Scientific Evidence)	
Therapy	Specific Therapeutic Use(s)
Boswellia (*Boswellia serrata* Roxb.)	Rheumatoid arthritis
Bromelain	Rheumatoid arthritis
Dehydroepiandrosterone (DHEA)	Systemic lupus erythematosus
Dong quai (*Angelica sinensis* [Oliv.] Diels), Chinese angelica	Arthritis
Evening primrose oil (*Oenothera biennis* L.)	Rheumatoid arthritis
Feverfew (*Tanacetum parthenium* L. Schultz-Bip.)	Rheumatoid arthritis
Ginger (*Zingiber officinale* Roscoe)	Rheumatic diseases (rheumatoid arthritis, osteoarthritis, arthralgias, muscle pain)
Glucosamine	Rheumatoid arthritis

Green tea (*Camellia sinensis*)	Arthritis
Guggul (*Commifora mukul*)	Rheumatoid arthritis
Omega-3 fatty acids, fish oil, alpha-linolenic acid	Lupus erythematosus
Propolis	Rheumatic diseases
Shark cartilage	Inflammatory joint diseases (rheumatoid arthritis, osteoarthritis)
Turmeric (*Curcuma longa* L.), curcumin	Rheumatoid arthritis

TRADITIONAL OR THEORETICAL USES THAT LACK SUFFICIENT EVIDENCE

Therapy	Specific Therapeutic Use(s)
Alfalfa (*Medicago sativa* L.)	Rheumatoid arthritis
Aloe (*Aloe vera*)	Arthritis
Aloe (*Aloe vera*)	Lupus erythematosus
Astragalus (*Astragalus membranaceus*)	Ankylosing spondylitis
Astragalus (*Astragalus membranaceus*)	Systemic lupus erythematosus
Belladonna (*Atropa belladonna* L. or its variety *A. acuminata* Royle ex Lindl)	Arthritis
Bilberry (*Vaccinium myrtillus*)	Arthritis
Bladderwrack (*Fucus vesiculosus*)	Arthritis
Bladderwrack (*Fucus vesiculosus*)	Rheumatism
Boron	Rheumatoid arthritis
Bromelain	Autoimmune disorders
Burdock (*Arctium lappa*)	Arthritis
Burdock (*Arctium lappa*)	Rheumatoid arthritis
Chamomile (*Matricaria recutita*, *Chamaemelum nobile*)	Arthritis
Chaparral (*Larrea tridentata* DC. Coville, *L. divaricata* Cav.), nordihydroguaiaretic acid (NDGA)	Arthritis
Chaparral (*Larrea tridentata* DC. Coville, *L. divaricata* Cav.), nordihydroguaiaretic acid (NDGA)	Rheumatic diseases
Dandelion (*Taraxacum officinale*)	Arthritis
Dandelion (*Taraxacum officinale*)	Rheumatoid arthritis

Continued

Devil's claw (*Harpagophytum procumbens* DC.)	Rheumatoid arthritis
Dehydroepiandrosterone (DHEA)	Rheumatic diseases
Dong quai (*Angelica sinensis* [Oliv.] Diels), Chinese angelica	Chilblains
Dong quai (*Angelica sinensis* [Oliv.] Diels), Chinese angelica	Rheumatic diseases
Echinacea (*Echinacea angustifolia* DC., *E. pallida*, *E. purpurea*)	Rheumatism
Essiac	Arthritis
Essiac	Systemic lupus erythematosus
Eucalyptus oil (*Eucalyptus globulus* Labillardiere, *E. fructicetorum* F. Von Mueller, *E. smithii* R.T. Baker)	Arthritis
Eucalyptus oil (*Eucalyptus globulus* Labillardiere, *E. fructicetorum* F. Von Mueller, *E. smithii* R.T. Baker)	Rheumatoid arthritis (applied to the skin)
Evening primrose oil (*Oenothera biennis* L.)	Systemic lupus erythematosus
Flaxseed and flaxseed oil (*Linum usitatissimum*)	Rheumatoid arthritis
Garlic (*Allium sativum* L.)	Arthritis
Globe artichoke (*Cynara scolymus* L.)	Arthritis
Globe artichoke (*Cynara scolymus* L.)	Rheumatoid arthritis
Goldenseal (*Hydrastis canadensis* L.), berberine	Arthritis
Goldenseal (*Hydrastis canadensis* L.), berberine	Lupus
Gotu kola (*Centella asiatica* L.), total triterpenic fraction of Centella asiatica (TTFCA)	Rheumatism
Gotu kola (*Centella asiatica* L.), total triterpenic fraction of *Centella asiatica* (TTFCA)	Systemic lupus erythematosus
Gymnema (*Gymnema sylvestre* R. Br.)	Rheumatoid arthritis
Hops (*Humulus lupulus* L.)	Rheumatic disorders
Horse chestnut (*Aesculus hippocastanum* L.)	Rheumatism
Horse chestnut (*Aesculus hippocastanum* L.)	Rheumatoid arthritis
Horsetail (*Equisetum arvense* L.)	Rheumatism
Kava (*Piper methysticum* G. Forst)	Arthritis
Lavender (*Lavandula angustifolia* Miller)	Rheumatism

Licorice (*Glycyrrhiza glabra* L.), deglycyrrhizinated licorice (DGL)	Rheumatoid arthritis
Lycopene	Inflammatory conditions
Maitake mushroom (*Grifola frondosa*), beta-glucan	Arthritis
Marshmallow (*Althaea officinalis* L.)	Arthritis
Marshmallow (*Althaea officinalis* L.)	Chilblains
Melatonin	Rheumatoid arthritis
Niacin (vitamin B_3, nicotinic acid), niacinamide, inositol hexanicotinate	Arthritis
Omega-3 fatty acids, fish oil, alpha-linolenic acid	Dermatomyositis
Omega-3 fatty acids, fish oil, alpha-linolenic acid	Systemic lupus erythematosus
Peppermint (*Mentha* x *piperita* L.)	Arthritis
Peppermint (*Mentha* x *piperita* L.)	Rheumatic pain
Polypodium leucotomos extract, Anapsos	Autoimmune diseases
Polypodium leucotomos extract, Anapsos	Rheumatic diseases
Propolis	Rheumatoid arthritis
Red clover (*Trifolium pratense*)	Arthritis
Seaweed, kelp, bladderwrack (*Fucus vesiculosus*)	Arthritis
Seaweed, kelp, bladderwrack (*Fucus vesiculosus*)	Rheumatism
Shark cartilage	Ankylosing spondylitis
Shark cartilage	Systemic lupus erythematosus
Slippery elm (*Ulmus rubra* Muhl. or *U. fulva* Michx.)	Rheumatic disorders
Soy (*Glycine max* L. Merr.)	Autoimmune diseases
Soy (*Glycine max* L. Merr.)	Rheumatoid arthritis
St. John's wort (*Hypericum perforatum* L.)	Rheumatism
Thyme (*Thymus vulgaris* L.), thymol	Arthritis
Thyme (*Thymus vulgaris* L.), thymol	Dermatomyositis
Thyme (*Thymus vulgaris* L.), thymol	Rheumatism
Valerian (*Valeriana officinalis* L.)	Arthritis
Valerian (*Valeriana officinalis* L.)	Rheumatic pain
Wild yam (*Dioscorea villosa*)	Rheumatic pain

SCHIZOPHRENIA AND RELATED CONDITIONS

Levels of Scientific Evidence for Specific Therapies

GRADE: C (Unclear or Conflicting Scientific Evidence)

Therapy	Specific Therapeutic Use(s)
Betel nut (*Areca catechu* L.)	Schizophrenia
Dehydroepiandrosterone (DHEA)	Schizophrenia
Melatonin	Schizophrenia (sleep disorders)
Omega-3 fatty acids, fish oil, alpha-linolenic acid	Schizophrenia

GRADE: D (Fair Negative Scientific Evidence)

Therapy	Specific Therapeutic Use(s)
Evening primrose oil (*Oenothera biennis* L.)	Schizophrenia

TRADITIONAL OR THEORETICAL USES THAT LACK SUFFICIENT EVIDENCE

Therapy	Specific Therapeutic Use(s)
American pennyroyal (*Hedeoma pulegioides* L.), European pennyroyal (*Mentha pulegium* L.)	Hallucinations
Chaparral (*Larrea tridentata* DC. Coville, *L. divaricata* Cav.), nordihydroguaiaretic acid (NDGA)	Hallucinations (including those due to LSD ingestion)
Coenzyme Q10	Psychiatric disorders
Ginkgo (*Ginkgo biloba* L.)	Schizophrenia
Ginseng (American ginseng, Asian ginseng, Chinese ginseng, Korean red ginseng, *Panax ginseng*: *Panax* spp. including *P. ginseng* C.C. Meyer and *P. quinquefolium* L., excluding *Eleutherococcus senticosus*)	Psychoasthenia
Gotu kola (*Centella asiatica* L.), total triterpenic fraction of *Centella asiatica* (TTFCA)	Mental disorders
Kava (*Piper methysticum* G. Forst)	Antipsychotic
Lavender (*Lavandula angustifolia* Miller)	Psychosis
Niacin (vitamin B_3, nicotinic acid), niacinamide, inositol hexanicotinate	Diagnostic test for schizophrenia
Niacin (vitamin B_3, nicotinic acid), niacinamide, inositol hexanicotinate	Drug-induced hallucinations

Niacin (vitamin B_3, nicotinic acid), niacinamide, inositol hexanicotinate	Psychosis
Niacin (vitamin B_3, nicotinic acid), niacinamide, inositol hexanicotinate	Schizophrenia
Oleander (*Nerium oleander*, *Thevetia peruviana*)	Psychiatric disorders
Pygeum (*Prunus africana*, *Pygeum africanum*)	Psychosis
Yohimbe bark extract (*Pausinystalia yohimbe* Pierre ex Beille)	Hallucinogenic
Yohimbe bark extract (*Pausinystalia yohimbe* Pierre ex Beille)	Schizophrenia

SEASICKNESS AND RELATED CONDITIONS

Levels of Scientific Evidence for Specific Therapies

GRADE: B (Good Scientific Evidence)

Therapy	Specific Therapeutic Use(s)
Ginger (*Zingiber officinale* Roscoe)	Nausea (due to chemotherapy)
Ginger (*Zingiber officinale* Roscoe)	Nausea and vomiting of pregnancy (hyperemesis gravidarum)

GRADE: C (Unclear or Conflicting Scientific Evidence)

Therapy	Specific Therapeutic Use(s)
Ginger (*Zingiber officinale* Roscoe)	Nausea and vomiting (after surgery)
Peppermint (*Mentha* x *piperita* L.)	Nausea

TRADITIONAL OR THEORETICAL USES THAT LACK SUFFICIENT EVIDENCE

Therapy	Specific Therapeutic Use(s)
Belladonna (*Atropa belladonna* L. or its variety *A. acuminata* Royle ex Lindl)	Motion sickness
Belladonna (*Atropa belladonna* L. or its variety *A. acuminata* Royle ex Lindl)	Nausea and vomiting during pregnancy
Black tea (*Camellia sinensis*)	Vomiting
Calendula (*Calendula officinalis* L.), marigold	Nausea

Continued

Chamomile (*Matricaria recutita*, *Chamaemelum nobile*)	Motion sickness
Chamomile (*Matricaria recutita*, *Chamaemelum nobile*)	Nausea
Chamomile (*Matricaria recutita*, *Chamaemelum nobile*)	Sea sickness
Chaparral (*Larrea tridentata* DC. Coville, *L. divaricata* Cav.), nordihydroguaiaretic acid (NDGA)	Vomiting
Clay	Vomiting
Clay	Vomiting/nausea during pregnancy
Clove (*Eugenia aromatica*)	Nausea or vomiting
Cranberry (*Vaccinium macrocarpon*)	Vomiting
Elder (*Sambucus nigra* L.)	Vomiting
Globe artichoke (*Cynara scolymus* L.)	Emesis
Lavender (*Lavandula angustifolia* Miller)	Motion sickness
Lavender (*Lavandula angustifolia* Miller)	Nausea
Lavender (*Lavandula angustifolia* Miller)	Vomiting
Marshmallow (*Althaea officinalis* L.)	Vomiting
Niacin (vitamin B_3, nicotinic acid), niacinamide, inositol hexanicotinate	Motion sickness
Oleander (*Nerium oleander*, *Thevetia peruviana*)	Vomiting
Valerian (*Valeriana officinalis* L.)	Nausea
White horehound (*Marrubium vulgare* L.)	Emetic
Wild yam (*Dioscorea villosa*)	E.metic

SEDATION AND RELATED CONDITIONS

Levels of Scientific Evidence for Specific Therapies

GRADE: C (UNCLEAR OR CONFLICTING SCIENTIFIC EVIDENCE)

Therapy	Specific Therapeutic Use(s)
Chamomile (*Matricaria recutita*, *Chamaemelum nobile*)	Sleep aid/sedation
Hops (*Humulus lupulus* L.)	Sedation
Lavender (*Lavandula angustifolia* Miller)	Hypnotic/sleep aid (lavender)

Melatonin	Preoperative sedation/ anxiolysis
Passionflower (*Passiflora incarnata* L.)	Sedation (agitation, anxiety, insomnia)

GRADE: D (Fair Negative Scientific Evidence)

Therapy	Specific Therapeutic Use(s)
Valerian (*Valeriana officinalis* L.)	Sedation

TRADITIONAL OR THEORETICAL USES THAT LACK SUFFICIENT EVIDENCE

Therapy	Specific Therapeutic Use(s)
American pennyroyal (*Hedeoma pulegioides* L.), European pennyroyal (*Mentha pulegium* L.)	Sedative
Belladonna (*Atropa belladonna* L. or its variety *A. acuminata* Royle ex Lindl)	Sedative
Devil's claw (*Harpagophytum procumbens* DC.)	Sedative
Dong quai (*Angelica sinensis* [Oliv.] Diels), Chinese angelica	Sedative
Elder (*Sambucus nigra* L.)	Sedative
Feverfew (*Tanacetum parthenium* L. Schultz-Bip.)	Tranquilizer
Garlic (*Allium sativum* L.)	Sedative
Ginseng (American ginseng, Asian ginseng, Chinese ginseng, Korean red ginseng, *Panax ginseng*: *Panax* spp. including *P. ginseng* C.C. Meyer and *P. quinquefolium* L., excluding *Eleutherococcus senticosus*)	Sedative
Goldenseal (*Hydrastis canadensis* L.), berberine	Sedative
Melatonin	Sedation
Niacin (vitamin B_3, nicotinic acid), niacinamide, inositol hexanicotinate	Sedative
Saw palmetto (*Serenoa repens* [Bartram] Small)	Sedation

SEIZURE DISORDER AND RELATED CONDITIONS

Levels of Scientific Evidence for Specific Therapies

GRADE: C (Unclear or Conflicting Scientific Evidence)

Therapy	Specific Therapeutic Use(s)
Melatonin	Seizure disorder (children)

TRADITIONAL OR THEORETICAL USES THAT LACK SUFFICIENT EVIDENCE

Therapy	Specific Therapeutic Use(s)
Chamomile (*Matricaria recutita*, *Chamaemelum nobile*)	Convulsions
Chamomile (*Matricaria recutita*, *Chamaemelum nobile*)	Seizure disorder
Elder (*Sambucus nigra* L.)	Epilepsy
Eyebright (*Euphrasia officinalis*)	Epilepsy
Ginseng (American ginseng, Asian ginseng, Chinese ginseng, Korean red ginseng, *Panax ginseng*: *Panax* spp. *including P. ginseng* C.C. Meyer and *P. quinquefolium* L., excluding *Eleutherococcus senticosus*)	Convulsions
Gotu kola (*Centella asiatica* L.), total triterpenic fraction of *Centella asiatica* (TTFCA)	Epilepsy
Kava (*Piper methysticum* G. Forst)	Seizures
Lavender (*Lavandula angustifolia* Miller)	Anticonvulsant
Niacin (vitamin B_3, nicotinic acid), niacinamide, inositol hexanicotinate	Seizure
Oleander (*Nerium oleander*, *Thevetia peruviana*)	Epilepsy (seizure)
Passionflower (*Passiflora incarnata* L.)	Anticonvulsant
Passionflower (*Passiflora incarnata* L.)	Generalized seizures
Thyme (*Thymus vulgaris* L.), thymol	Epilepsy
Turmeric (*Curcuma longa* L.), curcumin	Epilepsy
Valerian (*Valeriana officinalis* L.)	Anticonvulsive
Valerian (*Valeriana officinalis* L.)	Convulsions

SEXUAL DYSFUNCTION AND RELATED CONDITIONS

Levels of Scientific Evidence for Specific Therapies

GRADE: C (Unclear or Conflicting Scientific Evidence)

Therapy	Specific Therapeutic Use(s)
Arginine (L-arginine)	Erectile dysfunction
Clove (*Eugenia aromatica*)	Premature ejaculation
Dehydroepiandrosterone (DHEA)	Sexual function/libido/erectile dysfunction
Ephedra (*Ephedra sinica*)/ma huang	Sexual arousal
Ginkgo (*Ginkgo biloba* L.)	Decreased libido and erectile dysfunction (impotence)
Ginseng (American ginseng, Asian ginseng, Chinese ginseng, Korean red ginseng, *Panax ginseng*: *Panax* spp. including *P. ginseng* C.C. Meyer and *P. quinquefolium* L., excluding *Eleutherococcus senticosus*)	Erectile dysfunction
Yohimbe bark extract (*Pausinystalia yohimbe* Pierre ex Beille)	Erectile dysfunction (male impotence)
Yohimbe bark extract (*Pausinystalia yohimbe* Pierre ex Beille)	Libido (women)
Yohimbe bark extract (*Pausinystalia yohimbe* Pierre ex Beille)	Sexual side effects of selective serotonin reuptake inhibitor (SSRI) antidepressants
Yohimbe bark extract (*Pausinystalia yohimbe* Pierre ex Beille)	Male erectile dysfunction

TRADITIONAL OR THEORETICAL USES THAT LACK SUFFICIENT EVIDENCE

Therapy	Specific Therapeutic Use(s)
Betel nut (*Areca catechu* L.)	Aphrodisiac
Betel nut (*Areca catechu* L.)	Impotence
Black cohosh (*Cimicifuga racemosa* L. Nutt.)	Aphrodisiac
Burdock (*Arctium lappa*)	Aphrodisiac
Burdock (*Arctium lappa*)	Impotence
Fenugreek (*Trigonella foenum-graecum* L.)	Impotence

Continued

Garlic (*Allium sativum* L.)	Aphrodisiac
Ginger (*Zingiber officinale* Roscoe)	Aphrodisiac
Ginger (*Zingiber officinale* Roscoe)	Impotence
Ginseng (American ginseng, Asian ginseng, Chinese ginseng, Korean red ginseng, *Panax ginseng*: *Panax* spp. including *P. ginseng* C.C. Meyer and *P. quinquefolium* L., excluding *Eleutherococcus senticosus*)	Aphrodisiac
Ginseng (American ginseng, Asian ginseng, Chinese ginseng, Korean red ginseng, *Panax ginseng*: *Panax* spp. including *P. ginseng* C.C. Meyer and *P. quinquefolium* L., excluding *Eleutherococcus senticosus*)	Premature ejaculation
Ginseng (American ginseng, Asian ginseng, Chinese ginseng, Korean red ginseng, *Panax ginseng*: *Panax* spp. including *P. ginseng* C.C. Meyer and P. *quinquefolium* L., excluding *Eleutherococcus senticosus*)	Sexual arousal
Ginseng (American ginseng, Asian ginseng, Chinese ginseng, Korean red ginseng, *Panax ginseng*: *Panax* spp. including *P. ginseng* C.C. Meyer and *P. quinquefolium* L., excluding *Eleutherococcus senticosus*)	Sexual symptoms
Gotu kola (*Centella asiatica* L.), total triterpenic fraction of *Centella asiatica* (TTFCA)	Aphrodisiac
Gotu kola (*Centella asiatica* L.), total triterpenic fraction of *Centella asiatica* (TTFCA)	Libido
Gymnema (*Gymnema sylvestre* R. Br.)	Aphrodisiac
Hops (*Humulus lupulus* L.)	Aphrodisiac
Kava (*Piper methysticum* G. Forst)	Aphrodisiac
Lavender (*Lavandula angustifolia* Miller)	Aphrodisiac
Marshmallow (*Althaea officinalis* L.)	Aphrodisiac
Marshmallow (*Althaea officinalis* L.)	Impotence
Melatonin	Erectile dysfunction
Melatonin	Sexual activity enhancement
Niacin (vitamin B_3, nicotinic acid), niacinamide, inositol hexanicotinate	Orgasm improvement
Pygeum (*Prunus africana*, *Pygeum africanum*)	Aphrodisiac

Pygeum (*Prunus africana*, *Pygeum africanum*)	Impotence
Pygeum (*Prunus africana*, *Pygeum africanum*)	Sexual performance
Saw palmetto (*Serenoa repens* [Bartram] Small)	Aphrodisiac
Saw palmetto (*Serenoa repens* [Bartram] Small)	Impotence
Saw palmetto (*Serenoa repens* [Bartram] Small)	Sexual vigor
Sweet almond (*Prunus amygdalus dulcis*)	Aphrodisiac
Wild yam (*Dioscorea villosa*)	Libido
Yohimbe bark extract (*Pausinystalia yohimbe* Pierre ex Beille)	Aphrodisiac

SKIN CONDITIONS/RASH AND RELATED CONDITIONS

Levels of Scientific Evidence for Specific Therapies

GRADE: B (Good Scientific Evidence)

Therapy	Specific Therapeutic Use(s)
Aloe (*Aloe vera*)	Psoriasis vulgaris
Aloe (*Aloe vera*)	Seborrheic dermatitis (seborrhea, dandruff)
Evening primrose oil (*Oenothera biennis* L.)	Eczema (children and adults)
Evening primrose oil (*Oenothera biennis* L.)	Skin irritation (atopic dermatitis in children and adults)

GRADE: C (Unclear or Conflicting Scientific Evidence)

Therapy	Specific Therapeutic Use(s)
Calendula (*Calendula officinalis* L.), marigold	Skin inflammation
Chamomile (*Matricaria recutita*, *Chamaemelum nobile*)	Skin conditions (eczema/radiation damage/wound healing)
Evening primrose oil (*Oenothera biennis* L.)	Scalelike dry skin (ichthyosis vulgaris)
Marshmallow (*Althaea officinalis* L.)	Inflammatory skin conditions (eczema, psoriasis)
Omega-3 fatty acids, fish oil, alpha-linolenic acid	Eczema

Continued

Omega-3 fatty acids, fish oil, alpha-linolenic acid	Psoriasis
Polypodium leucotomos extract, Anapsos	Atopic dermatitis
Polypodium leucotomos extract, Anapsos	Psoriasis
Shark cartilage	Psoriasis
Thyme (*Thymus vulgaris* L.), thymol	Inflammatory skin disorders

GRADE: D (Fair Negative Scientific Evidence)

Therapy	Specific Therapeutic Use(s)
Boron	Psoriasis (boric acid ointment)
Evening primrose oil (*Oenothera biennis* L.)	Psoriasis

TRADITIONAL OR THEORETICAL USES THAT LACK SUFFICIENT EVIDENCE

Therapy	Specific Therapeutic Use(s)
Belladonna (*Atropa belladonna* L. or its variety *A. acuminata* Royle ex Lindl)	Rash
Belladonna (*Atropa belladonna* L. or its variety *A. acuminata* Royle ex Lindl)	Warts
Betel nut (*Areca catechu* L.)	Dermatitis (used on the skin)
Bilberry (*Vaccinium myrtillus*)	Dermatitis
Bitter melon (*Momordica charantia* L.) and MAP30	Psoriasis
Bladderwrack (*Fucus vesiculosus*)	Eczema
Bladderwrack (*Fucus vesiculosus*)	Psoriasis
Boron	Diaper rash (avoid because of case reports of death in infants from absorbing boron through skin or when taken by mouth)
Burdock (*Arctium lappa*)	Eczema
Burdock (*Arctium lappa*)	Ichthyosis (skin disorder)
Burdock (*Arctium lappa*)	Psoriasis
Burdock (*Arctium lappa*)	Skin disorders
Burdock (*Arctium lappa*)	Skin moisturizer
Burdock (*Arctium lappa*)	Warts
Calendula (*Calendula officinalis* L.), marigold	Diaper rash

Calendula (*Calendula officinalis* L.), marigold	Eczema
Calendula (*Calendula officinalis* L.), marigold	Warts
Chamomile (*Matricaria recutita*, *Chamaemelum nobile*)	Contact dermatitis
Chamomile (*Matricaria recutita*, *Chamaemelum nobile*)	Diaper rash
Chamomile (*Matricaria recutita*, *Chamaemelum nobile*)	Impetigo
Chamomile (*Matricaria recutita*, *Chamaemelum nobile*)	Psoriasis
Chaparral (*Larrea tridentata* DC. Coville, *L. divaricata* Cav.), nordihydroguaiaretic acid (NDGA)	Skin disorders
Dandelion (*Taraxacum officinale*)	Age spots
Dandelion (*Taraxacum officinale*)	Psoriasis
Dandelion (*Taraxacum officinale*)	Skin conditions
Dandelion (*Taraxacum officinale*)	Warts
Danshen (*Salvia miltiorrhiza*)	Eczema
Danshen (*Salvia miltiorrhiza*)	Psoriasis
Dehydroepiandrosterone (DHEA)	Psoriasis
Dong quai (*Angelica sinensis* [Oliv.] Diels), Chinese angelica	Dermatitis
Dong quai (*Angelica sinensis* [Oliv.] Diels), Chinese angelica	Eczema
Dong quai (*Angelica sinensis* [Oliv.] Diels), Chinese angelica	Psoriasis
Dong quai (*Angelica sinensis* [Oliv.] Diels), Chinese angelica	Skin pigmentation disorders
Echinacea (*Echinacea angustifolia* DC., *E. pallida*, *E. purpurea*)	Eczema
Echinacea (*Echinacea angustifolia* DC., *E. pallida*, *E. purpurea*)	Psoriasis
Elder (*Sambucus nigra* L.)	Psoriasis
Evening primrose pil (*Oenothera biennis* L.)	Skin conditions due to kidney failure in dialysis patients
Eyebright (*Euphrasia officinalis*)	Skin conditions
Fenugreek (*Trigonella foenum-graecum* L.)	Dermatitis
Fenugreek (*Trigonella foenum-graecum* L.)	Eczema

Continued

Feverfew (*Tanacetum parthenium* L. Schultz-Bip.)	Rash
Flaxseed and flaxseed oil (*Linum usitatissimum*)	Eczema
Flaxseed and flaxseed oil (*Linum usitatissimum*)	Psoriasis
Flaxseed and flaxseed oil (*Linum usitatissimum*)	Skin inflammation
Garlic (*Allium sativum* L.)	Psoriasis
Garlic (*Allium sativum* L.)	Warts
Ginger (*Zingiber officinale* Roscoe)	Psoriasis (topical)
Ginkgo (*Ginkgo biloba* L.)	Dermatitis
Ginkgo (*Ginkgo biloba* L.)	Eczema
Globe artichoke (*Cynara scolymus* L.)	Eczema
Glucosamine	Psoriasis
Goldenseal (*Hydrastis canadensis* L.), berberine	Eczema
Goldenseal (*Hydrastis canadensis* L.), berberine	Impetigo
Goldenseal (*Hydrastis canadensis* L.), berberine	Psoriasis
Goldenseal (*Hydrastis canadensis* L.), berberine	Seborrhea
Gotu kola (*Centella asiatica* L.), total triterpenic fraction of *Centella asiatica* (TTFCA)	Eczema
Gotu kola (*Centella asiatica* L.), total triterpenic fraction of *Centella asiatica* (TTFCA)	Skin diseases
Guggul (*Commifora mukul*)	Psoriasis
Hops (*Humulus lupulus* L.)	Dermatitis
Horse chestnut (*Aesculus hippocastanum* L.)	Skin conditions
Lactobacillus acidophilus	Diaper rash
Licorice (*Glycyrrhiza glabra* L.), deglycyrrhizinated licorice (DGL)	Eczema
Licorice (*Glycyrrhiza glabra* L.), deglycyrrhizinated licorice (DGL)	Inflammatory skin disorders
Licorice (*Glycyrrhiza glabra* L.), deglycyrrhizinated licorice (DGL)	Skin disorders
Marshmallow (*Althaea officinalis* L.)	Dermatitis (topical)
Melatonin	Hyperpigmentation

Milk thistle (*Silybum marianum*), silymarin	Psoriasis
Niacin (vitamin B_3, nicotinic acid), niacinamide, inositol hexanicotinate	Psoriasis
Niacin (vitamin B_3, nicotinic acid), niacinamide, inositol hexanicotinate	Skin disorders
Oleander (*Nerium oleander*, *Thevetia peruviana*)	Corns
Oleander (*Nerium oleander*, *Thevetia peruviana*)	Skin diseases
Oleander (*Nerium oleander*, *Thevetia peruviana*)	Skin eruptions
Oleander (*Nerium oleander*, *Thevetia peruviana*)	Warts
Polypodium leucotomos extract, Anapsos	Vitiligo (loss of pigment in the skin)
Propolis	Dermatitis
Propolis	Eczema
Propolis	Psoriasis
Psyllium (*Plantago ovata*, *P. ispaghula*)	Psoriasis
Red clover (*Trifolium pratense*)	Eczema
Red clover (*Trifolium pratense*)	Psoriasis
Seaweed, kelp, bladderwrack (*Fucus vesiculosus*)	Eczema
Seaweed, kelp, bladderwrack (*Fucus vesiculosus*)	Psoriasis
Shark cartilage	Contact dermatitis
Sorrel (*Rumex acetosa* L., *R. acetosella* L.), Sinupret	Nettle rash
Spirulina	Skin disorders
Spirulina	Warts
Tea tree oil (*Melaleuca alternifolia* [Maiden & Betche] Cheel)	Corns
Tea tree oil (*Melaleuca alternifolia* [Maiden & Betche] Cheel)	Eczema
Tea tree oil (*Melaleuca alternifolia* [Maiden & Betche] Cheel)	Impetigo
Tea tree oil (*Melaleuca alternifolia* [Maiden & Betche] Cheel)	Psoriasis
Tea tree oil (*Melaleuca alternifolia* [Maiden & Betche] Cheel)	Skin ailments

Continued

Tea tree oil (*Melaleuca alternifolia* [Maiden & Betche] Cheel)	Warts
Thyme (*Thymus vulgaris* L.), thymol	Dermatitis
Thyme (*Thymus vulgaris* L.), thymol	Eczema
Thyme (*Thymus vulgaris* L.), thymol	Warts
White horehound (*Marrubium vulgare* L.)	Skin conditions
White horehound (*Marrubium vulgare* L.)	Warts
Wild yam (*Dioscorea villosa*)	Rash

SLEEP DISORDERS/INSOMNIA/JET LAG AND RELATED CONDITIONS

Levels of Scientific Evidence for Specific Therapies

GRADE: A (Strong Scientific Evidence)

Therapy	Specific Therapeutic Use(s)
Melatonin	Jet lag

GRADE: B (Good Scientific Evidence)

Therapy	Specific Therapeutic Use(s)
Melatonin	Delayed sleep phase syndrome (DSPS)
Melatonin	Insomnia in the elderly
Melatonin	Sleep disturbances in children with neuropsychiatric disorders
Melatonin	Sleep enhancement in healthy people
Valerian (*Valeriana officinalis* L.)	Insomnia

GRADE: C (Unclear or Conflicting Scientific Evidence)

Therapy	Specific Therapeutic Use(s)
Hops (*Humulus lupulus* L.)	Insomnia/sleep quality
Lavender (*Lavandula angustifolia* Miller)	Hypnotic/sleep
Melatonin	Circadian rhythm entraining (in blind persons)

Melatonin	Insomnia (of unknown origin in the nonelderly)
Melatonin	Rapid eye movement (REM) sleep behavior disorder
Melatonin	Sleep disturbances due to pineal region brain damage
Melatonin	Work shift sleep disorder

TRADITIONAL OR THEORETICAL USES THAT LACK SUFFICIENT EVIDENCE

Therapy	Specific Therapeutic Use(s)
Astragalus (*Astragalus membranaceus*)	Insomnia
Black cohosh (*Cimicifuga racemosa* L. Nutt.)	Sleep disorders
Calendula (*Calendula officinalis* L.), marigold	Insomnia
Coenzyme Q10	Insomnia
Danshen (*Salvia miltiorrhiza*)	Sleep difficulties
Danshen (*Salvia miltiorrhiza*)	Stimulation of gamma-aminobutyric acid (GABA) release
Dehydroepiandrosterone (DHEA)	Sleep disorders
Elder (*Sambucus nigra* L.)	Insomnia
Eucalyptus oil (*Eucalyptus globulus* Labillardiere, *E. fructicetorum* F. Von Mueller, *E. smithii* R.T. Baker)	Snoring
Ginkgo (*Ginkgo biloba* L.)	Insomnia
Ginseng (American ginseng, Asian ginseng, Chinese ginseng, Korean red ginseng, *Panax ginseng*: *Panax* spp. including *P. ginseng* C.C. Meyer and *P. quinquefolium* L., excluding *Eleutherococcus senticosus*)	Insomnia
Hawthorn (*Crataegus laevigata*, *C. oxyacantha*, *C. monogyna*, *C. pentagyna*)	Insomnia
Kava (Piper methysticum G. Forst)	Jet lag
Niacin (vitamin B_3, nicotinic acid), niacinamide, inositol hexanicotinate	Insomnia
Passionflower (*Passiflora incarnata* L.)	Insomnia
St. John's wort (*Hypericum perforatum* L.)	Insomnia

Continued

Thyme (*Thymus vulgaris* L.), thymol	Insomnia
Thyme (*Thymus vulgaris* L.), thymol	Nightmares
Yohimbe bark extract (*Pausinystalia yohimbe* Pierre ex Beille)	Insomnia
Yohimbe bark extract (*Pausinystalia yohimbe* Pierre ex Beille)	Narcolepsy

SNAKE BITES AND RELATED CONDITIONS

Levels of Scientific Evidence for Specific Therapies

TRADITIONAL OR THEORETICAL USES THAT LACK SUFFICIENT EVIDENCE

Therapy	Specific Therapeutic Use(s)
American pennyroyal (*Hedeoma pulegioides* L.), European pennyroyal (*Mentha pulegium* L.)	Snake bites (venomous)
Black cohosh (*Cimicifuga racemosa* L. Nutt.)	Snake bites
Chaparral (*Larrea tridentata* DC. Coville, *L. divaricata* Cav.), nordihydroguaiaretic acid (NDGA)	Snakebite pain
Echinacea (*Echinacea angustifolia* DC., *E. pallida*, *E. purpurea*)	Snake bites
Ginger (*Zingiber officinale* Roscoe)	Poisonous snake bites
Globe artichoke (*Cynara scolymus* L.)	Snake bites
Gotu kola (*Centella asiatica* L.), total triterpenic fraction of *Centella asiatica* (TTFCA)	Antivenom
Gotu kola (*Centella asiatica* L.), total triterpenic fraction of *Centella asiatica* (TTFCA)	Snake bites
Gymnema (*Gymnema sylvestre* R. Br.)	Snake venom antidote
Milk thistle (*Silybum marianum*), silymarin	Snake bites
Oleander (*Nerium oleander*, *Thevetia peruviana*)	Snake bites
St. John's wort (*Hypericum perforatum* L.)	Snake bites

SPRAINS/STRAINS AND RELATED CONDITIONS

Levels of Scientific Evidence for Specific Therapies

TRADITIONAL OR THEORETICAL USES THAT LACK SUFFICIENT EVIDENCE

Therapy	Specific Therapeutic Use(s)
Bitter almond (*Prunus amygdalus* Batch var. *amara* DC. Focke), Laetrile	Muscle relaxant
Black cohosh (*Cimicifuga racemosa* L. Nutt.)	Muscle spasms
Boswellia (*Boswellia serrata* Roxb.)	Bursitis
Boswellia (*Boswellia serrata* Roxb.)	Tendonitis
Bromelain	Bursitis
Bromelain	Sports or other physical injuries
Bromelain	Tendonitis
Clove (*Eugenia aromatica*)	Muscle spasm
Devil's claw (*Harpagophytum procumbens* DC.)	Tendonitis
Dong quai (*Angelica sinensis* [Oliv.] Diels), Chinese angelica	Muscle relaxant
Eucalyptus oil (*Eucalyptus globulus* Labillardiere, *E. fructicetorum* F. Von Mueller, *E. smithii* R.T. Baker)	Muscle spasm
Eucalyptus oil (*Eucalyptus globulus* Labillardiere, *E. fructicetorum* F. Von Mueller, *E. smithii* R.T. Baker)	Strains/sprains (applied to the skin)
Garlic (*Allium sativum* L.)	Muscle spasms
Goldenseal (*Hydrastis canadensis* L.), berberine	Muscle spasm
Hops (*Humulus lupulus* L.)	Muscle and joint disorders
Hops (*Humulus lupulus* L.)	Muscle spasm
Lavender (*Lavandula angustifolia* Miller)	Muscle spasm
Lavender (*Lavandula angustifolia* Miller)	Sprains
Licorice (*Glycyrrhiza glabra* L.), deglycyrrhizinated licorice (DGL)	Muscle cramps
Marshmallow (*Althaea officinalis* L.)	Sprains
Niacin (vitamin B_3, nicotinic acid), niacinamide, inositol hexanicotinate	Bursitis

Continued

Omega-3 fatty acids, fish oil, alpha-linolenic acid	Tennis elbow
Peppermint (*Mentha* x *piperita* L.)	Tendonitis
Saw palmetto (*Serenoa repens* [Bartram] Small)	Muscle or intestinal spasms
Slippery elm (*Ulmus rubra* Muhl. or *U. fulva* Michx.)	Synovitis
St. John's wort (*Hypericum perforatum* L.)	Sprains
Thyme (*Thymus vulgaris* L.), thymol	Sprains
Valerian (*Valeriana officinalis* L.)	Muscle pain/spasm/tension

STROKE AND RELATED CONDITIONS

Levels of Scientific Evidence for Specific Therapies

GRADE: C (Unclear or Conflicting Scientific Evidence)

Therapy	Specific Therapeutic Use(s)
Betel nut (*Areca catechu* L.)	Stroke recovery
Danshen (*Salvia miltiorrhiza*)	Ischemic stroke
Melatonin	Stroke
Omega-3 fatty acids, fish oil, alpha-linolenic acid	Stroke prevention

GRADE: D (Fair Negative Scientific Evidence)

Therapy	Specific Therapeutic Use(s)
Ginkgo (*Ginkgo biloba* L.)	Stroke

TRADITIONAL OR THEORETICAL USES THAT LACK SUFFICIENT EVIDENCE

Therapy	Specific Therapeutic Use(s)
Arginine (L-arginine)	Ischemic stroke
Arginine (L-arginine)	Stroke
Astragalus (*Astragalus membranaceus*)	Stroke
Dong quai (*Angelica sinensis* [Oliv.] Diels), Chinese angelica	Stroke
Garlic (*Allium sativum* L.)	Stroke

Ginseng (American ginseng, Asian ginseng, Chinese ginseng, Korean red ginseng, *Panax ginseng*: *Panax* spp. including *P. ginseng* C.C. Meyer and *P. quinquefolium* L., excluding *Eleutherococcus senticosus*)	Strokes
Green tea (*Camellia sinensis*)	Ischemia–reperfusion injury protection
Green tea (*Camellia sinensis*)	Stroke prevention
Kava (*Piper methysticum* G. Forst)	Cerebral ischemia
Lycopene	Stroke prevention
Niacin (vitamin B_3, nicotinic acid), niacinamide, inositol hexanicotinate	Ischemia–reperfusion injury prevention

SUNBURN AND RELATED CONDITIONS

Levels of Scientific Evidence for Specific Therapies

GRADE: C (Unclear or Conflicting Scientific Evidence)

Therapy	Specific Therapeutic Use(s)
Green tea (*Camellia sinensis*)	Sun protection

TRADITIONAL OR THEORETICAL USES THAT LACK SUFFICIENT EVIDENCE

Therapy	Specific Therapeutic Use(s)
Aloe (*Aloe vera*)	Sunburn
American pennyroyal (*Hedeoma pulegioides* L.), European pennyroyal (*Mentha pulegium* L.)	Sunstroke
Gotu kola (*Centella asiatica* L.), total triterpenic fraction of *Centella asiatica* (TTFCA)	Sunstroke
Green tea (*Camellia sinensis*)	Sunburn
Peppermint (*Mentha* x *piperita* L.)	Sun block
Polypodium leucotomos extract, Anapsos	Sunburn protection
Propolis	Skin rejuvenant

SYSTEMIC LUPUS ERYTHEMATOSUS (LUPUS) AND RELATED CONDITIONS

Levels of Scientific Evidence for Specific Therapies

GRADE: B (Good Scientific Evidence)

Therapy	Specific Therapeutic Use(s)
Omega-3 fatty acids, fish oil, alpha-linolenic acid	Rheumatoid arthritis (fish oil)

GRADE: C (Unclear or Conflicting Scientific Evidence)

Therapy	Specific Therapeutic Use(s)
Boswellia (*Boswellia serrata* Roxb.)	Rheumatoid arthritis
Bromelain	Rheumatoid arthritis
Dehydroepiandrosterone (DHEA)	Systemic lupus erythematosus
Dong quai (*Angelica sinensis* [Oliv.] Diels), Chinese angelica	Arthritis
Evening primrose oil (*Oenothera biennis* L.)	Rheumatoid arthritis
Feverfew (*Tanacetum parthenium* L. Schultz-Bip.)	Rheumatoid arthritis
Ginger (*Zingiber officinale* Roscoe)	Rheumatic diseases (rheumatoid arthritis, osteoarthritis, arthralgias, muscle pain)
Glucosamine	Rheumatoid arthritis
Green tea (*Camellia sinensis*)	Arthritis
Guggul (*Commifora mukul*)	Rheumatoid arthritis
Omega-3 fatty acids, fish oil, alpha-linolenic acid	Lupus erythematosus
Propolis	Rheumatic diseases
Shark cartilage	Inflammatory joint diseases (rheumatoid arthritis, osteoarthritis)
Turmeric (*Curcuma longa* L.), curcumin	Rheumatoid arthritis

TRADITIONAL OR THEORETICAL USES THAT LACK SUFFICIENT EVIDENCE

Therapy	Specific Therapeutic Use(s)
Alfalfa (*Medicago sativa* L.)	Rheumatoid arthritis
Aloe (*Aloe vera*)	Arthritis

Aloe (*Aloe vera*)	Lupus erythematosus
Astragalus (*Astragalus membranaceus*)	Ankylosing spondylitis
Astragalus (*Astragalus membranaceus*)	Systemic lupus erythematosus
Belladonna (*Atropa belladonna* L. or its variety *A. acuminata* Royle ex Lindl)	Arthritis
Bilberry (*Vaccinium myrtillus*)	Arthritis
Bladderwrack (*Fucus vesiculosus*)	Arthritis
Bladderwrack (*Fucus vesiculosus*)	Rheumatism
Boron	Rheumatoid arthritis
Bromelain	Autoimmune disorders
Burdock (*Arctium lappa*)	Arthritis
Burdock (*Arctium lappa*)	Rheumatoid arthritis
Chamomile (*Matricaria recutita*, *Chamaemelum nobile*)	Arthritis
Chaparral (*Larrea tridentata* DC. Coville, *L. divaricata* Cav.), nordihydroguaiaretic acid (NDGA)	Arthritis
Chaparral (*Larrea tridentata* DC. Coville, *L. divaricata* Cav.), nordihydroguaiaretic acid (NDGA)	Rheumatic diseases
Dandelion (*Taraxacum officinale*)	Arthritis
Dandelion (*Taraxacum officinale*)	Rheumatoid arthritis
Devil's claw (*Harpagophytum procumbens* DC.)	Rheumatoid arthritis
Dehydroepiandrosterone (DHEA)	Rheumatic diseases
Dong quai (*Angelica sinensis* [Oliv.] Diels), Chinese angelica	Chilblains
Dong quai (*Angelica sinensis* [Oliv.] Diels), Chinese angelica	Rheumatic diseases
Echinacea (*Echinacea angustifolia* DC., *E. pallida*, *E. purpurea*)	Rheumatism
Essiac	Arthritis
Essiac	Systemic lupus erythematosus
Eucalyptus oil (*Eucalyptus globulus* Labillardiere, *E. fructicetorum* F. Von Mueller, *E. smithii* R.T. Baker)	Arthritis
Eucalyptus oil (*Eucalyptus globulus* Labillardiere, *E. fructicetorum* F. Von Mueller, *E. smithii* R.T. Baker)	Rheumatoid arthritis (applied to the skin)

Continued

Evening primrose oil (*Oenothera biennis* L.)	Systemic lupus erythematosus
Flaxseed and flaxseed oil (*Linum usitatissimum*)	Rheumatoid arthritis
Garlic (*Allium sativum* L.)	Arthritis
Globe artichoke (*Cynara scolymus* L.)	Arthritis
Globe artichoke (*Cynara scolymus* L.)	Rheumatoid arthritis
Goldenseal (*Hydrastis canadensis* L.), berberine	Arthritis
Goldenseal (*Hydrastis canadensis* L.), berberine	Lupus
Gotu kola (*Centella asiatica* L.), total triterpenic fraction of *Centella asiatica* (TTFCA)	Rheumatism
Gotu kola (*Centella asiatica* L.), total triterpenic fraction of *Centella asiatica* (TTFCA)	Systemic lupus erythematosus
Gymnema (*Gymnema sylvestre* R. Br.)	Rheumatoid arthritis
Hops (*Humulus lupulus* L.)	Rheumatic disorders
Horse chestnut (*Aesculus hippocastanum* L.)	Rheumatism
Horse chestnut (*Aesculus hippocastanum* L.)	Rheumatoid arthritis
Horsetail (*Equisetum arvense* L.)	Rheumatism
Kava (*Piper methysticum* G. Forst)	Arthritis
Lavender (*Lavandula angustifolia* Miller)	Rheumatism
Licorice (*Glycyrrhiza glabra* L.), deglycyrrhizinated licorice (DGL)	Rheumatoid arthritis
Lycopene	Inflammatory conditions
Maitake mushroom (*Grifola frondosa*), beta-glucan	Arthritis
Marshmallow (*Althaea officinalis* L.)	Arthritis
Marshmallow (*Althaea officinalis* L.)	Chilblains
Melatonin	Rheumatoid arthritis
Niacin (vitamin B_3, nicotinic acid), niacinamide, inositol hexanicotinate	Arthritis
Omega-3 fatty acids, fish oil, alpha-linolenic acid	Dermatomyositis
Omega-3 fatty acids, fish oil, alpha-linolenic acid	Systemic lupus erythematosus
Peppermint (*Mentha* x *piperita* L.)	Arthritis

Peppermint (*Mentha* x *piperita* L.)	Rheumatic pain
Polypodium leucotomos extract, Anapsos	Autoimmune diseases
Polypodium leucotomos extract, Anapsos	Rheumatic diseases
Propolis	Rheumatoid arthritis
Red clover (*Trifolium pratense*)	Arthritis
Seaweed, kelp, bladderwrack (*Fucus vesiculosus*)	Arthritis
Seaweed, kelp, bladderwrack (*Fucus vesiculosus*)	Rheumatism
Shark cartilage	Ankylosing spondylitis
Shark cartilage	Systemic lupus erythematosus
Slippery elm (*Ulmus rubra* Muhl. or *U. fulva* Michx.)	Rheumatic disorders
Soy (Glycine max L. Merr.)	Autoimmune diseases
Soy (*Glycine max* L. Merr.)	Rheumatoid arthritis
St. John's wort (*Hypericum perforatum* L.)	Rheumatism
Thyme (*Thymus vulgaris* L.), thymol	Arthritis
Thyme (*Thymus vulgaris* L.), thymol	Dermatomyositis
Thyme (*Thymus vulgaris* L.), thymol	Rheumatism
Valerian (*Valeriana officinalis* L.)	Arthritis
Valerian (*Valeriana officinalis* L.)	Rheumatic pain
Wild yam (*Dioscorea villosa*)	Rheumatic pain

THROMBOCYTOPENIA AND RELATED CONDITIONS

Levels of Scientific Evidence for Specific Therapies

GRADE: C (Unclear or Conflicting Scientific Evidence)

Therapy	Specific Therapeutic Use(s)
Dong quai (*Angelica sinensis* [Oliv.] Diels), Chinese angelica	Idiopathic thrombocytopenic purpura (ITP)
Melatonin	Thrombocytopenia (low platelets)

Continued

TRADITIONAL OR THEORETICAL USES THAT LACK SUFFICIENT EVIDENCE	
Therapy	Specific Therapeutic Use(s)
Astragalus (*Astragalus membranaceus*)	Low platelets
Black cohosh (*Cimicifuga racemosa* L. Nutt.)	Thrombocytopenia
Dong quai (*Angelica sinensis* [Oliv.] Diels), Chinese angelica	Immune cytopenias
Goldenseal (*Hydrastis canadensis* L.), berberine	Thrombocytopenia (low platelets)

THYROID DISORDERS AND RELATED CONDITIONS

Levels of Scientific Evidence for Specific Therapies

GRADE: C (Unclear or Conflicting Scientific Evidence)	
Therapy	Specific Therapeutic Use(s)
Bladderwrack (*Fucus vesiculosus*)	Goiter (thyroid disease)

TRADITIONAL OR THEORETICAL USES THAT LACK SUFFICIENT EVIDENCE	
Therapy	Specific Therapeutic Use(s)
Essiac	Thyroid disorders
Horsetail (*Equisetum arvense* L.)	Thyroid disorders
Niacin (vitamin B_3, nicotinic acid), niacinamide, inositol hexanicotinate	Hypothyroidism
Propolis	Thyroid disease
Seaweed, kelp, bladderwrack (*Fucus vesiculosus*)	Exophthalmos
Seaweed, kelp, bladderwrack (*Fucus vesiculosus*)	Goiter
Seaweed, kelp, bladderwrack (*Fucus vesiculosus*)	Myxedema

TINNITUS AND RELATED CONDITIONS

Levels of Scientific Evidence for Specific Therapies

GRADE: C (UNCLEAR OR CONFLICTING SCIENTIFIC EVIDENCE)	
Therapy	Specific Therapeutic Use(s)
Ginkgo (*Ginkgo biloba* L.)	Ringing in the ears (tinnitus)

TRADITIONAL OR THEORETICAL USES THAT LACK SUFFICIENT EVIDENCE	
Therapy	Specific Therapeutic Use(s)
Black cohosh (*Cimicifuga racemosa* L. Nutt.)	Ringing in the ears
Calendula (*Calendula officinalis* L.), marigold	Ringing in the ears
Dong quai (*Angelica sinensis* [Oliv.] Diels), Chinese angelica	Tinnitus (ringing in the ears)
Feverfew (*Tanacetum parthenium* L. Schultz-Bip.)	Ringing in the ears
Goldenseal (*Hydrastis canadensis* L.), berberine	Tinnitis (ringing in the ears)
Horse chestnut (*Aesculus hippocastanum* L.)	Ringing in the ears (tinnitus)
Melatonin	Tinnitus
Niacin (vitamin B_3, nicotinic acid), niacinamide, inositol hexanicotinate	Ear ringing

ULCERATIVE COLITIS AND RELATED CONDITIONS

Levels of Scientific Evidence for Specific Therapies

GRADE: C (Unclear or Conflicting Scientific Evidence)	
Therapy	Specific Therapeutic Use(s)
Barley (*Hordeum vulgare* L.), germinated barley foodstuff (GBF)	Ulcerative colitis
Betel nut (*Areca catechu* L.)	Ulcerative colitis
Boswellia (*Boswellia serrata* Roxb.)	Ulcerative colitis
Dandelion (*Taraxacum officinale*)	Colitis
Glucosamine	Inflammatory bowel disease
Licorice (*Glycyrrhiza glabra* L.), deglycyrrhizinated licorice (DGL)	Familial Mediterranean fever
Omega-3 fatty acids, fish oil, alpha-linolenic acid	Ulcerative colitis
Psyllium (*Plantago ovata*, *P. ispaghula*)	Inflammatory bowel disease

TRADITIONAL OR THEORETICAL USES THAT LACK SUFFICIENT EVIDENCE	
Therapy	Specific Therapeutic Use(s)
Aloe (*Aloe vera*)	Inflammatory bowel disease
Arginine (L-arginine)	Inflammatory bowel disease

Continued

Barley (*Hordeum vulgare* L.), germinated barley foodstuff (GBF)	Inflammatory bowel disorders
Belladonna (*Atropa belladonna* L. or its variety *A. acuminata* Royle ex Lindl)	Colitis
Belladonna (*Atropa belladonna* L. or its variety *A. acuminata* Royle ex Lindl)	Ulcerative colitis
Bromelain	Colitis
Bromelain	Ulcerative colitis
Calendula (*Calendula officinalis* L.), marigold	Ulcerative colitis
Dehydroepiandrosterone (DHEA)	Ulcerative colitis
Elder (*Sambucas nigra* L.)	Ulcerative colitis
Eucalyptus oil (*Eucalyptus globulus* Labillardiere, *E. fructicetorum* F. Von Mueller, *E. smithii* R.T. Baker)	Inflammatory bowel disease
Evening primrose oil (*Oenothera biennis* L.)	Ulcerative colitis
Flaxseed and flaxseed oil (*Linum usitatissimum*)	Ulcerative colitis
Ginkgo (*Ginkgo biloba* L.)	Ulcerative colitis
Ginseng (American ginseng, Asian ginseng, Chinese ginseng, Korean red ginseng, *Panax ginseng*: *Panax* spp. including *P. ginseng* C.C. Meyer and *P. quinquefolium* L., excluding *Eleutherococcus senticosus)*	Colitis
Glucosamine	Inflammatory bowel disease
Glucosamine	Ulcerative colitis
Goldenseal (*Hydrastis canadensis* L.), berberine	Colitis
Guggul (*Commifora mukul*)	Colitis
Lactobacillus acidophilus	Colitis
Lactobacillus acidophilus	Ulcerative colitis
Licorice (*Glycyrrhiza glabra* L.), deglycyrrhizinated licorice (DGL)	Colitis
Marshmallow (*Althaea officinalis* L.)	Colitis
Marshmallow (*Althaea officinalis* L.)	Inflammation of the small intestine
Marshmallow (*Althaea officinalis* L.)	Ulcerative colitis
Melatonin	Colitis

Propolis	Ulcerative colitis
Slippery elm (*Ulmus rubra* Muhl. or *U. fulva* Michx.)	Colitis
Slippery elm (*Ulmus rubra* Muhl. or *U. fulva* Michx.)	Ulcerative colitis
Spirulina	Colitis
Thyme (*Thymus vulgaris* L.), thymol	Inflammation of the colon

UPPER RESPIRATORY TRACT INFECTION/BRONCHITIS/ COMMON COLD/FLU AND RELATED CONDITIONS

Levels of Scientific Evidence for Specific Therapies

GRADE: B (Good Scientific Evidence)

Therapy	Specific Therapeutic Use(s)
Echinacea (*Echinacea angustifolia* DC., *E. pallida*, *E. purpurea*)	Upper respiratory tract infections: treatment

GRADE: C (Unclear or Conflicting Scientific Evidence)

Therapy	Specific Therapeutic Use(s)
Astragalus (*Astragalus membranaceus*)	Upper respiratory tract infection
Chamomile (*Matricaria recutita*, *Chamaemelum nobile*)	Common cold
Echinacea (*Echinacea angustifolia* DC., *E. pallida*, *E. purpurea*)	Upper respiratory tract infections: prevention
Elder (*Sambucus nigra* L.)	Bronchitis
Elder (*Sambucus nigra* L.)	Influenza
Garlic (*Allium sativum* L.)	Upper respiratory tract infection
Goldenseal (*Hydrastis canadensis* L.), berberine	Common cold/upper respiratory tract infection
Peppermint (*Mentha* x *piperita* L.)	Nasal congestion
Propolis	Prevention of colds
Slippery elm (*Ulmus rubra* Muhl. or *U. fulva* Michx.)	Sore throat
Sorrel (*Rumex acetosa* L., *R. acetosella* L.), Sinupret	Bronchitis

Continued

TRADITIONAL OR THEORETICAL USES THAT LACK SUFFICIENT EVIDENCE	
Therapy	Specific Therapeutic Use(s)
American pennyroyal (*Hedeoma pulegioides* L.), European pennyroyal (*Mentha pulegium* L.)	Chest congestion
American pennyroyal (*Hedeoma pulegioides* L.), European pennyroyal (*Mentha pulegium* L.)	Colds
American pennyroyal (*Hedeoma pulegioides* L.), European pennyroyal (*Mentha pulegium* L.)	Flu
American pennyroyal (*Hedeoma pulegioides* L.), European pennyroyal (*Mentha pulegium* L.)	Respiratory ailments
Arginine (L-arginine)	Cold prevention
Astragalus (*Astragalus membranaceus*)	Bronchitis
Barley (*Hordeum vulgare* L.), germinated barley foodstuff (GBF)	Bronchitis
Belladonna (*Atropa belladonna* L. or its variety *A. acuminata* Royle ex Lindl)	Colds
Belladonna (*Atropa belladonna* L. or its variety *A. acuminata* Royle ex Lindl)	Flu
Belladonna (*Atropa belladonna* L. or its variety *A. acuminata* Royle ex Lindl)	Sore throat
Betel nut (*Areca catechu* L.)	Respiratory stimulant
Bilberry (*Vaccinium myrtillus*)	Common cold
Bilberry (*Vaccinium myrtillus*)	Pharyngitis
Black cohosh (*Cimicifuga racemosa* L. Nutt.)	Bronchitis
Black cohosh (*Cimicifuga racemosa* L. Nutt.)	Sore throat
Black tea (*Camellia sinensis*)	Influenza
Bladderwrack (*Fucus vesiculosus*)	Sore throat
Blessed thistle (*Cnicus benedictus* L.)	Colds
Bromelain	Bronchitis
Bromelain	Common cold
Bromelain	Upper respiratory tract infection
Burdock (*Arctium lappa*)	Common cold

Burdock (*Arctium lappa*)	Respiratory infections
Burdock (*Arctium lappa*)	Tonsillitis
Calendula (*Calendula officinalis* L.), marigold	Influenza
Calendula (*Calendula officinalis* L.), marigold	Sore throat
Chaparral (*Larrea tridentata* DC. Coville, *L. divaricata* Cav.), nordihydroguaiaretic acid (NDGA)	Colds
Chaparral (*Larrea tridentata* DC. Coville, *L. divaricata* Cav.), nordihydroguaiaretic acid (NDGA)	Influenza
Chaparral (*Larrea tridentata* DC. Coville, *L. divaricata* Cav.), nordihydroguaiaretic acid (NDGA)	Respiratory tract infections
Dehydroepiandrosterone (DHEA)	Influenza
Dong quai (*Angelica sinensis* [Oliv.] Diels), Chinese angelica	Bronchitis
Dong quai (*Angelica sinensis* [Oliv.] Diels), Chinese angelica	Respiratory tract infection
Echinacea (*Echinacea angustifolia* DC., *E. pallida*, *E. purpurea*)	Tonsillitis
Elder (*Sambucus nigra* L.)	Colds
Ephedra (*Ephedra sinica*)/ma huang	Colds
Ephedra (*Ephedra sinica*)/ma huang	Flu
Ephedra (*Ephedra sinica*)/ma huang	Nasal congestion
Ephedra (*Ephedra sinica*)/ma huang infection	Upper respiratory tract
Eucalyptus oil (*Eucalyptus globulus* Labillardiere, *E. fructicetorum* F. Von Mueller, *E. smithii* R.T. Baker)	Bronchitis
Eucalyptus oil (*Eucalyptus globulus* Labillardiere, *E. fructicetorum* F. Von Mueller, *E. smithii* R.T. Baker)	Colds
Eucalyptus oil (*Eucalyptus globulus* Labillardiere, *E. fructicetorum* F. Von Mueller, *E. smithii* R.T. Baker)	Influenza
Eyebright (*Euphrasia officinalis*)	Bronchitis (chronic)
Eyebright (*Euphrasia officinalis*)	Common cold
Eyebright (*Euphrasia officinalis*)	Respiratory infections
Eyebright (*Euphrasia officinalis*)	Sore throat
Fenugreek (*Trigonella foenum-graecum* L.)	Bronchitis

Continued

Feverfew (*Tanacetum parthenium* L. Schultz-Bip.)	Colds
Flaxseed and flaxseed oil (*Linum usitatissimum*)	Sore throat
Flaxseed and flaxseed oil (*Linum usitatissimum*)	Upper respiratory tract infection
Garlic (*Allium sativum* L.)	Bronchitis
Garlic (*Allium sativum* L.)	Colds
Garlic (*Allium sativum* L.)	Influenza
Ginger (*Zingiber officinale* Roscoe)	Bronchitis
Ginger (*Zingiber officinale* Roscoe)	Colds
Ginger (*Zingiber officinale* Roscoe)	Flu
Ginkgo (*Ginkgo biloba* L.)	Bronchitis
Ginkgo (*Ginkgo biloba* L.)	Respiratory tract illnesses
Ginseng (American ginseng, Asian ginseng, Chinese ginseng, Korean red ginseng, *Panax ginseng*: *Panax* spp. including *P. ginseng* C.C. Meyer and *P. quinquefolium* L., excluding *Eleutherococcus senticosus*)	Influenza
Ginseng (American ginseng, Asian ginseng, Chinese ginseng, Korean red ginseng, *Panax ginseng*: *Panax* spp. including *P. ginseng* C.C. Meyer and *P. quinquefolium* L., excluding *Eleutherococcus senticosus*)	Upper respiratory tract infection
Goldenseal (*Hydrastis canadensis* L.), berberine	Bronchitis
Goldenseal (*Hydrastis canadensis* L.), berberine	Influenza
Goldenseal (*Hydrastis canadensis* L.), berberine	Tonsillitis
Gotu kola (*Centella asiatica* L.), total triterpenic fraction of *Centella asiatica* (TTFCA)	Bronchitis
Gotu kola (*Centella asiatica* L.), total triterpenic fraction of *Centella asiatica* (TTFCA)	Colds
Gotu kola (*Centella asiatica* L.), total triterpenic fraction of *Centella asiatica* (TTFCA)	Influenza
Gotu kola (*Centella asiatica* L.), total triterpenic fraction of *Centella asiatica* (TTFCA)	Tonsillitis
Guggul (*Commifora mukul*)	Sore throat
Hawthorn (*Crataegus laevigata*, *C. oxyacantha*, *C. monogyna*, *C. pentagyna*)	Sore throat

Kava (*Piper methysticum* G. Forst)	Colds
Lavender (*Lavandula angustifolia* Miller)	Bronchitis
Lavender (*Lavandula angustifolia* Miller)	Common cold
Licorice (*Glycyrrhiza glabra* L.), deglycyrrhizinated licorice (DGL)	Bronchitis
Licorice (*Glycyrrhiza glabra* L.), deglycyrrhizinated licorice (DGL)	Sore throat
Marshmallow (*Althaea officinalis* L.)	Bronchitis
Marshmallow (*Althaea officinalis* L.)	Sore throat
Milk thistle (*Silybum marianum*), silymarin	Bronchitis
Omega-3 fatty acids, fish oil, alpha-linolenic acid	Common cold
Peppermint (*Mentha* x *piperita* L.)	Bronchial spasm
Peppermint (*Mentha* x *piperita* L.)	Common cold
Peppermint (*Mentha* x *piperita* L.)	Influenza
Polypodium leucotomos extract, Anapsos	Upper respiratory tract infection
Psyllium (*Plantago ovata*, *P. ispaghula*)	Bronchitis
Red clover (*Trifolium pratense*)	Bronchitis
Saw palmetto (*Serenoa repens* [Bartram] Small)	Bronchitis
Saw palmetto (*Serenoa repens* [Bartram] Small)	Sore throat
Saw palmetto (*Serenoa repens* [Bartram] Small)	Upper respiratory tract infection
Seaweed, kelp, bladderwrack (*Fucus vesiculosus*)	Sore throat
Slippery elm (*Ulmus rubra* Muhl. or *U. fulva* Michx.)	Bronchitis
Sorrel (*Rumex acetosa* L., *R. acetosella* L.), Sinupret	Nasal inflammation
Sorrel (*Rumex acetosa* L., *R. acetosella* L.), Sinupret	Respiratory inflammation
Sorrel (*Rumex acetosa* L., *R. acetosella* L.), Sinupret	Sore throat
Spirulina	Influenza
St. John's wort (*Hypericum perforatum* L.)	Influenza
Tea tree oil (*Melaleuca alternifolia* [Maiden & Betche] Cheel)	Bronchial congestion

Continued

Tea tree oil (*Melaleuca alternifolia* [Maiden & Betche] Cheel)	Colds
Tea tree oil (*Melaleuca alternifolia* [Maiden & Betche] Cheel)	Sinus infections
Tea tree oil (*Melaleuca alternifolia* [Maiden & Betche] Cheel)	Sore throat
Tea tree oil (*Melaleuca alternifolia* [Maiden & Betche] Cheel)	Tonsillitis
Thyme (*Thymus vulgaris* L.), thymol	Flu
Thyme (*Thymus vulgaris* L.), thymol	Sore throat
Thyme (*Thymus vulgaris* L.), thymol	Tonsillitis
Thyme (*Thymus vulgaris* L.), thymol	Upper respiratory tract infection
White horehound (*Marrubium vulgare* L.)	Bronchitis
White horehound (*Marrubium vulgare* L.)	Respiratory (lung) spasms
White horehound (*Marrubium vulgare* L.)	Sore throat
White horehound (*Marrubium vulgare* L.)	Upper respiratory tract infection

URINARY INCONTINENCE AND RELATED CONDITIONS

Levels of Scientific Evidence for Specific Therapies

GRADE: C (Unclear or Conflicting Scientific Evidence)

Therapy	Specific Therapeutic Use(s)
Cranberry (*Vaccinium macrocarpon*)	Reduction of odor from incontinence/bladder catheterization
Saw palmetto (*Serenoa repens* [Bartram] Small)	Hypotonic neurogenic bladder

TRADITIONAL OR THEORETICAL USES THAT LACK SUFFICIENT EVIDENCE

Therapy	Specific Therapeutic Use(s)
Belladonna (*Atropa belladonna* L. or its variety *A. acuminata* Royle ex Lindl)	Bedwetting
Calendula (*Calendula officinalis* L.), marigold	Urinary retention
Ephedra (*Ephedra sinica*)/ma huang	Enuresis

Gotu kola (*Centella asiatica* L.), total triterpenic fraction of *Centella asiatica* (TTFCA)	Urinary retention
Horsetail (*Equisetum arvense* L.)	Urinary incontinence
Kava (*Piper methysticum* G. Forst)	Urinary incontinence
St. John's wort (*Hypericum perforatum* L.)	Bedwetting
Thyme (*Thymus vulgaris* L.), thymol	Enuresis

URINARY TRACT INFECTION AND RELATED CONDITIONS

Levels of Scientific Evidence for Specific Therapies

GRADE: B (Good Scientific Evidence)

Therapy	Specific Therapeutic Use(s)
Cranberry (*Vaccinium macrocarpon*)	Urinary tract infection prevention

GRADE: C (Unclear or Conflicting Scientific Evidence)

Therapy	Specific Therapeutic Use(s)
Bromelain	Urinary tract infection
Cranberry (*Vaccinium macrocarpon*)	Urinary tract infection treatment
Cranberry (*Vaccinium macrocarpon*)	Urine acidification
Peppermint (*Mentha* x *piperita* L.)	Urinary tract infection

GRADE: D (Fair Negative Scientific Evidence)

Therapy	Specific Therapeutic Use(s)
Cranberry (*Vaccinium macrocarpon*)	Chronic urinary tract infection prevention: children with neurogenic bladder

TRADITIONAL OR THEORETICAL USES THAT LACK SUFFICIENT EVIDENCE

Therapy	Specific Therapeutic Use(s)
Bilberry (*Vaccinium myrtillus*)	Urinary tract infections
Burdock (*Arctium lappa*)	Urinary tract infections

Continued

Chaparral (*Larrea tridentata* DC. Coville, *L. divaricata* Cav.), nordihydroguaiaretic acid (NDGA)	Urinary tract infections
Dandelion (*Taraxacum officinale*)	Urinary tract inflammation
Devil's claw (*Harpagophytum procumbens* DC.)	Urinary tract infections
Echinacea (*Echinacea angustifolia* DC., *E. pallida*, *E. purpurea*)	Urinary tract infections
Eucalyptus oil (*Eucalyptus globulus* Labillardiere, *E. fructicetorum* F. Von Mueller, *E. smithii* R.T. Baker)	Urinary tract infection
Flaxseed and flaxseed oil (*Linum usitatissimum*)	Urinary tract infection
Garlic (*Allium sativum* L.)	Urinary tract infections
Ginkgo (*Ginkgo biloba* L.)	Genitourinary disorders
Goldenseal (*Hydrastis canadensis* L.), berberine	Urinary tract disorders
Gotu kola (*Centella asiatica* L.), total triterpenic fraction of *Centella asiatica* (TTFCA)	Urinary tract infection
Horsetail (*Equisetum arvense* L.)	Urinary tract infection
Horsetail (*Equisetum arvense* L.)	Urinary tract inflammation
Kava (*Piper methysticum* G. Forst)	Urinary tract disorders
Marshmallow (*Althaea officinalis* L.)	Urinary tract infection
Saw palmetto (*Serenoa repens* [Bartram] Small)	Genitourinary tract disorders
Saw palmetto (*Serenoa repens* [Bartram] Small)	Urinary antiseptic
Slippery elm (*Ulmus rubra* Muhl. or *U. fulva* Michx.)	Urinary tract infections
Thyme (*Thymus vulgaris* L.), thymol	Urinary tract infection
Valerian (*Valeriana officinalis* L.)	Urinary tract disorders
Wild yam (*Dioscorea villosa*)	Urinary tract disorders

UTERINE DISORDERS AND RELATED CONDITIONS

Levels of Scientific Evidence for Specific Therapies

TRADITIONAL OR THEORETICAL USES THAT LACK SUFFICIENT EVIDENCE

Therapy	Specific Therapeutic Use(s)
Alfalfa (*Medicago sativa* L.)	Uterine stimulant
American pennyroyal (*Hedeoma pulegioides* L.), European pennyroyal (*Mentha pulegium* L.)	Preparation of uterus for labor

American pennyroyal (*Hedeoma pulegioides* L.), European pennyroyal (*Mentha pulegium* L.)	Uterine fibroids
Astragalus (*Astragalus membranaceus*)	Uterine bleeding
Astragalus (*Astragalus membranaceus*)	Uterine prolapse
Black cohosh (*Cimicifuga racemosa* L. Nutt.)	Uterine diseases and bleeding
Calendula (*Calendula officinalis* L.), marigold	Uterus problems
Ephedra (*Ephedra sinica*)/ma huang	Uterotonic
Eucalyptus oil (*Eucalyptus globulus* Labillardiere, *E. fructicetorum* F. Von Mueller, *E. smithii* R.T. Baker)	Urinary difficulties
Feverfew (*Tanacetum parthenium* L. Schultz-Bip.)	Uterine disorders
Goldenseal (*Hydrastis canadensis* L.), berberine	Uterus inflammation
Goldenseal (*Hydrastis canadensis* L.), berberine	Uterus stimulant
Kava (*Piper methysticum* G. Forst)	Uterus inflammation
Milk thistle (*Silybum marianum*), silymarin	Uterine complaints
Saw palmetto (*Serenoa repens* [Bartram] Small)	Uterine disorders

VERTIGO AND RELATED CONDITIONS

Levels of Scientific Evidence for Specific Therapies

GRADE: C (Unclear or Conflicting Scientific Evidence)

Therapy	Specific Therapeutic Use(s)
Ginkgo (*Ginkgo biloba* L.)	Vertigo

TRADITIONAL OR THEORETICAL USES THAT LACK SUFFICIENT EVIDENCE

Therapy	Specific Therapeutic Use(s)
American pennyroyal (*Hedeoma pulegioides* L.), European pennyroyal (*Mentha pulegium* L.)	Dizziness
Black cohosh (*Cimicifuga racemosa* L. Nutt.)	Dizziness
Calendula (*Calendula officinalis* L.), marigold	Dizziness
Echinacea (*Echinacea angustifolia* DC., *E. pallida*, *E. purpurea*)	Dizziness
Feverfew (*Tanacetum parthenium* L. Schultz-Bip.)	Dizziness

Continued

Ginkgo (*Ginkgo biloba* L.)	Dizziness
Ginseng (American ginseng, Asian ginseng, Chinese ginseng, Korean red ginseng, *Panax ginseng*: *Panax* spp. including *P. ginseng* C.C. Meyer and *P. quinquefolium* L., excluding *Eleutherococcus senticosus*)	Dizziness
Horse chestnut (*Aesculus hippocastanum* L.)	Dizziness
Kava (*Piper methysticum* G. Forst)	Dizziness
Lavender (*Lavandula angustifolia* Miller)	Dizziness
Niacin (vitamin B_3, nicotinic acid), niacinamide, inositol hexanicotinate	Vertigo
Turmeric (*Curcuma longa* L.), curcumin	Dizziness
Valerian (*Valeriana officinalis* L.)	Vertigo

VIRAL INFECTIONS AND RELATED CONDITIONS

Levels of Scientific Evidence for Specific Therapies

GRADE: C (Unclear or Conflicting Scientific Evidence)

Therapy	Specific Therapeutic Use(s)
Astragalus (*Astragalus membranaceus*)	Antiviral activity
Blessed thistle (*Cnicus benedictus* L.)	Viral infections
Cranberry (*Vaccinium macrocarpon*)	Antiviral, antifungal
Sorrel (*Rumex acetosa* L., *R. acetosella* L.), Sinupret	Antiviral

TRADITIONAL OR THEORETICAL USES THAT LACK SUFFICIENT EVIDENCE

Therapy	Specific Therapeutic Use(s)
Betel nut (*Areca catechu* L.)	Diphtheria
Calendula (*Calendula officinalis* L.), marigold	Antiviral
Chaparral (*Larrea tridentata* DC. Coville, *L. divaricata* Cav.), nordihydroguaiaretic acid (NDGA)	Antiviral
Clove (*Eugenia aromatica*)	Antiviral
Dandelion (*Taraxacum officinale*)	Antiviral
Dong quai (*Angelica sinensis* [Oliv.] Diels), Chinese angelica	Antiviral

Echinacea (*Echinacea angustifolia* DC., *E. pallida*, *E. purpurea*)	Diphtheria
Eucalyptus oil (*Eucalyptus globulus* Labillardiere, *E. fructicetorum* F. Von Mueller, *E. smithii* R.T. Baker)	Antiviral
Eyebright (*Euphrasia officinalis*)	Antiviral
Garlic (*Allium sativum* L.)	Antiviral
Garlic (*Allium sativum* L.)	Diphtheria
Ginger (*Zingiber officinale* Roscoe)	Antiviral
Goldenseal (*Hydrastis canadensis* L.), berberine	Diphtheria
Licorice (*Glycyrrhiza glabra* L.), deglycyrrhizinated licorice (DGL)	Coronavirus infection
Licorice (*Glycyrrhiza glabra* L.), deglycyrrhizinated licorice (DGL)	Epstein-Barr virus infection
Peppermint (*Mentha* x *piperita* L.)	Antiviral
Propolis	Viral infections
Spirulina	Antiviral
St. John's wort (*Hypericum perforatum* L.)	Antiviral
St. John's wort (*Hypericum perforatum* L.)	Epstein-Barr virus infection

VISION AND RELATED CONDITIONS

Levels of Scientific Evidence for Specific Therapies

GRADE: D (Fair Negative Scientific Evidence)

Therapy	Specific Therapeutic Use(s)
Bilberry (*Vaccinium myrtillus*)	Night vision

TRADITIONAL OR THEORETICAL USES THAT LACK SUFFICIENT EVIDENCE

Therapy	Specific Therapeutic Use(s)
Betel nut (*Areca catechu* L.)	Blindness from methanol poisoning
Flaxseed and flaxseed oil (*Linum usitatissimum*)	Vision improvement
Omega-3 fatty acids, fish oil, alpha-linolenic acid	Night vision enhancement
Valerian (*Valeriana officinalis* L.)	Vision

VOMITING AND RELATED CONDITIONS

Levels of Scientific Evidence for Specific Therapies

GRADE: B (Good Scientific Evidence)

Therapy	Specific Therapeutic Use(s)
Ginger (*Zingiber officinale* Roscoe)	Nausea (due to chemotherapy)
Ginger (*Zingiber officinale* Roscoe)	Nausea and vomiting of pregnancy (hyperemesis gravidarum)

GRADE: C (Unclear or Conflicting Scientific Evidence)

Therapy	Specific Therapeutic Use(s)
Ginger (*Zingiber officinale* Roscoe)	Nausea and vomiting (after surgery)
Peppermint (*Mentha* x *piperita* L.)	Nausea

TRADITIONAL OR THEORETICAL USES THAT LACK SUFFICIENT EVIDENCE

Therapy	Specific Therapeutic Use(s)
Belladonna (*Atropa belladonna* L. or its variety *A. acuminata* Royle ex Lindl)	Motion sickness
Belladonna (*Atropa belladonna* L. or its variety *A. acuminata* Royle ex Lindl)	Nausea and vomiting during pregnancy
Black tea (*Camellia sinensis*)	Vomiting
Calendula (*Calendula officinalis* L.), marigold	Nausea
Chamomile (*Matricaria recutita*, *Chamaemelum nobile*)	Motion sickness
Chamomile (*Matricaria recutita*, *Chamaemelum nobile*)	Nausea
Chamomile (*Matricaria recutita*, *Chamaemelum nobile*)	Sea sickness
Chaparral (*Larrea tridentata* DC. Coville, *L. divaricata* Cav.), nordihydroguaiaretic acid (NDGA)	Vomiting
Clay	Vomiting
Clay	Vomiting/nausea during pregnancy
Clove (*Eugenia aromatica*), clove oil (eugenol)	Nausea or vomiting

Cranberry (*Vaccinium macrocarpon*)	Vomiting
Elder (*Sambucus nigra* L.)	Vomiting
Globe artichoke (*Cynara scolymus* L.)	Emesis
Lavender (*Lavandula angustifolia* Miller)	Motion sickness
Lavender (*Lavandula angustifolia* Miller)	Nausea
Lavender (*Lavandula angustifolia* Miller)	Vomiting
Marshmallow (*Althaea officinalis* L.)	Vomiting
Niacin (vitamin B_3, nicotinic acid), niacinamide, inositol hexanicotinate	Motion sickness
Oleander (*Nerium oleander*, *Thevetia peruviana*)	Vomiting
Valerian (*Valeriana officinalis* L.)	Nausea
White horehound (*Marrubium vulgare* L.)	Emetic
Wild yam (*Dioscorea villosa*)	Emetic

WEIGHT REDUCTION AND RELATED CONDITIONS

Levels of Scientific Evidence for Specific Therapies

GRADE: A (Strong Scientific Evidence)

Therapy	Specific Therapeutic Use(s)
Ephedra (*Ephedra sinica*)/ma huang	Weight loss

GRADE: C (Unclear or Conflicting Scientific Evidence)

Therapy	Specific Therapeutic Use(s)
Bladderwrack (*Fucus vesiculosus*)	Weight loss
Evening primrose oil (*Oenothera biennis* L.)	Obesity/weight loss
Green tea (*Camellia sinensis*)	Weight loss
Guggul (*Commifora mukul*)	Obesity
Spirulina	Weight loss

Continued

TRADITIONAL OR THEORETICAL USES THAT LACK SUFFICIENT EVIDENCE	
Therapy	Specific Therapeutic Use(s)
Arginine (L-arginine)	Obesity
Astragalus (*Astragalus membranaceus*)	Weight loss
Barley (*Hordeum vulgare* L.), germinated barley foodstuff (GBF)	Appetite suppressant
Bladderwrack (*Fucus vesiculosus*)	Obesity
Bromelain	Appetite suppressant
Coenzyme Q10	Obesity
Dehydroepiandrosterone (DHEA)	Obesity
Ephedra (*Ephedra sinica*)/ma huang	Appetite suppressant
Evening primrose oil (*Oenothera biennis* L.)	Weight loss
Garlic (*Allium sativum* L.)	Obesity
Goldenseal (*Hydrastis canadensis* L.), berberine	Obesity
Guggul (*Commifora mukul*)	Obesity
Guggul (*Commifora mukul*)	Weight loss
Gymnema (*Gymnema sylvestre* R. Br.)	Obesity
Kava (*Piper methysticum* G. Forst)	Weight reduction
Licorice (*Glycyrrhiza glabra* L.), deglycyrrhizinated licorice (DGL)	Body fat reducer
Licorice (*Glycyrrhiza glabra* L.), deglycyrrhizinated licorice (DGL)	Obesity
Omega-3 fatty acids, fish oil, alpha-linolenic acid	Obesity
Psyllium (*Plantago ovata*, *P. ispaghula*)	Obesity
Red clover (*Trifolium pratense*)	Appetite suppressant
Seaweed, kelp, bladderwrack (*Fucus vesiculosus*)	Obesity
Thyme (*Thymus vulgaris* L.), thymol	Obesity
Yohimbe bark extract (*Pausinystalia yohimbe* Pierre ex Beille)	Obesity

WELL-BEING AND RELATED CONDITIONS

Levels of Scientific Evidence for Specific Therapies

GRADE: C (Unclear or Conflicting Scientific Evidence)	
Therapy	Specific Therapeutic Use(s)
Chamomile (*Matricaria recutita*, *Chamaemelum nobile*)	Quality of life in cancer patients

TRADITIONAL OR THEORETICAL USES THAT LACK SUFFICIENT EVIDENCE	
Therapy	Specific Therapeutic Use(s)
Essiac	Supportive care in advanced-cancer patients
Ginseng (American ginseng, Asian ginseng, Chinese ginseng, Korean red ginseng, *Panax ginseng*: *Panax* spp. including *P. ginseng* C.C. Meyer and *P. quinquefolium* L., excluding *Eleutherococcus senticosus*)	Qi deficiency and blood stasis syndrome in heart disease (Eastern medicine)
Ginseng (American ginseng, Asian ginseng, Chinese ginseng, Korean red ginseng, *Panax ginseng*: *Panax* spp. including *P. ginseng* C.C. Meyer and *P. quinquefolium* L., excluding *Eleutherococcus senticosus*)	Quality of life

WOUND HEALING AND RELATED CONDITIONS

Levels of Scientific Evidence for Specific Therapies

GRADE: C (Unclear or Conflicting Scientific Evidence)	
Therapy	Specific Therapeutic Use(s)
Arginine (L-arginine)	Wound healing
Calendula (*Calendula officinalis* L.), marigold	Wound and burn healing
Gotu kola (*Centella asiatica* L.), total triterpenic fraction of *Centella asiatica* (TTFCA)	Wound healing

GRADE: D (Fair Negative Scientific Evidence)	
Therapy	Specific Therapeutic Use(s)
Aloe (*Aloe vera*)	Infected surgical wounds

Continued

TRADITIONAL OR THEORETICAL USES THAT LACK SUFFICIENT EVIDENCE	
Therapy	**Specific Therapeutic Use(s)**
Aloe (*Aloe vera*)	Wound healing after cosmetic dermabrasion
Astragalus (*Astragalus membranaceus*)	Diabetic foot ulcers
Blessed thistle (*Cnicus benedictus* L.)	Skin ulcers
Blessed thistle (*Cnicus benedictus* L.)	Wound healing
Boswellia (*Boswellia serrata* Roxb.)	Cicatrizant (promoting scar formation)
Burdock (*Arctium lappa*)	Sores
Chamomile (*Matricaria recutita*, *Chamaemelum nobile*)	Abrasions
Chamomile (*Matricaria recutita*, *Chamaemelum nobile*)	Bed sores
Cranberry (*Vaccinium macrocarpon*)	Wound care
Devil's claw (*Harpagophytum procumbens* DC.)	Skin ulcers (used topically)
Dehydroepiandrosterone (DHEA)	Skin graft healing
Dong quai (*Angelica sinensis* [Oliv.] Diels), Chinese angelica	Skin ulcers
Echinacea (*Echinacea angustifolia* DC., *E. pallida*, *E. purpurea*)	Skin ulcers
Eucalyptus oil (*Eucalyptus globulus* Labillardiere, *E. fructicetorum* F. Von Mueller, *E. smithii* R.T. Baker)	Skin ulcers
Ginkgo (*Ginkgo biloba* L.)	Skin sores (ginkgo cream)
Goldenseal (*Hydrastis canadensis* L.), berberine	Anal fissures
Guggul (*Commifora mukul*)	Sores
Hawthorn (*Crataegus laevigata*, *C. oxyacantha*, *C. monogyna*, *C. pentagyna*)	Skin sores
Hops (*Humulus lupulus* L.)	Skin ulcers (hops used on the skin)
Lavender (*Lavandula angustifolia* Miller)	Sores
Licorice (*Glycyrrhiza glabra* L.), deglycyrrhizinated licorice (DGL)	Graft healing
Marshmallow (*Althaea officinalis* L.)	Vulnerary

Propolis	Skin rejuvenator
Shark cartilage	Wound healing
Slippery elm (*Ulmus rubra* Muhl. or *U. fulva* Michx.)	Abrasions
Slippery elm (*Ulmus rubra* Muhl. or *U. fulva* Michx.)	Anal fissures
Slippery elm (*Ulmus rubra* Muhl. or *U. fulva* Michx.)	Skin ulcer
Spirulina	Wound healing
St. John's wort (*Hypericum perforatum* L.)	Skin scrapes
White horehound (*Marrubium vulgare* L.)	Skin ulcers
White horehound (*Marrubium vulgare* L.)	Vulnerary

Index

P

S

T